Levels of Research Evidence

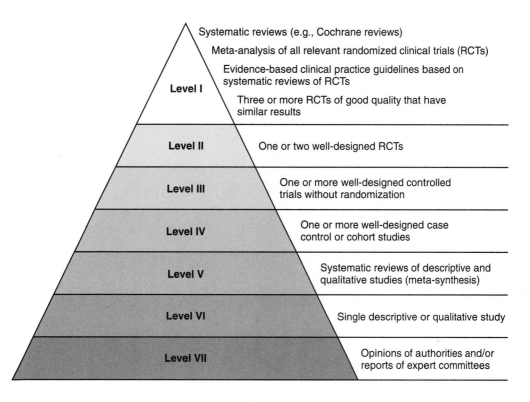

Level I — Systematic reviews (e.g., Cochrane reviews)
Meta-analysis of all relevant randomized clinical trials (RCTs)
Evidence-based clinical practice guidelines based on systematic reviews of RCTs
Three or more RCTs of good quality that have similar results

Level II — One or two well-designed RCTs

Level III — One or more well-designed controlled trials without randomization

Level IV — One or more well-designed case control or cohort studies

Level V — Systematic reviews of descriptive and qualitative studies (meta-synthesis)

Level VI — Single descriptive or qualitative study

Level VII — Opinions of authorities and/or reports of expert committees

Evidence-Based Nursing Care Guidelines

Medical-Surgical Interventions

Betty J. Ackley, MSN, EdS, RN
President, The Betty Ackley LLC;
Professor Emeritus
Jackson Community College
Jackson, Michigan

Beth Ann Swan, PhD, CRNP, FAAN
Associate Professor and Associate Dean,
    Graduate Program
Jefferson School of Nursing
Thomas Jefferson University
Philadelphia, Pennsylvania

Gail B. Ladwig, MSN, RN, CHTP
Professor Emeritus
Jackson Community College;
Co-owner and Nursing Consultant
Holistic Choices;
Healing Touch Practitioner
Jackson, Michigan

Sharon J. Tucker, PhD, RN
Nurse Administrator and Clinical Nurse
    Researcher
Division of Nursing Research
Department of Nursing
Mayo Clinic
Rochester, Minnesota

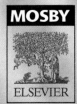

MOSBY

ELSEVIER

MOSBY
ELSEVIER

11830 Westline Industrial Drive
St. Louis, Missouri 63146

EVIDENCE-BASED NURSING CARE GUIDELINES: ISBN: 978-0-323-04624-4
MEDICAL-SURGICAL INTERVENTIONS
Copyright © 2008 by Mosby, Inc., an affiliate of Elsevier Inc.

Notice

Knowledge and best practice in this field are constantly changing. As new research and experience broaden our knowledge, changes in practice, treatment and drug therapy may become necessary or appropriate. Readers are advised to check the most current information provided (i) on procedures featured or (ii) by the manufacturer of each product to be administered, to verify the recommended dose or formula, the method and duration of administration, and contraindications. It is the responsibility of the practitioner, relying on their own experience and knowledge of the patient, to make diagnoses, to determine dosages and the best treatment for each individual patient, and to take all appropriate safety precautions. To the fullest extent of the law, neither the Publisher nor the Authors assumes any liability for any injury and/or damage to persons or property arising out of or related to any use of the material contained in this book.

Caution: The information that is offered in these guidelines should be applied using critical thinking to determine if it is applicable to the individual patient or to particular groups of patients. These guidelines may not be appropriate for a particular patient because of variations in patient conditions, situations, or settings. In addition, new information may have become available since publication, and an updated literature search by the practitioner may be necessary.

ISBN: 978-0-323-04624-4

Senior Editor: Lee Henderson
Senior Developmental Editor: Rae Robertson
Publication Services Manager: John Rogers
Senior Project Manager: Doug Turner
Designer: Margaret Reid

Printed in the United States of America

Last digit is the print number: 9 8 7 6 5 4 3 2

CONTRIBUTORS

Thomas Ahrens, DNSc, RN, FAAN
Research Scientist
Barnes-Jewish Hospital
St. Louis, Missouri
Hemorrhage Control
Shock Management
Shock Prevention

Julie Anderson, PhD, RN, CCRC
Associate Professor and Interim Associate
    Dean for Graduate Studies
College of Nursing
University of North Dakota
Grand Forks, North Dakota
Pressure Ulcer Care Stage I
Pressure Ulcer Prevention
Skin Surveillance

Keith A. Anderson, PhD
Assistant Professor
The Ohio State University
Columbus, Ohio
Family Involvement Promotion

Angelina A. Arcamone, DNSc, RN, CCE
Clinical Assistant Professor and Coordinator
    of Clinical Education
College of Nursing
Villanova University
Villanova, Pennsylvania
Pelvic Muscle Exercise
Perineal Care

Kristie B. Asimos, MSN, CRNP
Associate Course Director and Clinical
    Faculty
University of Pennsylvania
Philadelphia, Pennsylvania
Medication Administration

Jan Avakian-Kopatich, BSN, RN, CWON
School of Nursing
University of Wisconsin–Milwaukee
Milwaukee, Wisconsin;
School of Enterostomal Therapy
University of California–San Diego
San Diego, California
Wound Care
Wound Irrigation

**Elizabeth A. Ayello, PhD, RN, APRN-BC,
    FAPWCA, FAAN**
Faculty
School of Nursing
Excelsior College
Albany, New York
Pressure Ulcer Care Stage II
Pressure Ulcer Care Stage III
Pressure Ulcer Care Stage IV
Pressure Ulcer Prevention

L. Julia Ball, PhD, RN
Dean, School of Nursing
University of South Carolina—Aiken
Aiken, South Carolina
Dementia Management: Multisensory Therapy

Kathleen Gaskill Bappert, BSN, RN, MS
Instructor
College of Nursing
Michigan State University
East Lansing, Michigan
Mutual Goal-Setting
Patient Contracting

Lee Barks, PhD, ARNP, CDDN
Nurse Fellow
Patient Safety Center of Inquiry
Veterans Administration
James A. Haley VA Medical Center
Tampa, Florida
Positioning
Positioning: Wheelchair

Melissa M. Barth, MS, RN, CCRN
Nursing Education Specialist
Surgical Trauma ICU/PCU
Mayo Clinic
Rochester, Minnesota
Environmental Management: Noise Control

Cornelia Beck, PhD, RN, FAAN
Professor
College of Nursing;
Department of Geriatrics,
Department of Psychiatry and Behavioral
    Sciences
College of Medicine
University of Arkansas for Medical Sciences
Little Rock, Arkansas
Dressing
Self-Care Assistance: Dressing/Grooming

Mary P. Bennett, PhD, FNP, APRN
Assistant Dean and Professor
College of Nursing
Indiana State University
Terre Haute, Indiana;
Nurse Practitioner
Methodist Center for Occupational Health
Terre Haute, Indiana
Humor

Kathaleen C. Bloom, PhD, CNM
Professor
School of Nursing
University of North Florida
Jacksonville, Florida
Health Education
Learning Facilitation
Learning Readiness Enhancement
Teaching: Prescribed Medication

Cecilia Borden, EdD, RN, MSN
Assistant Professor, Medical-Surgical—
    Critical Care
College of Health Professions
Jefferson School of Nursing
Thomas Jefferson University
Philadelphia, Pennsylvania
Cognitive Stimulation

Judy Bradberry, PhD, RN
Professor
Department of Nursing
Brenau University
Gainesville, Georgia
Animal-Assisted Therapy

Susan Brust, MSN, CNS, APNP
Psychiatric Clinical Nurse Specialist
Psychiatric Nurse Practitioner
Reset My Soul, LLC
Rochester, Minnesota
Hallucination Management

**Janet L. Bryant, MSN, RN, CNS, CWCN,
    COCN**
Clinical Nurse Specialist
Wound Center
Akron General Medical Center
Akron, Ohio
Nail Care

Kathleen G. Burke, PhD, RN
Program Director, Nursing Administration/
    Health Care Leadership
Director, Center for Professional
    Development
School of Nursing
University of Pennsylvania
Philadelphia, Pennsylvania
Medication Administration

Lisa Burkhart, PhD, RN
Assistant Professor
Marcella Niehoff School of Nursing
Loyola University
Chicago, Illinois
Religious Ritual Enhancement
Spiritual Growth Facilitation
Spiritual Support

Barbara A. Caldwell, PhD, APRN-BC
Associate Professor
School of Nursing
University of Medicine & Dentistry of
    New Jersey
Newark, New Jersey
Presence

Claudia E. Campbell, BSN, RN-BC
Director of Clinical Operations
Intermountain Pain Center
Salt Lake City, Utah
Pain Management: Acute Pain

Virginia L. Carrieri-Kohlman, DNSc, RN,
    FAAN
Professor
Department of Physiological Nursing
University of California San Francisco
San Francisco, California
Dyspnea Management

Paulette C. Chiravalle, MSN, APRN-BC,
    CCRN
Nurse Practitioner
South Florida Center for Gynecologic
    Oncology
Boca Raton, Florida
Nausea Management: Postoperative Nausea
    and Vomiting

Misook Le Chung, PhD, RN
Assistant Professor
College of Nursing
University of Kentucky
Lexington, Kentucky
Cardiac Care: Rehabilitative

Jeannie P. Cimiotti, DNS, RN
Research Assistant Professor
University of Pennsylvania School of
    Nursing
Center for Health Outcomes & Policy
    Research
Philadelphia, Pennsylvania
Infection Control: Hand Hygiene

Angela P. Clark, PhD, RN, CNS, FAAN,
    FAHA
Associate Professor of Nursing
The University of Texas at Austin
Austin, Texas
Family Presence Facilitation

Kathleen A. Clark, MSN, RN, APN-BC
Nursing Instructor
Jefferson School of Nursing
Thomas Jefferson University;
Administrator on Duty
Friends Hospital
Philadelphia, Pennsylvania
Neurological Monitoring

Cheryl A. Cmiel, RN
Staff Registered Nurse
Mayo Clinic
Rochester, Minnesota
Environmental Management: Noise Control

Roseann Colosimo, PhD, RN
Education Consultant
Nevada State Board of Nursing
Las Vegas, Nevada
Behavior Management: Self-Harm

Rose E. Constantino, PhD, JD, RN, FAAN,
    FACFE
Associate Professor
School of Nursing
University of Pittsburgh
Pittsburgh, Pennsylvania
Abuse Protection Support
Environmental Management: Violence
    Prevention

Donna J. Corley, MEd, MSN, RN, CNE
Associate Professor of Nursing
Morehead State University
Morehead, Kentucky
Cardiac Care: Rehabilitative

Deborah Couture, PT, DPT, MS, OCS
Clinical Coordinator of Rehabilitation
  Services
Northeast Health Systems
Beverly, Massachusetts
Heat/Cold Application

Deborah L. Cox, PhD
Associate Professor, Counseling
Gender Studies Faculty
Missouri State University
Springfield, Missouri
Anger Control Assistance

Elizabeth A. Crago, MSN, RN
Research Associate
School of Nursing
University of Pittsburgh
Pittsburgh, Pennsylvania
Dysreflexia Management

**Patricia A. Crane, PhD, MSN, RN-C,
  WHNP**
Assistant Professor
School of Nursing
University of Texas Medical Branch
Galveston, Texas;
Forensic Nurse Consultant, Educator, and
  Expert Witness
Child Abuse and Forensic Services
Beaumont, Texas
Abuse Protection Support
*Environmental Management: Violence
  Prevention*

**Maryanne Crowther, MSN, RN, APNC,
  CCRN**
Guest Lecturer
Brookdale Community College
Lincroft, New Jersey;
APN Student Preceptor
Monmouth University
West Long Branch, New Jersey;
Rutgers University
Newark, New Jersey;
Seton Hall University
West Orange, New Jersey;
CHF Coordinator and Nurse Practitioner
Jersey Shore University Medical Center
Neptune, New Jersey
Deep Vein Thrombosis: Prevention
Deep Vein Thrombosis: Treatment

Kathleen Czekanski, PhD, RN, CNE
Nursing Instructor
Jefferson School of Nursing
Thomas Jefferson University
Philadelphia, Pennsylvania
Dying Care

Yvonne D'Arcy, MS, CRNP, CNS
Pain Management and Palliative Care Nurse
  Practitioner
Suburban Hospital
Bethesda, Maryland
Pain Management: Acute Pain
Pain Management: Chronic Pain
Procedural Pain Alleviation

**Ruth Davidhizar, DNS, RN, ARNP-BC,
  FAAN**
Dean of Nursing
School of Nursing
Bethel College
Mishawaka, Indiana
Active Listening

Joseph T. DeRanieri, MSN, RN, CPN, BCECR
Assistant Professor
Jefferson School of Nursing
Thomas Jefferson University
Philadelphia, Pennsylvania
Diet Staging
Nutrition Management
Nutritional Counseling
Nutritional Monitoring

Della J. Derscheid, MSN, RN, CNS
Clinical Nurse Specialist
Mayo Medical Center
Rochester, Minnesota
Resiliency Promotion

Suzanne L. Dibble, DNSc, RN
Professor Emerita
Institute of Health and Aging
University of California San Francisco
San Francisco, California
Nausea Management: Cancer

DorAnne Donesky-Cuenco, PhD, RN
Project Director
Assistant Adjunct Professor
Dyspnea Research Group
Department of Physiological Nursing
University of California
San Francisco, California
Dyspnea Management

Barbara L. Drew, PhD, APRN-BC
President, American Psychiatric Nurses Association;
Associate Professor
College of Nursing
Kent State University
Kent, Ohio
Suicide Prevention

Joyce A. Overman Dube, MS, RN
Nurse Administrator
Mayo Clinic
Rochester, Minnesota
Environmental Management: Noise Control

Wendy Duggleby, DSN, RN, AOCN
Professor
College of Nursing
University of Saskatchewan
Saskatoon, Saskatchewan
Hope Inspiration

Naomi E. Ervin, PhD, RN, APRN-BC, FAAN
Professor and Director
School of Nursing
Eastern Michigan University
Ypsilanti, Michigan
Decisional Control

Miriam O. Ezenwa, MS, RN
Doctoral Student
University of Wisconsin
Madison, Wisconsin
Preparatory Sensory Information: Cancer
Preparatory Sensory Information: Procedures
Preparatory Sensory Information: Surgery

Mary Fardy, MLS, MSW, LICSW, LADC
Social Worker and EAP Counselor
Healthcare for Homeless Veterans Program
Edith Nourse Rogers Veterans Hospital
Bedford, Massachusetts
Anger Control Assistance

Kathleen A. Fitzgerald, PhD, RN
Assistant Professor
School of Nursing
Lewis University
Romeoville, Illinois
Diarrhea Management
Diarrhea Management: Clostridium difficile
Diarrhea Management: Traveler's Diarrhea
Nasogastric Intubation
Tube Care: Gastrostomy
Tube Feeding (Enteral)

Andrea R. Fleiszer, RN, BN, BSc
Project Coordinator
School of Nursing
University of Ottawa
Ottawa, Ontario
Grief Work Facilitation

Judith A. Floyd, PhD, RN, FAAN
Associate Dean for Research
Director, Center for Health Research
Professor
College of Nursing
Wayne State University
Detroit, Michigan
Sleep Enhancement

Dorothy A. Forbes, PhD, RN
Associate Professor
School of Nursing, Faculty of Health
    Sciences
University of Western Ontario
London, Ontario
Reality Orientation
Validation Therapy

Susan K. Frazier, PhD, RN
Associate Professor
University of Kentucky
Lexington, Kentucky
Cardiac Care
Cardiac Care: Acute
Cardiac Precautions

Susan Froude, RN, MScN
Nurse Educator
Western Regional School of Nursing
Corner Brook, Newfoundland
Grief Work Facilitation

Phyllis Meyer Gaspar, PhD, RN
(with Dr. Gaspar's Spring 2006 Graduate
    Nursing Students)
Department of Nursing
Winona State University
Winona, Minnesota
Bowel Incontinence Care
Bowel Training

Joseph E. Gaugler, PhD
Assistant Professor
Center on Aging, Center for Gerontological
    Nursing
School of Nursing
University of Minnesota
Minneapolis, Minnesota
Family Involvement Promotion

Deborah Gavin-Dreschnack, PhD
Health Science Specialist
James A. Haley VA Patient Safety Research
    Center
Tampa, Florida
Positioning
Positioning: Wheelchair

Deborah L. Gentile, MSN, RN-BC
Nursing Education Specialist
Aurora Health Care
Milwaukee, Wisconsin
Teaching: Foot Care
Wound Care

Judith R. Gentz, RN, CS, NP
President
Nurse Practitioner Care, Inc.
Grass Lake, Michigan
Self-Esteem Enhancement

Angela J. Gillis, PhD, RN
Professor and Former Chair
School of Nursing
St. Francis Xavier University
Antigonish, Nova Scotia
Bed Rest Care

**Deborah R. Gillum, MSN, RN, ANP-C,
    FNP-C**
Assistant Professor of Nursing
Bethel College
Mishawaka, Indiana
Self-Responsibility Facilitation

Barbara Given, PhD, RN, FAAN
University Distinguished Professor
Associate Dean for Research
College of Nursing
Michigan State University
East Lansing, Michigan
Caregiver Support
Energy Management

Debra B. Gordon, MS, RN-C, APRN-BC,
  FAAN
Faculty Associate
School of Nursing
University of Wisconsin;
Senior Clinical Nurse Specialist
Pain Management
University of Wisconsin Hospital & Clinics
Madison, Wisconsin
Patient-Controlled Analgesia (PCA) Assistance

Lisa Gorski, MS, APRN-BC, CRNI, FAAN
Clinical Nurse Specialist
Wheaton Franciscan Home Health &
  Hospice
Milwaukee, Wisconsin
Intravenous Insertion
Intravenous Therapy
Peripherally Inserted Central Catheter Care
Total Parenteral Nutrition Administration

Deanna Gray-Miceli, DNSc, APRN,
  FAANP
Adjunct Assistant Professor
School of Nursing
University of Pennsylvania
Philadelphia, Pennsylvania
Fall Prevention

Margaret Griffiths, MSN, RN, CNE
Professor
Jefferson School of Nursing
Thomas Jefferson University
Philadelphia, Pennsylvania
Fever Treatment

Cathie E. Guzzetta, PhD, RN, AHN-BC,
  FAAN
Director, Holistic Nursing Consultants;
Nursing Research Consultant
Children's National Medical Center;
Associate Clinical Professor of Nursing
  Education
School of Medicine and Health Sciences
George Washington University
Washington, D.C.;
Nursing Research Consultant
Children's Medical Center Dallas
Dallas, Texas
Family Presence Facilitation

Mary E. Hagle, PhD, RN, AOCN
Adjunct Clinical Assistant Professor
University of Wisconsin—Milwaukee;
Regional Manager/Nursing Researcher
Aurora Health Care
Milwaukee, Wisconsin
Vital Signs Monitoring
Wound Care
Wound Irrigation

Margo A. Halm, PhD, RN, CCRN,
  APRN-BC
Adjunct Instructor
School of Nursing
University of Minnesota
Minneapolis, Minnesota;
Director of Nursing Research & Quality/
  Clinical Nurse Specialist
United Hospital
St. Paul, Minnesota
Family Presence Facilitation

Mary Beth Happ, PhD, RN
Associate Professor, Nursing
Associate Professor, Bioethics & Health
  Law
University of Pittsburgh
Pittsburgh, Pennsylvania;
Adjunct Faculty
School of Nursing
University of Pennsylvania
Philadelphia, Pennsylvania
*Communication Enhancement: Speech
  Deficit*

Seongkum Heo, PhD, RN
Assistant Professor
School of Nursing
Indiana University
Indianapolis, Indiana
Cardiac Care: Acute

Vicki L. Hicks, MSN, ARNP-CNS
Clinical Assistant Professor
School of Nursing
University of Kansas
Kansas City, Kansas
Substance Use Prevention

**Kathleen Higgins, RN, CCRN, CS, MSN,
  CRNP**
Coordinator, Acute Care Nurse Practitioner
  Program
School of Nursing
Thomas Jefferson University;
Cardiology Nurse Practitioner
University of Pennsylvania Presbyterian
  Hospital
Philadelphia, Pennsylvania
Circulatory Care: Arterial Insufficiency
Circulatory Care: Venous Insufficiency
Circulatory Precautions
Tube Care: Chest
*Venous Access Devices (VAD): Dressing
  Change*
Venous Access Devices (VAD): Flushing
Venous Access Device (VAD): Maintenance

Diane E. Holland, PhD, RN
Assistant Professor
Mayo Clinic College of Medicine;
Clinical Nurse Researcher
Mayo Clinic
Rochester, Minnesota
Discharge Planning
*Environmental Management: Home
  Preparation*
Home Maintenance Assistance

**Alicia Huckstadt, PhD, APRN-BC, FNP,
  GNP**
Graduate Program Director and Professor
School of Nursing
Wichita State University
Wichita, Kansas
Touch

Jean D. Humphries, MSN, RN
Doctoral Student
School of Nursing
Wayne State University
Detroit, Michigan
Sleep Enhancement

Debra A. Jansen, PhD, RN
Professor
College of Nursing and Health Sciences
University of Wisconsin—Eau Claire
Eau Claire, Wisconsin
Socialization Enhancement

Lynne A. Jensen, PhD, ARNP
Assistant Professor
Assoicate Director for Clinical Care
Center for the Advancement of Women's
  Health
University of Kentucky
Lexington, Kentucky
Cardiac Precautions

Mary Kay Jiricka, MSN, RN, APN-BC, CCRN
Staff Nurse
Cardiac Intensive Care Unit
Aurora St. Luke's Medical Center
Milwaukee, Wisconsin
Visitation Facilitation

Jean E. Johnson, PhD, FAAN
Professor Emerita
School of Nursing
University of Rochester
Rochester, New York
Preparatory Sensory Information: Cancer
Preparatory Sensory Information: Procedures
Preparatory Sensory Information: Surgery

Rebecca A. Johnson, PhD, RN, FAAN
Millsap Professor of Gerontological Nursing & Public Policy
Sinclair School of Nursing
University of Missouri—Columbia
Columbia, Missouri
Relocation Stress Reduction

Donald D. Kautz, PhD, RN, CNRN, CRRN-A
Assistant Professor of Nursing
University o†f North Carolina at Greensboro
Greensboro, North Carolina
Family Integrity Promotion

Teresa J. Kelechi, PhD, RN
Associate Professor
College of Nursing
Medical University of South Carolina
Charleston, South Carolina
Nail Care
Peripheral Sensation Management

Ruth M. Kleinpell, PhD, RN, FAAN, FAANP, FCCM
Professor
College of Nursing
Rush University;
Nurse Practitioner
Our Lady of the Resurrection Medical Center
Chicago, Illinois
Hemorrhage Control
Shock Management
Shock Prevention

Kathleen M. Kochanski, BSN, RN-BC
Nurse Clinician
Aurora St. Luke's Medical Center
Milwaukee, Wisconsin
Wound Care

Katharine Kolcaba, PhD, RN-C
Associate Professor
College of Nursing
University of Akron
Akron, Ohio
Hand Massage
Massage

JoAnne Konick-McMahan, RN, MSN, CCRN
Nursing Education Advisor
Pennsylvania State Board of Nursing
Harrisburg, Pennsylvania
Electrolyte Management: Hypomagnesemia
Electrolyte Management: Hyponatremia

†Lenore H. Kurlowicz, PhD, RN, CS, FAAN
Associate Professor of Geropsychiatric Nursing
School of Nursing
University of Pennsylvania;
Psychiatric Consultation-Liaison Nurse
University of Pennsylvania Medical Center
Philadelphia, Pennsylvania
Delirium Management

†Deceased

Judith Kutzleb, MSN, RN, CCRN, APN-C
Professor of Nursing
Fairleigh Dickinson University
Teaneck, New Jersey;
Professor of Nursing
William Patterson University
Wayne, New Jersey;
Nurse Practitioner, Trauma/Critical Care
    Service
Hackensack University Medical Center
Hackensack, New Jersey
Teaching: Disease Process
Teaching: Individual
Teaching: Prescribed Activity/Exercise

Andrea Maria Laizner, PhD, RN
Assistant Professor
McGill University School of Nursing;
Nursing Research Consultant
McGill University Health Centre;
Chercheure Associée
Centre de Recherche du CHU Sainte-Justine
Montreal, Quebec
Grief Work Facilitation

Scott Chisholm Lamont, BSN, RN, CCRN, CFRN
Master Clinician and Adjunct Clinical
    Lecturer
Emergency/Trauma Clinical Educator
College of Nursing
University of New Mexico Health Sciences
    Center
Albuquerque, New Mexico
Bathing
Self-Care Assistance: Bathing/Hygiene

Ariella Lang, PhD, RN
Canadian Institutes of Health Research
    Postdoctoral Fellow
School of Nursing
University of Ottawa
Ottawa, Ontario
Grief Work Facilitation

Diane K. Langemo, PhD, RN, FAAN
Fritz Distinguished Professor Emeritus
Adjunct Professor
College of Nursing
University of North Dakota;
President
Langemo & Associates
Grand Forks, North Dakota
Pressure Ulcer Care Stage I
Pressure Ulcer Prevention
Skin Surveillance

Marilyn L. Lanza, DNSc, ARNP, CS, FAAN
Associate Professor of Psychiatry
School of Medicine
Boston University
Boston, Massachusetts;
Nurse Researcher
Edith Nourse Rogers Memorial Veterans
    Hospital
Bedford, Massachusetts
Anger Control Assistance

Catherine E. Lein, MS, APRN, FNP-BC
Assistant Professor
College of Nursing
Michigan State University
East Lansing, Michigan
Mutual Goal-Setting
Patient Contracting

Terry A. Lennie, PhD, RN, FAHA
Associate Professor and Director, PhD
    Program
College of Nursing
University of Kentucky
Lexington, Kentucky
Cardiac Care
Cardiac Care: Acute
Cardiac Care: Rehabilitative
Cardiac Precautions

Cynthia K. Lewis, MSN, RN, APRN-BC
Surgical Clinical Nurse Specialist
Aurora St. Luke's Medical Center
Milwaukee, Wisconsin
Teaching: Preoperative
Teaching: Procedure/Treatment

Thomas James Loveless, MSN, CRNP
Nursing Faculty, Health Assessment
College of Health Professions
Thomas Jefferson University;
Adult Nurse Practitioner
Infectious Disease Associates, PC
Philadelphia, Pennsylvania
HIV Prevention
Infection Control
Infection Protection

Brenda MacDonald, MEd, MS, BN, RN
Assistant Professor
School of Nursing
St. Francis Xavier University
Antigonish, Nova Scotia
Bed Rest Care

Maria Marinelli, BSN, CNOR, RNFA
Perioperative Nursing Instructor
Jefferson School of Nursing
Thomas Jefferson University
Philadelphia, Pennsylvania;
Adjunct Faculty
Allied Health
Delaware County Community College
Media, Pennsylvania;
Registered Nurse First Assistant
Virtua Summit Surgical Centers
Marlton, New Jersey
Voorhees, New Jersey
Incision Site Care
Surgical Preparation

Carolyn Thompson Martin, PhD, RN, CFNP
Assistant Professor
California State University, Stanislaus
Turlock, California
Weight Gain Assistance

Marina Martinez-Kratz, MS, RN
Professor of Nursing
Jackson Community College;
Nurse Consultant, Behavioral Health
Foote Hospital
Jackson, Michigan
Weight Reduction Assistance

Ruth G. McCaffrey, DNP, ARNP-BC
Associate Professor
Christine E. Lynn College of Nursing
Florida Atlantic University
Boca Raton, Florida
Anxiety Reduction
Nausea Management: Postoperative Nausea
  and Vomiting

Patricia McCarthy, RN, MSc(A)
Clinical Nurse Specialist, Pediatric
  Oncology
Children's Hospital of Eastern Ontario;
Academic Consultant, Level 1
School of Nursing
University of Ottawa
Ottawa, Ontario
Grief Work Facilitation

Graham J. McDougall, Jr., PhD, RN, APRN-BC, FAAN
James R. Dougherty Jr. Centennial
  Professorship in Nursing
School of Nursing
University of Texas at Austin
Austin, Texas
Memory Training

Laura H. McIlvoy, PhD, RN, CCRN, CNRN
Assistant Professor
Division of Nursing
Indiana University Southeast
New Albany, Indiana
Cerebral Edema Management
Cerebral Perfusion Promotion

Ann McKay, MS, BSN
Assistant Professor of Nursing
Nursing Education Specialist
Mayo Clinic
Rochester, Minnesota
Substance Use Treatment: Alcohol Withdrawal

Janet C. Mentes, PhD, APRN-BC
Assistant Professor
School of Nursing
University of California Los Angeles
Los Angeles, California
Swallowing Therapy

Kimberly Meyer, MSN, RN, ACNP, CNRN
Neuroscience Clinician/TBI Specialist
Defense and Veterans Brain Injury Center
Washington, D.C.
Cerebral Edema Management
Cerebral Perfusion Promotion

Jill Milne, PhD, RN
Adjunct Assistant Professor
Faculty of Medicine
Department of Obstetrics & Gynecology
University of Calgary
Calgary, Alberta
Bladder Training

Annette R. Mitzel, MSN, RN, LMT, CNS
Instructor
College of Nursing
The University of Akron
Akron, Ohio
Hand Massage
Massage

Eloise Monzillo, PhD, RN, AHN-BC, CPHQ, QTTT
Former Adjunct Faculty and Consultant
Holistic Nurse Practitioner Program
Division of Nursing
New York University
New York, New York
Therapeutic Touch

Katherine N. Moore, PhD, RN, CCCN
Associate Dean of Graduate Studies
Faculty of Nursing;
Adjunct Professor
Faculty of Medicine, Division of Urology
University of Alberta
Edmonton, Alberta
Tube Care: Urinary
Urinary Catheterization
Urinary Catheterization: Intermittent

Alan R. Morse, PhD
Adjunct Professor of Ophthamology
Columbia University;
President and CEO
The Jewish Guild for the Blind
New York, New York
Communication Enhancement: Visual Deficit

Debra K. Moser, DNSc, RN, FAAN
Professor and Gill Endowed Chair of
    Nursing
College of Nursing
University of Kentucky
Lexington, Kentucky
Cardiac Care
Cardiac Care: Acute
Cardiac Care: Rehabilitative
Cardiac Precautions

Mary Muth, MS, RN, APNP, CEN
Advanced Practice Nurse
Aurora Quick Care;
Research Associate
Center for Nursing Research and Practice
St. Luke's South Shore
Aurora Health Care
Milwaukee, Wisconsin
Visitation Facilitation

Dale A. Nasby, MA, MS, RN, CNS
Assistant Professor
Graduate Nursing Program
Winona State University
Winona, Minnesota;
Nursing Research Administrative Specialist
Division of Nursing Research
Mayo Clinic
Rochester, Minnesota
Body Image Enhancement

Pamela J. Nelson, PhD(c), MS, RN, CNS
Nursing Research Specialist
Mayo Medical Center
Rochester, Minnesota
Behavior Modification

Leslie H. Nicoll, PhD, MBA, RN-BC
Maine Desk, LLC
Portland, Maine
Latex Precautions

Marci Lee Nilsen, BSN, RN
John A. Hartford Foundation BAGNC
    Scholar
School of Nursing
University of Pittsburgh;
Clinical Nurse
University of Pittsburgh Medical Center-
    Presbyterian Shadyside
Pittsburgh, Pennsylvania
Communication Enhancement: Speech Deficit

Barbara J. Olinzock, EdD, MSN, RN
Assistant Professor of Nursing
School of Nursing
Brooks College of Health
University of North Florida
Jacksonville, Florida
Health Education
Learning Facilitation
Learning Readiness Enhancement
Teaching: Prescribed Medication

Marianne E. Olson, PhD, RN
Education Specialist
Office for Human Research Protection
Mayo Clinic
Rochester, Minnesota
Chapter 2

Kathleen S. Oman, PhD, RN, CEN
Research Nurse Scientist
University of Colorado Hospital
Denver, Colorado
Chapter 3

Marybeth O'Neil, MS, RN, APRN-BC
Instructor of Nursing
College of Medicine;
Nursing Education Specialist
St. Mary's Hospital
Mayo Clinic
Rochester, Minnesota
Substance Use Treatment: Overdose

Karen A. Papastrat, MSN, RN
Assistant Dean and Instructor
Jefferson School of Nursing
Thomas Jefferson University
Philadelphia, Pennsylvania
Medication Administration: Intramuscular
Medication Administration: Subcutaneous

Kathleen L. Patusky, PhD, APRN-BC
Assistant Professor
School of Nursing
University of Medicine and Dentistry of New
    Jersey
Newark, New Jersey
Distraction
Security Enhancement

Susan T. Pierce, MSN, EdD, RN
Professor
College of Nursing;
Adjunct Professor
Master of Healthcare Administration
Northwestern State University of Louisiana
Shreveport, Louisiana
Chapter 4

Sherry H. Pomeroy, PhD, MS, RN
Assistant Professor
John A. Hartford Foundation BAGNC
    Postdoctoral Fellow
School of Nursing
University at Buffalo, The State University of
    New York
Buffalo, New York
Exercise Promotion: Motivational Techniques
Exercise Promotion: Strength Training
Exercise Promotion: Stretching
Exercise Therapy: Balance
Exercise Therapy: Cardiorespiratory (Aerobic)

Deborah Pool, MS, RN, CCRN
Instructor
Department of Nursing
Glendale Community College
Glendale, Arizona
Blood Products Administration
Hypothermia Treatment
Sepsis Prevention

William J. Puentes, DNSc, RN, CNS-BC
Assistant Professor
School of Nursing
University of Medicine and Dentistry of New
    Jersey
Stratford, New Jersey
Reminiscence Therapy

Rita Ray-Mihm, MS, APRN-BC
Nursing Education Specialist
St. Mary's Hospital
Mayo Clinic
Rochester, Minnesota
Substance Use Treatment: Drug Withdrawal

**Barbara Resnick, PhD, CRNP, FAAN,
    FAANP**
Professor
School of Nursing
University of Maryland;
General Nurse Practitioner
Roland Park Place
Baltimore, Maryland
Exercise Promotion: Motivational Techniques
Exercise Promotion: Strength Training
Exercise Promotion: Stretching
Exercise Therapy: Balance
Exercise Therapy: Cardiorespiratory (Aerobic)

**Lori M. Rhudy, PhD, RN, CNRN, CRRN,
    APRN-BC**
Nursing Research Specialist
Mayo Clinic;
Assistant Professor
Mayo Clinic College of Medicine;
Adjunct Faculty
School of Nursing
University of Minnesota
Rochester, Minnesota
Chapter 2
Unilateral Neglect Management

Florence B. Roberts, PhD, APRN-BC
Retired Professor of Nursing
Department of Nursing
Brenau University
Gainesville, Georgia
Animal-Assisted Therapy

Marilee Schmelzer, PhD, RN
Associate Professor
The University of Texas at Arlington
Arlington, Texas;
Research Consultant
Medical City Dallas Hospital
Dallas, Texas
Constipation Management
Enema Administration

Paula R. Sherwood, PhD, RN, CNRN
Assistant Professor
School of Nursing
School of Medicine, Department of
   Neurosurgery
University of Pittsburgh
Pittsburgh, Pennsylvania
Caregiver Support
Dysreflexia Management
Energy Management

Mary T. Shoemaker, MSN, RN, SANE
Assistant Professor of Nursing
Morehead State University
Morehead, Kentucky
Crisis Intervention

Valorie M. Shue, BA
Research Assistant
Department of Psychiatry and Behavioral
   Sciences
College of Medicine
University of Arkansas for Medical
   Sciences
Little Rock, Arkansas
Dressing
Self-Care Assistance: Dressing/Grooming

Stephanie A. Silver, MPH
Research Associate
Hebrew Home for the Aged at Riverdale
Riverdale, New York
Communication Enhancement: Visual Deficit

Sandra F. Simmons, PhD
Associate Professor
Center for Quality Aging
VA Medical Center
Geriatric Research, Education, and Clinical
   Center
Division of General Internal Medicine &
   Public Health
School of Medicine
Vanderbilt University
Nashville, Tennessee
Feeding
Weight Gain Assistance

Sheryl K. Sommer, PhD, RN
Director
Nursing Curriculum and Educational
   Services
Assessment Technologies Institute
Stilwell, Kansas
*Communication Enhancement: Hearing
   Deficit*

Elizabeth Speakman, EdD, RN, FANE, CDE
Associate Professor and Assistant Dean of
   RN Programs
Jefferson School of Nursing
Thomas Jefferson University
Philadelphia, Pennsylvania
Electrolyte Management: Hyperkalemia
Electrolyte Management: Hypokalemia

Sally D. Stabb, PhD
Professor of Counseling Psychology
Texas Woman's University
Denton, Texas
Anger Control Assistance

Elaine E. Steinke, PhD, ARNP
Professor of Nursing
School of Nursing
Wichita State University
Wichita, Kansas
Sexual Counseling

Jacqueline Sullivan, PhD, RN
Clinical Associate Professor
Jefferson School of Nursing
Thomas Jefferson University;
Vice President, Research & Quality
Department of Nursing
Thomas Jefferson University Hospital
Philadelphia, Pennsylvania
Chapter 5

Tracy A. Szirony, PhD, RN-C, CHPN
Associate Professor of Nursing
College of Nursing
University of Toledo
Toledo, Ohio;
Staff Nurse
Hospice of Northwest Ohio
Perrysburg, Ohio
Postmortem Care

Jeanne A. Teresi, EdD, PhD
Administrator and Director
Research Division
Hebrew Home for the Aged at Riverdale
Riverdale, New York;
Co-Director
Columbia University Resource Center for
    Minority Aging Research
Stroud Center & Faculty of Medicine
Columbia University
New York, New York;
Senior Research Scientist
New York State Psychiatric Institute
New York, New York
Communication Enhancement: Visual Deficit

Janelle M. Tipton, MSN, RN, AOCN
Adjunct Instructor
College of Nursing
University of Toledo;
Oncology Clinical Nurse Specialist
University of Toledo Medical Center
Toledo, Ohio
Nausea Management: Cancer

Elizabeth R. Van Horn, PhD, RN, CCRN
Assistant Professor
Adult Health Department
University of North Carolina at Greensboro
Greensboro, North Carolina
Family Integrity Promotion

Bonnie J. Wakefield, PhD, RN
Research Associate Professor
Sinclair School of Nursing
University of Missouri—Columbia;
Director, Health Services Research Program
Harry S. Truman Memorial Veterans'
    Hospital
Columbia, Missouri
Fluid Management

Sharon Wallace, MSN, RN, CCRN
Instructor
Assistant Dean, Senior Level
Jefferson School of Nursing
Jefferson College of Health Professions
Thomas Jefferson University
Philadelphia, Pennsylvania
Cultural Brokerage
Dysrhythmia Management

**Margaret I. Wallhagen, PhD, APRN-BC,
    GNP, AGSF**
Professor
Deparment of Physiological Nursing;
Director, John A. Hartford Center of
    Geriatric Nursing Excellence
School of Nursing
University of California—San Francisco;
Nurse Practitioner
Veterans Administration
San Francisco, California
*Communication Enhancement: Hearing
    Deficit*

Diane Wind Wardell, PhD, RN-C, AHN-BC
Associate Professor
Department of Integrative Nursing Care
School of Nursing
The University of Texas Health Science
    Center at Houston
Houston, Texas
Healing Touch

Dianna S. Weikel, RDH, MS
Associate Professor
Department of Pathology and Diagnostic
    Sciences
University of Maryland Dental School;
Dental Hygienist
Marlene and Stewart Greenebaum Cancer
    Center
University of Maryland
Baltimore, Maryland
Oral Health Maintenance
Oral Health Promotion
Oral Health Restoration

Linda Williams, MSN, RN-BC
Professor of Nursing
Jackson Community College
Jackson, Michigan
Self-Care Assistance: Bathing/Hygiene

Suzanne Lynn Williamson, BSN, RN, CDE
Diabetes Educator
Patient Education
Aurora Lakeland Medical Center
Elkhorn, Wisconsin
Foot Care

Celia E. Wills, PhD, RN
Associate Professor
College of Nursing
Michigan State University
East Lansing, Michigan
Mutual Goal-Setting
Patient Contracting

Jill M. Winters, PhD, RN
Director and Associate Professor
Office of Nursing Research and
    Scholarship
College of Nursing
Marquette University
Milwaukee, Wisconsin
Music Therapy

**Jean F. Wyman, PhD, APRN-BC, GNP,
    FAAN**
Professor and Cora Meidl Siehl Chair in
    Nursing Research;
Director, Center for Gerontological Nursing
School of Nursing
University of Minnesota
Minneapolis, Minnesota
Prompted Voiding
Urinary Habit Training
Urinary Stress Incontinence Care
Urinary Urge Incontinence Care

Christine A. Wynd, PhD, RN, CNAA
Dean and Strawbridge Professor of Nursing
The Breen School of Nursing
Ursuline College
Pepper Pike, Ohio
Guided Imagery

**Carolyn B. Yucha, PhD, RN, FAAN, CNE,
    BCIA**
Dean and Professor
School of Nursing
University of Nevada, Las Vegas
Las Vegas, Nevada
Autogenic Training
Progressive Muscle Relaxation

Kathleen K. Zarling, MSN, RN, APRN-BC
Adjunct Faculty
Nursing Program
Winona State University
Winona, Minnesota;
Cardiovascular Clinical Nurse Specialist
St. Mary's Hospital, Mayo Clinic
Rochester, Minnesota
Tobacco Cessation Assistance

Karen Zulkowski, DNS, RN, CWS
Associate Professor
College of Nursing
Montana State University—Bozeman
Bozeman, Montana
Pressure Ulcer Care Stage II
Pressure Ulcer Care Stage III
Pressure Ulcer Care Stage IV
Pressure Ulcer Prevention

PREFACE

Evidence-Based Nursing Care Guidelines: Medical-Surgical Interventions is written for you, the nurse—whether you are a nurse working in a hospital, an extended-care facility, a clinic, or a patient's home; a student nurse; a nurse educator; or a nurse who functions in any of the other diverse places where nurses give care in the twenty-first century. Whatever your role, you will find this groundbreaking new reference an indispensable guide to the state of research evidence for common medical-surgical nursing interventions.

Our goal in writing this book was to bring information on evidence-based nursing (EBN) to all nurses in a practical format. Physicians have multiple resources that define effective and ineffective treatments; we believe that nurses also need a convenient reference to effective and ineffective nursing interventions.

The first five chapters (Part One) introduce and explain EBN as a concept. Specific chapters are written to help nurses understand what EBN is, learn how to search the literature, use EBN as a student nurse, use EBN as a practicing nurse, and understand how EBN fits into a nursing organization.

The majority of the text (Part Two) is composed of 192 evidence-based guidelines for specific interventions, written by nurse experts based on research in the specific field. This compilation is the work of a large number of nurse researchers who have performed clinical studies on the effectiveness of nursing interventions. The focus is on medical-surgical, critical care, and geriatric nursing interventions—essentially those interventions that are in common use in a typical hospital.

Guidelines are identified by Nursing Interventions Classification (NIC) labels wherever appropriate. For each EBN care guideline, nursing activities are classified as Effective, Possibly Effective, Not Effective, or Possibly Harmful, based on the latest research evidence. Concise research summaries are provided for each nursing activity within each larger intervention. Easy-to-recognize icons classify references as nursing research ⓝⓡ, multidisciplinary research ⓜⓡ, or expert opinion ⓔⓞ. Each reference is also classified by level of evidence—from LOE I to LOE VII—to help the reader evaluate the importance of the relevant research. The abbreviation SP ⓢⓟ, for standard of practice, is used to designate an activity as effective, even though Level I or Level II research does not yet exist for that activity.

In order to link NIC interventions with Nursing Outcomes Classification (NOC) outcomes, NOC outcomes are provided for the majority of interventions. Because of space considerations, full NOC outcomes with outcome measures are presented only for the most commonly used outcomes, but readers are referred to the appropriate NOC outcome even where the full outcome statement could not be used. For comprehensive coverage of NOC outcomes, the reader is referred to Moorhead S, Johnson M, Maas M. (2004). *Iowa Outcomes Project: Nursing Outcomes Classification (NOC).* 3rd ed. St. Louis: Mosby. In addition to the identified NOC outcomes, other outcomes are also likely to be appropriate and important, depending on the particular patient, family, and setting. In such cases, nurses may write their own appropriate measurable outcomes.

NIC ⓝⓘⓒ and NOC ⓝⓞⓒ icons are included wherever NIC and NOC language is used.

An Evolve website is provided as an adjunct to the book and as a means to keep the content current between editions. The Evolve site includes resources to help nursing faculty and nurse educators in the health care facility introduce EBN into their environments. These resources include helpful handouts and worksheets on EBN concepts and processes, WebLinks for EBN search and information websites, PowerPoint lecture slides, and Content Updates that will include additional guidelines as they become available.

Just as nursing research is a work in progress, so too is this book. We hope that this work stimulates further research that will direct nursing care. Our goal was to find all of the relevant research and share it with the reader, but of course not everything could be included. We invite readers to share additional research findings and to develop additional guidelines that should be included in future editions or on Evolve. If you would like to recommend additional research findings for inclusion or are interested in developing additional guidelines, contact Betty Ackley at backley1108@aol.com.

A note to nursing students: The information in these guidelines can serve as excellent rationales for nursing interventions in your care plans. Also, the book can jumpstart your work on an EBN project or paper that may be required for completion of your nursing courses, as well as help ensure that you will give state-of-the-art nursing care after you graduate.

Thank you for purchasing this book and caring about the profession of nursing. The use of EBN will make nursing a more effective and powerful profession. This book is a step in that direction. The rest is up to all of us as nurses.

ACKNOWLEDGMENTS

Writing and editing this book meant that we contacted hundreds of nurses in many specialties. Over 150 nurses worked as contributors to this first edition. This represents a phenomenal amount of nursing intelligence and nursing experience, which these nurses were willing to share with all of us. It was a source of joy to interact with these dedicated nurses, who have devoted their lives to the profession. We are extremely grateful for their contributions.

We would also like to thank all the nurses who have taken part in developing the standardized nursing languages that we integrated into this book. Thanks to the Center for Nursing Classification for their work on the Nursing Interventions Classification (NIC) and the Iowa Outcomes Group for their work on the Nursing Outcomes Classification (NOC). To further the profession of nursing and simplify the collection of data, a common nursing language is paramount.

Betty J. Ackley, Gail B. Ladwig, Beth Ann Swan, Sharon J. Tucker

CONTENTS

PART ONE

Foundations for Evidence-Based Nursing

Chapter 1

EVIDENCE-BASED NURSING: WHAT IS IT?

Betty J. Ackley, MSN, EdS, RN; Gail B. Ladwig, MSN, RN, CHTP;
Beth Ann Swan, PhD, CRNP, FAAN; Sharon J. Tucker, PhD, RN

Welcome to the land of evidence-based nursing (EBN). We are excited that you are reading this text. Our goal is to bring information on EBN in a usable, timely format to all nurses and nursing students. It has been suggested that it may take up to 17 years before significant research findings are implemented in clinical practice (Balas & Boren, 2000). It is our hope that this time frame will be significantly reduced with the publication of this textbook.

This text is designed to help nurses:

- Make decisions about quality care of patients based on research evidence
- Design guidelines for practice and procedures based on research evidence
- See the research evidence that supports excellent nursing practice

Nurses need to base their care on evidence as it is available and appropriate for the patient. A question-and-answer format in this chapter is designed to facilitate use of this text by the busy nurse and nursing student. This text is designed not only for the practicing nurse but for nursing students as well. Nursing students will use the text to learn about EBN and to recognize how it will affect their future nursing practice. Physicians and those in other health-related disciplines have multiple resources that define effective and ineffective treatments. Nurses, as health care providers, also need convenient references on *nursing* interventions that are grounded in research evidence. It is the plan of the authors to provide a starting point for this effort with this textbook.

EVIDENCE-BASED NURSING

What Is It?

EBN is a systematic process that uses current evidence in making decisions about the care of patients, including evaluation of the quality and applicability of existing research, patients' preferences, costs, clinical expertise, and clinical settings (Fineout-Overholt & Melnyk, 2005). EBN is much more than critiquing research studies to determine what results to apply to nursing practice. The clinical reality can be very different from the research context (Thompson, 2004). Application of research findings that have emerged from a single study in a highly controlled environment can be unsafe. Clearly, the care of patients in actual clinical situations is very different and often cannot be controlled. It can be equally unsafe to take research done on people of one age or diagnosis and apply the results to patients of another age with multiple diagnoses

(Dracup & Bryan-Brown, 2006). It is important that the context in which the evidence will be used is considered. This includes the health care environment, the individual patient involved, the expertise of the nurse utilizing the intervention, and, of course, the cost. Using EBN is a complex but important process needed to facilitate quality care and optimal outcomes for patients.

Why Use EBN?

What is the best way to provide nursing care? The answer used to be, "This is how I was taught in nursing school or in orientation," or "That's the way we do it here." The answer now is, "We give care based on the evidence and how it applies to our facility and the individual patient." The EBN process leads to excellence in nursing; evidence-based practice is considered the "gold standard" of health care (Institute of Medicine, 2001).

Outcome measurement is built into the process so that the value of change, based on evidence, can be measured. A classic research study has shown that patients' outcomes were 28% better when nursing care was based on evidence rather than tradition or common sense (Heater et al., 1988). Hospitals that have Magnet Status, an accreditation process that signifies excellence in nursing care, use the EBN process to ensure quality of care (Goode et al., 2005; Turkel, 2005).

The use of EBN can reenergize nursing by helping nurses see the results of their nursing care using measurable outcomes. Nurses will know they are giving the best care possible based on the evidence that is available at the time. There is research on physicians that demonstrates that the use of evidence-based practice has increased work satisfaction (Dawes, 1996). It is predicted that nurses will have the same experience with the use of EBN. Thus, there are many reasons to use EBN, and *all* reasons are in the best interest of the nurse, the patient and family, the health care facility, and health care in general.

Nursing Research Utilization Versus EBN: What Is the Difference?

EBN has evolved from nursing research utilization. Nursing research utilization is a less complex concept; if the nurse finds some "good" research, he or she should evaluate it and put it into effect. EBN is much more complex. When using EBN, there are multiple variables for the nurse to evaluate, including strength of evidence, patient's preference, cost-effectiveness, staffing, clinician experiences, and environmental factors (Melnyk & Fineout-Overholt, 2005). Nursing takes place in a complex world where the patient's preference is now important, cost is a cruel reality, and evidence is needed to guide practice. Table 1-1 shows that EBN better reflects the complexity of today's health care environment than does nursing research utilization.

A Collaborative Approach: Why Is It Important for Health Care Professions to Work Together?

As you read this text, you will rapidly realize that we are utilizing more than nursing research. Medical research and research from many other professions such as psychology, gerontology, and social work are included in this text because many nursing interventions overlap with activities of other disciplines. It is essential that the professions work together to establish practice guidelines based on the best evidence available and interdisciplinary cooperation (Malloch & Porter-O'Grady, 2006). A limitation of EBN is the lack of research in some areas. Our goal for

TABLE 1-1	Evidence-Based Nursing versus Nursing Research Utilization
Evidence-Based Nursing	**Nursing Research Utilization**
Complex process	Less complex process
Newer concept—developed approximately 10 years ago	Older concept—used in the 1970s to early 1990s
Includes patient's preference	Patient's preference not included
Includes a system to grade or level the quality of the research	No defined system to evaluate research; may change practice based on one study
Includes evaluation of the evidence based on the clinical setting in which it will be applied	Clinical setting is not considered
Includes an evaluation of cost-effectiveness	Cost not addressed
Includes evaluation of staffing and expertise of staff	Staffing and expertise not addressed

Data from Melnyk BM, Fineout-Overholt E. (2005). *Evidence-based practice in nursing & healthcare.* Philadelphia: Mosby; University of Minnesota. (2001). *The evidence-based health care project.* Available online: http://evidence.ahc.umn.edu/ebn.htm. Retrieved on July 5, 2007.

this text is to link evidence bases of various professions into a meaningful guideline for nursing practice. We realize that this is an enormous undertaking and have done our best to achieve quality. We also recognize that new research is constantly evolving. You will need to search for newer research studies before applying the information given in this text.

The text also reflects collaboration among nursing practice, nursing administration, and nursing education. We come from education, administration, research, and practice backgrounds, as do the authors of the guidelines.

STANDARDIZED NURSING LANGUAGE: WHY USE IT?

Standardized nursing language is the use of three language components: nursing diagnoses, nursing outcomes, and nursing interventions. This text uses standardized nursing language, specifically nursing outcomes from Nursing Outcomes Classification (NOC) (Moorhead et al., 2004) and nursing interventions from Nursing Interventions Classification (NIC) (Dochterman & Bulechek, 2004). Standardized language for nursing can help the profession prove its worth and greatly facilitate EBN. It is a language to communicate nursing's unique functions. Using the same terms, nurses can speak the same language and share information more effectively (Goode, 2004). Standardized nursing language facilitates nursing research; once nursing phenomena are labeled, it becomes easier to collect data. Also, standardized nursing language becomes especially important as more health care facilities use electronic health records and access patients' charts on the computer. Standardized nursing language is the most effective way to include nursing in this process.

Nursing Diagnosis: What Is It?

Nursing diagnoses have been used since the 1970s. The diagnostic labels are from the North American Nursing Diagnosis Association, now an international organization (NANDA International [NANDA-I]). Nursing diagnoses are used in more than 20 countries throughout the world.

Generalist nurses cannot legally diagnose medical illness; nursing diagnosis is a way to identify and label patients' problems. For more information on nursing diagnoses, please refer to NANDA-International's *Nursing Diagnoses: Definitions & Classification 2007-2008*.

Nursing Outcomes: What Are They?

Nursing outcomes have been standardized by the Iowa Outcomes Project with the NOC. They are outcomes that are evaluated using a five-point Likert-type scale. We have included the appropriate nursing outcome, when available, for each intervention in this text to facilitate outcome evaluation. For more information, please refer to NOC (Moorhead et al., 2004).

Nursing Interventions: How Are They Used with Standardized Nursing Language?

Nursing interventions have been standardized by NIC (Dochterman & Bulechek, 2004). There are now over 514 interventions. These are actions that nurses use when providing nursing care. Each nursing intervention has nursing activities that constitute the intervention. This text uses NIC intervention labels and some of the NIC activity statements with an evaluation of the research that applies. Additional nursing interventions are included that are not NIC interventions. Box 1-1 is an example of the use of standardized nursing language.

Reasons for standardized nursing language include:

A language to communicate the unique function of nursing

Standardization of terms

A means to facilitate communication of the patient's plan of care

An easily attainable data source for research to improve nursing care (Goode, 2004)

BOX 1-1

Example of Standardized Nursing Language

Patient's Situation
A 56-year-old man who is 2 days postoperative from a colon resection. He has a smoking history of 60 pack-years (30 years × 2 packs per day). At present, he has course crackles in both lungs. His vital signs are: temperature 100.2, pulse 110, respirations 26, blood pressure 142/76, oxygen saturation 91%.
Nursing Diagnosis (NANDA-I): Ineffective airway clearance R/T shallow breathing associated with pain, decreased mobility, and smoking
Nursing Outcome (NOC): Respiratory status: Airway patency
Nursing Interventions (NIC):
Respiratory monitoring
Cough enhancement
Exercise therapy: Ambulation

R/T, Related to.
Data from Ackley B & Ladwig G. (2008). *Nursing diagnosis handbook: An evidence-based guide to planning care,* 8th ed. St. Louis: Mosby. Dochterman JM, Bulechek GM (Eds). (2004). *Nursing Interventions Classification (NIC),* 4th ed. St. Louis: Mosby; Moorhead S, Johnson M, Maas M (Eds). (2004). *Nursing Outcomes Classification (NOC),* 3rd ed. St. Louis: Mosby; NANDA-International: (2005). *Nursing diagnoses: Definitions and classification 2007-2008.* Philadelphia: NANDA International.

LEVELS OF EVIDENCE: EVALUATING QUALITY OF EXISTING RESEARCH

What Does *Levels of Evidence* Mean?

In this text, evidence for use of nursing activities ranges from rigorous to weak, and levels are assigned to rate the strength of the evidence to help assess the quality of the body of evidence. Melnyk (2004) have devised a rating scheme that has been adapted and used to rate the strength of the evidence supporting each intervention guideline in this book. The scheme includes seven levels of evidence (Table 1-2). *Level I* is the strongest evidence and is an analysis of many well-conducted randomized controlled studies (meta-analysis or systematic review of the literature). *Level VII* is the weakest evidence, usually consisting of non–research-based opinions of experts or published clinical articles that are not research based. For more information about research studies, please refer to the glossary in this text or to a text on nursing research. High levels of evidence may not exist for many clinical questions because of the nature of nursing problems and research and ethical limitations.

How Is Nursing Evidence Identified to Be Put into Practice?

In this text, we asked nursing experts to perform a systematic literature review and evaluate the meaning of existing research studies. To designate the meaning of the nursing activities read, the nurse experts classified nursing activities into four categories: *effective, possibly effective, not effective,* and *possibly harmful.* A further explanation of these labels follows.

Effective. Research validates the effectiveness of the nursing activity, preferably with level I evidence or with level 2 or less with expert opinion. Some activities have been deemed standards of practice (labeled *SP*) that should be performed even though there may not be an accessible research base supporting their use. An example of an SP regarding the nurse programming a patient-controlled analgesia (PCA) pump would be as presented at the top of p. 8.

TABLE 1-2	Levels of Evidence
Level and Quality of Evidence	**Type of Evidence**
Level I	Evidence from a systematic review or meta-analysis of all relevant randomized clinical trials (RCTs), or evidence-based clinical practice guidelines based on systematic reviews of RCTs or three or more RCTs of good quality that have similar results
Level II	Evidence obtained from at least one well-designed RCT
Level III	Evidence obtained from well-designed controlled trials without randomization
Level IV	Evidence from well-designed case-control or cohort studies
Level V	Evidence from systematic reviews of descriptive and qualitative studies (meta-synthesis)
Level VI	Evidence from a single descriptive or qualitative study
Level VII	Evidence from the opinion of authorities and/or reports of expert committees

Adapted from Melnyk BM. (2004). A focus on adult acute and critical care. *Worldviews Evid Based Nurs,* 1(3):194-197; modified from Guyatt & Rennie (2002), Harris et al. (2001).

■ ⓢⓟ *Double-check programming of the pump using the "second person separate*
     check" process (two professionals double-check the pump simultaneously).

This activity should be performed for patients' safety even though there is not enough research
to show unequivocally that it is effective.

Possibly Effective. There are some research studies that validate the effectiveness of the
nursing activity but not enough to recommend that nurses institute the activity at this time.
Generally, more research is needed. These are nursing activities that the nurse should watch for
more research to validate and recognize that the activity may be used in the future. In some settings, these activities may be implemented.

Not Effective. Research has shown that the nursing activity is not effective and generally
should not be used.

Possibly Harmful. There are some studies that show harm to patients when using the
nursing activity, and the nurse should evaluate carefully whether the activity is appropriate for
patients' care. As a general rule, the activity should no longer be performed. An example is adding
blue dye to tube feeding formula, as there have been reported cases of death caused by use of the
dye. (Please refer to the guideline on Tube Feeding for more information regarding this
activity.)

The authors of the guidelines sometimes were unable to find research relevant to all the
categories; the following wording was used in these circumstances: *No applicable published
research was found in this category.* After each nursing activity, you will find one- to two-sentence
descriptions of research studies that supported the activity. This information is helpful for the
nurse reader to learn where the research is found. We recommend that the reader obtain
full copies of the research before making major decisions in use of EBN. Thus, the guidelines
evaluate the existing research and give you beginning information on which to base nursing
practice.

To help ensure quality, each guideline was peer reviewed twice, once by the nurse author with
whom the contributor of the guideline was working and then again by an independent nurse
with expertise in the area.

MODELS OF EBN: WHAT ARE THEY?

EBN models are defined systems that are utilized to guide the use of EBN in health care facilities.
Many of these are highly prescriptive of how EBN can be instituted; others are more generalized
and provide nonspecific information.

What Are the More Commonly Used Models of EBN?

Multiple models exist of how EBN can be instituted in the health care setting. Some of the more
common are the Iowa model and the Stetler model. Refer to Table 1-3 for a brief explanation of
more frequently used models.

Chapter 3 provides an explanation of the model used at the University of Colorado Medical
Center to actualize EBN. The information shared will be helpful to any nurse who is attempting
to bring EBN to his or her health care facility.

A Cochrane review found that there has been no research performed that designates the
effectiveness or cost savings of an EBN model (Foxcroft & Cole, 2003). Again, the models are
concepts of how EBN can be actualized; there have been no empirical studies of their
effectiveness.

TABLE 1-3	Models for Application of Evidence-Based Nursing	
Conceptual Model	**Description**	**Source**
Advancing Research and Clinical Practice through Close Collaboration (ARCC)	A collaborative model of health care professions and also nursing education and practice working together to actualize EBP	Melnyk & Fineout-Overholt, 2002
Best Practice Health Care Map	A design model for planning and managing quality clinical care: improving population, system, and individual patient health outcomes through the incorporation of various forms of evidence	Brown, 2001
Evidence-Based Multidisciplinary Practice, University of Colorado Hospital	A conceptual model of multidisciplinary practice promoting EBN	Chapter 3 of this text
Iowa Model of Evidence-Based Practice to Promote Quality Care	A commonly used implementation model of EBN	Titler, 2006
Pathways of Research-Based Practice	An evidence appraisal model for clinical decision making based on the determination of the credibility, clinical significance, and applicability of the research evidence and a goal of quality improvement for the individual patient or practice	Brown, 1999
Rosswurm and Larrabee	An implementation model of EBN that includes the change process, similar to the nursing process	Rosswurm & Larrabee, 1999
Stetler Model of Research Utilization and Evidence-Based Practice	A commonly used implementation model that includes a five-phase process to appraise critically through theory and evidence and to determine if, when, and how to implement evidence	Stetler, 2001a, b

Data from University of Minnesota. (2001). The evidence-based health care project. Available online: http://evidence. ahc.umn.edu/ebn.htm. Retrieved on July 5, 2007. Melnyk BM, Fineout-Overholt E. (2005). *Evidence-based practice in nursing & healthcare*. Philadelphia: Lippincott Williams & Wilkins.

EBN AND QUALITY: HOW DO THEY FIT TOGETHER?

There are multiple quality initiatives affecting health care as a positive force at this time. Many forces are demanding quality care, including third-party payers, business, patients, and the government. All of the quality initiatives require collection of data, which is greatly facilitated by the health care facility having an EBN framework. One of these quality initiatives is from The Joint Commission (TJC). Others are voluntary but desirable for the facilities' well-being. These quality initiatives are summarized in Table 1-4.

TABLE 1-4	Quality Initiatives Affecting Health Care That Are Facilitated by Evidence-Based Nursing		
Quality Initiatives	Description	Core Measures	Mandatory or Voluntary
The Joint Commission (TJC), 2006	Organization dedicated to improve continuously the safety and quality of care provided to the public through the provision of health care accreditation and related services that support performance improvement in health care organizations (TJC, 2006)	Patient falls, skin breakdown, pneumonia, postoperative infections, upper gastrointestinal (GI) bleed, shock, cardiac arrest, urinary tract infections (UTIs), pain management	Mandatory
National Database of Nursing Quality Indicators (NDNQI, 2006)	Proprietary database of the American Nurses Association that collects and evaluates unit-specific nurse-sensitive data from hospitals in the United States (NDNQI, 2006)	Patient falls, skin breakdown, pneumonia, upper GI bleed, shock, cardiac arrest, UTIs, sepsis, deep vein thrombosis, failure to rescue	Voluntary
Magnet Status	Accreditation process from the American Nurses Credentialing Center that designates high-quality nursing care (ANCC, 2006)	Quality measures including nursing leadership, EBN, satisfaction of nurses in facility, hospital meets national safety goals	Voluntary
Institute for Health Care Improvement (IHI) 10,000 Lives Campaign, 2006	Campaign to save lives in American hospitals by applying evidence-based changes to patient care (IHI, 2006)	Deploy rapid response teams. Deliver reliable, evidence-based care for acute myocardial infarction. Prevent adverse drug events (ADEs). Prevent central line infections. Prevent surgical site infections. Prevent ventilator-associated pneumonia.	Voluntary

HOW DO I USE THIS TEXT?

The guidelines in this text are only a starting point for the use of EBN. They are an evaluation of the existing research by one or more nursing experts. Although the guidelines may seem prescriptive, there are multiple factors that must be considered before putting the findings into practice. To use the EBN process effectively, the nurse should:

Perform an updated literature search on the topic to see if there are any more current research findings in the area; it is always possible that newer findings may differ from the work found in this text.

Critically examine whether the guideline findings are appropriate for the particular patient.

Critically examine whether the guideline findings are appropriate for the health care facility in terms of costs, number of available staff, educational background, and abilities of the staff.

This is critical thinking at its finest to determine whether the recommendation is relevant in each situation. For more information on how to use EBN as a practicing nurse, please refer to Chapter 5. For information on how to use EBN as a student nurse, please refer to Chapter 4.

SUMMARY

EBN is an exciting new concept that will lead to improved quality of patients' care. It is based on research, but it is more. EBN is a logical blending of quality research, nursing expertise, patients' preference, and the health care reality. EBN is facilitated by use of standardized nursing language so that we are all using the same language, nationally and internationally. Everyone benefits from the practice of EBN: the patient, the nurse, other health care providers, and the health care environment. EBN, along with evidence-based practice with all health care professionals working in concert, will advance nursing into a new era of quality health care.

REFERENCES

American Nurses Credentialing Center (ANCC). (2006). Benefits of becoming a Magnet designated facility. Available online: http://www.nursingworld.org. Retrieved on July 5, 2007.

Balas EA, Boren SA. (2000). Managing clinical knowledge for health care improvements. In Schattauer V (Ed): *Yearbook of medical informatics.* St. Louis: Mosby, pp 65-70.

Brown SJ. (1999). *Knowledge for health care practice: A guide to using research evidence.* Philadelphia: Saunders.

Brown SJ. (2001). Managing the complexity of best practice health care. *J Nurs Care Qual,* 15(2):1-8.

Dawes M. (1996). On the need for evidence-based general and family practice. *Evid Based Med,* 1:68-69.

Dochterman JM, Bulechek GM. (Eds). (2004). *Nursing Interventions Classification (NIC),* 4th ed. St. Louis: Mosby.

Dracup K, Bryan-Brown CW. (2006). Evidence-based practice is wonderful . . . sort of. *Am J Crit Care,* 15(4):356-359.

Fineout-Overholt E, Melnyk B. (2005). Building a culture of best practice. *Nurse Leader,* 3(6):26-30.

Foxcroft DR, Cole N. (2003). Organisational infrastructures to promote evidence based nursing practice. *Cochrane Database Syst Rev,* (4):CD002212.

Goode CJ. (2004). Importance of using standardized language for the chief nursing officer and the nursing leadership. Presentation at the NANDA, NIC & NOC Conference. March 27, 2004.

Goode CJ, Krugman ME, Smith K, Diaz J, Edmonds S, Mulder J. (2005). The pull of magnetism: A look at the standards and the experience of a western academic medical center hospital in achieving and sustaining Magnet status. *Nurs Adm Q,* 29(3):202-213.

Guyatt G, Rennie D. (2002). *User's guides to the medical literature.* Washington, DC: American Medical Association Press.

Harris RP, Helfand M, Woolf SH, Lohr KN, Mulrow CD, Teutch SM et al. (2001). Current Methods of the US Preventive Services Task Force. A review of the process. *Am J Prev Med,* 20(3 Suppl):21-35.

Heater BS, Becker AM, Olson RK. (1988). Nursing interventions and patient outcomes: A meta-analysis of studies. *Nurs Res,* 37(5):303-307.

Institute for Health Care Improvement, 10,000 Lives Campaign. (2006). Overview. Available online: http://www.ihi.org/. Retrieved on July 5, 2007.

Institute of Medicine, Committee of Quality of Health Care in America. (2001). *Crossing the quality chasm: A new health system for the 21st century.* Washington, DC: National Academies Press.

The Joint Commission. (2006). Mission statement. Available online: http://www.jointcommission.org/. Retrieved on July 7, 2007.

Malloch K, Porter-O'Grady T. (2006). *Introduction to evidence-based practice.* Sudbury: Jones & Bartlett.

Melnyk BM. (2004). A focus on adult acute and critical care. *Worldviews Evid Based Nurs,* 1(3):194-197.

Melnyk BM, Fineout-Overholt E. (2002). Putting research into practice. Rochester ARCC. *Reflect Nurs Leadersh,* 28(2):22-25.

Melnyk BM, Fineout-Overholt E. (2005). *Evidence-based practice in nursing & healthcare.* Philadelphia: Lippincott Williams and Wilkins.

Moorhead S, Johnson M, Maas M. (Eds). (2004). *Nursing Outcomes Classification (NOC),* 3rd ed. St. Louis: Mosby.

National Database of Nursing Quality Indicators. (2006). Available online: http://www.nursingquality.org. Retrieved on July 5, 2007.

NANDA-International. (2005). *Nursing diagnoses: Definitions and classification 2005-2006.* Philadelphia: NANDA International.

Rosswurm MA, Larrabee J. (1999). A model for change to evidence-based practice. *Image J Nurs Sch,* 31(4):317-322.

Stetler CB. (2001a). Updating the Stetler model of research utilization to facilitate evidence-based practice. *Nurs Outlook,* 49:272-278.

Stetler CB. (2001b). *Evidence-based practice and the use of research: A synopsis of basic strategy and concepts to improve care.* Washington, DC: Nova Fdn.

Thompson C. (2004). Fortuitous phenomena: On complexity, pragmatic randomized controlled trials, and knowledge for evidence-based practice. *Worldviews Evid Based Nurs,* 1(1):9-17.

Titler MG. (2006). Use of research in practice. In LoBiondo-Wood G, Haber J (Eds). *Nursing research: Methods and critical appraisal for evidence-based practice,* 6th ed. St Louis: Mosby.

Turkel MC. (2005). An essential component of the magnet journey: Fostering an environment for evidence-based practice and nursing research. *Nurs Adm Q,* 29(3):254-262.

University of Minnesota. (2001). *The evidence-based health care project.* Available online: http://evidence.ahc.umn.edu/ebn.htm. Retrieved on July 5, 2007.

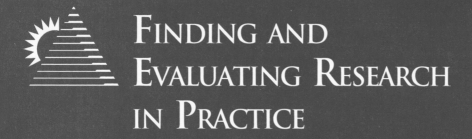

Chapter 2

FINDING AND EVALUATING RESEARCH IN PRACTICE

Sharon J. Tucker, PhD, RN; Marianne E. Olson, PhD, RN;
Lori M. Rhudy, PhD, RN, CNRN, CRRN, APBN-BC

Finding and evaluating research evidence for professional nursing practice are critical activities in evidence-based practice (EBP). This chapter offers a practical approach to the identification, organization, and critique of such evidence. The specific objective of this chapter is to provide examples, tools, and resources to assist in finding and evaluating evidence to support nursing practice within the confines of limited resources, time, and experience. The chapter is organized according to the five-step process of EBP suggested by Melnyk (Melnyk & Fineout-Overholt, 2005).

STEP ONE: ASKING THE QUESTION

Searching for research evidence requires a structured approach. When a problem or question has been identified, it must be phrased as a question that can be answered. The question or questions asked guide the selection of tools used to locate the evidence and the terms used to search a database; key considerations in developing the question are given in Box 2-1. For example, a nurse might wonder whether placing items such as call bells and urinals in a stroke patient's unaffected visual field is more effective than placing them in the affected visual field.

STEP TWO: LOCATING RESOURCES

When a clinical question is formulated, the search for answers begins with locating resources that will provide the evidence to address the clinical question. A number of skills and actions are necessary for achieving this step, including acquiring a basic set of skills and obtaining access to a number of resources. These skills and resources are discussed.

Required Skills

In today's electronic environment, computer skills and resources are essential tools for nurses. At a minimum, the nurse must possess the skill to search relevant and credible websites as well as access electronic libraries and databases. A variety of approaches can be used to gain the necessary skills to perform these activities, including completing independent learning modules or tutorials, attending classes, and consulting with experts for one-on-one education or guidance. Many health care organizations and nursing programs not only provide access to electronic resources but also employ individuals skilled in using electronic tools and databases to provide training and support. Librarians (especially medical librarians), information technology (IT) support, online and telephone help-desk services, and faculty in computer education are some of the experts who can aid in developing the skills needed for locating evidence.

Library Resources

There is perhaps no more valuable asset in the search for evidence than a medical reference librarian. Medical reference librarians complete specialized education in health care information. They are knowledgeable about each of the many health care databases (discussed subsequently) and can provide valuable insight in search strategies. Medical reference librarians are employed by many health care organizations and academic institutions. If an agency does not employ a medical reference librarian, a nurse can make contact or partner with a local university colleague to find a medical librarian.

Electronic Databases

Electronic databases are web-based tools that allow one to search, navigate, and personalize searches for thousands of textbooks, journals, and articles. Examples include the Ovid databases (CINAHL, MEDLINE, and PsycINFO) and PubMed; brief descriptions of these and other databases are provided in Table 2-1. Although content from these databases may overlap, each has a specific focus and audience in mind. When used in combination, they can provide an extensive search for information specific to a topic of interest.

Internet Resources

Internet resources provide the most efficient and effective way to find research evidence. Internet resources include not only websites about EBP and specific problems or practices but also databases such as PubMed and Ovid that allow searching for research publications on a specific topic. There are many websites focused on EBP. These websites serve four purposes: (1) to learn about EBP in general; (2) to identify the processes and tools for EBP; (3) to provide links to evidence in the form of clinical guidelines, integrative reviews, or consensus statements; and (4) to provide links to databases in which the nurse can search for evidence on a specific topic. Examples of the most referenced EBP websites are listed in Box 2-2. These websites offer links to research evidence and many helpful tools and tips for finding evidence.

Access to some databases housed within EBP websites is limited to subscribers. Generally, subscriptions can be held by an organization (usually through library services) or by an individual. When trying to access information that requires subscription, prompts with information about subscribing usually appear. Before subscribing individually, consultation with a librarian is recommended to determine whether a subscription exists for one's organization.

TABLE 2-1	Electronic Databases
Database	**Description**
Ovid MEDLINE	Literature in the fields of medicine, nursing, dentistry, veterinary medicine, and the preclinical sciences.
Ovid CINAHL (Cumulative Index of Nursing and Allied Health Literature)	Literature related to nursing and the allied health disciplines including medical records, physical and occupational therapy, medical/laboratory technology, respiratory therapy, biomedicine, behavioral sciences, management, and more. Also provides access to book chapters, dissertations, selected conference proceedings, standards of professional practice, educational software, and audiovisual materials related to nursing and allied health.
OVID PsycINFO	Professional and academic literature in psychology and related disciplines including medicine, psychiatry, nursing, sociology, education, pharmacology, physiology, linguistics, allied health, and other areas.
Ovid Embase	Biomedical and pharmaceutical database that contains selective coverage for nursing, dentistry, veterinary medicine, psychology, and alternative medicine.
ERIC	U.S. Department of Education database of education publications and research reports.
PubMed	The U.S. National Library of Medicine (NLM) database of biomedical citations and abstracts that is searchable on the Web (http://pubmed.gov) at no cost. MEDLINE is the largest component of PubMed.
ISI Web of Knowledge • Arts & Humanities Citation Index • Science Citation Index Expanded • Social Science Citation Index	Institute for Scientific Information (ISI) citation databases of international journals in the arts and humanities; leading scholarly science and technical journals (including agriculture, biology, chemistry, computer science, engineering, medicine, physics, and veterinary science); and the world's leading scholarly social sciences journals.
Cochrane Library	A collection of databases designed to supply high-quality evidence to inform people providing and receiving care.
Cochrane Database of Systematic Reviews	Full text articles reviewing the effects of health care. The reviews are highly structured and systematic, with evidence included or excluded on the basis of explicit quality criteria to minimize bias.
ClinicalTrials.gov	A review of clinical studies sponsored by the National Institutes of Health, other federal agencies, and private industry on a wide range of diseases and conditions.
National Guideline Clearinghouse	An initiative of the Agency for Healthcare Research and Quality (AHRQ) and the U.S. Department of Health and Human Services that provides a public resource for evidence-based clinical practice guidelines.
Sigma Theta Tau International (STTI) Registry of Nursing Research	Searchable database of nursing research studies from Sigma Theta Tau International, the International Honor Society of Nursing.

BOX 2-2

Evidence-Based Practice Websites

Academic Center for Evidence-Based Nursing
http://www.acestar.uthscsa.edu/About.htm
(The University of Texas Health Science Center at San Antonio)
This site introduces a model for understanding the cycles, nature, and characteristics of knowledge that are used in various aspects of evidence-based practice (EBP). The ACE Star Model places nursing's previous scientific work within the context of EBP, serves as an organizer for examining and applying EBP, and mainstreams nursing into the formal network of EBP.

The Iowa Model for Evidence-Based Practice
http://www.uihealthcare.com/depts/nursing/rqom/evidencebasedpractice/iowamodel.html
(University of Iowa Hospitals and Clinics)
This comprehensive site introduces the Iowa Model, which has several distinct advantages: it provides a guide for clinical decision making, it provides details regarding implementation of EBP, and it includes both the practitioner and organizational perspective.

The Joanna Briggs Institute
http://www.joannabriggs.edu.au/about/home.php
(The University of Adelaide)
This site describes a collaborative approach to the evaluation of evidence derived from a diverse range of sources, including experience, expertise, and all forms of rigorous research and the translation, transfer, and use of the "best available" evidence into practice.

Healthlinks at University of Washington
http://healthlinks.washington.edu/
(University of Washington)
This comprehensive site includes links to Find the Evidence, Evidence Calculators, EBP Statistics, EBP Research Centers, Learn about EBP, and EBP Literature.

Teaching/Learning Resources for Evidence-Based Practice
http://www.mdx.ac.uk/www/rctsh/ebp/main.htm
(Middlesex University Research Centre for Transcultural Studies in Health)
This is a collection of tools for identifying, assessing, and applying relevant evidence for better health care decision making.

Resources for Evidence-Based Nursing at McMaster University
http://hsl.lib.mcmaster.ca/education/nursing/ebn/index.htm
(McMaster University)
This comprehensive site outlines a process for asking the practice question with supporting links to finding the evidence, EBP literature, and learning more about EBP.

Tips for Searching Electronic Databases

Locating EBP websites and databases is followed by navigating these sites to find the evidence related to a particular aspect of nursing care. This process requires a systematic search and many times involves some trial-and-error learning to find the best terms to use. Seldom is one term enough (Box 2-3). Each database has its own search mechanism. As a result, searching methods within databases may vary. Nearly all of the databases provide tutorials or help-related search strategies. It is worth the time and effort to explore these resources in order to make more efficient and effective searches (Box 2-4).

Many electronic databases allow searches not only by term but also by author, journal, or title. These features allow a search for a specific paper, which is useful when a citation is given. For example, one might want to read the first in a series of two studies but have only the second

---

BOX 2-3

Case in Point: Search Terms

One intervention activity for the management of unilateral neglect (inattention to one side of the body or visual field) is to give frequent reminders to cue the patient in the environment. To examine the evidence underlying this information, the Ovid CINAHL and MEDLINE databases were searched with the following key terms entered:
- Unilateral neglect
- Unilateral neglect and management

  Results from this search consisted of several studies related to therapies for patients with unilateral neglect, but none of the abstracts discussed environmental cues. The search was then refined to:
- Unilateral neglect and environment
- Environmental and scan

  Then further to:
- Unilateral neglect and scan and environment

  This refined the search, which resulted in identification of a series of papers related to interventions used in the treatment of unilateral neglect.

  In addition, review of the literature suggested that a suitable synonym for unilateral neglect is visuospatial neglect. Based on clinical experience, the nurse asking the question knew that homonymous visuospatial neglect hemianopsia is frequently associated with visual perceptual alterations. The search was repeated using these terms, which provided additional literature for consideration.

BOX 2-4

Expanding and Limiting Searches

One way to search for evidence is to use symbols to expand or limit your search. Exploding search terms is useful when you want to include variations on terms. In the example in Box 2-3, one might want to include not only the word environment but also "environmental," "environ," or similar mutations of the term. By using the explode features of a database, entering "envir" and a character ("$" in CINAHL) allows searching all terms at once. Identifying limits for the search can also be helpful in managing a search. Common limits that can be applied are publication date, language, research, and abstract or full text available. Search limits generally decrease the number of citations identified, and the search is thus a little less overwhelming than when thousands of citations are found.

---

paper. Using the citation as a guide, it is possible to search for that particular first paper. Perhaps a particular author is known to have published extensively on a topic, but the citations are not available. In this case, a search by author name can be helpful. Finally, perhaps a colleague may say something like, "Wasn't there an article on that in (a recent journal)?" In this case, a journal search might help locate the paper.

Other electronic sources of evidence include nursing organization websites and electronic journals. Browsing the websites of specialty organizations for references, resources, and evidence related to the specialty area of practice can be useful. Specialty websites can help to identify experts in a specialty area. There are also a number of electronic journals that are focused on EBP; some of the most widely recognized are listed in Box 2-5.

> ### BOX 2-5
>
> #### Evidence-Based Practice Online Nursing Journals
>
> *Clinical Effectiveness in Nursing*
> *Evidence-Based Nursing*
> *Evidence-Based Healthcare*
> *Bandolier*
> *EBM Online*
> *Worldviews on Evidence-Based Nursing*

> ### BOX 2-6
>
> #### Using Favorites and Bookmarks
>
> Choose "Favorites" or "Bookmark" from the toolbar on your web browser (Internet Explorer, Netscape, etc.) to return quickly to a website. As with placing a bookmark in a book, the site's Internet address is stored as a link. Some tips for using Favorites and Bookmarks:
> - After selecting "Add to Favorites" or "Bookmark," change the name of the Favorite to something that will help you remember where the link leads to.
> - Bookmarks or Favorites will sometimes link only to a main or home page of a website. To find desired information, you may have to navigate through additional links.
> - As websites are updated, links to desired information may change, and so too must your Favorites list.

Sharing Resources

Nurses may choose to collaborate in locating the best evidence for a practice question, especially because it is common for nurses to observe similar concerns or issues related to nursing care and specialty interventions or practices. Given the concentrated and focused shift responsibilities of nurses, there is often very limited time for one nurse to explore a clinical question comprehensively. Creating forums to discuss these questions and search for evidence to provide the answers can maximize use of resources and allow full exploration of the question. Sharing of resources is thus important in these collaborative endeavors.

Using "Favorites" on the home page of the website is often one easy way to access and share frequently visited sites. In settings where computers are shared, well-defined (intuitive) labels for these sites are important to be most efficient (Box 2-6). Shared electronic folders are another option for settings where either computers or networks are shared among users. These folders could be storage for documents downloaded from a website or documents generated by the users at the site. Similarly, shared libraries on work units can store documents, articles, or books that include important evidence or sources of evidence that support nursing interventions or practices. It is recommended that guidelines be drafted for generating and modifying the shared resource or that one person be specifically assigned, perhaps in a rotating fashion, to create and update the guidelines and any indexes. Thus, accuracy, completeness, consistency, and up-to-date evidence will more likely be maintained. Nurses with minimal computer skills will be wise to attend a basic computer skills class or complete an online tutorial to be able to

---

BOX 2-7

Current Topics and E-mail Alerts: Keeping Current on the Evidence

A helpful service that many libraries offer is current topics. In this type of service, the library forwards a copy of the table of contents from selected current issues of journals. After an article of interest has been identified, paper or electronic copies of it can be requested from a library. Check with the librarians at one's organization to find out if this type of service is available. Similar alerts are offered by publishers and can be accessed by registering on the publisher's website. Although the disadvantage is that these alerts are limited to publications of the particular publisher, the advantage is the opportunity to receive alerts, not only by journal but also by author or topic. These alerts are typically sent by e-mail with links to specific articles that can be accessed when desired.

---

participate in the discussions related to clinical questions and in the search for the evidence to provide answers and solutions to questions about the best practices. An additional resource that nurses can share and that is available through many libraries is current topics and e-mail alerts (Box 2-7).

In summary, locating and organizing references that can address a question about the evidence supporting a nursing practice require time, skills, and access to resources. Multiple tools are available to assist nurses in this process, many of which are available at low or no cost. When the evidence is located, it must be critically reviewed and appraised. The next section outlines this process and suggests resources to assist nurses in this sophisticated process.

STEP THREE: CRITICALLY APPRAISING THE EVIDENCE

When the research evidence has been located, it must be critically appraised for its strength. This process was completed by the numerous contributors who created the guidelines found in this book. A critical appraisal process involves reviewing each relevant reference or article and rating the type and level of the evidence. Use of a guiding table such as that in Figure 2-1 provides a systematic approach to compiling and comparing research studies to draw conclusions about the overall level of evidence supporting a particular nursing intervention or practice. A decision can then be made about whether a particular intervention should be implemented, applied universally, applied only under specific circumstances, or eliminated if ineffective or possibly even harmful to patients. How quickly action should be taken is an important consideration in making a decision about a practice change. As noted by Guyatt and colleagues (2001), a decision about initiating a preventive or therapeutic regimen requires consideration of the patient or public benefits in comparison with the toxicity, cost, and administrative burden to patients and providers. Hence, clinicians do not administer all treatments judged to be effective by a positive outcome to all patients eligible for the treatment (Guyatt et al., 2001).

Leveling of Evidence

Leveling of evidence is based largely on the study design and methods, although a number of other factors should be considered in evaluating the evidence, such as the study sample characteristics, setting, magnitude of treatment or intervention effects, strengths, limitations, and clinical relevance. Systematic reviews, evidence-based guidelines, and meta-analyses are often

Source	Purpose/ Problem	Sample	Framework	Concepts	Design	Instruments	Results	Implications	Comments
Tham & Kielhofner (2003)	Gain understanding of social environmental influences on occupational experience and performance over the course of rehabilitation	Four women with unilateral neglect in Sweden	Phenomenological philosophy	Unilateral neglect; inattention to stimuli or one half of one's body; interaction with daily environment and others in environment	Qualitative phenomenology *Phenomenology (use noun, not adj)*	Interviews – 5-7 over 16 weeks of rehab services	Participants identified that professionals and relatives used a sequence of strategies for helping them deal with the neglect, allowing the patients to regain the neglected half of the world; participants learned to incorporate others as extensions of themselves	More careful attention to the lived body and the life-world of such persons; more systematically adapt the social environment to adapt a comprehension of the left world Changing levels of support as neglect improves	Small sample of Swedish women Occupational therapy literature

FIG 2-1 • Example format of organized research. (Adapted from Burns NB, Grove SK. [2005]. *The practice of nursing research*, 5th ed. St. Louis: Saunders, Table 6-5, p. 106.)

organized together as the highest type and level of evidence, followed by single randomized controlled trials (RCTs), observation, and descriptive studies. Each of these types of evidence is summarized subsequently.

Evidence-Based Clinical Practice Guidelines. Evidence-based clinical practice guidelines provide the strongest level of support to guide practice, as they are based on rigorous reviews of the best research on specific topic areas (Melnyk, 2004). The National Guideline Clearinghouse (NGC) is probably the best known comprehensive database of evidence-based clinical practice guidelines and related documents. NGC is an initiative of the Agency for Healthcare Research and Quality (AHRQ), U.S. Department of Health and Human Services. "NGC was originally created by AHRQ in partnership with the American Medical Association and the American Association of Health Plans (now America's Health Insurance Plans [AHIP]). . . . The NGC mission is to provide physicians, nurses, other health professionals, health care providers, health plans, integrated delivery systems, purchasers, and others with an accessible mechanism for obtaining objective, detailed information on clinical practice guidelines and to further their dissemination, implementation, and use" (AHRQ, 2007). These guidelines are published and endorsed only after a rigorous and exhaustive review of the research evidence.

Systematic Reviews. A systematic review is a summary of evidence on a particular topic that uses a rigorous process for retrieving, critically appraising, and synthesizing studies in order to answer a question about a burning clinical issue (Melnyk, 2004). The Cochrane Database is perhaps the most outstanding resource to identify and retrieve systematic reviews. The Cochrane Collaboration is an international, nonprofit, independent organization established to ensure that up-to-date, accurate information about the effects of health care interventions is readily available worldwide (Cochrane Library, 2007). It produces and disseminates systematic reviews of health care interventions and promotes the search for evidence in the form of clinical trials and other studies of the effects of interventions. The Cochrane Collaboration prepares Cochrane reviews and aims to update them regularly with the latest scientific evidence. Members of the organization (mostly volunteers) work together to provide evidence to help people make decisions about health care. The Cochrane Collaboration website provides information on a variety of ways of registering interest or becoming directly involved.

Meta-Analyses. A meta-analysis is a type of data analysis wherein the results of several studies, none of which need find anything of statistical significance, are pooled together and analyzed as if they were the results of one large study. In order to summarize results of comparative experiments, the dependent variable in a meta-analysis is converted to a standardized measure of effect size. The effect size must be standardized as the independent variables and their scales differ from study to study (Wikipedia, 2007). "The usual effect size indicator is the standardized mean difference *(d),* which is the standard score equivalent to the difference between means, or an odds ratio if the outcome of the experiments is a dichotomous variable (success versus failure)" (Wikipedia, 2007). A meta-analysis can also be performed on correlational studies, whereby the correlation coefficients are the indicator of the effect size. Additionally, the method can be performed on a collection of studies without restricting to those in which one or more variables are defined as "dependent."

Randomized Clinical Trials. The RCT is considered the "gold standard" of research methods when evaluating the strength of the study findings (i.e., evidence) because no other study design can provide the same safeguards against bias. For example, if an investigator were interested in studying the effects of a home visiting program (delivered by nurses) on infant and maternal health outcomes, it would be important not only to have a control group (a group that does not receive the nurse home visits) but also to assign randomly (by chance) participants to an intervention or control group so as to eliminate other explanations for why outcomes were superior in one group. "Blinding" participants to treatment or control group assignment is even more robust in terms of linking differences in group outcomes to the intervention and maximally reducing alternative explanations for differences in group outcomes. However, in many nursing intervention trials, such as a home visiting trial, blinding participants and providers to group assignment is not possible.

Level I. Multiple RCTs yielding consistent findings on the effects of a nursing intervention constitute level I evidence. When findings are inconsistent among multiple RCTs, other factors need to be evaluated before making a conclusion about an intervention. Factors that could account for inconsistent findings are differences in the study samples, fidelity of intervention implementation, outcomes measured, procedures for measuring outcomes, the overall study procedures, and the effects of chance. Guyatt and colleagues (2001) proposed that studies be compared and evaluated statistically to determine whether or not the differences in findings can be explained in a way that provides evidence of the intervention effectiveness under specific circumstances.

Level II. When only *one* RCT on the effects of an intervention exists, the evidence is rated as level II. Such findings must be viewed through a cautious lens before considering a practice change.

Level III. Level III studies may include well-designed controlled (control or comparison group) trials but without randomization. Such studies have less internal validity, given that the participants cannot be assumed to be equal in terms of other demographic and clinical variables.

Level IV. Level IV studies include well-designed case-control and cohort studies where there may be measurement of naturalistic events or exposures but no manipulation of variables or random assignment of participants to different conditions.

Levels V and VI. Levels V and VI consist of findings obtained from descriptive, observational, and/or qualitative research designs. These types of designs are important in nursing research for generating information and knowledge of various phenomena. Multiple qualitative or descriptive studies on the same intervention may be summarized in a systematic review, which provides a higher level of evidence than a single study.

Level VII. Level VII evidence is the lowest level of evidence and consists of the opinion of clinical experts.

Knowledge and understanding of these five levels and knowledge of basic and advanced research methods are required to rate effectively the research evidence related to nursing interventions. Staff nurses and student nurses who have limited knowledge and training in these areas are strongly encouraged to seek consultation from nurses with advanced research and statistical training as well as statisticians to provide the best review of the existing research evidence. Multiple resources are also available to assist nurses in the review process, such as an article published by Melnyk and Fineout-Overholt (2005) that offers a guideline for rapid critical appraisal of RCTs. They propose three questions for a nurse to consider:

Are the findings valid (i.e., as close to the truth as possible)?

Are the findings important? (That is, what is the impact of the intervention? What is the size or the extent to which the intervention or treatment worked?)

Are the findings clinically relevant or applicable to the patients for whom I am caring?

In addition to existing published and Internet resources for reviewing research articles, Table 2-2 presents a number of factors to consider when evaluating the quality of research articles.

TABLE 2-2	Factors to Consider When Evaluating Research Evidence
Factor	**Evaluation Questions**
Study design	Did the study include random assignment, a control group, and repeated measures? Was it a descriptive study or observational design?
Population/sample	Who is the population under study, what was the sample, and how was the sample selected? Were participants randomly assigned to treatment or control group?
Inclusion/exclusion criteria	What criteria did participants need to meet to be included in the study and what factors excluded people from participating?
Time frame of study and intervention/ treatment	What was the full span of time for the study including the specific time of the treatment?
Intervention/treatment	Was the intervention/treatment described in detail? Was there a detailed manual for behavioral interventions? Can the intervention be replicated in practice or another study?
Blinding	Was the assignment to the condition/group blinded? Was it double-blinded? If observational measures were used, were blinded coders included in the measurement process?
Data collection	Were the variables, dependent and independent, clearly defined?
Data analysis	Were the data analysis techniques clearly defined?
Results/findings	Were the results reported in terms of research questions/hypotheses? Did the results make sense and address the questions/hypotheses?
Conclusions	Were conclusions clearly stated and consistent with the results presented?
Limitation	Were study limitations identified including randomization problems, missing data, dropouts, and treatment fidelity problems?

STEP FOUR: INTEGRATING INFORMATION TO IMPLEMENT A DECISION

The final step in the process of evidence-based nursing is to consider the research evidence in light of clinical experience and patient-related factors and preferences. A decision can then be made about whether to reject, implement, or adapt the intervention for the population of patients and the setting.

Clinical Experience

There are numerous nursing interventions that are standard nursing practices but are based in tradition rather than on research evidence (Rodgers, 2005). Nurses are thus challenged to ask questions about their practices and search for existing evidence to support the best nursing care and promote optimal outcomes for patients. When no research evidence exists, nurses must evaluate a practice in light of what is believed to be the current standard of practice, what benefits are believed to exist for patients with the current standards, and what consequences (risks) are likely if the practice is not implemented. This is the case for many of the guidelines in this book. For example, ensuring that items such as urinals and call bells are in the unaffected motor and visual fields for patients with unilateral neglect is not evidence based, yet staff nurses are taught to offer this intervention as a part of the usual care for this problem (Hinkle et al., 2004; Howard, 2000). On the other hand, even when evidence does exist on the effectiveness of a nursing intervention, nurses must consider their experiences with implementing the intervention with a particular population and setting and decide whether and how the intervention will work with a particular patient. Even then, a nurse's decision to implement an intervention can be overruled by a patient and his or her preferences or wishes.

Patients' Preferences

Patients often have preferences that influence the types of nursing activities implemented. For example, a patient who has been managing a colostomy stoma for many years in a certain fashion may struggle to change to a new care system despite evidence that the new system is more effective or easier to use. A patient with very limited resources may need antihypertensive medicine but must choose one month between paying rent or purchasing the medications and other health services. Thus, nurses have to work realistically with patients to select the interventions and activities that are most likely to work for the patients and promote positive or the best outcomes.

Making a Decision

Integrating the research evidence, clinical experience, and patients' preferences to make a decision about a practice change can be an enormous undertaking. Burns and Grove (2005) stated appropriately that it is unlikely that one could identify every relevant source in the literature to develop a specific guideline and that the most extensive literature retrievals are those where funding allowed someone to dedicate time and effort to an exhaustive literature search. A staff nurse may want to identify a nursing partner with advanced training and education to help sift through the evidence review process and come up with a recommendation for practice. These partners might be from other settings such as academic settings or larger clinical agencies when resources are limited in smaller settings. Staff nurses can also make direct contact with authors-investigators or other experts in the field who can help summarize the available evidence and put forward recommendations. Library resources, interdisciplinary colleagues, and journal groups might be additional resources for identifying practices to adopt, continue, or eliminate when little research evidence exists or research exists that suggests possible harm from the intervention. Finally, textbooks as resources should be used with caution and a critical eye for the citation of recent research references supporting the recommended nursing practices.

STEP FIVE: EVALUATING THE OUTCOMES

When a decision has been made regarding a recommendation for practice, the next step is to identify a strategy for presenting the recommendation, implementing the intervention or practice change, and evaluating the outcomes. Chapter 3 discusses the importance of organizational culture and key stakeholders for facilitating change to evidence-based care in health care systems. Implementation models that include evaluation components are discussed along with key characteristics and programs used by health care systems to support and develop evidence-based practice.

SUMMARY

Locating and evaluating the evidence for EBP can be challenging. This chapter has provided an overview of resources and tools to assist in locating and evaluating evidence. EBP websites and library resources including librarians and electronic databases are tools that can aid in locating resources. When the evidence is located, it must be evaluated and rated for the strength or level of evidence. Only then can a decision be made about maintaining or adopting an existing practice, implementing a new practice, or eliminating a practice. Implementation of evidence-based nursing is examined in Chapter 3.

REFERENCES

Agency for Healthcare Research and Quality. (2007). *National Clearinghouse Mission Statement*. Retrieved April 9, 2007, from http://www.guideline.gov/about/mission.aspx

Burns NB, Grove SK. (2005). *The practice of nursing research: Conduct, critique, and utilization*, 5th ed. St. Louis: Saunders.

Cochrane Library. (2007). *About Cochrane*. Retrieved April 9, 2007, from http://www3.interscience.wiley.com/cgi-bin/mrwhome/106568753/AboutCochrane.html

Guyatt GH, Sinclair JC, Hayward R, Cook DJ, & Cook RJ. (2001). *Method for grading healthcare recommendations*. Retrieved June 29, 2006, from http://www.cche.net/usersguides/recommend.asp#36

Hinkle JL, Guanci MM, Bowman L, Hermann L, McGinty LB, Rose J. (2004). Cerebrovascular events of the nervous system. In Bader MK, Littlejohns LR (Eds): *AANN core curriculum for neuroscience nursing*. St. Louis: Saunders.

Howard CJ. (2000). Stroke. In Edwards PA (Ed): *The specialty practice of rehabilitation nursing: A core curriculum*, 4th ed. Glenview, IL: Association of Rehabilitation Nurses.

Melnyk BM. (2004). Integrating levels of evidence into clinical decision making. *Pediatr Nurs*, 30(4):323-325.

Melnyk BM & Fineout-Overholt E. (2005). *Evidence-based practice in nursing & healthcare: A guide to best practice*. Philadelphia: Lippincott Williams & Wilkins.

Rodgers B. (2005). Developing nursing knowledge: Philosophical traditions and influences. New York: Lippincott Williams & Wilkins.

Wikipedia. (2007). *Meta-analysis*. Retrieved April 9, 2007, from http://en.wikipedia.org/wiki/Meta-analysis

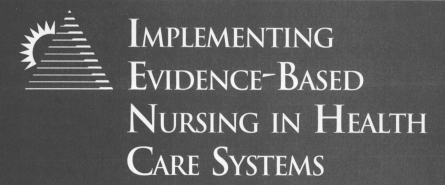

Chapter 3

IMPLEMENTING EVIDENCE-BASED NURSING IN HEALTH CARE SYSTEMS

Kathleen S. Oman, PhD, RN, CEN

REALITY OF HEALTH CARE AND EVIDENCED-BASED NURSING

Today's health care environment is complex, rapidly changing, and fraught with staffing short-ages, cost reductions, workplace redesign, and very sick patients. Professionals are constantly balancing their obligation to provide excellent care for patients with the competing demands of organizational change. Although nurses value the use of research and scientific evidence to guide practice, they frequently lack the resources and skills to achieve an evidence-based practice (EBP). There is sufficient evidence describing the barriers to using research in practice (Bryar et al., 2003; Hommelstad & Ruland, 2004; Pravikoff et al., 2005; Fink et al., 2005; Hutchinson & Johnston, 2006), which include:

  Lack of administrative support and mentorship
  Nurses' beliefs that they lack the authority to change practice
  Lack of basic knowledge about research and statistics
  Inability to analyze critically research reports
  Insufficient time in the clinical setting to implement change

Creating an organizational culture that supports EBP is critical to promoting positive out-comes and quality care for patients (Goode, 2003) and is probably the most critical strategy in facilitating the change to evidence-based care (Melnyk, 2002). This chapter identifies some key characteristics and programs used by health care systems to support and develop EBP.

ORGANIZATIONAL STRUCTURE

Health care systems need to have certain elements of structure in place to foster evidence-based nursing (EBN). Chief nurse executives and the leadership staff set the expectation and create the culture for EBN (Stetler et al., 1998; Sams et al., 2004). There are three key areas to consider when creating the foundation for EBN: (1) philosophy, values, mission, and organizational model; (2) strategic plan; and (3) performance expectations.

Philosophy, Values, Mission, and Organizational Model

It is important that the philosophy, values, mission, and organizational model of the organization (or patient services division) reflect a commitment to providing evidence-based care. Examples of statements include the following:

> *We, the registered nurses at University of Colorado Hospital, participate in the hospital's mission to deliver comprehensive health services, to support the education of health professionals, to acquire new knowledge through research, and to provide service to the university, community, state, and region. . . . We are encouraged to actively participate in research. We believe that research arises from inquiry, and research outcomes become the foundation for nursing practice.*
> **—Excerpt of University of Colorado Philosophy of Nursing statement**

Organizational models may also depict the foundational relationships between EBN and patients' care. At the University of Colorado Hospital, the shared governance model (Fig. 3-1) incorporates their nursing theory, philosophy of nursing care, and structural organization and visually exemplifies EBP's importance as the surrounding influence of all aspects of the model. These statements or models lay the foundation for integrating EBN throughout the organization.

Strategic Planning

Nursing leaders integrating EBN in their organization must be willing to (1) establish a culture based on the use of evidence, (2) create the capacity for organizational change, and (3) sustain that shift in the health care system's infrastructure (Stetler et al., 1998). Organizational infrastructure needed to support EBN includes interventions related to work patterns, skill mix, research support, clinical supervision, communication systems, management structure, quality improvement, and staff development (Foxcroft & Cole, 2003). Securing these resources requires planning and persistence.

The regulatory influences in the health care environment, including (1) The Joint Commission National Patient Safety Goals (2008), (2) the Institute for Healthcare Improvement (IHI) Five Million Lives campaign (2006), and (3) the Institute of Medicine (IOM) patients' safety recommendations, are evidence-based initiatives that can be used as leverage in budgeting for resources and training to establish an organizational culture supportive of EBN (IOM, 2001). The quest for Magnet hospital designation has fostered additional emphasis on EBN and the environment to support it (Willson et al., 2004).

Examples of strategic EBN planning initiatives include processes for staff education, new employee orientation, developing or hiring research and EBN mentors, budgeting to support work patterns to include time for EBN activities, and targeting unit or hospital-based implementation projects.

Creating a culture supportive of EBN is not an overnight endeavor. Strategic planning initiatives will most likely take years to accomplish. As part of the process, Melnyk (2005) recommended conducting a SWOT (strengths, weaknesses, opportunities, threats) analysis, which will:

1. Identify the strengths in the organization to support EBN
2. Identify the weaknesses in the organization that may hinder the initiative
3. Outline the opportunities for success
4. Delineate the threats or barriers to the initiative, with strategies to overcome them

Action, persistence, and patience are additional essential elements for success (Melnyk, 2005).

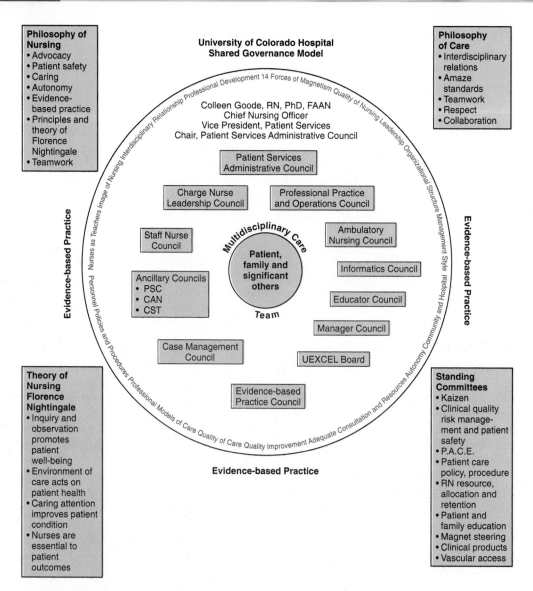

FIG 3-1 • University of Colorado Hospital shared governance model. (Used with permission from the University of Colorado Hospital.)

Performance Expectations

For EBN to be evident in everyday work, critical behaviors must be identified and performance expectations explicated. It is important that expectations be identified for every level of nursing practice including bedside nurses, advanced practice nurses, and nurses in administrative and managerial roles, each having a specific set of expectations reflective of their position and scope of responsibility (Table 3-1).

TABLE 3-1	Sample EBN Performance Criteria for Nursing Roles			
Bedside Nurse	Advanced Practice Nurse	Nurse Manager	Nursing Director	Chief Nursing Officer
Critically thinks through patient care practice issues Questions current practices Participates in implementing practice changes based on evidence Reads evidence related to practice Participates in QI activities Suggests resolutions for clinical issues based on evidence	Serves as coach and mentor in EBN Locates and/or synthesizes the evidence Uses evidence to write/modify practice standards Role-models and/or teaches use of evidence in practice Facilitates system changes to support use of evidence	Creates or supports a culture that values interdisciplinary quality improvement based on evidence Allocates human and fiscal resources to support bedside nurses in EBN activities Challenges staff to seek out evidence to resolve clinical issues Role-models EBN Uses performance criteria for EBN in staff evaluations	Hires and retains nurses with knowledge and skills in EBN Provides learning environment for EBN Uses evidence in leadership decisions; sets strategic directions for EBN Provides human and fiscal vision to resources for EBN Integrates EBN processes into governance structure	Ensures that governance structure reflects EBN in councils and committees Assigns accountability for EBN Ensures organizational and department commitment to EBN Modifies mission and include EBN terminology Provides human and fiscal resources to support EBN by direct care providers Provides access to consultants for data management and statistical analysis Articulates value of EBN to CEO and governing board Role-models EBN in administrative decision making

QI, Quality improvement. Adapted with permission from Titler MG. (2006). Developing an evidence-based practice. In LoBiondo-Wood G, Haber J (Eds). *Nursing research: Methods and critical appraisal for evidence-based practice,* 6th ed. St. Louis: Mosby, pp. 472-473.

BOX 3-1

Clinical Levels of Registered Nurse Practice: EBN Expectations

Level I Expectations
- Orients to *Research Manual,* EBN models
- Completes EBN course (residency curriculum)
- Completes annual outcomes competency
- Orients to the National Database of Nursing Quality Indicators (NDNQI)—unit-based nurse-sensitive outcomes (falls and pressure ulcer prevalence) are reported and benchmarked.
- Orients to the University of Colorado Hospital Quality model FOCUS-PDCA (Find a process to improve, Organize a team, Clarify current knowledge, Understand sources of process variation, Select the process improvement, Plan, Do, Check, Act)
- Other research conducted in practice area

Level II Expectations
- Accesses and uses *Research Manual*
- Completes annual outcomes competency
- Participates in one journal club
- Identifies nurse-sensitive outcomes for unit
- Verbalizes what FOCUS-PDCA means

Level III Expectations
- Acts as co-leader in a FOCUS-PDCA project
- Actively participates in journal club
- Attends one EBN course
- Communicates/improves nurse-sensitive indicator outcomes
- Disseminates annual research outcomes competency
- Takes the "Quality and Outcomes Tools" class

Level IV Expectations
- Takes the "Clinical Research: Getting Started" class
- Leads one evidence-based or quality project
- Conducts literature review and facilitates group discussion
- Communicates outcomes/findings by formal presentation
- Leads journal club; guides staff
- Leads a practice change initiative based on data analysis

Used with permission of the University of Colorado Hospital.

Clinical Ladders

Organizations with clinical ladders may decide to delineate EBN expectations at the various levels of clinical nursing practice. For example, the University of Colorado Hospital clinical ladder system is based on Benner's (1984) work. It includes four levels of registered nurse practice, from entry to expert with job descriptions, performance appraisals, and standards for each level (Box 3-1).

IMPLEMENTING EVIDENCE-BASED NURSING

Models

Models help to describe and visualize a process and can serve as a guide for nurses and other health care professionals in their quest to provide evidence-based care. There are several EBN and research utilization models described in the health care literature. Some are conceptual models (Kitson et al., 1998; Logan & Graham, 1998; Goode & Piedalue, 1999; DiCenso et al., 2005), and others are implementation models (Rosswurm & Larrabee, 1999; Stetler, 2001; Titler

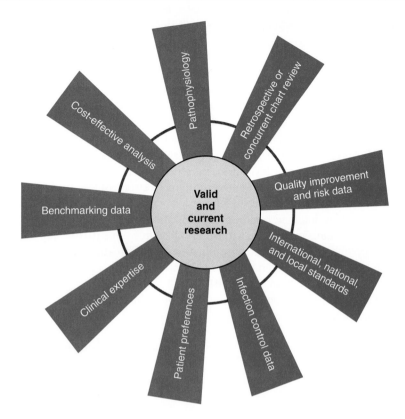

Evidence-based Multidisciplinary Practice Model©
University of Colorado Hospital

FIG 3-2 • University of Colorado Hospital evidence-based model. (Used with permission from the University of Colorado Hospital.)

et al., 2001; Pape, 2003). The evidence-based multidisciplinary practice model (Fig. 3-2) at the University of Colorado Hospital (Goode & Piedalue, 1999) depicts the various sources of evidence clinicians use to make practice decisions.

Valid and current research forms the core of the model, and the circle linking the evidence sources indicates that evidence is connected from any of the sources to establish the evidence base. The more sources of evidence added to the research core, the stronger the evidence.

In conjunction with this conceptual model, an implementation model such as the Iowa model (Titler et al., 2001) or the Stetler model (Stetler, 2001) is useful to help outline the process and steps of making a practice change based on evidence.

Computer Resources

One of the key steps in EBP is being able to find and use current evidence. Access to the Internet and search engines of medical databases are essential resources an organization must provide for health care providers. It is also important to provide this access at the clinical site of patients' care; whether it be the nursing unit, the clinic, or the patients' examination room, the clinicians must have timely access to find evidence to support their care decisions for patients (Bakken, 2001). Organizations need to provide computers and software programs or library links as a fundamental building block of EBN.

Given the complexity and time constraints involved in care delivery, finding the right information at the right time is increasingly difficult. Traditionally, nurses rely on their peers and personal experience rather than print or online resources to answer questions about patients' care (Estabrooks et al., 2003; Pravikoff et al., 2005). This may be the result of inadequate computer and information skills. Computer and information literacy is critical to EBN, and nursing programs are lacking in their preparation of practitioners who are fully competent in these areas (McNeil et al., 2003, 2006; Pravikoff et al., 2003). Also, nurses who were born before the mid-1960s did not grow up in the computer age and may need additional assistance to participate in EBP. Nurses need to assess their own level of competence and implement personal strategies to become more information literate. Hospitals and health care organizations need to provide access to resources for training and education. Both nurses and patients benefit from a partnership with librarians. Librarians can provide point-to-point dissemination of information, watch communities of practice for information pearls, and monitor the literature and other sources of information for nurses and administrators (Willson et al., 2004).

Examples of courses that may be offered in your library include:
Answering clinical questions
Finding full text online
Ovid (learn search techniques for the online Ovid databases, focusing on MEDLINE)
Ovid tips and tricks
PubMed (learn to search MEDLINE through the National Library of Medicine's Entrez search engine)
Searching for the evidence
If such courses are not available, the Denison Memorial Library at the University of Colorado at Denver Health Sciences Center can provide information on starting such a class.

Educational Resources

Classes and Conferences

The process of EBN can be taught so that nurses can develop the knowledge and skills needed to implement evidence-based care of patients. The content required in these educational offerings includes (1) how to ask searchable questions, (2) how to search for the best evidence, (3) how to critique and appraise the literature, and (4) implementing the evidence in the clinical arena (Melnyk, 2002).

Multiple strategies have been used to teach EBN to the professional patient care providers at the University of Colorado Hospital. Formal continuing education courses in a three-part series are offered three times a year, starting with an introduction to EBN that includes a collaborative library session taught by the medical librarians on searching for the evidence. An intermediate course titled "Evidence-Based Practice: Beyond the Basics" focuses on how evidence is used in organizational change and clinical decision making. The final course, "Clinical Research: Getting Started," is an overview of the research process. More informal "brown bag" sessions are offered yearly and provide individualized mentoring offered by a research nurse scientist to nurses implementing EBN projects in their clinical areas. These are examples of courses that have proved successful in an academic teaching clinical environment and can be found at the University of Colorado website www.UCH.edu/professionalresources/. Maljanian and colleagues (2002) describe the use of research roundtables that are designed with collaboration between the health care institutions and university faculty to teach EBN skills to practicing nurses and nursing students. The roundtables are a four-part series offered yearly that cover searching for the literature, critiquing the literature (two sessions), and methods and application of EBN. The series increases nurses' knowledge and skills, demystifies the research process, provides role models, demonstrates managerial and collegial support, and provides library, fiscal, and other resource support to complete EBN projects.

Conferences are another strategy used to enhance EBN knowledge and skills. The University of Iowa Hospitals and Clinics, the Center for Research and Evidence-Based Practice at the University of Rochester School of Nursing, and the University of Colorado Hospital and Denver affiliates, to name a few, all hold annual research and EBP conferences.

Mentorship and Internship Programs

Education alone is not sufficient to change practice. Mentorship and internship programs have been shown to be effective in assisting nurses to integrate EBN skills in the complex care delivery systems in which they practice. Thurston and King (2004) described a mentorship program designed to enable nurses in the clinical community to understand and implement an evidence-based approach to practice. The program was a partnership between a Canadian regional health authority and university nursing faculty who recognized an opportunity to share resources and maximize collaboration. Groups met monthly for over a year and were provided with in-depth education and mentoring to plan and implement practice changes based on evidence. The authors reported the results of 10 successful change projects and discussed implications for future directions for the program.

The University of Iowa Hospitals and Clinics have developed a competitive internship program in which staff nurse interns work with their peers to promote adoption of an EBN change (Cullen & Titler, 2004). The program includes coursework, team meetings, and facilitated project work time to accomplish the following goals: (1) promote innovative thinking by staff nurses, (2) facilitate the development and integration of a clinically relevant EBN project, (3) expand understanding and use of the Iowa Model of Evidence-Based Practice to Promote Quality Care (Titler et al., 2001), and (4) promote professional growth and development of staff nurses. This program provides a process to address practice questions through implementing, evaluating, and integrating practice changes.

Journal Clubs

Reading current research or other sources of evidence is the precursor to EBP, and clinical nurses benefit from a structure and process to accomplish this. Journal clubs are an excellent strategy that can be implemented in the clinical setting without intense resources (Melnyk, 2002). Journal clubs involve nurses who are willing to commit to a regularly scheduled forum in which they review and discuss current research, systematic reviews, or evidence-based protocols. Journal club interactions improve critical thinking skills and serve as a powerful tool for education (Hagman & Krugman, 2003).

Using a consistent approach for critiquing a research article provides a structured format that helps improve critical appraisal skills. There are many examples of critique forms that can be used to review research articles and guide discussion in a journal club. Figure 3-3 illustrates the research report critique form currently in use at the University of Colorado Hospital. The general

**UNIVERSITY OF COLORADO HOSPITAL
RESEARCH CRITIQUE GUIDE***

Bring completed critiques to your journal club discussion.

Note: This form includes questions for *both* quantitative and qualitative studies; questions assessed specifically for qualitative studies are noted. Mark non-applicable questions N/A.

Name: _____ *Date:* _____

Reference: APA format: Authors. (Year). Title. *Journal, volume* (issue), pages. _____

Research Problem and Purpose

❑ What is the purpose/problem of the study? Is it clearly identified? _____

❑ Are/is there a research question(s) and/or hypotheses? List, or if not stated, formulate them from the author's statements regarding the purpose of the study. _____

❑ If hypotheses, are they directional or nondirectional? _____

❑ Identify why the phenomenon requires a qualitative format. *(Qualitative)* _____

❑ Identify the philosophic underpinnings of the research. *(Qualitative)* _____

❑ Is the research question one that tries to explore, describe, or expand knowledge about how reality is experienced? *(Qualitative)* _____

Review of Literature and Background

❑ Do the authors specify a theoretical/conceptual framework guiding the study (do they provide a "word picture" or visual image of the framework)? Specify the framework/conceptual model used. _____
_____

❑ Is the literature reviewed relevant to the study purpose? _____

❑ Is the review logically and clearly organized? _____

❑ Does the review primarily use current literature? _____

❑ Were primary sources used? _____

Research Design and Methods

❑ What type of design(s) was (were) used? Circle all that apply:

None specified	Quasi-experimental	Hermeneutics	Descriptive
Experimental	Phenomenology	Grounded Theory	Survey
Nonexperimental	Ethnography	Historical	Other:

❑ Does the study method make sense in light of the research purpose/questions/hypotheses? _____

❑ Identify and describe the population: _____
_____
_____

❑ Is the sample (size, selection, representativeness) adequate and appropriate? N = _____

❑ What type of sampling method was used?

• Probability (simple random, stratified random, cluster, systematic sampling)

• Nonprobability (quota, convenience, purposive)

❑ List the inclusion and exclusion criteria: _____

❑ What is the context/setting for the study? _____

*Adapted from the CU School of Nursing Student Journal Club Critique Form.

FIG 3-3 • Research critique guide. (Used with permission from the University of Colorado Hospital.)

❑ List key variables (dependent and independent) and level of measurement (nominal, ordinal, interval, ratio) for each: _____
_____

❑ Are any variables left undefined? If so, what are they? _____
_____

❑ Was institutional review board (IRB) approval obtained? _____
_____

Data Collection, Measurement, and Analysis

❑ Describe the methods of data collection: _____
_____

❑ List the instruments/tools used and note how reliability (consistency) and validity (accuracy) were established for each: _____
_____

❑ Describe the procedures for analyzing the data. Are they understandable? _____
_____

❑ List the statistics used to analyze data. Are they appropriated for the questions/hypotheses and levels of measurement? _____
_____

For qualitative data collection

❑ Credibility: Does the researcher describe going back to the participants to validate the findings? _____
_____

❑ Auditability: Are enough examples given that the reader can follow the researcher's reasoning process throughout the study? Is the research process described step-by-step? _____
_____

❑ Fittingness: Are the findings described in enough detail to be useful to practice, research, and/or theory? Are the results useful for guiding your practice? _____
_____

❑ Is the saturation of data described? _____

Findings/Results and Conclusions

❑ Are the tables and figures clear and relevant? _____
❑ Are the results organized logically and presented clearly? _____
❑ Briefly describe the results and the conclusions drawn from them. Are the conclusions consistent with the results? Do the answers make sense? _____
_____

❑ Are the conclusions discussed in relation to the theoretical/conceptual framework? Give an example: _____
_____

❑ Does the researcher place the report in the context of what is already known about the phenomenon (e.g., other studies, philosophies)? Give an example: _____
_____

❑ Are there answers to the all research question(s)/hypotheses asked in this study? If not, which one(s) were left unanswered? _____
_____

❑ Do the themes/theory/process presented make sense in light of the data provided? *(Qualitative)*
_____

FIG 3-3 *Continued*

❑ List the strengths, limitations, and biases: _____

_____

❑ Are the limitations/biases concerning enough to cause you to question the validity of the results? _____

_____

❑ Are suggestions for future research included? If so, what are they? _____

_____

Professional Context:

❑ Are the implications for practice clearly stated (i.e., how do the conclusions of the study affect my practice)? List
  the implications: _____

_____

❑ Is this study significant to nursing (i.e., will this study have an impact on nursing practice)? If so, how is it
  significant? _____

_____

How do you rate this study as a whole? _____ **(scale of 1-5) (1 = low scientific merit; 5 = high scientific merit)**
What is your rationale for behind this rating? _____

_____

Personal Growth and Development

  Check box if you agree with the statement:

  ❑ I have increased my knowledge of _____ from
    reading this article.

  ❑ I understand the steps of the research process better from reading, critiquing, and discussing this article.

  ❑ I have a greater understanding of how to apply research findings to practice from reading and discussing this
    article.

❑ List at least one thing you learned/relearned from reading this article: _____

_____

❑ List at least one way that YOU could apply the findings of this study to your nursing practice:_____

_____

FIG 3-3 *Continued*

elements of quantitative study critique forms are similar and include purpose and/or problem statement, literature review, hypotheses and/or research questions, research methodology/design, variables, data collection and measurement, data analysis, results, clinical implications, and limitations (Oman, 2003). Critique criteria for qualitative studies include auditability (or confirmability), credibility, and fit (or transferability) (Sandelowski, 1993; Beck, 1993; Mays & Pope, 2000).

Setting the expectation for journal club participation (i.e., in performance evaluation criteria) helps nurses and managers prioritize the activity into the clinical work schedule.

Annual EBN Competency

Yearly skills laboratories that test and maintain clinical skill competency are commonplace in the hospital nursing structure. Testing and teaching EBN skills in the form of a yearly competency are equally important and send the very notable message that EBN skills are as important as clinical skills.

For a number of years, the University of Colorado Hospital has had the directive that its policy and procedures be evidence based, but there was no formal mechanism to accomplish this until 2005. In 2005, the EBN Council developed a step-by-step algorithm approach to an EBN policy revision (or development) (Box 3-2) and incorporated assigning levels of evidence to the process. For more information regarding levels of evidence, please refer to Chapter 1.

It became the focus of a yearly EBN competency to communicate this process of developing policies and procedures based on evidence with the clinical nurses. This competency was introduced to the nursing staff in grand rounds presentations followed by a self-learning module and post-test. To fulfill the competency, nurses either attended grand rounds or completed the self-learning module and post-test and returned it to their supervisor before their performance evaluation.

Other examples of yearly competencies include (1) searching for the evidence: a web-based module presented by the medical librarians, (2) reading and critiquing a research report, and (3) journal club participation.

▊ FACILITATION

Education about EBN is necessary but inadequate alone to change practice. In fact, facilitating change in practice is the most difficult challenge that nurse administrators and educators face (Kitson et al., 1998; Cullen & Titler, 2004). Getting evidence into practice is complex and does not follow a prescribed and logical path (Rycroft-Malone et al., 2004). In general, for EBN to become mainstream in an institution, the organizational culture must support EBN and nurses must have the authority to change practice. Mentors and role models should be available and accessible to facilitate the practice.

Mentors and Role Models

Mentors and role models may be research nurse scientists, clinical nurse specialists, or champions of change. Mentors and role models are agents who are instrumental to support an evidence-based enterprise. Establishing an EBN committee or council is a key component of facilitation. An EBN council should include representatives from all levels of nursing practice and multiple disciplines. Champions of change might be staff nurses who promote EBN in their clinical areas and are mentored by the research nurse scientists, EBN council members, and nursing faculty from the school of nursing who active initiate EBP projects and promote journal clubs (Fink et al., 2005). The role of facilitation with the champions of change model is a significant strategy in successful EBN implementation (Flynn & Fink, 2001; Titler & Everett, 2001; Rycroft-Malone et al., 2004; Willson et al., 2004).

Partnering with Schools of Nursing and Health Care Facilities

Partnering or collaboration is another successful strategy used to foster and develop an EBN program. Collaborative exchange between academic and service/practice settings is one such partnering relationship that enhances the hospital EBN culture. Educational programs in the form of conferences, roundtables, "author talks," internship programs, and mentorship programs are examples of the result of such collaboration (Caramanica et al., 2002; Maljanian et al., 2002; Cullen & Titler, 2004; Thurston & King, 2004; Engelke & Marshburn, 2006). These initiatives have provided opportunities for practicing nurses to learn and implement EBN projects in their clinical settings. They have also been instrumental in bridging the gap between nursing practice and nursing education (Engelke & Marshburn, 2006).

> ## BOX 3-2
>
> **Process for Revising and Developing Evidence-Based Policy and Procedure—Developed by EBN Council June 2005, Revised February 2006**
>
> 1. *Select the policy for revision.* Routine review or changes in practice; this process is also applicable for new policies.
> 2. *Search for evidence* (suggested approaches and sites)
>   a. Literature review for research evidence
>   i. CINAHL and MEDLINE databases or PubMed if no access to library
>   ii. Cochrane library
>   iii. ACP Pier, a product of the American College of Physicians, is a web-based evidence-based guide of disease modules and current best practices.
>   b. National Guideline Clearinghouse (www.guideline.gov)
>   c. Professional association guidelines/standards of care
>   d. Turning Research into Practice (TRIP) (www.tripdatabase.com) provides access to health care publications relevant to clinical practice in one place. Evidence-based publications are searched monthly by experts and indexed fully before being presented in an easy-to-use format with access to full-text articles, medical images, patient leaflets, and more.
>   e. University Health Consortium (UHC) for other academic hospital policies/procedures
>   f. Local standards or policies
>   g. Expert opinion/clinical expertise
>   i. Clinical articles
>   ii. Web search
>   iii. Clinical experts
> 3. *Systematic evaluation of the evidence*
>   a. Critique of research
>   b. Assign level of evidence: a method of evaluating the strength of the evidence
>   c. Consider a mechanism for organization of evidence (table)
> 4. *Compare evidence to current policy and make a decision.*
>   • *Decision point*
>   a. Make no changes.
>   b. Make language more precise or update references.
>   c. Revise policy to incorporate new evidence.
>   d. Develop new P&P based on evidence if indicated.
>   e. Retire or delete policy if no longer effective for quality patient care.
>   *Final policy should include references and levels of evidence.*
> 5. *Policy review by stakeholders/experts*
> 6. *Make revisions based on stakeholder/experts' comments*
> 7. *Obtain P&P sign-off list* to determine who needs to review and approve it (consider legal/risk management review if appropriate) and obtain approval signatures (e-mail approval is acceptable).
> 8. *Submit policy to patient care policy and procedure subcommittee for final recommendations and approval.*
> 9. *Staff education as needed*
> 10. *Final policy published on intranet*

P&P, Policy and procedure.
Used with permission of the University of Colorado Hospital.

Melnyk and Fineout-Overholt (2002) have developed an organizational model of collaboration involving an academic health center and community leaders. The Advancing Research and Clinical practice through close Collaboration (ARCC) model is an excellent example of how research evidence is translated into best practices.

Partnering with other hospitals is another successful strategy that strengthens EBN initiatives. For example, the University of Colorado Hospital has effectively partnered with four area hospitals and the University of Colorado Health Sciences Center School of Nursing along with the Denver Sigma Theta Tau International chapter in sponsoring a yearly research and EBN conference. This partnership has been very productive in providing educational sessions and sharing regionally conducted research and EBN projects. The conference, with nationally prominent nursing keynote speakers, has approximately 400 participants over the two daily sessions and continues to grow. The successful collaboration has enhanced the quality and content of the conference.

Rewarding Behaviors

It takes a great deal of effort, persistence, and patience to make practice changes based on the evidence, and nurses who accomplish this ought to be recognized for their efforts. The recognition may take many forms, including:

- Journal publication of the project
- Presentation of projects at local, national, or international EBN conferences
- Acknowledgment from professional organizations that have recognition programs for excellence in EBN (e.g., Sigma Theta Tau International)
- Poster presentations of projects on the clinical nursing unit or at hospital-based recognition events (e.g., Nurses' Week, Hospital Week)
- Use of EBN activities in clinical ladder programs when available
- Awarding release or administrative time from patients' care duties for EBN activities

Recognition by peers and nursing administrators is an important aspect of organizational structure that supports and strengthens an EBN environment (Titler, 2006).

SUMMARY

Creating an organizational culture that supports EBP requires a comprehensive approach. Nurse executives and nurses in leadership positions responsible for creating this culture have many components of organizational structure to consider. Essential components that support EBN include incorporating the language of EBN into mission, value, and philosophy of care statements; strategic planning to ensure the variety of resources needed for EBN; incorporating EBN expectations into performance expectations; and recognizing the successful efforts of nurses who choose to implement evidence in their nursing practice. When nurses are taught and supported to practice from an evidence-based model, patients' outcomes will improve. When nurses are empowered to evaluate the evidence and make practice changes, patients benefit, the nursing practice environment is enhanced, and quality of care improves.

REFERENCES

Bakken S. (2001). An informatics infrastructure is essential for evidence-based practice. *J Am Med Inform Assoc,* 8(3):199-201.

Beck CT. (1993). Qualitative research: The evaluation of its credibility, fittingness, and auditability. *West J Nurs Res,* 15(2):263-266.

Benner P. (1984). *From novice to expert: Excellence and poser in clinical nursing practice.* Menlo Park, CA: Addison-Wesley.

Bryar RM, Closs SJ, Baum G, Cooke J, Griffiths J, Hostick T, et al. (2003). The Yorkshire BARRIERS project: Diagnostic analysis of barriers to research utilisation. *Int J Nurs Stud,* 40(1):73-84.

Caramanica L, Maljanian R, McDonald D, Taylor SK, MacRae JB, Beland DK. (2002). Evidence-based nursing practice, Part 1: A hospital and university collaborative. *J Nurs Adm,* 32(1):27-30.

Cullen L, Titler MG. (2004). Promoting evidence-based practice: An internship for staff nurses. *Worldviews Evid Based Nurs,* 1(4):215-223.

DiCenso A, Cullum N, Ciliska D, et al. (2005). Introduction to evidence-based nursing. In DiCenso A, et al (Eds): *Evidence-based nursing: A guide to clinical practice.* Philadelphia: Saunders.

Engelke MK, Marshburn DM. (2006). Collaborative strategies to enhance research and evidence-based practice. *J Nurs Adm,* 36(3):131-135.

Estabrooks CA, O'Leary KA, Ricker KL, Humphrey CK. (2003). The internet and access to evidence: How are nurses positioned? *J Adv Nurs,* 42(1):73-81.

Fink R, Thompson CJ, Bonnes D. (2005). Overcoming barriers and promoting the use of research in practice. *J Nurs Adm,* 35(3):121-129.

Flynn MB, Fink R. (2001). Committing to evidence-based skin care practice. *Crit Care Nurs Clin North Am,* 13(4):555-568.

Foxcroft DR, Cole N. (2003). Organisational infrastructures to promote evidence based nursing practice. *Cochrane Database Syst Rev,* (4):CD002212.

Goode CJ. (2003). Evidence-based practice. In Oman K, Krugman M, Fink R (Eds): *Nursing research secrets.* Philadelphia: Hanley & Belfus.

Goode CJ, Piedalue F. (1999). Evidence-based clinical practice. *J Nurs Adm,* 29(6):15-21.

Hagman J, Krugman ME. (2003). Journal clubs. In Oman K, Krugman M, Fink R (Eds): *Nursing research secrets.* Philadelphia: Hanley & Belfus.

Hommelstad J, Ruland CM. (2004). Norwegian nurses' perceived barriers and facilitators to research use. *AORN J,* 79(3):621-634.

Hutchinson AM, Johnston L. (2006). Beyond the BARRIERS Scale: Commonly reported barriers to research use. *J Nurs Adm,* 36(4):189-199.

Institute for Healthcare Improvement (IHI). (2006). *Five Million Lives Campaign.* Available online: http://www.ihi.org. Retrieved on July 5, 2007.

Institute of Medicine. Committee on Quality of Health Care in America. (2001). *Crossing the quality chasm: A new health system for the 21st century.* Washington, DC: National Academy Press.

The Joint Commission. (2008). *National patient safety goals.* Available online: http://www.jointcommission.org/Patientsafety/NationalSafetyGoals/ Retrieved on July 5, 2007.

Kitson A, Harvey G, McCormack B. (1998). Enabling the implementation of evidence based practice: A conceptual framework. *Qual Health Care,* 7(3):149-158.

Logan J, Graham ID. (1998). Toward a comprehensive interdisciplinary model of health care research use. *Sci Commun,* 20(2):227-246.

Maljanian R, Caramanica L, Taylor SK, MacRae JB, Beland DK. (2002). Evidence-based nursing practice, Part 2: Building skills through research roundtables. *J Nurs Adm,* 32(2):85-90.

Mays N, Pope C. (2000). Qualitative research in health care. Assessing quality in qualitative research. *BMJ,* 320(7226):50-52.

McNeil BJ, Elfrink V, Beyea SC, Pierce ST, Bickford CJ. (2006). Computer literacy study: Report of qualitative findings. *J Prof Nurs,* 22(1):52-59.

McNeil BJ, Elfrink VL, Bickford CJ, Pierce ST, Beyea SC, Averill C, et al. (2003). Nursing information technology knowledge, skills, and preparation of student nurses, nursing faculty, and clinicians: A US survey. *J Nurs Educ,* 42(8):341-349.

Melnyk BM. (2002). Strategies for overcoming barriers in implementing evidence-based practice. *Pediatr Nurs,* 28(2):159-161.

Melnyk BM. (2005). Creating a vision: Motivating a change to evidence-based practice in individuals and organizations. In Melnyk B, Fineout-Overholt E (Eds): *Evidence-based practice in nursing and healthcare: A guide to best practice.* Philadelphia: Lippincott Williams & Wilkins.

Melnyk BM, Fineout-Overholt E. (2002). Putting research into practice. *Reflect Nurs Leadersh,* 28(2):22-25, 45.

Oranta O, Routasalo P, Hupli M. (2002). Barriers to and facilitators of research utilization among Finnish registered nurses. *J Clin Nurs,* 11(2):205-213.

Pape TM. (2003). Evidence-based nursing practice: To infinity and beyond. *J Contin Educ Nurs,* 34(4):154-161.

Pravikoff DS, Pierce S, Tanner A. (2003). Are nurses ready for evidence-based practice? *Am J Nurs,* 103(5):95-96.

Pravikoff DS, Tanner AB, Pierce ST. (2005). Readiness of U.S. nurses for evidence-based practice. *Am J Nurs,* 105(9):40-51.

Rosswurm MA, Larrabee JH. (1999). A model for change to evidence-based practice. *Image J Nurs Scholarsh,* 31(4):317-322.

Rycroft-Malone J, Harvey G, Seers K, Kitson A, McCormack B, Titchen A. (2004). An exploration of the factors that influence the implementation of evidence into practice. *J Clin Nurs,* 13(8):913-924.

Sams L, Penn BK, Facteau L. (2004). The challenge of using evidence-based practice. *J Nurs Adm,* 34(9):407-414.

Sandelowski M. (1993). Rigor or rigor mortis: The problem of rigor in qualitative research revisited. *ANS Adv Nurs Sci,* 16(2):1-8.

Stetler CB. (2001). Updating the Stetler Model of research utilization to facilitate evidence-based practice. *Nurs Outlook,* 49(6):272-279.

Stetler CB, Brunell M, Giuliano KK, Morsi D, Prince L, Newell-Stokes V. (1998). Evidence-based practice and the role of nursing leadership. *J Nurs Adm,* 28(7-8):45-53.

Tham K, Kielhofner G. (2003). Impact of the social environment on occupational experience and performance among persons with unilateral neglect. *Am J Occup Ther,* 57(4):403-412.

Thurston NE, King KM. (2004). Implementing evidence-based practice: Walking the talk. *Appl Nurs Res,* 17(4):239-247.

Titler MG. (2006). Developing an evidence-based practice. In LoBiondo-Wood G, Haber J (Eds). *Nursing research: Methods and critical appraisal for evidence-based practice,* 6th ed. St. Louis: Mosby.

Titler MG, Everett LQ. (2001). Translating research into practice. Considerations for critical care investigators. *Crit Care Nurs Clin North Am,* 13(4):587-604.

Titler MG, Kleiber C, Steelman VJ, Rakel BA, Budreau G, Everett LQ, et al. (2001). The Iowa Model of Evidence-Based Practice to Promote Quality Care. *Crit Care Nurs Clin North Am,* 13(4):497-509.

Willson P, Madary A, Brown J, Gomez L, Martin J, Molina T. (2004). Using the forces of magnetism to bridge nursing research and practice. *J Nurs Adm,* 34(9):393-394.

Chapter 4

USE OF EVIDENCE-BASED NURSING AS A NURSING STUDENT

Betty J. Ackley, MSN, EdS, RN; Susan Pierce, EdD, MSN, RN;
Beth Ann Swan, PhD, CRNP, FAAN

STUDENT CASE STUDY 1

Student nurse Kate worked as a CNA on the surgical floor of the local hospital for 5 years and continued to work there part-time while in nursing school. She was taught in her Fundamentals of Nursing class that indwelling urinary catheters should always be secured to the thigh (Wong & Hooton, 1981; SUNA, 2006). On the unit, she always secured urinary catheters using the method available. She found that the tube pulled off the thigh in 1 to 2 hours, and the tape was "flying in the wind" around the tubing. She noticed that most nurses did not bother with securing catheters. This meant that the Centers for Disease Control and Prevention (CDC) guidelines were not being followed where she worked. Kate was frustrated; she had been taught a principle for best care but had difficulty practicing it in the clinical area because of the ineffective function of the adhesive method available. Because she was learning about evidence-based nursing (EBN) in school, she decided to investigate methods to secure urinary catheters effectively as her senior EBN project.

EBN AND THE NURSING STUDENT: IT'S YOUR EXCITING FUTURE!

EBN is a trend to improve the quality of care. By developing skills to provide EBN, a nurse, including you as a student or new graduate, is empowered to give the best care possible, promote professional nursing practice, and increase pride in being a nurse. In an environment where EBN is practiced, there is continuous evaluation of the quality of care and ongoing innovation to provide better care. You will not be bored—there will always be something changing and something new to learn.

In Chapter 1, you learned what EBN is and why it is done. In Chapter 2, you learned about resources for accessing research evidence and about models for EBN. In this chapter, the information is put together in an action plan to demonstrate how an individual student or nurse might solve a problem using the EBN process and how evidence-based practice fits into the profession of nursing as you already know it. You will see how EBN and the nursing process are related. The examples used are typical of what you encounter in clinical settings.

There are multiple guidelines on how EBN practice should be done. Here is a simplified version that is designed to help you remember essential steps. The steps are Ask, Search, thinK, Measure, Evaluate. An acronym to remember these steps is "ASKME."

THE FIVE STEPS OF EBN: ASKME

Step 1—Ask the Burning Question

EBN begins with a student or nurse observing practice, questioning the status quo, trying to solve a problem, or learning about new evidence that should be used in the nursing practice. Practicing nurses say that they need information many times a day and most often seek that information by asking a peer. Often the question is, "How do we . . .?" and the answer is "We always. . . ." Instead, you should learn to ask, "Why do we do it this way?" or "How could we do this better?"

With more thought, the question becomes more complex and helps begin the process of EBN. A well-framed question leads to a more thorough search for evidence and, subsequently, a better evidence-based outcome.

PICO is another acronym that can be used to help further define the elements of the question so that you are able to locate the best evidence to answer the question. PICO is defined as (University of Washington, 2007; Melnyk & Fineout-Overholt, 2005):

Patient population of interest/disease: Decide what group of patients you will be studying, for example, elderly female patients with diabetes.

Intervention of interest or exposure of patient to a new experience: This is the change you want to make in practice, for example, a structured teaching intervention such as a series of group learning sessions.

Comparison of interest: This is the comparison, existing treatment, or status quo in the situation or, if doing research, the control (for example, the usual teaching method such as a brochure).

Outcome of interest: Determine the change in the patient's present reality you hope to have happen (the outcome). Make sure the patient's outcome is measurable, for example, improved glycemic control as measured by hemoglobin A_{1c} stability.

Step 2—Search and Collect Evidence

The next step is to identify and retrieve all of the best available and most current research evidence relevant to answering your question. To do this, you need to conduct a thorough search of the literature in the area. As a student, you need to develop strong information literacy skills of your own, but remember that you will find medical librarians most helpful. Critical information literacy skills include how to conduct the search and evaluate the literature. Basic computer skills are essential to search the nursing/medical literature (Pierce, 2005). These skills are competencies for the beginning nurse identified by the American Nurses Association (ANA, 2001) and, as such, should be learned as part of your nursing education. For changes in nursing practice, it can be helpful to find out how nurses are providing similar care in other hospitals by talking to colleagues and reviewing policy and procedure manuals.

Step 3—Think Critically

Next, it is important to appraise the evidence for validity (credibility), clinical importance (clinical significance), and applicability to your patient or practice environment. This step requires some knowledge and understanding of the research process. You must first evaluate the quality of the evidence you find. You must decide whether research is credible—in other words, did the researcher follow the "rules" of research so that you can trust the findings of the study? A research text and your instructor can help you with this. If the research is credible, you need to think critically about the clinical importance of the intervention to clinical practice. Ask, "Will it make a difference?" Remember, the fact that something is statistically significant does not mean that it is clinically significant (for example, is it cost-effective?). If you determine that the evidence is both credible and clinically significant, you are ready to make a decision about integrating the intervention into your practice. To do this, you must use your knowledge and experience as a nurse to "interpret" the evidence for practice. In other words, is it right for the individual patient or population of patients in your setting when considered in light of the patient's preferences, the values in the situation, and the policies in the facility?

Step 4—Measure the Outcomes

Utilize the outcome measurements determined as part of PICO, and always measure the patients' outcomes before and after widely instituting a change in practice. Otherwise, there is no way to determine whether the change is effective in your practice setting. Generally, a pilot study on a smaller population is done before any institution-wide change in practice is made. The results of the pilot study become part of the evidence for the larger decision. As part of measurement, it is important to determine whether it is an evidence-based project or a research study that would require application to the human subjects board of the institution to conduct the study.

Step 5—Evaluate the Practice Decision or Change

Evaluation is the process to determine whether the change made a significant difference. What were the results of the pilot study? Was the change in practice effective in improving patients' outcomes? Even if it did make a difference, was the difference worth any extra cost or time?

To help you understand this process, let us see how Kate, the student nurse in Case Study 1, used the steps of EBN.

CASE STUDY 1, CONTINUED

Step 1—Ask the Burning Question

Kate identified a problem through her observations. She noted that either catheters were not secured or the method used to secure them was not effective because they did not remain intact over time. She asked nurses about the securement options and kept hearing, "This is what we always do even though it doesn't work too well." Kate decided to gather all the information she could to investigate solutions to the problem. She first devised a plan for collecting the "evidence." She gathered policy and procedures from area facilities and used her critical thinking skills to develop a thorough search strategy for locating relevant research studies. To guide her search, she developed a clinical question "How can we keep catheters secured?" But then Kate had to focus her question. Using PICO, the question evolved.

> Population: Kate decided to focus on adult postsurgical patients because this matched the patients on her unit.
>
> Intervention: The intervention was an effective method for catheter securement. She defined "effective" as comfortable and functional.
>
> Comparison: The comparison was the ineffective securement method that was currently being used.

Outcome: Effective catheter securement. Kate thought of many outcomes—no blood in the urine, fewer urinary tract infections, no catheters becoming pulled out, and more. But she was not sure she could measure all of these. So she simplified measurement of the outcomes to the length of time the catheter remained secured and the degree of comfort described by the patients.

The burning question now with the use of PICO is, for adult postsurgical patients, will the use of another method for catheter securement versus the existing method maintain the catheter more effectively than the current method used? This is a broad question that allows Kate to search for evidence about different securement methods and determine the method most applicable to her population of patients. This, then, would become the intervention she would test.

At this time Kate decided to put together a team. She recruited two other nursing students, the clinical specialist on the surgical unit, the research specialist at the hospital, the most respected registered nurse on the unit, and a CENA who was highly respected, had oriented Kate to the unit, and had worked in the surgical unit for 25 years. Kate chose these people carefully, recognizing that they were stakeholders in the change and would be influential to make the change happen on the unit. (For more information about making a change in an organization, please refer to Chapter 5, Use of Evidence-Based Nursing as a Practicing Nurse.)

Step 2—Search and Collect Evidence

Working with the other students, Kate did a thorough literature review with the help of the hospital librarian. She especially looked for state-of-the-science studies, including Cochrane studies, meta-analyses, and clinical practice guidelines, and she searched for single randomized controlled trials. There was one article that was especially helpful on techniques for stabilizing urinary catheters (Hanchett, 2002). She found out how catheters were secured in nearby hospitals, asking her fellow students in the program or calling the surgical floor of the hospital and asking to talk with a nurse. Kate also obtained several of the more recommended securement methods for close examination.

Step 3—Think Critically

Kate and her student team members wrote a review of the literature and created an evidence table summarizing the appraisals of the evidence sources with the help of her instructor. Using critical thinking and their nursing knowledge and expertise, they evaluated the credibility and clinical importance evidence as it applied to the patients' characteristics, values, and preferences and the characteristics of the organization (e.g., attitudes toward change, cost impact) and made a practice decision of which securement method to try.

At a scheduled meeting with the unit manager of the surgical unit, Kate gave a brief overview of the project and asked for her support for a pilot project of the evidence-based intervention selected for comparison with the standard practice.

Step 4—Measure the Outcomes

Working together, the team devised a plan to measure specific aspects of the current reality of patients with catheters, such as the frequency of resecuring catheters, the duration of securement, and the patients' perception of comfort across time of use (e.g., using a comfort

Continued

scale of 1 to 10 at daily intervals). Then Kate and her team tried the new method on 30 patients and measured the same aspects for comparison.

Step 5—Evaluate the Practice Decision or Change

The results of the EBN study demonstrated that patients with the new securement method were more comfortable and the catheter securement method kept the catheter in place for as long as the patients had a catheter. A decision was made by the nursing practice committee to use the securement method throughout the hospital.

Epilogue

Kate received a 4.0 for her work on EBN in her capstone course. After graduation, she became a staff nurse on the surgical unit and continued her interest in EBN. Kate became so knowledgeable about how to search the literature that most of the staff on her unit came to her with questions, which she usually could answer after a computer search. She was nicknamed "AskmeKate." Currently she is working on another EBN project on pain with the research coordinator. Kate is also back in school working towards a masters of science in nursing degree. And guess what? The catheters on her surgical unit are consistently secured to the thigh and *stay* secured to the thigh.

The student case study will not be realistic in some situations. Kate was able to change nursing practice because she was respected on that nursing unit, she had an existing power base, and she selected additional powerful people to support her in this EBN change. It is sometimes not realistic that a student nurse can come into an environment and change practice unless he or she is already known and respected with an established power base.

EBN AND CRITICAL THINKING: HOW DO THEY FIT TOGETHER?

Critical thinking is an essential element for EBN (Profetto-McGrath, 2005). Using logical, purposeful thinking, a key component of critical thinking (Alfaro-LeFevre, 2004), is how evidence-based care is accomplished.

Critical thinking includes questioning the status quo (Loy et al., 2004) which is the beginning of the evidence-based process. In the case study, Kate questioned the status quo of the reality in the hospital and found it needed change. Questions abound in EBN; the "who," "what," "when," "where," "why," and "how" must all be addressed. Example questions that should be asked include:

Who: Which patient(s) will be involved?

What: What is the change in practice?

When: When should the intervention be offered?

Where: Where is the intervention appropriate?

Why: Why should the change be made?

How: How should the change be made?

In fact, the model for evidence-based practice given in this chapter, ASKME, begins with:

Asking the burning question. Determining PICO is critical thinking; this template is helpful in designing a clinical question in a way that makes the search effective in the least amount of time.

For example:

What is the effect *of* (nursing intervention) *on* (patient outcome) *compared with* (current practice) *in* (population)?

The variables you select become your initial search terms in the electronic database you use to find the research evidence. Remember, the question drives the search and the search focuses the question.

Searching also requires critical thinking. The nurse must know what to search for, how to search, and how to obtain the information. These are information literacy skills that you need. It is important to keep in mind that you should always *translate* your "natural language" search terms, the ones in your question, into the "controlled vocabulary" of the selected database. Use subject headings in the CINAHL database and MeSH headings in the MEDLINE/PubMed database to do this. Controlled vocabulary use ensures that you will find the most relevant evidence to answer your question.

Critical thinking is both left-brain logical thinking and right-brain creative thinking. Making a conceptual map of an EBN project, a right-brain way of thinking, can be very helpful to stimulate formation of new ideas that apply to the EBN process.

Analysis of information is also a significant part of critical thinking (Profetto-McGrath, 2005), just as it is an essential part of evidence-based practice. Analysis is the thinking (**K**) portion of the EBN process. Here a nurse analyzes large amounts of information including the present reality, the quality of the evidence, and the relevance of the findings to a particular situation.

As part of analysis, the nurse must make a large number of decisions to implement EBN effectively and appropriately, and decision making is critical thinking. These include the following:

Is the research credible (valid and reliable)?

Is this EBN change appropriate for this patient?

Can the hospital afford to make this change?

Are the nursing staff sufficiently educated and motivated to make the change?

Measurement of the effects of EBN is critical thinking. The nurse must decide what outcomes to measure, how to measure them, when to measure them, on whom the measurements should be made, and more.

Evaluation is critical thinking. The nurse analyzes the outcome measures and makes decisions about the significance of the results.

The bottom line is that EBN is based on evidence and critical thinking throughout the process. This is what makes EBN so exciting; it is the nurse's logical and creative thinking plus availability of evidence that makes it happen.

CASE STUDY 2

Student nurse Ben was assigned to care for an elderly male cerebrovascular accident patient who was receiving continual tube feedings. The patient was confused and thought Ben was his son. He was frequently incontinent of stool, the buttock area was reddened and denuded, and the patient cried out when he cleansed the area. Ben was told there was a physician's order to insert an indwelling catheter.

Does EBN provide any guidelines on how Ben should care for this patient? You bet it does. Suggestions for care of this patient are included throughout the remainder of this chapter, based on EBN.

HOW DOES EBN DIRECT BASIC NURSING CARE?

EBN affects all aspects of nursing, including basic care such as washing patients, feeding patients, giving oral care, positioning, communicating, encouraging sleep, and more.

CASE STUDY 2, CONTINUED

Let us help Ben with his challenging patient. He wants to give his patient the very best care possible. To do that, he needs to know how EBN can help ensure he gives quality care.

Question: How should Ben position his patient receiving tube feedings?

Answer: Using information from EBN, Ben should keep the head of the bed elevated 30 to 45 degrees to help decrease regurgitation and aspiration of the tube feeding formula. (Please refer to the guideline on Tube Feeding.)

Question: What should Ben do about the redness in the rectal area?

Answer: Ben should use a barrier cream on the rectal area to protect the skin from contact with stool, after washing carefully, preferably with a nonionic cleaner. (Please refer to the guideline on Bowel Incontinence Care.)

Question: How should Ben respond to the patient when he calls him his son?

Answer: Ben should gently tell him that he is a nursing student and not his son. Then he should tell him the date and time and find him a calendar. This is an intervention called reality orientation, and there is good evidence that it is effective. (Please refer to the guideline on Reality Orientation.)

EBN AND PERFORMING PROCEDURES

Nurses perform many procedures, and they should be done in the most effective way possible for improved patients' outcomes, safety, and comfort. Many procedures are invasive and can cause pain. An example is insertion of an indwelling catheter (Foley) into a male patient, which Ben was assigned to perform on his patient. The procedure manual and textbook, *Lippincott manual of nursing practice* (Nattina, 2005), directs that the catheter be inserted 6 to 8 inches until urine is obtained and then inserted further.

CASE STUDY 2, CONTINUED

Question: How far should Ben insert the indwelling catheter into the urethra of the male patient?

Answer: Research has demonstrated that the catheter should be inserted to the "Y" bifurcation of the catheter and then allowed to come back as it does naturally. In a male, the catheter will drain urine if it is in the urethra; obtaining urine does not mean that the catheter is in the bladder (Daneshgari et al., 2002). (Please refer to the guideline on Urinary Catheterization.)

EBN AND THE NURSING PROCESS: HOW DO THEY FIT TOGETHER?

All aspects of the nursing process are affected by EBN.

Assessment and EBN. How, when, who, and why we assess are all affected by research. For example, obtaining a patient's temperature is part of assessment. Research has demonstrated that

TABLE 4-1	Evidence-Based Nursing versus the Nursing Process
EBN Steps/ASKME	**Nursing Process Steps/ADPIE**
Ask the question	**A**ssess the patient
Search the literature	**D**iagnose
Thin**k**	**P**lan = Determine desired outcomes and interventions
Measure before and after	**I**mplement interventions
Evaluate the outcomes and how effective the change in intervention was	**E**valuate the outcomes and the effectiveness of the interventions

Note that EBN and the nursing process begin and end in the same way.

axillary temperatures are not very accurate. (Please refer to the guideline on Hypothermia Treatment.) Also, there is a rhythm that often dictates when the patient will have a fever. Have you ever noticed that you generally do not have a fever until late afternoon, and it is usually highest in the evening?

Nursing Diagnosis. Nursing diagnoses were developed on the basis of research and are approved only after extensive reviews of the literature are completed.

Nursing Outcomes. Outcomes are preferably measured using standardized scales of measurement based on research. An example is the Oral Mucositis Assessment Scale, which is based on research and has been shown to be valid.

Nursing Interventions. Interventions should be based on evidence—what works best. This text is an evaluation of 192 interventions and how they should be done most effectively based on evidence.

Nursing Rationale. The best rationale for an intervention is nursing research that shows how it should be done most effectively or demonstrates that the intervention is effective. The research studies that are included in this text can be ideal rationales for your care plans to explain why or how an intervention should be done.

Evaluation. Evaluation should be done using researched outcome measurements as mentioned before; Nursing Outcomes Classification (NOC) outcomes, which are explained in Chapter 1; or written outcome statements that are individualized for the patient (Table 4-1).

IS EBN RELEVANT FOR PHYSICIAN-ORDERED DEPENDENT INTERVENTIONS?

EBN is relevant for all nursing care, whether dependent or independent. For example, if the physician orders an intravenous (IV) solution of 5% dextrose in 0.45 normal saline to be given at 100 mL per hour, the nurse decides what size IV Angiocath to insert to administer the solution, whether to put the IV solution on a pump or let it drip in without a pump, how often the tubing should be changed, how often the IV site should be changed, whether there are problems with the IV administration with infiltration or inflammation at the site, and other matters such as whether it is appropriate to stop the infusion temporarily so that the patient can take a shower. Thus, in this case, the physician orders only the kind of solution and the rate; the nurse makes all the other decisions and ideally uses evidence to guide decision making. (Please refer to the guideline on Intravenous Therapy.)

HOW EBN PROMOTES INDEPENDENT NURSING INTERVENTIONS

Nurses have much more power than we think. When we think of nausea treatment, we think of medication that is ordered by a physician. But we can do more. There is good evidence that stimulation of the P6 point can help decrease nausea without the side effects associated with most antiemetics. (Please refer to the guidelines on Nausea Management: Cancer and Nausea Management: Postoperative Nausea and Vomiting.)

Another example is helping patients with anxiety. There are many things nurses can do to decrease anxiety. Research has demonstrated that telling patients what they will experience before a procedure can decrease anxiety. (Please refer to the guideline on Sensory Preparation: Procedures.) Sometimes, use of the patient's preferred music can help with anxiety. (Please refer to the guideline on Music Therapy.) Other ways of helping with anxiety are hand massage, touch, therapeutic touch, active listening, distraction, guided imagery, use of humor, use of presence, progressive muscle relaxation, and more. (There are guidelines for each of these methods, including a guideline on Anxiety Reduction.) As nurses, we now have many ways of helping patients that do not require a physician's order and do not involve medication, and there is research that validates the effectiveness of these interventions.

CONCLUSION

EBN is new and exciting. It will be your future as a nurse, and it will be a fascinating one. The next generation of nursing, of which you are a part, will change how nursing is done, and those of us from previous generations will be proud of your contributions to nursing and the excellence in patient care that you will provide based on evidence.

REFERENCES

Alfara-LeFevre R. (2004). *Critical thinking and clinical judgment: A practical approach.* St. Louis: Saunders.

American Nurses Association (ANA). (2001). *Scope and standards of nursing informatics practice.* Washington, DC: American Nurses Publishing.

Daneshgari F, Krugman M, Bahn A, Lee RS. (2002). Evidence-based multidisciplinary practice: Improving the safety and standards of male bladder catheterization. *Medsurg Nurs,* 11(5):236-241, 246.

Hanchett M. (2002). Techniques for stablizing urinary catheters. Tape may be the oldest method, but it's not the only one. *AJN,* 102(3):44-48.

Loy GL, Gelula MH, Vontver LA. (2004). Teaching students to question. *Am J Obstet Gynecol,* 191(5):1752-1756.

Melnyk BM, Fineout-Overholt E. (2005). *Evidence-based practice in nursing & healthcare: A guide to best practice.* Philadelphia: Lippincott Williams & Wilkins.

Nattina SM. (2005). *The Lippincott manual of nursing practice,* 8th ed. Philadelphia: Lippincott Williams & Wilkins.

Pierce ST. (2005). Integrating evidence-based practice into nursing curricula. *Annu Rev Nurs Educ,* 3:233-248.

Profetto-McGrath J. (2005). Critical thinking and evidence-based practice. *J Prof Nurs,* 21(6):364-371.

Society of Urologic Nurses and Associates (SUNA) Clinical Practice Guidelines Task Force. (2006). Care of the patient with an indwelling catheter. *Urol Nurs,* 26(1):80-81.

University of Washington. (2007). Construct well-built clinical questions using PICO. *HealthLinks.* Available online: http://healthlinks.washington.edu. Retrieved July 5, 2007.

Wong ES, Hooten TM. (1981). Guideline for prevention of catheter-associated urinary tract infection. Center for Disease Control and Prevention. Available http://www.fen.ufg.br/documentos/nucleos/TratoUrinario.pdf. Retrieved June 30, 2007.

Chapter 5

USE OF EVIDENCE-BASED NURSING AS A PRACTICING NURSE

Beth Ann Swan, PhD, CRNP, FAAN; Jacqueline Sullivan, PhD, RN;
Betty J. Ackley, MSN, EdS, RN

As a nurse, you make hundreds of clinical decisions every day. We predict that many of these decisions are currently influenced by organizational clinical practices together with professional knowledge and personal values (Swan et al., 2004). At this time, the majority of nursing care is minimally based on research findings because of factors such as limited access to research resources, minimal knowledge about evidence-based nursing (EBN), limited competencies and skills in implementing evidence-based practice, and misperceptions and negative attitudes about research (Melnyk et al., 2004; Fineout-Overholt et al., 2005; Pravikoff et al., 2005; Thompson et al., 2005). Therefore, the provision of most nursing care interventions is opinion-based decision making with limited attention to evidence-based decision making. This will change in the near future as there is more emphasis on providing evidence-based care. EBN is a process you can use to increase the quality of your individual nursing care, improve nursing practice in your health care facility, and promote nursing professionalism. These topics and more are discussed in this chapter. The goal of this text is to help you, as a nurse, use EBN as a process to improve your own nursing care and the quality of care given in your health care facility.

INDEPENDENT VERSUS DEPENDENT NURSING INTERVENTIONS: WHAT IS THE DIFFERENCE?

As you learn of evidence-based findings that affect your nursing practice, you may or may not be able to put the findings into practice immediately. Ideally, before making any change in practice, you need to do a systematic review of the literature. The guidelines in this text are prescriptive in specifying which nursing activities are effective, but the findings should be verified.

As a general rule, nursing interventions that are independent in nature do not require an order from a physician and can sometimes be implemented in a timely fashion by the nurse. Many of the guidelines in this text are independent nursing interventions. Examples include active listening, use of reality orientation, use of preparatory sensory information, hope instillation, and many more independent interventions. Timeliness in adopting changes in independent care suggested by the guidelines is not absolute. Teaching is an independent intervention, but nurses should follow the guidelines of the facility at which they are employed.

Dependent interventions, or collaborative interventions, are those that are ordered by a physician and carried out by the nurse. Examples include insertion of a catheter, a dressing change, and medication administration. For these interventions, the nurse must follow a defined hospital policy and procedure. To make changes in dependent interventions, the nurse must follow a defined process with support from the nurses in education and administration to institute a change in nursing practice based on evidence. It is not appropriate for you as a nurse to make the change individually in isolation. Sometimes the change is impossible because the prescribed supplies are not available, or there is not enough staff to carry out the change, or you may not be aware of other variables that affect how or whether the change based on evidence should be made. This process of making an evidence-based change in nursing practice as an individual nurse is explained further in the next section.

MAKING AN EBN CHANGE IN PRACTICE

There are five steps to the process. You will find the process challenging and intellectually stimulating.

Step 1: Formulate Your Clinical Question

The first step in your journey is to ask a question about a nursing intervention that you are interested in, a change in nursing practice, or a new nursing practice that may have consequences for patients.

Example

> Why must I use 2% chlorhexidine to cleanse the skin before inserting an angiocatheter? I have used povidone-iodine (Betadine) for the last 20 years. What's the big deal?
> To identify the best evidence about your question, it is important to consider these four factors:
> Population of patients in which you are interested (Z)
> Nursing intervention you are concerned about (X)
> Comparison of interest (XX)
> Patient outcome(s) you would like to examine (Y)
> Another way to think of your question is to ask, what is the effect of some intervention X on some outcome Y in a given population of patients Z? Or what is the effect of some intervention X on some outcome Y compared with XX intervention in a given population of patients Z?

Example

> What is the effect of 2% chlorhexidine skin preparation (X intervention) on decreasing the risk of catheter-related bloodstream infections (Y outcome) compared with povidone-iodine skin preparation (XX intervention) in peripheral intravenous catheters (IVs) in general medical and surgical patients (Z population)?

Step 2: Search, Identify, and Gather Your Evidence

Guided by your focused question, you will begin your search of the literature using concepts and terms from your question and querying a variety of databases described in Chapter 2. You will need access to a library and the Internet. If this is your first time conducting a search, it is recommended that you seek out the expertise of a reference librarian. If you have Internet access, you can go to http://www.pubmed.gov and begin your search without charge.

Example

For our question, the initial search terms would include 2% chlorhexidine, skin preparation, peripheral IVs, catheter-related bloodstream infections, povidone-iodine, Betadine, and medical and surgical patients.

These terms can be combined using Boolean operators AND, OR, NOT (or AND NOT), and NEAR. Boolean operators tell search engines which keywords you want your results to include or exclude and whether you require that your keywords appear close to each other. Depending on the outcome of your initial search, you may want to include the term "research" or "evidence" or "guidelines." If your search yields few articles, you may want to check your terms with MeSH subject headings. MeSH is the National Library of Medicine's controlled vocabulary thesaurus. It consists of sets of terms naming descriptors in a hierarchical structure that permits searching at various levels of specificity. When conducting a search, always remember to save your searches so that you have a history or paper trail for future work.

When you are ready to print your search results, print the view that includes the abstracts for your citations. A review of the abstracts will help you identify the articles that apply to your question and narrow your search. Some of the articles may be available free online through pubmed.gov or some other database. Others you may need to request from interlibrary loan. For this reason, you want to be sure you select the best articles that pertain to your question and topic of interest in order to identify and gather the best evidence. Once you have all your articles in hand, it is time to evaluate the evidence.

Step 3: Evaluate Your Evidence

You should read each article with a critical eye, subjecting each publication to a systematic critique and review for the purpose of evaluating and categorizing its level of evidence and research rigor. There are several strategies you can use when reviewing your evidence or articles. You can code each article in the margin for applicability to your question, design, sample size, strengths, weaknesses, and validity of the evidence. Some clinicians may write a short summary or annotate each article. Other clinicians use an Excel spreadsheet to create a table of evidence and abstract the coding onto a spreadsheet. This facilitates the synthesis and evaluation of the evidence. Rating the level of evidence and determining the level of rigor is an essential step in the literature review process in evidence-based practice because it influences decisions regarding readiness for translation and adaptation of research-driven practice recommendations. Many schemas exist for rating the strength and quality of research and evidence (Swan & Boruch, 2004). The schema used in this book and described in Chapter 1 is the rating system for the level of evidence (Melnyk & Fineout-Overholt, 2005). Refer to Chapter 1 for a complete discussion of this rating system.

You can use the information in this text as a beginning point to learn what evidence is available, but you must also obtain the articles and follow the process to ensure that newer research does not refute what this text recommends.

Step 4: Apply the Evidence to Your Question

Following the evaluation of your evidence, you must decide whether a change in practice is supported by the evidence. Please ask yourself a series of questions:
1. Is the evidence valid? Is it evidence or research of the nursing practice or nursing intervention that you are interested in?
2. If the evidence is valid, is the evidence important? Are the valid results of this evidence and research important?

3. If the evidence and research are valid and important, can you apply this evidence in caring for your patient, patients, or population of patients? Do these results apply to your patient(s)? Is your patient(s) so different from those described that its results cannot help you? How great would the potential benefit of this intervention actually be for your individual patient(s) or population of patients?
4. Are your patient's values and preferences satisfied by the intervention and its benefits versus its consequences? Do you and your patients have a clear assessment of their (the patients') values and preferences? Are they met by this nursing intervention or nursing practice and its consequences?

After you answer each of these questions, you must decide whether a change in practice is supported. If it is, when the practice change is implemented, a plan must be in place to evaluate the practice change. This plan should be developed in conjunction with the change in practice.

Step 5: Evaluate Change in Practice

The process to evaluate change in an EBN practice is the same as any quality improvement process. For example, the Lang model for quality assurance in nursing took the form of a continuous feedback loop, much the same as the EBN process described here (Lang, 1975). The feedback loop begins with the formation of values, informed by societal and professional values and scientific knowledge. Next, criteria for nursing care (diagnoses, interventions, outcomes) are established. The degree of discrepancy between the current practice and the potential evidence-based practice change is assessed, followed by selecting and implementing an evidence-based alternative for changing practice, ultimately leading to improving practice (Swan et al., 2004).

INSTITUTING EBN IN YOUR ORGANIZATION OR HEALTH CARE SYSTEM

To be successful in implementing and evaluating EBN, it is essential for you to have access to support resources and consultation, such as Internet access to search databases, reference librarians, and search experts (Fineout-Overholt et al., 2005). This environment can be cultivated in academic health care centers as well as community hospital settings through development of an infrastructure driven by an evidence-based practice framework. Chapter 3 provides a detailed description of implementing EBN in health care systems.

ADDITIONAL RESOURCES/SUPPORT

There are several clinical research resources and supports available to help you institute EBN after identifying your question, including (1) clinical practice guidelines, (2) review and critique of the research literature, and (3) best practice consensus decisions. Clinical practice guidelines, if available and appropriate for your specific clinical practice issue or question, are critically evaluated before translating into practice. Experts review the evidence that supports the guidelines; they evaluate the rigor of the supporting evidence and research and its applicability and feasibility within the targeted population of patients and clinical environment. When the strength, applicability, and feasibility of the evidence are confirmed, the guideline is adapted into practice with the goal of changing and improving the quality of patients' care. Following clinical practice adaptation, the effectiveness and success of outcomes resulting from guideline use are critically evaluated and measured both quantitatively and qualitatively.

If clinical practice guidelines do not exist for a specific clinical practice issue or if the guidelines reviewed are insufficient in currency, strength, applicability, or feasibility, you can pursue a second approach. This approach consists of a comprehensive review and critique of the literature as described previously. Using this strategy, the state of the science for a particular clinical initiative is assessed and evaluated. Current available research literature is identified through multiple systematically conducted electronic database searches (e.g., MEDLINE, CINAHL, PubMed). Refer to Chapter 2 for a detailed discussion of finding and evaluating research for practice. Ideally, dedicated expert staff conduct these electronic database searches on request as well as instruct staff nurses and nurse leaders on effective database search techniques. When the current state of the science is identified, this literature is accessed through online acquisition, through hard-copy retrieval from library resources on site, or, when necessary, from other libraries through interlibrary loan. Library services should include assistance with current literature searches using multiple diverse databases. Ideally, in a dedicated data-driven environment, electronic database search access is immediately available to clinical staff nurses desiring to conduct electronic literature searches while delivering care to patients.

When the available research literature has been reviewed and classified based on level of strength, this evidence is synthesized into a compilation of practice recommendations with a listing of the number of citations, sources of citations, and classification of level of supporting evidence. Research-based clinical practice recommendations resulting from evidentiary data review and synthesis processes are then subjected to further evaluation based on determining the clinical applicability and feasibility for specific populations of patients and clinical practice settings. Finally, prior to implementation into clinical practice, the effectiveness and success of outcomes resulting from evidence-based clinical practice adaptations are critically evaluated and measured using both quantitative and qualitative methods.

In cases where clinical practice guidelines and research literature reviews yield insufficient results in terms of quantity, currency, strength, applicability, or feasibility, a third strategy may be pursued. This strategy involves developing, implementing, and evaluating best practice consensus decisions. The best practice decision is developed after consulting a variety of institutional, regional, national, and international clinical and research experts for consensus recommendations in a specific clinical area of interest. Once developed, the best practice decision is uniformly and simultaneously implemented in the targeted population of patients and clinical setting. Best practice decisions result when the state of the science is insufficient for developing evidence-based clinical practice recommendations; hence, they are the least stable of all three approaches and are subject to frequent modification necessitated by new research developments and changes in practice standards. Despite these limitations, best practice consensus decisions are advantageous in that they prevent paralysis of practice or inconsistencies in practice based on habit, ritual, or myth, which otherwise might result in the absence of available evidence. As with each of the evidence-based practice approaches, effectiveness and success of best practice recommendations are also subjected to systematic evaluation using both quantitative and qualitative research methods. Refinements of best practice decisions and recommendations often occur after reviewing outcome variables measured in the evaluation process.

THE CHANGE PROCESS

For any change in nursing practice to be effective, it is helpful to use some version of the change process to make it happen. There are many theories on how to make change effectively in industry and health care. Figure 5-1 illustrates how to combine EBN with the change process. This change

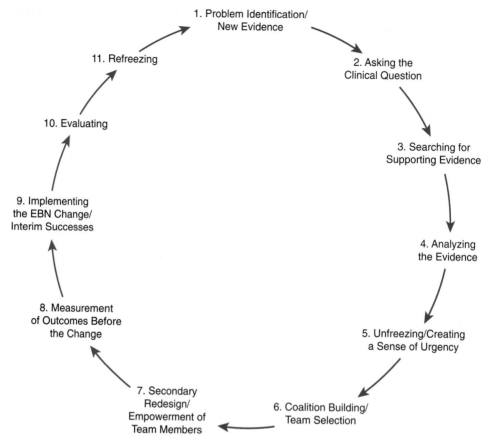

FIG 5-1 • The change process with evidence-based nursing in a health care institution.

process is circular and never stops. All health care facilities are involved in nonstop change, some initiated by staff and administration change also comes from key forces outside the organization. These stages of change with EBN are explained in Table 5-1.

CONCEPT OF CHAMPIONS OF CHANGE

There is often one nurse who leads the change. Because you are reading this chapter, that nurse might be *you*. The nurse may be designated a "champion" for the change. This is a term that comes from the business world (Peters & Waterman, 2004), but it is also useful in health care (Everett & Titler, 2006). Some hospitals now identify specialized nurses as champions. At the University of Colorado (Goode, 2004), this designation is used for specialized nurses who, for example, are "Pain Champions of Change" and also "Skin Champions of Change." These nurses are passionate about their specialty; they teach, role model, promote quality, and serve as consultants in their area. The title of champion increases the nurse's status and increases ownership and learning in the area.

TABLE 5-1	Explanation of Stages of Change with an Evidence-Based Nursing Change in Practice*
Stage	**Explanation**
1. Problem identification/ new evidence	A problem is identified that needs a solution, or new research evidence is available that necessitates a change in nursing practice.
2. Asking the clinical question	The clinical question should be formulated preferably using a system such as PICO (Population, Intervention, Comparison, Outcome). Please refer to Chapter 4.
3. Searching for supporting evidence	A thorough literature search should be done. For many changes, it is helpful to find out how it is done in other health care facilities.
4. Analyzing the evidence	The evidence must be thoroughly analyzed to determine whether it is significant and whether the results apply to the present situation.
5. Unfreezing/creating a sense of urgency	The process where the change agent works to get people questioning the current reality; he or she talks to everyone about the problem or new evidence and creates a sense of urgency for changes to happen.
6. Coalition building/team selection	The change agent looks for support for the change from stakeholders, key people with power in the unit or organization. At times this may be someone with informal power only (e.g., the licensed practical nurse who has been working on the unit for 20 years and is highly respected). The priority for team selection is to have a coalition of powerful supportive people who want the change. This team will ideally work together to make the change happen.
7. Secondary redesign/ empowerment of team members	The stakeholders are able to have input into how the change is made or into the actual change itself. As people are able to do this, the change becomes their own and they will more strongly help "sell" the change to others. This process is part of empowerment, which is giving power to others.
8. Measurement of outcomes before the change	The change agents must decide on what outcomes measures will be used and then measure the patients' outcomes before the change is instituted.
9. Implementing the EBN change/interim successes	The change is implemented, often as a pilot test on one unit in a hospital. This is to have short-term successes that support the change.
10. Evaluating	The outcomes are measured again after implementation of the change, and a determination is made of whether the outcomes are significant enough to justify a permanent change in practice that can be used by the entire medical center.
11. Refreezing	The change in practice is locked into the organization by being part of a policy and procedure or clinical practice guideline. The changed practice becomes part of orientation for new staff. Everyone knows "this is how we do this here and it is based on evidence."

*This is a simplified version of the change process, and the order of the process may need to change based on the situation. Also, implementing a change is an important step that involves more than teaching everyone about the change. Disseminating information should be done creatively, using many strategies. Examples include use of a poster, rewarding those who utilize the change, and providing computer-assisted instruction and competency testing (Everett & Titler, 2006).

Data from Lewin K. (1951). *Field theory in social sciences: Selected theoretical papers.* New York: Harper & Row; Kotter JP, Cohen DS. (2002). *The heart of change. Real-life stories of how people change their organizations.* Boston: Harvard Business School Press; Olade RA. (2004). Strategic collaborative model for evidence-based nursing practice. *Worldviews Evid Based Nurs,* 1(1):60-68; Rogers E. (1983). *Diffusions of innovation,* 3rd ed. New York: The Free Press; Rosswurm MA, Larrabee JH. (1999). A model for change to evidence-based practice. *Image J Nurs Scholarsh,* 31(4):317-322.

EXAMPLE OF CHANGE IN NURSING PRACTICE

Going back to the example question presented previously, what is the effect of 2% chlorhexidine skin preparation on decreasing the risk of catheter-related bloodstream infections compared with povidone-iodine skin preparation for peripheral IVs in medical and surgical patients? You can use this book as a resource in your clinical setting. The question is focused on a nursing intervention related to skin preparation and peripheral IV insertion. Please refer to the guideline on Intravenous (IV) Insertion.

Example

What is the Best Evidence That Exists That Supports the Nursing Activity?

Using 2% chlorhexidine–based preparation for disinfection of the intended venipuncture site to reduce the risk of infection when performing venipuncture. Level of evidence = I.

Following a search and review of the literature, the level of evidence that supports this nursing activity is rated at level I. According to Melnyk and Fineout-Overholt's (2005) schema, level I is "evidence from a systematic review or meta-analysis of all relevant randomized controlled trials (RCTs), or evidence-based clinical practice guidelines based on systematic reviews of RCTs" (p. 10).

What is the Level I Evidence?

A multidisciplinary meta-analysis of studies ($N = 8$ studies involving 4143 catheters of which 1361 were peripheral IV catheters) comparing chlorhexidine gluconate with povidone-iodine solutions for catheter site care found that the incidence of bloodstream infections is significantly reduced when chlorhexidine gluconate is used (CDC, 2002; Chaiyakunapruk et al., 2002). Level I is the highest level of evidence or the "gold standard" to support this change in practice. When a nurse colleague asks, "Why do I have to use 2% chlorhexidine? I used povidone-iodine or Betadine for the last 20 years," you can confidently answer with the best evidence to support the practice. This book provides the best evidence for almost 200 nursing interventions used in everyday practice when caring for hospitalized medical and surgical patients.

REWARDS FOR UTILIZING EBN

The most important reward in utilizing EBN is knowing that you are giving the best care possible. With this comes pride in professional practice; you are empowered because you have control over your nursing practice and can influence others as needed. You will be treated with respect because you can cite research findings to explain your practice, and you are more likely to have compliance when you ask for an order from a physician or when you delegate to others. You will be the nurse whom others come to when they have a question. Who are they going to ask? It is *you.*

There are even more advantages to being an expert on using EBN. Because of your experiences with EBN, you will know how to make change effectively in an organization. Many EBN nurses find their EBN experiences a stepping-stone to further professional practice. It is likely that you will be on professional practice committees or other powerful committees in your facility. Many health care facilities have clinical ladders. Work on EBN can be rewarded by heading further up the ladder. Depending on your facility, you may become actively involved in the Magnet process that supports the quality of nursing given in a hospital. We predict that you will want to further your career and seek further education in nursing as a result of being an EBN nurse. We invite you to share with us the personal and professional rewards you have experienced when initiating or being a part of EBN. Please send us an e-mail at beth.swan@jefferson.edu and Backley1108@aol.com.

In summary, the EBN process starts with your curiosity, enthusiasm, and questioning of the status quo. You can successfully complete an EBN project with support from an appropriate research staff, meaningful clinical research education, active engagement of nurse colleagues, and ongoing mentorship. Administrative commitment and institutional allocation of dedicated resources greatly contribute to clinical staff nurse participation in a climate of clinical inquiry leading to data-driven, patient-centered quality of care. Your active engagement as a staff nurse working with a supportive team to promote EBN leads to the best outcomes for patients, with the result of giving the best nursing care possible.

REFERENCES

Centers for Disease Control and Prevention (CDC), Department of Health and Human Services. (2002). Services Fact Sheet (2002). Guidelines for isolation precautions in hospitals. *MMWR* 51(42):RR-16.

Chaiyakunapruk N, Veenstra DL, Lipsky BA, Saint S. (2002). Cholorhexidine compared with povidone-iodine solution for vascular catheter sight care: A meta-analysis. *Ann Intern Med,* 136(11):792-801.

Everett LQ, Titler MG. (2006). Making EBP part of clinical practice: The Iowa model. In Levin RF, Feldman HR (Eds): *Teaching evidence-based practice in nursing.* New York: Springer.

Fineout-Overholt E, Melnyk BM, Schultz A. (2005). Transforming health care from the inside out: Advancing evidence-based practice in the 21st century. *J Prof Nurs,* 21(6):335-344.

Goode CJ. (2004). Importance of using standardized language for the chief nursing officer and the nursing leadership. Presentation at the NANDA, NIC & NOC Conference, "Working Together for Quality Nursing Care: Striving Toward Harmonization," Chicago, March 27, 2004.

Kotter JP, Cohen DS. (2002). *The heart of change. Real-life stories of how people change their organizations.* Boston: Harvard Business School Press.

Lang NM. (1975). Quality assurance in nursing. *AORN J,* 22(4):180-186.

Lewin K. (1951). *Field theory in social sciences: Selected theoretical papers.* New York: Harper & Row.

Melnyk BM, Fineout-Overholt E. (2005). *Evidence-based practice in nursing and healthcare.* Philadelphia: Lippincott Williams & Wilkins.

Melnyk BM, Fineout-Overholt E, Feinstein NF, Li H, Small L, Wilcox L, et al. (2004). Nurses' perceived knowledge, beliefs, skills, and needs regarding evidence-based practice: Implications for accelerating the paradigm shift. *Worldviews Evid Based Nurs,* 1(3):185-193.

Mohide EA, Coker E. (2005). Toward clinical scholarship: Promoting evidence-based practice in the clinical setting. *J Prof Nurs,* 21(6):372-379.

Olade RA. (2004). Strategic collaborative model for evidence-based nursing practice. *Worldviews Evid Based Nurs,* 1(1):60-68.

Peters T, Waterman RH Jr. (2004). *In search of excellence.* New York: Harper Collins Business Essentials.

Pravikoff DS, Tanner AB, Pierce ST. (2005). Readiness of U.S. nurses for evidence-based practice. *Am J Nurs,* 105(9):40-51.

Rogers E. (1983). *Diffusions of innovation,* 3rd ed. New York: The Free Press.

Rosswurm MA, Larrabee JH. (1999). A model for change to evidence-based practice. *Image J Nurs Scholarsh,* 31(4):317-322.

Swan BA, Boruch RF. (2004). Quality of evidence: Usefulness in measuring the quality of health care. *Med Care,* 42(2 Suppl):II12-II20.

Swan BA, Lang NM, McGinley AM. (2004). Access to quality health care: Links between evidence, nursing language, and informatics. *Nurs Econ,* 22(6):325-332.

Thompson C, McCaughan D, Cullum N, Sheldon T, Raynor P. (2005). Barriers to evidence-based practice in primary care nursing—Why viewing decision-making as context is helpful. *J Adv Nurs,* 52(4):432-444.

PART TWO

GUIDELINES FOR EVIDENCE-BASED NURSING

ABUSE PROTECTION SUPPORT

Rose E. Constantino, PhD, JD, RN, FAAN, FACFE;
Patricia A. Crane, PhD, MSN, RN-C, WHNP

NIC **Definition:** Identification of high-risk dependent relationships and actions to prevent further infliction of physical or emotional harm (Dochterman & Bulechek, 2004).

NURSING ACTIVITIES

Effective

■ *Screen for risk factors associated with domestic abuse and symptoms of a history of domestic violence and provide support to empower victims to take action and make changes to prevent further victimization.* **LOE = I**

NR In a two-arm RCT with 360 abused women who assessed positive for physical or sexual abuse within the preceding 12 months, two interventions were tested: (1) providing a wallet-sized referral card and (2) a 20-minute nurse case management protocol. Results demonstrated that both interventions resulted in significantly fewer threats of abuse, assaults, danger risks for homicide, and events of work harassment (McFarlane et al., 2006).

NR In a two-group, systematically allocated repeated-measures study, telephone intervention for 75 women who were victims of intimate partner violence compared with 75 women in the usual care control group ($N = 150$) showed efficacy for 18 months. Participants were systematically allocated to either the treatment group or the control group based on the week of enrollment in the study to minimize sampling bias. Further, the women in the intervention group practiced significantly more safety-promoting behaviors than they had at the time of intake than the women in the control group (McFarlane et al., 2004).

NR In a pilot study of feasibility of the intervention, a two-group by two-repeated-measures randomized control design was used to evaluate a group intervention program in comparison with a no-treatment control in women ($N = 24$) who were first-time residents of a domestic violence shelter. Results showed that the treatment group had greater improvement in psychological distress and social support and less health care utilization than the control group (Constantino et al., 2005).

NR A qualitative phenomenological pilot study that explored the feasibility of e-mail–mediated interaction in survivors of abuse between six mother and child pairs who received a protection from abuse order within the last six months and a nurse e-mail facilitator suggests that e-mail is a feasible source of safety information, follow-up referrals, and social support (Constantino et al., 2007).

MR A review of published studies from 1966 to 1999 containing original research with a primary focus on screening for intimate partner violence showed that interventions were likely to be more effective if they included strategies (providing specific screening questions) in addition to provider education (Waalen et al., 2000).

MR The experimental social innovation and dissemination (ESID) model was used as an intervention to reduce intimate partner violence against women. Women ($N = 278$) who had

---

NR = Nursing Research, **MR** = Multidisciplinary Research, **SP** = Standard of Practice, **EO** = Expert Opinion, **LOE** = Level of Evidence

exited a domestic violence shelter program were randomly assigned to the experimental or control condition. Women who received the intervention reported less violence over time as well as higher social support and perceived quality of life (Sullivan, 2003).

(MR) An experimental study of a community-based advocacy program for 284 women with abusive partners demonstrated positive change in the lives of women even more than 2 years after the intervention (Bybee & Sullivan, 2002).

(MR) A descriptive study employed quantitative and qualitative methods through semi-structured interviews and a series of exploratory and confirmatory focus groups with women ($N = 24$) who experienced abuse. Results showed that survivors of abuse needed community interventions that facilitated choices and enhanced their successes (Lutenbacher et al., 2003).

(EO) Interventions reduce harm to children when child abuse or neglect has been assessed (USPSTF, 2004).

Possibly Effective

■ *Listen to individuals talk about their own problems, provide positive affirmation of worth, and encourage expression of concerns and feelings.* **LOE = IV**

(MR) In a study using a qualitative approach through semistructured personal interviews, 41 women who experienced intimate partner violence described what they wanted from interventions provided to them and how they wished to receive these interventions. Characteristics of the interventions included not requiring disclosure or identification as intimate partner victims, multiple-option intervention, and preserving respect for individual autonomy (Chang et al., 2005).

(MR) Using an interpersonal protection model of abuse, psychotherapeutic intervention strategies for specific cases of adult survivors of child abuse were implemented. In a case study format, four cases were used as examples of intervention strategies in caring for survivors of abuse. Effective strategies included active remembering, mixed feedback and dissociation, trances and time out, subselves and internal criticism, alliances with inner critics, and reconstruction of trauma memories (Thomas, 2005).

(MR) In a study that used a matched, yoked, and randomized design, 10 pairs of psychologically abused women were randomly assigned to forgiveness therapy (FT) and an alternative treatment (AT) and met individually with the intervener for almost 8 months (mean = 7.95 months). Results showed that the FT participants had significantly greater improvement in depression, trait anxiety, post-traumatic stress symptoms, self-esteem, forgiveness, environmental mastery, and finding meaning in suffering than AT participants (Reed & Enright, 2006).

(EO) The need for violence prevention in children is great because even the impact of child witness to violence is cumulative, affecting both mental and physical health as adults and increasing the risk for the children to be in a violent relationship as adults, perpetuating the cycle of violence (Ernst, 2006).

■ *Assist individuals and families to evaluate objectively strengths and weaknesses of relationships.* **LOE = II**

(MR) A quasi-experimental design study examined outcomes of a domestic violence-focused treatment program for couples who chose to stay together after mild to moderate violence had occurred. Forty-two couples were randomly assigned to individual couple treatment and multicouple group treatment, and a group of nine volunteer couples participated as a comparison group. Results showed that male recidivism rates 6 months after treatment were significantly lower for the multicouple group (25%) than the individual couple treatment group (43%) and the comparison group (66%), indicating that couple treatment (multiple or single) could be a useful way to help couples with mild to moderate violence who freely choose to stay together (Stith et al., 2004).

Note: As a practicing clinician and expert in the area of domestic violence, the author of this guideline cautions against couples therapy outside a formal domestic violence-focused treatment program.

■ *Monitor elder patient-caretaker interactions and record observations, consult with community resources for information, and report suspected elder abuse or neglect to proper authorities.* **LOE = II**

(MR) A field experiment on an intervention to reduce repeated incidents of elder abuse involved randomly selecting public housing projects to receive educational material on elder abuse. Thirty of 60 public housing projects were randomly assigned to receive public education and home visits by a team of a police officer and a domestic violence counselor. Households that received home visits and educational material on elder abuse prevention called the police significantly more often and reported significantly higher levels of elder abuse than the control group who received home visits only (Davis & Medina-Ariza, 2001).

(EO) The Division of Clinical Forensic Medicine (CFM), part of the Office of the Kentucky Chief Medical Examiner and the University of Louisville Division of Forensic Pathology, provided important and practical expert suggestions on elder maltreatment screening questions for six areas of elderly vulnerability: general situational, generalized health and well-being, specifics about activities of daily living, specifics about injury, financial status, and emotional and psychological status. Suggested screening questions in the general situational vulnerability area included (1) Do you feel safe where you live?, (2) Are you having difficulties with the living condition?, (3) How are you getting along with _____?, (4) Are you getting out with your friends?, and (5) Are you afraid of ____? Also suggested were assessing for signs and symptoms that could be gathered from medical records and physical examination as potential indicators of elder abuse (Shryock et al., 2005).

(NR) A concept paper/report described the roles of nurses on collaborative, interprofessional elder maltreatment teams. In addition to common nursing roles that included assessment, screening, mandatory reporting, direct care, and complaint investigation, nurses gave expert opinion, educated team members, and provided case consultation (Baker & Heitkemper, 2005).

Not Effective

No applicable published research was found in this category.

Possibly Harmful

No applicable published research was found in this category.

OUTCOME MEASUREMENT

ABUSE PROTECTION NOC

Definition: Protection of self or dependent others from abuse.

Abuse Protection as evidenced by the following selected NOC indicators:

- Plan for leaving situation
- Safety of self
- Safety of children
- Limitation of contact with abuser by means of a restraining order
- Self-advocacy
- Safety of residence
- Plan for avoiding abuse
- Facilitation of abuser obtaining counseling
- Withdrawal when relationship is unsafe
- Severance of relationship as needed

(Rate each indicator of **Abuse Protection**: 1 = not adequate, 2 = slightly adequate, 3 = moderately adequate, 4 = substantially adequate, 5 = totally adequate) (Moorhead et al., 2004).

REFERENCES

Baker MW, Heitkemper MM. (2005). The roles of nurses on interpersonal teams to combat elder mistreatment. *Nurs Outlook,* 53(5):253-259.

Bybee DI, Sullivan CM. (2002). The process through which an advocacy intervention resulted in positive change for battered women over time. *Am J Community Psychol,* 30(1):103-132.

Chang JC, Cluss PA, Ranieri L, Hawker L, Buranosky R, Dado D, et al. (2005). Health care interventions for intimate partner violence: What women want. *Womens Health Issues,* 15(1):21-30.

Constantino R, Crane PA, Noll BS, Doswell WM, Braxter B. (2007). Exploring the feasibility of email-mediated interaction in survivors of abuse. *J Psychiatr Ment Health Nurse,* 14(3):291-301.

Constantino R, Kim Y, Crane PA. (2005). Effects of a social support intervention on health outcomes in residents of a domestic violence shelter: A pilot study. *Issues Ment Health Nurs,* 26(6):575-590.

Davis RC, Medina-Ariza J. (2001). Results from an elder abuse prevention experiment in New York City. US Department of Justice, National Institute of Justice. *Res Brief,* 1-7.

Dochterman JM, Bulechek GM (Eds). (2004). *Nursing Interventions Classification (NIC),* 4th ed. St. Louis: Mosby.

Ernst AA. (2006). Intimate partner violence: Steps for future generations. *Ann Emerg Med,* 47(2):200-202.

Lutenbacher M, Cohen A, Mitzel J. (2003). Do we really help? Perspectives of abused women. *Public Health Nurs,* 20(1):56-64.

McFarlane J, Malecha A, Gist J, Watson K, Batten E, Hall I, et al. (2004). Increasing the safety-promoting behaviors of abused women. *Am J Nurs,* 104(3):40-50.

McFarlane JM, Groff JY, O'Brien JA, Watson K. (2006). Secondary prevention of intimate partner violence: A randomized controlled trial. *Nurs Res,* 55(1):52-61.

Moorhead M, Johnson M, Maas M (Eds). (2004). *Nursing Outcomes Classification (NOC),* 3rd ed. St. Louis: Mosby.

Reed GL, Enright RD. (2006). The effects of forgiveness therapy on depression, anxiety, and posttraumatic stress for women after spousal emotional abuse. *J Consult Clin Psychol,* 74(5):920-929.

Shryock S, Hunsaker DM, Corey TS, Weakley-Jones B. (2005). Forensic evaluation of the elderly. *J Ky Med Assoc,* 103(9):451-455.

Stith SM, Rosen KH, McCollum EE, Thomsen CJ. (2004). Treating intimate partner violence within intact couple relationships: Outcomes of multi-couple versus individual couple therapy. *J Marital Fam Ther,* 30(3):305-318.

Sullivan CM. (2003). Using the ESID model to reduce intimate male violence against women. *Am J Community Psychol,* 32(3-4):295-303.

Thomas PM. (2005). Dissociation and internal models of protection: Psychotherapy with child abuse survivors. *Psychotherapy,* 42(1):20-36.

US Preventive Services Task Force (USPSTF). (2004). Screening for family and intimate partner violence: Recommendation statement. *Ann Intern Med,* 140(5):382-386.

Waalen J, Goodwin MM, Spitz AM, Petersen R, Saltzman LE. (2000). Screening for intimate partner violence by health care providers: Barriers and interventions. *Am J Prev Med,* 19(4):230-237.

 # ACTIVE LISTENING

Ruth Davidhizar, DNS, RN, ARNP-BC, FAAN

NIC **Definition:** Attending closely to and attaching significance to a patient's verbal and nonverbal messages (Dochterman & Bulechek, 2004).

NURSING ACTIVITIES

Effective

■ *To become a better listener, understand that listening is not easy.* **LOE = VII**

   EO It is important to appreciate behaviors necessary for effective listening and to work to develop active listening skills (Giger & Davidhizar, 2004).

■ *Realize that to listen to another sincerely and actively is the ultimate compliment and communicates the respect that is central to the therapeutic relationship (Cornn, 2003).* **LOE = VII**

   EO Culture designates what we pay attention to and what we ignore. It is our culture that provides structure for the world and filters for what we react to. Research on the silent language provides a research base (LOE = I) for much of what is common interpersonal theory today (Hall, 1959, 1976).

■ *Use listening to assist the insecure patient, to gain trust from the patient who fears lack of acceptance, to work collaboratively on a plan of care, and to encourage returning for further care.* **LOE = VII**

   EO The most critical skill in effective communication is the ability to listen (Davidhizar, 2004; Giger & Davidhizar, 2004).

   EO Active listening is a universal care construct or, in other words, a universal concept of communication that crosses cultures (Leininger, 1995).

■ *Assess people with whom communication occurs, whether they be patient, family, or members of the health care team.* **LOE = VII**

   EO Only by careful assessment can behavior be personalized so that effective communication can occur and behaviors that block communication be avoided. The stronger the cultural

NR = Nursing Research, **MR** = Multidisciplinary Research, **SP** = Standard of Practice, **EO** = Expert Opinion, **LOE** = Level of Evidence

filters, the more likely that there are forms of bias in listening that are beyond personal awareness (Egan, 1994).

■ *Recognize that listening is an interpersonal skill basic to all effective interactions.* **LOE = VII**

(EO) Listening is one of six ways to make people like another person. Listening is strategic to effective nursing because being able to listen is important, not only to assess a patient adequately but also to develop patient- and family-focused care. Listening is a critical nursing strategy that transcends culture (Carnegie, 1936).

■ *Actively listen to appear interested and encourage further elaboration. This may include nodding; the suggestion to "go on"; encouraging further expression of feelings, thoughts, and concerns; and other facilitated nonverbal and verbal techniques.* **LOE = I**

(EO) Active listening can be achieved by stating back to the patient what has been said (giving feedback) and asking further questions to encourage elaboration. It is also important to listen for inconsistencies or things that the patient says that may need clarification (Giger & Davidhizar, 2004).

Possibly Effective

■ *Use or do not use eye contact as appropriate to the patient and the patient's culture.* **LOE = VII**

(EO) In some cultures, individuals communicate that they are listening by eye contact. In other cultures, an individual who maintains eye contact can be considered rude or aggressive. For example, people from Chinese or Vietnamese cultures reserve eye contact for individuals whom they view as being in the same social class. If a person is seen as having authority, eye contact may be avoided (Bonder et al., 2002).

■ *Show genuine listening and respect by turning the ear to the individual, as appropriate to the patient and the patient's culture (Giger & Davidhizar, 2004).* **LOE = VII**

(EO) A paranoid, shy, or embarrassed patient may feel more comfortable talking to the provider who stands at a slight angle and avoids constant eye contact (Wehlage, 2000).

■ *Promote hesitancy to speak about health care concerns as appropriate to the patient's cultural and unique needs.* **LOE = VII**

(EO) For example, some American Indians who have grown up with the Ojibway tradition are hesitant to talk to Westerners about personal needs. The Ojibway may avoid oral questioning by health care workers and consider questions a violation of dignity and space. Rather than cooperating, the patient who values noninterference may leave the health care setting when questioned and not return for further care that the health care worker deems necessary (Reimer & Redskye, 1998).

RCT = Randomized Controlled (Clinical) Trial, **NIC** = Nursing Interventions Classification, **NOC** = Nursing Outcomes Classification

■ *Utilize selective and careful use of silence.* **LOE = VII**

(EO) Silence may be useful to facilitate communication and at other times may be frightening to the patient (Schulman, 1974).

(EO) Silence among some African Americans may be related to anger, insulted feelings, or acknowledgment of the nurse's lack of sensitivity. Giving the "silent treatment" in some societies communicates rejection and is a hurtful type of communication (Ingram, 1991).

Not Effective

■ *Listening for too short a time, talking about self, and interrupting.* **LOE = VII**

(EO) "If you want to persuade someone to your point of view, make him feel like somebody. Put yourself in his shoes. Don't talk—listen to his problems and concerns. Show that you are genuinely interested. Don't argue—respect the opinions of others. Lavish praise for the merest achievement or improvement" (Carnegie, 1936).

Possibly Harmful

■ *Minimizing feelings, offering easy solutions, interrupting, talking about self, premature closure, and communicating prejudice and bias.* **LOE = I**

(EO) Active listening necessitates avoidance of communication techniques that are commonly perceived as barriers to communication (Giger & Davidhizar, 2004).

■ *Misinterpreting communication techniques.* **LOE = VII**

(EO) Because everyone is unique and has a personal style of communication and perception of interpersonal behavior in light of their cultural orientation, almost any communication technique may be misinterpreted. In communication intended to be positive, verbal and nonverbal techniques useful in one situation may actually be harmful in another. Thus, it is essential that the nurse assess the communication of others in an ongoing manner and monitor personal behavior so that optimal communication can occur (Giger & Davidhizar, 2004).

OUTCOME MEASUREMENT

COMMUNICATION (NOC)

Definition: Reception, interpretation, and expression of spoken, written, and nonverbal messages.

Communication as evidenced by the following selected NOC indicators:
- Acknowledgement of messages received
- Accurate interpretation of messages received
- Exchanges messages accurately with others

(Rate each indicator of **Communication:** 1 = severely compromised, 2 = substantially compromised, 3 = moderately compromised, 4 = mildly compromised, 5 = not compromised) (Moorhead et al., 2004).

REFERENCES

Bonder B, Martin L, Miracle A. (2002). *Culture in clinical care.* St. Louis: Slack.

Carnegie D. (1936). *How to win friends and influence people.* New York: Simon and Schuster.

Cornn K. (2003). Can you hear me now: A nurse's perspective on the importance of listening. *NurseLife*, 1(9):2.

Davidhizar R. (2004). Listening—A nursing strategy to transcend culture. *J Pract Nurs*, 54(2):22-24.

Dochterman JM, Bulechek GM (Eds). (2004). *Nursing Interventions Classification (NIC)*, 4th ed. St. Louis: Mosby.

Egan G. (1994). *The skilled helper.* Pacific Grove, CA: Brooks/Cole.

Giger J, Davidhizar R. (2004). *Transcultural nursing: Assessment and intervention.* St. Louis: Mosby.

Hall ET. (1959). *The silent culture.* Westport, CT: Greenwood Press.

Hall ET. (1976). *Beyond culture.* Garden City, NJ: Anchor Press.

Ingram C. (1991). How can we become more aware of culturally specific body language and use this awareness therapeutically? *J Psychosoc Nurs Ment Health Serv*, 29(11):38-41.

Leininger M. (1995). *Transcultural nursing: Concepts, theories, research and practices.* New York: McGraw-Hill.

Moorhead M, Johnson M, Maas M (Eds). (2004). *Nursing Outcomes Classification (NOC)*, 3rd ed. St. Louis: Mosby.

Reimer J, Redskye C. (1998). The Canadian Ojibwa. In Davidhizar R, Giger J (Eds). *Canadian transcultural nursing: Assessment and intervention.* St. Louis: Mosby.

Schulman ED. (1974). *Intervention in human services.* St. Louis: Mosby.

Wehlage D. (2000). Personal conversation.

 ## ANGER CONTROL ASSISTANCE   NIC

Marilyn L. Lanza, DNSc, ARNP, CS, FAAN; Sally D. Stabb, PhD; Deborah L. Cox, PhD; Mary Fardy, MLS, MSW, LICSW, LADC

NIC   **Definition:** Facilitation of the expression of anger in an adaptive, nonviolent manner (Dochterman & Bulechek, 2004).

NURSING ACTIVITIES

Effective

■ *Use multimodal/combined interventions for short-term and long-term regulation of anger expression and control.* **LOE = I**

(MR) A meta-analytic review of 23 studies indicated that combinations of cognitive, behavioral, social skills, and relaxation interventions effected both anger expression and control in positive directions (Del Vecchio & O'Leary, 2004).

(MR) A meta-analytic review of 50 studies indicated that treatments produced both a decrease in negative affect and an increase in positive behaviors (DiGiuseppe & Tafrate, 2003).

(MR) A systematic review of the literature indicated that multitheoretical approaches to treating anger were effective, especially those that build in new alternative behaviors (DiGiuseppe, 1999).

RCT = Randomized Controlled (Clinical) Trial, **NIC** = Nursing Interventions Classification, **NOC** = Nursing Outcomes Classification

■ *Use cognitive-behavioral therapy for short-term and long-term regulation of anger expression and control.* **LOE = I**

(MR) A systematic review of treatment literature from 1995 to 2001 indicated that cognitive, behavioral, or combination treatments yielded the greatest success (DiGiuseppe & Tafrate, 2001).

(MR) A meta-analytic review of 50 studies found that cognitive-behavioral treatment for the management of anger resulted in grand mean weighted effect sizes of 0.70, indicating that a treated individual was better off than 76% of those who did not receive treatment, and that effects were consistent across studies (Beck & Fernandez, 1998).

(MR) A review of systematic desensitization, cognitive-behavioral techniques, social skills training, and problem-solving skills found that they resulted in positive gains for anger expression and control (Sharkin, 1988).

(MR) A single RCT evaluating cognitive-behavioral anger management for intellectually disabled clients ($N = 14$) indicated effectiveness of cognitive-behavioral assertiveness and coping skills (Willner et al., 2002). **LOE = II**

■ (NIC) *Instruct on the use of calming measures (e.g., time outs and deep breaths).* **LOE = I**

(MR) A meta-analytic review of 23 studies found that relaxation treatments were the most effective intervention for those in a current state of anger as evidenced by a large effect size of 1.20 (Del Vecchio & O'Leary, 2004).

(MR) A meta-analytic review of 50 studies found medium to large effect sizes for relaxation and systemic desensitization, showing that those who received this treatment had moderate or significant improvement compared with the untreated participants (DiGiuseppe & Tafrate, 2003).

(MR) A meta-analysis of 18 studies found that relaxation treatments produced a large effect size and seemed to effect the most change in the anger experience (Edmondson & Conger, 1996).

(MR) A systematic review of nine studies found that these treatments yielded a large overall effect size (1.16), with systemic desensitization producing the highest rating of 1.63 (Tafrate, 1995).

■ (NIC) *Assist in developing appropriate methods of expressing anger to others (e.g., assertiveness and use of feeling statements).* **LOE = I**

(MR) A meta-analytic review of 23 studies found that approaches in the category deemed "other" treatments, which included social skills training and process group counseling, were most effective in treating those with difficulties in controlling their anger (Del Vecchio & O'Leary, 2004).

(MR) A meta-analytic review of 50 studies found large effect sizes for anger management training and problem solving (DiGiuseppe & Tafrate, 2003).

(MR) A meta-analysis of 18 studies found that social skills treatments, teaching individuals appropriate skills for handling anger in social situations, produced a large effect size (Edmondson & Conger, 1996).

(MR) A systematic review of nine studies found that these treatments yielded a large overall effect size (1.16), with systemic desensitization producing the highest rating of 1.63 (Tafrate, 1995).

NR = Nursing Research, **MR** = Multidisciplinary Research, **SP** = Standard of Practice, **EO** = Expert Opinion, **LOE** = Level of Evidence

■ **NIC** *Use external controls (e.g., physical or manual restraint, time outs, and seclusion) as needed to calm a patient who is expressing anger in a maladaptive manner.* **LOE = V**

MR A descriptive study reported on a program to reduce the use of physical restraint on three psychiatric units of a university hospital. During the first two quarters after implementation of the program, physical restraint rates declined significantly, and they continued to be low on all three units for the remainder of the year after implementation (Jonikas et al., 2004).

MR A quantitative study was conducted to reduce the use of restraint in a public psychiatric inpatient service that served an economically disadvantaged urban population. There was a significant decrease in the rate of restraint use after the restraint reduction initiatives were implemented (McCue et al., 2004).

MR A systematic review examined the use of seclusion and mechanical restraint from 1990 to 2000 and the rate of staff injuries from patient assaults from 1998 to 2000 in the Pennsylvania State Hospital system. The rate and duration of seclusion and mechanical restraint decreased dramatically from 1990 to 2000. No significant changes were seen in rates of staff injuries (Smith et al., 2005).

MR A systematic review summarized recent research on the use of seclusion and restraint and measures taken to reduce their use. Several innovative programs succeeded in controlling and reducing their use (Sailas & Wahlbeck, 2005).

Possibly Effective

■ **NIC** *Monitor the potential for inappropriate aggression and intervene before its expression.* **LOE = III**

MR A quasi-experimental study using an interrupted time series design (N = 30) found that community meetings held twice a week on the ward reduced assaults about 30% from pretest to treatment weeks and almost 50% from pretest to post-test (Lanza, 2005).

■ *Use cognitive-behavioral anger management treatment for forensic/court/ inmate/prison populations.* **LOE = III**

MR A pretest/post-test comparison group treatment study (N = 180) of anger management treatment for clients in court-mandated programs compared with undergraduates led to short-term gains in anger control and expression (Lench, 2004).

MR A pretest/post-test comparison group study of women inmates (N = 33) found that anger management treatment that included relaxation techniques resulted in decreases in anger, hostility, aggression, and rumination (Eamon et al., 2001).

■ *Use cognitive-behavioral anger management treatment for other specific populations.* **LOE = III**

MR A pretest/post-test study with a control group (N = 27) of substance-abusing women in a residential setting found anger management effective in helping women to gain better control over their actions, to comply with treatment, and to reduce the tendency to suppress angry feelings (Briscoe, 2001).

MR A one-group pretest/post-test investigation of patients with acquired brain injury (N = 16) given anger management therapy after experiencing post-traumatic onset of anger problems showed significant decreases in externalized anger maintained at 2-month follow-up, although actual anger scores remained somewhat high (Medd & Tate, 2000).

RCT = Randomized Controlled (Clinical) Trial, **NIC** = Nursing Interventions Classification, **NOC** = Nursing Outcomes Classification

(MR) A pretest/post-test study with a control group ($N = 15$) of Vietnam War veterans suffering from combat-related post-traumatic stress disorder treated with cognitive-behavioral techniques showed reduction in symptoms and better cognitive anger regulation (Chemtob et al., 1997).

Not Effective

▨ *Use of debrief counseling.* **LOE = III**

(MR) A quasi-experimental control study found that unavailability of debriefing counseling was associated with increased reports of post-traumatic stress among employees, yet found no difference between those who had received counseling and those who had access to counseling but chose not to enroll (Mathews, 1998).

Possibly Harmful

▨ *No intervention.* **LOE = V**

(MR) A descriptive national study showed that when verbal aggression was left untreated, physical aggression could increase (Gerberich et al., 2004; Lanza et al., 2006; Nachreiner et al., 2005).

▨ *Use of debrief counseling.* **LOE = III**

(MR) A quasi-experimental study specifically tested debriefing of assault victims using one or two sessions. The results were that psychological stress was not reduced and that the counseling did not prevent the onset of post-traumatic stress disorder. Assault victims were generally no better with than without debriefing, and if there was a change, the assault victims were worse off than when they started (Wessely et al., 2000).

▨ *Use of restraints.* **LOE = IV**

(NR) A quasi-experimental study assessed the effect of an intervention designed to reduce the use of seclusion and restraint on reported episodes of patient-related violence on an acute inpatient psychiatric service. Results showed a significant decrease in the total number of episodes of seclusion and restraint in the 12 months before and after the intervention. However, the number of episodes of assault on patients and staff increased significantly. Efforts to decrease seclusion and restraint may be accompanied by an increased risk of harm to psychiatric patients and staff (Khadivi et al., 2004).

▨ *Use of cathartic treatments in which the expression of anger is encouraged through means of aggressive verbal and/or physical activity such as screaming, hitting, and venting.* **LOE = V**

(MR) A systematic review noted that although no controlled outcome studies of the effectiveness of cathartic activities have been conducted, the experimental studies that have been done found that using these interventions led to more, not less, anger, aggression, hostile attitudes, and behavior (Tafrate, 1995).

(MR) A single RCT ($N = 600$) demonstrated with small to moderate effects that venting (fueling aggressive thoughts and feelings) increased aggressive responding (Bushman, 2002).

(MR) A meta-analysis of 23 studies confirmed Tafrate's 1995 findings and called for further study of the potential harm of cathartic treatments (Del Vecchio & O'Leary, 2004).

NR = Nursing Research, **MR** = Multidisciplinary Research, **SP** = Standard of Practice, **EO** = Expert Opinion, **LOE** = Level of Evidence

OUTCOME MEASUREMENT

AGGRESSION SELF-CONTROL NOC

Definition: Self-restraint of assaultive, combative, or destructive behaviors toward others.

Aggression Self-Control as evidenced by the following selected NOC indicators:

- Identifies when angry
- Identifies when frustrated
- Identifies when feeling aggressive
- Identifies alternatives to aggression
- Identifies alternatives to verbal outbursts
- Communicates needs appropriately
- Communicates feelings appropriately
- Refrains from verbal outbursts
- Uses specific techniques to control anger
- Uses specific techniques to control frustration

(Rate each indicator of **Aggression Self-Control:** 1 = never demonstrated, 2 = rarely demonstrated, 3 = sometimes demonstrated, 4 = often demonstrated, 5 = consistently demonstrated) (Moorhead et al., 2004).

REFERENCES

Beck R, Fernandez E. (1998). Cognitive-behavioral therapy in the treatment of anger: A meta-analysis. *Cognit Ther Res,* 22(1):63-74.

Briscoe YB. (2001). *A cognitive behavioral anger management intervention for women with histories of substance abuse.* San Francisco: University of San Francisco.

Bushman BJ. (2002). Does venting anger feed or extinguish the flame? Catharsis, rumination, distraction, anger, and aggressive responding. *Pers Soc Psychol Bull,* 28(6):724-731.

Chemtob CM, Novaco RW, Hamada RS, Gross DM. (1997). Cognitive-behavioral treatment for severe anger in posttraumatic stress disorder. *J Consult Clin Psychol,* 65(1):184-189.

Del Vecchio T, O'Leary KD. (2004). Effectiveness of anger treatments for specific anger problems: A meta-analytic review. *Clin Psychol Rev,* 24(1):15-34.

DiGiuseppe R. (1999). End piece: Reflections on the treatment of anger. *J Clin Psychol,* 55(3):365-379.

DiGiuseppe R, Tafrate RC. (2001). A comprehensive treatment model for anger disorders. *Psychotherapy,* 38(3):262-271.

DiGiuseppe R, Tafrate RC. (2003). Anger treatment for adults: A meta-analytic review. *Clin Psychol,* 10(1):70-84.

Dochterman JM, Bulechek GM (Eds). (2004). *Nursing Interventions Classification (NIC),* 4th ed. St. Louis: Mosby.

Eamon KC, Munchua MM, Reddon JR. (2001). Effectiveness of an anger management program for women inmates. *J Offender Rehabil,* 34(1):45-60.

Edmondson CB, Conger JC. (1996). A review of treatment efficacy for individuals with anger problems: Conceptual, assessment, and methodological issues. Clin Psychol Rev, *16(3):*251-275.

Gerberich SG, Church TR, McGovern PM, Hansen HE, Nachreiner NM, Geisser MS, et al. (2004). An epidemiological study of the magnitude and consequences of work related violence: The Minnesota Nurses' Study. *Occup Environ Med,* 61(6):495-503.

Jonikas JA, Cook JA, Rosen C, Laris A, Kim JB. (2004). A program to reduce use of physical restraint in psychiatric inpatient facilities. *Psychiatr Serv,* 55(7):818-820.

Khadivi AN, Patel RC, Atkinson AR, Levine JM. (2004). Association between seclusion and restraint and patient-related violence. *Psychiatr Serv,* 55(11):1311-1312.

Lanza M. (2005). *Community meeting protocol for assault prevention.* Paper presented at the 2005 Annual Meeting of the American Group Psychotherapy Association, New York.

Lanza ML, Zeiss RA, Rierdan J. (2006). Non-physical violence: A risk factor for physical violence in health care settings. American Association of Occupational Health Nurses Journal, 54(9):397-402.

Lench HC. (2004). Anger management: Diagnostic differences and treatment implications. *J Soc Clin Psychol,* 23(4):512-531.

Mathews LR. (1998). Effect of staff debriefing on posttraumatic stress symptoms after assaults by community housing residents. *Psychiatr Serv,* 49(2):207-212.

McCue RE, Urcuyo L, Lilu Y, Tobias T, Chambers MJ. (2004). Reducing restraint use in a public psychiatric inpatient service. *J Behav Health Serv Res,* 31(2):217-224.

Medd J, Tate RL. (2000). Evaluation of an anger management therapy programme following acquired brain injury: A preliminary study. *Neuropsychol Rehabil,* 10(2):185-201.

Moorhead M, Johnson M, Maas M (Eds). (2004). *Nursing Outcomes Classification (NOC),* 3rd ed. St. Louis: Mosby.

Nachreiner NM, Gerberich SG, McGovern PM, Church TR, Hansen HE, Geisser MS, et al. (2005). Relation between policies and work related assault: Minnesota Nurses' Study. *Occup Environ Med,* 62(10):675-681.

Sailas E, Wahlbeck K. (2005). Restraint and seclusion in psychiatric inpatient wards. *Curr Opin Psychiatry,* 18(5):555-559.

Sharkin BS. (1988). The measurement and treatment of client anger in counseling. *J Couns Dev,* 66:361-365.

Smith GM, Davis RH, Bixler EO, Lin HM, Altenor A, Altenor RJ, et al. (2005). Pennsylvania State Hospital system's seclusion and restraint reduction program. *Psychiatr Serv,* 56(9):1115-1122.

Tafrate RC. (1995). Evaluation of treatment strategies for adult anger disorders. In Kassinove H (Ed): Anger disorders: Definition, diagnosis, and treatment. Washington, DC: Taylor & Francis, pp 109-130.

Wessely S, Rose S, Bisson J. (2000). Brief psychological interventions ("debriefing") for trauma-related symptoms and the prevention of post traumatic stress disorder. *Cochrane Database Syst Rev,* (2): CD000560.

Willner P, Jones J, Tams R, Green G. (2002). A randomized controlled trial of the efficacy of a cognitive behavioural anger management group for clients with learning disabilities. *J Appl Res Intellect Disabil,* 15(3):224-235.

ANIMAL-ASSISTED THERAPY   NIC

Florence B. Roberts, PhD, APRN-BC; Judy Bradberry, PhD, RN

NIC   Definition: Purposeful use of animals to provide affection, attention, diversion, and relaxation (Dochterman & Bulechek, 2004).

NURSING ACTIVITIES

Effective

■ **NIC** *Provide therapy animals for the patient, such as dogs, cats, horses, snakes, turtles, gerbils, guinea pigs, and birds.* **LOE = II**

 Cognitively intact elderly residents of a nursing home ($N = 144$) were randomly divided into three groups. One group received a canary, one a plant, and one nothing. The intervention lasted 3 months with before-and-after testing. The canary group had fewer depressed symptoms and an increased perception of quality of life (Colombo et al., 2006).

NR = Nursing Research, **MR** = Multidisciplinary Research, **SP** = Standard of Practice, **EO** = Expert Opinion, **LOE** = Level of Evidence

Possibly Effective

- **NIC** *Determine the patient's acceptance of animals as therapeutic agents.*
  LOE = II

MR Patients of long-term care facilities ($N = 3$ facilities; $N = 45$ subjects) were randomly vassigned to three groups: one with a 30-minute session of animal-assisted therapy (AAT) per week, one with three 30-minute sessions of AAT per week, and a control group with no AAT. The results showed that the best predictor of desire for pet therapy was experience of having pets prior to entering the facilities (Banks & Banks, 2002).

EO An activity coordinator reported that only 6 of 125 residents of a mental health facility showed disinterest in a resident dog. Those who were not interested did not have previous positive interactions with pets (Parshall, 2003).

- *Determine staff acceptance of animals as therapeutic agents.* **LOE = IV**

MR Two cross-sectional surveys of administrators, doctors, nurses, and therapists at a children's hospital ($N = 224$) indicated that the staff thought a dog visitation program was worthwhile and that the ward was a happier place after the dog visits. There was less concern about negative aspects (e.g., bites, damage to equipment) after the intervention. Acceptance was higher among administrative and nonclinical staff and lower for doctors and nurses (Moody et al., 2002).

- *Determine potential risks to the patient of the use of animals (allergies, zoonoses, accidents, dog bites).* **LOE = VII**

MR A literature review determined that risks in well-controlled health care environments were minimal compared with benefits (Brodie et al., 2002).

EO An expert citing a 1997 study that determined no known cases of transmission of diseases from animals to humans also stated that none were found in 2002 (Stanley-Hermanns & Miller, 2002).

- **NIC** *Enforce standards for screening, training, and grooming of animals in a therapy program.* **LOE = VII**

EO "Handlers must wash their hands with soap and water between patients. Animals must be clean (bathed within 24 hours), currently vaccinated, [sic] and free of disease and parasites. Animals must always be kept on a leash or in a basket and under handler's complete control" (Stanley-Hermanns & Miller, 2002, p. 7).

- **NIC** *Encourage the patient to feed/groom animals.* **LOE = III**

MR A quasi-experimental study with a time series design (N = 15, mean age of 86 years) introduced a dog for therapeutic recreation (e.g., subjects could talk to, touch, play with the dog) for 1 hour a day 5 days per week for 3 weeks for elderly patients with dementia. Social interactions among the patients increased (Richeson, 2003).

MR Weekly 50-minute group sessions for 9 months in a before-and-after quasi-experimental design ($N = 7$) with chronically ill schizophrenic patients found that there was improvement in domestic and health-related activities following the AAT (Kovacs et al., 2004).

RCT = Randomized Controlled (Clinical) Trial, **NIC** = Nursing Interventions Classification, **NOC** = Nursing Outcomes Classification

■ **NIC** *Provide therapy animals for the patient such as dogs, cats, horses, snakes, turtles, gerbils, guinea pigs, and birds.* **LOE = II**

MR Chronic schizophrenic individuals ($N = 20$) were randomly assigned to experimental and control groups for weekly 3-hour sessions for 12 months, focused on "ADL modeling activities" (e.g., petting, feeding, grooming) with a provided dog or cat according to the patient's choice. Control-group patients participated in reading and discussion of current events during the experimental group meetings. The AAT group had significantly increased social functioning (Barak et al., 2001).

NR A qualitative study ($N = 6$) involved abused women in therapeutic interaction with horses. Participants reported increased self-esteem, increased empowerment, decreased depression, a new ability to do things that they had previously been unable to do (e.g., work, move to new places), and an increased ability to cope with anxiety (Meinersmann et al., 2006). **LOE = VI**

Not Effective

■ *Providing therapy animals for some patients.* **LOE = III**

NR A quasi-experimental study ($N = 30$) of the presence of a dog during discharge teaching following open heart surgery to determine the effect on teaching illustrated that the presence of the dog had a negative effect on patients' learning (Miller et al., 2003).

Possibly Harmful

■ *Potential risks to the patient of the use of animals (allergies, zoonoses, accidents, dog bites).* **LOE = VII**

EO Contraindications to the use of animals were "allergy to animal, open wounds or burns, open tracheostomy, immunosuppression, agitation or aggression, isolation of any kind, fear of animals" (Stanley-Hermanns & Miller, 2002, p. 7).

EO Consideration must be given to psychological damage caused by removal of pet therapy animals from people who have become attached to them (Parshall, 2003).

■ **NIC** *Avoid animal visits with unpredictable or violent patients.* **LOE = VI**

MR An observational study ($N = 14$) indicated that horses exhibited a greater mean number of stress-related behaviors when ridden by at-risk children compared with physically or psychologically handicapped riders, special education children, or recreational riders (Kaiser et al., 2006).

■ *Poor health maintenance of animals.* **LOE = VI**

MR A multiple baseline study of children with multiple disabilities ($N = 14$) for two 30-minute sessions weekly for 8 weeks with a dog found that the dog was suffering from Cushing's syndrome, often seen in chronic stress. The research was stopped after two

NR = Nursing Research, **MR** = Multidisciplinary Research, **SP** = Standard of Practice, **EO** = Expert Opinion, **LOE** = Level of Evidence

groups of seven students participated, although three groups had been planned (Heimlich, 2001).

EO An expert described two dogs that were significantly overfed by residents at a mental health facility. One dog died of congestive heart failure secondary to obesity (Parshall, 2003).

OUTCOME MEASUREMENT

COPING   **NOC**

Definition: Personal actions to manage stressors that tax an individual's resources.

Coping as evidenced by the following selected NOC indicators:
- Reports decrease in stress
- Identifies multiple coping strategies
- Uses effective coping strategies

(Rate each indicator of **Coping:** 1 = never demonstrated, 2 = rarely demonstrated, 3 = sometimes demonstrated, 4 = often demonstrated, 5 = consistently demonstrated) (Moorhead et al., 2004).

REFERENCES

Banks MR, Banks WA. (2002). The effects of animal-assisted therapy on loneliness in an elderly population in long-term care facilities. *J Gerontol A Biol Sci Med Sci*, 57(7):M428-M432.

Barak Y, Savorai O, Mavashev S, Beni A. (2001). Animal-assisted therapy for elderly schizophrenic patients. *Am J Geriatr Psychiatry*, 9(4):439-442.

Brodie SJ, Biley FC, Shewring M. (2002). An exploration of the potential risks associated with using pet therapy in healthcare settings. *J Clin Nurs*, 11(4):444-456.

Colombo G, Buono MD, Smania K, Raviola R, De Leo D. (2006). Pet therapy and institutionalized elderly: A study on 144 cognitively unimpaired subjects. *Arch Gerontol Geriat*, 42(2):207-216.

Dochterman JM, Bulechek GM (Eds). (2004). *Nursing Interventions Classification (NIC)*, 4th ed. St. Louis: Mosby.

Heimlich K. (2001). Animal-assisted therapy and the severely disabled child: A quantitative study. *J Rehabil*, 67(4):48-54.

Kaiser L, Heleski CR, Siegford J, Smith KA. (2006). Stress-related behaviors among horses used in a therapeutic riding program. *J Am Vet Med Assoc*, 228(1):39-45.

Kovacs Z, Kis R, Rozsa S, Rozsa L. (2004). Animal-assisted therapy for middle-aged schizophrenic patients living in a social institution: A pilot study. *Clin Rehabil*, 18(5):483-486.

Meinersmann K, Bradberry J, Roberts F. (2006). *Lived experience of equine facilitated psychotherapy among adult women survivors of abuse.* Lecture presented at the Nursing Network on Violence Against Women, International (meeting), Portland, Oregon, April 8, 2006.

Miller J, Connor K, Deal B, Duke GW, Stanley-Hermanns M, Varnell G, et al. (2003). How animal-assisted therapy affects discharge teaching: A pilot study. *Nurs Manage*, 34(8 Suppl):36-40.

Moody WJ, King R, O'Rourke S. (2002). Attitudes of paediatric medical ward staff to a dog visitation programme. *J Clin Nurs*, 11(4):537-544.

Moorhead M, Johnson M, Maas M (Eds). (2004). *Nursing Outcomes Classification (NOC)*, 3rd ed. St. Louis: Mosby.

Parshall DP. (2003). Research and reflection: Animal-assisted therapy in mental health settings. *Couns Values*, 48(1):47-56.

Richeson NE. (2003). Effects of animal-assisted therapy on agitated behaviors and social interactions of older adults with dementia. *Am J Alzheimers Dis Other Demen*, 18(6):353-358.

Stanley-Hermanns M, Miller J. (2002). Animal-assisted therapy. *Am J Nurs*, 102(10):69-76.

RCT = Randomized Controlled (Clinical) Trial, **NIC** = Nursing Interventions Classification, **NOC** = Nursing Outcomes Classification

ANXIETY REDUCTION

Ruth G. McCaffrey, DNP, ARNP-BC

NIC **Definition:** Minimizing apprehension, dread, foreboding, or uneasiness related to an unidentified source of anticipated danger (Dochterman & Bulechek, 2004).

NURSING ACTIVITIES

Effective

■ *Administer selective serotonin reuptake inhibitors (SSRIs) that are effective for many types of anxiety.* **LOE = I**

(MR) An RCT placebo study of 128 children 6 to 17 years old with social phobia, separation anxiety disorder, and general anxiety disorder (GAD) was undertaken over a 5-year period in five separate medical facilities. Based on the pediatric anxiety scale 8 weeks after the initiation of either fluvoxamine or placebo, the fluvoxamine group had significantly lower anxiety and social phobia. It was concluded that fluvoxamine is an effective treatment for children and adolescents with social phobia, separation anxiety disorder, or generalized anxiety disorder (Walkup et al., 2001).

(MR) In several large-scale placebo-controlled studies of obsessive-compulsive disorder, SSRI medications have demonstrated efficacy and tolerability in relieving the anxiety associated with obsessive-compulsive disorder (Pigott & Seay, 1999).

(MR) An RCT ($N = 248$) demonstrated the effectiveness of paroxetine, an SSRI for GAD, in reducing the symptoms associated with GAD and improving self-directedness and decreased harm avoidance (Zohar & Westenberg, 2000).

(MR) An RCT ($N = 1266$) studying several types of SSRIs versus placebo demonstrated that SSRIs in general were effective in the treatment of panic disorder. In a meta-analysis, SSRIs were proved to be superior to imipramine and alprazolam for the treatment of panic disorder and were better tolerated with fewer side effects (Figgitt & McClellan, 2000).

■ *Administer buspirone to reduce anxiety in patients with GAD without impeding balance or causing withdrawal symptoms.* **LOE = I**

(MR) In an RCT ($N = 1180$), patients with GAD were given buspirone 15 mg twice daily or placebo. Those in the buspirone group had reduced anxiety as measured by the state anxiety inventory (Sramek et al., 1996).

■ *Use music as an effective intervention for anxiety.* **LOE = I**

(NR) A review of the literature demonstrated that music was effective in reducing anxiety prior to diagnostic cardiac catheterization (McCaffrey & Taylor, 2005).

(NR) In a two-group, pretest/post-test repeated measures RCT ($N = 64$), a single music therapy session was found to be effective for decreasing anxiety and promoting relaxation as indicated by heart rate and respiratory rate in a sample of patients receiving ventilatory assistance (Chlan, 2000).

NR = Nursing Research, **MR** = Multidisciplinary Research, **SP** = Standard of Practice, **EO** = Expert Opinion, **LOE** = Level of Evidence

(MR) In an RCT ($N = 140$), patients undergoing hysterosalpingography who listened to music during the procedure had lower scores on the State Anxiety measure than a control group (Agwu & Okoye, 2007).

(MR) In an RCT ($N = 220$), two groups of women undergoing colposcopy were tested. Those who listened to music during the procedure had less pain and lower anxiety than women in the nonmusic group (Chan et al., 2003).

(MR) In an RCT ($N = 98$), patients who listened to music had decreased mean arterial pressures, improved oxygen saturation, and less anxiety on the State Trait Anxiety measure (Yilmaz et al., 2003).

■ *Use guided imagery as an effective intervention for anxiety.* **LOE = II**

(NR) In an RCT, 30 individuals in rehabilitation for anterior cruciate ligament reconstruction who participated in 10 guided imagery sessions had improved knee strength and less anxiety and pain than those who participated in 10 encouragement and support sessions and those who did not participate in any sessions (Cupal & Brewer, 2001).

(NR) A quasi-experimental design study ($N = 60$) found that men who listened to music while recovering from transurethral resection of the prostate had lower blood pressure levels and better anxiety scores on state anxiety measures than a group who did not listen to music (Yung et al., 2002).

■ *Encourage mindfulness meditation to reduce anxiety.* **LOE = II**

(NR) In an RCT to evaluate the usefulness of mindfulness meditation, 20 women were randomly divided into two groups. All participants had been diagnosed with cardiac diseases including angina, hypertension, and valvular disorders. The experimental group completed a mindfulness meditation course for stress reduction that met for 2 hours weekly over 16 weeks. Findings of the study demonstrated that those who completed the mindfulness meditation course had significantly lower state anxiety scores than the control group 20 weeks after the study began (Tacon et al., 2003).

■ *Use certain types of aromatherapy for anxiety reduction.* **LOE = III**

(MR) In an RCT ($N = 200$), the effects of orange and lavender aroma were tested on participants in the dental office. These two aromatherapies demonstrated the ability to decrease anxiety and improve the mood of people undergoing dental procedures (Lehrner et al., 2005).

■ *Encourage physical exercise to decrease anxiety and reduce sensitivity to stress.* **LOE = I**

(NR) In a qualitative study ($N = 45$), men and women diagnosed with anxiety disorders were provided with an anaerobic exercise regimen for 6 weeks. Qualitative analysis of interview data presented the following themes from participants: locus of control, feeling of achievement, social support, self-esteem, and reflecting on the body image (Morrissey, 1997).

(MR) In an RCT ($N = 428$), regular exercise demonstrated the ability to reduce anxiety in people with mental illness and depression (Tkackuk & Martin, 1999).

(MR) In an RCT ($N = 48$), female individuals who participated in brisk walking and Tai Chi were found to have reduced salivary cortisol levels, heart rate, blood pressure, and urinary catecholamines (Jin, 1992).

RCT = Randomized Controlled (Clinical) Trial, **NIC** = Nursing Interventions Classification, **NOC** = Nursing Outcomes Classification

(MR) RCT participants ($N = 22$) with obsessive-compulsive disorder had either a five-times-a-week yoga intervention or a meditation intervention. The 12 participants in the yoga group had a 20% to 35% lower rating on the Yale-Brown obsessive-compulsive scale (Kirkwood et al., 2005).

■ *Use programmed relaxation including breathing techniques and progressive muscle relaxation training to reduce anxiety.* **LOE = II**

(MR) In an RCT ($N = 110$), anxiety and depression had a prevalence of 30% in pregnant women. In a study of married primigravida pregnant women, applied relaxation training consisting of breathing techniques and muscle relaxation significantly reduced state and trait anxiety scores as well as perceived stress (Bastani et al., 2005).

■ *Use massage and reflexology to reduce anxiety.* **LOE = I**

(NR) In an RCT, reflexology foot massage was shown to reduce anxiety in hospitalized cancer patients ($N = 68$) undergoing chemotherapy treatments. Using the state anxiety measure, there was a significant difference between patients who received reflexology foot massage and a control group who did not receive the massage (Quattrin et al., 2006).

(NR) In a quasi-experimental study, 102 elderly participants were randomly allocated to a control group or a group who received slow stroke back massage for seven consecutive evenings. The back massage group had reduced levels of pain and anxiety, improved systolic and diastolic blood pressures, and improved heart rates compared with the control group (Mok & Woo, 2004).

(NR) A one-group pretest/post-test quasi-experimental study with random assignment ($N = 14$) measured the effects of aromatherapy massage with music on anxiety in emergency room nurses. Those who received the massage intervention had reduced anxiety levels (Davis et al., 2005).

(NR) In an RCT ($N = 60$), primiparous women were randomly assigned to a control group or an experimental group who received massage. Based on the visual analogue scale for anxiety, the experimental group had significantly lower pain reactions in the latent, active, and transitional phases of labor. Anxiety levels were lower in the experimental group during the latent phase of labor (Chang et al., 2002).

Possibly Effective

■ *Use kava kava for the treatment of anxiety. (Note: Kava kava has been shown to cause liver problems, and a patient's liver enzymes should be monitored while administering this product.)* **LOE = I**

(MR) A double-blind placebo-controlled RCT ($N = 141$) observed the effect of 150 mg of kava kava WS 1490 on adult male and female patients with anxiety. Findings of this study demonstrated that kava kava WS 1490 was well tolerated with no influence on liver function tests and only one adverse event (tiredness) attributable to the study drug (Gastpar & Klimm, 2003).

(MR) A Cochrane systematic review of 12 double-blind RCTs on the use of kava kava for anxiety found that, compared with placebo, kava kava extract was an effective treatment for anxiety. However, the effect lacked robustness and was based on relatively small sample sizes. Adverse effects as reported in the reviewed trials were mild, transient, and infrequent (Pittler & Ernst, 2000).

NR = Nursing Research, **MR** = Multidisciplinary Research, **SP** = Standard of Practice, **EO** = Expert Opinion, **LOE** = Level of Evidence

■ *Use passion flower to relieve GAD.* **LOE = II**

MR A double-blind placebo-controlled trial involving outpatients with GAD ($N = 36$) was conducted. Over a 4-week course, passion flower 45 drops daily was prescribed for 18 patients, and oxazepam 30 mg was prescribed for the other 18 participants. Results demonstrated that although oxazepam had a more rapid onset of relief from GAD, it also produced greater side effects such as fatigue, loss of concentration, and impaired job performance. At the end of 4 weeks, both groups had the same levels of improvement in GAD measures (Akhondzadeh et al., 2001).

■ *Use gotu kola to reduce anxiety.* **LOE = II**

MR In an RCT ($N = 1200$), the startle responses in healthy (nonanxious) individuals were studied and gotu kola reduced the startle response in those who took 60 mg twice daily for 3 weeks. However, more research is needed before evidence-based therapeutic recommendations can be made (Bradwejn et al., 2000).

■ *Use lavender as aromatherapy for the treatment of anxiety.* **LOE = II**

NR A descriptive study showed that cancer hospice patients ($N = 17$) using humidified essential lavender oil aromatherapy expressed a slight transient improvement of anxiety levels and an increased sense of well-being (Louis & Kowalski, 2002).

NR In a quasi-experimental study ($N = 25$), the effects of passively diffused lavender aromatherapy on anxiety and sleep quality in coronary care were studied. The study used a repeated measures design with the State Trait Anxiety Inventory immediately before treatment and then 30 to 60 minutes after treatment. Passively diffused aromatherapy using lavender on a cotton ball did not significantly affect anxiety levels (Borromeo, 1998).

Not Effective

No applicable published research was found in this category.

Possibly Harmful

No applicable published research was found in this category.

OUTCOME MEASUREMENT

ANXIETY SELF-CONTROL NOC

Definition: Personal actions to eliminate or reduce feelings of apprehension, tension, or uneasiness from an unidentifiable source.

Anxiety Self-Control as evidenced by the following selected NOC indicators:

• Controls anxiety response
• Plans coping strategies for stressful situations
• Uses effective coping strategies

(Rate each indicator of **Anxiety Self-Control:** 1 = never demonstrated, 2 = rarely demonstrated, 3 = sometimes demonstrated, 4 = often demonstrated, 5 = consistently demonstrated) (Moorhead et al., 2004).

RCT = Randomized Controlled (Clinical) Trial, **NIC** = Nursing Interventions Classification, **NOC** = Nursing Outcomes Classification

REFERENCES

Agwu KK, Okoye IJ. (2007). The effect of music on the anxiety levels of patients undergoing hysterosalpin-gography. *Radiography,* 12(2):38-43.

Akhondzadeh S, Naghavi HR, Vazirian M, Shayeganpour A, Rashidi H, Khani M. (2001). Passionflower in the treatment of generalized anxiety: A pilot double-blind randomized controlled trial with oxazepam. *J Clin Pharm Ther,* 26(5):363-369.

Bastani F, Hidarnia A, Kazemnejad, Vafaei M, Kashanian M. (2005). A randomized controlled trial of the effects of applied relaxation training on reducing anxiety and perceived stress in pregnant women. *J Midwifery Womens Health,* 50(4):e36-e40.

Borromeo A. (1998). *The effects of aromatherapy on the patient outcomes of anxiety and sleep quality in coronary care unit patients.* Unpublished doctoral dissertation. Texas Woman's University.

Bradwejn J, Zhou Y, Koszycki D, Shlik J. (2000). A double-blind, placebo-controlled study on the effects of Gotu Kola (*Centella asiatica*) on acoustic startle response in healthy subjects. *J Clin Psychopharmacol,* 20(6):680-684.

Chan YM, Lee PW, Ng TY, Ngan HY, Wong LC. (2003). The use of music to reduce anxiety for patients undergoing colposcopy: A randomized trial. *Gynecol Oncol,* 91(1):213-217.

Chang MY, Wang SY, Chen CH. (2002). Effects of massage on pain and anxiety during labor: A randomized controlled trial in Taiwan. *J Adv Nurs,* 38(1):68-73.

Chlan LL. (2000). Music therapy as a nursing intervention for patients supported by mechanical ventilation. *AACN Clin Issues,* 11(1):128-138.

Cupal DD, Brewer BW. (2001). Effects of relaxation and guided imagery on knee strength, re-injury anxiety, and pain following anterior cruciate ligament reconstruction. *Rehabil Psychol,* 46(1):28-43.

Davis C, Cooke M, Holzhauser K, Jones M, Finucane J. (2005). The effect of aromatherapy massage with music on the stress and anxiety levels of emergency nurses. *Aust Emerg Nurs J,* 8(1-2):43-50.

Dochterman JM, Bulechek GM (Eds). (2004). *Nursing Interventions Classification (NIC),* 4th ed. St. Louis: Mosby.

Figgitt DP, McClellan KJ. (2000). Fluvoxamine: An updated review of its use in the management of adults with anxiety disorders. *Drugs,* 60(4):925-954.

Gastpar M, Klimm HD. (2003). Treatment of anxiety, tension and restlessness states with Kava special extract WS 1490 in general practice: A randomized placebo-controlled double-blind multicenter trial. *Phytomedicine,* 10(8):631-639.

Jin P. (1992). Efficacy of Tai Chi, brisk walking, meditation, and reading in reducing mental and emotional stress. *J Psychosom Res,* 36(4):361-370.

Kirkwood G, Rampes H, Tuffrey V, Richardson J, Pilkington K. (2005). Yoga for anxiety: A systematic review of the research evidence. *Br J Sports Med,* 39(12):884-891.

Lehrner J, Marwinski G, Lehr S, Johren P, Deecke L. (2005). Ambient odors of orange and lavender reduce anxiety and improve mood in a dental office. *Physiol Behav,* 86(1-2):92-95.

Louis M, Kowalski SD. (2002). Use of aromatherapy with hospice patients to decrease pain, anxiety, and depression and to promote an increased sense of well-being. *Am J Hosp Palliat Care,* 19(6): 381-386.

McCaffrey R, Taylor N. (2005). Effective anxiety treatment prior to diagnostic cardiac catheterization. *Holist Nurs Pract,* 19(2):70-73.

Mok E, Woo CP. (2004). The effects of slow-stroke back massage on anxiety and shoulder pain in elderly stroke patients. *Complement Ther Nurs Midwifery,* 10(4):209-216.

Moorhead M, Johnson M, Maas M (Eds). (2004). *Nursing Outcomes Classification (NOC),* 3rd ed. St. Louis: Mosby.

Morrissey M. (1997). Mood enhancement and anxiety reduction using physical exercise in a clinical sample. *Int J Psychiatr Nurs,* 3(2):336-344.

Pigott TA, Seay SM. (1999). A review of the efficacy of selective serotonin reuptake inhibitors in obsessive-compulsive disorder. *J Clin Psychiatr,* 60(2):101-106.

Pittler MH, Ernst E. (2000). Efficacy of kava extract for treating anxiety: Systematic review and meta-analysis. *J Clin Psychopharmacol,* 20(1):84-89.

Quattrin R, Zanini A, Buchini S, Turello D, Annunziata MA, Vidotti C, et al. (2006). Use of reflexology foot massage to reduce anxiety in hospitalized cancer patients in chemotherapy treatment: Methodology and outcomes. *J Nurs Manag,* 14(2):96-105.

Sramek J, Tansman M, Suri A, Hornig-Rohan M, Amsterdam JD, Stahl SM, et al. (1996). Efficacy of bus-pirone in generalized anxiety disorder with coexisting mild depressive symptoms. *J Clin Psychiatry*, 57(7):287-291.

Tacon AM, McComb J, Caldera Y, Randolph P. (2003). Mindfulness meditation, anxiety reduction, and heart disease: A pilot study. *Fam Community Health*, 26(1):25-33.

Tkackuk GA, Martin GL. (1999). Exercise therapy for patients with psychiatric disorders: Research and clinical implications. *Prof Psychol Res Pr*, 30(3):275-282.

Walkup J, Labellarte M, Riddle M, Pine D, Greenhill L, Klein R, et al. (2001). Fluvoxamine for the treatment of anxiety disorders in children and adolescents. The Research Unit on Pediatric Psychopharmacology Anxiety Study Group. *N Engl J Med*, 344(17):1279-1285.

Yilmaz E, Ozcan S, Basar M, Basar H, Batislam E, Ferhat M. (2003). Music decreases anxiety and provides sedation in extracorporeal shock wave lithotripsy. *Urology*, 61(2):282-286.

Yung PM, Chui-Kam S, French P, Chan TM. (2002). A controlled trial of music and pre-operative anxiety in Chinese men undergoing transurethral resection of the prostate. *J Adv Nurs*, 39(4):352-359.

Zohar J, Westenberg HG. (2000). Anxiety disorders: A review of tricyclic antidepressants and selective serotonin reuptake inhibitors. *Acta Psychiatr Scand Suppl*, 403:39-49.

AUTOGENIC TRAINING

Carolyn B. Yucha, PhD, RN, FAAN, CNE, BCIA

NIC **Definition:** Assisting with self-suggestions about feelings of heaviness and warmth for the purpose of inducing relaxation (Dochterman & Bulechek, 2004).

NURSING ACTIVITIES

Effective

■ *Use autogenic training (AT) to improve clinical outcomes.* **LOE = I**

MR A meta-analysis of 60 studies (35 RCTs) showed AT to be better than nothing for tension headache/migraine, hypertension, coronary heart disease, asthma, Raynaud's disease, pain, anxiety, depression, and sleep disorders (Stetter & Kupper, 2002).

■ *Use AT to reduce anxiety.* **LOE = I**

NR An RCT involving women with breast cancer (*N* = 31) showed that those receiving AT during a home visit had statistically significant improvements in anxiety and depression in comparison with those who received only a home visit (Hidderley & Holt, 2004).

NR A controlled study of patients with cancer (*N* = 18) showed that a 10-week course of AT reduced anxiety and increased "fighting spirit" with an improved sense of coping and sleep (Wright et al., 2002).

MR An RCT comparing AT with standard care in patients undergoing coronary angioplasty (*N* = 59) showed a significant reduction in anxiety 2 months after the procedure (Kanji et al., 2004).

MR A controlled study of high school students (*N* = 139) in postwar Kosovo showed that a 6-week program of mind-body skills that included AT significantly reduced post-traumatic stress scores. The effect of AT could not be distinguished from that of other program components (Gordon et al., 2004).

RCT = Randomized Controlled (Clinical) Trial, **NIC** = Nursing Interventions Classification, **NOC** = Nursing Outcomes Classification

(MR) An RCT involving adult cancer patients comparing progressive muscle relaxation ($N = 80$) with AT ($N = 71$) and a control group ($N = 78$) showed that both treatment groups had moderate to large-scale improvements in sleep latency, duration, efficiency, and quality (Simeit et al., 2004).

(MR) A systematic review of the literature showed that evidence to support the use of AT for generalized anxiety was limited (Jorm et al., 2004).

■ *Use AT to reduce chronic pain.* **LOE = II**

(MR) A controlled study of women ($N = 12$) with pure migraine or a combination of migraine and tension-type headache showed that thermal biofeedback with AT reduced headache activity and medication taken for headaches (Blanchard & Kim, 2005).

(MR) An RCT comparing Internet-delivered combination therapy (progressive muscle relaxation, biofeedback, AT, and stress management) with waitlist control in those with chronic headache ($N = 86$) showed a significant reduction in headache symptoms and associated medication usage (Devineni & Blanchard, 2005).

(MR) A controlled study examining the drug consumption of patients with migraine, tension, or mixed headaches ($N = 25$) showed that AT practiced daily for 4 months led to a reduction in headache frequency and consumption of anxiolytic and analgesic drugs (Zsombok et al., 2003).

(MR) A controlled study in patients with phantom limb pain ($N = 9$) showed that thermal biofeedback coupled with AT over 4 to 6 weeks led to a 20% to 30% reduction in pain in the phantom limb (Harden et al., 2005).

(MR) An RCT of patients with myofascial pain disorder ($N = 40$) comparing AT, use of an occlusal appliance, and minimal treatment showed that AT was more effective in reducing the subjective report of pain (Winocur et al., 2002).

Possibly Effective

■ *Use AT to reduce behavioral and emotional problems.* **LOE = III**

(MR) An RCT of children aged 6 to 15 years with internalizing symptoms and/or some aggressive, impulsive, or attention deficit symptoms showed that those assigned to the AT group ($N = 35$) had improvements in stress, behavior, and psychosomatic complaints compared with the waitlist control group ($N = 15$) (Goldbeck & Schmid, 2003).

(MR) In an RCT comparing AT with control in patients with multiple sclerosis ($N = 22$), the AT group reported more energy and vigor (Sutherland et al., 2005).

■ *Use AT for irritable bowel syndrome (IBS).* **LOE = IV**

(MR) A controlled study comparing patients with IBS ($N = 19$) using a home treatment version of a scripted hypnosis protocol with matched patients not using the protocol ($N = 57$) found that 53% of the experimental group reported more than 50% reduction in IBS severity compared with 26% of control patients (Palsson et al., 2006).

(MR) A case study of a patient with refractory IBS treated with hypnotherapy in the office and at home through audiotapes showed a 38% reduction in IBS symptoms as well as reduction in depression and anxiety (Galovski & Blanchard, 2002).

NR = Nursing Research, **MR** = Multidisciplinary Research, **SP** = Standard of Practice, **EO** = Expert Opinion, **LOE** = Level of Evidence

■ *Use AT to reduce blood pressure.* **LOE = IV**

(NR) A controlled study of biofeedback including AT in hypertensive people ($N = 54$) showed that this combination resulted in a small reduction in systolic and diastolic blood pressure. The effect of AT could not be distinguished from that of other program components (Yucha et al., 2005).

(MR) A controlled study of AT in hypertensive people ($N = 11$) showed that it lowered excessive BP variability (Watanabe et al., 2003).

Not Effective

■ *Use of AT to reduce pain in labor.* **LOE = I**

(MR) A systematic review of 12 trials involving acupuncture, biofeedback, hypnosis, massage, and AT showed insufficient evidence to support the use of any of these measures to reduce labor pain (Huntley et al., 2004).

■ *Use of AT in bronchial asthma.* **LOE = I**

(MR) A systematic review of the literature on complementary and alternative medicine in bronchial asthma showed that AT might have a small effect in selected cases but was not proved to be superior to placebo (Gyorik & Brutsche, 2004).

Possibly Harmful

No applicable published research was found in this category.

OUTCOME MEASUREMENT

PERSONAL WELL-BEING (NOC)

Definition: Extent of positive perception of one's health status and life circumstances.
Personal Well-Being as evidenced by the following selected NOC indicators:
• Psychological health
• Physical health
• Ability to cope
• Ability to relax
(Rate each indicator of **Personal Well-Being:** 1 = not at all satisfied, 2 = somewhat satisfied, 3 = moderately satisfied, 4 = very satisfied, 5 = completely satisfied) (Moorhead et al., 2004.)

REFERENCES

Blanchard EB, Kim M. (2005). The effect of the definition of menstrually-related headache on the response to biofeedback treatment. *Appl Psychophysiol Biofeedback,* 30(1):53-63.

Devineni T, Blanchard EB. (2005). A randomized controlled trial of an internet-based treatment for chronic headache. *Behav Res Ther,* 43(3):277-292.

Dochterman JM, Bulechek GM (Eds). (2004). *Nursing Interventions Classification (NIC),* 4th ed. St. Louis: Mosby.

Galovski TE, Blanchard EB. (2002). Hypnotherapy and refractory irritable bowel syndrome: A single case study. *Am J Clin Hypn,* 45(1):31-37.

RCT = Randomized Controlled (Clinical) Trial, **NIC** = Nursing Interventions Classification, **NOC** = Nursing Outcomes Classification

Goldbeck L, Schmid K. (2003). Effectiveness of autogenic relaxation training on children and adolescents with behavioral and emotional problems. *J Am Acad Child Adolesc Psychiatry,* 42(9):1046-1054.

Gordon JS, Staples JK, Blyta A, Bytyqi M. (2004). Treatment of posttraumatic stress disorder in postwar Kosovo high school students using mind-body skills groups: A pilot study. *J Trauma Stress,* 17(2):143-147.

Gyorik SA, Brutsche MH. (2004). Complementary and alternative medicine for bronchial asthma: Is there new evidence? *Curr Opin Pulm Med,* 10(1):37-43.

Harden RN, Houle TT, Green S, Remble TA, Weinland SR, Colio S, et al. (2005). Biofeedback in the treatment of phantom limb pain: A time-series analysis. *Appl Psychophysiol Biofeedback,* 30(1): 83-93.

Hidderley M, Holt M. (2004). A pilot randomized trial assessing the effects of autogenic training in early stage cancer patients in relation to psychological status and immune system responses. *Eur J Oncol Nurs,* 8(1):61-65.

Huntley AL, Coon JT, Ernst E. (2004). Complementary and alternative medicine for labor pain: A systematic review. *Am J Obstet Gynecol,* 191(1):36-44.

Jorm AF, Christensen H, Griffiths KM, Parslow RA, Rodgers B, Blewitt KA. (2004). Effectiveness of complementary and self-help treatments for anxiety disorders. *Med J Aust,* 181(7 Suppl):S29-S46.

Kanji N, White AR, Ernst E. (2004). Autogenic training reduces anxiety after coronary angioplasty: A randomized clinical trial. *Am Heart J,* 147(3):E10.

Moorhead M, Johnson M, Maas M (Eds). (2004). *Nursing Outcomes Classification (NOC),* 3rd ed. St. Louis: Mosby.

Palsson OS, Turner MJ, Whitehead WE. (2006). Hypnosis home treatment for irritable bowel syndrome: A pilot study. *Int J Clin Exp Hypn,* 54(1):85-99.

Simeit R, Deck R, Conta-Marx B. (2004). Sleep management training for cancer patients with insomnia. *Support Care Cancer,* 12(3):176-183.

Stetter F, Kupper S. (2002). Autogenic training: A meta-analysis of clinical outcome studies. *Appl Psychophysiol Biofeedback,* 27(1):45-98.

Sutherland G, Andersen MB, Morris T. (2005). Relaxation and health-related quality of life in multiple sclerosis: The example of autogenic training. *J Behav Med,* 28(3):249-256.

Watanabe Y, Cornelissen G, Watanabe M, Watanabe F, Otsuka K, Ohkawa S, et al. (2003). Effects of autogenic training and antihypertensive agents on circadian and circaseptan variation of blood pressure. *Clin Exp Hypertens,* 25(7):405-412.

Winocur E, Gavish A, Emodi-Perlman A, Halachmi M, Eli I. (2002). Hypnorelaxation as treatment for myofascial pain disorder: A comparative study. *Oral Surg Oral Med Oral Pathol Oral Radiol Endod,* 93(4):429-434.

Wright S, Courtney U, Crowther D. (2002). A quantitative and qualitative pilot study of the perceived benefits of autogenic training for a group of people with cancer. *Eur J Cancer Care,* 11(2):122-130.

Yucha CB, Tsai P, Calderon KS, Tian L. (2005). Biofeedback assisted relaxation training for essential hypertension: Who is most likely to benefit? J Cardiovasc Nurs, 20(3):198-205.

Zsombok T, Juhasz G, Budavari A, Vitrai J, Bagdy G. (2003). Effect of autogenic training on drug consumption in patients with primary headache: An 8-month follow-up study. *Headache,* 43(3):251-257.

BATHING

Scott Chisholm Lamont, BSN, RN, CCRN, CFRN

NIC **Definition:** Cleaning of the body for the purposes of relaxation, cleanliness, and healing (Dochterman & Bulechek, 2004).

NR = Nursing Research, **MR** = Multidisciplinary Research, **SP** = Standard of Practice, **EO** = Expert Opinion, **LOE** = Level of Evidence

NURSING ACTIVITIES

Effective

■ ⓢⓟ *Promote routine bathing or showering for physical and psychological health.* **LOE = VII**

ⓔⓞ Bathing removes contaminants from the skin while providing a sense of relaxation and refreshment (Perry & Potter, 2006).

■ ⓢⓟ *Apply moisturizers or creams to the skin within 3 minutes of exiting the shower or bath.* **LOE = VII**

ⓔⓞ Applying moisturizers before the skin completely dries helps trap moisture in the upper layers of skin, reducing skin dryness and irritation (AAD, 2002).

■ ⓢⓟ *Recognize that bathing practices may have culturally specific significance and support social well-being for members of that culture.* **LOE = V**

ⓜⓡ A qualitative review regarding the provision of bathing assistance as a social service for long-term care in Japan noted the importance of cultural considerations in both individual and policy level decision making in long-term care (Traphagan, 2004).

Possibly Effective

■ *Add lavender oil to bathwater to improve psychological well-being.* **LOE = III**

ⓜⓡ A two-part, single-blind RCT involving female volunteers ($N = 80$) compared the effect of placebo oil and lavender oil added to bathwater upon two aspects of psychological well-being. Results demonstrated psychologically positive mood changes in the first study group ($N = 40$) and reduced negative responses regarding the future in the second study group ($N = 40$) (Morris, 2002).

■ *Use passive body heating with warm (40°C) bathwater to assist with sleep onset, duration, and quality in elderly people.* **LOE = V**

ⓜⓡ A systematic review of three controlled studies, all using a randomized crossover design, of the effect on sleep of passive heating by bathing among participants 60 years old and over ($N = 53$) found that participants had improved subjective quality of sleep and quantitative measures of sleep. However, because results for males and females were not reported separately in the one mixed-gender study, results could be considered definitively positive only for females (Liao, 2002).

■ *Recognize that a brief immersion in a 40°C hot tub is as safe for stable, treated hypertensive people as for normotensive people.* **LOE = IV**

ⓜⓡ A case-control descriptive study ($N = 44$) comparing blood pressure and heart rate changes during and following a 10-minute immersion in a public hot tub found that although diastolic blood pressure fell and heart rate increased in both the hypertensive and normotensive groups, no adverse symptoms were reported. The study concluded that brief bathing in hot tubs should be safe for most treated hypertensive people (Shin et al., 2003).

RCT = Randomized Controlled (Clinical) Trial, **NIC** = Nursing Interventions Classification, **NOC** = Nursing Outcomes Classification

■ *Clean shower facilities immediately before use for immunocompromised patients.* **LOE = III**

(MR) A pretest/post-test descriptive study of randomly selected patients' shower facilities (*N* = 11) on a bone marrow transplantation unit found a significant reduction in the concentration of airborne filamentous fungi, including pathogenic species, even if only the floor of the shower was cleaned (Anaissie et al., 2002).

Not Effective

No applicable published research was found in this category.

Possibly Harmful

■ *Exposing central venous catheters to hospital tap water in the course of bathing or showering.* **LOE = VII**

(NR) A case-control study of bone marrow transplant and oncology patients (*N* = 18) following an outbreak of *Mycobacterium mucogenicum* bacteremias found a DNA match between isolates from one patient's blood and the shower in that patient's room and found *Mycobacterium* isolates from numerous water sources in the facility. Poststudy follow-up of recommendations to protect central venous catheters from water during bathing showed a reduction of *Mycobacterium* bacteremia cases from six in a 4-month period to one in a 30-month period (Kline et al., 2004).

■ *Use of shower gel, antiseptic agents, or shampoo in the bath by women being treated for bacterial vaginosis.* **LOE = VII**

(EO) The British Association for Sexual Health and HIV recommends that this population avoid these products (Hay, 2006).

■ *Tap water exposure for patients at risk for infection, including those who are immunocompromised or have open wounds.* **LOE = V**

(NR) A systematic review of selected literature on bathwater as a source of infection concluded that following recommendations such as using sterile water for drinking and sterile sponges for bathing, educating staff and families on infection control practices related to waterborne infections, targeted surveillance, and following CDC guidelines to suppress organisms present in water systems may improve patients' outcomes. However, significantly more study is needed to determine best practices (John, 2006).

■ *Bathing or showering in hot water as opposed to warm water.* **LOE = VII**

(EO) Hot water strips the skin of oils that help maintain skin moisture, resulting in increased dryness and irritation (AAD, 2002).

■ *Prolonged bathing in hot water (40°C or greater).* **LOE = V**

(MR) A descriptive study comparing young men (*N* = 9) with older men (*N* = 9) found that heart rate variability changed after 4 minutes of immersion in 40°C water, possibly reflecting decreased sympathetic tone and risk for syncope (Nagasawa et al., 2001).

NR = Nursing Research, **MR** = Multidisciplinary Research, **SP** = Standard of Practice, **EO** = Expert Opinion, **LOE** = Level of Evidence

(MR) A descriptive study of heart rate variability experienced by young men bathing in 38°C and 41°C water ($N = 14$) led the authors to conclude that immersion time should be limited to 10 minutes at 38°C or 5 minutes at 41°C (Kataoka & Yoshida, 2005).

OUTCOME MEASUREMENT

CLIENT SATISFACTION: PHYSICAL CARE (NOC)

Definition: Extent of positive perception of nursing care to maintain body functions and cleanliness.

Client Satisfaction: Physical Care as evidenced by the following selected NOC indicators:

• Assistance with bath or shower
• Assistance with hair care
• Assistance with nail care
• Special skin care needs followed

(Rate each indicator of **Client Satisfaction: Physical Care:** 1 = not at all satisfied, 2 = somewhat satisfied, 3 = moderately satisfied, 4 = very satisfied, 5 = completely satisfied) (Moorhead et al., 2004.)

REFERENCES

American Academy of Dermatology (AAD). (2002). *Protecting your skin as the snow flies: Separating the myth from the fact about dry winter skin.* Available online: http://www.aad.org/. Retrieved on April 4, 2007.

Anaissie EJ, Stratton SL, Dignani MC, Lee CK, Mahfouz TH, Rex JH, et al. (2002). Cleaning patient shower facilities: A novel approach to reducing patient exposure to aerosolized *Aspergillus* species and other opportunistic molds. *Clin Infect Dis,* 35(8):E86-E88.

Dochterman JM, Bulechek GM (Eds). (2004). *Nursing Interventions Classification (NIC),* 4th ed. St. Louis: Mosby.

Hay P. (2006). National guideline for the management of bacterial vaginosis. Clinical Effectiveness Group, British Association for Sexual Health and HIV. Available online: http://www.bashh.org. Retrieved on April 4, 2007.

John LD. (2006). Nosocomial infections and bath water: Any cause for concern? *Clin Nurse Spec,* 20(3):119-123.

Kataoka Y, Yoshida F. (2005). The change of hemodynamics and heart rate variability on bathing by the gap of water temperature. *Biomed Pharmacother,* 59(Suppl 1):S92-S99.

Kline S, Cameron S, Streifel A, Yakrus MA, Kairis F, Peacock K, et al. (2004). An outbreak of bacteremias associated with *Mycobacterium mucogenicum* in a hospital water supply. *Infect Control Hosp Epidemiol,* 25(12):1042-1049.

Liao WC. (2002). Effects of passive body heating on body temperature and sleep regulation in the elderly: A systematic review. *Int J Nurs Stud,* 39(8):803-810.

Moorhead M, Johnson M, Maas M (Eds). (2004). *Nursing Outcomes Classification (NOC),* 3rd ed. St. Louis: Mosby.

Morris N. (2002). The effects of lavender (*Lavendula angusifolium*) baths on psychological well-being: Two exploratory randomised control trials. *Complement Ther Med,* 10(4):223-228.

Nagasawa Y, Komori S, Sato M, Tsuboi Y, Umetani K, Watanabe Y, et al. (2001). Effects of hot bath immersion on autonomic activity and hemodynamics: Comparison of the elderly patient and the healthy young. *Jpn Circ J,* 65(7):587-592.

Perry AG, Potter PA. (2006). *Clinical nursing skills & techniques,* 6th ed. St. Louis: Mosby.

Shin TW, Wilson M, Wilson TW. (2003). Are hot tubs safe for people with treated hypertension? *CMAJ,* 169(12):1265-1268.

RCT = Randomized Controlled (Clinical) Trial, **NIC** = Nursing Interventions Classification, **NOC** = Nursing Outcomes Classification

Traphagan JW. (2004). Culture and long-term care: The bath as social service in Japan. *Care Manag J*, 5(1):53-60.

 # Bed Rest Care

Angela J. Gillis, PhD, RN; Brenda MacDonald, MEd, MS, BN, RN

NIC **Definition:** Promotion of comfort and safety and prevention of complications for a patient unable to get out of bed (Dochterman & Bulechek, 2004).

NURSING ACTIVITIES

Effective

■ **SP** *Use range-of-motion (ROM) exercises to maintain joint mobility and muscle integrity.* **LOE = VII**

MR An RCT ($N = 16$) found that 20 days of bed rest increased the stiffness of tendon structures in the knee extensors and that resistance exercises (leg-press exercises) prevented these changes (Kubo et al., 2004).

MR An RCT involving 120 patients who received a total knee arthroplasty found that postoperative rehabilitation regimens that focused on early mobilization of the patient with standardized exercises were effective in attaining a satisfactory level of knee ROM and function. Adjunct continuous passive motion exercises or slider board therapy did not alter postoperative recovery (Beaupre et al., 2001).

EO Unless contraindicated, three repetitions of passive ROM exercises should be performed on each joint at a minimum of twice daily (*Nursing*, 2006).

EO Early initiation and maintenance of ROM exercises during acute care of the patient with a spinal cord injury are recommended (Fries, 2005).

■ **SP** *Assess the skin daily and monitor for any changes, especially over bony prominences, on a regular basis.* **LOE = VII**

EO Patients who are restricted to bed care should have their skin condition monitored daily and be assessed for pressure, friction, and shear in all positions as well as during lifting, turning, and repositioning (RNAO, 2005).

EO The Institute for Clinical Systems Improvement (ICSI) Pressure Ulcer Risk Assessment and Skin Inspection Protocol is recommended to identify patients who require skin safety plans (ICSI, 2006).

MR A systematic literature review recommended that skin risk assessment should occur on admission to the unit, following a significant clinical event or change in condition, and at regular intervals (Wiechula, 1997).

■ *Conduct a risk assessment and classify patients as "at high risk," "at risk," or "not at risk" for development of pressure ulcers.* **LOE = I**

MR A systematic review demonstrated that bed care patients with limited ability to reposition themselves should be monitored as their condition warrants, and a risk assessment should be performed using a risk assessment tool. Risk assessment scales such as the Braden and Norton scales are valuable tools to support clinical judgment in assessing risks of skin breakdown but should not replace clinical judgment (AHCPR, 1992).

(EO) The validity of the Braden scale to predict the development of pressure ulcers has been tested extensively. Its validity increases when combined with the Norton scale. Interrater reliability between 0.83 and 0.99 has been reported (Ayello, 2003).

■ (NIC) *Apply antiembolism stockings.* **LOE = I**

(MR) A Cochrane review of 16 RCTs determined the effectiveness of graduated compression stockings in diminishing the risk of deep vein thrombosis (DVT) in hospitalized patients (Amaragiri & Lees, 2000).

(MR) A systematic literature review demonstrated that patients with DVTs who received graduated elastic compression stockings had greater reductions in the incidence of any or severe post-thrombotic syndrome than those who received a control intervention (Elton, 2004).

(MR) An evidence-based literature review concluded that above-the-knee graduated compression stockings were effective for the prevention of postoperative DVT in moderate-risk surgical patients (Evans & Read, 2001).

■ *Use pressure-relieving devices on the bed.* **LOE = I**

(EO) As a minimum provision, patients vulnerable to pressure ulcers should be placed on a high-specification foam mattress with pressure-relieving properties (NICE, 2003).

(MR) A review of 13 clinical studies demonstrated that the incidence of pressure ulcers in at-risk patients was consistently lower for patients cared for on pressure-reducing devices than those cared for on a hospital mattress, according to a standardized protocol (AHCPR, 1992).

(MR) A systematic review of evidence suggested that pressure support devices were more effective than standard hospital beds in reducing the incidence of pressure sore development and that dynamic devices such as large-cell alternating mattresses may be superior to low-pressure support surfaces (Wiechula, 1997).

Possibly Effective

■ *Perform resistance exercises to prevent deconditioning and functional decline during bed rest.* **LOE = II**

(EO) The Gerontological Nursing Interventions Research Center recommends three workouts per week with a minimum of three sets per exercise for approximately 30- to 40-minute intervals without discomfort (Mobily & Mobily, 2004).

(EO) Moderate weight-lifting exercise (60% to 80% of one resistance movement [RM]) does not cause adverse effects in patients with heart disease; there is improved cardiac muscle strength and endurance and favorable alterations in skeletal muscle (King, 2001).

(MR) A Cochrane systematic review found that progressive resistance strength training for physical disability in older individuals was an effective intervention to increase muscle strength. In addition, it provided some improvement in gait speed of older hospitalized patients. There was no evidence that it had an effect in reducing overall disability (i.e., completion of more complex daily activities) (Latham et al., 2003).

(MR) An RCT ($N = 39$) found that using a standardized and simple exercise regimen (a maximum of three sets per exercise three times a week) enabled older hospitalized adults to perform resistance exercises. Further research is required to determine whether resistance

---

RCT = Randomized Controlled (Clinical) Trial, **NIC** = Nursing Interventions Classification, **NOC** = Nursing Outcomes Classification

exercises can prevent or treat hospital-related deterioration in mobility and function (Mallery et al., 2003).

(MR) A case study ($N = 3$) demonstrated that exercising with In-Bed Exercise (IBEX) several times a day offered a possible method for reducing functional decline in frail elderly people following illness or injury. Further studies are needed to establish the efficacy of using the device (Deneen et al., 2002).

Use a risk assessment tool to predict the risk of developing pressure sores. LOE = VI

(EO) Risk assessment tools such as the Norton scale or Braden scale illustrate factors that should be considered when determining risk and planning care. It was concluded that no tool can be confidently held to be superior to the rest in all settings with all levels of staff or more effective than clinical judgment in the prediction of pressure sore development (AHCPR, 1992; Wiechula, 1997).

(MR) A multisite prospective cohort descriptive study with a sample of 322 pediatric patients on bed rest for at least 24 hours concluded that the Braden Q scale, with three subscales, provided a tool that was shorter than, yet comparable to, the Braden scale for predicting pressure ulcer risk in pediatric patients (Curley et al., 2003).

(NR) A prospective comparative study of 530 adult medical-surgical patients identified risk factors associated with pressure ulcer development. It confirmed that bed rest is a risk factor for pressure ulcer development in hospitalized patients and concluded that the Risk Assessment Pressure Sore scale may be useful for prediction of pressure ulcer development in clinical practice (Lindgren et al., 2004).

Use knee-length versus thigh-length antiembolism stockings in bed rest care. LOE = V

(NR) A literature review of four studies (an RCT, a control study, and two other studies) concluded that knee-length antiembolism stockings were as effective as thigh-length antiembolism stockings in preventing DVT in immobilized medical-surgical patients. In addition, the former stockings received better compliance from patients and were more cost effective. However, the author concluded that more research was needed to assess the effectiveness of both lengths of stockings in preventing DVT in medical-surgical patients (Ingram, 2003).

Use pressure-relieving devices (mattresses, overlays, both high and low technology) with bed care patients assessed at risk for pressure ulcers. LOE = VII

(EO) Use of alternating pressure or other high-technology pressure-relieving systems when patients are at high risk for pressure ulcers is recommended. However, pressure-relieving mattresses and overlays were not found to be more effective than high-specification (low-technology) foam mattresses and overlays (NICE, 2003; Wiechula, 1997).

Not Effective

Use of high-technology pressure-relieving devices (dynamic systems) versus low-technology pressure-relieving devices (conforming support systems that redistribute body weight) on the bed. LOE = I

(MR) A panel review of three RCTs, each testing two types of pressure-reducing devices (air mattress versus water mattress, alternating pressure pad versus silicone mattress overlay, foam

NR = Nursing Research, MR = Multidisciplinary Research, SP = Standard of Practice, EO = Expert Opinion, LOE = Level of Evidence

overlay versus alternating pressure mattress), concluded that pressure-reducing devices decreased the incidence of pressure ulcers, but there was no evidence that one type of pressure-reducing device was more effective than another in preventing pressure ulcers (AHCPR, 1992).

Possibly Harmful

■ *Encouraging bed rest as a treatment.* LOE = II

(NR) A descriptive longitudinal study ($N = 141$ mothers) lasting 5 years found that antepartum bed rest treatment was ineffective for improving the mother's or infant's weight during a high-risk pregnancy. Future research is needed in completing a randomized trial (Maloni, 2003).

(NR) A descriptive longitudinal study ($N = 126$ mothers) found that women who were prescribed bed rest during pregnancy had unresolved psychological and physical symptoms 6 weeks following delivery (Maloni et al., 2004).

(MR) An RCT involving 250 patients with sciatica for less than 1 month found that continuing activities of daily living was as effective as bed rest or physiotherapy in decreasing pain, disability, and surgery (Wiener, 2002).

(MR) A systematic review of 39 RCTs of bed rest for 15 different conditions ($N = 5777$) found that bed rest was overprescribed, and evidence demonstrated that bed rest may delay the patient's recovery or have harmful effects. Further research is needed with a focus on the strictness and the duration of bed rest (Allen et al., 1999).

(MR) A prospective cohort study of elderly hospitalized patients 70 years of age or older ($N = 498$) showed bed rest to be a risk factor for a variety of adverse outcomes including death (Brown et al., 2004).

(MR) A prospective cohort study of community-living elderly people ($N = 680$) concluded that there was a direct relationship between bed rest and a decline in a variety of functional measures (Gill et al., 2004).

■ *Allowing compression stockings to bunch up and form a constricting band that can decrease circulation and cause skin damage.* LOE = IV

(EO) Compression stockings should be removed at least once daily for skin care and checked regularly to ensure correct placement and fit and that no bunching or restrictions to circulation are caused by the stockings (Evans & Read, 2001).

(NR) A validation study of published research on the use of graduated compression stockings and their implementation in practice concluded that although the use of graduated compression stockings may seem without risk, this intervention is associated with hidden dangers such as ill-fitting and improperly applied stockings that can lead to pressure ulcers and DVT (Hayes et al., 2002).

(MR) In a descriptive study of 112 stroke patients, Doppler assessment was used to evaluate the feasibility and tolerability of graduated compression stockings on a stroke unit. Although 84% of the patients had no contraindications to the stockings, leg edema, venous ulceration, and skin intolerance were reported for 16% of the sample. Graduated compression stockings should not be used in patients with peripheral vascular insufficiency without Doppler assessment (Scholten et al., 2000).

RCT = Randomized Controlled (Clinical) Trial, **NIC** = Nursing Interventions Classification, **NOC** = Nursing Outcomes Classification

OUTCOME MEASUREMENT

BEDREST CARE

Definition: Presence of comfort, safety, and absence of complications.

Bedrest Care as evidenced by the following indicators:

- Ability to change body position
- Maintenance of physiological and psychocognitive functioning
- Tissue integrity
- Pain level
- Mobility level

(**Note:** This is not a NOC outcome.)

REFERENCES

Agency for Healthcare Policy and Research (AHCPR). (1992). Pressure ulcers in adults: Prediction and prevention. Agency for Healthcare Policy and Research. *Clin Pract Guidel Quick Ref Guide Clin,* 3:1-15.

Allen C, Glasziou P, Del Mar C. (1999). Bed rest: A potentially harmful treatment needing more careful evaluation. *Lancet,* 354(9186):1229-1233.

Amaragiri SV, Lees TA. (2000). Elastic compression stockings for prevention of deep vein thrombosis. *Cochrane Database Syst Rev,* (2):CD001484.

Ayello EA. (2003). Predicting pressure ulcer sore risk. *Medsurg Nurs,* 12(2):130-131.

Beaupre LA, Davies DM, Jones CA, Cinats JG. (2001). Exercise combined with continuous passive motion or slider board therapy compared with exercise only: A randomized controlled trial of patients following total knee arthroplasty. *Phys Ther,* 81(4):1029-1037.

Braden BJ, Bergstrom N. (1987). A conceptual schema for the study of the etiology of pressure sores. *Rehabil Nurs,* 12(1):8-12.

Braden BJ, Bergstrom N. (1989). Clinical utility of the Braden scale for Predicting Pressure Sore Risk. *Decubitus,* 2(3):44-46, 50-51.

Braden BJ, Bryant R. (1990). Innovations to prevent and treat pressure ulcers. *Geriatr Nurs,* 11(4): 182-186.

Brown CJ, Friedkin RJ, Inouye SK. (2004). Prevalence and outcomes of low mobility in hospitalized older patients. *J Am Geriatr Soc,* 52(8):1263-1270.

Curley MA, Razmus IS, Roberts KE, Wypij D. (2003). Predicting pressure ulcer risk in pediatric patients: The Braden Q Scale. *Nurs Res,* 52(1):22-33.

Deneen EK, Banerjee S, Heermans AG, Dean RC. (2002). Bedside exercise for mobility-limited nursing home residents: A case study. *J Geriatr Phys Ther,* 25(2):12-19.

Dochterman JM, Bulechek GM (Eds). (2004). *Nursing Interventions Classification (NIC),* 4th ed. St. Louis: Mosby.

Elton G. (2004). Review: Elastic compression stockings prevent the post thrombotic syndrome in patients with deep venous thrombosis. *Evid Based Nurs,* 7(3):86.

Evans D, Read K. (2001). Graduated compression stockings for the prevention of post-operative venous thromboembolism. *Best Pract,* 5(2):1-6.

Fries JM. (2005). Critical rehabilitation of the patient with spinal cord injury. *Crit Care Nurs Q,* 28(2):179-187.

Gill TM, Allore H, Guo Z. (2004). The deleterious effects of bed rest among community-living older persons. *J Gerontol,* 59(7):755-761.

Hayes JM, Lehman CA, Castonguay P. (2002). Graduated compression stockings: Updating practice, improving compliance. *Medsurg Nurs,* 11(4):163-166.

Ingram JE. (2003). A review of thigh-length vs knee-length antiembolism stockings. *Br J Nurs,* 12(14):845-851.

Institute for Clinical Systems Improvement (ICSI). (2006). Pressure ulcer prevention protocol and skin safety plan. 1:1-20. Available online: http://www.icsi.org. Retrieved on July 5, 2007.

King L. (2001). The effects of resistance exercise on skeletal muscle abnormalities in patients with advanced heart failure. *Prog Cardiovasc Nurs,* 16(4):142-151.

Kubo K, Akima H, Ushiyama J, Tabata I, Fukuoka H, Kanehisa H, et al. (2004). Effects of resistance training during bed rest on the viscoelastic properties of tendon structures in the lower limb. *Scand J Med Sci Sports,* 14(5):296-302.

Latham N, Anderson C, Bennett D, Stretton C. (2003). Progressive resistance strength training for physical disability in older people. *Cochrane Database Syst Rev,* (2):CD002759.

Lindgren M, Unosson M, Fredrikson M, Ek AC. (2004). Immobility—A major risk factor for the development of pressure ulcers among adult hospitalized patients: A prospective study. *Scand J Caring Sci,* 18(1):57-64.

Mallery LH, MacDonald EA, Hubley-Kozey CL, Earl ME, Rockwood K, MacKnight C. (2003). The feasibility of performing resistance exercise with acutely ill hospitalized older adults. *BMC Geriatr,* 3:3.

Maloni JA. (2003). *Postpartum symptoms of recovery from antepartum bed rest.* Abstract from the Midwest Nursing Research Society Conference. Available online: http://www.nursinglibrary.org. Retrieved on July 5, 2007.

Maloni JA, Alexander GR, Schluchter MD, Shah DM, Park S. (2004). Antepartum bed rest: Maternal weight change and infant birth weight. *Biol Res Nurs,* 5(3):177-186.

Mobily K, Mobily P. (2004). *Progressive resistance training.* University of Iowa Gerontological Nursing Interventions Research Center, Research Dissemination Core, February 28, 2004. Iowa City, Iowa.

National Institute for Clinical Excellence (NICE). (2003). *Pressure ulcer prevention.* Clinical Guideline B. Available online: http://www.nice.org.uk. Retrieved on July 5, 2007.

Nursing. (2006). Performing passive range-of-motion exercises. *Nursing,* 36(3)50-51.

Registered Nurses' Association of Ontario (RNAO). (2005). *Risk assessment and prevention of pressure ulcers.* (Revised). Toronto, Canada: RNAO.

Scholten P, Bever A, Turner K, Warburton L. (2000). Graduated elastic compression stockings on a stroke unit: A feasibility study. *Age Aging,* 29(4):357-359.

Wiechula R. (1997). Pressure sores—Part 1: Prevention of pressure related damage. *Best Pract,* 1(1): 1-6.

Wiener SL. (2002). Bed rest, physiotherapy, and continuation of activities of daily living were equally effective for sciatica. *ACP J Club,* 137(2):66.

 # BEHAVIOR MANAGEMENT: SELF-HARM

Roseann Colosimo, PhD, RN

NIC **Definition:** Assisting the patient to decrease or eliminate self-mutilating or self-abusive behaviors (Dochterman & Bulechek, 2004).

NURSING ACTIVITIES

Effective

No applicable published research was found in this category.

RCT = Randomized Controlled (Clinical) Trial, **NIC** = Nursing Interventions Classification, **NOC** = Nursing Outcomes Classification

Possibly Effective

■ **NIC** *Administer medications as appropriate to decrease anxiety, stabilize mood, and decrease self-stimulation.* **LOE = I**

MR A small quasi-experimental study involving a pretest/post-test design showed a decrease in acute states of aversive inner tension, dissociative symptoms, and the urge to commit self-injurious acts with administration of clonidine (Philipsen et al., 2004).

MR A cohort study with nested case control looked at suicides within 120 days of being ordered an antidepressant. Age, gender, and preexisting depression or suicidal ideation were important confounders in observational studies of the association between antidepressants and suicide or self-harm. Paroxetine was a significant risk factor for suicide on univariate analysis but not when corrected for age, gender, and depression or suicidal ideation (Didham et al., 2005).

■ *Assess the patient for history of self-injury behaviors, including method used and known triggers.* **LOE = V**

NR A controlled study found the Self-Injury Questionnaire to be a reliable and valid measure for research in an acute self-harming population (Santa Mina et al., 2006).

NR A qualitative study discussed the assessment of risk for adolescents who struggled with self-harm behavior. Assessment of risk depended on the nurse's ability to establish a relationship with the youth and understand self-harm behavior in the context of family and social experience (Murray & Wright, 2006).

MR In a community sample with 934 participants, young females underwent a clinical interview to assess for self-injurious behaviors. Twenty-four percent of the sample reported self-injurious behavior (Favaro et al., 2007).

MR A descriptive national 5-year study evaluated 412,000 annual emergency department visits, representing 0.4% of all emergency department visits, for attempted suicide and self-inflicted injury. The most common method of injury was poisoning (68%), followed by cutting or piercing (20%) (Doshi et al., 2005).

MR A meta-analysis examined whether the Beck hopelessness scale could be used to predict suicide and nonfatal self-harm. The standard cutoff on the Beck scale was capable of identifying those who were at risk for future self-harm (McMillan et al., 2007).

Additional research: Hawton et al., 2003, 2006; Karila et al., 2007.

■ **NIC** *Place the patient in a more protective environment (e.g., area restriction and seclusion) if self-harmful impulses/behaviors escalate.* **LOE = VII**

NR A qualitative research study using the grounded theory approach found that environmental factors as well as the nurses' knowledge and skills and the type of support patients received affected the advancement of suicide nursing care (Sun et al., 2006a).

NR A descriptive study of 31 cases of suicide or serious self-harm in people in receipt of inpatient care highlighted environmental factors in which there was considerable variation in the content and quality of the observation policy (Gournay & Bowers, 2000).

■ *Provide therapeutic nursing caring communication.* **LOE = V**

NR A qualitative study of experiences of patients during inpatient care in Sweden following a suicide attempt revealed that verbal contacts with staff were seen as essential to the process of healing and for the desire to go on living (Samuelsson et al., 2000).

NR = Nursing Research, **MR** = Multidisciplinary Research, **SP** = Standard of Practice, **EO** = Expert Opinion, **LOE** = Level of Evidence

(NR) A qualitative study with a grounded theory design involved 15 patients with suicidal ideas or attempt. The provision of safe and compassionate care through the channel of the therapeutic relationship emerged as an important theme (Sun et al., 2006b).

(NR) A small qualitative study based on hermeneutic interpretation of 10 narrative interviews with biographical information found themes helpful to nurses' understanding. The themes were life on the edge, the struggle for health and dignity—a balance act on a slack wire over a volcano, and good and bad acts of psychiatric care in the drama of suffering (Perseius et al., 2005).

(EO) Clinicians who understand self-mutilating behavior as a means of self-preservation and emotional regulation are better able to provide supportive and empathetic care (Starr, 2004).

- (NIC) *Instruct the patient in coping strategies (e.g., assertiveness training, impulse control training, and progressive muscle relaxation), as appropriate.* **LOE = V**

(MR) A controlled study indicated that treatments for deliberate self-harm with repeated episodes should include problem solving (McAuliffe et al., 2006).

(MR) A systematic review of three RCTs, four clinical control trials, and three quasi-experimental studies found that the evidence base for treatments designed to reduce the repetition of self-harm in adolescents was very limited (Burns et al., 2005).

(MR) A small quasi-experimental study examining a group intervention on acceptance-based emotion regulation showed promising results, but larger randomized control group research is needed (Gratz & Gunderson, 2006).

(MR) A quasi-experimental small study of treatment as usual compared with manual assisted cognitive treatment for patients who self-harmed showed a decrease in frequency and severity but not suicidal ideation or time to repeat (Weinberg et al., 2006).

Not Effective

- (NIC) *Contract with the patient, as appropriate, for "no self-harm."* **LOE = IV**

(NR) A controlled study did not show statistical significance in the incidence of self-harm episodes after implementation of a safety agreement. Registered nurses did perceive numerous positive effects of agreements (Potter et al., 2005).

(NR) A descriptive study of retrospective medical records examined whether no-suicide contracting affected the likelihood of self-harm behavior in psychiatric inpatient settings. The study showed no evidence of prevention of self-harm behaviors by using no-suicide contracting (Drew, 2001).

Possibly Harmful

No applicable published research was found in this category.

OUTCOME MEASUREMENT

SELF-MUTILATION RESTRAINT   (NOC)

(Please refer to *Nursing Classifications Outcome* [Moorhead et al., 2004] for the **Self-Mutilation Restraint** outcome.)

RCT = Randomized Controlled (Clinical) Trial, **NIC** = Nursing Interventions Classification, **NOC** = Nursing Outcomes Classification

REFERENCES

Burns J, Dudley M, Hazell P, Patton G. (2005). Clinical management of deliberate self-harm in young people: The need for evidence-based approaches to reduce repetition. *Aust N Z J Psychiatry,* 39(3):121-128.

Didham RC, McConnell DW, Blair HJ, Reith DM. (2005). Suicide and self-harm following prescription of SSRIs and other antidepressants: Confounding by indication. *Br J Clin Pharmacol,* 60(5):519-525.

Dochterman JM, Bulechek GM (Eds). (2004). *Nursing Interventions Classification (NIC),* 4th ed. St. Louis: Mosby.

Doshi A, Boudreaux ED, Wang N, Pelletier AJ, Camargo CA Jr. (2005). National Study of US emergency department visits for attempted suicide and self-inflicted injury, 1997-2001. *Ann Emerg Med,* 46(4):369-375.

Drew BL. (2001). Self-harm behavior and no-suicide contracting in psychiatric inpatient settings. *Arch Psychiatr Nurs,* 15(3):99-106.

Favaro A, Ferrara S, Santonastaso P. (2007). Self-injurious behavior in a community sample of young women: Relationship with childhood abuse and other types of self-damaging behaviors. *J Clin Psychiatry,* 68(1):122-131.

Gournay K, Bowers L. (2000). Suicide and self-harm in inpatient psychiatric units: A study of nursing issues in 31 cases. *J Adv Nurs,* 32(1):124-131.

Gratz KL, Gunderson JG. (2006). Preliminary data on an acceptance-based emotion regulation group intervention for deliberate self-harm among women with borderline personality disorder. *Behav Ther,* 37(1):25-35.

Hawton K, Harriss L, Zahl D. (2006). Deaths from all causes in a long-term follow-up study of 11,583 deliberate self-harm patients. *Psychol Med,* 36(3):397-405.

Hawton K, Zahl D, Weatherall R. (2003). Suicide following deliberate self-harm: Long-term follow-up of patients who presented to a general hospital. *Br J Psychiatry,* 182:537-542.

Karila L, Ferreri M, Coscas S, Cottencin O, Benyamina A, Reynaud M. (2007). Self-mutilation induced by cocaine abuse: The pleasure of bleeding. *Presse Med,* 36(2 Pt 1):235-237.

McAuliffe C, Corcoran P, Keeley HS, Arensman E, Bille-Brahe U, De Leo D, et al. (2006). Problem-solving ability and repetition of deliberate self-harm: A multicentre study. *Psychol Med,* 36(1):45-55.

McMillan D, Gilbody S, Beresford E, Neilly L. (2007). Can we predict suicide and non-fatal self-harm with the Beck Hopelessness Scale? A meta-analysis. *Psychol Med,* 1-10 [E-pub].

Moorhead M, Johnson M, Maas M (Eds). (2004). *Nursing Outcomes Classification (NOC),* 3rd ed. St. Louis: Mosby.

Murray BL, Wright K. (2006). Integration of a suicide risk assessment and intervention approach: The perspective of youth. *J Psychiatr Ment Health Nurs,* 13(2):157-164.

Perseius KI, Ekdahl S, Asberg M, Samuelsson M. (2005). To tame a volcano: Patients with borderline personality disorder and their perceptions of suffering. *Arch Psychiatr Nurs,* 19(4):160-168.

Philipsen A, Richter H, Schmahl C, Peters J, Rusch N, Bohus M, et al. (2004). Clonidine in acute aversive inner tension and self-injurious behavior in female patients with borderline personality disorder. *J Clin Psychiatry,* 65(10):1414-1419.

Potter ML, Vitale-Nolen R, Dawson AM. (2005). Implementation of safety agreements in an acute psychiatric facility. *J Am Psychiatr Nurses Assoc,* 11(3):144-155.

Samuelsson M, Wiklander M, Asberg M, Saveman BI. (2000). Psychiatric care as seen by the attempted suicide patient. *J Adv Nurs,* 32(3):635-643.

Santa Mina EE, Gallop R, Links P, Heslegrave R, Pringle D, Wekerle C, et al. (2006). The Self-Injury Questionnaire: Evaluation of the psychometric properties in a clinical population. *J Psychiatr Ment Health Nurs,* 13(2):221-227.

Starr DL. (2004). Understanding those who self mutilate. *J Psychosoc Nurs Ment Health Serv,* 42(6):32-40.

Sun FK, Long A, Boore J, Tsao LI. (2006a). Patients and nurses' perceptions of ward environmental factors and support systems in the care of suicidal patients. *J Clin Nurs,* 15(1):83-92.

Sun FK, Long A, Boore J, Tsao LI. (2006b). A theory for the nursing care of patients at risk for suicide. *J Adv Nurs,* 53(6):680-690.

Weinberg I, Gunderson JG, Hennen J, Cutter CJ Jr. (2006). Manual assisted cognitive treatment for deliberate self-harm in borderline personality disorder patients. *J Personal Disord,* 20(5):482-492.

 # BEHAVIOR MODIFICATION

Pamela J. Nelson, PhD(c), MS, RN, CNS

NIC **Definition:** Promotion of a behavior change (Dochterman & Bulechek, 2004).

NURSING ACTIVITIES

Effective

■ *Implement a behavior change program for cancer patients.* **LOE = II**

NR In an RCT, cognitive-behavioral therapy (CBT) delivered through five telephone sessions over an 8-week period in addition to conventional care was found to be more effective than conventional care alone in improving symptom management in patients with advanced cancer (Sherwood et al., 2005).

MR A qualitative study of women with breast cancer who participated in a cognitive-behavioral group found that participants enjoyed the social and interpersonal aspects of the group and also found the CBT components beneficial (Edelman et al., 2005).

MR In an RCT, group CBT offered over 10 sessions in 18 weeks reduced symptom limitation (the degree to which symptoms interfered with one's life) more than conventional care for people with a new diagnosis of solid tumor cancer (*N* = 137) (Doorenbos et al., 2005).

■ *Implement a behavior change program for chronic pain patients.* **LOE = I**

MR A systematic review of behavior therapy in the treatment of chronic low back pain and sciatica showed a significant treatment effect on reductions of pain, improved functional ability, and behavioral outcomes compared with no treatment, placebo, and waitlist control groups (van Tulder & Koes, 2003).

■ *Implement a behavior change program for smoking cessation.* **LOE = I**

NR A Cochrane systematic review of nursing interventions for smoking cessation determined that this intervention was more effective than control or usual care (Rice & Stead, 2004).

MR A Cochrane systematic review of interventions for cessation of smokeless tobacco use showed that behavioral interventions were more effective than pharmacological interventions (Ebbert et al., 2004).

MR In a Cochrane systematic review, group therapy was a more effective intervention than self-help to assist individuals in smoking cessation (Stead & Lancaster, 2005).

■ *Determine the cystic fibrosis patient's motivation to change.* **LOE = I**

(MR) A Cochrane systematic review demonstrated that behavioral interventions could improve emotional outcomes in people with cystic fibrosis as well as their caregivers (Glasscoe & Quittner, 2003).

■ (NIC) *Communicate an intervention plan and modifications to the treatment team on a regular basis. Facilitate the involvement of other health care providers in the modification process, as appropriate.* **LOE = I**

(NR) Several RCTs were reviewed in which nurse practitioners acted as case managers on an outpatient basis in augmenting the care and communicating with cardiac care providers by initiating and providing case management to patients in need of cholesterol-lowering interventions. The interventions of the case managers, including telephone counseling, outpatient counseling, and prescription of lipid-lowering medication, were more effective than follow-up by primary care providers (Allen, 2000).

Possibly Effective

■ *Implement a behavior change program for incontinence patients.* **LOE = I**

(NR) A systematic literature review found evidence to support the use of three different types of behavioral treatments for patients who are incontinent: (1) lifestyle modifications (change in dietary factors, obesity, smoking, constipation, and physical activity); (2) scheduled voiding regimens, especially in women; and (3) use of pelvic floor muscle training in stress, urge, and mixed incontinence in older women (Wyman, 2003, 2005).

(NR) A systematic review of the literature showed modest evidence for the effectiveness of behavioral treatment using pelvic floor muscle training on short-term continence in men with radical prostatectomy (Milne, 2004).

(MR) A systematic review of the literature was conducted to outline the behavioral treatment methods of fluid management, bladder retraining, and pelvic floor rehabilitation for older adults with stress or urge incontinence. Behavioral treatment resulted in improvement rates from 78% to 94% (Khan & Tariq, 2004).

(MR) A Cochrane systematic review of the effects of fixed intervals in toileting assistance in the management of urinary incontinence in adults was inconclusive because of the lack of data and poor quality of the studies reviewed (Ostaszkiewicz et al., 2004).

■ *Implement a behavior change program for individuals who are obese.* **LOE = I**

(MR) Systematic reviews and subsequent RCTs found evidence that a combination of diet, exercise, and behavioral therapy for weight loss was more effective than diet or exercise alone in treating obesity (Thorogood et al., 2004; Orzano & Scott, 2004).

(MR) A Cochrane review of many high-quality RCTs found that use of behavioral weight reduction strategies in overweight or obese individuals resulted in significantly greater weight loss than placebo (Shaw et al., 2005).

(MR) A Cochrane systematic review was conducted to assess the effectiveness of nonpharmacological interventions for weight loss in adults with type 2 diabetes mellitus. Findings indicated that only small between-group improvements existed between weight loss strategies using dietary, physical activity, or behavioral interventions (Norris et al., 2005).

NR = Nursing Research, **MR** = Multidisciplinary Research, **SP** = Standard of Practice, **EO** = Expert Opinion, **LOE** = Level of Evidence

■ *Implement a behavior change program for individuals with insomnia.* LOE = I

(NR) A systematic review of RCTs regarding the efficacy of CBT for primary insomnia indicated that CBT was superior to any single-component treatment, including stimulus control, relaxation training, education, or other control conditions. CBT was primarily provided by psychiatrists rather than nurses (Wang et al., 2005).

(MR) CBT was found in an RCT to be a more effective treatment for insomnia in patients with fibromyalgia ($N = 47$) than either usual care or an alternative behavioral therapy that included sleep hygiene instructions (Edinger et al., 2005).

(MR) In an RCT that compared two behavioral interactions—sleep hygiene instructions plus relaxation tape or sleep hygiene instructions plus stimulus control (behavioral prescriptions to use the bed and bedroom only for sleep activities)—there were no significant differences in treatment effect for older adults with insomnia (Pallesen et al., 2003).

(MR) In a Cochrane systematic review of cognitive-behavioral interventions for insomnia in older adults, only a mild effect was demonstrated (Montgomery & Dennis, 2003).

(MR) A meta-analysis comparing pharmacotherapy and behavior therapy for chronic insomnia found no differences between the two strategies and suggested that behavioral therapy be considered the first-line treatment for chronic insomnia (Perlis et al., 2003).

■ *Implement a behavior change program for multiple sclerosis patients.* LOE = III

(NR) In a quasi-experimental study examining the effectiveness of CBT, significant improvements in perceived health competence, coping, and psychological well-being in women with multiple sclerosis were reported (Sinclair & Scroggie, 2005).

■ *Implement a behavior change program for individuals with dysmenorrhea.* LOE = II

(MR) In two RCTs, there was insufficient evidence for the effects of behavioral interventions for dysmenorrhea (Proctor & Farquhar, 2006).

■ *Implement a behavior change program for human immunodeficiency virus (HIV)-positive patients.* LOE = II

(MR) In an RCT, a behavioral group intervention using social cognitive theory significantly improved HIV risk reduction behavior in HIV-positive people compared with a social support group (total $N = 181$) (Kalichman et al., 2001).

■ *Implement a behavior change program for individuals with acute myocardial infarction.* LOE = II

(MR) An individualized educational behavioral rehabilitation program delivered by cardiac nurses to patients after acute myocardial infarction was shown in an RCT ($N = 114$) to be more effective than usual care (Mayou et al., 2002).

■ (NIC) *Determine the patient's motivation to change.* LOE = II

(MR) A meta-analysis of 26 RCTs using interventions that included motivational interviewing (MI), a therapeutic strategy intended to assist clients in addressing and resolving their ambivalence about behavior change, found strong support (moderate effect size from 0.25 to 0.57)

RCT = Randomized Controlled (Clinical) Trial, **NIC** = Nursing Interventions Classification, **NOC** = Nursing Outcomes Classification

for the use of MI in treating problem drinking and diet and exercise. Less conclusive support was found for its effectiveness in the treatment of smoking, drug addiction, and HIV risk behaviors (Burke et al., 2003).

NR An RCT involving 137 patients with cancer studied the effects on smoking cessation of a MI intervention, including a visit with a smoking cessation counselor, providing smoking cessation booklets, nicotine replacement therapy, family advice to quit, and an in-person or telephone follow-up delivered over a 3-month period. At 6 months follow-up there was no difference in biochemically confirmed 3-month prevalence quit rates between the intervention (5%) and control (6%) groups (Wakefield et al., 2004).

NR A quasi-experimental research study using a one-group pretest/post-test design in 62 pregnant women tested a brief counseling session for smoking cessation provided by nurses that included empowerment techniques, MI, stress management, and educational materials during the antepartum, intrapartum, and postpartum periods. Relapse to smoking occurred in 52% of women by the second week after delivery. Chi-square analysis showed no significant difference between the intervention and control groups in smoking relapse (Suplee, 2005).

NR A case study was conducted to show how integration of the transtheoretical model of readiness for change into initial and follow-up assessments of patients with diabetes significantly promoted wound healing (Rivera et al., 2000).

■ **NIC** *Establish a baseline occurrence of the behavior before initiating change. Encourage the patient to participate in recording behaviors.* **LOE = II**

MR An RCT ($N = 139$) demonstrated that patients with chronic benign headache receiving Internet-delivered behavioral therapy (consisting of logging a daily headache diary 2 weeks before and during treatment, progressive relaxation, modified biofeedback with autogenic training, and stress management) showed significant improvement in pain symptoms and functional impairment compared with patients randomly assigned to symptom monitoring alone (Devineni & Blanchard, 2005).

■ **NIC** *Introduce the patient to persons (or groups) who have successfully undergone the same experience.* **LOE = VI**

MR A qualitative study matched peers successfully coping with diabetes with individuals struggling with diabetic management. Participants reported in focus groups the usefulness of coaching in making behavior changes related to diet, exercise, and blood glucose monitoring (Joseph et al., 2001).

■ **NIC** *Administer positive reinforcers with behaviors that are to be increased. Coordinate a token or point system of reinforcement for complex or multiple behaviors.* **LOE = II**

MR In an RCT with difficult-to-treat cigarette smokers ($N = 102$), participants were randomly allocated to four conditions that provided monetary incentives for smoking abstinence. Different percentile schedules were used to "shape" reductions in breath CO levels during study visits. All four of the contingency management conditions reduced breath CO levels gradually over the 3-month study period, indicating the importance of shaping for difficult-to-treat smokers (Lamb et al., 2004).

NR = Nursing Research, **MR** = Multidisciplinary Research, **SP** = Standard of Practice, **EO** = Expert Opinion, **LOE** = Level of Evidence

EO Positive reinforcers are recommended as components of a model of behavior modification interventions for health care in the future, incorporating telehealth, e-health, and incentive-based strategies. Such delivery systems will require that health care professionals develop a relationship with consumers in order to foster and support behavior change (Ratner, 2002).

■ **NIC** *Offer positive reinforcement for the patient's independently made decisions.* **LOE = VII**

EO Self-monitoring of target behaviors by patients and meaningful, positive feedback offered by health care providers are recommended strategies to increase the likelihood of successful change in eating and exercise behavior (Burgard & Gallagher, 2006).

■ **NIC** **SP** *Assist the patient to identify strengths, and reinforce these. Give feedback in terms of feelings when the patient is noted to be free of symptoms and looks relaxed. Avoid showing rejection or belittlement as the patient struggles with changing behavior.* **LOE = VII**

EO These activities are interventions consistent with theories of behavioral change and are considered key strategies in best practices to increase physical activities for adults older than 50 years (ACSM, 2004).

Not Effective

No applicable published research was found in this category.

Possibly Harmful

No applicable published research was found in this category.

OUTCOME MEASUREMENT

HEALTH-SEEKING BEHAVIOR   **NOC**

Definition: Personal actions to promote optimal wellness, recovery, and rehabilitation.
Health-Seeking Behavior as evidenced by the following selected NOC indicators:
• Seeks assistance from health care professionals when indicated
• Describes strategies to eliminate unhealthy behavior
• Adheres to self-developed strategies to eliminate unhealthy behavior
• Performs prescribed health behavior when indicated
• Seeks current health-related information
• Describes strategies to maximize health
• Adheres to self-developed strategies to maximize health
(Rate each indicator of **Health-Seeking Behavior:** 1 = never demonstrated, 2 = rarely demonstrated, 3 = sometimes demonstrated, 4 = often demonstrated, 5 = consistently demonstrated) (Moorhead et al., 2004.)

RCT = Randomized Controlled (Clinical) Trial, **NIC** = Nursing Interventions Classification, **NOC** = Nursing Outcomes Classification

REFERENCES

Allen JK. (2000). Cholesterol management: An opportunity for nurse case managers. *J Cardiovasc Nurs*, 14(2):50-58.

American College of Sports Medicine (ACSM). (2004). Physical activity programs and behavior counseling in older adult populations. *Med Sci Sports Exerc*, 36(11):1997-2003.

Burgard M, Gallagher KI. (2006). Self-monitoring: Influencing effective behavior change in your clients. *ACSMS Health Fitness J*, 10(1):14-19, 37-39.

Burke BL, Arkowitz H, Menchola M. (2003). The efficacy of motivational interviewing: A meta-analysis of controlled clinical trials. *J Consult Clin Psychol*, 71(5):843-861.

Devineni T, Blanchard EB. (2005). A randomized controlled trial of an internet-based treatment for chronic headache. *Behav Res Ther*, 43(3):277-292.

Dochterman JM, Bulechek GM (Eds). (2004). *Nursing Interventions Classification (NIC)*, 4th ed. St. Louis: Mosby.

Doorenbos A, Given B, Given C, Verbitsky N, Cimprich B, McCorkle R. (2005). Reducing symptom limitations: A cognitive behavioral intervention randomized trial. *Psychooncology*, 14(7):574-584.

Ebbert JO, Rowland LC, Montori V, Vickers KS, Erwin PC, Dale LC, et al. (2004). Interventions for smokeless tobacco use cessation. *Cochrane Database Syst Rev*, (3):CD004306.

Edelman S, Lemon J, Kidman A. (2005). Group cognitive behavior therapy for breast cancer patients: A qualitative evaluation. *Psychol Health Med*, 10(2):139-144.

Edinger JD, Wohlgemuth WK, Krystal AD, Rice JR. (2005). Behavioral insomnia therapy for fibromyalgia patients: A randomized clinical trial. *Arch Intern Med*, 165(21):2527-2535.

Glasscoe CA, Quittner AL. (2003). Psychological interventions for cystic fibrosis. *Cochrane Database Syst Rev*, (3):CD003148.

Johnson M, Bulechek G., Butcher H, Dochterman JM, Maas M, Moorhead S, et al (Eds). (2006). *NANDA, NOC, and NIC linkages*, 2nd ed. St. Louis: Mosby.

Joseph DH, Griffin M, Hall RF, Sullivan ED. (2001). Peer coaching: An intervention for individuals struggling with diabetes. *Diabetes Educ*, 27(5):703-710.

Kalichman SC, Rompa D, Cage M, DiFonzo K, Simpson D, Austin J, et al. (2001). Effectiveness of an intervention to reduce HIV transmission risks in HIV-positive people. *Am J Prev Med*, 21(2):84-92.

Khan IJ, Tariq SH. (2004). Urinary incontinence: Behavioral modification therapy in older adult. *Clin Geriatr Med*, 20(3):499-509.

Lamb RJ, Morral AR, Kirby K, Iguchi MY, Galbicka G. (2004). Shaping smoking cessation using percentile schedules. *Drug Alcohol Depend*, 76(3):247-259.

Mayou RA, Thompson DR, Clements A, Davies CH, Goodwin SJ, Normington K, et al. (2002). Guideline-based early rehabilitation after myocardial infarction. A pragmatic randomized controlled trial. *J Psychosom Res*, 52(2):89-95.

Milne J. (2004). Behavioral therapies at the primary care level: The current state of knowledge. *J Wound Ostomy Continence Nurs*, 31(6):367-376.

Montgomery P, Dennis J. (2003). Cognitive-behavioural interventions for sleep problems in adults aged 60+. *Cochrane Database Syst Rev*, (1):CD003161.

Moorhead M, Johnson M, Maas M (Eds). (2004). *Nursing Outcomes Classification (NOC)*, 3rd ed. St. Louis: Mosby.

Norris SL, Zhang X, Avenell A, Gregg E, Brown TJ, Schmid CH, et al. (2005). Long-term non-pharmacological weight loss interventions for adults with type 2 diabetes mellitus. *Cochrane Database Syst Rev*, (2):CD004095.

Orzano AJ, Scott JG. (2004). Diagnosis and treatment of obesity in adults: An applied evidence-based review. *J Am Board Fam Pract*, 17(5):359-369.

Ostaszkiewicz J, Johnston L, Roe B. (2004). Timed voiding for the management of urinary incontinence in adults. *Cochrane Database Syst Rev*, (1):CD002802.

Pallesen S, Nordhus IH, Kvale G, Nielsen GH, Havik OE, Johnsen BH, et al. (2003). Behavioral treatment of insomnia in older adults: An open clinical trial comparing two interventions. *Behav Res Ther*, 41(1):31-48.

Perlis ML, Smith MT, Cacialli DO, Nowakowski S, Orff H. (2003). On the comparability of pharmacotherapy and behavior therapy for chronic insomnia. Commentary and implications. *J Psychosom Res*, 54(1):51-59.

Proctor ML, Farquhar CM. (2006). Dymenorrhoea. *Clin Evid*, (15):2429-2448.

Ratner D. (2002). The triangulation of telehealth, e-health and incentive-based behavioral modification: A model for the future. *Care Management*, 8(2):36-39.

Rice VH, Stead LF. (2004). Nursing interventions for smoking cessation. *Cochrane Database Syst Rev*, (1): CD001188.

Rivera E, Walsh A, Bradley M. (2000). Using behavior modification to promote wound healing. *Home Healthc Nurse*, 18(9):579-586.

Shaw K, O'Rourke P, Del Mar C, Kenardy J. (2005). Psychological interventions for overweight or obesity. *Cochrane Database Syst Rev*, (2):CD003818.

Sherwood P, Given BA, Champion VL, Doorenbos AZ, Kozachik S, Wagler-Ziner K, et al. (2005). A cognitive behavioral intervention for symptom management in patients with advanced cancer. *Oncol Nurs Forum*, 32(6):1190-1198.

Sinclair VG, Scroggie J. (2005). Effects of a cognitive-behavioral program for women with multiple sclerosis. *J Neurosci Nurs*, 37(5):249-257, 276.

Stead LF, Lancaster T. (2005). Group behaviour therapy programmes for smoking cessation. *Cochrane Database Syst Rev*, (2):CD001007.

Suplee PD. (2005). The importance of providing smoking relapse counseling during the postpartum hospitalization. *J Obstet Gynecol Neonatal Nurs*, 34(6):703-712.

Thorogood M, Hillsdon M, Summerbell C. (2004). Cardiovascular disorders. Changing behaviour. *Clin Evid*, (12):85-114.

van Tulder M, Koes B. (2003). Low back pain and sciatica (chronic). *Clin Evid*, (10):1359-1376.

Wakefield M, Olver I, Whitford H, Rosenfeld E. (2004). Motivational interviewing as a smoking cessation intervention for patients with cancer: Randomized controlled trial. *Nurs Res*, 53(6):396-405.

Wang M, Wang S, Tsai P. (2005). Cognitive behavioral therapy for primary insomnia: A systematic review. *J Adv Nurs*, 50(5):553-564.

Wyman JF. (2003). Treatment of urinary incontinence in men and older women: The evidence shows the efficacy of a variety of techniques. *Am J Nurs*, (Suppl):26-35.

Wyman JF. (2005). Behavioral interventions for the patient with overactive bladder. *J Wound Ostomy Continence Nurs*, 32(3 Suppl 1):S11-S15.

BLADDER TRAINING

Jill Milne, PhD, RN

Definition: Voiding according to a progressive schedule that gradually increases the interval between voids, ideally until a voiding pattern of every 3 to 4 hours is reached.

Although bladder training is generally used to treat symptoms of overactive bladder (frequency, urgency, urge incontinence), bladder training may also be helpful for stress and mixed incontinence (Wallace et al., 2004; Wyman et al., 1998).

NURSING ACTIVITIES

Effective

■ *Teach individuals who are motivated and cognitively intact to void according to a schedule (whether they feel the need to empty their bladders or not) to reflect initially their maximum voiding interval at baseline. Gradually increase the time between voidings, often by 30 minutes per week, as tolerated. Use*

*urge suppression strategies, such as counting backward from 100 by 7
and performing five quick contractions of the pelvic floor muscles, self-
monitoring with a voiding diary, and education about healthy bladder habits.*
LOE = II

(NR) A Cochrane systematic review to assess the impact of bladder training on urinary incontinence found that the strategy appeared to be helpful, but reviewers noted that trials have been limited and sample sizes have been small (Wallace et al., 2004).

(NR) In a quasi-experimental study involving 16 community-dwelling women with urinary incontinence aged 64 to 88 years who participated in 4 weeks of bladder training, voiding schedules were individualized on the basis of pretreatment voiding diaries. Participants received weekly phone calls from researchers to assess progress. There was a significant reduction in incontinent episodes at treatment completion, which was maintained at 6-month follow-up (Publicover & Bear, 1997).

(MR) In an RCT of women aged 55 years and older with urethral sphincter incompetence ($N = 88$) or overactive bladder ($N = 35$), bladder training reduced the frequency of incontinence by approximately 57% and reduced the amount of urine lost by approximately 54% (Fantl et al., 1991).

(MR) An RCT compared the effects of a 12-week program of (1) bladder training, (2) pelvic floor muscle exercise, and (3) combined therapy in women with stress incontinence, detrusor instability, or both. Based on the number of incontinence episodes per week, 69% of women in the bladder training group were cured or at least 50% improved at treatment completion and 57% had maintained this improvement at 3-month follow-up. Those in the pelvic floor exercise group had comparable results. Although significantly more women who received the combined therapy were cured or improved at treatment end, this difference was not maintained at the 3-month follow-up. Of particular note, adherence to scheduled voidings decreased from 85% at treatment completion to 44% at 3-month follow-up in the bladder training group (Wyman et al., 1998).

(MR) In a quasi-experimental trial in which women with overactive bladders were randomly assigned to groups receiving medication (oxybutynin) ($N = 42$) or bladder training ($N = 39$), after 6 weeks of treatment the majority in both groups were clinically cured (74% and 73%, respectively). However, 70% of women in the bladder training group had maintained this improvement 6 months later compared with only 42% of the medication group (Colombo et al., 1995).

Possibly Effective

No applicable published research was found in this category.

Not Effective

No applicable published research was found in this category.

Possibly Harmful

No applicable published research was found in this category.

NR = Nursing Research, **MR** = Multidisciplinary Research, **SP** = Standard of Practice, **EO** = Expert Opinion, **LOE** = Level of Evidence

OUTCOME MEASUREMENT

URINARY CONTINENCE

Definition: Control of elimination of urine from the bladder.

Urinary Continence as evidenced by the following selected NOC indicators:

- Maintains predictable pattern of voiding
- Responds to urge in timely manner
- Gets to toilet between urge and passage of urine
- Starts and stops stream
- Ingests adequate amount of fluid

(Rate each indicator of **Urinary Continence:** 1 = never demonstrated, 2 = rarely demonstrated, 3 = sometimes demonstrated, 4 = often demonstrated, 5 = consistently demonstrated) (Moorhead et al., 2004).

REFERENCES

Colombo M, Zanzetta G, Scalambrino S, Milani R. (1995). Oxybutynin and bladder training in the management of female urinary urge incontinence: A randomized study. *Int Urogynecol J,* 6(2):63-67.

Fantl JA, Wyman JF, McClish DK, Harkins SW, Elswick RK, Taylor JR, et al. (1991). Efficacy of bladder training in older women with urinary incontinence. *JAMA,* 265(5):609-613.

Moorhead M, Johnson M, Maas M (Eds). (2004). *Nursing Outcomes Classification (NOC),* 3rd ed. St. Louis: Mosby.

Publicover C, Bear M. (1997). The effect of bladder training on urinary incontinence in community-dwelling older women. *J Wound Ostomy Continence Nurs,* 24(6):319-324.

Wallace SA, Roe B, Williams K, Palmer M. (2004). Bladder training for urinary incontinence in adults. *Cochrane Database Syst Rev,* (1):CD001308.

Wyman JF, Fantl JA, McClish DK, Bump RC. (1998). Comparative efficacy of behavioral interventions in the management of female urinary incontinence. Continence Program for Women Research Group. *Am J Obstet Gynecol,* 179(4):999-1007.

 # BLOOD PRODUCTS ADMINISTRATION   NIC

Deborah Pool, MS, RN, CCRN

NIC Definition: Administration of blood or blood products and monitoring of patient's response (Dochterman & Bulechek, 2004).

NURSING ACTIVITIES

Effective

■ **NIC** **SP** *Verify the physician's orders.* **LOE = VII**

 Recheck the physician's order, and verify any special processing (i.e., leukocyte reduction) if required (Wooldridge-King, 2005; Davis et al., 2006).

RCT = Randomized Controlled (Clinical) Trial, **NIC** = Nursing Interventions Classification, **NOC** = Nursing Outcomes Classification

■ **NIC** **SP** *Obtain the patient's transfusion history.* **LOE = VII**

EO Patients who have received multiple blood transfusions or who have experienced transfusion reactions previously are more likely to experience a transfusion reaction than patients who have received few or no transfusions (Wooldridge-King, 2005; Bradbury & Cruickshank, 2000; McConnell, 1997).

■ **NIC** **SP** *Obtain or verify the patient's informed consent.* **LOE = IV**

EO Recipients of blood products (nonemergently) are required to be educated about the risks and benefits of transfusions, and written consent is required before administration of blood products (JCAHO, 2003; Simmons, 2003; CDHS, 1999).

MR In a prospective cohort study ($N = 61$), 53 participants indicated that written information about transfusion therapy was helpful in understanding the procedure (Wargon et al., 2002).

■ **NIC** **SP** *Assemble the administration system with the filter appropriate for the blood product and the recipient's immune status. Prime the administration system with isotonic saline.* **LOE = VII**

EO Intravenous solutions other than isotonic saline may result in hemolysis (dextrose-containing solutions) or alterations in coagulation (lactated Ringer's solution) (Cheever et al., 2006; Wooldridge-King, 2005).

■ **SP** *Change the administration set and filter every 12 hours or after every fourth unit of blood.* **LOE = VII**

EO Change the administration set at least every 12 hours or more frequently if blood is administered in a very warm climate (WHO, 2002).

■ **SP** *Perform venipuncture using an 18- to 20-gauge catheter as appropriate to administer blood.* **LOE = VII**

EO Blood products may be administered through peripheral intravenous sites or central lines, but catheters less than 20 gauge result in slow transfusion rates (Fitzpatrick & Fitzpatrick, 1997; McConnell, 1997).

■ **NIC** **SP** *Verify the correct patient, blood type, Rh type, unit number, and expiration date; and record per agency protocol.* **LOE = V**

EO Final identification check of blood products should be at the bedside of the patient and should be done by two RNs comparing patient's identity, date of birth, blood type, and gender against both the blood product and the patient's wristband from the blood bank. Identifying information on the blood product label must be identical to the information on the wristband of the recipient (Davis et al., 2006; Wooldridge-King, 2005; Beyea & Majewski, 2003; WHO, 2002; Gray & Murphy, 2000).

MR In two nonrandomized quality improvement studies consisting of questionnaires and observations in 217 institutions ($N = 1,757,730$), errors in wristband identification were found in 45,197 wristbands—a mean error rate of 7.4%. The most common error (71%) was the absence of a blood bank wristband (Howanitz et al., 2002).

MR An audit of all transfusion errors related to administration of blood to other than the intended recipient reported in New York from 1990 to 1998 found that 1.8 million transfusions were administered with 92 cases of erroneous transfusions; 43% of instances were due

NR = Nursing Research, **MR** = Multidisciplinary Research, **SP** = Standard of Practice, **EO** = Expert Opinion, **LOE** = Level of Evidence

to failure to identify the patient prior to transfusion. Remaining errors were related to the phlebotomist (11%), the blood bank (25%), or other hospital services (Linden et al., 2000).

(MR) In two separate nonrandomized quality improvement audit studies in 1994 and 2000, 16,494 total transfusions in 660 hospitals were audited by blood bank personnel. Four components of identification were reviewed. In 1994, all four were present in 62.3% of transfusions, and in 2000, they were present in 25.04%. The most likely error was lack of comparison of the recipient's stated name and the identification wristband (Novis et al., 2003).

(MR) In a continuous quality improvement study performed for 3 months at one site, all transfusion episodes ($N = 85$) were evaluated to determine whether procedures were being followed; 16 of 85 instances were noted to have variance in identification of the recipients (as noted in the hospital policy) at the bedside (Shulman et al., 1999).

■ (SP) ***Administer the blood product within 30 minutes of its retrieval from the blood bank. If a delay occurs, return the product to the blood bank. Do not store in the refrigerator on the nursing unit.* LOE = VII**

(EO) Blood bank refrigeration units are calibrated and closely maintained to prevent bacterial growth in blood products. Improper refrigeration or storage may result in contamination, excess hemolysis, and sepsis. Blood not maintained properly should be discarded (Wooldridge-King, 2005; WHO, 2002; Fitzpatrick & Fitzpatrick, 1997; Nursing, 1996).

■ (NIC) (SP) ***Refrain from administering IV medications or fluids, other than isotonic saline, into the blood or blood product lines.* LOE = VII**

(EO) Another intravenous line should be started to administer other fluids or medications while blood products are being infused (Simmons, 2003; WHO, 2002).

■ (NIC) (SP) ***Refrain from transfusing product removed from controlled refrigeration for more than 4 hours.* LOE = VII**

(EO) The risk of bacterial proliferation, loss of red blood cell function, or increased hemolysis increases with the length of time the blood product is at ambient temperature. If the transfusion is not completed within 4 hours, the remainder of the unit should be discarded (Wooldridge-King, 2005; Simmons, 2003; WHO, 2002).

■ (SP) ***Monitor the patient for transfusion reactions such as urticaria, flushing, chills, fever, change in level of consciousness, chest or flank pain, tachycardia, hypotension, new-onset cough, difficulty breathing, or signs of fluid overload. In the event a transfusion reaction is suspected, immediately remove the blood product and all IV tubing; replace with isotonic saline utilizing new tubing, and infuse to keep the vein open; notify the blood bank and the physician immediately. With minor reactions such as fever or headache, stop the infusion and notify the blood bank and physician for further direction.* LOE = VII**

(EO) Acute reactions occur in 1% to 2% of transfused patients. Severe transfusion reactions are most likely to occur during the first 15 minutes of infusion. Patients should be monitored closely during this time to facilitate early recognition of potentially life-threatening complications (Gray et al., 2005; Simmons, 2003; WHO, 2002; Young, 2000; Sazama et al., 2000).

(MR) A meta-analysis suggested that the incidence of blood transfusion reactions was 43.2 per 100,000 red blood cells ($N = 337$ recipients); the most likely severe reactions were acute hemolytic transfusion reaction and volume overload (Kleinman et al., 2003).

RCT = Randomized Controlled (Clinical) Trial, **NIC** = Nursing Interventions Classification, **NOC** = Nursing Outcomes Classification

■ (SP) *Monitor vital signs immediately before administering blood, baseline, 15 minutes after initiation of transfusion, every 15 to 60 minutes during the infusion of the blood product, when the infusion is completed, and 4 hours after completion of the transfusion.* **LOE = VII**

(EO) Begin the transfusion slowly; the first 20 to 30 mL of blood should be given over a 15-minute period. The most likely time for a reaction to occur is during the first 15 minutes after beginning the transfusion. Immediate reactions are the cause of more than 50% of transfusion-related deaths. The infusion of 10 to 15 mL of blood may be sufficient to initiate a potentially life-threatening reaction (Gray et al., 2005; WHO, 2002; Bradbury & Cruickshank, 2000).

■ (SP) *Document the date and time the infusion was started, the staff member who verified the recipient's identification, the blood product administered, the amount administered, the time the transfusion was completed, and the patient's response to the treatment.* **LOE = VII**

(EO) It is crucial to document each step of the transfusion process for both the patient's safety and verification of blood products. Transfusion reactions may occur as long as 5 to 10 days after the transfusion, and documentation is key in determining the events. Careful documentation also allows monitoring of transfusion therapy, which is mandated by regulatory agencies such as The Joint Commission (WHO, 2002; Bradbury & Cruickshank, 2000; Gray & Murphy, 2000; Fitzpatrick & Fitzpatrick, 1997).

■ (SP) *Use a blood warmer as ordered for large transfusions in adults (>50 mL/kg/ hr) or patients with significant cold agglutinins.* **LOE = VII**

(EO) At rapid infusion rates (>100 mL/min), the cold temperature of the blood may contribute to cardiac dysrhythmia or arrest. There is no evidence that warming the blood is beneficial at slower transfusion rates. Blood should be warmed only in a blood warmer specifically designed for this purpose; the warmer has a visible thermometer and temperature alarm. Use of non-regulated devices such as a water bath or microwave may result in hemolysis (Simmons, 2003; WHO, 2002; Sazama et al., 2000; Nerlich, 1998).

■ (SP) *Instruct the recipient to notify nursing staff at once if he or she experiences any untoward reaction to the transfusion such as chills, fever, headache, backache, chest pain, itching, difficulty breathing, or palpitations.* **LOE = VII**

(EO) Recipients may experience subjective symptoms of an acute hemolytic transfusion reaction or allergic-type reaction before there is a change in vital signs. This may be an early indicator of a possibly life-threatening condition (WHO, 2002; McConnell, 1997; Gray et al., 2005).

Possibly Effective

No applicable published research was found in this category.

Not Effective

No applicable published research was found in this category.

NR = Nursing Research, **MR** = Multidisciplinary Research, **SP** = Standard of Practice, **EO** = Expert Opinion, **LOE** = Level of Evidence

Possibly Harmful

No applicable published research was found in this category.

OUTCOME MEASUREMENT

BLOOD TRANSFUSION REACTION NOC

(Please refer to *Nursing Outcomes Classifications* [Moorhead et al., 2004] for the **Blood Transfusion Reaction** outcome.)

REFERENCES

Beyea SC, Majewski C. (2003). Blood transfusion in the OR—Are you practicing safely? *AORN J*, 78(6):1007-1010.

Bradbury M, Cruickshank JP. (2000). Blood transfusion: Crucial steps in maintaining safe practice. *Br J Nurs*, 9(3):134-138

California Department of Health Services (CDHS) in conjunction with Medical Technical Advisory Committee of the Blood Centers of California. (1999). *A Patient's Guide to Blood Transfusions Information Sheet*. Sacramento, California.

Cheever KH, Dooling E, Hagler D, Hodges M, Keuth J, Pool D, et al. (2006). Therapeutic modalities. In Stillwell SB (Ed): *Mosby's Critical Care Nursing Reference*, 4th ed. St. Louis: Mosby, pp 585-590.

Davis K, Hui CH, Quested B. (2006). Transfusing safely: A 2006 guide for nurses. *Aust Nurs J*, 13(6):17-20.

Dochterman JM, Bulechek GM (Eds). (2004). *Nursing Outcomes Classification (NIC)*, 4th ed. St. Louis: Mosby.

Fitzpatrick L. (2002). Blood products. *Nursing*, 32(5):36-42.

Fitzpatrick L, Fitzpatrick T. (1997). Blood transfusion: Keeping your patient safe. *Nursing*, 27(8):34-41.

Gray A, Howell C, Pirie E. (2005). Improving blood transfusion: A patient-centred approach. *Nurs Stand*, 19(26):38-42.

Gray S, Murphy M. (2000). Guidelines for administering blood and blood components. *Nurs Stand*, 14(13-15):36-39.

Howanitz PJ, Renner SW, Walsh MK. (2002). Continuous wristband monitoring over 2 years decreases identification errors: A College of American Pathologists Q-Tracks Study. *Arch Pathol Lab Med*, 126(7):809-815.

Joint Commission for the Accreditation of Healthcare Organizations (JCAHO). (2003). *Comprehensive Accreditation Manual*. Oakbrook Terrace, IL: JCAHO.

Kleinman S, Chan P, Robillard P. (2003). Risks associated with transfusion of cellular blood components in Canada. *Transfus Med Rev*, 17(2):120-162.

Linden JV, Wagner K, Voytovich AE, Sheehan J. (2000). Transfusion errors in New York State: An analysis of 10 years' experience. *Transfusion*, 40(10):1207-1213.

McConnell EA. (1997). Safely administering a blood transfusion. *Nursing*, 27(6):30.

Moorhead M, Johnson M, Maas M (Eds). (2004). *Nursing Outcomes Classification (NOC)*, 3rd ed. St. Louis: Mosby

Nerlich S. (1998). Blood transfusion. *Aust Nurs J*, 5(11):Suppl i-iv.

Novis DA, Miller KA, Howanitz PJ, Renner SW, Walsh MK, College of American Pathologists. (2003). Audit of transfusion procedures in 660 hospitals: A College of American Pathologists Q-Probes study of patient identification and vital sign monitoring frequencies in 16,494 transfusions. *Arch Pathol Lab Med*, 127(5):541-548.

Sazama K, DeChristopher PJ, Dodd R, Harrison CR, Shulman IA, Cooper ES, et al. (2000). Practice parameter for recognition, management and prevention of adverse consequences of blood transfusion. *Arch Pathol Lab Med*, 124(1):61-70.

Shulman IA, Saxena S, Ramer L. (1999). Assessing blood administration practices. *Arch Pathol Lab Med,* 123(7):595-598.

Simmons P. (2003). A primer for nurses who administer blood products. *Medsurg Nurs,* 12(3):184-190.

Wargon C, Kunz V, Pibarot ML, Ozier Y, Rieux C, Benbunan M, et al. (2002). Evaluation of an information document about patients and transfusion. *Ann Fr Anesth Reanim,* 21(3):198-204.

Wooldridge-King M. (2005). Blood and blood component administration. In Wiegand DJ, Carlson KK (Eds): *AACN Procedure Manual for Critical Care,* 5th ed. St. Louis: Saunders.

World Health Organization (WHO). (2002). *The Clinical Use of Blood Handbook.* Geneva: WHO Blood Transfusion Safety, p 77.

Young J. (2000). Transfusion reaction. *Nursing,* 30(12):33.

BODY IMAGE ENHANCEMENT

Dale A. Nasby, MA, MS, RN, CNS

> NIC **Definition:** Improving a patient's conscious and unconscious perceptions and attitudes toward his/her body (Dochterman & Bulechek, 2004).

NURSING ACTIVITIES

Effective

■ *Engage in regular physical activity.* **LOE = I**

 A meta-analysis (*N* = 121) found that exercise was associated with a more positive body image and people who exercised regularly had a better body image than nonexercisers. Furthermore, participants in studies who received an exercise intervention reported an improvement in body image whereas the control groups did not (Hausenblas & Fallon, 2006).

 A pretest/post-test quasi-experimental study (*N* = 44) found that both men and women who participated in a 12-week strength training program experienced a statistically significant improvement in body image satisfaction (Ginis et al., 2005).

 A systematic review (*N* = 34) examined the effectiveness of exercise in improving the psychological well-being (including body image) of cancer patients during and after treatment and found that cancer patients may benefit from physical exercise, although the specific benefits of exercise may vary as a function of the stage of the illness, the nature of the medical treatment received, and the lifestyle of the patient (Knols et al., 2005).

 A randomized crossover control study found that a movement and dance program improved quality of life, body image, and shoulder function in women with breast cancer (Sandel et al., 2005).

 A descriptive study (*N* = 56) found a positive relationship between regular participation in physical activity and body image among lower limb amputees (Wetterhahn et al., 2002).

■ *Provide cognitive-behavioral therapy (CBT).* **LOE = V**

 A meta-analysis (*N* = 19) found that CBT was effective in improving body image (Jarry & Ip, 2005).

NR = Nursing Research, **MR** = Multidisciplinary Research, **SP** = Standard of Practice, **EO** = Expert Opinion, **LOE** = Level of Evidence

Possibly Effective

■ *Actively listen and encourage the patient's input to promote the patient's decision making and enhance coping with altered body image.* **LOE = V**

(NR) A systematic review of nursing literature ($N = 14$) regarding the psychological and social impact of a stoma on people's lives led to the following recommendations: nurses should provide opportunities for open and honest communication with patients, encourage them to express their feelings, refer them to counseling if needed, and promote patients' participation in decision making to improve coping with an altered body image (Brown & Randle, 2005).

(MR) A longitudinal cohort study ($N = 563$) of women with stage 1 or 2 breast cancer found that women who participated in the decision-making process regarding their treatment had a better body image than those who did not. However, if a woman's preference for treatment was different from the type of treatment actually received, body image was adversely affected (Figueiredo et al., 2004).

■ *Provide support and reassurance to patients to improve coping with altered body image.* **LOE = VI**

(NR) A qualitative study described nursing practices regarding when and how patients look at their burn injuries and identified the qualitative themes that influenced patients' responses to this event. The themes that emerged included reading and waiting for patients' nonverbal cues indicating that the patients were ready to look at wounds; using silence, presence of self, encouragement, and emotional support to help patients deal with the injury; and responding to patients in a positive, honest, and hopeful manner (Birdsall & Weinberg, 2001).

(NR) A review of the nursing literature described the psychosocial issues (including altered body image) in women with ovarian cancer and recommended that nurses educate patients on the potential impact of the visible side effects of chemotherapy, listen to patients' stories and experiences, and refer patients to a support group or other counseling as needed (Fitch, 2003).

Not Effective

■ *Use of videotape intervention on body image and self-esteem for patients with chemotherapy-induced alopecia.* **LOE = II**

(NR) In a prospective randomized study ($N = 136$), women with chemotherapy-induced alopecia, a mean age of 57.7 years, and advanced disease at study entry were allocated randomly to view a videotape intervention on body image and self-esteem. The study results support prior studies that have reported changes in body image as a result of chemotherapy-induced alopecia. The intervention employed (a videotape) was not effective (Nolte et al., 2006).

Possibly Harmful

No applicable published research was found in this category.

RCT = Randomized Controlled (Clinical) Trial, **NIC** = Nursing Interventions Classification, **NOC** = Nursing Outcomes Classification

OUTCOME MEASUREMENT

BODY IMAGE

(Please refer to *Nursing Outcomes Classification* [Moorhead et al., 2004] for the **Body Image** outcome.)

REFERENCES

Birdsall C, Weinberg K. (2001). Adult patients looking at their burn injuries for the first time. *J Burn Care Rehabil*, 22(5):360-364.

Brown H, Randle J. (2005). Living with a stoma: A review of the literature. *J Clin Nurs*, 14(1):74-81.

Dochterman JM, Bulechek GM (Eds). (2004). *Nursing Interventions Classification (NIC)*, 4th ed. St. Louis: Mosby.

Figueiredo MI, Cullen J, Hwang YT, Rowland JH, Mandelblatt JS. (2004). Breast cancer treatment in older women: Does getting what you want improve your long-term body image and mental health? *J Clin Oncol*, 22(19):4002-4009.

Fitch MI. (2003). Psychosocial management of patients with recurrent ovarian cancer: Treating the whole patient to improve quality of life. *Semin Oncol Nurs*, 19(3 Suppl 1):40-53.

Ginis KA, Eng JJ, Arbour KP, Hartman JW, Phillips SM. (2005). Mind over muscle? Sex differences in the relationship between body image change and subjective and objective physical changes following a 12-week strength-training program. *Body Image*, 2(4):363-372.

Hausenblas HA, Fallon EA. (2006). Exercise and body image: A meta-analysis. *Psychol Health*, 21(1):33-47.

Jarry JL, Ip K. (2005). The effectiveness of stand-alone cognitive behavioural therapy for body image: A meta-analysis. *Body Image*, 2(4):317-331.

Knols R, Aaronson NK, Uebelhart D, Fransen J, Aufdemkampe G. (2005). Physical exercise in cancer patients during and after medical treatment: A systematic review of randomized and controlled clinical trials. *J Clin Oncol*, 23(16):3830-3842.

Moorhead M, Johnson M, Maas M (Eds). (2004). *Nursing Outcomes Classification (NOC)*, 3rd ed. St. Louis: Mosby.

Nolte S, Donnelly J, Kelly S, Conley P, Cobb R. (2006). A randomized clinical trial of a videotape intervention for women with chemotherapy-induced alopecia: A gynecologic oncology group study, *Oncol Nurs Forum*, 33(2):305-311.

Sandel SL, Judge JO, Landry N, Faria L, Ouellette R, Majczak M. (2005). Dance and movement program improves quality-of-life measures in breast cancer survivors. *Cancer Nurs*, 28(4):301-309.

Wetterhahn KA, Hanson C, Levy CE. (2002). Effect of participation in physical activity on body image of amputees. *Am J Phys Med Rehabil*, 81(3):194-201.

BOWEL INCONTINENCE CARE

Phyllis Meyer Gaspar, PhD, RN

Co-Authors: Students Enrolled in the Master's Program in Nursing at Winona State University—Erin Anderson, Katrina Beckman, Debra Coy, Virginia Darling, Jennifer Drier, Kevin Elker, Amanda Hanson, Nancy Harris, Andrea Hauser, Danyel Helgeson, Adam Holland, Sarah Hunt, Patricia Jensen, Mary Kasel, Tanya Kehren, Chelsey Kolbet, Elizabeth Larsen, John Laymon, Hilaree Lore, Mark Outzen, Denise Rollmann, Jeremy Ronneberg, Kelly Scherger, Melinda Seifers, Lisa Stark, Katie Young, Rebekah Zinnecker

NIC **Definition:** Promotion of bowel continence and maintenance of perianal skin integrity (Dochterman & Bulechek, 2004).

NR = Nursing Research, **MR** = Multidisciplinary Research, **SP** = Standard of Practice, **EO** = Expert Opinion, **LOE** = Level of Evidence

NURSING ACTIVITIES

Effective

- ■ *Use barrier products on perianal area after cleansing.* **LOE = II**

  (NR) A prospective randomized study ($N = 40$) demonstrated that 3M barrier film (Cavilon NSBF) was more cost effective and resulted in faster healing rates than zinc oxide oil among incontinent adults (Baatenburg de Jong & Admiraal, 2004).

  (NR) A quasi-experimental pretest/post-test study ($N = 136$) demonstrated a significant reduction in stage I and II pressure ulcers with the use of body wash and protectant (Hunter et al., 2003).

  (NR) A review of 20 published studies (only two specific to the use of barrier creams) demonstrated support for the use of barrier creams (Hughes, 2002).

  (NR) A prospective descriptive study ($N = 31$) demonstrated that nonrinse cleanser and barrier cream were more effective for skin conditions related to urinary and bowel incontinence than soap, water, and lotion, but the results were not statistically significant (Lewis-Byers & Thayer, 2002).

  (NR) A quasi-experimental noncontrolled design ($N = 19$) demonstrated that a cleanser-protectant combination was effective in lessening pain and erythema after 7 days and cost effective for breakdown in low-risk incontinent patients (Warshaw et al., 2002).

  Additional research: Nix & Ermer-Seltun, 2004; Byers et al., 1995.

- ■ *Use incontinence pads, diapers, and/or sanitary pads as appropriate.* **LOE = II**

  (NR) A descriptive survey ($N = 242$ elderly people) reported that the most common self-care practice for fecal incontinence was wearing a sanitary panty liner, pad, or brief (Bliss et al., 2005).

  (NR) A laboratory model experiment showed that smoothed absorbent pads placed patients at less risk for pressure ulcers than wrinkled or wet pads (Fader et al., 2004).

  (NR) A crossover design study ($N = 78$ women older than 65) reported no differences in erythema or pH with pad changing frequency. However, less frequent pad changes resulted in more risk for pressure ulcers (Fader et al., 2003).

  (NR) A literature review of a number of controlled trials reported that continence aids helped reduce skin problems and promote quality of life for vulnerable adults (Hughes, 2002).

  (MR) A meta-analysis (Cochrane systematic review) of six randomized and quasi-randomized controlled trials ($N = 415$) reported that disposable products may be more effective for fecal incontinence management, but data and quality limited evidence (Brazzelli et al., 2002).

  Additional research: Brown, 1994; Leiby & Shanahan, 1994.

- ■ **NIC** **SP** *Keep bed and clothing clean.* **LOE = II**

  (NR) A controlled, prospective RCT ($N = 107$) supported the idea that a clean, dry environment was possible and contributed to skin integrity (Leiby & Shanahan, 1994).

- ■ **SP** *Monitor defecation and bowel patterns.* **LOE = VII**

  (EO) A "defecation diary" that includes volume, consistency, time, and voluntary or involuntary nature of stools may be helpful (Demata, 2000).

RCT = Randomized Controlled (Clinical) Trial, **NIC** = Nursing Interventions Classification, **NOC** = Nursing Outcomes Classification

(NR) A prospective study ($N = 152$) found fecal incontinence a common problem among hospitalized patients who were acutely ill, but the condition was not associated with a specific cause, indicating the need for frequent assessment (Bliss et al., 2000).

(EO) To help patients achieve and maintain their personal maximum fecal continence, use sensory retraining and have the patient keep a diary of output as well as factors influencing output (Bentsen & Braun, 1996).

Possibly Effective

■ (SP) *Provide the patient or caregiver with education on etiology, bowel management procedures, and expected outcomes that reflect mutually agreed-on goals.* **LOE = III**

(NR) A quasi-experimental study of home caregivers ($N = 40$) of patients with dementia demonstrated that education intervention was effective in increasing low levels of knowledge related to strategies for management of fecal incontinence (Clemesha & Davies, 2004).

(NR) A review of the literature indicated that it was the nurse's responsibility to provide support and information to patients with fecal incontinence and their families and to ensure that they understood the causes and treatment regimens available (Boyd-Carson, 2003).

(EO) Set mutually agreed-upon goals and outcomes with the patient and family, and include an education component for all aspects of the management approach (Demata, 2000).

(EO) To help patients achieve and maintain their personal maximum fecal continence, use sensory retraining including education on the neurophysiology and pathophysiology of incontinence, purpose of the retraining program, and procedures (Bentsen & Braun, 1996).

(MR) An RCT to evaluate the effect of a nursing educational/assessment session that included targeted education for stroke patients ($N = 146$) found the intervention effective in improving symptoms of bowel dysfunction, changing bowel-modifying lifestyle behaviors, and influencing patients' interaction with health care providers (Harari et al., 2004).

■ (NIC) *Use nonionic detergent preparations, such as Peri-Wash, for cleansing, as appropriate.* **LOE = III**

(NR) An RCT ($N = 93$) demonstrated that soap and water maintained skin integrity in 37% of patients and Clinisan maintained skin integrity in 66% of patients (Cooper & Gray, 2001).

(NR) A controlled design study ($N = 29$) indicated that Clinisan was superior to Triple Care and soap and water for cleansing as it improved skin condition, saved time, and was cost saving (Whittingham & May, 1998).

■ (NIC) *Implement a bowel training program as appropriate.* **LOE = III**

(MR) An RCT demonstrated that a nursing educational/assessment session for stroke patients ($N = 146$) was effective in improving symptoms of bowel dysfunction, changing bowel-modifying lifestyle behaviors, and influencing patients' interaction with health care providers, but there was no difference in frequency of fecal incontinence (Harari et al., 2004).

(EO) A bowel management program should be implemented in patients with persistent constipation or bowel incontinence (DVA/DOD, 2003).

(MR) A descriptive study ($N = 498$) demonstrated that only danthron (laxative) was positively associated with fecal incontinence and enemas and suppositories were negatively associated with fecal incontinence (Brocklehurst et al., 1999).

NR = Nursing Research, **MR** = Multidisciplinary Research, **SP** = Standard of Practice, **EO** = Expert Opinion, **LOE** = Level of Evidence

(MR) A controlled study using a one-group pretest/post-test design (*N* = 165) demonstrated that prompted voiding intervention resulted in an increase in continent bowel movements among nursing home residents (Ouslander & Schnelle, 1995; Demata, 2000).

■ (NIC) *Monitor for adequate bowel evacuation.* **LOE = III**

(EO) A suppository or a tap water enema every morning to cleanse the rectum and distal colon of feces is effective for patients who do not have an abnormally rapid intestinal transit time (Rudolph & Galandiuk, 2002).

(MR) A prospective randomized study (*N* = 206) demonstrated that patients who had complete rectal emptying had 35% fewer episodes of fecal incontinence and 42% fewer incidents of soiled laundry than the rest of the group (Chassagne et al., 2000).

(MR) A descriptive study (*N* = 498) demonstrated that only use of danthron (stimulant laxative) was positively associated with fecal incontinence and enemas and suppositories diminished the occurrence of fecal incontinence (Brocklehurst et al., 1999).

■ *Ensure dietary fiber intake that facilitates continence for the individual.* **LOE = II**

(NR) A phenomenological research methodology design study (*N* = 10) of approaches women used to manage fecal incontinence identified increasing fiber and water intake, eating yogurt, and taking over-the-counter digestive enzymes as effective. Caffeine was shown to increase incontinence by 60% (Hansen et al., 2006).

(NR) A prospective, single-blind RCT (*N* = 39) demonstrated that supplementation with dietary fiber containing psyllium or gum Arabic was associated with a decrease in percentage of incontinent stools and an improvement in stool consistency (Bliss et al., 2001).

■ (NIC) (SP) *Monitor for side effects of medication administration.* **LOE = IV**

(MR) A prospective survey of the prevalence of fecal incontinence (*N* = 6099) identified 585 patients as having fecal incontinence with the odds for fecal incontinence higher if they were taking psychoactive medications (Quander et al., 2005).

(MR) A cohort (*N* = 1187) and case-control study (*N* = 94) found that the use of proton pump inhibitors was independently associated with an increased risk of *Clostridium difficile* diarrhea, with the risk greater among patients taking low-risk antibiotics such as cefazolin than patients taking high-risk antibiotics (Dial et al., 2004).

(MR) A descriptive study (*N* = 498) demonstrated that only danthron was positively associated with decreased fecal incontinence and enemas and suppositories were negatively associated with fecal incontinence (Brocklehurst et al., 1999).

■ *Use intra-anal devices (rectal/anal tubes, trumpets, or plugs) as ordered and appropriate.* **LOE = I**

(MR) A meta-analysis (Cochrane systematic review) of four RCTs and quasi-randomized controlled trials, including crossovers, demonstrated that patients (*N* = 136 age older than 4) with fecal incontinence using the anal plug achieved pseudocontinence if compliant. With a polyurethane plug there was less soiling, a higher feeling of security, and a lower incidence of losing the plug than with a polyvinyl alcohol plug. High dropout rates related to discomfort, not liking the idea, or losing the plug were documented (Deutekom & Dobben, 2005).

RCT = Randomized Controlled (Clinical) Trial, **NIC** = Nursing Interventions Classification, **NOC** = Nursing Outcomes Classification

(MR) A symposium report ($N = 140$ burn patients) indicated that the Zassi BMS system (an invasive tube/balloon and drainage device) was effective for stool containment, decreased rate of infection, increased comfort and dignity, cost savings, and better use of staff time (Echols et al., 2004).

(MR) A clinical trial ($N = 7$) of the Procon incontinence device (a pluglike tube with an occlusive balloon connected to a flatus vent and a sensor that alerts ambulatory users to impending evacuation) demonstrated significant differences in pre- and postincontinence scores and quality of life scores as well as odor control with use. A high attrition rate (61%) was noted (Giamundo et al., 2002).

(MR) A descriptive clinical trial (no statistical analysis) ($N = 32$ age older than 16) of a continent anal plug (a rectal tube–like device used for bedridden patients with intractable diarrhea) showed that it resulted in better fecal containment and improvement in skin integrity (Kim et al., 2001).

Additional research: Grogan & Kramer, 2002; Doherty, 2004.

■ *Use extra-anal devices (rectal pouches or anal bags) as appropriate.* **LOE = V**

(NR) A literature review reported that rectal pouches were noninvasive but could cause dermatitis and could be difficult to adhere (Newman et al., 2004).

(MR) A product evaluation of an anal bag (prospective one-group post-test) ($N = 120$) demonstrated patients' approval of the device as it was comfortable, there was no pain with application, and the patients experienced decreased anxiety about fecal incontinence even when ambulating (Palmieri et al., 2005).

(MR) A methodological report ($N = 5$) demonstrated that stool excretion was contained half the time, serious dermatitis was eliminated, odor control improved for patients, and contact with pressure ulcers decreased with the intermittent use of an anal bag on bedridden patients with pressure ulcers, which was applied after a suppository was given and removed after bowel evacuation (Fujii et al., 2004).

Not Effective

No applicable published research was found in this category.

Possibly Harmful

■ (NIC) *Wash the perianal area with soap and water and dry it thoroughly after each stool.* **LOE = III**

(NR) A prospective descriptive study ($N = 31$) compared the use of soap and water followed by a moisturizing lotion with that of no-rinse liquid cleanser. The results demonstrated that the use of no-rinse cleanser was time and cost effective, and it increased skin improvement and decreased worsening of skin (Lewis-Byers & Thayer, 2002).

(NR) A controlled study ($N = 93$) compared two skin care regimens: (1) soap and water and (2) Clinisan. The study demonstrated that soap and water maintained skin integrity in 37% of the patients and Clinisan maintained skin integrity in 66% of the patients (Cooper & Gray, 2001).

(NR) A crossover control design study ($N = 10$) indicated that a regimen of soap and water alone was less effective than a no-rinse cleanser. Skin effects improved when a moisture barrier was added, but the regimen was not better than a no-rinse cleanser alone (Byers et al., 1995).

NR = Nursing Research, **MR** = Multidisciplinary Research, **SP** = Standard of Practice, **EO** = Expert Opinion, **LOE** = Level of Evidence

OUTCOME MEASUREMENT

BOWEL CONTINENCE (NOC)

(Please refer to *Nursing Outcomes Classification* [Moorhead et al., 2004] for the **Bowel Continence** outcome.)

REFERENCES

Baatenburg de Jong H, Admiraal H. (2004). Comparing cost per use of 3M Cavilon No Sting Barrier Film with zinc oxide oil in incontinent patients. *J Wound Care*, 13(9):398-400.

Bentsen D, Braun JW. (1996). Controlling fecal incontinence with sensory restraining managed by advanced practice nurses. *Clin Nurse Spec*, 10(4):171-5.

Bliss DZ, Fischer LR, Savik K. (2005). Managing fecal incontinence: Self-care practices of older adults. *J Gerontol Nurs*, 31(7):35-44.

Bliss DZ, Johnson S, Savik K, Clabots CR, Gerding DN. (2000). Fecal incontinence in hospitalized patients who are acutely ill. *Nurs Res*, 49(2):101-108.

Bliss DZ, Jung H, Savik K, Lowry A, LeMoine M, Jensen L, et al. (2001). Supplementation with dietary fiber improves fecal incontinence. *Nurs Res*, 50(4):203-213.

Boyd-Carson W. (2003). Faecal incontinence in adults. *Nurs Stand*, 18(8):45-51.

Brazzelli M, Shirran E, Vale L. (2002). Absorbent products for containing urinary and/or fecal incontinence in adults. *J Wound Ostomy Continence Nurs*, 29(1):45-54.

Brocklehurst J, Dickinson E, Windsor J. (1999). Laxatives and faecal incontinence in long-term care. *Nurs Stand*, 13(52):32-36.

Brown DS. (1994). Diapers and underpads, part 1: Skin integrity outcomes. *Ostomy Wound Manage*, 40(9):20-22, 24-26, 28 passim.

Byers PH, Ryan PA, Regan MB, Shields A, Carta SG. (1995). Effects of incontinence care cleansing regimens on skin integrity. *J Wound Ostomy Continence Nurs*, 22(4):187-192.

Chassagne P, Jego A, Gloc P, Capet C, Trivalle C, Doucet J, et al. (2000). Does treatment of constipation improve faecal incontinence in institutionalized elderly patients? *Age Ageing*, 29(2):159-164.

Clemesha L, Davies E. (2004). Educating home carers on faecal continence in people with dementia. *Nurs Stand*, 18(34):33-40.

Cooper P, Gray D. (2001). Comparison of two skin care regimes for incontinence. *Br J Nurs*, 10(6 Suppl): S6, S8, S10 passim.

Demata EU. (2000). Faecal incontinence: Part 3: Nursing management. *World Counc Enterostom Therapists J*, 20(2):12-16.

Department of Veterans Affairs/Department of Defense (DVA/DOD). (2003). *VA/DOD clinical practice guideline for the management of stroke rehabilitation in the primary care setting.* Washington, DC, Department of Veterans Affairs. Available online: www.guideline.gov/.

Deutekom M, Dobben A. (2005). Plugs for containing faecal incontinence. *Cochrane Database Syst Rev*, (3): CD005086.

Dial S, Alrasadi K, Manoukian C, Huang A, Menzies D. (2004). Risk of Clostridium difficile diarrhea among hospital inpatients prescribed proton pump inhibitors: Cohort and case control studies. *CMAJ*, 171(1):33-38.

Dochterman JM, Bulechek GM (Eds). (2004). *Nursing Interventions Classification (NIC)*, 4th ed. St. Louis: Mosby.

Doherty W. (2004). Managing faecal incontinence or leakage: The Peristeen Anal Plug. *Br J Nurs*, 13(21):1293-1297.

Echols J, Friedman B, Mullins RF, Still JM. (2004). *Initial experience with a new system for the control and containment of fecal output for the protection of patients in a large burn center.* Symposium conducted at the meeting of the Jothn A. Boswick, MD, Burn and Wound Care Symposium, Augusta, GA, February 2004.

Fader M, Bain D, Cottenden A. (2004). Effects of absorbent incontinence pads on pressure management mattresses. *J Adv Nurs,* 48(6):569-574.

Fader M, Clarke-O'Neill S, Cook D, Dean G, Brooks R, Cottenden A, et al. (2003). Management of night-time urinary incontinence in residential settings for older people: An investigation into the effects of different pad changing regimes on skin health. *J Clin Nurs,* 12(3):374-386.

Fujii M, Sato TN, Ohrui T, Sato T, Sasaki H. (2004). Interanal stool bag for the bedridden elderly with pressure ulcer. *Geriatr Gerontol Int,* 4:120-122.

Giamundo P, Welber A, Weiss EG, Vernava AM 3rd, Noqueras JJ, Wexner SD. (2002). The procon incontinence device: A new nonsurgical approach to preventing episodes of fecal incontinence. *Am J Gastroenterol,* 97(9):2328-2332.

Grogan TA, Kramer DJ. (2002). The rectal trumpet: Use of a nasopharyngeal airway to contain fecal incontinence in critically ill patients. *J Wound Ostomy Continence Nurs,* 29(4):193-201.

Hansen JL, Bliss DZ, Peden-McAlpine C. (2006). Diet strategies used by women to mange facial incontinence. *J Wound Ostomy Continence Nurs,* 33(1):52-61.

Harari D, Norton C, Lockwood L, Swift C. (2004). Treatment of constipation and fecal incontinence in stroke patients: Randomized controlled trial. *Stroke,* 35(11):2549-2555.

Hughes S. (2002). Do incontinence aids help to maintain skin integrity? *J Wound Care,* 11(6):235-239.

Hunter S, Anderson J, Hanson D, Thompson P, Langemo D, Klug M. (2003). Clinical trial of a prevention and treatment protocol for skin breakdown in two nursing homes. *J Wound Ostomy Continence Nurs,* 30(5):250-258.

Kim J, Shim M, Choi B, Ahn SH, Jang SH, Shin HJ. (2001). Clinical application of continent anal plug in bedridden patients with intractable diarrhea. *Dis Colon Rectum,* 44(8):1162-1167.

Leiby D, Shanahan N. (1994). Clinical study: Assessing the performance and environments of two reusable underpads. *Ostomy Wound Manage,* 40(8):30-32, 34-37.

Lewis-Byers K, Thayer D. (2002). An evaluation of two incontinence skin care protocols in a long-term care setting. *Ostomy Wound Manage,* 48(12):44-51.

Moorhead M, Johnson M, Maas M (Eds). (2004). *Nursing Outcomes Classification (NOC).* 3rd ed. St. Louis: Mosby.

Newman DK, Fader M, Bliss DZ. (2004). Managing incontinence using technology, devices, and products: Directions for research. *Nurs Res,* 53(6 Suppl):S42-S48.

Nix D, Ermer-Seltun J. (2004). A review of perineal skin care protocols and skin barrier product use. *Ostomy Wound Manage,* 50(12):59-67.

Ouslander JG, Schnelle JF. (1995). Incontinence in the nursing home. *Ann Intern Med,* 122(6):438-449.

Palmieri B, Benuzzi G, Bellini N. (2005). The anal bag: A modern approach to fecal incontinence management. *Ostomy Wound Manage,* 51(12):44-52.

Quander CR, Morris MC, Melson J, Bienias JL, Evans DA. (2005). Prevalence of and factors associated with fecal incontinence in a large community study of older individuals. *Am J Gastroenterol,* 100(4):905-909.

Rudolph W, Galandiuk S. (2002). A practical guide to the diagnosis and management of fecal incontinence. *Mayo Clin Proc,* 77(3):271-275.

Warshaw E, Nix D, Kula J, Markon CE. (2002). Clinical and cost effectiveness of a cleanser protectant lotion for treatment of perineal skin breakdown in low-risk patients with incontinence. *Ostomy Wound Manage,* 48(6):44-51.

Whittingham K, May S. (1998). Cleansing regimens for continence care. *Prof Nurse,* 14(3):167-172.

 # BOWEL TRAINING   NIC

Phyllis Meyer Gaspar, PhD, RN

NIC Definition: Assisting the patient to train the bowel to evacuate at specific intervals (Dochterman & Bulechek, 2004).

NR = Nursing Research, **MR** = Multidisciplinary Research, **SP** = Standard of Practice, **EO** = Expert Opinion, **LOE** = Level of Evidence

NURSING ACTIVITIES

Effective

■ **NIC** **SP** *Provide foods high in bulk and/or that have been identified as assistive by the patient.* **LOE = III**

EO Dietary fiber intake should be 25 to 30 g of dietary fiber per day with a gradual increase to this level when fluid intake is between 1500 and 2000 mL per day (RNAO, 2005).

EO An adult's diet should include 20 to 35 g of fiber per day to maintain normal bowel function and prevent constipation, but this may be inappropriate for terminally ill patients (Folden, 2002).

MR A literature review recommended that symptoms of constipation may improve with an increase in dietary fiber intake to 25 to 30 g daily (Hsieh, 2005).

MR A controlled study using a one-group pretest/post-test design ($N = 114$) demonstrated that adding processed pea hull fiber to the diet increased the number of bowel movements and decreased the administration of prune-based laxative (Dahl et al., 2003).

Additional research: Lembo & Camilleri, 2003; Hinrichs & Huseboe, 2001; Locke et al., 2000.

Possibly Effective

■ *Administer laxatives when ordered based on the bowel elimination pattern ensuring short-term and time-limited use.* **LOE = VII**

NR A systematic review demonstrated that appropriate prescription of a laxative required an understanding of how the different drugs worked, the effectiveness of the drug when it was tested in research, and the common risks associated with drug use (Folden, 2002).

NR An evidence-based review of constipation recommended a stepwise progression of laxative treatment when necessary (Hinrichs & Huseboe, 2001).

EO A pharmacological stepwise approach is recommended as part of the treatment plan for constipation (Locke et al., 2000).

■ **SP** *Monitor effectiveness of the pharmacological laxative step program to ensure short-term and time-limited use.* **LOE = VII**

EO Excessive use of laxatives may cause colonic damage and adds to the incidence of drug-drug interactions and cost to the patient. Assessment of the need for laxatives is recommended (Folden, 2002).

EO If laxative use is necessary, a prioritized approach should be instituted with monitoring to avoid chronic laxative use (Hinrichs & Huseboe, 2001).

EO A pharmacological stepwise approach is recommended as part of the treatment plan for constipation (Locke et al., 2000).

■ *Perform digital rectal dilatation for spinal cord injury patient.* **LOE = VII**

EO A literature review indicated that digital stimulation was a suitable rectal intervention for bowel management for those with a spinal cord injury with reflex or mixed neurogenic bowel dysfunction (Ash, 2005).

RCT = Randomized Controlled (Clinical) Trial, **NIC** = Nursing Interventions Classification, **NOC** = Nursing Outcomes Classification

■ **SP** *Teach the patient with spinal cord injury digital rectal dilatation.*
LOE = VII

NR A literature review indicated that digital stimulation was an inexpensive approach to stimulated defecation. Lack of patients' acceptance of the technique may limit its success (Doughty, 1996).

NR A literature review indicated that ideally the individual (with spinal cord injury) should learn the skills to manage bowel care independently, which would include digital rectal dilatation as appropriate (Ash, 2005).

■ **NIC** **SP** *Plan a bowel program with the patient and appropriate others.*
LOE = VII

NR A literature review indicated that an individualized plan for the patient was necessary with consideration of each of the contributing factors (Doughty & Jensen, 2006).

MR An RCT to evaluate the effect of one nursing educational/assessment session for stroke patients ($N = 146$) found the intervention effective in improving symptoms of bowel dysfunction, changed bowel-modifying lifestyle behaviors, and influenced patients' interaction with the health care provider (Harari et al., 2004).

■ **NIC** **SP** *Teach the patient/family the principles of bowel training.* **LOE = VII**

EO Comprehensive education programs aimed at reducing constipation and promoting bowel health organized and delivered by specialist nurses or adult nurse practitioners should be aimed at all levels of providers, clients, and family caregivers (RNAO, 2005).

MR A literature review presented the need to educate patients regarding principles of bowel training and nonpharmacological interventions (Hsieh, 2005).

MR An RCT to evaluate the effect of one nursing educational/assessment session for stroke patients ($N = 146$) found the intervention effective in improving symptoms of bowel dysfunction, changed bowel-modifying lifestyle behaviors, and influenced patients' interaction with the health care provider (Harari et al., 2004).

■ **NIC** **SP** *Ensure adequate fluid intake.* **LOE = V**

EO Fluid intake should be between 1500 and 2000 mL per day (RNAO, 2005).

EO Insufficient amounts of fluid predispose to constipation; a fluid intake of at least 1.5 L per day is recommended (Hinrichs & Huseboe, 2001).

MR According to a literature review, evidence to support the lack of fluid intake as a risk factor for constipation was lacking (Hsieh, 2005).

MR A systematic review reported that an increase in fluid intake, except in patients who were dehydrated, did not relieve chronic constipation (Lembo & Camilleri, 2003).

■ **SP** *Ensure sufficient exercise that is tailored to the individual's abilities.*
LOE = VII

EO Physical activity should be tailored to the individual's abilities with a walking program if possible (RNAO, 2005).

EO An exercise program should be a component of the plan to prevent and treat constipation, although conclusive evidence is lacking (Folden, 2002).

NR = Nursing Research, **MR** = Multidisciplinary Research, **SP** = Standard of Practice, **EO** = Expert Opinion, **LOE** = Level of Evidence

(EO) Exercise individualized for the patient in combination with other interventions is beneficial in the management of constipation (Hinrichs & Huseboe, 2001).

(EO) Physical activity should be encouraged to improve bowel regularity (Hsieh, 2005).

■ *Establish a routine toileting pattern.* LOE = III

(EO) Promote regular consistent toileting each day based on the client's triggering meal (RNAO, 2005).

(EO) Setting a regular time for defecation, usually after a meal, that is consistent with the person's usual time for defection and his or her everyday living demands is effective (Folden, 2002).

(EO) A routine pattern for toileting 5 to 15 minutes after meals and as needed should be established, especially after breakfast, when the gastrocolic reflex is strongest (Hinrichs & Huseboe, 2001).

(EO) Patients should be encouraged to attempt to have a bowel movement soon after waking in the morning or 30 minutes after meals to take advantage of the gastrocolic reflex (Hsieh, 2005).

(MR) A controlled study ($N = 165$) demonstrated that prompted voiding intervention resulted in an increase in continent bowel movements among nursing home residents (Ouslander et al., 1996).

■ (NIC) (SP) *Ensure privacy.* LOE = VII

(EO) A client's visual and auditory privacy when toileting should be safeguarded (RNAO, 2005).

(EO) Provide visual, olfactory, and auditory privacy as much as possible (Folden, 2002).

■ *Encourage promptly responding to the urge to defecate.* LOE = VII

(EO) Patients should be encouraged to respond promptly to the urge to defecate, as the reflex diminishes after a few minutes (Folden, 2002).

■ (NIC) (SP) *Modify the bowel program as needed.* LOE = VII

(EO) Evaluate the patient's response and need for ongoing interventions and the patient's perception of goal achievement related to bowel patterns (RNAO, 2005).

(EO) Outcome measures should be carried out frequently throughout use of the protocol (Hinrichs & Huseboe, 2001).

■ (SP) *Position patients upright for bowel evacuation.* LOE = VII

(EO) A squat position (or simulated left-side lying position while bending the knees toward the abdomen) is recommended to facilitate the defecation process (RNAO, 2005).

(EO) Sitting upright is beneficial; if expelling feces is difficult, have the patient simulate a squatting position (Folden, 2002).

(EO) An upright position for toileting facilitates bowel evacuation (Hinrichs & Huseboe, 2001).

RCT = Randomized Controlled (Clinical) Trial, **NIC** = Nursing Interventions Classification, **NOC** = Nursing Outcomes Classification

Not Effective

No applicable published research was found in this category.

Possibly Harmful

No applicable published research was found in this category.

OUTCOME MEASUREMENT

BOWEL ELIMINATION NOC

Definition: Formation and evacuation of stool.

Bowel Elimination as evidenced by the following selected NOC indicators:

- Elimination pattern
- Control of bowel movements
- Stool color
- Stool amount for diet
- Stool soft and formed
- Ease of stool passage
- Comfort of stool passage
- Passage of stool without aids

(Rate each indicator of **Bowel Elimination:** 1 = severely compromised, 2 = substantially compromised, 3 = moderately compromised, 4 = mildly compromised, 5 = not compromised) (Moorhead et al., 2004).

REFERENCES

Ash D. (2005). Sustaining safe and acceptable bowel care in spinal cord injured patients. *Nurs Stand,* 20(8): 55-64.

Dahl WJ, Whiting SJ, Healey A, Zello GA, Hildebrandt SL. (2003). Increased stool frequency occurs when finely processed pea hull fiber is added to usual foods consumed by elderly residents in long-term care. *J Am Diet Assoc,* 103(9):1199-1202.

Dochterman JM, Bulechek GM (Eds). (2004). *Nursing Interventions Classification (NIC),* 4th ed. St. Louis: Mosby.

Doughty D. (1996). A physiologic approach to bowel training. *J Wound Ostomy Continence Nurs,* 23(1):46-56.

Doughty D, Jensen L. (2006). Assessment and management of the patient with fecal incontinence and related bowel dysfunction. In Doughty D (Ed): *Urinary and fecal incontinence: Current management concepts.* St. Louis: Mosby, pp 457-490.

Folden SL. (2002). Practice guidelines for the management of constipation in adults. *Rehabil Nurs,* 27(5):169-175.

Harari D, Norton C, Lockwood L, Swift C. (2004). Treatment of constipation and fecal incontinence in stroke patients: Randomized controlled trial. *Stroke,* 35(11):2549-2555.

Hinrichs M, Huseboe J. (2001). Research-based protocol. Management of constipation. *J Gerontol Nurs,* 27(2):17-28.

Hsieh C. (2005). Treatment of constipation in older adults. *Am Fam Physician,* 72(11):2277-2284.

Lembo A, Camilleri M. (2003). Chronic constipation. *N Engl J Med,* 349(14):1360-1368.

Locke GR, Pemberton JH, Phillips SF. (2000). American Gastroenterological Association Medical Position Statement: Guidelines on constipation. *Gastroenterology,* 119(6):1761-1766.

NR = Nursing Research, **MR** = Multidisciplinary Research, **SP** = Standard of Practice, **EO** = Expert Opinion, **LOE** = Level of Evidence

Moorhead M, Johnson M, Maas M (Eds). (2004). *Nursing Outcomes Classification (NOC)*, 3rd ed. St. Louis: Mosby.

Ouslander JG, Simmons S, Schnelle J, Fingold S. (1996). Effects of prompted voiding on fecal continence among nursing home residents. *J Am Geriatr Soc*, 44(4):424-428.

Registered Nurses Association of Ontario (RNAO). (2005). Prevention of constipation in the older adult population. Toronto, Ontario: RNAO. Available online: http://www.guideline.gov/. Retrieved on May 6, 2007.

 ## CARDIAC CARE

Debra K. Moser, DNSc, RN, FAAN; Terry A. Lennie, PhD, RN, FAHA; Susan K. Frazier, PhD, RN

> **NIC** **Definition:** Limitation of complications resulting from an imbalance between myocardial oxygen supply and demand for a patient with symptoms of impaired cardiac function (Dochterman & Bulechek, 2004).

NURSING ACTIVITIES

(See also guidelines on Cardiac Precautions, Cardiac Care: Acute, and Cardiac Care: Rehabilitative.)

Effective

■ *Refer patients with heart failure who are at risk for hospitalization for heart failure exacerbation to a comprehensive heart failure disease management program that includes a flexible, individualized approach; an in-hospital phase of care (especially with elderly patients); intensive education of patients; promotion of self-care; optimization of medical therapy; vigilant and ongoing follow-up to detect early deterioration; and active involvement of a cardiac nurse and cardiologist.* **LOE = I**

(MR) In a meta-analysis of 21 RCTs of heart failure disease management programs, such programs were found to be effective in reducing rehospitalization or mortality in older adults when they included a flexible, individualized approach; an in-hospital phase of care; intensive education of patients; promotion of self-care; optimization of medical therapy; vigilant and ongoing follow-up to detect early deterioration; and active involvement of a cardiac nurse and cardiologist (Yu et al., 2006).

(MR) The most recent interdisciplinary, evidence-based heart failure management guideline from the Heart Failure Society of America recommends referral of high-risk patients with heart failure to comprehensive heart failure disease management programs (HFSA, 2006).

(NR) In an RCT, a total of 106 patients with heart failure were randomly assigned to heart failure disease management or usual care and observed for 12 months. Patients in the heart failure disease management group demonstrated better survival, fewer hospitalizations for heart failure, and better self-care behaviors (Stromberg et al., 2003).

(NR) In an RCT (*N* = 358 patients with heart failure), a nurse-delivered heart failure disease management program based on telephone case management resulted in lower rehospitalization rates, fewer heart failure hospital days, fewer multiple readmissions, and lower health care costs, even factoring in the cost of the intervention (Riegel et al., 2002).

RCT = Randomized Controlled (Clinical) Trial, **NIC** = Nursing Interventions Classification, **NOC** = Nursing Outcomes Classification

■ *In elderly cardiac patients at risk for readmission, use a transitional care model that includes discharge planning and home follow-up to improve outcomes.*
LOE = II

(NR) An RCT study of a transitional care intervention, which focused on needs of older adults with heart failure ($N = 239$) and their caregivers, use of quality care management strategies, implementation of evidence-based guidelines delivered by advanced practice nurses, and home follow-up for 3 months, demonstrated an increased length of time between hospital discharge and readmission or death, decreased total hospitalizations, and lower health care costs (Naylor et al., 2004).

(NR) In an RCT ($N = 363$) of nurse-centered comprehensive discharge planning and home follow-up for hospitalized elders at risk for poor outcomes, elders in the intervention group had fewer readmissions, longer times to readmission, and decreased health care costs (Naylor et al., 1999).

■ *Educate patients (of all ages, genders, ethnicities, and socioeconomic status) about the signs and symptoms of acute coronary syndrome and stroke and about the appropriate actions to take (i.e., calling 911 and being transported by ambulance and not by friends or relatives to the hospital) when they experience them.* **LOE = V**

(MR) A systematic review of the literature on treatment-seeking delay in patients with signs and symptoms of acute coronary syndrome and stroke documented that patients' delay in seeking treatment remained the number one cause of failure to receive definitive treatment in a timely manner that would reduce morbidity and mortality. Although knowledge of signs and symptoms alone was not sufficient to promote rapid treatment seeking, it was a necessary baseline (Moser et al., 2006).

(MR) Because timely access to definitive cardiac treatment is partially dependent on early recognition of symptoms of acute coronary syndrome, public recognition of major heart attack symptoms (i.e., pain or discomfort in the jaw, neck, back; feeling weak, lightheaded, faint; chest pain or discomfort; pain or discomfort in the arms or shoulder; shortness of breath) was assessed in a descriptive study of 61,018 participants in 17 states and the U.S. Virgin Islands. Although 95% recognized chest pain as a symptom, only 11% correctly classified all symptoms and knew to call 911; moreover, knowledge was lower among men than women, people of various ethnic groups than whites, younger and older people than middle-aged people, and people with less education (Greenlund et al., 2004).

(MR) A descriptive study of 1294 adults in 20 U.S. communities revealed that although most respondents knew that chest pain or discomfort was a major symptom of heart attack, very few knew other common symptoms. Knowledge was lower among ethnic minorities, older and younger individuals compared with middle-aged people, and individuals of lower socioeconomic status (Goff et al., 1998).

■ *Inform all individuals (regardless of gender, age, ethnicity, or socioeconomic status) of the cardiac risk factors they have and provide education about reduction of these risk factors.* **LOE = V**

(MR) In a descriptive study using a nationally representative sample of 1008 women selected through random digit dialing, the rate of awareness of heart disease as the leading cause of death doubled since 1997 and correlated with increased physical activity and weight loss.

NR = Nursing Research, **MR** = Multidisciplinary Research, **SP** = Standard of Practice, **EO** = Expert Opinion, **LOE** = Level of Evidence

Although less than half the sample were aware of healthy levels of risk factors, awareness that personal risk level was not healthy was associated with action to decrease personal risk level (Mosca et al., 2006).

(MR) In their evidence-based guideline for the management of ST-segment elevation myocardial infarction, the American College of Cardiology/American Heart Association strongly advocated for identifying all patients with risk factors, informing patients of their risk, and instituting risk factor modification appropriate to the level of risk. This recommendation is based on the importance of primary and secondary prevention because of the high morbidity and mortality from myocardial infarction, the well-documented and large benefit of preventing myocardial infarction by attending to risk factors, and the well-documented effectiveness of risk factor modification (Antman et al., 2004).

(MR) Despite beliefs by many health care providers and lay people to the contrary, the vast majority—at least 90%—of people who die from coronary heart disease have one or more of the three major modifiable risk factors: hypertension, dyslipidemia, or smoking (Mensah et al., 2005).

■ *Advocate for referral to a cardiac rehabilitation program after an acute cardiac event.* **LOE = I**

(Refer to the guideline on Cardiac Care: Rehabilitative.)

■ *Promote secondary prevention that focuses on reduction of modifiable risk factors (e.g., smoking, hypertension, dyslipidemias, sedentary lifestyle, diet) for recurrent cardiac events or for progression of disease and on control of comorbidities (e.g., diabetes, chronic kidney disease) that increase the risk of recurrent cardiac events or progression of disease.* **LOE = I**

(Refer to the guideline on Cardiac Care: Rehabilitative.)

■ *Advocate for evidence-based guideline-driven care for patients with acute coronary syndrome and with heart failure.* **LOE = I**

(MR) A number of evidence-based guidelines have been written and are regularly updated by specialty professional societies and government agencies in which the evidence bases for management of acute coronary syndrome and heart failure have been evaluated and summarized for use by all health care practitioners in order to optimize patients' outcomes. Use of these guidelines is associated with improved patients' outcomes compared with usual care (Antman et al., 2004; Braunwald et al., 2002; HFSA, 2006; Hunt et al., 2005; Smith et al., 2006).

(MR) In a descriptive study of 3754 patients presenting with acute coronary syndrome, compliance with American College of Cardiology/American Heart Association guidelines for acute coronary syndrome was associated with a better prognosis regardless of patients' risk scores (Gulati et al., 2004).

(NR) In a quasi-experimental study of the impact of a multifaceted intervention designed to improve adherence to the American College of Cardiology/American Heart Association practice guidelines for heart failure (and including reminders and other methods of advocating for use of guidelines), the intervention significantly improved clinician adherence with addressing all self-management categories in the electronic medical record and adherence with self-management education given to the patient in writing at discharge (Dykes et al., 2005).

RCT = Randomized Controlled (Clinical) Trial, **NIC** = Nursing Interventions Classification, **NOC** = Nursing Outcomes Classification

■ *Involve family members, significant others, and/or caregivers or support people in patients' education and counseling activities.* **LOE = VII**

(MR) Because most care for heart failure patients is provided by patients and their family members or caregivers at home and because of the complexities of self-care for patients with heart failure, the Heart Failure Society of America in their evidence-based guideline for the management of heart failure recommended that all teaching be delivered to both patients and their families or caregivers. Their recommendation was based on a systematic review of the literature (HFSA, 2006).

■ *Promote self-care (also known as self-management).* **LOE = I**

(MR) In a meta-analysis of 21 RCTs of heart failure disease management programs, such programs were found to be effective in reducing rehospitalization or mortality in older adults when they included a flexible, individualized approach; an in-hospital phase of care; intensive education of patients; promotion of self-care; optimization of medical therapy; vigilant and ongoing follow-up to detect early deterioration; and active involvement of a cardiac nurse and cardiologist. A major mechanism for the effectiveness of disease management is the promotion of patients' self-care (Yu et al., 2006).

(NR) In an RCT ($N = 358$ patients with heart failure), a nurse-delivered heart failure disease management program designed to enhance patients' self-care resulted in lower rehospitalization rates, fewer heart failure hospital days, fewer multiple readmissions, and lower health care costs, even factoring in the cost of the intervention (Riegel et al., 2002).

(MR) Based on a systematic review of the literature, the Heart Failure Society of America noted that most care for heart failure patients is provided by patients and their family members or caregivers at home and that strategies aimed to increase patients' self-care abilities improved patients' adherence and clinical outcomes. As a result, they recommend promotion of self-care as the basic care model (HFSA, 2006).

■ *Assess for social isolation or inadequate social support.* **LOE = IV**

(MR) In a systematic review, social isolation or lack of adequate social support (along with depression and anxiety) was shown to influence strongly and negatively the course of cardiac disease. Thus, routine screening for social support (and other psychosocial factors), referral for patients with severe psychological distress to behavioral specialists, and directly treating those with milder distress using targeted interventions are advocated (Rozanski et al., 2005).

(MR) In this cohort study of 292 elderly patients with heart failure, lack of emotional support was independently associated with 1-year risk of fatal and nonfatal cardiovascular outcomes (Krumholz et al., 1998).

(MR) A cohort study of 1503 post–myocardial infarction patients demonstrated that low perceived social support predicted death and recurrent myocardial infarction upon follow-up (Burg et al., 2005).

■ *Assess anxiety status.* **LOE = V**

(Refer to the guideline on Cardiac Care: Acute.)

■ *Assess for symptoms of depression.* **LOE = V**

(Refer to the guideline on Cardiac Care: Acute.)

NR = Nursing Research, **MR** = Multidisciplinary Research, **SP** = Standard of Practice, **EO** = Expert Opinion, **LOE** = Level of Evidence

■ *Increase level of perceived control through education and counseling that reframes an acute cardiac event from an out-of-control crisis to a chronic condition that can be controlled with adherence to recommended therapy and lifestyle changes.* **LOE = IV**

(Refer to the guideline on Cardiac Care: Acute.)

Possibly Effective

No applicable published research was found in this category.

Not Effective

■ *Vitamin E supplementation to prevent recurrent cardiac events.* **LOE = I**

MR An RCT of 400 international units daily of vitamin E supplementation versus placebo conducted among 9542 patients at high risk (i.e., older than 55 years plus cardiovascular disease or diabetes and one other risk factor) for recurrent cardiac events (i.e., myocardial infarction, stroke, death from cardiovascular causes, unstable angina, congestive heart failure, revascularization or amputation, complications of diabetes, or death from any cause) revealed no impact of vitamin E supplementation on cardiovascular outcomes (Yusuf et al., 2000).

MR In a 7-year follow-up of the RCT reported previously, there was still no positive impact of vitamin E supplementation on cardiovascular events, but participants had a higher risk for the development of heart failure and hospitalization for heart failure (Lonn et al., 2005).

MR The impact of vitamin E supplementation on cardiovascular outcomes was examined in an RCT of 993 individuals with renal insufficiency as evidenced by elevated serum creatinine and at high risk for cardiovascular events. There was no difference in the development of cardiac events between the two groups (Mann et al., 2004).

Possibly Harmful

No applicable published research was found in this category.

OUTCOME MEASUREMENT

CARDIAC PUMP EFFECTIVENESS

Definition: Adequacy of blood volume ejected from the left ventricle to support systemic perfusion pressure.

Cardiac Pump Effectiveness as evidenced by the following selected NOC indicators:
- Systolic blood pressure
- Diastolic blood pressure
- Apical heart rate
- Cardiac index
- Ejection fraction
- Activity tolerance
- Peripheral pulses

Continued

RCT = Randomized Controlled (Clinical) Trial, **NIC** = Nursing Interventions Classification, **NOC** = Nursing Outcomes Classification

OUTCOME MEASUREMENT—*cont'd*

- Skin color
- Urinary output
- Cognitive status

(Rate each indicator of **Cardiac Pump Effectiveness:** 1 = severely compromised, 2 = substantially compromised, 3 = moderately compromised, 4 = mildly compromised, 5 = not compromised) (Moorhead et al., 2004).

CARDIAC DISEASE SELF-MANAGEMENT   NOC

Definition: Personal actions to manage heart disease and prevent disease progression.
Cardiac Disease Self-Management as evidenced by the following selected NOC indicators:

- Reports symptoms of worsening disease
- Performs treatment regimen as prescribed
- Monitors symptom onset
- Uses warning signs to seek health care
- Limits sodium intake
- Limits fat and cholesterol intake
- Follows recommended diet
- Participates in smoking cessation regimen
- Participates in recommended exercise program

(Rate each indicator of **Cardiac Disease Self-Management:** 1 = never demonstrated, 2 = rarely demonstrated, 3 = sometimes demonstrated, 4 = often demonstrated, 5 = consistently demonstrated) (Moorhead et al., 2004).

REFERENCES

Antman EM, Anbe DT, Armstrong PW, Bates ER, Green LA, Hand M, et al. (2004). ACC/AHA guidelines for the management of patients with ST-elevation myocardial infarction; a report of the American College of Cardiology/American Heart Association Task Force on Practice Guidelines (Committee to Revise the 1999 Guidelines for the Management of Patients with Acute Myocardial Infarction). *J Am Coll Cardiol*, 44(3):E1-E211.

Braunwald E, Antman EM, Beasley JW, Califf RM, Cheitlin MD, Hochman JS, et al. (2002). ACC/AHA guideline update for the management of patients with unstable angina and non-ST-segment elevation myocardial infarction—2002: Summary article: A report of the American College of Cardiology/American Heart Association Task Force on Practice Guidelines (Committee on the Management of Patients with Unstable Angina). *Circulation*, 106(14):1893-1900.

Burg MM, Barefoot J, Berkman L, Catellier DJ, Czajkowski S, Saab P, et al. (2005). Low perceived social support and post-myocardial infarction prognosis in the enhancing recovery in coronary heart disease clinical trial: The effects of treatment. *Psychosom Med*, 67(6):879-888.

Dochterman JM, Bulechek GM (Eds). (2004). *Nursing Interventions Classification (NIC)*, 4th ed. St. Louis: Mosby.

Dykes PC, Acevedo K, Boldrighini J, Boucher C, Frumento K, Gray P, et al. (2005). Clinical practice guideline adherence before and after implementation of the HEARTFELT (HEART Failure Effectiveness & Leadership Team) intervention. *J Cardiovasc Nurs*, 20(5):306-314.

Goff DC Jr, Sellers DE, McGovern PG, Meischke H, Goldberg RJ, Bittner V, et al. (1998). Knowledge of heart attack symptoms in a population survey in the United States: The REACT Trial. Rapid Early Action for Coronary Treatment. *Arch Intern Med*, 158(21):2329-2338.

NR = Nursing Research, **MR** = Multidisciplinary Research, **SP** = Standard of Practice, **EO** = Expert Opinion, **LOE** = Level of Evidence

Greenlund KJ, Keenan NL, Giles WH, Zheng ZJ, Neff LJ, Croft JB, et al. (2004). Public recognition of major signs and symptoms of heart attack: Seventeen states and the US Virgin Islands, 2001. *Am Heart J,* 147(6):1010-1016.

Gulati M, Patel S, Jaffe AS, Joseph AJ, Calvin JE Jr. (2004). Impact of contemporary guideline compliance on risk stratification models for acute coronary syndromes in the Registry of Acute Coronary Syndromes. *Am J Cardiol,* 94(7):873-878.

Heart Failure Society of America (HFSA). (2006). HFSA 2006 Comprehensive Heart Failure Practice Guideline. *J Card Fail,* 12(1):e1-e2.

Hunt SA; American College of Cardiology; American Heart Association Task Force on Practice Guidelines. (2005). ACC/AHA 2005 guideline update for the diagnosis and management of chronic heart failure in the adult. A report of the American College of Cardiology/American Heart Association Task Force on Practice Guidelines (Writing Committee to Update the 2001 Guidelines for the Evaluation and Management of Heart Failure). *J Am Coll Cardiol,* 46(6):e1-e82.

Krumholz HM, Butler J, Miller J, Vaccarino V, Williams CS, Mendes de Leon CF, et al. (1998). Prognostic importance of emotional support for elderly patients hospitalized with heart failure. *Circulation,* 97(10):958-964.

Lonn E, Bosch J, Yusuf S, Sheridan P, Pogue J, Arnold JM, et al. (2005). Effects of long-term vitamin E supplementation on cardiovascular events and cancer: A randomized controlled trial. *JAMA,* 293(11):1338-1347.

Mann JF, Lonn EM, Yi Q, Gerstein HC, Hoogwerf BJ, Pogue J, et al. (2004). Effects of vitamin E on cardiovascular outcomes in people with mild-to-moderate renal insufficiency: Results of the HOPE study. *Kidney Int,* 65(4):1375-1380.

Mensah GA, Brown DW, Croft JB, Greenlund KJ. (2005). Major coronary risk factors and death from coronary heart disease: Baseline and follow-up mortality data from the Second National Health and Nutrition Examination Survey (NHANES II). *Am J Prev Med,* 29(5 Suppl 1):68-74.

Moorhead S, Johnson M, Maas M (Eds). (2004). *Nursing Outcomes Classification (NOC),* 3rd ed. St. Louis: Mosby.

Mosca L, Mochari H, Christian A, Berra K, Taubert K, Mills T, et al. (2006). National study of women's awareness, preventive action, and barriers to cardiovascular health. *Circulation,* 113(4):525-534.

Moser DK, Kimble LP, Alberts MJ, Alonzo A, Croft JB, Dracup K, et al. (2006). Reducing delay in seeking treatment by patients with acute coronary syndrome and stroke: A scientific statement from the American Heart Association Council on Cardiovascular Nursing and Stroke Council. *Circulation,* 114(2):168-182.

Naylor MD, Brooten D, Campbell R, Jacobsen BS, Mezey MD, Pauly MV, et al. (1999). Comprehensive discharge planning and home follow-up of hospitalized elders: A randomized clinical trial. *JAMA,* 281(7):613-620.

Naylor MD, Brooten DA, Campbell RL, Maislin G, McCauley KM, Schwartz JS. (2004). Transitional care of older adults hospitalized with heart failure: A randomized, controlled trial. *J Am Geriatr Soc,* 52(5):675-684.

Riegel B, Carlson B, Kopp Z, LePetri B, Glaser D, Unger A. (2002). Effect of a standardized nurse case-management telephone intervention on resource use in patients with chronic heart failure. *Arch Intern Med,* 162(6):705-712.

Rozanski A, Blumenthal JA, Davidson KW, Saab PG, Kubzansky L. (2005). The epidemiology, pathophysiology, and management of psychosocial risk factors in cardiac practice: The emerging field of behavioral cardiology. *J Am Coll Cardiol,* 45(5):637-651.

Smith SC Jr, Allen J, Blair SN, Bonow RO, Brass LM, Fonarow GC, et al. (2006). AHA/ACC guidelines for secondary prevention for patients with coronary and other atherosclerotic vascular disease: 2006 update: Endorsed by the National Heart, Lung, and Blood Institute. *Circulation,* 113(19):2363-2372.

Stromberg A, Martensson J, Fridlund B, Levin LA, Karlsson JE, Dahlstrom U. (2003). Nurse-led heart failure clinics improve survival and self-care behaviour in patients with heart failure. Results from a prospective, randomised trial. *Eur Heart J,* 24(11):1014-1023.

Yu DS, Thompson DR, Lee DT. (2006). Disease management programmes for older people with heart failure: Crucial characteristics which improve post-discharge outcomes. *Eur Heart J,* 27(5):596-612.

Yusuf S, Dagenais G, Pogue J, Bosch J, Sleight P. (2000). Vitamin E supplementation and cardiovascular events in high-risk patients. The Heart Outcomes Prevention Evaluation Study Investigators. *N Engl J Med,* 342(3):154-160.

RCT = Randomized Controlled (Clinical) Trial, **NIC** = Nursing Interventions Classification, **NOC** = Nursing Outcomes Classification

CARDIAC CARE: ACUTE

Susan K. Frazier, PhD, RN; Terry A. Lennie, PhD, RN, FAHA;
Seongkum Heo, PhD, RN; Debra K. Moser, DNSc, RN, FAAN

> **NIC** **Definition:** Limitation of complications for a patient recently experiencing an episode of an imbalance between myocardial oxygen supply and demand resulting in impaired cardiac function (Dochterman & Bulechek, 2004).

NURSING ACTIVITIES

(Please also refer to the guideline on Cardiac Precautions.)

Effective

■ *Perform uninterrupted cardiac rhythm monitoring by a dedicated "monitor watcher."* **LOE = II**

(NR) A controlled study comparing the accuracy of detection of cardiac dysrhythmias in a telemetry unit for a period with and without a dedicated monitor watcher found that the use of a monitor watcher resulted in significantly greater detection of clinically important and life-threatening rhythm disturbances (Stukshis et al., 1997).

(MR) A systematic review and practice guideline recommended continuous cardiac monitoring beginning upon arrival to the emergency department and continuing for a minimum of 24 hours in patients with uncomplicated acute myocardial infarction, for 24 hours after complications have been resolved, and for 24 hours after resolution of ischemia in patients with transient ST-segment changes and/or symptoms of myocardial ischemia (Drew et al., 2004).

■ *Monitor multiple ECG leads including V1 when capability is present to maximize P-wave size, QRS interval, and morphology.* **LOE = III**

(MR) A controlled study of cardiac patients ($N = 46$) undergoing electrophysiological testing to determine the best electrocardiographic lead for diagnosis of aberrant supraventricular tachycardia from ventricular ectopy determined that leads MCL1 and V1 were superior to MCL6 and V6 (Drew et al., 1991).

(MR) A controlled study of the diagnosis of episodes of wide QRS tachycardia ($N = 133$) in cardiac patients undergoing electrophysiological testing determined that multiple leads are necessary for accurate evaluation of QRS width and identified V1 as the most sensitive lead for distinguishing ventricular tachycardia from an aberrant supraventricular tachycardia (Drew & Scheinman, 1995).

■ *Evaluate and document QT interval corrected for heart rate (QT$_c$) in one consistent lead at least every 8 hours for detection of proarrhythmia.* **LOE = IV**

(MR) A systematic review and practice standards recommended monitoring of the QT interval corrected for heart rate, particularly in patients who receive an antidysrhythmic agent known to cause torsades de pointes and in those who present with a new-onset bradyarrhythmia,

NR = Nursing Research, **MR** = Multidisciplinary Research, **SP** = Standard of Practice, **EO** = Expert Opinion, **LOE** = Level of Evidence

severe hypokalemia, severe hypomagnesemia, or following an overdose with a potentially proarrhythmic drug (Drew et al., 2004).

(MR) A cohort study of Medicare patients aged 65 and older ($N = 5888$) found that a QT_c interval greater than 450 milliseconds doubled the mortality rate for those with coronary heart disease within 10 years of electrocardiographic measurement (Robbins et al., 2003).

(MR) A descriptive study of patients who experienced a myocardial infarction ($N = 481$) determined that QT length measures independently predicted mortality in the 3 years following infarction (Jensen et al., 2005).

Implement an open visiting policy. LOE = II

(NR) An RCT evaluating a patient-controlled device to manage visiting times for coronary care patients (N = 60) found that patients' control of family visiting produced greater perceived control over visits and rest between visits and lower heart rate and diastolic blood pressure, with slightly greater appraisal of visit stress for those who used the device to manage visiting time (Lazure & Baun, 1995).

(NR) An RCT of cardiac care patients and their responses to investigator interviews and family visits while in the cardiac care unit found no significant differences in systolic or diastolic blood pressure, heart rate, or prevalence of premature ventricular contractions between the interview time and the visiting time but significantly lower systolic and diastolic blood pressure during the family visit (Simpson & Shaver, 1990).

(MR) An RCT comparing critical care patients' responses ($N = 111$) to unrestricted visiting hours with those from patients ($N = 115$) who experienced a restrictive policy found that unrestricted visiting was significantly associated with lower anxiety scores, lower cardiovascular complications, and less change in thyroid-stimulating hormone from admission to discharge (Fumagalli et al., 2006).

Initiate patients' education/discharge planning. LOE = I

(NR) A controlled study of patients with myocardial infarction ($N = 252$) found that a standardized audiovisual education program produced an increase in knowledge and optimism about future abilities, reduced mortality at 6 weeks, reduced fear about myocardial infarction, resulted in a more rapid resumption of physical activities, and generated fewer consultations with physicians during the first 6 weeks after discharge. There were no differences in long-term survival (Maeland & Havik, 1987).

(MR) A meta-analysis of studies ($N = 191$) of the effects of psychosocial and educational interventions on recovery time, severity of postsurgical pain, and level of psychological distress of adult surgical patients identified small to moderate beneficial effects on recovery time, postoperative pain level, and psychological distress (Devine, 1992).

(MR) An RCT of a 1-hour, one-on-one teaching session with a nurse educator at discharge in patients with systolic heart failure ($N = 223$) found that patients who received the education had fewer hospital days and a lower mortality rate during the follow-up period, and the costs of care, including the cost of the intervention, were lower in patients in the education intervention group by $2823 per patient (Koelling et al., 2005).

(MR) An RCT of specialized counseling from staff nurses for male patients ($N = 60$) admitted for the first time to a coronary care unit with an acute myocardial infarction found that those who received counseling reported statistically significantly less anxiety and depression, and these lower levels were still evident 6 months after discharge (Thompson & Meddis, 1990).

RCT = Randomized Controlled (Clinical) Trial, NIC = Nursing Interventions Classification, NOC = Nursing Outcomes Classification

■ *Provide music therapy to improve psychological and physiological state.* **LOE = I**

(NR) An RCT of the impact of 20 minutes of music therapy on anxiety, pain, and physiological indicators in patients undergoing cardiac surgery ($N = 86$) found that in those who received music, anxiety and pain levels were reduced without changes in heart rate and systolic or diastolic blood pressure (Sendelbach et al., 2006).

(NR) An RCT of the impact of 30 minutes of music therapy on psychological distress, pain, and physiological indicators in patients with cardiac disease on bed rest ($N = 140$) identified a reduction in psychological distress, blood pressure, and respiratory rate after music therapy (Cadigan et al., 2001).

(NR) An RCT of the effects of music therapy, relaxation therapy, and standard care in patients with a presumptive acute myocardial infarction ($N = 80$) found reduction in apical heart rate, increase in peripheral temperature, and fewer cardiac complications in the music and relaxation therapy groups (Guzzetta, 1989).

■ *Ambulate after bed rest for 2 hours following cardiac catheterization.* **LOE = I**

(MR) An RCT of patients receiving a cardiac catheterization ($N = 201$) and a meta-analysis of three similar published studies determined that ambulation 2 hours after cardiac catheterization using a 6 F catheter was not associated with increased complication rates compared with 6 hours of bed rest after catheterization (Logemann et al., 1999).

(MR) A controlled study of patients receiving a cardiac catheterization ($N = 98$) found that 1.5 to 2 hours of bed rest following catheterization did not increase complication rates in comparison with 4 to 5 hours of bed rest after the procedure (Rosenstein et al., 2004).

(MR) An RCT of patients receiving percutaneous coronary intervention ($N = 354$) determined that ambulation after 2 hours of bed rest after the procedure produced no increase in complications compared with bed rest for 4 and 6 hours (Vlasic et al., 2001).

Possibly Effective

■ *Monitor ST-segment ischemia for a minimum of 24 hours and until event free for 12 to 24 hours.* **LOE = III**

(NR) A controlled study of patients ($N = 422$) with unstable coronary syndromes found that routine monitoring of leads V1 and II had low sensitivity for episodes of ischemia in these patients (33%) and that monitoring leads identified with coronary occlusion during an angioplasty also had less than ideal sensitivity (58%) (Drew et al., 1998).

(MR) A controlled study of patients ($N = 149$) following elective surgery who received ST-segment monitoring simultaneously by standard monitoring (5 electrodes, 2 leads) and by 12-lead electrocardiogram obtained every 2 minutes found that standard monitoring had low sensitivity (12%) for ST-segment evidence of a first episode of myocardial ischemia and even lower sensitivity for all episodes of ischemia (3%) compared with 12-lead electrocardiogram monitoring (Martinez et al., 2003).

(MR) A controlled study of patients ($N = 40$) during elective coronary angioplasty found that maximal ST-segment elevation occurred in lead V3 for left anterior descending artery occlusion, in lead V2 for occlusion of the left circumflex artery, and in lead III for occlusion of the right coronary artery during myocardial ischemia induced by angioplasty balloon inflation (Persson et al., 2006).

NR = Nursing Research, **MR** = Multidisciplinary Research, **SP** = Standard of Practice, **EO** = Expert Opinion, **LOE** = Level of Evidence

■ *Achieve hemostasis following cardiac catheterization using mechanical compression or an arterial closure device.* **LOE = II**

NR An RCT of patients ($N = 100$) following cardiac catheterization found that mechanical compression was as safe and effective as manual compression in achieving hemostasis after the procedure (Jones & McCutcheon, 2003).

MR An RCT of patients ($N = 122$) following percutaneous coronary intervention determined that those randomly assigned to a vascular sealing device ambulated more rapidly and experienced less pain with identical rates of complication compared with those who had a mechanical compression device after the procedure (Juergens et al., 2004).

MR An RCT of patients ($N = 167$) following percutaneous angioplasty found that the use of a percutaneous suture device that closed the femoral puncture immediately after the procedure produced a similar rate of vascular complications compared with manual compression (Tron et al., 2003).

■ *Offer family presence during cardiopulmonary resuscitation.* **LOE = V**

NR A systematic review of studies ($N = 28$), primarily descriptive surveys, found that there was no evidence that family presence during resuscitation was disruptive or psychologically traumatic for either the family member or clinicians involved in the resuscitative effort (Halm, 2005).

(Please refer to the guideline on Family Presence Facilitation for more research on family presence during resuscitation.)

■ *Administer supplementary oxygen.* **LOE = III**

MR A controlled study of patients ($N = 17$) following acute anterior transmural myocardial infarction who received oxygen for an average of 66 minutes described an average reduction of 16% in the magnitude and extent of ischemic injury with the application of oxygen therapy (Madias et al., 1976).

MR A controlled laboratory study ($N = 15$) found that administration of oxygen ($FiO_2 = 0.40$) during an experimental coronary artery occlusion reduced ischemic injury and eventual degree of muscle necrosis (Maroko et al., 1975).

MR A systematic review and practice guideline recommended the use of supplemental oxygen therapy with evaluation of oxygenation by pulse oximetry until stable (>90% saturation) for 6 hours followed by consideration of discontinuation (Antman et al., 2004).

■ *Administer NPO or clear liquids only when the patient is nauseated or the infarction size is large.* **LOE = VI**

MR A descriptive study of patients ($N = 265$) admitted to an acute coronary care unit found that 55% of patients with an acute myocardial infarction reported nausea and vomiting; the presence of nausea or vomiting was most strongly associated with the size of the infarction, and there was no relationship between the location of the infarction and the incidence of nausea and vomiting (Herlihy et al., 1987).

■ *Assess anxiety status.* **LOE = V**

NR A descriptive study of patients ($N = 76$) with myocardial infarction found that patients who were anxious within the first week of hospital admission had more cardiac events (cardiovascular death, myocardial infarction, and revascularization) during the 31 months of

RCT = Randomized Controlled (Clinical) Trial, **NIC** = Nursing Interventions Classification, **NOC** = Nursing Outcomes Classification

follow-up, and these events happened earlier than those in nonanxious patients (Benning-hoven et al., 2006).

(MR) A descriptive study of patients ($N = 288$) with myocardial infarction determined that anxiety and depression during hospitalization did not predict mortality but did predict quality of life at 4 months (Lane et al., 2000).

(MR) A descriptive study of patients ($N = 222$) with myocardial infarction found that anxiety during hospitalization increased the likelihood of cardiac events (recurrences of acute coronary syndromes, dysrhythmic events) 3.13 times more than in nonanxious patients (Frasure-Smith et al., 1995).

■ *Assess for symptoms of depression.* **LOE = V**

(MR) A descriptive study of patients ($N = 222$) with myocardial infarction found that depression during hospitalization increased the likelihood of cardiac events (recurrences of acute coronary syndromes, dysrhythmic events) 3.32 times more than in nondepressed patients. Major depression and history of major depression also affected the occurrence of cardiac events (Frasure-Smith et al., 1995).

(MR) A descriptive study of patients ($N = 196$) with myocardial infarction found that those who had depression during the first 2 to 5 days following admission reported poorer baseline quality of life and quality of life at 4 months than nondepressed patients (Fauerbach et al., 2005).

(MR) A descriptive study of patients ($N = 347$) with myocardial infarction found that patients who were distressed (anxious and/or depressed) within 3 days after admission reported worse quality of life and greater functional impairment at 3 months and 1 year than nondistressed patients. Baseline distress did not predict mortality at either 6 or 18 months (Mayou et al., 2000).

■ *Increase the level of perceived control through education and counseling that reframes an acute cardiac event from an out-of-control crisis to a chronic condition that can be controlled with adherence to recommended therapy and lifestyle changes.* **LOE = IV**

(NR) A descriptive study of patients admitted for an acute myocardial infarction and/or who had received coronary artery bypass grafts ($N = 176$) found that patients with high levels of perceived control ($N = 85$) had lower anxiety, depression, and hostility and a better overall psychosocial adjustment to illness than those with low perceived control ($N = 91$) at 3 and 6 months after discharge (Moser & Dracup, 1995).

(NR) A descriptive study of patients ($N = 536$) hospitalized for an acute myocardial infarction found that those with higher anxiety levels had more complications (ventricular tachycardia and fibrillation, reinfarction, ischemia), and the level of perceived control moderated the effect of anxiety on complications. Patients with the highest anxiety and lowest perceived control had the most complications (Moser et al., 2007).

■ *Take thermodilution cardiac output measurements with the patient in one consistent position using 5 or 10 mL of room temperature solution.* **LOE = II**

(NR) A controlled study of patients ($N = 50$) with low ejection fraction (<35%) in a cardiac care unit determined that thermodilution cardiac output measurements made with 5 or 10 mL of iced solution did not differ (McCloy et al., 1999).

(NR) A controlled study of patients ($N = 50$) with low cardiac index (<2.5 L/m^2/min) found that thermodilution measures made with iced solution and room temperature solution were not different (Kiely et al., 1998).

NR = Nursing Research, **MR** = Multidisciplinary Research, **SP** = Standard of Practice, **EO** = Expert Opinion, **LOE** = Level of Evidence

(NR) A controlled study of patients (N = 30) in two intensive care units determined that thermodilution measures made in a 45-degree upright position were significantly lower than those made in the supine position (Driscoll et al., 1995).

■ *Provide a quiet, restful environment with uninterrupted periods (>2 hours) of sleep.* **LOE = III**

(NR) A controlled study of the effect of critical care unit sound on sleep in healthy women (N = 70) found that women exposed to critical care unit noise during sleep achieved significantly less REM sleep (Topf & Davis, 1993).

(NR) A controlled study of the effect of critical care sound in healthy women (N = 60) determined that exposure to critical care unit noise during sleep resulted in a longer time to achieve sleep, less sleep time, a greater number of awakenings during the night, and overall poorer sleep quality by self-report (Topf et al., 1996).

(MR) A descriptive study of patients (N = 203) from different critical care units (cardiac, cardiac step-down, medical, and surgical) determined that sleep in the units was significantly poorer than sleep at home, daytime sleepiness was a significant problem, and sleep interruption resulting from diagnostic testing and human intervention was as disruptive as environmental noise (Freedman et al., 1999).

Not Effective

■ *Monitoring hemodynamic status with a pulmonary artery catheter.* **LOE = I**

(MR) A multicenter RCT evaluating the clinical effectiveness of clinical management guided by a pulmonary artery catheter in adult intensive care patients (N = 1041) found no clear evidence that management guided by a pulmonary artery catheter was either beneficial or harmful (Harvey et al., 2005).

(MR) A meta-analysis of 13 RCTs (N = 5051 patients) evaluating the safety and efficacy of pulmonary artery catheterization in critically ill patients found no substantive evidence that the use of a pulmonary artery catheter either improved outcomes or increased mortality or hospital days (Shah et al., 2005).

(MR) A multicenter RCT evaluating the safety and efficacy of pulmonary artery catheter–guided therapy in patients with severe, recurrent heart failure (N = 433) did not detect significant differences in mortality or hospital length of stay but did find more in-hospital adverse events for those with a pulmonary artery catheter (Binanay et al., 2005).

Possibly Harmful

No applicable published research was found in this category.

OUTCOME MEASUREMENT

CARDIAC PUMP EFFECTIVENESS

Definition: Adequacy of blood volume ejected from the left ventricle to support systemic perfusion pressure.

Continued

RCT = Randomized Controlled (Clinical) Trial, **NIC** = Nursing Interventions Classification, **NOC** = Nursing Outcomes Classification

OUTCOME MEASUREMENT—*cont'd*

Cardiac Pump Effectiveness as evidenced by the following selected NOC indicators:
- Systolic blood pressure
- Diastolic blood pressure
- Apical heart rate
- Cardiac index
- Ejection fraction
- Activity tolerance
- Peripheral pulses
- Skin color
- Urinary output
- Cognitive status

(Rate each indicator of **Cardiac Pump Effectiveness:** 1 = severely compromised, 2 = substantially compromised, 3 = moderately compromised, 4 = mildly compromised, 5 = not compromised) (Moorhead et al., 2004).

REFERENCES

Antman EM, Anbe DT, Armstrong PW, et al. (2004). ACC/AHA guidelines for the management of patients with ST-elevation myocardial infarction–executive summary. A report of the American College of Cardiology/American Heart Association Task Force on Practice Guidelines, *J Am Coll Cardiol* 44(3): 671-719.

Benninghoven D, Kaduk A, Wiegand U, Specht T, Kunzendorf S, Jantschek G. (2006). Influence of anxiety on the course of heart disease after acute myocardial infarction—Risk factor or protective function? *Psychother Psychosom,* 75(1):56-61.

Binanay C, Califf RM, Hasselblad V, O'Connor CM, Shah MR, Sopko G, et al. (2005). Evaluation study of congestive heart failure and pulmonary artery catheterization effectiveness: The ESCAPE trial. *JAMA,* 294(13):1625-1633.

Cadigan ME, Caruso NA, Haldeman SM, McNamara ME, Noyes DA, Spadafora MA, et al. (2001). The effects of music on cardiac patients on bed rest. *Prog Cardiovasc Nurs,* 16(1):5-13.

Devine EC. (1992). Effects of psychoeducational care for adult surgical patients: A meta-analysis of 191 studies. *Patient Educ Couns,* 19(2):129-142.

Dochterman JM, Bulechek GM (Eds). (2004). *Nursing Interventions Classification (NIC)*, 4th ed. St. Louis: Mosby.

Drew BJ, Califf RM, Funk M, Kaufman ES, Krucoff MW, Laks MM, et al. (2004). Practice standards for electrocardiographic monitoring in hospital settings: An American Heart Association scientific statement from the Councils on Cardiovascular Nursing, Clinical Cardiology, and Cardiovascular Disease in the Young: Endorsed by the International Society of Computerized Electrocardiology and the American Association of Critical-Care Nurses. *Circulation,* 110(17):2721-2746.

Drew BJ, Pelter MM, Adams MG, et al. (1998). 12-lead ST-segment monitoring vs single-lead maximum ST-segment monitoring for detecting ongoing ischemia in patients with unstable coronary syndromes, *Am J Crit Care,* 7(5): 355-363.

Drew BJ, Scheinman MM. (1995). ECG criteria to distinguish between aberrantly conducted supraventricular tachycardia and ventricular tachycardia: Practical aspects for the immediate care setting. *Pacing Clin Electrophysiol,* 18(12 Pt 1):2194-2208.

Drew BJ, Scheinman MM, Dracup K. (1991). MCL1 and MCL6 compared to V1 and V6 in distinguishing aberrant supraventricular from ventricular ectopic beats. *Pacing Clin Electrophysiol,* 14(9):1375-1383.

Driscoll A, Shanahan A, Crommy L, Foong S, Gleeson A. (1995). The effect of patient position on the reproducibility of cardiac output measurements. *Heart Lung*, 24(1):38-44.

Fauerbach JA, Bush DE, Thombs BD, McCann UD, Fogel J, Ziegelstein RC. (2005). Depression following acute myocardial infarction: A prospective relationship with ongoing health and function. *Psychosomatics*, 46(4):355-361.

Frasure-Smith N, Lesperance F, Talajic M. (1995). The impact of negative emotions on prognosis following myocardial infarction: Is it more than depression? *Health Psychol*, 14(5):388-398.

Freedman NS, Kotzer N, Schwab RJ. (1999). Patient perception of sleep quality and etiology of sleep disruption in the intensive care unit. *Am J Respir Crit Care Med*, 159(4 Pt 1):1155-1162.

Fumagalli S, Boncinelli L, Lo Nostro A, Valoti P, Baldereschi G, Di Bari M, et al. (2006). Reduced cardio-circulatory complications with unrestrictive visiting policy in an intensive care unit: Results from a pilot, randomized trial. *Circulation*, 113(7):946-952.

Guzzetta CE. (1989). Effects of relaxation and music therapy on patients in a coronary care unit with presumptive acute myocardial infarction. *Heart Lung*, 18(6):609-616.

Halm MA. (2005). Family presence during resuscitation: A critical review of the literature. *Am J Crit Care*, 14(6):494-511.

Harvey S, Harrison DA, Singer M, Ashcroft J, Jones CM, Elbourne D, et al. (2005). Assessment of the clinical effectiveness of pulmonary artery catheters in management of patients in intensive care (PAC-Man): A randomised controlled trial. *Lancet*, 366(9484):472-477.

Herlihy T, McIvor ME, Cummings CC, Siu CO, Alikahn M. (1987). Nausea and vomiting during acute myocardial infarction and its relation to infarct size and location. *Am J Cardiol*, 60(1):20-22.

Jensen BT, Abildstrom SZ, Larroude CE, Agner E, Torp-Pedersen C, Nyvad O, et al. (2005). QT dynamics in risk stratification after myocardial infarction. *Heart Rhythm*, 2(4):357-364.

Jones T, McCutcheon H. (2003). A randomised controlled trial comparing the use of manual versus mechanical compression to obtain haemostasis following coronary angiography. *Intensive Crit Care Nurs*, 19(1):11-20.

Juergens CP, Leung DY, Crozier JA, Wong AM, Robinson JT, Lo S, et al. (2004). Patient tolerance and resource utilization associated with an arterial closure versus an external compression device after percutaneous coronary intervention. *Catheter Cardiovasc Interv*, 63(2):166-170.

Kiely M, Byers LA, Greenwood R, Carroll E, Carroll D. (1998). Thermodilution measurement of cardiac output in patients with low output: Room-temperature versus iced injectate. *Am J Crit Care*, 7(6):436-438.

Koelling TM, Johnson ML, Cody RJ, Aaronson KD. (2005). Discharge education improves clinical outcomes in patients with chronic heart failure. *Circulation*, 111(2):179-185.

Lane D, Carroll D, Ring C, Beevers DG, Lip GY. (2000). Effects of depression and anxiety on mortality and quality-of-life 4 months after myocardial infarction. *J Psychosom Res*, 49(4):229-238.

Lazure LL, Baun MM. (1995). Increasing patient control of family visiting in the coronary care unit. *Am J Crit Care*, 4(2):157-164.

Logemann T, Luetmer P, Kaliebe J, Olson K, Murdock DK. (1999). Two versus six hours of bed rest following left-sided cardiac catheterization and a meta-analysis of early ambulation trials. *Am J Cardiol*, 84(4):486-488, A10.

Madias JE, Madias NE, Hood WB Jr. (1976). Precordial ST-segment mapping. Effects of oxygen inhalation on ischemic injury in patients with acute myocardial infarction. *Circulation*, 53(3):411-417.

Maeland JG, Havik OE. (1987). The effects of an in-hospital educational programme for myocardial infarction patients. *Scand J Rehabil Med*, 19(2):57-65.

Maroko PR, Radvany P, Braunwald E, Hale SL. (1975). Reduction of infarct size by oxygen inhalation following acute coronary occlusion. *Circulation*, 52(3):360-368.

Martinez EA, Kim LJ, Faraday N, Rosenfeld B, Bass EB, Perler BA, et al. (2003). Sensitivity of routine intensive care unit surveillance for detecting myocardial ischemia. *Crit Care Med*, 31(9):2302-2308.

Mayou RA, Gill D, Thompson DR, Day A, Hicks N, Volmink J, et al. (2000). Depression and anxiety as predictors of outcome after myocardial infarction. *Psychosom Med*, 62(2):212-219.

McCloy K, Leung S, Belden J, Castenada J, Erickson V, Koch K, et al. (1999). Effects of injectate volume on thermodilution measurements of cardiac output in patients with low ventricular ejection fraction. *Am J Crit Care*, 8(2):86-92.

Moorhead S, Johnson M, Maas M (Eds). (2004). *Nursing outcomes classification (NOC)*, 3rd ed. St. Louis: Mosby.

Moser DK, Dracup K. (1995). Psychosocial recovery from a cardiac event: The influence of perceived control. *Heart Lung*, 24(4):273-280.

Moser DK, Riegel B, McKinley S, Doering LV, An K, Sheahan S. (2007). Impact of anxiety and perceived control on in-hospital complications after acute myocardial infarction. *Psychosom Med*, 69:10-16.

Persson E, Pettersson J, Ringborn M, Sornmo L, Warren SG, Wagner GS, et al. (2006). Comparison of ST-segment deviation to scintigraphically quantified myocardial ischemia during acute coronary occlusion induced by percutaneous transluminal coronary angioplasty. *Am J Cardiol*, 97(3):295-300.

Robbins J, Nelson J, Rautaharju PM, Gottdiener JS. (2003). The association between the length of the QT interval and mortality in the Cardiovascular Health Study. *Am J Med*, 115(9):689-694.

Rosenstein G, Cafri C, Weinstein JM, Yeroslavtsev S, Abuful A, et al. (2004). Simple clinical risk stratification and the safety of ambulation two hours after 6 French diagnostic heart catheterization. *J Invasive Cardiol*, 16(3):126-128.

Sendelbach SE, Halm MA, Doran KA, Miller EH, Gaillard P. (2006). Effects of music therapy on physiological and psychological outcomes for patients undergoing cardiac surgery. *J Cardiovasc Nurs*, 21(3):194-200.

Shah MR, Hasselblad V, Stevenson LW, Binanay C, O'Connor CM, Sopko G, et al. (2005). Impact of the pulmonary artery catheter in critically ill patients. Meta-analysis of randomized clinical trials. *JAMA*, 294(13):1664-1670.

Simpson T, Shaver J. (1990). Cardiovascular responses to family visits in coronary care unit patients. *Heart Lung*, 19(4):344-351.

Stukshis I, Funk M, Johnson CR, Parkosewich JA. (1997). Accuracy of detection of clinically important dysrhythmias with and without a dedicated monitor watcher. *Am J Crit Care*, 6(4):312-317.

Thompson DR, Meddis R. (1990). A prospective evaluation of in-hospital counselling for first time myocardial infarction men. *J Psychosom Med*, 34(3):237-248.

Topf M, Bookman M, Arand D. (1996). Effects of critical care unit noise on the subjective quality of sleep. *J Adv Nurs*, 24(3):545-551.

Topf M, Davis JE. (1993). Critical care unit noise and rapid eye movement (REM) sleep. *Heart Lung*, 22(3):252-258.

Tron C, Koning R, Eltchaninoff H, Douillet R, Chassaing S, Sanchez-Giron C, et al. (2003). A randomized comparison of a percutaneous suture device versus manual compression for femoral artery hemostasis after PTCA. *J Interv Cardiol*, 16(3):217-221.

Vlasic W, Almond D, Massel D. (2001). Reducing bedrest following arterial puncture for coronary interventional procedures–impact on vascular complications: The BAC Trial. *J Invasive Cardiol*, 13(12):788-792.

 # CARDIAC CARE: REHABILITATIVE

Terry A. Lennie, PhD, RN, FAHA; Misook Lee Chung, PhD, RN;
Donna J. Corley, MEd, MSN, RN, CNE, Debra K. Moser, DNSc, RN, FAAN

> **NIC** **Definition:** Promotion of maximum functional activity level for a patient who has experienced an episode of impaired cardiac function that resulted from an imbalance between myocardial oxygen supply and demand (Dochterman & Bulechek, 2004).

NURSING ACTIVITIES

(Note: Please refer to the guidelines on Cardiac Care: Acute, Cardiac Care, and Cardiac Precautions.)

NR = Nursing Research, **MR** = Multidisciplinary Research, **SP** = Standard of Practice, **EO** = Expert Opinion, **LOE** = Level of Evidence

Effective

■ *Advocate for referral to a cardiac rehabilitation/secondary prevention program when available.* LOE = I

(MR) A meta-analysis of 48 trials of exercise-based cardiac rehabilitation programs that included a total of 8940 patients with coronary heart disease showed that patients in rehabilitation programs had a reduction in all-cause mortality, cardiac mortality, reduced total serum cholesterol and triglycerides, lower systolic blood pressure, and lower rates of self-reported smoking (Taylor et al., 2004).

(MR) A meta-analysis of 63 RCTs of secondary prevention programs that included a total of 21,295 patients with a history of acute myocardial infarction, heart failure, angina, or bypass grafts demonstrated that patients enrolled in prevention programs had decreased all-cause mortality and a 17% lower risk of myocardial infarction at 12 months. There were no differences in the effectiveness of programs that offered exercise alone, risk factor education and counseling alone, or combined interventions (Clark et al., 2005).

(MR) A meta-analysis of nine RCTs of exercise training that included a total of 801 patients with heart failure demonstrated that exercise training significantly reduced mortality and readmissions compared with the control group with no increase in adverse events (Piepoli et al., 2004).

■ *Provide smoking cessation advice and counseling when appropriate.* LOE = II

(Note: Please also refer to the guideline on Tobacco Cessation Assistance.)

(MR) A meta-analysis of 12 cohort studies involving 5878 patients from six countries who were discharged after an acute myocardial infarction showed a significant reduction in risk for all-cause mortality (odds ratios = 0.54) in patients who quit smoking compared with patients who continued smoking (Wilson et al., 2000).

(MR) A prospective cohort study of 2579 patients discharged after an acute myocardial infarction found that patients who quit smoking had a 61% reduction in risk for all-cause mortality after 1 year compared with patients who continued to smoke. The greatest risk was in continuing smokers who had a history of prior myocardial infarction (Kinjo et al., 2005).

■ *Encourage lifestyle changes and facilitate treatment for hypercholesterolemia according to current guidelines when appropriate.* LOE = I

(MR) An expert panel systematic review of all RCTs and relevant meta-analyses examining the effectiveness of treating hypercholesterolemia for secondary prevention of coronary heart disease and myocardial infarction showed that treatment significantly reduced the risk of fatal and nonfatal reinfarction and cardiovascular deaths (NCEP, 2002).

■ *Encourage lifestyle changes according to current guidelines for patients with blood pressures ≥120/80 mm Hg, and facilitate treatment for hypertension for patients with blood pressures ≥140/90 or ≥130/80 if patients have diabetes or chronic renal disease.* LOE = I

(MR) A systematic review of 15 RCTs that included a total of 74,696 participants showed that treatment of hypertension reduced the risk of myocardial infarction or cardiac death by 20% to 30% in patients with preexisting cardiovascular disease (Neal et al., 2000).

(MR) Based on a systematic review of available research studies, the American College of Cardiology/American Heart Association Task Force on Practice Guidelines recommended

RCT = Randomized Controlled (Clinical) Trial, **NIC** = Nursing Interventions Classification, **NOC** = Nursing Outcomes Classification

lifestyle changes (weight reduction, regular physical activity, sodium restriction, diets low in fat and high in fruits and vegetables) for patients with blood pressures above 120/80 mm Hg with the addition of antihypertensive drug treatment for blood pressures above 140/90 or 130/80 in patients with diabetes or chronic renal disease as secondary prevention measures after ST-segment elevation myocardial infarction (Antman et al., 2004).

■ *Encourage lifestyle changes and facilitate treatment using current guidelines to maintain tight blood glucose control (HbA$_{1c}$ <7%).* **LOE = II**

(MR) A stratified RCT in which 10-year outcomes were compared between an intensive glucose control group ($N = 2729$, median HbA$_{1c}$ = 7%) and a conventional treatment group ($N = 1138$, median HbA$_{1c}$ = 7.9%) of patients with type 2 diabetes showed that tight glucose control was associated with a 16% reduction in risk for fatal and nonfatal myocardial infarction (UK Prospective Diabetes Study Group, 1998).

(MR) Post hoc analysis of an RCT in which mortality rates were compared among 9020 patients stratified by their blood glucose levels during hospitalization for acute coronary syndrome showed that glucose levels above 157 mg/dL during hospitalization were an independent predictor of death at 10 months after discharge, placing these patients at 1.7 times higher risk of death than patients with blood glucose levels below 101 mg/dL (Bhadriraju et al., 2006).

Possibly Effective

■ *Encourage lifestyle changes that promote weight loss in patients who are obese, particularly patients with abdominal obesity.* **LOE = IV**

(Note: Please also refer to the guideline on Weight Reduction Assistance.)

(MR) A case-control study involving 52 countries in which the body mass index and waist-to-hip-ratio of 12,461 participants experiencing a first myocardial infarction were compared with those of 14,637 age- and sex-matched control subjects showed that obesity was a significant risk factor (odds ratio 1.33) for myocardial infarction in participants with the highest waist-to-hip ratio (abdominal obesity) after controlling for other risk factors (Yusuf et al., 2005).

■ *Encourage a minimum of 30 to 60 minutes of activity (walking, jogging, cycling, or aerobic exercise) preferably daily but at least 3 days per week in addition to normal daily activities, particularly for low-risk patients who do not have access to a cardiac rehabilitation program.* **LOE = I**

(MR) Based on a systematic review of available research studies, the American College of Cardiology/American Heart Association Task Force on Practice Guidelines recommended that patients discharged after ST-segment elevation myocardial infarction engage in regular physical activity such as walking, jogging, cycling, or other aerobic activity preferably daily but at least 3 days per week in addition to increased routine daily activities such as housework and gardening as a secondary prevention measure (Antman et al., 2004).

■ *Assess for anxiety and depression and facilitate referral for treatment.* **LOE = VI**

(MR) A descriptive study of 347 patients admitted for myocardial infarction showed that patients with symptoms of anxiety and depression during hospitalization and at 3 months after discharge experienced more symptoms of chest pain, made more visits to their primary care provider, reported a lower quality of life, and were less likely to have made recommended lifestyle changes at 1 year after discharge than nondistressed patients (Mayou et al., 2000).

NR = Nursing Research, **MR** = Multidisciplinary Research, **SP** = Standard of Practice, **EO** = Expert Opinion, **LOE** = Level of Evidence

(NR) A descriptive study of 86 patients admitted for acute myocardial infarction in which anxiety levels were assessed within 48 hours of admission demonstrated that patients with higher levels of anxiety were 4.9 times more likely to experience in-hospital complications (reinfarction, new-onset ischemia, ventricular fibrillation, sustained ventricular tachycardia, or in-hospital death) than patients with lower levels of anxiety (Moser & Dracup, 1996).

■ *Assess for potential barriers, involve spouse or family members, obtain a formal written commitment, and provide postdischarge telephone counseling on the importance of participation as methods to promote adherence to cardiac rehabilitation/secondary prevention programs and to medication regimen.*
LOE = III

(MR) A systematic review of 12 studies testing methods to improve adherence to cardiac rehabilitation programs showed that written commitments by patients increased attendance by 12% and telephone counseling/persuasion improved attendance slightly compared with controls (Beswick et al., 2005).

(NR) A quasi-experimental study of the effect of 58 patient-spouse dyad counseling programs on adherence found that patient-spouse dyads who received the counseling intervention demonstrated lowered blood pressure and significant differences in body fat compared with controls. Although not significant, the patient-spouse intervention group trended toward having the highest adherence to the exercise program (Dracup et al., 1984).

■ *Provide education and counseling about lifestyle changes and medication treatment for secondary prevention to patients and family members using verbal, written, and audiovisual formats beginning at admission, intensifying at discharge, and continuing after discharge.* **LOE = II**

(MR) Based on a systematic review of available research studies, the American College of Cardiology/American Heart Association Task Force on Practice Guidelines recommended instruction of patients using verbal, written, and audiovisual formats that begins at admission, is enhanced at discharge, and continues through rehabilitation programs as a means of improving adherence to prescribed treatments (Antman et al., 2004).

(NR) An RCT of education and psychological support programs related to recovery from a myocardial infarction for 60 wives of patients with first-time myocardial infarction found that wives who received counseling were significantly less anxious than usual care wives (Thompson & Meddis, 1990).

■ *Advise patients and family to learn about automatic electronic defibrillator devices and cardiopulmonary resuscitation, and refer to a cardiopulmonary resuscitation training program, preferably one with a social support component.*
LOE = V

(Note: Please also refer to the guideline on Cardiac Care: Acute.)

(MR) Based on a systematic review of available data, patients discharged after an ST-segment elevation myocardial infarction are four to six times more likely to experience sudden death, most cardiac arrests occur within the first 18 months after discharge, and chances of surviving a witnessed cardiac arrest are higher if cardiopulmonary resuscitation is initiated. The American College of Cardiology/American Heart Association Task Force on Practice Guidelines recommended that patients and family members receive information about automatic electronic defibrillator devices and be referred to cardiopulmonary resuscitation training

RCT = Randomized Controlled (Clinical) Trial, **NIC** = Nursing Interventions Classification, **NOC** = Nursing Outcomes Classification

programs, ideally ones that include a social support component, which has been shown to improve psychosocial adjustment and decrease anxiety and hostility (Antman et al., 2004).

   (NR) An RCT of cardiopulmonary resuscitation training of spouses ($N = 196$) of patients recovering from acute coronary syndrome found that perceived control, which decreases anxiety, was significantly increased in spouses after receiving training (Moser & Dracup, 2000).

■ *Educate all patients, regardless of age, gender, ethnicity, or socioeconomic status, about the signs and symptoms of acute coronary syndrome and stroke and the appropriate actions to take (i.e., calling 911 and transport by ambulance to the hospital) when they experience them.* **LOE = V**

(Note: Please refer to the guideline on Cardiac Care.)

Not Effective

No applicable published research was found in this category.

Possibly Harmful

No applicable published research was found in this category.

OUTCOME MEASUREMENT

CARDIAC DISEASE SELF-MANAGEMENT (NOC)

Definition: Personal actions to manage heart disease and prevent disease progression. **Cardiac Disease Self-Management** as evidenced by the following selected NOC indicators:

- Reports symptoms of worsening disease
- Performs treatment regimen as prescribed
- Limits sodium intake
- Follows recommended diet
- Participates in smoking cessation regimen
- Participates in recommended exercise program
- Uses warning signs to seek health care

(Rate each indicator of **Cardiac Disease Self-Management:** 1 = never demonstrated, 2 = rarely demonstrated, 3 = sometimes demonstrated, 4 = often demonstrated, 5 = consistently demonstrated) (Moorhead et al., 2004).

Additional non-NOC indicators:

- Monitors symptoms
- Limits saturated fat intake
- Limits trans-fatty acids intake

REFERENCES

Antman EM, Anbe DT, Armstrong PW, Bates ER, Green LA, Hand M, et al. (2004). ACC/AHA guidelines for the management of patients with ST-elevation myocardial infarction: A report of the American College of Cardiology/American Heart Association task force on practice guidelines (Committee to revise the 1999 guidelines for the management of patients with acute myocardial infarction). *Circulation,* 110(9):e82-e292.

Beswick AD, Rees K, West RR, Taylor FC, Burke M, Griebsch I, et al. (2005). Improving uptake and adherence in cardiac rehabilitation: Literature review. *J Adv Nurs,* 49(5):538-555.

Bhadriraju S, Ray KK, DeFranco AC, Barber K, Bhadriraju P, Murphy SA, et al. (2006). Association between blood glucose and long-term mortality in patients with acute coronary syndromes in the OPUS-TIMI 16 trial. *Am J Cardiol,* 97(11):1573-1577.

Clark AM, Hartling L, Vandermeer B, McAlister FA. (2005). Meta-analysis: Secondary prevention programs for patients with coronary artery disease. *Ann Intern Med,* 143(9):659-672.

Dochterman JM, Bulechek GM (Eds). (2004). *Nursing Interventions Classification (NIC),* 4th ed. St. Louis: Mosby.

Dracup K, Meleis AI, Clark S, Clyburn A, Shields L, Staley M. (1984). Group counseling in cardiac rehabilitation: Effect on patient compliance. *Patient Educ Couns,* 6(4):169-177.

Kinjo K, Sato H, Sakata Y, Nakatani D, Mizuno H, Shimizu M, et al. (2005). Impact of smoking status on long-term mortality in patients with acute myocardial infarction. *Circ J,* 69(1):7-12.

Mayou RA, Gill D, Thompson DR, Day A, Hicks N, Volmink J, et al. (2000). Depression and anxiety as predictors of outcome after myocardial infarction. *Psychosom Med,* 62(2):212-219.

Moorhead S, Johnson M, Maas M (Eds). (2004). *Nursing Outcomes Classification (NOC),* 3rd ed. St. Louis: Mosby.

Moser DK, Dracup K. (1996). Is anxiety early after myocardial infarction associated with subsequent ischemic and arrhythmic events? *Psychosom Med,* 58(5):395-401.

Moser DK, Dracup K. (2000). Impact of cardiopulmonary resuscitation training on perceived control in spouses of recovering cardiac patients. *Res Nurs Health,* 23(4):270-278.

National Cholesterol Education Program (NCEP) Expert Panel on Detection, Evaluation, and Treatment of High Blood Cholesterol in Adults (Adult Treatment Panel III). (2002). Third report of the National Cholesterol Education Program (NCEP) expert panel on detection, evaluation, and treatment of high blood cholesterol in adults (Adult Treatment Panel III) final report. *Circulation,* 106(25):3143-3421.

Neal B, MacMahon S, Chapman N. (2000). Effects of ACE inhibitors, calcium antagonists, and other blood-pressure-lowering drugs: Results of prospectively designed overviews of randomised trials. Blood Pressure Lowering Treatment Trialists' Collaboration. *Lancet,* 356(9246):1955-1964.

Piepoli MF, Davos C, Francis DP, Coats AJ. (2004). Exercise training meta-analysis of trials in patients with chronic heart failure (ExTraMATCH). *BMJ,* 328(7433):189.

Taylor RS, Brown A, Ebrahim S, Jolliffe J, Noorani H, Rees K, et al. (2004). Exercise-based rehabilitation for patients with coronary heart disease: Systematic review and meta-analysis of randomized controlled trials. *Am J Med,* 116(10):682-692.

Thompson DR, Meddis R. (1990). Wives' responses to counselling early after myocardial infarction. *J Psychosom Res,* 34(3):249-258.

UK Prospective Diabetes Study Group. (1998). Intensive blood-glucose control with sulphonylureas or insulin compared with conventional treatment and risk of complications in patients with type 2 diabetes (UKPDS 33). UK Prospective Diabetes Study (UKPDS) Group. *Lancet,* 352(9131):837-853.

Wilson K, Gibson N, Willan A, Cook D. (2000). Effect of smoking cessation on mortality after myocardial infarction: Meta-analysis of cohort studies. *Arch Intern Med,* 160(7):939-944.

Yusuf S, Hawken S, Ounpuu S, Bautista L, Franzosi MG, Commerford P, et al. (2005). Obesity and the risk of myocardial infarction in 27,000 participants from 52 countries: A case-control study. *Lancet,* 366(9497):1640-1649.

 # CARDIAC PRECAUTIONS

Susan K. Frazier, PhD, RN; Terry A. Lennie, PhD, RN, FAHA; Lynne Jensen, PhD, ARNP; Debra K. Moser, DNSc, RN, FAAN

NIC **Definition:** Prevention of an acute episode of impaired cardiac function by minimizing myocardial oxygen consumption or increasing myocardial oxygen supply (Dochterman & Bulechek, 2004).

RCT = Randomized Controlled (Clinical) Trial, **NIC** = Nursing Interventions Classification, **NOC** = Nursing Outcomes Classification

NURSING ACTIVITIES

Effective

- ☐ SP *Avoid or treat excessive anxiety.* **LOE = V**

  NR A descriptive study of patients ($N = 86$) within 48 hours of acute myocardial infarction found higher complication rates (reinfarction, recurrent myocardial ischemia, sustained ventricular tachycardia, ventricular fibrillation, or in-hospital death) following infarction in patients with high anxiety than patients with low anxiety (Moser & Dracup, 1996).

  MR A descriptive study of patients ($N = 204$) within 1 week of acute myocardial infarction suggested that reduced cardiac baroreflex control was associated with level of anxiety after controlling for age, blood pressure, and respiratory frequency (Watkins et al., 2002).

  MR A descriptive study of patients ($N = 246$) treated for acute myocardial infarction at hospital discharge identified anxiety and emotional sensitivity as significant predictors of mortality at 8 years after acute myocardial infarction (Carpeggiani et al., 2005).

Possibly Effective

No applicable published research found in this category.

Not Effective

- ☐ *Restricting caffeinated beverages.* **LOE = I**

  MR An RCT comparing caffeine and placebo in patients ($N = 70$) within 1 week of onset of acute myocardial infarction demonstrated no significant difference in the occurrence or severity of ventricular dysrhythmias (Myers et al., 1987).

  MR An RCT comparing caffeine restriction, caffeinated coffee, and decaffeinated coffee intake in patients with symptomatic frequent idiopathic ventricular premature beats ($N = 13$) found no significant association between plasma caffeine levels and frequency of ventricular dysrhythmias or detected palpitations (Newby et al., 1996).

  MR A multicenter cohort study of patients ($N = 1902$) after acute myocardial infarction found no overall association between self-reported caffeine consumption and postinfarction mortality (Mukamal et al., 2004).

- ☐ *Restricting beverages warmer than 160°F (70°C) or colder than 45°F (7°C).* **LOE = III**

  MR A controlled study of patients ($N = 20$) admitted with an acute myocardial infarction and a comparison group of patients ($N = 11$) admitted with angina or chest wall syndrome observed no change in cardiac rhythm or increase in ectopy during or after ingestion of warm (>70°C) or cold liquids (<7°C) within 36 hours of admission (Cohen et al., 1977).

- ☐ NIC *Refrain from taking rectal temperatures.* **LOE = III**

  MR In a controlled study of patients with acute myocardial infarction who underwent a digital rectal examination 6 to 12 hours after admission ($N = 160$), patients with acute myocardial infarction ($N = 155$) who were resting, and intensive care patients with nonacute myocardial infarction who underwent a digital rectal examination 6 to 12 hours after admission ($N = 165$), there were no sustained dysrhythmias or change in vital signs during the examination (Akhtar et al., 2000).

NR = Nursing Research, **MR** = Multidisciplinary Research, **SP** = Standard of Practice, **EO** = Expert Opinion, **LOE** = Level of Evidence

Possibly Harmful

■ *Bed rest for 12 to 24 hours for stable patients following ST-elevation myocardial infarction.* **LOE = VII**

(MR) A systematic review and practice guideline suggested that even short-term bed rest and the absence of regular orthostatic stress produced by ambulation may result in orthostatic hypotension and/or syncope during the initial ambulation following acute myocardial infarction (Antman et al., 2004).

(MR) A meta-analysis (15 RCTs) that compared short (2 to 12 days) versus prolonged (5 to 28 days) bed rest after uncomplicated acute myocardial infarction found no difference in mortality, reinfarction rate, postinfarction angina, or thromboembolic events (Herkner et al., 2003).

■ *Restricting caffeinated beverages in patients who are caffeine tolerant (regularly drink caffeinated beverages).* **LOE = III**

(MR) A controlled study of the cardiovascular, behavioral, and subjective effects of caffeine withdrawal in healthy male and female (50%), nonsmoking individuals ($N = 120$) determined that caffeine withdrawal in persons who were caffeine tolerant produced increased heart rate, reduced motor activity, decreased reported daytime wakefulness, negative mood in the afternoons, and a higher incidence of headache with greater analgesic use (Hofer & Battig, 1994).

■ *The Valsalva maneuver (straining during defecation, cough, lifting self onto bedpan, or lifting self in bed).* **LOE = II**

(NR) A controlled study of healthy men and women ($N = 32$) studied the effects of a Valsalva maneuver of 40 mm Hg for 10 seconds in five random chair and bed positions and found that the greatest alteration in systolic blood pressure occurred with the head of the bed elevated more than 30 degrees and in the chair positions (Metzger & Therrien, 1990).

(MR) A controlled study of patients ($N = 22$) during cardiac catheterization (7 normal, 5 normal wall motion after myocardial infarction, 10 abnormal wall motion) found that action potential duration alterations that could generate dysrhythmias occurred during the strain and unloading phases of the Valsalva, and these changes were influenced by wall motion abnormalities (Taggart et al., 1992).

OUTCOME MEASUREMENT

CARDIAC PUMP EFFECTIVENESS   (NOC)

Definition: Adequacy of blood volume ejected from the left ventricle to support systemic perfusion pressure.

Cardiac Pump Effectiveness as evidenced by the following selected NOC indicators:
- Systolic blood pressure
- Diastolic blood pressure
- Apical heart rate
- Cardiac index

Continued

OUTCOME MEASUREMENT—*cont'd*

- Ejection fraction
- Activity tolerance
- Peripheral pulses
- Skin color
- Urinary output
- Cognitive status

(Rate each indicator of **Cardiac Pump Effectiveness:** 1 = severely compromised, 2 = substantially compromised, 3 = moderately compromised, 4 = mildly compromised, 5 = not compromised) (Moorhead et al., 2004).

REFERENCES

Akhtar AJ, Moran D, Ganesan K, Akanno J, Tran T, Wu R, et al. (2000). Safety and efficacy of digital rectal examination in patients with acute myocardial infarction. *Am J Gastroenterol,* 95(6):1463-1465.

Antman EM, Anbe DT, Armstrong PW, Bates ER, Green LA, Hand M, et al. (2004). ACC/AHA guidelines for the management of patients with ST-elevation myocardial infarction; a report of the American College of Cardiology/American Heart Association Task Force on Practice Guidelines (Committee to Revise the 1999 Guidelines for the Management of Patients with Acute Myocardial Infarction). *Circulation,* 110(9):e82-e292.

Carpeggiani C, Emdin M, Bonaguidi F, Landi P, Michelassi C, Trivella MG, et al. (2005). Personality traits and heart rate variability predict long-term cardiac mortality after myocardial infarction. *Eur Heart J,* 26(16):1612-1617.

Cohen IM, Alpert JS, Francis GS, Vieweg WV, Hagan AD. (1977). Safety of hot and cold liquids in patients with acute myocardial infarction. *Chest,* 71(4):450-452.

Dochterman JM, Bulechek GM (Eds). (2004). *Nursing Interventions Classification (NIC),* 4th ed. St. Louis: Mosby.

Herkner H, Thoennissen J, Nikfardjam M, Koreny M, Laggner AN, Mullner M. (2003). Short versus prolonged bed rest after uncomplicated acute myocardial infarction: A systematic review and meta-analysis. *J Clin Epidemiol,* 56(8):775-781.

Hofer I, Battig K. (1994). Cardiovascular, behavioral, and subjective effects of caffeine under field conditions. *Pharmacol Biochem Behav,* 48(4):899-908.

Metzger BL, Therrien B. (1990). Effect of position on cardiovascular response during the Valsalva maneuver. *Nurs Res,* 39(4):198-202.

Moorhead S, Johnson M, Maas M (Eds). (2004). *Nursing Outcomes Classification (NOC),* 3rd ed. St. Louis: Mosby.

Moser DK, Dracup K. (1996). Is anxiety early after myocardial infarction associated with subsequent ischemic and arrhythmic events? *Psychosom Med,* 58(5):395-401.

Mukamal KJ, Maclure M, Muller JE, Sherwood JB, Mittleman MA. (2004). Caffeinated coffee consumption and mortality after acute myocardial infarction. *Am Heart J,* 147(6):999-1004.

Myers MG, Harris L, Leenen FH, Grant DM. (1987). Caffeine as a possible cause of ventricular arrhythmias during the healing phase of acute myocardial infarction. *Am J Cardiol,* 59(12):1024-1028.

Newby DE, Neilson JM, Jarvie DR, Boon NA. (1996). Caffeine restriction has no role in the management of patients with symptomatic idiopathic ventricular premature beats. *Heart,* 76(4):355-357.

Taggart P, Sutton P, John R, Lab M, Swanton H. (1992). Monophasic action potential recordings during acute changes in ventricular loading induced by the Valsalva manoeuvre. *Br Heart J,* 67(3):221-229.

Watkins LL, Blumenthal JA, Carney RM. (2002). Association of anxiety with reduced baroreflex cardiac control in patients after acute myocardial infarction. *Am Heart J,* 143(3):460-466.

NR = Nursing Research, **MR** = Multidisciplinary Research, **SP** = Standard of Practice, **EO** = Expert Opinion, **LOE** = Level of Evidence

CAREGIVER SUPPORT   NIC

Barbara Given, PhD, RN, FAAN; Paula R. Sherwood, PhD, RN, CNRN

NIC **Definition:** Provision of the necessary information, advocacy, and support to facilitate primary patient care by someone other than a health care professional (Dochterman & Bulechek, 2004).

NURSING ACTIVITIES

Effective

- ***Implement training programs for caregivers that focus on skill building, education, and problem solving. LOE = I***

  (MR) In an RCT of 127 caregivers of people with Alzheimer's disease, an intervention focused on skill building, education, and problem solving resulted in decreased days assisting with activities of daily living (ADLs), decreased upset with memory-related behaviors, improved affect, and improved task management strategies (Gitlin et al., 2005).

  (MR) Skill training in an RCT of 169 female caregivers of people with dementia resulted in decreased anger, hostility, and depressive symptoms and improved self-efficacy (Coon et al., 2003).

  (NR) In an RCT of 74 caregivers of people who had a stroke, although caregiver burden was not affected, a home visit followed by phone calls for 2½ months led to improved problem-solving skills, preparedness, vitality, social functioning, and mental health (Grant et al., 2002).

  (NR) In an RCT of 237 caregivers of people with Alzheimer's disease, an in-home psychoeducational intervention led to improved response to care recipients' memory problems (Gerdner et al., 2002).

  (NR) In an RCT of 354 caregivers of people with cancer in hospice, an intervention to improve coping skills led to improved quality of life and lower levels of burden (McMillan et al., 2006).
  Additional research: Hepburn et al., 2003; Kuzu et al., 2005.

- ***Develop individual and group counseling sessions for caregivers. LOE = I***

  (MR) In an RCT of 406 spousal caregivers of people with Alzheimer's disease, individual and family counseling sessions followed by group sessions resulted in decreased caregiver distress over 4 years (Mittelman et al., 2004).

  (MR) In a systematic review of 22 interventions for caregivers of people with stroke, counseling programs (approximately 8 hours) appeared to have the most positive outcome, although most interventions were given on a fixed schedule versus on demand from the caregiver (Visser-Meily et al., 2005).

  (MR) In an RCT of 312 spousal caregivers of people with Alzheimer's disease, individual and family counseling was associated with a higher number of support persons and satisfaction with support network (Roth et al., 2005).

RCT = Randomized Controlled (Clinical) Trial, **NIC** = Nursing Interventions Classification, **NOC** = Nursing Outcomes Classification

(MR) In an RCT of 225 caregivers of people with Alzheimer's disease, family therapy plus a computer telephone integrated system resulted in a reduced number of depressive symptoms (Eisdorfer et al., 2003).

■ *Prescribe, or encourage a health care provider to prescribe, cholinesterase inhibitors for the care recipient with dementia as indicated.* **LOE = I**

(NR) In a systematic review of 10 studies with caregivers of people with dementia, the use of cholinesterase inhibitors in the care recipient was associated with decreased caregiver burden and decreased time spent caring (Lingler et al., 2005).

(MR) In an RCT of 290 caregivers of people with Alzheimer's disease, prescribing donepezil to the care recipient was associated with caregivers who spent less time helping with ADLs, although no impact was seen on time helping with instrumental ADLs (Feldman et al., 2003).

■ *Design interventions that incorporate multiple components such as education and counseling.* **LOE = I**

(MR) In a meta-analysis involving 73 studies of caregivers of people with dementia, multicomponent interventions were effective at reducing caregiver burden (Acton & Kang, 2001).

(MR) In a meta-analysis of 127 intervention studies involving caregivers of people with dementia, multicomponent interventions reduced the risk for institutionalization. Psychoeducational interventions involving active caregiver participation had the broadest impact (Pinquart & Sorensen, 2006).

■ *Identify sociodemographic characteristics of the caregiver that can be used to tailor interventions.* **LOE = I**

(MR) Data from multiple interventions with caregivers of people with Alzheimer's disease demonstrated that interventions aimed at lowering caregiver burden varied by ethnicity, gender, and relationship to the care recipient (Gitlin et al., 2001, 2003).

(MR) In an RCT of 257 caregivers of people with stroke, group counseling sessions rather than individual sessions were preferred by caregivers with higher levels of burden and those whose care recipient had higher levels of psychological handicap (Schure et al., 2006).

(MR) In an RCT of 225 caregivers of people with Alzheimer's disease, caregivers who were Cuban American and those who were the husband or daughter of the care recipient gained particular benefit from family therapy plus a computer telephone integrated system (Eisdorfer et al., 2003).

■ *Identify personality characteristics of the caregiver that can be used to tailor interventions.* **LOE = I**

(MR) Counseling sessions in an RCT of 320 spousal caregivers of people with Alzheimer's disease were more effective in lowering levels of depression with caregivers who reported low levels of neuroticism (Jang et al., 2004).

(MR) In an RCT of 100 caregivers of people with Alzheimer's disease, caregivers' level of mastery affected response to an automated interactive voice intervention (Mahoney et al., 2003).

(MR) In a descriptive study involving 233 caregivers of individuals with cancer, caregivers' level of mastery and optimism served as a buffer to subjective caregiver stress; intrinsic feelings of optimism moderated caregiver distress (Gaugler et al., 2005).

Possibly Effective

Identify people in the community to assist the caregiver. **LOE = II**

(NR) In an RCT of 95 caregivers of people with Alzheimer's disease, using trained community consultants to help caregivers resulted in decreased depression and anxiety (Teri et al., 2005).

Identify a caregiver advocate. **LOE = II**

(MR) In a cohort study of 56 caregivers of people with brain injury, social work support at and after discharge was associated with decreased burden and improved mastery and satisfaction (Albert et al., 2002).

(MR) In an RCT of 205 caregivers of people with stroke, a family support organizer during hospitalization and home visits up to 9 months after discharge were not found to affect caregiver burden (Lincoln et al., 2003).

Provide telephone support. **LOE = II**

(NR) In a qualitative study of eight caregivers of people with dementia, telephone support met caregivers' needs for information and education, referral and assistance for navigating the health care system, and emotional support (Salfi et al., 2005).

(MR) In an RCT of 100 caregivers of people with Alzheimer's disease, year-long access to an automated interactive voice response system improved caregiver bother and depressive symptoms in selected caregivers (Mahoney et al., 2003).

(MR) In a descriptive study involving 41 Caucasian and Cuban caregivers of people with Alzheimer's disease, telecommunication technology had a positive effect as measured by increased knowledge skills and satisfaction (Bank et al., 2006).

Develop a formal partnership with the caregiver. **LOE = III**

(NR) In a quasi-experimental study of 185 caregivers of people with dementia, a partnership agreement with the caregiver followed by orientation to the facility and educational programs resulted in fewer feelings of loss, captivity, and negative feelings toward staff and improved perceptions of care from staff (Maas et al., 2004).

Teach the caregiver creative arts. **LOE = III**

(NR) In a quasi-experimental study of 40 caregivers of people with cancer, an intervention involving creative arts activities resulted in reduced stress, lower anxiety, and increased positive emotions 1 hour after the activity (Walsh et al., 2004).

Teach the caregiver relaxation techniques. **LOE = III**

(NR) In a quasi-experimental study of 36 caregivers of people with Alzheimer's disease, a 6-week relaxation training program was associated with improved self-efficacy in controlling anxiety stemming from care recipient behaviors (Fisher & Laschinger, 2001).

(MR) In a quasi-experimental study of 12 caregivers of people with Alzheimer's disease, an intervention involving six sessions of yoga was associated with reduced anxiety and depressive symptoms and improved self-efficacy (Waelde et al., 2004).

(NR) In an RCT involving 42 spouses of people with cancer, an intervention involving a 20-minute therapeutic back massage had a positive effect on mood and perceived stress (Goodfellow, 2003).

RCT = Randomized Controlled (Clinical) Trial, **NIC** = Nursing Interventions Classification, **NOC** = Nursing Outcomes Classification

■ *Implement interventions focused on improving sleep.* **LOE = II**

(MR) In an RCT of 36 caregivers of people with Alzheimer's disease, an intervention focused on sleep hygiene including daily walking and light exposure resulted in improved sleep time and fewer waking periods per hour (McCurry et al., 2005).

Not Effective

■ *Minimal home visits.* **LOE = I**

(MR) In an RCT of 39 caregivers of people with dementia, no change in time spent caring or caregiver stress occurred as a result of a home visit by a psychologist and occupational therapist (Nobili et al., 2004).

(NR) In an RCT of 106 caregivers of people with advanced cancer, a psychoeducational intervention delivered during two home visits with one follow-up phone call did not affect preparedness, self-efficacy, competence, or anxiety (Hudson et al., 2005).

■ *Cognitive-behavioral interventions.* **LOE = I**

(MR) In an RCT of 237 caregivers of people with cancer, a cognitive-behavioral intervention focused on symptom management and reducing emotional distress did not affect caregivers' depressive symptoms (Kurtz et al., 2005).

(MR) In an RCT of 89 caregivers of people with cancer, a cognitive-behavioral intervention focusing on symptom management and reducing emotional distress did not affect caregivers' depressive symptoms (Kozachik et al., 2001).

Possibly Harmful

No applicable published research was found in this category.

OUTCOME MEASUREMENT

CAREGIVER WELL-BEING   (NOC)

Definition: Extent of positive perception of primary care provider's health status and life circumstances.

Caregiver Well-Being as evidenced by the following selected NOC indicators:

• Psychological health
• Physical health
• Performance of usual roles
• Ability to cope

(Rate each indicator of **Caregiver Well-Being:** 1 = not at all satisfied, 2 = somewhat satisfied, 3 = moderately satisfied, 4 = very satisfied, 5 = completely satisfied) (Moorhead et al., 2004).

Additional non-NOC indicators:

• Social supports are available and in place
• Reports low or no feelings of burden/distress
• Mastery of the care situation

REFERENCES

Acton GJ, Kang J. (2001). Interventions to reduce the burden of caregiving for an adult with dementia: A meta-analysis. *Res Nurs Health,* 24(5):349-360.

Albert SM, Im A, Brenner L, Smith M, Waxman R. (2002). Effect of a social work liaison program on family caregivers to people with brain injury. *J Head Trauma Rehabil,* 17(2):175-189.

Bank AL, Arguelles S, Rubert M, Eisdorfer C, Czaja SJ. (2006). The value of telephone support groups among ethnically diverse caregivers of persons with dementia. *Gerontologist,* 46(1):134-138.

Coon DW, Thompson L, Steffen A, Sorocco K, et al. (2003). Anger and depression management: Psycho-educational skill training interventions for women caregivers of a relative with dementia. *Gerontologist,* 43(5):678-689.

Dochterman JM, Bulechek GM (Eds). (2004). *Nursing Interventions Classification (NIC),* 4th ed. St. Louis: Mosby.

Eisdorfer C, Czaja SJ, Loewenstein DA, Rubert MP, Arquelles S, Mitrani VB, et al. (2003). The effect of a family therapy and technology-based intervention on caregiver depression. *Gerontologist,* 43(4): 521-531.

Feldman H, Gauthier S, Hecker J, Vellas B, Emir B, Mastey V, et al. (2003). Efficacy of donepezil on maintenance of activities of daily living in patients with moderate to severe Alzheimer's disease and the effect on caregiver burden. *J Am Geriatr Soc,* 51(6):737-744.

Fisher PA, Laschinger HS. (2001). A relaxation training program to increase self-efficacy for anxiety control in Alzheimer family caregivers. *Holist Nurs Pract,* 15(2):47-58.

Gaugler JE, Hanna N, Linder J, Given CW, Tolbert V, Kataria R, et al. (2005). Cancer caregiving and subjective stress: A multi-site, multi-dimensional analysis. *Psychooncology,* 14(9):771-785.

Gerdner LA, Buckwalter KC, Reed D. (2002). Impact of a psychoeducational intervention on caregiver response to behavioral problems. *Nurs Res,* 51(6):363-374.

Gitlin LN, Belle SH, Burgio LD, Czaja SJ, Mahoney D, Gallagher-Thompson D, et al. (2003). Effect of multicomponent interventions on caregiver burden and depression: The REACH multisite initiative at 6-month follow up. *Psychol Aging,* 18(3):361-374.

Gitlin LN, Corcoran M, Winter L, Boyce A, Hauck WW. (2001). A randomized, controlled, trial of a home environmental intervention: Effect on efficacy and upset in caregivers and on daily function of persons with dementia. *Gerontologist,* 41(1):4-14.

Gitlin LN, Hauck WW, Dennis MP, Winter L. (2005). Maintenance of effects of the home environmental skill-building program for family caregivers and individuals with Alzheimer's disease and related disorders. *J Gerontol A Biol Sci Med Sci,* 60(3):368-374.

Goodfellow LM. (2003). The effects of therapeutic back massage on psychophysiologic variables and immune function in spouses of patients with cancer. *Nurs Res,* 52(5):318-328.

Grant JS, Elliott TR, Weaver M, Bartolucci AA, Giger JN. (2002). Telephone intervention with family caregivers of stroke survivors after rehabilitation. *Stroke,* 33(8):2060-2065.

Hepburn KW, Lewis M, Sherman CW, Tornatore J. (2003). The savvy caregiver program: Developing and testing a transportable dementia family caregiver training program. *Gerontologist,* 43(6):908-915.

Hudson PL, Aranda S, Hayman-White K. (2005). A psycho-educational intervention for family caregivers of patients receiving palliative care: A randomized controlled trial. *J Pain Symptom Manage,* 30(4):329-341.

Jang Y, Clay OJ, Roth DL, Haley WE, Mittelman MS. (2004). Neuroticism and longitudinal change in caregiver depression: Impact of a spouse-caregiver intervention program. *Gerontologist,* 44(3): 311-317.

Kozachik SL, Given CW, Given BA, Pierce SJ, Azzouz F, Rawl SM, et al. (2001). Improving depressive symptoms among caregivers of patients with cancer: Results of a randomized clinical trial. *Oncol Nurs Forum,* 28(7):1149-1157.

Kurtz ME, Kurtz JC, Given CW, Given B. (2005). A randomized, controlled trial of a patient/caregiver symptom control intervention: Effects on depressive symptomatology of caregivers of cancer patients. *J Pain Symptom Manage,* 30(2):112-122.

Kuzu N, Beser N, Zencir M, Sahiner T, Nesrin E, Ahmet E, et al. (2005). Effects of a comprehensive educational program on quality of life and emotional issues of dementia patient caregivers. *Geriatr Nurs,* 26(6):378-386.

Lincoln NB, Francis VM, Lilley SA, Sharma JC, Summerfield M. (2003). Evaluation of a stroke family support organiser: A randomized controlled trial. *Stroke,* 34(1):116-121.

Lingler JH, Martire LM, Schulz R. (2005). Caregiver-specific outcomes in antidementia clinical drug trials: A systematic review and meta-analysis. *J Am Geriatr Soc,* 53(6):983-990.

Maas ML, Reed D, Park M, Specht JP, Schutte D, Kelley LS, et al. (2004). Outcomes of family involvement in care intervention for caregivers of individuals with dementia. *Nurs Res,* 53(2):76-86.

Mahoney DF, Tarlow BJ, Jones RN. (2003). Effects of an automated telephone support system on caregiver burden and anxiety: Findings from the REACH for TLC intervention study. *Gerontologist,* 43(4): 556-567.

Moorhead M, Johnson M, Maas M (Eds). (2004). *Nursing Outcomes Classification (NOC),* 3rd ed. St. Louis: Mosby.

McCurry SM, Gibbons LE, Logsdon RG, Vitiello MV, Teri L. (2005). Nighttime insomnia treatment and education for Alzheimer's disease: A randomized, controlled trial. *J Am Geriatr Soc,* 53(5):793-802.

McMillan SC, Small BJ, Weitzner M, Schonwetter R, Tittle M, Moody L, et al. (2006). Impact of coping skills intervention with family caregivers of hospice patients with cancer: A randomized clinical trial. *Cancer,* 106(1):214-222.

Mittelman MS, Roth DL, Haley WE, Zarit SH. (2004). Effects of a caregiver intervention on negative caregiver appraisals of behavior problems in patients with Alzheimer's disease: Results of a randomized trial. *J Gerontol B Psychol Sci Soc Sci,* 59(1):P27-P34.

Nobili A, Riva E, Tettamanti M, Lucca U, Liscio M, Petrucci B, et al. (2004). The effect of a structured intervention on caregivers of patients with dementia and problem behaviors: A randomized controlled pilot study. *Alzheimer Dis Assoc Discord,* 18(2):75-82.

Pinquart M, Sorensen S. (2006). Helping caregivers of persons with dementia: Which interventions work and how large are their effects? *Int Psychogeriatr,* 18(4):577-595.

Roth DL, Mittelman MS, Clay OJ, Madan A, Haley WE. (2005). Changes in social support as mediators of the impact of a psychosocial intervention for spouse caregivers of persons with Alzheimer's disease. *Psychol Aging,* 20(4):634-644.

Salfi J, Ploeg J, Black ME. (2005). Seeking to understand telephone support for dementia caregivers. *West J Nurs Res,* 27(6):701-721.

Schure LM, van den Heuvel ET, Stewart RE, Sanderman R, de Witte LP, Meyboom-de Jong B. (2006). Beyond stroke: Description and evaluation of an effective intervention to support family caregivers of stroke patients. *Patient Educ Couns,* 62(1):46-55.

Teri L, McCurry SM, Logsdon R, Gibbons LE. (2005). Training community consultants to help family members improve dementia care: A randomized controlled trial. *Gerontologist,* 45(6):802-811.

Visser-Meily A, van Heugten C, Post M, Schepers V, Lindeman E. (2005). Intervention studies for caregivers of stroke survivors: A critical view. *Patient Educ Couns,* 56(3):257-267.

Waelde LC, Thompson L, Gallagher-Thompson D. (2004). A pilot study of a yoga and meditation intervention for dementia caregiver stress. *J Clin Psychol,* 60(6):677-687.

Walsh SM, Martin SC, Schmidt LA. (2004). Testing the efficacy of a creative-arts intervention with family caregivers of patients with cancer. *J Nurs Scholarsh,* 36(3):214-219.

 # CEREBRAL EDEMA MANAGEMENT

Laura H. McIlvoy, PhD, RN, CCRN, CNRN; Kimberly Meyer, MSN, RN, ACNP, CNRN

NIC **Definition:** Limitation of secondary cerebral injury resulting from swelling of brain tissue (Dochterman & Bulechek, 2004).

NR = Nursing Research, **MR** = Multidisciplinary Research, **SP** = Standard of Practice, **EO** = Expert Opinion, **LOE** = Level of Evidence

NURSING ACTIVITIES

Effective

■ **NIC** *Position with head of bed up 30 degrees or greater.* **LOE = II**

NR A systematic review demonstrated that ICP decreased with 30-degree elevation compared with 0-degree elevation in 9 of 11 studies of brain-injured individuals (Fan, 2004).

NR A randomized crossover trial involving patients with traumatic brain injury ($N = 8$) demonstrated that head of bed elevation of 30 degrees significantly improved ICP (Winkelman, 2000).

MR A controlled trial of middle cerebral artery stroke patients ($N = 18$) demonstrated that ICP decreased significantly with backrest elevations of 15 and 30 degrees (Schwarz et al., 2002b).

MR A controlled trial of patients with traumatic brain injury ($N = 38$) demonstrated that ICP was significantly lower at 30 degrees than 0 degrees head elevation (Ng et al., 2004).

■ *Remove/loosen rigid cervical collars.* **LOE = III**

MR A controlled trial of patients with traumatic brain injury ($N = 30$) demonstrated that ICP increased significantly and was sustained during the 5-minute period a rigid cervical collar was on and immediately decreased to baseline following removal of the collar (Hunt et al., 2001).

MR A controlled trial of head-injured patients ($N = 10$) demonstrated that ICP rose significantly in 9 out of 10 patients following application of a hard cervical collar (Mobbs et al., 2002).

■ **NIC** *Give sedation, as needed.* **LOE = II**

MR An RCT of 42 traumatic brain injury patients demonstrated that patients receiving a propofol infusion compared with a morphine infusion had significantly lower ICP by treatment day 3; required less neuromuscular blocking agents, benzodiazepam, pentobarbital, and cerebrospinal fluid drainage; and had better outcomes in terms of disability and mortality at 6 months (Kelly et al., 1999).

MR A controlled trial of traumatic brain injury patients ($N = 17$) demonstrated that ICP increased significantly higher with endotracheal suctioning in patients who were inadequately sedated versus those who were well sedated (Gemma et al., 2002).

■ *Administer mannitol per order.* **LOE = I**

EO Mannitol is effective for control of raised ICP after severe head injury (Brain Trauma Foundation & American Association of Neurological Surgeons, 2000).

MR A Cochrane systematic review found that administration of high-dose mannitol resulted in reduced mortality and morbidity compared with conventional dose mannitol in patients with severe traumatic brain injury (Wakai et al., 2005).

■ *Administer hypertonic saline per order to decrease ICP in refractory intracranial hypertension.* **LOE = II**

MR An RCT of traumatic brain injury patients ($N = 20$) demonstrated that the mean number of intracranial hypertension episodes per day and the duration of the episodes were significantly lower in patients receiving hypertonic saline than in patients receiving the conventional dose of mannitol (Vialet et al., 2003).

(MR) A controlled trial of stroke patients ($N = 8$) with 22 episodes of intracranial hypertension after failure of conventional treatment with mannitol demonstrated that hypertonic saline decreased ICP in all episodes and lasted for 4 hours (Schwarz et al., 2002a).

(MR) An RCT of acute liver failure patients ($N = 30$) demonstrated a significant decrease in ICP in patients who received hypertonic saline titrated to maintain sodium levels at 145 to 155 mmol/L compared with patients who received the normal standard of care. Patients receiving the normal care had a significantly higher number of episodes of intracranial hypertension than those receiving hypertonic saline (Murphy et al., 2004).

(MR) A randomized controlled crossover trial of brain injury patients with intracranial hypertension ($N = 9$) demonstrated that treatment with mannitol over 5 minutes and a hypertonic saline/dextran solution reduced ICP, but the hypertonic saline mix caused a significantly greater decrease in ICP that lasted longer than the mannitol effect (Battison et al., 2005).

■ (SP) *Administer steroids per order to control cerebral edema in brain tumor patients.* **LOE = III**

(MR) A controlled trial of brain tumor patients with intracranial hypertension ($N = 76$) demonstrated that the administration of dexamethasone reduced ICP in 90% of brain tumor patients within 12 to 18 hours after beginning therapy, with maximum improvement obtained within 4 days (French & Galicich, 1964).

(MR) A controlled trial of patients with cerebral tumors ($N = 10$) found that dexamethasone treatment decreased cerebral blood flow and blood volume as measured by positron emission tomography scans before and after treatment (Leenders et al., 1985).

■ (SP) *Perform cerebral spinal fluid drainage per order.* **LOE = III**

(NR) A controlled trial of traumatic brain injury patients ($N = 58$) demonstrated that a 3-mL withdrawal of cerebral spinal fluid resulted in a 10.1% decrease in ICP sustained for 10 minutes (Kerr et al., 2001).

■ *Allow auditory stimuli (quiet family voices and music), recognizing that the stimuli do not affect ICP.* **LOE = II**

(NR) A controlled trial of traumatic brain injury patients ($N = 15$) demonstrated that there was no significant change in ICP when patients experienced the auditory stimulation of ear plugs, music tapes, or a tape of environmental noise (Schinner et al., 1995).

(NR) A controlled trial of comatose patients ($N = 10$) demonstrated that taped messages by family members caused no significant change in ICP (Walker et al., 1998).

Possibly Effective

■ *Administer barbiturates per order for refractory intracranial hypertension in traumatic brain injury patients.* **LOE = II**

(EO) High-dose barbiturate therapy may be considered in hemodynamically stable salvageable severe head injury patients with intracranial hypertension refractory to maximal medical and

---

NR = Nursing Research, **MR** = Multidisciplinary Research, **SP** = Standard of Practice, **EO** = Expert Opinion, **LOE** = Level of Evidence

surgical ICP-lowering therapy (Brain Trauma Foundation & American Association of Neurological Surgeons, 2000).

(MR) A Cochrane systematic review found that barbiturate decreased ICP in two studies of traumatic brain injury patients, but for every four patients treated, one developed clinically significant hypotension (Roberts et al., 2004).

▨ *Induce moderate hypothermia per order for refractory intracranial hypertension.* LOE = III

(MR) A controlled trial of traumatic brain injury patients with ICP refractory to barbiturate therapy ($N = 64$) demonstrated that induced hypothermia of 32° to 34°C markedly decreased ICP in all patients during cooling (Polderman et al., 2002).

(MR) A controlled trial of traumatic brain injury patients with Glasgow Coma Scale score ≥5 ($N = 31$) demonstrated that induced hypothermia of 33°C significantly decreased the incidence of intracranial hypertension, with ICP decreasing significantly at 36°C and decreasing further at 35°C, but with no further decrease below 35°C (Tokutomi et al., 2003).

(MR) A controlled trial of patients with acute liver failure and refractory intracranial hypertension ($N = 13$) demonstrated that inducing hypothermia to 32° to 33°C significantly reduced ICP for 24 hours, bridging all 13 patients to successful orthotopic liver transplantation with complete neurologic recovery (Jalan et al., 2004).

▨ (NIC) *Maintain normothermia.* LOE = V

(MR) A descriptive study of brain injury patients ($N = 20$) found that an increase in brain temperature was associated with a significant rise in ICP; as fever ebbed, there was a significant decrease in ICP (Rossi et al., 2001).

▨ *Administer pain medications to control pain and maintain normal ICP.* LOE = III

(MR) A controlled study of postcraniotomy patients ($N = 35$) demonstrated that tramadol did not significantly change ICP, with satisfactory analgesia obtained in 50% of patients receiving smaller doses and in 88% of patients receiving larger doses (Ferber et al., 2000).

(MR) A controlled study of traumatic brain injury patients sedated with propofol and sufentanil ($N = 20$) demonstrated that a bolus of remifentanil followed by a continuous infusion for 20 minutes did not significantly change ICP in sedated traumatic brain injury patients (Englehard, Reeker, Kochs, & Werner, 2004).

▨ *Apply positive end-expiratory pressure (PEEP) as ordered to ensure adequate cerebral oxygenation and maintain normal ICP.* LOE = III

(MR) A controlled trial of traumatic brain injury patients ($N = 20$) demonstrated that increasing PEEP levels to 5, 10, and 15 cm H_2O decreased ICP (Huynh et al., 2002).

(MR) A controlled trial of ventilated acute stroke patients ($N = 16$) demonstrated that varying I/E ratios and PEEP of 5.3 and 10.6 cm H_2O produced no significant changes in ICP (Georgiadis et al., 2001).

(MR) A controlled trial of patients requiring ICP monitoring ($N = 20$) demonstrated that PEEP levels of 5, 10, and 15 cm H_2O produced a significant increase in ICP but did not approach intracranial hypertension (Videtta et al., 2002).

RCT = Randomized Controlled (Clinical) Trial, **NIC** = Nursing Interventions Classification, **NOC** = Nursing Outcomes Classification

Not Effective

No applicable published research was found in this category.

Possibly Harmful

▪ *Use of steroids to control cerebral edema in traumatic brain injury patients.*
LOE = I

> (MR) A multicenter RCT of traumatic brain injury patients ($N = 10,008$) found that the risk of death from all causes within 2 weeks was higher in the group allocated corticosteroids than that receiving placebo (Roberts et al., 2004).
> (EO) The use of steroids is not recommended for improving outcome or reducing ICP in patients with severe head injury (Bullock et al., 2001).

▪ *Use of routine hyperventilation to prevent increased ICP.* **LOE = I**

> (MR) An RCT of traumatic brain injury patients with paCO$_2$ 35 mm Hg versus $N = 36$ traumatic brain injury patients with paCO$_2$ 25 mm Hg for 5 days ($N = 41$) found that patients with initial Glasgow Coma Scale motor score of 4 or 5 had significantly better outcomes at 3 and 6 months when they were *not* hyperventilated (Muizelaar et al., 1991).
> (EO) In the absence of increased ICP, chronic prolonged hyperventilation therapy (PaCO$_2$ of 25 mm Hg or less) should be avoided after severe traumatic brain injury (Bullock et al., 2001).

▪ *Use of prolonged endotracheal suctioning. Limit suction passes to two to limit ICP increase.* **LOE = III**

> (NR) A systematic review demonstrated that endotracheal suctioning in acute head injury patients may increase ICP, causing intracranial hypertension in patients with a spiking ICP pattern, and these changes may be cumulative with each suction pass (Joanna Briggs Institute, 2000).

OUTCOME MEASUREMENT

NEUROLOGICAL STATUS

Definition: Ability of the peripheral and central nervous system to receive, process, and respond to internal and external stimuli.

Neurological Status as evidenced by the following selected NOC indicators:
- Consciousness
- Intracranial pressure
- Pupil size
- Pupil reactivity
- Eye movement pattern

(Rate each indicator of **Neurological Status:** 1 = severely compromised, 2 = substantially compromised, 3 = moderately compromised, 4 = mildly compromised, 5 = not compromised) (Moorhead et al., 2004).

NR = Nursing Research, **MR** = Multidisciplinary Research, **SP** = Standard of Practice, **EO** = Expert Opinion, **LOE** = Level of Evidence

REFERENCES

Battison C, Andrews PJ, Graham C, Petty T. (2005). Randomized, controlled trial on the effect of a 20% mannitol solution and a 7.5% saline/6% dextran solution on increased intracranial pressure after brain injury. *Crit Care Med*, 33(1):196-202.

Brain Trauma Foundation (BTF) & American Association of Neurological Surgeons (AANS). (2000). Management and prognosis of severe traumatic brain injury. *J Neurosurg*, 17:449-467.

Bullock R, Chestnut R, Clifton G. (2001). Management and prognosis of severe traumatic brain injury. *J Neurotrauma*, 17(6 & 7):451-627.

Dochterman JM, Bulechek GM (Eds). (2004). *Nursing Interventions Classification (NIC)*, 4th ed. St. Louis: Mosby.

Engelhard K, Reeker W, Kochs E, Werner C. (2004). Effect of remifentanil on intracranial pressure and cerebral blood flow velocity in patients with head trauma. *Acta Anaesthesiol Scand*, 48(4):396-399.

Fan JY. (2004). Effect of backrest position on intracranial pressure and cerebral perfusion pressure in individuals with brain injury: A systematic review. *J Neurosci Nurs*, 36(5):278-288.

Ferber J, Juniewicz H, Glogowska E, Wronski J, Abraszko R, Mierzwa J. (2000). Tramadol for postoperative analgesia in intracranial surgery. Its effect on ICP and CPP. *Neurol Neurochir Pol*, 34(6 Suppl):70-79.

French L, Galicich J. (1964). The use of steroids for control of cerebral edema. *Clin Neurosurg*, 10:212-223.

Gemma M, Tommasino C, Cerri M, Giannotti A, Piazzi B, Borghi T. (2002). Intracranial effects of endotracheal suctioning in the acute phase of head injury. *J Neurosurg Anesthesiol*, 14(1):50-54.

Georgiadis D, Schwarz S, Baumgartner R, Veltkamp R, Schwab S. (2001). Influence of positive end-expiratory pressure on intracranial pressure and cerebral perfusion pressure in patients with acute stroke. *Stroke*, 32(9):2088-2092.

Hunt K, Hallworth S, Smith M. (2001). The effects of rigid collar placement on intracranial and cerebral perfusion pressures. *Anaesthesia*, 56(6):511-513.

Huynh T, Messer M, Sing RF, Miles W, Jacobs DG, Thomason MH. (2002). Positive end-expiratory pressure alters intracranial and cerebral perfusion pressure in severe traumatic brain injury. *J Trauma*, 53(3): 488-493.

Jalan R, Olde Damink SW, Deutz NE, Hayes PC, Lee A. (2004). Moderate hypothermia in patients with acute liver failure and uncontrolled intracranial hypertension. *Gastroenterology*, 127(5):1338-1346.

Joanna Briggs Institute (JBI). (2000). Tracheal suctioning of adults with an artificial airway. *Best Pract*, 4(4):1-6.

Kelly DF, Goodale DB, Williams J, Herr DL, Chappell ET, Rosner MJ, et al. (1999). Propofol in the treatment of moderate and severe head injury: A randomized, prospective double-blinded pilot trial. *J Neurosurg*, 90(6):1042-1052.

Kerr ME, Weber BB, Sereika SM, Wilberger J, Marion DW. (2001). Dose response to cerebrospinal fluid drainage on cerebral perfusion in traumatic brain-injured adults. *Neurosurg Focus*, 11(4):E1.

Leenders KL, Beaney RP, Brooks DJ, Lammertsma AA, Heather JD, McKenzie CG. (1985). Dexamethasone treatment of brain tumor patients: Effects on regional cerebral blood flow, blood volume, and oxygen utilization. *Neurology*, 35(11):1610-1616.

Mobbs RJ, Stoodley MA, Fuller J. (2002). Effect of cervical hard collar on intracranial pressure after head injury. *ANZ J Surg*, 72(6):389-391.

Moorhead M, Johnson M, Maas M (Eds). (2004). *Nursing Outcomes Classification (NOC)*, 3rd ed. St. Louis: Mosby.

Muizelaar JP, Marmarou A, Ward JD, Kontos HA, Choi SC, Becker DP, et al. (1991). Adverse effects of prolonged hyperventilation in patients with severe head injury: A randomized clinical trial. *J Neurosurg*, 75(5):731-739.

Murphy N, Auzinger G, Bernel W, Wendon J. (2004). The effect of hypertonic sodium chloride on intracranial pressure in patients with acute liver failure. *Hepatology*, 39(2):464-470.

Ng I, Lim J, Wong H. (2004). Effects of head posture on cerebral hemodynamics: Its influences on intracranial pressure, cerebral perfusion, and cerebral oxygenation. *Neruosurgery*, 54(3):593-597.

Polderman KH, Tjong Tjin Joe R, Peerdeman SM, Vandertop WP, Girbes AR. (2002). Effects of therapeutic hypothermia on intracranial pressure and outcome in patients with severe head injury. *Intensive Care Med*, 28(11):1563-1573.

RCT = Randomized Controlled (Clinical) Trial, **NIC** = Nursing Interventions Classification, **NOC** = Nursing Outcomes Classification

Roberts I, Yates D, Sandercock P, Farrell B, Wasserberg J, Lomas G, et al. (2004). Effect of intravenous corticosteroids on death within 14 days in 10,008 adults with clinically significant head injury (MRC CRASH trial): Randomised placebo-controlled trial. *Lancet*, 364(9442):1321-1328.

Rossi S, Zanier ER, Mauri I, Columbo A, Stocchetti N. (2001). Brain temperature, body core temperature, and intracranial pressure in acute cerebral damage. *J Neurol Neurosurg Psychiatry*, 71(4):448-454.

Schinner KM, Chisholm AH, Grap MJ, Siva P, Hallinan M, LaVoice-Hawkins AM. (1995). Effects of auditory stimuli on intracranial pressure and cerebral perfusion pressure in traumatic brain injury. *J Neurosci Nurs*, 27(6):348-354.

Schwarz S, Georgiadis D, Aschoff A, Schwab S. (2002a). Effects of body position on intracranial pressure and cerebral perfusion in patients with large hemispheric stroke. *Stroke*, 33(2):497-501.

Schwarz S, Georgiadis D, Aschoff A, Schwab S. (2002b). Effects of hypertonic (10%) saline in patients with raised intracranial pressure after stroke. *Stroke*, 33(1):136-140.

Tokutomi T, Morimoto K, Miyagi T, Yamaguchi S, Ishikawa K, Shigemori M. (2003). Optimal temperature for the management of severe traumatic brain injury: Effect of hypothermia on intracranial pressure, systemic and intracranial hemodynamics, and metabolism. *Neurosurgery*, 52(1):102-111.

Vialet R, Albanese J, Thomachot L, Antonini F, Bourgouin A, Alliez B, et al. (2003). Isovolume hypertonic solutes (sodium chloride or mannitol) in the treatment of refractory posttraumatic intracranial hypertension: 2 mL/kg 7.5% saline is more effective than 2 mL/kg 20% mannitol. *Crit Care Med*, 31(6):1683-1687.

Videtta W, Villarejo F, Cohen M, Domeniconi G, Santa Cruz R, Pinillos O, et al. (2002). Effects of positive end-expiratory pressure on intracranial pressure and cerebral perfusion pressure. *Acta Neurochir Suppl*, 81:93-97.

Wakai A, Roberts I, Schierhout G. (2005). Mannitol for acute traumatic brain injury. *Cochrane Database Syst Rev*, (4):CD001049.

Walker JS, Eakes GG, Siebelink E. (1998). The effects of familial voice interventions on comatose head-injured patients. *J Trauma Nurs*, 5(2):41-45.

Winkelman C. (2000). Effect of backrest position on intracranial and cerebral perfusion pressures in traumatically brain-injured adults. *Am J Crit Care*, 9(6):373-380.

 # CEREBRAL PERFUSION PROMOTION

Laura H. McIlvoy, PhD, RN, CCRN, CNRN; Kimberly Meyer, MSN, RN, ACNP, CNRN

NIC **Definition:** Promotion of adequate perfusion and limitation of complications for a patient experiencing or at risk for inadequate cerebral perfusion (Dochterman & Bulechek, 2004).

NURSING ACTIVITIES

Effective

■ *Control ICP.* **LOE = I**

(Please refer to the guideline on Cerebral Edema Management.)

■ *Maintain CPP at or above 60 mm Hg.* **LOE = I**

EO CPP should be maintained at a minimum of 60 mm Hg. In the absence of cerebral ischemia, aggressive attempts to maintain CPP above 70 mm Hg with fluids and pressor should be avoided because of the risk of adult respiratory distress syndrome (BTF & AANS, 2003).

NR = Nursing Research, **MR** = Multidisciplinary Research, **SP** = Standard of Practice, **EO** = Expert Opinion, **LOE** = Level of Evidence

■ *Administer norepinephrine as ordered to raise MAP as needed to maintain adequate CPP.* **LOE = III**

(MR) A controlled trial of patients with severe head injury ($N = 16$) determined that noradrenaline was more effective than dopamine and that increasing MAP effectively increased CPP without changes in ICP (Biestro et al., 1998).

(MR) A prospective randomized crossover trial of head injury patients ($N = 10$) demonstrated that norepinephrine led to predictable and significant increases in cerebral blood flow for each step of CPP increase (65, 75, 85 mm Hg) compared with inconsistent cerebral blood flow when dopamine was used (Steiner et al., 2004).

(MR) A controlled trial of stroke patients ($N = 19$) with a total of 47 monitoring sessions demonstrated that norepinephrine raised MAP, raising CPP, augmenting peak mean flow velocity of the middle cerebral arteries, and slightly increasing ICP (Schwarz et al., 2002).

■ *Maintain euvolemia to prevent decreases in CPP.* **LOE = II**

(MR) An RCT demonstrated that a fluid balance lower than −594 mL was associated with poor outcome, independent of ICP, MAP, or CPP (Clifton et al., 2002).

■ *Administer hypertonic saline to increase CPP as ordered.* **LOE = III**

(MR) A controlled trial of critically ill patients with subarachnoid hemorrhage ($N = 7$) demonstrated that an infusion of hypertonic saline in hydroxyethyl starch during 20 minutes in 20 episodes of intracranial hypertension decreased ICP and achieved a peak increase in CPP of 26% (Bentsen et al., 2004).

(MR) A controlled trial of poor-grade patients with subarachnoid hemorrhage ($N = 9$) demonstrated that an infusion of hypertonic saline significantly increased arterial blood pressure and CPP (Al-Rawi et al., 2005).

(MR) A controlled trial of stroke patients ($N = 8$), with 22 episodes of intracranial hypertension after conventional treatment with mannitol failed, demonstrated that 75 mg of 20% hypertonic saline consistently increased CPP with the effect lasting 4 hours (Schwarz et al., 2002).

Possibly Effective

■ *Apply positive end-expiratory pressure (PEEP) as ordered to ensure adequate oxygenation and maintain adequate CPP.* **LOE = III**

(MR) A controlled trial of traumatic brain injury patients ($N = 20$) demonstrated that on increasing PEEP levels to 5, 10, and 15 cm H_2O, ICP decreased and CPP improved (Huynh et al., 2002).

(MR) A controlled trial of ventilated acute stroke patients ($N = 20$) demonstrated that PEEP as high as 12 cm H_2O did not adversely affect CPP as long as MAP was maintained (Schwarz et al., 2002).

■ (NIC) *Consult with physician to determine optimal head of bed (HOB) placement (e.g., 0, 15, or 30 degrees) and monitor the patient's responses to head positioning.* **LOE = III**

(NR) A systematic review demonstrated that CPP showed no statistical significance in the magnitude of change from a flat position to 30-degree elevation in five of nine studies of brain-injured individuals (Fan, 2004).

RCT = Randomized Controlled (Clinical) Trial, **NIC** = Nursing Interventions Classification, **NOC** = Nursing Outcomes Classification

(NR) A randomized crossover trial of traumatic brain injury patients ($N = 8$) demonstrated that head of bed elevation of 30 degrees resulted in significant and clinically important improvements in CPP (Winkelman, 2000).

(MR) A controlled trial of middle cerebral artery stroke patients ($N = 18$) demonstrated that CPP was highest at 0 degrees compared with 15 and 30 degrees during periods of normal ICP (Schwarz et al., 2002).

■ *Institute hypertension as ordered as a prevention/treatment for vasospasm in subarachnoid hemorrhage patients.* **LOE = V**

(MR) A retrospective descriptive study of patients with subarachnoid hemorrhage ($N = 45$) found that moderate hypertension (CPP 80 to 120 mm Hg) in normovolemic, hemodiluted patients was an effective method of improving cerebral oxygenation and was associated with a lower complication rate than hypervolemia (Raabe et al., 2005).

■ *Institute cerebrospinal fluid (CSF) drainage as ordered for control of low CPP.* **LOE = V**

(MR) A controlled trial of traumatic brain injury patients ($N = 26$) demonstrated that receiving CSF drainage as a treatment for low CPP was as effective as mannitol administration, and patients who received CSF drainage received less crystalloid infusion (Kinoshita et al., 2006).

Not Effective

No applicable published research was found in this category.

Possibly Harmful

■ *Head of bed elevations greater than 30 degrees.* **LOE = III**

(MR) A controlled trial of comatose patients with intracranial lesions ($N = 37$) demonstrated that head elevations between 30 and 45 degrees significantly decreased CPP (Moraine et al., 2000).

OUTCOME MEASUREMENT

TISSUE PERFUSION: CEREBRAL (NOC)

Definition: Adequacy of blood flow through the cerebral vasculature to maintain brain function.

Tissue Perfusion: Cerebral as evidenced by the following selected NOC indicators:
• Neurological function
• Intracranial pressure
• Systolic blood pressure
• Diastolic blood pressure

(Rate each indicator of **Tissue Perfusion: Cerebral:** 1 = severely compromised, 2 = substantially compromised, 3 = moderately compromised, 4 = mildly compromised, 5 = not compromised) (Moorhead et al., 2004).

NR = Nursing Research, **MR** = Multidisciplinary Research, **SP** = Standard of Practice, **EO** = Expert Opinion, **LOE** = Level of Evidence

REFERENCES

Al-Rawi PG, Zygun D, Tseng MY, Hutchinson PJ, Matta BF, Kirkpatrick PJ. (2005). Cerebral blood flow augmentation in patients with severe subarachnoid haemorrhage. *Acta Neurochir Suppl*, 95:123-127.

Bentsen G, Breivik H, Lundar T, Stubhaug A. (2004). Predictable reduction of intracranial hypertension with hypertonic saline hydroxyethyl starch: A prospective clinical trial in critically ill patients with subarachnoid haemorrhage. *Acta Anaesthesiol Scand*, 48(9):1089-1095.

Biestro A, Barrios E, Baraibar J, Puppo C, Lupano D, Cancela M, et al. (1998). Use of vasopressors to raise cerebral perfusion pressure in head injured patients. *Acta Neurochir Suppl*, 71:5-9.

Bullock RM, Chestnut RM, Clifton G, et al. (2000). Guidelines for the Management of Severe Traumatic Brain Injury: Cerebral Perfusion Pressure. *J Neurotrauma*, 17:449-554.

Clifton GL, Miller ER, Choi SC, Levin HS. (2002). Fluid thresholds and outcome from severe brain injury. *Crit Care Med*, 30(4):739-745.

Dochterman JM, Bulechek GM (Eds). (2004). *Nursing Interventions Classification (NIC)*, 4th ed. St. Louis: Mosby.

Fan JY. (2004). Effect of backrest position on intracranial pressure and cerebral perfusion pressure in individuals with brain injury: A systematic review. *J Neurosci Nurs*, 36(5):278-288.

Huynh T, Messer M, Sing RF, Miles W, Jacobs DG, Thomason MH. (2002). Positive end-expiratory pressure alters intracranial and cerebral perfusion pressure in severe traumatic brain injury. *J Trauma*, 53(3):488-493.

Kinoshita K, Sakurai A, Utagawa A, Ebihara T, Furukawa M, Moriya T, et al. (2006). Importance of cerebral perfusion pressure management using cerebrospinal drainage in severe traumatic brain injury. *Acta Neurochir Suppl*, 96:37-39.

Moorhead M, Johnson M, Maas M (Eds). (2004). *Nursing Outcomes Classification (NOC)*, 3rd ed. St. Louis: Mosby.

Moraine JJ, Berre J, Melot C. (2000). Is cerebral perfusion pressure a major determinant of cerebral blood flow during head elevation in comatose patients with severe intracranial lesions? *J Neurosurg*, 92(4):606-614.

Raabe A, Beck J, Keller M, Vatter H, Zimmermann M, Seifert V. (2005). Relative importance of hypertension compared with hypervolemia for increasing cerebral oxygenation in patients with cerebral vasospasm after subarachnoid hemorrhage. *J Neurosurg*, 103(6):974-981.

Schwarz S, Georgiadis D, Aschoff A, Schwab S. (2002). Effects of body position on intracranial pressure and cerebral perfusion in patients with large hemispheric stroke. *Stroke*, 33(2):497-501.

Steiner LA, Johnston AJ, Czosnyka M, Chatfield DA, Salvador R, Coles JP, et al. (2004). Direct comparison of cerebrovascular effects of norepinephrine and dopamine in head-injured patients. *Crit Care Med*, 32(4):1049-1054.

Winkelman C. (2000). Effect of backrest position on intracranial and cerebral perfusion pressures in traumatically brain-injured adults. *Am J Crit Care*, 9(6):373-380.

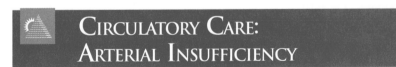

CIRCULATORY CARE: ARTERIAL INSUFFICIENCY

NIC

Kathleen Higgins, RN, CCRN, CS, MSN, CRNP

NIC   **Definition:** Promotion of arterial circulation (Dochterman & Bulechek, 2004).

NURSING ACTIVITIES

Effective

■ *Encourage the patient to exercise as tolerated.* **LOE = I**

RCT = Randomized Controlled (Clinical) Trial, **NIC** = Nursing Interventions Classification, **NOC** = Nursing Outcomes Classification

(MR) A Cochrane systematic review of patients with intermittent claudication demonstrated that a three-times-weekly exercise therapy program significantly improved maximal walking time and overall walking ability in patients with leg pain (Leng et al., 2000).

(MR) An RCT (N = 31 patients) demonstrated an improvement in claudication walking distances and walking economy at 6 and 12 months in older patients with intermittent claudication despite a progressively decreasing exercise rehabilitation program (Gardner et al., 2002).

(MR) An RCT (N = 61 patients) demonstrated that exercise rehabilitation in older patients with peripheral artery occlusive disease increased treadmill claudication distance, which increased daily physical activity and improved patients' independent function (Gardner et al., 2001).

■ (NIC) *Determine the ankle brachial index (ABI) as appropriate.* **LOE = II**

(MR) An RCT (N = 50 patients) demonstrated the relationship between ABI and venoarteriolar response (VAR) in patients with peripheral artery disease (PAD) and correlated the presence and severity of PAD with abnormal ABI and VAR (Otah et al., 2005).

(MR) A case-control study (N = 131 patients) assessed brachial artery flow-mediated dilation and plasma levels of inflammatory markers in a control group, asymptomatic PAD patients, and symptomatic PAD patients and found that ABI correlated positively with flow-mediated dilation and negatively with inflammatory markers (Brevetti et al., 2003).

(MR) A multicenter, cross-sectional descriptive study (N = 6979 patients) indicated that ABI was a simple and effective method to identify patients with recognized and unrecognized PAD (Hirsch et al., 2001).

■ *Educate the family and patient on the procedures and plan of care.* **LOE = IV**

(MR) A case-control study (N = 381 patients) using a 38-year follow-up of the Framingham Heart Study determined that identifying patients with a profile of high-risk factors was essential and a beneficial tool toward patient education and risk factor modification (Murabito et al., 1997).

(EO) The nurse should educate the patient, caregiver, or legally authorized representative relative to the prescribed therapy and plan of care including, but not limited to, potential complications associated with treatment or therapy and risks and benefits (Johnson & Psustian, 2005).

■ *Obtain a comprehensive history and physical examination for peripheral arterial circulation assessment.* **LOE = IV**

(MR) A multicenter, case-control study (N = 6979 patients) demonstrated the need for health care providers to assess for PAD and the prevalence of PAD in primary care practice where patients were not identified and not treated (Hirsch et al., 2001).

(EO) The nurse should perform an assessment of the peripheral circulation including assessment of pain in the arms and legs; history of pain in the calf with exercise and relieved with rest; sensitivity to temperature changes; cold limbs, numbness, tingling in limbs, color pallor, or limbs with loss of hair; color and pain in fingers and toes with cold; swelling in calves, legs, or feet; and swelling with redness or tenderness in limbs (Bickley & Szilagyi, 2003).

(EO) The nurse should recognize the normal aging changes related to the peripheral circulation (thinning skin, dry skin, decreased nail growth, decreased hair growth on lower extremities) and should differentiate these from abnormal changes (decrease or absence of pulse, swelling, extremity pain, ulcers, cyanosis, hyperpigmentation, and focal warmth) (Bickley & Szilagyi, 2003).

NR = Nursing Research, **MR** = Multidisciplinary Research, **SP** = Standard of Practice, **EO** = Expert Opinion, **LOE** = Level of Evidence

(MR) A descriptive cross-sectional study ($N = 2174$ patients) found that the prevalence of PAD in adults older than 40 in the United States was positively associated with increasing age, black race/ethnicity, current smoking, diabetes, hypertension, hypercholesterolemia, and low kidney function (Selvin & Erlinger, 2004).

■ *Identify patients who have risk factors for PAD so that they can be treated.* **LOE = IV**

(MR) A retrospective, cross-sectional study determined the risk factors for poor collateral development in patients ($N = 45$) with claudication as diabetes and short duration of symptoms in the multivariate analysis (De Vivo et al., 2005).

(MR) A case-control study ($N = 381$ patients) using a 38-year follow-up of the Framingham Heart Study determined that identifying patients with a profile of high-risk factors was essential and a beneficial tool toward patient education and risk factor modification (Murabito et al., 1997).

(EO) The nurse should identify factors that contribute to PAD and document these findings, including tobacco use, diabetes, hypertension, hyperlipidemia, and cardiovascular or cerebrovascular disease (Bickley & Szilagyi, 2003).

■ (NIC) *Administer antiplatelet or anticoagulant medications, as appropriate.* **LOE = I**

(MR) A Cochrane systematic review to determine which antithrombotic drug would reduce recurrent arterial obstruction revealed that results were occlusion specific: aspirin combined with dipyridamole improved patency after femoropopliteal angioplasty; low-molecular-weight heparin before intervention resulted in a decrease in femoropopliteal obstruction restenosis rate; data on clopidogrel and abciximab need further study; and aspirin started before femoropopliteal intervention was determined the most effective and safe therapy for patients (Dorffler-Melly et al., 2005).

(MR) A meta-analysis of randomized trials regarding antiplatelet regimens demonstrated the benefit of antiplatelet therapy in most types of patients at increased risk for occlusive vascular events (arterial occlusions and venous thromboembolism) (Antithrombotic Trialists' Collaboration, 2002).

(MR) A meta-analysis of randomized trials regarding antiplatelet regimens by the American College of Chest Physicians gave a grade 1 recommendation for aspirin for patients with lifelong chronic limb ischemia (Clagett et al., 2004).

■ *Apply intermittent compression therapy modalities as appropriate.* **LOE = V**

(MR) A systematic review of the literature indicated that an intermittent pneumatic compression program was appropriate therapy for patients with severe peripheral arterial disease who were not candidates for revascularization (Labropoulos et al., 2002).

■ *Apply an appropriate dressing or device for the wound size and type.* **LOE = II**

(MR) A randomized trial ($N = 10$ patients) compared the rate of wound healing with traditional moisture gauze dressings and a vacuum-assisted closure (VAC) device and demonstrated that wounds treated with the VAC system decreased in length/width and depth more effectively than those with traditional dressings (Eginton et al., 2003).

(MR) An RCT ($N = 22$ patients) compared the VAC system with traditional gauze soaked in Ringer's solution three times a day and found that the VAC system was as effective as the traditional method, cost less, and was more comfortable for patients (Wanner et al., 2003).

RCT = Randomized Controlled (Clinical) Trial, **NIC** = Nursing Interventions Classification, **NOC** = Nursing Outcomes Classification

(MR) An RCT of diabetic patients with foot ulcers ($N = 162$ patients) demonstrated that the rate of wound healing was greater in the group that received negative-pressure wound therapy than those who received standard moist wound care according to current consensus guidelines (Armstrong et al., 2005).

(MR) A retrospective study ($N = 14$ patients) demonstrated that vacuum-assisted wound closure was beneficial in achieving early wound closure in abdominal trauma patients (Garner et al., 2001).

Possibly Effective

■ (NIC) *Instruct the patient on factors that interfere with circulation (e.g., smoking, restrictive clothing, exposure to cold temperatures, and crossing of legs and feet).* **LOE = VI**

(NR) A randomized intervention study measured the nursing interventions of education and reinforcement of hygienic-dietary measures in patients 65 years or older with stage I-II Fontaine scale intermittent claudication and found that only hygiene tended to improve in the intervention group (Pujol Campini et al., 2004).

(EO) The guidelines of the Wound Ostomy and Continence Nurses Society recommend that patients should be educated on smoking cessation, compliance with medications, and neutral or dependent position for legs (Bonham & Flemister, 2002).

(EO) The guidelines of the Wound Ostomy and Continence Nurses Society recommend that patients should be educated on avoidance of chemical trauma, thermal trauma, hot soaks, heating pads, medicated corn pads, moisture between toes, friction, constrictive clothing, going barefoot, and leg crossing (Bonham & Flemister, 2002).

(EO) The guidelines of the Wound Ostomy and Continence Nurses Society recommend that patients should be educated on professional care for toenails, corns, and calluses (Bonham & Flemister, 2002).

(EO) The guidelines of the Wound Ostomy and Continence Nurses Society recommend that patients should be educated on the use of properly fitting footwear and the necessity of wearing socks or hose with shoes (Bonham & Flemister, 2002).

(EO) The guidelines of the Wound Ostomy and Continence Nurses Society recommend that patients should be educated on pressure reduction for heels, toes, and other bony prominences (Bonham & Flemister, 2002).

■ (NIC) *Implement wound care as appropriate.* **LOE = I**

(MR) A Cochrane systematic review found that there was insufficient evidence to determine whether the choice of topical agent or dressing affected wound healing of arterial leg ulcers (Nelson & Bradley, 2003).

(EO) The guidelines of the Wound Ostomy and Continence Nurses Society recommend topical antiseptic for dry, stable ischemic wounds to decrease the bioburden on the wound surface (Bonham & Flemister, 2002).

(EO) The guidelines of the Wound Ostomy and Continence Nurses Society recommend choosing dressings for arterial wounds that permit frequent visualization inspection (Bonham & Flemister, 2002).

(EO) The guidelines of the Wound Ostomy and Continence Nurses Society recommend a trial with moist dressing, which may benefit open, draining wounds (Bonham & Flemister, 2002).

NR = Nursing Research, **MR** = Multidisciplinary Research, **SP** = Standard of Practice, **EO** = Expert Opinion, **LOE** = Level of Evidence

■ **NIC** *Protect the extremity from injury (e.g., sheepskin under feet and lower legs, footboard/bed cradle at foot of bed).* **LOE = I**

MR A Cochrane systematic review found that consideration should be given to the use of higher specification foam mattresses rather than standard hospital foam mattresses in high-risk patients (Cullum et al., 2001).

MR A Cochrane systematic review found that there was insufficient evidence to support the value of seat cushions, limb protectors, and various constant low-pressure devices as pressure ulcer prevention strategies (Cullum et al., 2004).

MR An RCT ($N = 1772$ patients) evaluated the effectiveness of two risk assessment scales (Braden and Norton); 314 patients were randomly placed in a "turning group," who were turned either every 2 or 4 hours with a pressure-reducing mattress, and a "nonturn group," who received care based on clinical judgment. Although the risk assessment scales' effectiveness was low, it was superior to nursing clinical judgment (Defloor & Grypdonck, 2005).

■ **NIC** *Instruct the patient on proper foot care.* **LOE = I**

MR A systematic review of the literature on diabetic patients demonstrated that all patients with diabetes should be assessed for the risk of foot ulcers and considered for possible beneficial interventions, including patients' education, prescription footwear, intensive podiatric care, and evaluation for surgical intervention (Singh et al., 2005).

■ **NIC** *Inspect skin for arterial ulcers or tissue breakdown.* **LOE = II**

MR An RCT ($N = 1772$ patients) evaluated the effectiveness of two risk assessment scales (Braden and Norton); 314 patients were randomly placed in a "turning group," who were turned either every 2 or 4 hours with a pressure-reducing mattress, and a "nonturn group," who received care based on clinical judgment. Although the risk assessment scales' effectiveness was low, it was superior to nursing clinical judgment (Defloor & Grypdonck, 2005).

Not Effective

No applicable published research was found in this category.

Possibly Harmful

No applicable published research was found in this category.

OUTCOME MEASUREMENT

TISSUE PERFUSION: PERIPHERAL NOC

Definition: Adequacy of blood flow through the small vessels of the extremities to maintain tissue function.

Tissue Perfusion: Peripheral as evidenced by the following selected NOC indicators:

• Capillary refill toes
• Sensation

Continued

RCT = Randomized Controlled (Clinical) Trial, **NIC** = Nursing Interventions Classification, **NOC** = Nursing Outcomes Classification

OUTCOME MEASUREMENT—*cont'd*

- Skin color
- Skin integrity
- Pedal pulse rate (left)
- Pedal pulse rate (right)

(Rate each indicator of **Tissue Perfusion: Peripheral:** 1 = severely compromised, 2 = substantially compromised, 3 = moderately compromised, 4 = mildly compromised, 5 = not compromised) (Moorhead et al., 2004).

REFERENCES

Antithrombotic Trialists' Collaboration. (2002). Collaborative meta-analysis of randomised trials of antiplatelet therapy for prevention of death, myocardial infarction, and stroke in high risk patients. *BMJ*, 324(7329):71-86.

Armstrong DG, Lavery LA; Diabetic Foot Study Consortium. (2005). Negative pressure wound therapy after partial diabetic foot amputation: A multicentre, randomised controlled trial. *Lancet*, 366(9498): 1704-1710.

Bickley LS, Szilagyi PG. (2003). *Bates' guide to physical examination and history taking*, 8th ed. Philadelphia: Lippincott Williams & Wilkins.

Bonham P, Flemister B. (2002). Guidelines for Management of Wounds in Patients with Lower Extremity Arterial Disease. *Clinical practice guidelines* (Series No. 1). Glenview, IL: Wound Ostomy Continence Nurses Society.

Brevetti G, Silvestro A, Schiano V, Chiariello M. (2003). Endothelial dysfunction and cardiovascular risk prediction in peripheral arterial disease: Additive value of flow-mediated dilation to ankle-brachial pressure index. *Circulation*, 108(17):2093-2098.

Clagett GP, Sobel M, Jackson MR, Lip GYH, Tangelder M, Verhaeghe R. (2004). Antithrombotic therapy in peripheral arterial occlusive disease: The Seventh ACCP Conference on Antithrombotic and Thrombolytic Therapy. *Chest*, 126(3 Suppl):609S-626S.

Cullum N, McInnes E, Bell-Syer SE, Legood R. (2004). Support surfaces for pressure ulcer prevention. *Cochrane Database Syst Rev*, (3):CD001735.

Cullum N, Nelson EA, Fletcher AW, Sheldon TA. (2001). Compression for venous leg ulcers. *Cochrane Database Syst Rev*, (2):CD000265.

Defloor T, Grypdonck MF. (2005). Pressure ulcers: Validation of two risk assessment scales. *J Clin Nurs*, 14(3):373-382.

De Vivo S, Palmer-Kazen U, Kalin B, Wahlberg E. (2005). Risk factors for poor collateral development in claudication. *Vasc Endovascular Surg*, 39(6):519-524.

Dochterman JM, Bulechek GM (Eds). (2004). *Nursing Interventions Classification (NIC)*, 4th ed. St. Louis: Mosby.

Dorffler-Melly J, Koopman MM, Prins MH, Buller HR. (2005). Antiplatelet and anticoagulant drugs for prevention of restenosis/reocclusion following peripheral endovascular treatment. *Cochrane Database Syst Rev*, (1):CD002071.

Eginton MT, Brown KR, Seabrook GR, Towne JB, Cambria RA. (2003). A prospective randomized evaluation of negative-pressure wound dressings for diabetic foot wounds. *Ann Vasc Surg*, 17(6): 645-649.

Gardner AW, Katzel LI, Sorkin JD, Bradham DD, Hochberg MC, Flinn WR, et al. (2001). Exercise rehabilitation improves functional outcomes and peripheral circulation in patients with intermittent claudication: A randomized controlled trial. *J Am Geriatr Soc*, 49(6):755-762.

Gardner AW, Katzel LI, Sorkin JD, Goldberg AP. (2002). Effects of long-term exercise rehabilitation on claudication distances in patients with peripheral arterial disease: A randomized controlled trial. *J Cardiopulm Rehabil*, 22(3):192-198.

Garner GB, Ware DN, Cocanour CS, Duke JH, McKinley BA, Kozar RA, et al. (2001). Vacuum-assisted wound closure provides early fascial reapproximation in trauma patients with open abdomens. *Am J Surg*, 182(6):630-638.

Hirsch AT, Criqui MH, Treat-Jacobson D, Regensteiner JG, Creager MA, Olin JW, et al. (2001). Peripheral arterial disease detection, awareness, and treatment in primary care. *JAMA*, 286(11): 1317-1324.

Johnson JJ, Psustian C. (2005). Guidelines for Management of Wounds in Patients with Lower Extremity Venous Disease. *Clinical practice guidelines* (Series No. 4). Glenview, IL: Wound Ostomy and Continence Nurses Society.

Labropoulos N, Wierks C, Suffoletto B. (2002). Intermittent pneumatic compression for the treatment of lower extremity arterial disease: A systematic review. *Vasc Med*, 7(2):141-148.

Leng GC, Fowler B, Ernst E. (2000). Exercise for intermittent claudication. *Cochrane Database Syst Rev*, (2):CD000990.

Moorhead M, Johnson M, Maas M (Eds). (2004). *Nursing Outcomes Classification (NOC)*, 3rd ed. St. Louis: Mosby.

Murabito JM, D'Agostino RB, Silbershatz H, Wilson WF. (1997). Intermittent claudication. A risk profile from the Framingham Heart Study. *Circulation*, 96(1):44-49.

Nelson EA, Bradley MD. (2003). Dressings and topical agents for arterial leg ulcers. *Cochrane Database Syst Rev*, (1):CD001836.

Otah KE, Clark LT, Salifu MO. (2005). Relationship of lower extremity skin blood flow to the ankle brachial index in patients with peripheral arterial disease and normal volunteers. *Int J Cardiol*, 103(1):41-46.

Pujol Campi E, Nolla Benavent M, Olona M, Berga C. (2004). Health education reinforcement in patients aged more than 65 years with intermittent claudication. *Enferm Clinica*, 14(1):7-11.

Selvin E, Erlinger TP. (2004). Prevalence of and risk factors for peripheral arterial disease in the United States: Results from the National Health and Nutrition Examination Survey, 1999-2000. *Circulation*, 110(6):738-743.

Singh N, Armstrong DG, Lipsky BA. (2005). Preventing foot ulcers in patients with diabetes. *JAMA*, 293(2):217-228.

Wanner MB, Schwarzl F, Strub B, Zaech GA, Pierer G. (2003). Vacuum-assisted wound closure for cheaper and more comfortable healing of pressure sores: A prospective study. *Scand J Plast Reconstr Surg Hand Surg*, 37(1):28-33.

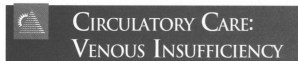

CIRCULATORY CARE: VENOUS INSUFFICIENCY

NIC

Kathleen Higgins, RN, CCRN, CS, MSN, CRNP

NIC **Definition:** Promotion of venous circulation (Dochterman & Bulechek, 2004).

NURSING ACTIVITIES

Effective

■ **NIC** *Encourage passive or active range-of-motion exercises, especially of the lower extremities, during bed rest.* **LOE = III**

MR A prospective controlled study demonstrated that supervised isotonic exercise of the calf could improve venous calf hemodynamics and function by increasing muscular endurance, efficacy, and power (Kan & Delis, 2001).

RCT = Randomized Controlled (Clinical) Trial, **NIC** = Nursing Interventions Classification, **NOC** = Nursing Outcomes Classification

SP The patient should perform a regular exercise program daily, including brisk walking and isotonic calf muscle, tiptoe, and ankle flexion exercises, to decrease venous congestion and venous reflux (Johnson & Psustian, 2005).

■ *Thoroughly assess peripheral vascular circulation and identify risk factors that lead to venous insufficiency.* **LOE = IV**

MR A prospective study of patients with confirmed deep vein thrombosis (DVT) ($N = 5451$ patients) identified the most frequent comorbidities as hypertension, surgery within 3 months, immobility within 30 days, cancer, and obesity (Goldhaber & Tapson, 2004).

■ NIC *Instruct the patient on proper foot care.* **LOE = V**

MR A systematic review of diabetic patients' literature demonstrated that all patients with diabetes should be assessed for the risk of foot ulcers and considered for possible beneficial interventions, including patients' education, prescription footwear, intensive podiatric care, and evaluation for surgical intervention (Singh et al., 2005).

■ NIC *Administer antiplatelet or anticoagulation medications, as appropriate.* **LOE = I**

MR A meta-analysis addressed the duration of anticoagulation after venous thromboembolism (VTE) and demonstrated that there was benefit of long-term anticoagulation in patients with VTE to reduce recurrent thrombotic events. In addition, a clinical benefit in the reduction of recurrent VTE risk was seen up to at least 6 months after the therapy was stopped. The analysis also suggested that prescribers should consider risk stratification when considering the course length of anticoagulation (Ost et al., 2005).

MR A Cochrane systematic review found that for the initial treatment of DVT, low-molecular-weight heparin (LMWH) was more effective than unfractionated heparin. Also, LMWH significantly reduced the occurrence of major hemorrhage during the initial treatment phase. The authors suggested that this should be adopted as the standard therapy for DVT (van Dongen et al., 2004).

MR A meta-analysis of RCTs of antiplatelet regimens revealed that antiplatelet drugs were protective in most types of patients who were at increased risk for vascular events, arterial occlusions, or VTE events (ATC, 2002).

MR An RCT ($N = 134$ patients) demonstrated the clinical benefit associated with extending the duration of anticoagulant therapy to 1 year; however, this benefit was not maintained after the therapy was discontinued (Agnelli et al., 2001).

■ NIC *Apply compression therapy modalities (short-stretch or long-stretch bandages) as appropriate.* **LOE = I**

MR A Cochrane systematic review demonstrated that graduated compression stockings (GCSs) were effective in diminishing the risk of DVT in hospitalized patients and that GCSs and DVT prophylactics were more effective than just GCSs (Amaragiri & Lees, 2000).

MR A Cochrane systematic review demonstrated that in venous ulcers, compression increased healing rates compared with no compression, multilayer systems were more effective than single-layer systems, and higher compression was more effective than low compression (Cullum et al., 2001).

MR A Cochrane systematic review demonstrated that the use of elastic compression stockings (ECSs) reduced the occurrence of post-thrombotic syndrome, which was characterized by chronic pain, swelling, and skin changes in the affected limb. It was not clear whether ECSs should be applied immediately in the acute phase of DVT or after compression bandaging (Kolbach et al., 2003, 2004).

■ *Apply intermittent compression therapy modalities as appropriate.* **LOE = I**

(MR) A review and analysis of the literature indicated that all the major types of intermittent compression systems were successful in emptying deep veins of the lower limb and were effective in preventing stasis and DVT (Morris & Woodcock, 2004).

■ (NIC) *Apply a dressing appropriate for wound size and type as appropriate.*
    LOE = II

(MR) An RCT (*N* = 162 patients) demonstrated that negative-pressure wound therapy using the vacuum-assisted closure (VAC) therapy system was safe and effective in the treatment of complex diabetic foot wounds by increasing healing rates, and the frequency and severity of adverse events were similar in both treatment groups (Armstrong & Lavery, 2005).

(MR) A retrospective study demonstrated that vacuum-assisted wound closure was beneficial in achieving early wound closure in abdominal trauma patients (Garner et al., 2001).

(MR) A prospective randomized study (*N* = 8) concluded that the VAC therapy system in diabetic foot wounds resulted in decreased wound dimension length and width, which were increased in the moist dressing group (Eginton et al., 2003).

(MR) An RCT (*N* = 22 patients) proved that the VAC therapy system was as effective as gauze soaked with Ringer's solution and was superior in cost effectiveness and patients' comfort (Wanner et al., 2003).

■ (NIC) *Perform a comprehensive appraisal of peripheral circulation (e.g., check peripheral pulses, edema, capillary refill, color, and temperature).* **LOE = IV**

(MR) In a prospective study of patients with confirmed DVT (*N* = 5451 patients), the most frequent comorbidities found were hypertension, surgery within 3 months, immobility within 30 days, cancer, and obesity (Goldhaber & Tapson, 2004).

Possibly Effective

No applicable published research was found in this category.

Not Effective

■ (NIC) *Protect the extremity from injury (e.g., sheepskin, under feet and lower legs, footboard/bed cradle at foot of bed; well-fitted shoes).* **LOE = I**

(MR) A Cochrane systematic review found that there was insufficient evidence to support the value of seat cushions, limb protectors, and various constant low-pressure devices as pressure ulcer prevention strategies (Cullum et al., 2004).

■ *Using adjunctive therapy for wound healing.* **LOE = I**

(MR) A Cochrane systematic review found that electromagnetic therapy offered no benefit in healing venous ulcers (Flemming & Cullum, 2001).

RCT = Randomized Controlled (Clinical) Trial, **NIC** = Nursing Interventions Classification, **NOC** = Nursing Outcomes Classification

Possibly Harmful

■ **NIC** *Apply compression therapy modalities (short-stretch or long-stretch bandages), as appropriate.* **LOE = VII**

EO The Wound Ostomy and Continence Nurses Society guidelines state that compression should not be applied if the ankle brachial index is less than 0.5 (Johnson & Psustian, 2005).

OUTCOME MEASUREMENT

TISSUE PERFUSION: PERIPHERAL **NOC**

Definition: Adequacy of blood flow through the small vessels of the extremities to maintain tissue function.

Tissue Perfusion: Peripheral as evidenced by the following selected NOC indicators:
- Capillary refill toes
- Sensation
- Skin color
- Skin integrity
- Pedal pulse rate (left)
- Pedal pulse rate (right)

(Rate each indicator of **Tissue Perfusion: Peripheral:** 1 = severely compromised, 2 = substantially compromised, 3 = moderately compromised, 4 = mildly compromised, 5 = not compromised) (Moorhead et al., 2004).

REFERENCES

Agnelli G, Prandoni P, Santamaria MG, Bagatella P, Iorio A, Bazzan M, et al. (2001). Three months versus one year of oral anticoagulant therapy for idiopathic deep venous thrombosis. Warfarin Optimal Duration Italian Trial Investigators. *N Engl J Med,* 345(3):165-169.

Amaragiri SV, Lees TA. (2000). Elastic compression stockings for prevention of deep vein thrombosis. *Cochrane Database Syst Rev,* (3):CD001484.

Antithrombotic Trialists' Collaboration (ATC). (2002). Collaborative meta-analysis of randomised trials of antiplatelet therapy for prevention of death, myocardial infarction, and stroke in high risk patients. *BMJ,* 324(7329):71-86.

Armstrong DG, Lavery LA; Diabetic Foot Study Consortium. (2005). Negative pressure wound therapy after partial diabetic foot amputation: A multicentre, randomised controlled trial. *Lancet,* 366(9498):1704-1710.

Cullum N, McInnes E, Bell-Syer SE, Legood R. (2004). Support surfaces for pressure ulcer prevention. *Cochrane Database Syst Rev,* (3):CD001735.

Cullum N, Nelson EA, Fletcher AW, Sheldon TA. (2001). Compression for venous leg ulcers. *Cochrane Database Syst Rev,* (2):CD000265.

Dochterman JM, Bulechek GM (Eds). (2004). *Nursing Interventions Classification (NIC),* 4th ed. St. Louis: Mosby.

Eginton MT, Brown KR, Seabrook GR, Towne JB, Cambria RA. (2003). A prospective randomized evaluation of negative-pressure wound dressings for diabetic foot wounds. *Ann Vasc Surg,* 17(6): 645-649.

Flemming K, Cullum N. (2001). Electromagnetic therapy for the treatment of venous leg ulcers. *Cochrane Database Syst Rev,* (1):CD002933.

Garner GB, Ware DN, Cocanour CS, Duke JH, McKinley BA, Kozar RA, et al. (2001). Vacuum-assisted wound closure provides early fascial reapproximation in trauma patients with open abdomens. *Am J Surg,* 182(6):630-638.

Goldhaber SZ, Tapson VF; DVT FREE Steering Committee. (2004). A prospective registry of 5,451 patients with ultrasound-confirmed deep vein thrombosis. *Am J Cardiol,* 93(2):259-262.

Johnson JJ, Psustian C. (2005). Guidelines for management of wounds in patients with lower extremity venous disease. In *Clinical practice guidelines* (Series No. 4). Glenview, IL: Wound Ostomy and Continence Nurses Society.

Kan YM, Delis KT. (2001). Hemodynamic effects of supervised calf muscle exercise in patients with venous leg ulceration: A prospective controlled study. *Arch Surg,* 136(12):1364-1369.

Kolbach DN, Sandbrink MW, Hamulyak K, Neumann HA, Prins MH. (2004). Non-pharmaceutical measures for prevention of post-thrombotic syndrome. *Cochrane Database Syst Rev,* (1):CD004174.

Kolbach DN, Sandbrink MW, Neumann HA, Prins MH. (2003). Compression therapy for treating stage I and II (Widmer) post-thrombotic syndrome. *Cochrane Database Syst Rev,* (4):CD004177.

Moorhead M, Johnson M, Maas M (Eds). (2004). *Nursing Outcome Classifications (NOC),* 3rd ed. St. Louis: Mosby.

Morris RJ, Woodcock JP. (2004). Evidence-based compression: Prevention of stasis and deep vein thrombosis. *Ann Surg,* 239(2):162-171.

Ost D, Tepper J, Mihara H, Lander O, Heinzer R, Fein A. (2005). Duration of anticoagulation following venous thromboembolism: A meta-analysis. *JAMA,* 294(6):706-715.

Singh N, Armstrong DG, Lipsky BA. (2005). Preventing foot ulcers in patients with diabetes. *JAMA,* 293(2):217-228.

van Dongen CJ, van den Belt AG, Prins MH, Lensing AW. (2004). Fixed dose subcutaneous low molecular weight heparins versus adjusted dose unfractionated heparin for venous thromboembolism. *Cochrane Database Syst Rev,* (4):CD001100.

Wanner MB, Schwarzl F, Strub B, Zaech GA, Pierer G. (2003). Vacuum-assisted wound closure for cheaper and more comfortable healing of pressure sores: A prospective study. *Scand J Plast Reconstr Surg Hand Surg,* 37(1):28-33.

 ## CIRCULATORY PRECAUTIONS

Kathleen Higgins, RN, CCRN, CS, MSN, CRNP

NIC **Definition:** Protection of a localized area with limited perfusion (Dochterman & Bulechek, 2004).

NURSING ACTIVITIES

Effective

■ *Apply an appropriate dressing or device for the size and type of the wound.*
LOE = III

(MR) A randomized trial (*N* = 10 patients) compared the rate of wound healing with traditional moisture gauze dressings and a vacuum-assisted closure (VAC) device and demonstrated that wounds treated with the VAC system decreased in length, width, and depth more effectively than those with traditional dressings (Eginton et al., 2003).

(MR) A prospective RCT (*N* = 22 patients) compared the VAC system with traditional gauze soaked in Ringer's solution three times a day and found that the VAC system was as effective as the traditional method, cost less, and was more comfortable for patients (Wanner et al., 2003).

RCT = Randomized Controlled (Clinical) Trial, **NIC** = Nursing Interventions Classification, **NOC** = Nursing Outcomes Classification

(MR) An RCT of diabetic patients with foot ulcers ($N = 162$ patients) demonstrated that the rate of wound healing was greater in the group who received negative-pressure wound therapy than in those who received standard moist wound care according to current consensus guidelines (Armstrong & Lavery, 2005).

(MR) A retrospective study demonstrated that vacuum-assisted wound closure was beneficial in achieving early wound closure in abdominal trauma patients (Gardner et al., 2002).

■ (SP) *Educate the family and patient on procedures and plan of care.* **LOE = IV**

(MR) A case-control study ($N = 381$ patients) using a 38-year follow-up of the Framingham Heart Study determined that identifying patients with a profile of high-risk factors was essential and a beneficial tool toward patients' education and risk factor modification (Murabito et al., 1997).

(EO) The nurse should educate the patient, caregiver, or legally authorized representative relative to the prescribed therapy and plan of care including, but not limited to, potential complications associated with treatment or therapy and risks and benefits (Johnson & Psustian, 2005).

■ (NIC) (SP) *Perform a comprehensive appraisal of peripheral circulation (e.g., check peripheral pulses, edema, capillary refill, color, and temperature of extremity).* **LOE = IV**

(EO) Guidelines from the Wound Ostomy and Continence Nurses Society recommend that a comprehensive health history be obtained, including risk factors for arterial and venous disease, wound history, pain history, and prescription and over-the-counter pharmacological history (Johnson & Paustian, 2005).

■ (SP) *Perform a circulatory physical assessment.* **LOE = IV**

(MR) A multicenter, case-control study ($N = 6979$ patients) demonstrated the need for health care providers to assess for peripheral artery disease (PAD) and the prevalence of PAD in primary care practice where patients are not identified and not treated (Hirsch et al., 2001).

(EO) The nurse should perform an assessment of the peripheral circulation, including assessment of pain in the arms and legs; history of pain in the calf with exercise and relieved with rest; sensitivity to temperature changes; cold limbs, numbness, tingling in limbs, color pallor, or limbs with loss of hair; color and pain in fingers and toes with cold; swelling in calves, legs, or feet; and swelling with redness or tenderness in limbs (Bickley & Szilagyi, 2003).

(EO) The nurse should recognize the normal aging changes related to the peripheral circulation (thinning skin, dry skin, decreased nail growth, decreased hair growth on lower extremities) and should differentiate these from abnormal changes (decrease or absence of pulse, swelling, extremity pain, ulcers, cyanosis, hyperpigmentation, and focal warmth) (Bickley & Szilagyi, 2003).

(MR) A descriptive cross-sectional study ($N = 2174$ patients) found that the prevalence of PAD in adults older than 40 in the United States was positively associated with increasing age, black race/ethnicity, current smoking, diabetes, hypertension, hypercholesterolemia, and low kidney function (Selvin & Erlinger, 2004).

NR = Nursing Research, **MR** = Multidisciplinary Research, **SP** = Standard of Practice, **EO** = Expert Opinion, **LOE** = Level of Evidence

■ **NIC** **SP** *Prevent infection in wounds.* **LOE = IV**

EO Guidelines from the Wound Ostomy and Continence Nurses Society recommend a short course of topical antimicrobial therapy for wounds with a high level of bacterial load (Johnson & Paustian, 2005).

■ *Instruct and encourage the patient on the benefit of exercise.* **LOE = I**

MR A Cochrane systematic review found that exercise therapy for patients with intermittent claudication three times a week significantly improved maximal walking time and overall walking ability in patients with leg pain (Leng et al., 2000).

■ *Perform a comprehensive circulation assessment.* **LOE = IV**

MR In a prospective study of patients with confirmed deep vein thrombosis ($N = 5451$ patients), the most frequent comorbidities found were hypertension, surgery within 3 months, immobility within 30 days, cancer, and obesity (Goldhaber & Tapson, 2004).

MR An RCT ($N = 31$ patients) demonstrated an improvement in claudication walking distances and walking economy at 6 and 12 months in older patients with intermittent claudication despite a progressively decreasing exercise rehabilitation program (Gardner et al., 2002).

MR An RCT ($N = 61$ patients) demonstrated that exercise rehabilitation in older patients with peripheral artery occlusive disease increased treadmill claudication distances, which increased daily physical activity and improved patients' independent function (Gardner et al., 2001a).

MR A controlled clinical trial study demonstrated that in older individuals with PAD ($N = 19$ patients), 6 months of exercise rehabilitation improved ambulatory function (Brendle et al., 2001).

■ *Screen for patients at risk and instruct on proper care of the feet.* **LOE = V**

MR A systematic review of diabetic patients' literature demonstrated that all patients with diabetes should be assessed for the risk of foot ulcers and considered for possible beneficial interventions, including patients' education, prescription footwear, intensive podiatric care, and evaluation for surgical intervention (Singh et al., 2005).

Possibly Effective

■ **NIC** *Avoid injury to affected area.* **LOE = I**

MR A Cochrane systematic review found that consideration should be given to the use of higher specification foam mattresses rather than standard hospital foam mattresses in high-risk patients (Cullum et al., 2001).

Not Effective

No applicable published research was found in this category.

Possibly Harmful

No applicable published research was found in this category.

RCT = Randomized Controlled (Clinical) Trial, **NIC** = Nursing Interventions Classification, **NOC** = Nursing Outcomes Classification

OUTCOME MEASUREMENT

TISSUE PERFUSION: PERIPHERAL (NOC)

Definition: Adequacy of blood flow through the small vessels of the extremities to maintain tissue function.

Tissue Perfusion: Peripheral as evidenced by the following selected NOC indicators:

- Capillary refill toes
- Sensation
- Skin color
- Skin integrity
- Pedal pulse rate (left)
- Pedal pulse rate (right)

(Rate each indicator of **Tissue Perfusion: Peripheral:** 1 = severely compromised, 2 = substantially compromised, 3 = moderately compromised, 4 = mildly compromised, 5 = not compromised) (Moorhead et al., 2004).

REFERENCES

Armstrong DG, Lavery LA; Diabetic Foot Study Consortium. (2005). Negative pressure wound therapy after partial diabetic foot amputation: A multicentre, randomised controlled trial. *Lancet*, 366(9498):1704-1710.

Bickley LS, Szilagyi PG. (2003). *Bates' guide to physical examination and history taking*, 8th ed. Philadelphia: Lippincott Williams & Wilkins.

Brendle DC, Joseph LJ, Corretti MC, Gardner AW, Katzel LI. (2001). Effects of exercise rehabilitation on endothelial reactivity in older patients with peripheral arterial disease. *Am J Cardiol*, 87(3):324-329.

Cullum N, Nelson EA, Fletcher AW, Sheldon TA. (2001). Compression for venous leg ulcers. *Cochrane Database Syst Rev*, (2):CD000265.

Dochterman JM, Bulechek GM (Eds). (2004). *Nursing Interventions Classification (NIC)*, 4th ed. St. Louis: Mosby.

Eginton MT, Brown KR, Seabrook GR, Towne JB, Cambria RA. (2003). A prospective randomized evaluation of negative-pressure wound dressings for diabetic foot wounds. *Ann Vasc Surg*, 17(6):645-649.

Gardner AW, Katzel LI, Sorkin JD, Bradham DD, Hochberg MC, Flinn WR, et al. (2001a). Exercise rehabilitation improves functional outcomes and peripheral circulation in patients with intermittent claudication: A randomized controlled trial. *J Am Geriatr Soc*, 49(6):755-762.

Gardner AW, Katzel LI, Sorkin JD, Goldberg AP. (2002). Effects of long-term exercise rehabilitation on claudication distances in patients with peripheral arterial disease: A randomized controlled trial. *Journal of Cardiopulmonary Rehabilitation*, 22:192-198.

Gardner GB, Ware DN, Cocanour CS, Duke JH, McKinley BA, Kozar RA, et al. (2001b). Vacuum-assisted wound closure provides early fascial reapproximation in trauma patients with open abdomens. *Am J Surg*, 182(6):630-638.

Goldhaber SZ, Tapson VF; DVT FREE Steering Committee. (2004). A prospective registry of 5,451 patients with ultrasound-confirmed deep vein thrombosis. *Am J Cardiol*, 93(2):259-262.

Hirsch AT, Criqui MH, Treat-Jacobson D, Regensteiner JG, Creager MA, Olin JW, et al. (2001). Peripheral arterial disease detection, awareness, and treatment in primary care. *JAMA*, 286(11):1317-1324.

Johnson JJ, Paustian C. (2005). Guidelines for management of wounds in patients with lower extremity venous disease. In *Clinical practice guidelines* (Series No. 4). Glenview, IL: Wound Ostomy and Continence Nurses Society.

Leng GC, Fowler B, Ernst E. (2000). Exercise for intermittent claudication. *Cochrane Database Syst Rev*, (2): CD000990.

Moorhead M, Johnson M, Maas M (Eds). (2004). *Nursing Outcomes Classification (NOC)*, 3rd ed. St. Louis: Mosby.

Murabito JM, D'Agostino RB, Silbershatz H, Wilson WF. (1997). Intermittent claudication. A risk profile from the Framingham Heart Study. *Circulation*, 96(1):44-49.

Selvin E, Erlinger TP. (2004). Prevalence of and risk factors for peripheral arterial disease in the United States: Results from the National Health and Nutrition Examination Survey, 1999-2000. *Circulation*, 110(6):738-743.

Singh N, Armstrong DG, Lipsky BA. (2005). Preventing foot ulcers in patients with diabetes. *JAMA*, 293(2):217-228.

Wanner MB, Schwarzl F, Strub B, Zaech GA, Pierer G. (2003). Vacuum-assisted wound closure for cheaper and more comfortable healing of pressure sores: A prospective study. *Scand J Plast Reconstr Surg Hand Surg*, 37(1):28-33.

 # COGNITIVE STIMULATION

Cecilia Borden, EdD, MSN, RN

NIC **Definition:** Promotion of awareness and comprehension of surroundings by utilization of planned stimuli (Dochterman & Bulechek, 2004).

NURSING ACTIVITIES

Effective

■ *Perform screening baseline and ongoing cognitive assessment.* **LOE = VI**

(MR) A cross-sectional study (*N* = 81) with blinded assessments performed on consecutive elderly patients (>70 years) demonstrated that the Confusion Assessment Method (CAM) seemed to be an acceptable in-hospital screening instrument (Laurila et al., 2002).

(NR) A prospective descriptive study assessed the diagnostic validity of the CAM (*N* = 641 paired observations), SENS (sensitive method), and SPEC (specific method) when administered by staff RNs. The CAM SENS tool had the greatest diagnostic accuracy. Staff nurses' identification of delirium was less accurate than that of trained research personnel, indicating a need for more formalized teaching regarding the tool (Lemiengre et al., 2006).

■ *Address the patient by name, speaking clearly, slowly, and with respect.* **LOE = V**

(NR) A review of three RCTs, three controlled studies, and one before-and-after study concluded that nurses should play a pivotal role in utilizing reality orientation techniques when caring for older adults (Milisen et al., 2005).

■ *Engage in positive, caring communication.* **LOE = VI**

(NR) A qualitative descriptive study was used to answer the question, "What is the meaning of the experience of being listened to for older adults?" Twenty residents ages 70 to 90 years participated in the study and demonstrated that the quality of life of the older adult improved with feelings of contentment, respect, and care (Jonas-Simpson et al., 2006).

■ *Provide reassurance and reorientation.* **LOE = VII**

(EO) A geriatric symposium held at the Mayo Clinic recommended therapeutic approaches when caring for and orienting older adults (Rummans et al., 1995).

RCT = Randomized Controlled (Clinical) Trial, **NIC** = Nursing Interventions Classification, **NOC** = Nursing Outcomes Classification

■ *Review all medications with the patient and family.* **LOE = VII**

(EO) A nursing outcomes evaluation reiterated that reviewing medication profiles for drugs that caused or contributed to delirium (i.e., medications with anticholinergic or sedative effects) was critical when assessing older adults' cognitive orientation (St. Pierre, 1998).

■ *Provide appropriate sensory stimulation (e.g., memory cues, calendars, clocks, familiar objects).* **LOE = V**

(NR) A systematic review of the literature revealed that nonpharmacological therapies improved cognitive orientation in confused and demented patients (Douglas et al., 2004).

■ *Make sensory aids available and in working order.* **LOE = VI**

(MR) A prospective study was done to evaluate a multicomponent strategy involving 852 patients 70 years or older. When sensory aids were available and working, 87% of patients had significant improvement in the degree of cognitive orientation (Inouye et al., 1999).

■ (SP) *Avoid using physical restraints.* **LOE = VII**

(MR) A review of the literature and Joint Committee guidelines documented the need to limit and/or eliminate restraints to decrease adverse events (Park et al., 2005).

■ *Provide ambulation two to three times daily and/or range-of-motion exercises twice daily, and maintain normal sleep patterns.* **LOE = V**

(MR) A prospective cohort study (N = 422 patients) showed that, following an intervention aimed at orientation activities, mobility, sleep, hearing, and vision, patients' orientation improved by 86% (Inouye et al., 2003).

■ *Decrease or eliminate excessive noise.* **LOE = VII**

(NR) A systematic review of current practices revealed that a quiet, nonstimulating environment supported cognitive orientation (Irving & Foreman, 2006).

■ *Encourage visits from family and friends and provide consistency in nursing care.* **LOE = VII**

(NR) A literature review revealed that consistency could enhance cognitive orientation (Rigney, 2006).

Possibly Effective

No applicable published research was found in this category.

Not Effective

No applicable published research was found in this category.

Possibly Harmful

No applicable published research was found in this category.

NR = Nursing Research, **MR** = Multidisciplinary Research, **SP** = Standard of Practice, **EO** = Expert Opinion, **LOE** = Level of Evidence

OUTCOME MEASUREMENT

COGNITIVE ORIENTATION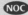

Definition: Ability to identify person, place, and time accurately.

Cognitive Orientation as evidenced by the following selected NOC indicators:

- Identifies self
- Identifies significant other
- Identifies current place
- Identifies significant current events

(Rate each indicator of **Cognitive Orientation:** 1 = severely compromised, 2 = substantially compromised, 3 = moderately compromised, 4 = mildly compromised, 5 = not compromised) (Moorhead et al., 2004).

REFERENCES

Dochterman JM, Bulechek GM (Eds). (2004). *Nursing Interventions Classification (NIC)*, 4th ed. St. Louis: Mosby.

Douglas S, James I, Ballard C. (2004). Non-pharmacological interventions in dementia. *Adv Psychiatr Treat,* 10(3):171-177.

Inouye SK, Bogardus ST Jr, Charpentier PA, Leo-Summers L, Acampora D, Holford TR, et al. (1999). A multicomponent intervention to prevent delirium in hospitalized older patients. *N Engl J Med,* 340(9):669-676.

Inouye SK, Bogardus ST Jr, Williams CS, Leo-Summers L, Agostini JV. (2003). The role of adherence on the effectiveness of nonpharmacologic interventions: Evidence from the delirium prevention trial. *Arch Intern Med,* 163(8):958-964.

Irving K, Foreman M. (2006). Delirium, nursing practice and the future. *Int J Older People Nurs,* 1(2):121-127.

Jonas-Simpson C, Mitchell G, Fisher A, Jones G, Linscott J. (2006). The experience of being listened to: A qualitative study of older adults in long-term care settings. *J Gerontol Nurs,* 32(1):46-53.

Laurila JV, Pitkala KH, Strandberg TE, Tilvis RS. (2002). Confusion assessment method in the diagnostics of delirium among aged hospital patients: Would it serve better in screening than as a diagnostic instrument? *Int J Geriatr Psychiatry,* 17(12):1112-1119.

Lemiengre J, Nelis T, Joosten E, Braes T, Foreman M, Gastmans C, et al. (2006). Detection of delirium by bedside nurses using the confusion assessment method. *J Am Geriatr Soc,* 54(4):685-694.

Milisen K, Lemiengre J, Braes T, Foreman M. (2005). Multicomponent intervention strategies for managing delirium in hospitalized older adults: Systematic review. *J Adv Nurs,* 52(1):79-90.

Moorhead M, Johnson M, Maas M (Eds). (2004). *Nursing Outcomes Classification (NOC)*, 3rd ed. St. Louis, Mosby.

Park M, Hsiao-Chen Tang J, Ledford L. (2005). *Changing the practice of physical restraint use in acute care.* Iowa City, IA: University of Iowa Gerontological Nursing Interventions Research Center, Research Translation and Dissemination Core. Available online: http://www.guideline.gov. Retrieved on July 18, 2006.

Rigney T. (2006). Delirium in the hospitalized elder and recommendations for practice. *Geriatr Nurs,* 27(3):151-157.

Rummans TA, Evans JM, Krahn LE, Fleming KC. (1995). Delirium in elderly patients: Evaluation and management. *Mayo Clin Proc,* 70(10):989-998.

St Pierre J. (1998). Functional decline in hospitalized elders: Preventive nursing measures. *AACN Clin Issues,* 9(1):109-118.

COMMUNICATION ENHANCEMENT: HEARING DEFICIT

Sheryl K. Sommer, PhD, RN; Margaret I. Wallhagen, PhD, APRN-BC, GNP, AGSF

Definition: Facilitation of effective communication with hearing-impaired individuals.

NURSING ACTIVITIES

Effective

■ **SP** *Ask patients about the preferred communication approach.* **LOE = VI**

MR A descriptive study ($N = 26$) of hearing-impaired and deaf individuals reported that they would benefit from health care providers asking for the preferred communication approach (Iezzoni et al., 2004).

EO Asking which mode of communication and assistive devices a hearing-impaired individual prefers promotes more effective communication (Sommer & Sommer, 2002).

■ **SP** *Demonstrate patience.* **LOE = VII**

EO Patience on the part of the speaker facilitates relaxation in the hearing-impaired person, increasing confidence and aiding concentration (Slaven, 2003).

■ **NIC** *Face the client directly, speak slowly, clearly, and concisely. Do not cover your mouth, smoke, talk with a full mouth, or chew gum when speaking.* **LOE = II**

NR In a descriptive study ($N = 359$) from the United Kingdom, previously hospitalized, hearing-impaired individuals reported studying lip movements, facial expressions, and other body language to receive messages (Hines, 2000).

EO Hearing-impaired individuals interpret speech based on what they can hear and on lip reading, body language, and the context of the conversation. Because they may not hear inflections clearly, they look to nonverbal forms of communication to judge the tone in which words are being used (Sommer & Sommer, 2002).

MR An RCT demonstrated that when a male spouse of a hearing-impaired person was taught how to use clear speech, current hearing aid–using people with acquired hearing loss ($N = 15$, Xage = 54) and normal hearing individuals ($N = 15$, Xage = 38.2) recognized words and sentences in the presence of noise more easily. Participants were not randomized; rather, the sentences were randomized in their presentation to participants (Caissie et al., 2005).

MR In an RCT ($N = 30$) of hearing impaired people, speaking more slowly and clear articulation were associated with improved speech recognition (Caissie et al., 2005).

MR A descriptive study of prelingually ($N = 10$, Xage = 23.6 years) and postlingually ($N = 10$, Xage = 40.5 years) profoundly hearing-impaired individuals reported that the understanding of words within sentences (contextualized) surpassed the perception of isolated but meaningful words (Most & Adi-Bensaid, 2001).

NR = Nursing Research, **MR** = Multidisciplinary Research, **SP** = Standard of Practice, **EO** = Expert Opinion, **LOE** = Level of Evidence

(MR) In a descriptive study (N = 43) of hearing-impaired individuals, speech accents and surgical masks were obstacles to good communication (Bain et al., 2004).

(MR) In a nonrandom study using a convenience sample of 40 participants divided into four groups of varying ages and stages of hearing loss, it was found that comprehension accuracy decreased in hearing-impaired participants, especially in the older participants, when speech rate was more rapid, although it remained above 85% when the sentences were simple syntactically. Comprehension accuracy declined further when sentences were more syntactically complex, and this decline was exacerbated when speech rate was increased, especially in the hearing-impaired older adults (Wingfield et al., 2006).

■ (SP) *Use a sign language interpreter as appropriate.* **LOE = VI**

(NR) In a descriptive study of a convenience sample (N = 28) of deaf adults who were raised using spoken language, 26% noted that they frequently used sign language, some out of frustration and some as their first or preferred language (McAleer, 2006).

■ (SP) *Face the client directly when speaking.* **LOE = VI**

(NR) A descriptive study (N = 359) of hearing-impaired individuals who had been hospitalized within the past 3 years found that being able to see the face of the speaker facilitated understanding of speech (Hines, 2000).

(EO) The speaker should face the hearing-impaired individual at all times, making sure that the mouth is visible and not covered by a hand or mask (Sommer & Sommer, 2002).

(MR) In a descriptive study (N = 43) of hearing-impaired individuals, communication was facilitated when the speaker's face was visible (Bain et al., 2004).

(MR) In a descriptive focus group study of deaf (N = 14; ages 23 to 51) and hard-of-hearing (N = 12; ages 30 to 74) people, participants "noted difficulties understanding words when lip reading, especially when physicians speak quickly, turn away, bow heads, have foreign accents, or wear beards or masks" (Iezzoni et al., 2004).

■ (SP) *Keep background noise to a minimum when communicating. Turn off televisions and radios. If feasible, take the person to a private room.* **LOE = VI**

(EO) Hearing aids amplify all sounds; when other conversation or sounds in the background are present, it becomes very difficult for aided individuals to understand oral communication (Sommer & Sommer, 2002).

(MR) In a nonrandomized study of 30 individuals (15 controls with normal hearing [NH] and 15 people with sensory neural hearing loss [SNHL]), speech recognition was assessed in the presence of two types of background interference/masking (speech and noise). Both types of masking resulted in impaired hearing; the greater the number of maskers, the worse the hearing for both NH and hearing-impaired, but significantly more so for those with SNHL, and multiple speech maskers contributed additional masking over and above that of noise (Hornsby et al., 2006).

■ (SP) *Encourage verbalization of questions and concerns.* **LOE = VI**

(MR) A qualitative study of deaf (N = 14) and hearing-impaired (N = 13) women reported having communication difficulty with medical professionals. The women often did not ask questions or make complaints because they did not want to "make a fuss or they were afraid of further embarrassment" (Ubido et al., 2002).

RCT = Randomized Controlled (Clinical) Trial, **NIC** = Nursing Interventions Classification, **NOC** = Nursing Outcomes Classification

(EO) Encouragement to interrupt conversation and seek clarification may be assistive (Sommer & Sommer, 2002).

■ (SP) *Periodically ask patients about the effectiveness of communication by asking them to repeat what was said and request suggestions to rectify unsatisfactory situations. If hearing-impaired individuals have difficulty understanding verbal communication, first try repeating what was said. If the individual continues to have difficulty understanding a message, try rephrasing rather than repeating exact words.* **LOE = VI**

(NR) A descriptive study ($N = 359$) of hearing-impaired individuals who had been hospitalized during the previous 3 years reported that communication problems were often overcome by having the nurse verify the patient's understanding (Hines, 2000).

(MR) In a descriptive survey ($N = 866$) of deaf and hard-of-hearing people who responded to their experiences following general practitioner visits, surgeries, and hospitalizations, difficulty communicating with staff was reported by 42% of respondents, and over one third (35%) of deaf or hard-of-hearing people reported being left unclear about their condition because of communication problems with health care providers (RNID, 2003).

(EO) Some individuals with hearing impairments may smile, nod, and appear to understand the information they are being given, even if they do not, out of fear of appearing stupid or taxing another's patience (Sommer & Sommer, 2002).

(EO) The speaker should check frequently to ensure that the recipient of the message has understood what was said (Slaven, 2003).

■ (NIC) (SP) *Use paper, pencil, or computer communication when necessary.* **LOE = VI**

(NR) A descriptive study ($N = 359$) of hearing-impaired individuals hospitalized in the previous 3 years reported that printed information helped ensure that information was fully understood (Hines, 2000).

(EO) Deaf people often use communication support systems. The availability of a TTY telephone, closed-caption television, and access to a computer for e-mail may reduce feelings of isolation (McAleer, 2006).

(EO) When there is uncertainty regarding whether a message was understood, try writing it down for the individual to read (Sommer & Sommer, 2002).

■ (SP) *Implement the use of assistive listening devices (ALDs).* **LOE = VI**

(MR) A descriptive study ($N = 43$) of hearing-impaired individuals reported that ALDs such as hearing aids, cochlear implants, amplifiers, and closed-caption television facilitated effective communication (Bain et al., 2004).

■ (SP) *Use pictures or diagrams depicting tests/procedures.* **LOE = VI**

(MR) A descriptive study ($N = 26$) of hearing-impaired and deaf individuals reported that pictures and diagrams may be helpful in detailed discussions about health care issues such as surgical procedures (Iezzoni et al., 2004).

■ (SP) *Watch for signs of depression in hearing-impaired people, and refer for further assessment and treatment as needed.* **LOE = VI**

(MR) A descriptive survey ($N = 2300$) of hearing-impaired adults age 50 and older found that "those with untreated hearing loss were more likely to report depression, anxiety, and para-

NR = Nursing Research, **MR** = Multidisciplinary Research, **SP** = Standard of Practice, **EO** = Expert Opinion, **LOE** = Level of Evidence

noia, and were less likely to participate in organized social activities, compared to those who wear hearing aids" (Senior Research Group, 1999).

NR A descriptive study (*N* = 2442) of adults with both vision and hearing impairment demonstrated decreased mental health with major depressive episodes and decreased social functioning in participants even with mild hearing loss (Wallhagen et al., 2001).

Possibly Effective

■ *Use Talking Mats as an interview tool.* **LOE = VI**

MR A descriptive study (*N* = 10) of elderly patients recently entering a care home found that participants were able to express views on subjects such as activities and the nursing home environment using the Talking Mats (Murphy et al., 2005).

Not Effective

No applicable published research was found in this category.

Possibly Harmful

■ NIC *Refrain from shouting at the patient with communication disorders.* **LOE = VI**

NR A descriptive study (*N* = 359) of hearing-impaired individuals who had experienced hospitalization in the past 3 years identified shouting as an obstacle to effective communication (Hines, 2000).

EO Shouting can result in exaggerated lip movements that impede understanding (Slaven, 2003).

EO Shouting distorts the voice and makes it more difficult for hearing-impaired individuals to identify words. Also, you can appear to be angry and cause embarrassment to the person. An increased volume can be painful for deaf and hearing-impaired people, especially if they wear a hearing aid (RNID, 2006).

■ *Presence of background noise when communicating with a hearing-impaired person.* **LOE = VI**

EO Beeping alarms, ringing telephones, and other people's conversations may make communication difficult for hearing-impaired individuals (Sommer & Sommer, 2002).

MR In a nonrandomized study of 30 individuals (15 controls with NH and 15 people with SNHL), speech recognition was assessed in the presence of two types of background interference/masking (speech and noise). Both types of masking resulted in impaired hearing; the greater the number of maskers, the worse the hearing for both NH and hearing-impaired, but significantly more so for those with SNHL, and multiple speech maskers contributed additional masking over and above that of noise (Hornsby et al., 2006).

OUTCOME MEASUREMENT

HEARING COMPENSATION BEHAVIOR   NOC

(Please refer to *Nursing Classifications Outcome* [Moorhead et al., 2004] for the **Hearing Compensation Behavior** outcome.)

RCT = Randomized Controlled (Clinical) Trial, **NIC** = Nursing Interventions Classification, **NOC** = Nursing Outcomes Classification

REFERENCES

Bain L, Scott S, Steinberg AG. (2004). Socialization experiences and coping strategies of adults raised using spoken language. *J Deaf Stud Deaf Educ,* 9(1):120-128.

Caissie R, Campbell MM, Frenette WL, Scott L, Howell I, Roy A. (2005). Clear speech for adults with a hearing loss: Does intervention with communication partners make a difference? *J Am Acad Audiol,* 16(3):157-171.

Hines J. (2000). Communication problems of hearing-impaired patients. *Nurs Stand,* 14(19):33-37.

Hornsby BW, Ricketts TA, Johnson EE. (2006). The effects of speech and speechlike maskers on unaided and aided speech recognition in persons with hearing loss. *J Am Acad Audiol,* 17(6):432-447.

Iezzoni LI, O'Day BL, Killeen M, Harker H. (2004). Communicating about health care: Observations from persons who are deaf or hard of hearing. *Ann Intern Med,* 140(5):356-362.

McAleer M. (2006). Communicating effectively with deaf patients. *Nurs Stand,* 20(19):51-54.

Moorhead M, Johnson M, Maas M (Eds). (2004). *Nursing Outcomes Classification (NOC),* 3rd ed. St. Louis: Mosby.

Most T, Adi-Bensaid A. (2001). The influence of contextual information on the perception of speech by postlingually and prelingually profoundly hearing-impaired Hebrew-speaking adolescents and adults. *Ear Hear,* 22(3):252-263.

Murphy J, Tester S, Hubbard G, Downs M, MacDonald C. (2005). Enabling frail older people with a communication difficulty to express their views: The use of Talking Mats as an interview tool. *Health Soc Care Community,* 13(2):95-107.

Royal National Institute for Deaf People (RNID). (2003). *A simple cure survey.* Available online: http://www.rnid.org.uk. Retrieved on May 27, 2006.

Royal National Institute for Deaf People (RNID). (2006). *Five common myths about deafness and deaf and hard of hearing people.* Available online: http://www.rnid.org.uk/. Retrieved on May 27, 2006.

Slaven A. (2003). Communication and the hearing-impaired patient. *Nurs Stand,* 18(12):39-41.

Sommer SK, Sommer NW. (2002). When your patient is hearing impaired. *RN,* 65(12):28-32.

Ubido J, Huntington J, Warburton D. (2002). Inequalities in access to healthcare faced by women who are deaf. *Health Soc Care Community,* 10(4): 247-253.

Wallhagen MI, Strawbridge WJ, Shema SJ, Kurata J, Kaplan GA. (2001). Comparative impact of hearing and vision impairment on subsequent functioning. *J Am Geriatr Soc,* 49(8):1086-1092.

Wingfield A, McCoy SL, Peelle JE, Tun PA, Cox LC. (2006). Effects of adults' aging and hearing loss on comprehension of rapid speech varying in syntactic complexity. *J Am Acad Audiol,* 17(7):487-497.

 # COMMUNICATION ENHANCEMENT: SPEECH DEFICIT

Marci Lee Nilsen, BSN, RN; Mary Beth Happ, PhD, RN

NIC Definition: Assistance in accepting and learning alternate methods for living with impaired speech (Dochterman & Bulechek, 2004).

Speech deficit can be caused by structural (e.g., tracheostomy, laryngectomy, endotracheal tube, maxillofacial surgery), neuromuscular (e.g., amyotrophic lateral sclerosis, Parkinson's disease), or cognitive impairments (e.g., aphasia/brain injury). Nursing interventions for speech deficit must be individualized from a careful assessment of the patient's cognitive and motor function (Garrett et al., 2007). The nursing interventions presented in the following sections are intended to guide nurses in communicating with *cognitively intact* patients who are speech impaired *without the use of electronic aids.* Collaboration with a speech-language

NR = Nursing Research, **MR** = Multidisciplinary Research, **SP** = Standard of Practice, **EO** = Expert Opinion, **LOE** = Level of Evidence

pathologist is recommended when planning communication interventions for all patients with speech deficit, cognitively impaired patients with speech deficit, and those who use electronic speech generating devices. Expert opinion and clinical practice experience provide additional support for the use of these techniques with nonspeaking patients (Beukelman et al., 2007).

NURSING ACTIVITIES

Effective

No applicable published research was found in this category.

Possibly Effective

■ *Face the patient and make eye contact.* **LOE=III**

(MR) In a controlled study of nurse-patient interaction in the ICU (*N*=18 nurses and 120 patients), facing the patient and making eye contact were components of a multifaceted intensive training program for nurses that demonstrated an increase in positive nurse inter-actional behaviors and patients' satisfaction and a decrease in perceived pain and modal length of stay (de los Rios Castillo & Sanchez-Sosa, 2002).

■ (NIC) *Use simple words and short sentences, as appropriate.* **LOE=VI**

(NR) In a descriptive study of the communication needs of mechanically ventilated, critically ill patients (*N*=29), patients reported that asking simple questions that could be answered with yes or no enhanced communication and required minimal amounts of energy to respond to (Patak et al., 2004).

■ *Use an alphabet board.* **LOE=VI**

(MR) A controlled study of adults with cerebral palsy accompanied by dysarthria (*N*=3) and listeners (*N*=144) demonstrated that alphabet cues (indicating the first letter on an alphabet board while simultaneously speaking) increased intelligibility for the listener (Hustad & Garcia, 2005).

(MR) A controlled single case study of a 24-year-old woman diagnosed with quadriplegia and anarthria following a motor vehicle accident at 16 years old showed that training of both the patient and staff on the use of an alphabet board improved communication more than train-ing the patient alone (Calculator & Luchko, 1983).

(MR) A qualitative study of patients with acute severe neuromuscular disease who received prolonged mechanical ventilation in the ICU (*N*=5) reported that the alphabet board was a satisfactory method of communication. However, simple, direct instructions for family members and patients were needed to increase the benefit and understanding of how to use the technique (Fried-Oken et al., 1991).

(MR) In a descriptive study involving 50 temporarily nonspeaking ICU patients who received augmentative and alternative communication consultation during a 2-year period, electrolar-ynx/tracheostomy occlusion was recommended most frequently, but direct selection (eye gaze, word, picture, or alphabet boards) and natural speaking approaches (writing, mouthing words, gesture) had much better success rates (Dowden et al., 1986).

RCT = Randomized Controlled (Clinical) Trial, **NIC** = Nursing Interventions Classification, **NOC** = Nursing Outcomes Classification

■ **NIC** *Use a picture board, if appropriate.* **LOE=VI**

NR A controlled study of subjects who underwent cardiac surgery (*N*=48) and cardiac surgical ICU nurses (*N*=22) comparing an experimental group who received a picture board method with a usual care control group demonstrated a significant increase in patients' satisfaction with communication in the group using the picture board method (Stovsky et al., 1988).

MR In a descriptive study involving 50 temporarily nonspeaking ICU patients who received AAC consultation during a 2-year period, electrolarynges/tracheostomy occlusion was recommended most frequently, but direct selection (eye gaze, word, picture or alphabet boards) and natural speaking approaches (writing, mouthing words, gesture) had much better success rates (Dowden et al., 1986).

■ **NIC** *Use hand gestures, as appropriate.* **LOE=VI**

MR A controlled study of adults with cerebral palsy accompanied by dysarthria (*N*=3) and listeners (*N*=144) demonstrated that speaker-initiated iconic gestures (natural hand movements that add or illustrate content words) increased intelligibility for listeners when combined with alphabet cues (Hustad & Garcia, 2005).

NR A descriptive study of gestural communication among mechanically ventilated surgical and trauma ICU patients showed that nonspeaking ICU patients used some highly recognizable gestures for communication and that "mirroring," or nurse replication of patient-initiated gestures to affirm their meaning, was a technique leading to increased frequency of gestural communication by patients (Connolly, 1992).

MR In a descriptive study involving 50 temporarily nonspeaking ICU patients who received AAC consultation during a 2-year period, electrolarynges/tracheostomy occlusion was recommended most frequently, but direct selection (eye gaze, word, picture, or alphabet boards) and natural speaking approaches (writing, mouthing words, gesture) had much better success rates (Dowden et al., 1986).

■ *Provide writing materials.* **LOE=VI**

NR A descriptive study of the communication needs of mechanically ventilated, critically ill patients (*N*=29) reported that practitioners who provided writing materials and read the words aloud as patients wrote enhanced communication by allowing the patient to verify the nurse's interpretation (Patak et al., 2004).

MR In a descriptive study involving 50 temporarily nonspeaking ICU patients who received AAC consultation during a 2-year period, electrolarynges/tracheostomy occlusion was recommended most frequently, but direct selection (eye gaze, word, picture or alphabet boards) and natural speaking approaches (writing, mouthing words, gesture) had much better success rates (Dowden et al., 1986).

NR In a qualitative study involving patients who required mechanical ventilation for a minimum of 6 hours (*N*=22), patients reported a preference for simple methods of communication including body language, touch, and paper and pen as most effective (Wojnicki-Johansson, 2001).

NR = Nursing Research, **MR** = Multidisciplinary Research, **SP** = Standard of Practice, **EO** = Expert Opinion, **LOE** = Level of Evidence

■ *Provide written choice communication strategy, which involves the nurse simultaneously saying the choice while pointing to the written word, then allowing the patient to choose from the written array of three to five options.* **LOE=III**

(MR) A controlled single case study of a male subject who was not able to communicate at a functional level 1 year and 5 months after a left cerebral vascular accident demonstrated that the written choice techniques improved comprehensibility and accuracy (Garrett & Beukelman, 1995).

(MR) A controlled study of adults with severe aphasia compared the standard written choice strategy with two variations (auditory-only and visual-only format). All patients performed with the most accuracy when using the standard written choice strategy (Lasker et al., 1997).

■ (NIC) *Provide positive reinforcement and praise, as appropraite.* **LOE=VI**

(NR) A descriptive study of communication needs of mechanically ventilated, critically ill patients ($N=29$) reported that practitioners who provided reassurance and had a kind or patient demeanor enhanced communication (Patak et al., 2004).

Not Effective

■ *Use of a phrase board.* **LOE=VI**

(MR) A qualitative study of patients diagnosed with acute severe neuromuscular disease and requiring admission to the ICU for prolonged mechanical ventilation ($N=5$) reported that messages on the phrase board were too limited and therefore did not aid sufficiently in expression (Fried-Oken et al., 1991). More research is needed to determine the effectiveness of phrase boards. However, clinical practice experience, particularly in the use of handwritten phrases generated by patients and/or their families, supports the use of this technique with selected patients (Beukelman et al., 2007).

Possibly Harmful

No applicable published research was found in this category.

OUTCOME MEASUREMENT

COMMUNICATION (NOC)

Definition: Reception, interpretation, and expression of spoken, written, and nonverbal messages.

Communication as evidenced by the following selected NOC indicators:

• Use of written language
• Use of spoken language
• Use of pictures and drawings
• Use of nonverbal language
• Acknowledgment of messages received

Continued

RCT = Randomized Controlled (Clinical) Trial, **NIC** = Nursing Interventions Classification, **NOC** = Nursing Outcomes Classification

OUTCOME MEASUREMENT—*cont'd*

- Accurate interpretation of messages received
- Exchanges messages accurately with others

(Rate each indicator of **Communication:** 1=severely compromised, 2=substantially compromised, 3=moderately compromised, 4=mildly compromised, 5=not compromised) (Moorhead et al., 2004).

REFERENCES

Beukelman DR, Garrett KL, Yorkston KM (Eds). (2007). *Augmentative communication strategies for adults with acute or chronic medical conditions.* Baltimore: Brookes.

Calculator S, Luchko CD. (1983). Evaluating the effectiveness of a communication board training program. *J Speech Hear Disord,* 48(2):185-191.

Connolly M. (1992). Temporarily nonvocal trauma patients and their gestures: A descriptive study. Unpublished doctoral dissertation. Rush University, Chicago, IL. UMI# 9224758.

de los Rios Castillo JL, Sanchez-Sosa JJ. (2002). Well-being and medical recovery in the critical care unit: The role of the nurse-patient interaction. *Salud Mental,* 25(2), 21-31.

Dochterman JM, Bulechek GM (Eds). (2004). *Nursing Interventions Classification (NIC),* 4th ed. St. Louis: Mosby.

Dowden P, Beukelman DR, Lossing C. (1986). Serving nonspeaking patients in acute care settings: Intervention outcomes. *Augmentatitve Altern Commun,* 2(2):38-44.

Fried-Oken M, Howard JM, Stewart SR. (1991). Feedback on AAC Intervention from adults who are temporarily unable to speak. *Augmentative Altern Commun,* 7(1):43-50.

Garrett KL, Beukelman DR. (1995). Changes in the interaction patterns of an individual with severe aphasia given three types of partner support. *Clin Aphasiol Conf,* 23(1):237-251.

Garrett KL, Happ MB, Costello J, Fried-Oken M. (2007). Intensive care contexts (and transient conditions). In Beukelman DR, Garrett KL, Yorkston KM (Eds): *Augmentative communication strategies for adults with acute or chronic medical conditions.* Baltimore: Brookes.

Hustad KC, Garcia JM. (2005). Aided and unaided speech supplement strategies: Effect of alphabet cues and ionic hand gestures on dysarthric speech. *J Speech Lang Hear Res,* 48(5):996-1012.

Lasker J, Hux K, Garrett KL, Moncrief EM, Eischeid TJ. (1997). Variations on the written choice communication strategy for individuals with severe aphasia. *Augmentative Altern Commun,* 13(2):108-116.

Moorhead M, Johnson M, Maas M (Eds). (2004). *Nursing Outcomes Classification (NOC),* 3rd ed. St. Louis: Mosby.

Patak L, Gawlinski A, Fung NI, Doering L, Berg J. (2004). Patients' reports of health care practitioner interventions that are related to communication during mechanical ventilation. *Heart Lung,* 33(5):308-320.

Stovsky B, Rudy E, Dragonette P. (1988). Comparison of two types of communication methods used after cardiac surgery with patients with endotracheal tubes. *Heart Lung,* 17(3):281-289.

Wojnicki-Johansson G. (2001). Communication between nurse and patient during mechanical ventilator treatment: Patient reports and RN evaluations. *Intensive Crit Care Nurs,* 17(1):29-39.

COMMUNICATION ENHANCEMENT: VISUAL DEFICIT

 NIC

Jeanne A. Teresi, EdD, PhD; Alan R. Morse, PhD; Stephanie A. Silver, MPH

NIC **Definition:** Assistance in accepting and learning alternate methods for living with diminished vision (Dochterman & Bulechek, 2004).

NR = Nursing Research, **MR** = Multidisciplinary Research, **SP** = Standard of Practice, **EO** = Expert Opinion, **LOE** = Level of Evidence

NURSING ACTIVITIES

Effective

■ *Use self-management programs to improve function of visually impaired patients.* **LOE=II**

(MR) An RCT (*N*=214) of people with macular degeneration demonstrated sustained improvement in emotional function, self-efficacy, and physical function for those in the self-management program (Brody et al., 2005).

(MR) An RCT (*N*=64) demonstrated that patients with age-related macular degeneration (AMD) who received five 1-hour training sessions in using low-vision devices had significantly improved reading accuracy and reading rates at 5- and 12-week follow-up and reported better self-rated eyesight than controls at 12-week follow-up (Scanlan & Cuddeford, 2004).

(MR) A three-armed longitudinal RCT of nursing home residents (*N*=166) demonstrated that residents in the staff training and visual aid group showed significant improvement in affect over controls and over those receiving visual aids alone (Teresi et al., 2003).

(MR) A three-armed longitudinal RCT (*N*=106) demonstrated a significant improvement in function for the group that received eyeglasses, reinforcement of their use, and staff training; some decline was shown in the group that received eyeglasses without staff training and reinforcement; the control group showed the most decline in function (Teresi et al., 2005).

(MR) An RCT (*N*=187) of AMD patients who participated in either a health education program promoting self-efficacy in activities of daily living or a traditional intervention program demonstrated that the self-efficacy group reported significantly greater perceived security in performing activities of daily living (Dahlin Ivanoff et al., 2002).

(MR) A controlled study of patients attending interdisciplinary low-vision service clinics (*N*=71) demonstrated significantly less fear of deteriorating vision, concern about safety at home, and problems coping with everyday life and significantly improved vision-related quality of life at 6 months after the visit (Hinds et al., 2003).

(MR) The intervention arm (*N*=29) of an RCT that received vision rehabilitation services (including visual aids and orientation and mobility training) demonstrated significantly greater improvement in the living skills inventory and better goal attainment than controls (Pankow et al., 2004).

Additional research: Brody et al., 2002, 1999; McCabe et al., 2000; Wolffsohn & Cochrane, 2000.

■ *Help patients obtain needed visual aids including eyeglasses, magnifiers, filters, or electronic vision enhancement systems as needed.* **LOE=II**

(MR) An RCT (*N*=111) of community-dwelling elderly persons demonstrated that those who received a prescription for free eyeglasses and/or a magnifier showed significantly better vision-specific quality of life and perceived visual acuity at 3-month follow-up than the control group (Coleman et al., 2006).

(MR) In a controlled study of four electronic vision enhancement systems (EVESs), subjects (*N*=70) were able to read faster using a stand EVES with monitor, but standard optical magnification was equivalent in terms of speed for some tasks (Peterson et al., 2003).

RCT = Randomized Controlled (Clinical) Trial, **NIC** = Nursing Interventions Classification, **NOC** = Nursing Outcomes Classification

(MR) A controlled trial (N=100) demonstrated that near vision devices and, for those with acuity less than 6/18, standard spectacles and telescopes improved visual acuity (Khan et al., 2002).

(MR) A cross-sectional study of a convenience sample of bioptic drivers (N=58) showed that most drivers found the use of a bioptic telescope helpful (Bowers et al., 2005).

(MR) A case-control study (N=38) of subjects using their preferred filter to view colored pictures of natural scenes demonstrated that they preferred filters with lower gains and that unsharp masking and Peli adaptive enhancement provided significantly improved perceived visibility for some images (Leat et al., 2005).

Additional research: Margrain, 2000; Shuttleworth et al., 1995.

Possibly Effective

- *Use a system such as a prefilled medication organizer with large lettering or three-dimensional markers to help the visually impaired patient take medications.* **LOE=VII**

  (EO) Working with patients with macular degeneration to help them use devices for safety in taking medications can help them maintain a better quality of life (McGrory & Remington, 2004).

  (MR) A descriptive study (N=492) found that 9.4% of a random sample of community-based and institutionalized elderly participants could not read the label on a standard medicine bottle (Beckman et al., 2005).

  (MR) In a cross-sectional descriptive study, a representative sample of disabled participants aged 73 to 82 years (N=335) were evaluated with respect to the ability to take medications using the Hopkins Medication Schedule (HMS) Pillbox Component as well as vision, including contrast sensitivity, stereopsis, and visual acuity. Almost half of this cohort made medication management errors. Vision measures were significantly related to performance on the HMS measure. Cognition was a modifier of this relationship (Windham et al., 2005).

- *Institute fall precaution interventions for the visually impaired patient.* **LOE=IV**

  (MR) A case-control study of hospitalized patients aged 60+ (N=911 cases; 910 controls) demonstrated that decreased visual acuity and self-report of impaired vision were significantly associated with increased risk of hip fracture (Ivers et al., 2000).

  (MR) A case-control study of in-hospital hip fractures in patients aged ≥65 years (N=129 with fracture; 234 controls) demonstrated that impaired vision was one of six factors associated with fracture; existence of multiple factors increased risk for fracture (Lichtenstein et al., 1994).

  (MR) A systematic review of well-designed, sufficiently powered studies in which confounders were controlled demonstrated a significant relationship between visual acuity and falls (Legood et al., 2002).

Not Effective

- *Home visits by a rehabilitation officer as part of a visual rehabilitation program.* **LOE=II**

  (MR) An RCT (N=194) demonstrated no significant effects of enhanced low-vision rehabilitation (ELVR) over conventional low-vision rehabilitation (CLVR) and CLVR enhanced by

---

NR = Nursing Research, **MR** = Multidisciplinary Research, **SP** = Standard of Practice, **EO** = Expert Opinion, **LOE** = Level of Evidence

rehabilitation officer home visits (ECLVR). Statistically significant differences were found between CLVR and ECLVR only on measures of physical and mental function; however, differences favored the usual (CLVR) care group. No effects were observed for CLVR enhanced by a community care worker (Reeves et al., 2004).

■ *Use of prism glasses by visually impaired patients.* LOE=II

MR An RCT of patients with AMD ($N=225$) assigned participants to one of three study arms: (1) nonprism glasses, (2) standard prisms, and (3) custom prisms. No significant differences in any outcomes (including visual acuity and words read per minute) were observed for those patients wearing prism lenses versus those wearing standard lenses (Smith et al., 2005).

Possibly Harmful

No applicable published research was found in this category.

OUTCOME MEASUREMENT

VISION COMPENSATION BEHAVIOR   NOC

(Please refer to *Nursing Outcomes Classification* [Moorhead et al., 2004] for the **Vision Compensation Behavior** outcome.)

REFERENCES

Beckman AG, Parker MG, Thorslund M. (2005). Can elderly people take their medicine? *Patient Educ Couns,* 59(2):186-191.

Bowers AR, Apfelbaum DH, Peli E. (2005). Bioptic telescopes meet the needs of drivers with moderate visual acuity loss. *Invest Ophthalmol Vis Sci,* 46(1):66-74.

Brody BL, Roch-Levecq AC, Gamst AC, Maclean K, Kaplan RM, Brown SI. (2002). Self-management of age-related macular degeneration and quality of life: A randomized controlled trial. *Arch Ophthalmol,* 120(11):1477-1483.

Brody BL, Roch-Levecq AC, Thomas RG, Kaplan RM, Brown SI. (2005). Self-management of age-related macular degeneration at the 6-month follow-up: A randomized controlled trial. *Arch Ophthalmol,* 123(1):46-53.

Brody BL, Williams RA, Thomas RG, Kaplan RM, Chu RM, Brown SI. (1999). Age-related macular degeneration: A randomized clinical trial of a self-management intervention. *Ann Behav Med,* 21(4):322-329.

Coleman AL, Yu F, Keeler E, Mangione CM. (2006). Treatment of uncorrected refractive error improves vision-specific quality of life. *J Am Geriatr Soc,* 54(6):883-890.

Dahlin Ivanoff S, Sonn U, Svensson E. (2002). A health education program for elderly persons with visual impairments and perceived security in the performance of daily occupations: a randomized study. *Am J Occup Ther,* 56(3):322-330.

Dochterman JM, Bulechek GM (Eds). (2004). *Nursing Interventions Classification (NIC),* 4th ed. St. Louis: Mosby.

Hinds A, Sinclair A, Park J, Suttie A, Paterson H, Macdonald M. (2003). Impact of an interdisciplinary low vision service on the quality of life of low vision patients. *Br J Ophthalmol,* 87(11):1391-1396.

Ivers RQ, Norton R, Cumming RG, Butler M, Campbell AJ. (2000). Visual impairment and risk of hip fracture. *Am J Epidemiol,* 152(7):633-639.

RCT = Randomized Controlled (Clinical) Trial, **NIC** = Nursing Interventions Classification, **NOC** = Nursing Outcomes Classification

Khan SA, Das T, Kumar SM, Nutheti R. (2002). Low vision rehabilitation in patients with age-related macular degeneration at a tertiary eye care centre in southern India. *Clin Experiment Ophthalmol,* 30(6):404-410.

Leat SJ, Omoruyi G, Kennedy A, Jernigan E. (2005). Generic and customized digital image enhancement filters for the visually impaired. *Vision Res,* 45(15):1991-2007.

Legood R, Scuffham P, Cryer C. (2002). Are we blind to injuries in the visually impaired? A review of the literature. *Inj Prev,* 8(2):155-160.

Lichtenstein MJ, Griffin MR, Cornell JE, Malcolm E, Ray WA. (1994). Risk factors for hip fractures occurring in the hospital. *Am J Epidemiol,* 140(9):830-838.

Margrain TH. (2000). Helping blind and partially sighted people to read: The effectiveness of low vision aids. *Br J Ophthalmol,* 84(8):919-921.

McCabe P, Nason F, Demers Turco P, Friedman D, Seddon JM. (2000). Evaluating the effectiveness of a vision rehabilitation intervention using an objective and subjective measure of functional performance. *Ophthalmic Epidemiol,* 7(4):259-270.

McGrory A, Remington R. (2004). Optimizing the functionality of clients with age-related macular degeneration. *Rehabil Nurs,* 29(3):90-94.

Moorhead M, Johnson M, Maas M (Eds). (2004). *Nursing Outcomes Classification (NOC),* 3rd ed. St. Louis: Mosby.

Pankow L, Luchins D, Studebaker J, Chettleburgh D. (2004). Evaluation of a vision rehabilitation program for older adults with visual impairment. *Top Geriatr Rehabil,* 20(3):223-232.

Peterson RC, Wolffsohn JS, Rubinstein M, Lowe J. (2003). Benefits of electronic vision enhancement systems (EVES) for the visually impaired. *J Ophthalmol,* 136(6):1129-1135.

Reeves BC, Harper RA, Russell WB. (2004). Enhanced low vision rehabilitation for people with age related macular degeneration: A randomised controlled trial. *Br J Ophthalmol,* 88(11):1443-1449.

Scanlan JM, Cuddeford JE. (2004). Low vision rehabilitation: A comparison of traditional and extended teaching programs. *J Vis Impair Blind,* 98(10):601-611.

Shuttleworth GN, Dunlop A, Collins JK, James CR. (1995). How effective is an integrated approach to low vision rehabilitation? Two year follow up results from south Devon. *Br J Ophthalmol,* 79(8):719-723.

Smith HJ, Dickinson CM, Cacho I, Reeves BC, Harper RA. (2005). A randomized controlled trial to determine the effectiveness of prism spectacles for patients with age-related macular degeneration. *Arch Ophthalmol,* 123(8):1042-1050.

Teresi JA, Morse AR, Holmes D, Yatzkan ES, Ramirez M, Rosenthal B, et al. (2003). The impact of a low vision intervention on affective state among nursing home residents. *J Ment Health Aging,* 9(2): 73-84.

Teresi J, Morse AR, Holmes D, Yatzkan ES, Ramirez M, Rosenthal B, et al. (2005). Impact of a vision intervention on the functional status of nursing home residents. *J Vis Impair Blind,* 99(2):96-108.

Windham BG, Griswold ME, Fried LP, Rubin GS, Xue QL, Carlson MC. (2005). Impaired vision and the ability to take medications. *J Am Geriatr Soc,* 53(7):1179-1190.

Wolffsohn JS, Cochrane AL. (2000). Design of the low vision quality-of-life questionnaire (LVQOL) and measuring the outcome of low-vision rehabilitation. *Arch Ophthalmol,* 130(6):793-802.

 # Constipation Management

Marilee Schmelzer, PhD, RN

Definition: Prevention and alleviation of constipation.

NURSING ACTIVITIES

Effective

No applicable published research was found in this category.

NR = Nursing Research, **MR** = Multidisciplinary Research, **SP** = Standard of Practice, **EO** = Expert Opinion, **LOE** = Level of Evidence

Possibly Effective

■ *Provide 20 g of dietary fiber daily in a form that the individual finds palatable. Make sure that the individual is well hydrated before increasing the amount of fiber, and increase the amount of fiber gradually. Cereal grains are particularly effective for increasing stool size, and extra fluids are needed when dietary fiber is added to the diet.* **LOE=II**

(MR) In a comparative study with analysis of survey data from a subset of women (N=62,036) in the Nurses' Health Study ages 36 to 61 years, it was found that the women in the highest quintile of dietary fiber intake (median intake 20 g/day) were less likely to experience constipation than the women in the lowest quintile (median intake 7 g/day) (Dukas et al., 2003).

(MR) An RCT was conducted with elderly patients (N=111) admitted for orthopedic surgery or orthopedic injury that required bed rest and opiates. Those receiving either pear juice (150 mL twice daily) or a fiber supplement (bran, prune, oats, apple, and coconut mixture) had no greater bowel movement frequency and no less laxative use than the control group, perhaps because they had difficulty ingesting adequate amounts of dietary fiber and fluids (Stumm et al., 2001).

(MR) A Cochrane systematic review found that daily supplements of dietary fiber in the form of bran or wheat fiber were safe and effective for women complaining of constipation during pregnancy (Jewell & Young, 2001).

(NR) A 3-year quality improvement study using a protocol that included high-fiber cookies and muffins that had been tested for palatability with hospitalized, immobilized, vascular surgery patients resulted in a reduction in the incidence of constipation from 59% to 9%, a reduction in the use of laxatives from 59% to about 8%, and the elimination of impactions (N=66). Patients were also encouraged to drink 1500 mL of fluids daily (Hall et al., 1995).

(MR) A two-by-two factorial design found that rye bread significantly shortened intestinal transit time, softened the feces, and increased the ease of defecation in healthy women with self-reported constipation (N=59). Yogurt lessened the bloating and flatulence resulting from rye bread ingestion (Hongisto et al., 2006).

(NR) A systematic review of 20 studies reporting the effectiveness of dietary fiber on constipation found that only 8 met the review criteria, 2 were double-blinded RCT studies, 5 of 6 studies found a decline in laxative use, and contradictory results were reported for comfort with defecation. The reviewers concluded that a lack of strong or consistent evidence for the effectiveness of dietary fiber was partly due to poor study design (Kenny & Skelly, 2001).

Additional research: Ouellet et al., 1996; Benton et al., 1997; Dahl et al., 2003; Hall et al., 1995.

■ *Provide prunes or prune juice daily.* **LOE=VII**

(EO) Through conventional wisdom and common experience, the laxative effects of dried prunes and prune juice are widely accepted, but no research studies were found to support their use (Stacewicz-Sapuntzakis et al., 2001).

RCT = Randomized Controlled (Clinical) Trial, **NIC** = Nursing Interventions Classification, **NOC** = Nursing Outcomes Classification

■ *Encourage patients to resume walking as soon as possible if they have been on bed rest or restricted mobility and to perform their activities of daily living as independently as possible. (Bed rest and decreased mobility lead to constipation, but additional exercise does not help the constipated person who is already mobile.)* **LOE=II**

(MR) In a classic clinical study, researchers applied pelvic girdle and leg casts to four healthy young men to study the effects of immobility. Two of the four developed constipation, but the other two routinely used a bedpan every evening and did not become constipated (Deitrick et al., 1948).

(MR) In a comparative study with analysis of survey data from a subset of women in the Nurses' Health Study (N=62,036), it was found that women who reported daily physical activity had a lower prevalence of constipation (Dukas et al., 2003).

(MR) An experimental study with six healthy dogs found that physical exercise increased colonic motor activity after a meal and stimulated defecation and mass movements in the colon in both the fasting and fed states (Dapoigny & Sarna, 1991).

(MR) In a descriptive study, a comparison of colon transit times using radiopaque markers found no differences in large bowel transit times between 11 young male soccer players who regularly engaged in intensive physical exercise and nine healthy, young, male radiology technicians who did not engage in physical activity (Sesboüe et al., 1995).

(MR) A randomized crossover design involving sedentary patients with chronic constipation (N=43) found that 12 weeks of physical activity (twice weekly walking and daily strength and flexibility exercises) significantly decreased symptoms of constipation and difficulty defecating. Transit time decreased only in those whose transit time was increased before starting the exercise program (De Schryver et al., 2005).

■ *Provide privacy for defecation; assist the patient to the bathroom and close the door unless contraindicated.* **LOE=VII**

(EO) Defecation is a private act in Western cultures and lack of privacy inhibits defecation (Weeks et al., 2000).

■ *Assist the patient to the toilet or commode at the same time every day, based on usual bowel habits. If the individual routinely defecated in the morning, schedule toileting time within 30 to 40 minutes following breakfast. If the individual routinely defecated in the evening, schedule toileting time for 30 to 40 minutes following the evening meal. Allow the patient distraction-free time (up to 15 to 20 minutes) to sit on the toilet.* **LOE=II**

(NR) In a quasi-experimental study, after initiation of a bowel program that included adequate hydration, dietary fiber, and regular toileting, 26 of 30 continuing-care patients had normal bowel elimination patterns without laxatives, and the other four patients required fewer laxatives (Benton et al., 1997).

(NR) An RCT of patients (N=46) receiving bowel retraining following a stroke demonstrated that patients who were scheduled for defecation in the morning after breakfast attained regular bowel elimination patterns faster than those scheduled for evening defecation. Patients whose defecation was scheduled to coincide with bowel patterns before the stroke also returned to their normal bowel elimination patterns significantly faster (Venn et al., 1992).

NR = Nursing Research, **MR** = Multidisciplinary Research, **SP** = Standard of Practice, **EO** = Expert Opinion, **LOE** = Level of Evidence

■ *Encourage the use of a commode or toilet for proper squatting posture, and encourage the individual to lean forward.* **LOE=II**

(MR) An experimental study with healthy, young men (*N*=10) determined that flexing the hip to 90 degrees or more straightened the angle between the anus and the rectum and pulled the anal canal open to decrease the resistance to the movement of feces from the rectum and the amount of pressure needed to empty the rectum. Hip flexion was greatest when squatting or when leaning forward while sitting (Tagart, 1966).

(EO) The upright position allows gravity to assist with defecation (Weeks et al., 2000).

■ *Teach the patient to respond to the defecation urge promptly.* **LOE=III**

(MR) A controlled trial of healthy male volunteers (*N*=12) determined that the defecation urge could be delayed (three participants delayed for 3 days) and that suppression of constipation led to decreased bowel movement frequency, decreased stool weight, and decreased colon transit times (Klauser et al., 1990).

Not Effective

No applicable published research was found in this category.

Possibly Harmful

No applicable published research was found in this category.

OUTCOME MEASUREMENT

BOWEL ELIMINATION (NOC)

Definition: Formation and evacuation of stool.
Bowel Elimination as evidenced by the following selected NOC indicators:
• Elimination pattern
• Stool soft and formed
• Passage of stool without aids
• Ease of stool passage
(Rate each indicator of **Bowel Elimination:** 1=severely compromised, 2=substantially compromised, 3=moderately compromised, 4=mildly compromised, 5=not compromised) (Moorhead et al., 2004).

REFERENCES

Benton JM, O'Hara PA, Chen H, Harper DW, Johnston SF. (1997). Changing bowel hygiene practice successfully: A program to reduce laxative use in a chronic care hospital. *Geriatr Nurs,* 18(1):12-17.

Dahl WJ, Whiting SJ, Healey A, Zello GA, Hildebrandt SL. (2003). Increased stool frequency occurs when finely processed pea hull fiber is added to usual foods consumed by elderly residents in long-term care. *J Am Diet Assoc,* 103(9):1199-1202.

Dapoigny M, Sarna SK. (1991). Effects of physical exercise on colonic motor activity. *Am J Physiol,* 260(4 Pt 1):G646-G652.

Deitrick JE, Whedon GD, Shorr E. (1948). Effects of immobilization upon various metabolic and physiologic functions of normal men. *Am J Med,* 4(1):3-36.

RCT = Randomized Controlled (Clinical) Trial, **NIC** = Nursing Interventions Classification, **NOC** = Nursing Outcomes Classification

De Schryver AM, Keulemans YC, Peters HP, Akkermans LM, Smout AJ, De Vries WR, et al. (2005). Effects of regular physical activity on defecation pattern in middle-aged patients complaining of chronic constipation. *Scand J Gastroenterol,* 40(4):422-429.

Dukas L, Willett WC, Giovannucci EL. (2003). Association between physical activity, fiber intake, and other lifestyle variables and constipation in a study of women. *Am J Gastroenterol,* 98(8):1790-1796.

Hall GR, Karstens M, Rakel B, Swanson E, Davidson A. (1995). Managing constipation using a research-based protocol. *Medsurg Nurs,* 4(1):11-18.

Hongisto SM, Paajanen L, Saxelin M, Korpela R. (2006). A combination of fibre-rich rye bread and yoghurt containing Lactobacillus GG improves bowel function in women with self-reported constipation. *Eur J Clin Nutr,* 60(3):319-324.

Jewell DJ, Young G. (2001). Interventions for treating constipation in pregnancy. *Cochrane Database Syst Rev,* (2):CD001142.

Kenny KA, Skelly JM. (2001). Dietary fiber for constipation in older adults: A systematic review. *Clin Effect Nurs,* 5(3):120-128.

Klauser AG, Voderholzer WA, Heinrich CA, Schindlbeck NE, Muller-Lissner SA. (1990). Behavioral modification of colonic function. Can constipation be learned? *Dig Dis Sci,* 35(10):1271-1275.

Moorhead M, Johnson M, Maas M (Eds). (2004). *Nursing Outcomes Classification (NOC),* 3rd ed. St. Louis: Mosby.

Ouellet LL, Turner TR, Pond S, McLaughlin H, Knorr S. (1996). Dietary fiber and laxation in postop orthopedic patients. *Clin Nurs Res,* 5(4):428-440.

Sesboüe B, Arhan P, Devroede G, Lecointe-Besancon I, Congard P, Bouchoucha M, et al. (1995). Colonic transit in soccer players. *J Clin Gastroenterol,* 20(3):211-214.

Stacewicz-Sapuntzakis M, Bowen PE, Hussain EA, Damayanti-Wood BI, Farnsworth NR. (2001). Chemical composition and potential health effects of prunes: A functional food? *Crit Rev Food Sci Nutr,* 41(4):251-286.

Stumm RE, Thomas MS, Coombes J, Greenhill J, Hay J. (2001). Managing constipation in elderly orthopaedic patients using either pear juice or a high fibre supplement. *Aust J Nutr Diet,* 58(3):181-185.

Tagart RE. (1966). The anal canal and rectum: Their varying relationship and its effect on anal continence. *Dis Colon Rectum,* 9(6):449-452.

Venn MR, Taft L, Carpentier B, Applebaugh G. (1992). The influence of timing and suppository use on efficiency and effectiveness of bowel training after a stroke. *Rehabil Nurs,* 17(3):116-120.

Weeks SK, Hubbartt E, Michaels TK. (2000). Keys to bowel success. *Rehabil Nurs,* 25(2):66-69, 79-80.

 # CRISIS INTERVENTION

Mary T. Shoemaker, MSN, RN, SANE

NIC **Definition:** Use of short-term counseling to help the patient cope with a crisis and resume a state of functioning comparable to or better than the precrisis state (Dochterman & Bulechek, 2004).

NURSING ACTIVITIES

Effective

■ **NIC** *Provide an atmosphere of support.* **LOE=I**

EO There is general consensus among many crisis clinicians, researchers, and administrators that relief programs, disaster mental health initiatives, crime victim services, and community mental health–based crisis intervention units grew out of a fervent desire to lessen the suffering and aid in the recovery of all people affected by crises (Roberts & Everly, 2006).

NR = Nursing Research, **MR** = Multidisciplinary Research, **SP** = Standard of Practice, **EO** = Expert Opinion, **LOE** = Level of Evidence

- **NIC** *Determine whether the patient presents a safety risk to self or others.* LOE=VII

    FO When a patient verbalizes a suicidal threat and the plan to use a lethal method, it is imperative that the patient be involuntarily committed for a minimum of 48 to 72 hours for assessment and observation, including one-on-one observation (Yeager et al., 2005).

- **NIC** *Initiate necessary precautions to safeguard the patient or others at risk for physical harm.* LOE=VII

    FO Rapid assessment, timely crisis intervention, medication stabilization, and placement in a secure facility with architectural barriers to suicide should be mandatory for all people at imminent risk of suicide (Yeager et al., 2005).

- **NIC** *Encourage the expression of feelings in a nondestructive manner.* LOE=I

    MR An exploratory meta-analysis examined 36 studies providing high average effect sizes demonstrating that adults in acute crisis or with trauma symptoms and abusive families in acute crisis could be helped with intensive crisis intervention and multicomponent Critical Incident Stress Management in a large number of cases (Roberts & Everly, 2006).

- **NIC** *Assist in identification of the precipitants and dynamics of the crisis.* LOE=VII

    FO Applying Roberts' seven-stage crisis intervention model can facilitate the clinician's effective intervention by emphasizing rapid assessment of the client's problem and resources, collaborating on goal selection and attainment, finding alternative coping methods, developing a working alliance, and building upon the client's strengths (Roberts & Ottens, 2005).

- **NIC** *Assist in identification of personal strengths and abilities that can be used in resolving the crisis.* LOE=VII

    FO Regularly monitor clients in high-stress jobs in whom unexpected events or critical incidents have an emotional impact that overwhelms their usual coping skills and may cause significant distress in otherwise healthy people (Caine & Ter-Bagdasarian, 2003).

- **NIC** *Assist in identification of available support systems.* LOE=III

    NR In a qualitative technique analysis, 26 patients who were awaiting heart surgery identified that the support they felt was from people who were more or less close to them. The patients experienced very strong support and encouragement from next of kin and close friends who were considerate and good listeners (Ivarsson et al., 2004).

- **NIC** *Provide guidance about how to develop and maintain support system(s).* LOE=II

    NR In a qualitative technique analysis, 26 patients learned from and were inspired by the experience and support of people close to them who had already had heart surgery (Ivarsson et al., 2004).

- **NIC** *Introduce the patient to persons (or groups) who have successfully undergone the same experience.* LOE=VII

    FO Experts identify the importance of using group process techniques that are comfortable and appropriate for participants (Lim et al., 2000).

RCT = Randomized Controlled (Clinical) Trial, **NIC** = Nursing Interventions Classification, **NOC** = Nursing Outcomes Classification

(NR) A quality assurance audit reviewing 406 cases identified the importance of using group process techniques that were comfortable and appropriate for the participants (Webster & Harrison, 2004).

Possibly Effective

■ (NIC) *Plan with the patient how adaptive coping skills can be used to deal with crises in the future.* **LOE=VII**

(EO) The therapeutic values of mental health nurses relate that it is not about blaming and dwelling on the past but developing awareness about the factors that have brought the person to the present. If we ignore people's valuable stories and what has brought them to the present, we are in effect showing disregard for their personhood (Hurley et al., 2006).

■ (NIC) *Assist in formulating a time frame for implementation of a chosen course of action.* **LOE=VII**

(EO) Experts in the field of community crisis resolution have developed, modified, and implemented a program to provide support and give time to people referred and accepted to the support group, promote their recovery, and maintain them in their community environment. This program helps the service user to gain access to resources, provides information on health promotion, and helps to identify early warning signs to prevent a relapse. This team effort also assists the team coordinator and mental health practitioners in assessing, planning, implementing, and evaluating crisis care plans (Uddin et al., 2006).

Not Effective

No applicable published research was found in this category.

Possibly Harmful

No applicable published research was found in this category.

OUTCOME MEASUREMENT

COPING · (NOC)

Definition: Personal actions to manage stressors that tax an individual's resources.
Coping as evidenced by the following selected NOC indicators:
• Reports decrease in stress
• Identifies multiple coping strategies
• Uses effective coping strategies
(Rate each indicator of **Coping:** 1=never demonstrated, 2=rarely demonstrated, 3=sometimes demonstrated, 4=often demonstrated, 5=consistently demonstrated) (Moorhead et al., 2004).

REFERENCES

Caine RM, Ter-Bagdasarian L. (2003). Early identification and management of critical incident stress. *Crit Care Nurse,* 23(1):59-65.

NR = Nursing Research, **MR** = Multidisciplinary Research, **SP** = Standard of Practice, **EO** = Expert Opinion, **LOE** = Level of Evidence

Dochterman JM, Bulechek GM (Eds). (2004). *Nursing Interventions Classification (NIC)*, 4th ed. St. Louis: Mosby.

Hurley J, Barrett P, Reet P. (2006). "Let a hundred flowers blossom, let a hundred schools of thought contend": A case for therapeutic pluralism in mental health nursing. *J Psychiatr Ment Health Nurs*, 13(2):173-179.

Ivarsson B, Larsson S, Sjoberg T. (2004). Patients' experiences of support while waiting for cardiac surgery. A critical incident technique analysis. *Eur J Cardiovasc Nurs*, 3(2):183-191.

Lim JJ, Childs J, Gonsalves K. (2000). Critical incident stress management. *AAOHN J*, 48(10):487-497.

Moorhead M, Johnson M, Maas M (Eds). (2004). *Nursing Outcomes Classification (NOC)*, 3rd ed. St. Louis: Mosby.

Roberts AR, Everly Jr GS. (2006). A meta-analysis of 36 crisis intervention studies. *Brief Treat Crisis Interven*, 6(1):10-21.

Roberts AR, Ottens AJ. (2005). The seven-stage crisis intervention model: A road map to goal attainment, problem solving, and crisis resolution. *Brief Treat Crisis Interven*, 5(4):329-339.

Uddin MS, Pankhania T, Rudkin C. (2006). Resolving crisis within the community: The role of the support, time and recovery (STR) workers. *Ment Health Pract*, 9(7):14-18.

Webster S, Harrison L. (2004). The multidisciplinary approach to mental health crisis management: An Australian example. *J Psychiatr Ment Health Nurs*, 11(1):21-29.

Yeager KR, Saveanu R, Roberts AR, Reissland G, Mertz D, Cirpili A, et al. (2005). Measured response to identified suicide risk and violence. *Brief Treat Crisis Interven*, 5(2):121-141.

CULTURAL BROKERAGE NIC

Sharon Wallace, MSN, RN, CCRN

NIC **Definition:** The deliberate use of culturally competent strategies to bridge or mediate between the patient's culture and the biomedical health care system (Dochterman & Bulechek, 2004).

NURSING ACTIVITIES

Effective

■ *Determine the nature of the conceptual differences that the patient and nurse have of the health problem or treatment plan.* **LOE=VI**

 In a qualitative study of aging and frail rural African-American women (*N*=41), study participants (mean age=84 years) described functional aging as being "worn out." Health problems were referred to as "inconveniences" rather than concerns. Participants took medications if they remembered but did not follow a special diet. Advantages of aging were identified. For example, they were guaranteed a comfortable seat at church. Overall, chronological aging was perceived to be a cause for celebration (Jett, 2003).

In a qualitative study, Kanadier Mennonite women (*N*=45) were interviewed about knowledge, beliefs, and practices related to pregnancy and childbirth to determine the importance of beliefs and practices held in Mexico. Findings identified that prenatal care was not routine. Childbearing was a private topic and typically not discussed. A variety of beliefs regarding miscarriage, breast feeding, diet, and activity were found to differ. For example, of women interviewed, only one mother followed the hospital's advice for cord care (Kulig et al., 2004).

RCT = Randomized Controlled (Clinical) Trial, **NIC** = Nursing Interventions Classification, **NOC** = Nursing Outcomes Classification

(NR) In a qualitative study of physical disability and factors affecting meaning of life for Korean adolescents ($N=88$), findings suggested that the meaning of life was derived from helping others, which created value and usefulness in their lives. Relationships with people and recognition by others, adapting to become a member of society, and achieving goals also contributed to a meaningful life. Conversely, traumatic experiences were described as being useless, not having meaning, and resulting in financial hardship (Kim & Kang, 2003).

(NR) In a qualitative study, an open-ended self-report questionnaire exploring perceptions of death and expected help was administered to fourth-year Bachelor of Science in Nursing (BSN) students ($N=110$) attending college in Taiwan. Thematic analysis identified six types of expected help: quality physical care, respect for dignity of patient and family, support and companionship between patient and family, maintaining communication, fostering a peaceful mind, and help to be free of guilt or shame while dying. It was also noted that help with making the transition to an afterlife was expected (Shih et al., 2006).

■ (NIC) *Negotiate, when conflicts cannot be resolved, an acceptable compromise regarding treatment based on biomedical knowledge, knowledge of the patient's belief systems, and ethical standards.* **LOE=VII**

(EO) It is important to understand the meaning behind a custom or practice to facilitate choice. If a choice poses a risk, negotiate compromise by providing information in a nonjudgmental manner. Explain potential risks and harm associated with a practice or custom and whether ethical or legal implications are present (College of Nurses of Ontario [CNO], 2005).

(NR) To provide education regarding end-of-life care, it is important to understand the basis for ethical differences in health care. In American health care systems, autonomy and individual control are highlighted in ethical dilemmas, which is not consistent with the interdependent or family-focused values found in many cultures and ethnic groups. Distinct differences can be found with regard to choices surrounding death and use of advanced directives (Valente, 2004).

■ (NIC) *Arrange for cultural accommodation (e.g., late kitchen during Ramadan).* **LOE=VI**

(NR) In a case study of a Filipino patient with cancer, findings suggested that cultural accommodation would include obliging extended family (e.g., additional chairs in room); open visiting hours; meeting with family members to discuss disclosure of diagnosis; teaching about pain management; importance of nonverbal pain cues in pain assessment; recognizing that support groups might not be beneficial; acknowledging association among faith, health, and destiny; and providing opportunity for spiritual and/or religious support (Schmit, 2005).

■ (NIC) *Appear relaxed and unhurried in interactions with the patient.* **LOE=VI**

(NR) In a qualitative study, older Taiwanese Americans ($N=100$) were screened for depression using a Geriatric Depression Scale to explore somatization as a symptom of depression. It was found that 7% of the participants screened experienced depressive symptoms. Findings suggest that if participants were given enough time to express themselves, somatic symptoms decreased and participants were able to report sadness, anger, loneliness, helplessness, and hopelessness (Suen & Tusaie, 2004).

NR = Nursing Research, **MR** = Multidisciplinary Research, **SP** = Standard of Practice, **EO** = Expert Opinion, **LOE** = Level of Evidence

■ **NIC** *Facilitate intercultural communication (e.g., use of a translator, bilingual written materials/media, accurate nonverbal communication, avoid stereotyping).* **LOE=VII**

EO Use of interpreters facilitates two-way communication. To work effectively with an interpreter, obtain consent for use of an interpreter, identify factors that influence communication (e.g., dialect), address confidentiality, and talk to and maintain eye contact with the patient (not the interpreter). Additional recommendations can also be found in the guideline (CNO, 2005).

EO The National Standards on Culturally and Linguistically Appropriate Services was developed to assist health care organizations apply 14 standards to various aspects of communication including the use of interpreters. Standards 4 to 6 indicate that health care organizations must provide language assistance services free of cost and around the clock, inform patients of the right to language assistance services, and ensure the competence of interpreters (Office of Minority Health, 2000).

EO JCAHO Standard RI.2.100 addresses the requirement for appropriate interpreter and translation services in the provision of culturally competent care (The Joint Commission, 2006).

NR In a descriptive study exploring the reliability and validity of content using a translation-retrotranslation process in an instrument adapted to measure quality of nursing care by emergency department patients ($N=102$), it was found that the adapted version had good internal consistency and construction validity (Cunado et al., 2002).

EO Communication in health care is increasingly important, particularly in a culturally and ethnically diverse society. Recommendations include research to examine effective communication strategies and the development of science-based interventions (Institute of Medicine, 2002a).

■ **NIC** *Provide information to other health care providers about the patient's culture.* **LOE=II**

NR In a quasi-experimental design study to explore cultural competency of RN-BSN undergraduate students ($N=13$) using pretest and post-test, students were paired with public health nurses during a 16-week clinical component of community health. Students also participated in workshops regarding clinical judgment and vulnerable populations as well as clinical post conferences. Post-test results indicated a statistically significant improvement in cultural competency scores (Doutrich & Storey, 2004).

NR An RCT explored the effects of cultural sensitivity training in health care providers ($N=114$) and patients' ($N=133$) outcomes. Health care providers ($N=50$) assigned to the experimental group received cultural sensitivity training. Data were collected and compared with baseline data. Results indicated an increased sensitivity score for health care providers in the experimental group. Differences between experimental and control groups were statistically significant. Patients' outcomes did not indicate statistically significant differences in satisfaction, mental health, physical health, or activities of daily living. In the category of social resources and economic resources, statistically significant outcomes were identified (Majumdar et al., 2004).

■ **NIC** *Alter the therapeutic environment by incorporating appropriate cultural elements.* **LOE=VI**

NR A case study of an Amish birthing center described a therapeutic environment that was a blend of Amish culture and modern health care. The birthing center was funded by the

RCT = Randomized Controlled (Clinical) Trial, **NIC** = Nursing Interventions Classification, **NOC** = Nursing Outcomes Classification

surrounding community. The site provided an alternative to hospital delivery and associated costs while recognizing the value of skilled care. A flat fee was charged for birth and 72 hours of care, and midwife and physician fees were separate; barter was an option. Labor, delivery, postpartum, and newborn care all occurred in the patient's room. Rooms were without television and telephone, hitching posts and a barn for lodging horses were provided, and families were allowed to bring food. A red bag placed on the barn roof indicated to neighbors that additional help was needed (Lemon, 2002).

(NR) An old order Amish elder with Alzheimer's disease and the caregiver participated in a case study that comprised visits and observation conducted over a period of 9 months. Themes identified included respect for the elderly, an unrestricted environment that included assistance and direction, and companionship of extended family (Crist et al., 2002).

■ (NIC) *Modify typical interventions (e.g., patient teaching) in culturally competent ways.* **LOE=II**

(MR) In an ongoing RCT comparing Becoming a Responsible Team (BART), a community-based translation of an HIV risk reduction intervention found to be effective in other populations, with a standard health promotion condition in adolescent Haitian males and females aged 14 to 17 years, important preliminary data suggested that to reduce stigma associated with HIV for the Haitian population, HIV care needed to be addressed within the context of overall health and well-being and not HIV alone (Malow et al., 2004).

(NR) In a systematic review of nursing research ($N=167$) pertaining to race, ethnicity, and culture, it was found that the majority of conducted studies assessed the fitness of an instrument related to culture. A recommendation for future research included an increase in intervention studies and studies to examine translation of theoretical frameworks (Jacobson et al., 2004).

(NR) Case studies documented misdiagnosis and harmful outcomes associated with culturally incongruent interventions. Interventions to promote cultural competency in forensic nursing were described. For example, Leininger's short cultural assessment could be used to identify beliefs and practices that affect care (Crane, 2005).

■ *Provide culturally congruent care.* **LOE=VI**

(EO) Incorporate ethnopharmacological knowledge into the plan of care and recognize that pharmacokinetics and pharmacodynamics are influenced by genetic and cultural factors (Muñoz & Hilgenberg, 2005).

(MR) Using a quasi-experimental design, reliability of the Cultural Competence Assessment instrument was evaluated. Hospice respondents ($N=51$) were compared with nonhospice health care providers ($N=405$). Study results indicated that the instrument detected differences in levels of cultural competency. Statistically significant differences were found between those who reported cultural diversity training and those who reported no training (Doorenbos et al., 2005). **LOE=IV**

(EO) Research findings indicated disparities in health status across racial and ethnic groups. A growing body of research indicates an association between culturally congruent care and reducing health disparities. To this end, states can promote cultural competency by sponsoring education and training initiatives for senior state health officials (AHCPR, 1999).

(EO) Increased awareness of racial and ethnic disparities by health care providers is recommended. The use of evidence-based guidelines can help to promote equity (Institute of Medicine, 2002b).

NR = Nursing Research, **MR** = Multidisciplinary Research, **SP** = Standard of Practice, **EO** = Expert Opinion, **LOE** = Level of Evidence

Possibly Effective

No applicable published research was found in this category.

Not Effective

No applicable published research was found in this category.

Possibly Harmful

No applicable published research was found in this category.

OUTCOME MEASUREMENT

CLIENT SATISFACTION: CULTURAL NEEDS FULFILLMENT (NOC)

Definition: Extent of positive perception of integration of cultural beliefs, values, and social structures into nursing care.

Client Satisfaction: Cultural Needs Fulfillment as evidenced by the following selected NOC indicators:

- Respect for cultural beliefs
- Respect for cultural health behaviors
- Respect for background and traditions
- Care consistent with cultural beliefs

(Rate each indicator of **Client Satisfaction: Cultural Needs Fulfillment:** 1=not at all satisfied, 2=somewhat satisfied, 3=moderately satisfied, 4=very satisfied, 5=completely satisfied) (Moorhead et al., 2004).

REFERENCES

Agency for Health Care Policy and Research (AHCPR). (1999). Providing care to diverse populations: State strategies for promoting cultural competency in health systems. Workshop summary, June 9-11. User Liaison Program, Rockville, MD. Available online: http://www.ahrq.gov. Retrieved on January 14, 2007.

College of Nurses of Ontario (CNO). (2005). Practice guideline: Culturally sensitive care. Available online: www.cno.org. Retrieved on January 14, 2007.

Crane P. (2005). Cultural competence and the advanced practice forensic nurse. *Topics Emerg Med,* 27(2):157-162.

Crist J, Armer J, Radina ME. (2002). A study in cultural diversity: Caregiving for the old order Amish elder with Alzheimer's disease. *J Multicult Nurs Health,* 8(3):78-81.

Cunado BA, Garcia CB, Rial CC, Garcia LF. (2002). Spanish validation of an instrument to measure the quality of nursing care in hospital emergency units. *J Nurs Care Qual,* 16(3):13-23.

Dochterman JM, Bulechek GM (Eds). (2004). *Nursing Interventions Classification (NIC),* 4th ed. St. Louis: Mosby.

Doorenbos AZ, Schim SM, Benkert R, Borse NN. (2005). Psychometric evaluation of the cultural competence assessment instrument among healthcare providers. *Nurs Res,* 54(5):324-331.

Doutrich D, Storey M. (2004). Education and practice: Dynamic partners for improving cultural competence in public health. *Fam Community Health,* 27(4):298-307.

Institute of Medicine. (2002a). Speaking of health: Assessing health communication strategies for diverse populations. Available online: www.iom.edu. Retrieved on January 14, 2007.

Institute of Medicine. (2002b). Unequal treatment: Confronting racial and ethnic disparities in health care. Available online: www.iom.edu. Retrieved on January 14, 2007.

Jacobson S, Lin-Lin Chu N, Pascucci M, Gaskins S. (2004). Characteristics of nursing research on race, ethnicity, and culture. *J Multicult Nurs Health*, 10(3):6-10.

Jett KF. (2003). The meaning of aging and the celebration of years among rural African-American women. *Geriatr Nurs*, 24(5):290-293, 320.

The Joint Commission. (2006). Joint Commission 2006 Requirements Related to the Provision of Culturally and Linguistically Appropriate Health Care. Available online: http://www.jointcommission.org/. Retrieved on January 14, 2007.

Kim S, Kang K. (2003). Meaning of life for adolescents with a physical disability in Korea. *J Adv Nurs*, 43(2):155-157.

Kulig JC, Hall BL, Babcock R, Campbell R, Wall M. (2004). Childbearing practices in Kanadier Mennonite women. *Can Nurse*, 100(8):34-37.

Lemon B. (2002). Amish health care beliefs and practices in an obstetrical setting. *J Multicult Nurs Health*, 8(3):72-76.

Majumdar B, Browne G, Roberts J, Carpio B. (2004). Effects of cultural sensitivity training on health care provider attitudes and patient outcomes. *J Nurs Scholarsh*, 36(2):161-166.

Malow R, Jean-Gilles M, Devieux J, Rosenburg R, Russell A. (2004). Increasing access to preventive health care through cultural adaptation of effective HIV prevention intervention: A brief report from the HIV prevention in Haitian youths study. *ABNFJ*, 15(6):127-132.

Moorhead M, Johnson M, Maas M (Eds). (2004). *Nursing Outcomes Classification (NOC)*, 3rd ed. St. Louis: Mosby.

Muñoz C, Hilgenberg C. (2005). Ethnopharmacology: understanding how ethnicity can affect drug response is essential to providing culturally competent care. *Am J Nurs*, 105(8):40-48.

Office of Minority Health. (2000). National Standards on Culturally and Linguistically Appropriate Services. U.S. Department of Health & Human Services. Available online: www.hhs.gov. Retrieved on January 14, 2007.

Schmit K. (2005). Nursing implications for treating "kanser" in Filipino patients. *J Hosp Palliat Nurs*, 7(6):345-349.

Shih FJ, Gau ML, Lin YS, Pong SJ, Lin HR. (2006). Death and help expected from nurses when dying. *Nurs Ethics*, 13(4):360-375.

Suen LJ, Tusaie K. (2004). Is somatization a significant depressive symptom in older Taiwanese Americans? *Geriatr Nurs*, 25(3):157-163.

Valente S. (2004). End of life and ethnicity. *J Nurses Staff Dev*, 20(6):285-293.

DECISIONAL CONTROL

Naomi E. Ervin, PhD, RN, APRN-BC, FAAN

Definition: A process that results in a decision, satisfactory to the patient and supportive of health, made from a patient's knowledge and skill base and from a number of options within an interactive relationship in a specific environment (Appleyard, 1989; Averill, 1973; Cox, 1982; Ervin & Pierangeli, 2005; Smith et al., 1984).

NURSING ACTIVITIES

Effective

■ *Use decision aids to facilitate informed choice about prostate-specific-antigen (PSA) screening.* **LOE=I**

 An RCT of 421 men demonstrated that participants receiving an evidence-based booklet compared with men who received a video or leaflet scored higher at post-test on knowledge and required detailed information about the pros and cons of PSA screening in order to make an informed decision (Gattellari & Ward, 2005).

(MR) An RCT of 248 men resulted in greater knowledge scores about PSA and lower levels of decisional conflict for men receiving the evidence-based booklet compared with men who received a government-published pamphlet. Decisional control preference (passive, active, or collaborative) was not negatively affected by the evidence-based information (Gattellari & Ward, 2003).

(MR) An RCT ($N=100$) demonstrated that men given information before a health examination had a significantly more active role (decisional control) in making a screening decision for prostate cancer (Davison et al., 1999).

Possibly Effective

■ *Use a computer program for assessing and providing information to men newly diagnosed with prostate cancer and their partners.* **LOE=IV**

(MR) A controlled study using a one-group ($N=74$ couples), pretest/post-test design demonstrated that men reported having more active roles (decisional control) in decision making than originally intended and partners had more passive roles (decisional control) than intended. All participants had lower levels of psychological distress at 4 months after study (Davison et al., 2003).

■ *Use an information sheet prompting patients to ask questions of their physicians.* **LOE=II**

(MR) An RCT of 233 patients diagnosed with cancer showed that the intervention of providing an information sheet to patients was not effective in prompting patients to ask physicians about their disease, prognosis, and treatment. Results showed that failure to achieve preferred decisional control roles appeared to adversely affect patients' emotional well-being (Gattellari et al., 2001).

■ *Use a computer-assisted intervention to enhance communication between physicians and women with breast cancer.* **LOE=II**

(NR) An RCT of 749 women with breast cancer used an intervention of encouraging the use of information and decision preference profiles generated by a computer program. A significantly higher proportion of women in the intervention group reported playing a more passive role (decisional control) than originally planned. Both groups reported high satisfaction levels (Davison & Degner, 2002).

Not Effective

No applicable published research was found in this category.

Possibly Harmful

No applicable published research was found in this category.

RCT = Randomized Controlled (Clinical) Trial, **NIC** = Nursing Interventions Classification, **NOC** = Nursing Outcomes Classification

OUTCOME MEASUREMENT

DECISIONAL CONTROL

Definition: A process that results in a decision, satisfactory to the patient and supportive of health, made from a patient's knowledge and skill base and from a number of options within an interactive relationship in a specific environment (Appleyard, 1989; Averill, 1973; Cox, 1982; Ervin & Pierangeli, 2005; Smith et al., 1984).

Decisional Control as evidenced by the following indicators:

Client states:

- Psychological equilibrium
- Decisional resolution
- Decision is supportive of client's health
- Satisfaction with decision
- Satisfaction with health care

(Note: This is not a NOC outcome.)

REFERENCES

Appleyard JA. (1989). Decisional control in the client-provider relationship: An exploratory investigation in a primary care setting. Unpublished doctoral dissertation, University of Illinois at Chicago.

Averill JR. (1973). Personal control over aversive stimuli and its relationship to stress. *Psychol Bull,* 80:286-303.

Cox CL. (1982). An interaction model of client health behavior: Formulation and test. Unpublished doctoral dissertation, University of Rochester, Rochester, NY.

Davison BJ, Degner LF. (2002). Feasibility of using a computer-assisted intervention to enhance the way women with breast cancer communicate with their physicians. *Cancer Nurs,* 25(6):417-424.

Davison BJ, Goldenberg SL, Gleave ME, Degner LF. (2003). Provision of individualized information to men and their partners to facilitate treatment decision making in prostate cancer. *Oncol Nurs Forum,* 30(1):107-114.

Davison BJ, Kirk P, Degner LF, Hassard TH. (1999). Information and patient participation in screening for prostate cancer. *Patient Educ Couns,* 37(3):255-263.

Ervin NE, Pierangeli LT. (2005). The concept of decisional control: Building the base for evidence-based nursing practice. *Worldviews Evid Based Nurs,* 2(1):16-24.

Gattellari M, Butow PN, Tattersall MH. (2001). Sharing decisions in cancer care. *Soc Sci Med,* 52(12):1865-1878.

Gattellari M, Ward JE. (2003). Does evidence-based information about screening for prostate cancer enhance consumer decision-making? A randomised controlled trial. *J Med Screen,* 10(1):27-39.

Gattellari M, Ward JE. (2005). A community-based randomised controlled trial of three different educational resources for men about prostate cancer screening. *Patient Educ Couns,* 57(2):168-182.

Smith RA, Wallston BS, Wallston KA, Forsberg PR, King JE. (1984). Measuring desire for control of health care processes. *J Pers Soc Psychol,* 47(2):415-426.

 # DEEP VEIN THROMBOSIS: PREVENTION

Maryanne Crowther, MSN, RN, APNC, CCRN

Definition: Prevention of deep vein thrombosis (DVT).

NR = Nursing Research, **MR** = Multidisciplinary Research, **SP** = Standard of Practice, **EO** = Expert Opinion, **LOE** = Level of Evidence

NURSING ACTIVITIES

Effective

■ *Use early ambulation and exercise after surgical procedures as prophylaxis for patients against DVT.* **LOE=I**

> (EO) Early and persistent ambulation is recommended for low-risk general surgery patients undergoing minor procedures who are younger than 40 years and have no additional risk factors for DVT (Geerts et al., 2004).

> (MR) A controlled study of healthy males (*N*=20) demonstrated that femoral vein peak blood flow velocity was greatest with deep breathing combined with ankle exercises and most useful to prevent venous stasis in this group (Kwon et al., 2003).

■ *Use elastic compression stockings in combination with another prophylaxis for patients at risk for developing DVT.** **LOE=I**

> (EO) Mechanical methods of prophylaxis may be used for patients as an adjunct to anticoagulant-based prophylaxis (Geerts et al., 2004).

> (MR) A Cochrane systematic review (*N*=111) found that a combination of graded compression stockings and unfractionated heparin is better than heparin alone in preventing DVT and/or pulmonary embolus (PE) for those undergoing colorectal surgery (Wille-Jorgensen et al., 2003).

> (MR) A Cochrane systematic review (*N*=1184) found an overall effect of favoring treatment with graduated compression stockings on the background of another DVT prophylaxis for hospitalized medical and surgical patients (Amaragiri & Lees, 2000).

> (MR) A systematic review by the Health Technology Assessment Programme (*N*=1120) found that graduated compression stockings in combination with another method of prophylaxis produced a highly significant reduction (60%) in DVT (Roderick et al., 2005).

■ *Administer unfractionated heparin as ordered for patients at risk for developing DVT.* **LOE=I**

> (EO) Unfractionated heparin is recommended as one option for pharmacological prophylaxis for moderate- or high-risk patients and others with risk factors (in the absence of contraindications) for DVT/PE, such as those undergoing general surgery, major vascular surgery, major gynecological surgery, extensive surgery for malignancy, urologic surgery, laparoscopic procedures, elective spinal surgeries, or neurosurgery; stabilized burn patients; and acutely ill medical patients (Geerts et al., 2004).

> (MR) A Cochrane systematic review (*N*=292) demonstrated that unfractionated heparin gave better prophylaxis than no treatment or placebo against DVT/PE in patients who underwent colorectal surgery (Wille-Jorgensen et al., 2003).

---

*No mechanical option of DVT prophylaxis has been shown to reduce risk of death or pulmonary embolism. Special caution must be used when interpreting risk reduction ascribed to mechanical prophylaxis because most trials were not blinded; studies that used I-fibrinogen leg scanning assessments may have lower false-positive rates solely in the treatment groups; and poor clinical compliance with mechanical devices probably does not parallel the compliance used in the research studies (Geerts et al., 2004).

RCT = Randomized Controlled (Clinical) Trial, **NIC** = Nursing Interventions Classification, **NOC** = Nursing Outcomes Classification

(MR) A Cochrane systematic review of patients following hip fracture surgery (N=826) found that use of unfractionated heparin was effective in reducing the incidence of lower limb DVT (Handoll et al., 2002).

■ Administer low-molecular-weight heparin as ordered for prophylaxis for patients at risk for DVT/PE. **LOE=I**

(EO) Low-molecular-weight heparin (LMWH) is recommended as one option for pharmacological prophylaxis for moderate- or high-risk patients and those with risk factors (in the absence of contraindications) for DVT/PE, such as those undergoing general surgery, vascular surgery, major gynecological surgery, extensive surgery for malignancy, urological surgery, laparoscopic surgery, elective hip arthroplasty, elective knee arthroplasty, hip fracture surgery, major orthopedic surgery, or postoperative neurosurgery; trauma patients; those with acute spinal cord injuries; stabilized burn patients; acutely ill medical patients; and as a single dose prior to long-distance air travel (Geerts et al., 2004).

(MR) A Cochrane systematic review (N=349) demonstrated that LMWH gave better prophylaxis than no treatment or placebo against DVT/PE in patients who underwent colorectal surgery (Wille-Jorgensen et al., 2003).

(MR) A Cochrane systematic review of patients following hip fracture surgery (N=373) found that use of LMWH was effective in reducing the incidence of lower limb DVT (Handoll et al., 2002).

(MR) A case-control study of acutely ill medical hospitalized inpatients (N=3719) found 70% lower risk of DVT/PE in those receiving LMWH than those without prophylaxis (McGarry & Thompson, 2004).

(MR) A qualitative study (N=28) of advanced cancer inpatients receiving palliative care unanimously found LMWH to be an acceptable intervention that had a positive impact on quality of life (Noble et al., 2006).

■ Administer fondaparinux as ordered for prophylaxis for patients at risk for DVT/PE. **LOE=I**

(EO) Fondaparinux is recommended as one option for prophylaxis against DVT/PE in patients undergoing elective hip arthroplasty, elective knee arthroplasty, and hip fracture surgery (Geerts et al., 2004).

(MR) A systematic review (N=5385) found that fondaparinux was consistently more effective than enoxaparin in preventing DVT/PE in patients undergoing major orthopedic surgery (Turpie et al., 2004).

■ Administer oral anticoagulation as ordered for prophylaxis for patients at risk for developing DVT/PE. **LOE=I**

(EO) Vitamin K antagonists are recommended as one alternative for patients who have undergone elective hip arthroplasty, elective knee arthroplasty, or hip fracture surgery and in the rehabilitation phase for post-trauma and spinal cord injuries (Geerts et al., 2004).

(MR) A systematic review by the Health Technology Assessment Programme (N=1624) found that use of oral anticoagulants resulted in a significant reduction (50%) in DVT (Roderick et al., 2005).

NR = Nursing Research, **MR** = Multidisciplinary Research, **SP** = Standard of Practice, **EO** = Expert Opinion, **LOE** = Level of Evidence

Possibly Effective

■ *Use elastic compression stockings as sole prophylaxis for patients at risk for developing DVT.**LOE=I

(EO) Mechanical methods of prophylaxis may be used primarily in patients who are at high risk for bleeding (Geerts et al., 2004).

(MR) A Cochrane systematic review (N=1027) found an overall effect of favoring treatment with graduated compression stockings over no treatment to prevent DVT in medical and surgical hospitalized patients (Amaragiri & Lees, 2000).

(MR) A systematic review by the Health Technology Assessment Programme (N=1292) found that use of graduated compression stockings resulted in a highly significant reduction in DVT (Roderick et al., 2005).

(NR) A systematic review (N=2472) of RCTs demonstrated the effectiveness of medium compression pressure, below-knee graduated compression stockings in preventing flight-related DVT in low-, medium-, or high-risk participants (Hsieh & Lee, 2005).

(NR) A review of studies (N=710) indicated that knee-length elastic compression stockings were equally effective, were associated with better patients' compliance, and were more cost effective than thigh-high elastic compression stockings (Ingram, 2003).
Additional research: Morris & Woodcock, 2004; Scurr, 2002; Nagahiro et al., 2004.

■ *Use intermittent compression devices as sole prophylaxis for patients at risk for developing DVT.**LOE=I

(EO) Mechanical methods of prophylaxis may be used primarily in patients who are at high risk for bleeding (Geerts et al., 2004).

(MR) A systematic review by the Health Technology Assessment Programme (N=2255) found that use of intermittent compression devices resulted in a highly significant reduction (66%) in DVT (Roderick et al., 2005).

(MR) A small RCT of healthy adult males (N=10) found no advantage of plantar-calf sequential compression devices over intermittent pneumatic compression (Iwama et al., 2004).

(MR) An RCT of trauma patients (N=442) demonstrated that intermittent pneumatic compression devices were as effective as LMWH in prevention of DVT/PE (Ginzburg et al., 2003).

(MR) A controlled study (N=200) found that intermittent pneumatic compression was as effective for prophylaxis against DVT/PE for 100 patients undergoing single-level anterior corpectomy/fusion and 100 having circumferential procedures as existing therapies (mini-heparin and low-dose heparin) without risk of hemorrhage (Epstein, 2005).

(MR) A controlled study of four pneumatic compression devices (N=4350) found no difference in DVT incidence based on length of intermittent compression device or method of compression (Proctor et al., 2001).

(MR) A controlled study of trauma patients (N=33) found that a miniaturized pneumatic compression device with a battery component led to better compliance than traditional intermittent pneumatic compression devices (Murakami et al., 2003).

---

*See footnote on p 207.

RCT = Randomized Controlled (Clinical) Trial, **NIC** = Nursing Interventions Classification, **NOC** = Nursing Outcomes Classification

(EO) All intermittent compression systems produce changes in femoral vein velocity, yet of the five length varieties that exist, evidence remains unclear to determine one superior over another (Morris & Woodcock, 2004).

■ *Use intermittent compression devices in combination with another prophylaxis for patients at risk for developing DVT.* **LOE=I**

(EO) Mechanical methods of prophylaxis may be used as an adjunct to anticoagulant-based prophylaxis (Geerts et al., 2004).

(MR) An RCT of patients who underwent total knee arthroplasty ($N=423$) demonstrated that the use of rapid inflation, asymmetrical calf compression gave a significantly lower rate of DVT/PE than a sequential circumferential compression device on the background of single-dose acetylsalicylic acid prior to the procedure (Lachiewicz et al., 2004).

(MR) A prospective controlled trial ($N=200$) found that mechanical compression with an intermittent compression device in conjunction with pharmacological prophylaxis was effective in reducing DVT/PE in patients undergoing hip fracture surgery (Westrich et al., 2005).

■ *Use sequential compression devices for patients at risk for developing DVT.** **LOE=I**

(EO) Mechanical methods of prophylaxis may be used primarily in patients who are at high risk for bleeding (Geerts et al., 2004).

(MR) A case-control study ($N=168$) of women undergoing gynecological surgeries for malignancies found that sequential compression devices alone were as effective as sequential compression devices combined with low-dose unfractionated heparin (Ailawadi & Del Priore, 2001).

(MR) A case-control study of patients who underwent thoracic surgery ($N=706$) found that a sequential pneumatic compression device effectively prevented postoperative PE compared with no treatment (Nagahiro et al., 2004).

(MR) A controlled study of patients undergoing hip arthroplasty ($N=50$) found that sequential compression devices with feedback loops that allow dynamic control of each chamber's pressure improved compression 88% of the time (Masri et al., 2004).

■ *Use foot pumps as sole prophylaxis for patients at risk for developing DVT.** **LOE=I**

(MR) A systematic review by the Health Technology Assessment Programme ($N=126$) found that foot pumps appeared to produce a highly significant reduction (77%) in DVT (Roderick et al., 2005).

(EO) Foot compression requires substantially higher pressures than calf compression to achieve adequate venous peak velocities, and this may adversely effect compliance with use (Morris & Woodcock, 2004).

Not Effective

■ *Administration of aspirin for VTE prophylaxis.* **LOE=I**

(EO) The use of aspirin alone as prophylaxis against VTE for any group of patients is not recommended (Geerts et al., 2004).

---

*See footnote on p 207.

NR = Nursing Research, **MR** = Multidisciplinary Research, **SP** = Standard of Practice, **EO** = Expert Opinion, **LOE** = Level of Evidence

Possibly Harmful

■ *Administration of anticoagulation for patients undergoing neuraxial anesthesia or analgesia.* **LOE=I**

(EO) Special caution should be observed when using anticoagulation in this population of patients (Geerts et al., 2004).

■ *Routine use of inferior vena cava filters as primary pulmonary embolism prophylaxis for trauma and acute spinal cord injury patients.* **LOE=I**

(EO) The use of inferior vena cava filters as primary prophylaxis against pulmonary embolism is not recommended (Geerts et al., 2004).

OUTCOME MEASUREMENT

TISSUE PERFUSION: PERIPHERAL (NOC)

Definition: Adequacy of blood flow through the small vessels of the extremities to maintain tissue function.

Tissue Perfusion: Peripheral as evidenced by the following selected NOC indicators:
• Peripheral edema
• Localized extremity pain

(Rate each indicator of **Tissue Perfusion: Peripheral:** 1=severe, 2=substantial, 3=moderate, 4=mild, 5=none) (Moorhead et al., 2004).

REFERENCES

Ailawadi M, Del Priore G. (2001). A comparison of thromboembolism prophylaxis in gynecologic oncology patients. *Int J Gynecol Cancer,* 11(5):354-358.

Amaragiri SV, Lees TA. (2000). Elastic compression stockings for prevention of deep vein thrombosis. *Cochrane Database Syst Rev,* (3):CD001484.

Epstein NE. (2005). Intermittent pneumatic compression stocking prophylaxis against deep venous thrombosis in anterior cervical spinal surgery: A prospective efficacy study in 200 patients and literature review. *Spine,* 30(22):2538-2543.

Geerts WH, Pineo GF, Heit JA, Bergqvist D, Lassen MR, Colwell CW, et al. (2004). Prevention of venous thromboembolism: The Seventh ACCP Conference on Antithrombotic and Thrombolytic Therapy. *Chest,* 126(3 Suppl):338S-400S.

Ginzburg E, Cohn SM, Lopez J, Jackowski J, Brown M, Hameed SM; Miami Deep Vein Thrombosis Study Group. (2003). Randomized clinical trial of intermittent pneumatic compression and low molecular weight heparin in trauma. *Br J Surg,* 90(11):1338-1344.

Handoll HH, Farrar MJ, McBirnie J, Tytherleigh-Strong G, Milne AA, Gillespie WJ. (2002). Heparin, low molecular weight heparin and physical methods for preventing deep vein thrombosis and pulmonary embolism following surgery for hip fractures. *Cochrane Database Syst Rev,* (4):CD000305.

Hsieh HF, Lee FP. (2005). Graduated compression stockings as prophylaxis for flight-related venous thrombosis: Systematic literature review. *J Adv Nurs,* 51(1):83-98.

Ingram JE. (2003). A review of thigh-length vs knee-length antiembolism stockings. *Br J Nurs,* 12(14):845-851.

Iwama H, Obara S, Ohmizo H. (2004). Changes in femoral vein blood flow velocity by intermittent pneumatic compression: Calf compression device versus plantar-calf sequential compression device. *J Anesth,* 18(3):232-233.

Kwon OY, Jung DY, Kim Y, Cho SH, Yi CH. (2003). Effects of ankle exercise combined with deep breathing on blood flow velocity in the femoral vein. *Aust J Physiother,* 49(4):253-258.

Lachiewicz PF, Kelley SS, Haden LR. (2004). Two mechanical devices for prophylaxis of thromboembolism after total knee arthroplasty. A prospective, randomized study. *J Bone Joint Surg Br,* 86(8):1137-1141.

Masri B, Dunlop D, McEwen J, Garbuz D, Duncan C. (2004). Can a new design of pneumatic compression device reduce variations in delivered therapy for the mechanical prophylaxis of thromboembolic disease after total hip arthroplasty? *Can J Surg,* 47(4):263-269.

McGarry LJ, Thompson D. (2004). Retrospective database analysis of the prevention of venous thromboembolism with low-molecular-weight heparin in acutely ill medical inpatients in community practice. *Clin Ther,* 26(3):419-430.

Moorhead M, Johnson M, Maas M (Eds). (2004). *Nursing Outcomes Classification (NOC),* 3rd ed. St. Louis: Mosby.

Morris RJ, Woodcock JP. (2004). Evidence-based compression: Prevention of stasis and deep vein thrombosis. *Ann Surg,* 239(2):162-171.

Murakami M, McDill TL, Cindrick-Pounds L, Loran DB, Woodside KJ, Mileski WJ, et al. (2003). Deep venous thrombosis prophylaxis in trauma: Improved compliance with a novel miniaturized pneumatic compression device. *J Vasc Surg,* 38(5):923-927.

Nagahiro I, Andou A, Aoe M, Sano Y, Date H, Shimizu N. (2004). Intermittent pneumatic compression is effective in preventing symptomatic pulmonary embolism after thoracic surgery. *Surg Today,* 34(1):6-10.

Noble SI, Nelson A, Turner C, Finlay IG. (2006). Acceptability of low molecular weight heparin thromboprophylaxis for inpatients receiving palliative care: Qualitative study. *BMJ,* 332(7541):577-580.

Proctor MC, Greenfield LJ, Wakefield TW, Zajkowski PJ. (2001). A clinical comparison of pneumatic compression devices: The basis for selection. *J Vasc Surg,* 34(3):459-464.

Roderick P, Ferris G, Wilson K, Halls H, Jackson D, Collins R, et al. (2005). Towards evidence-based guidelines for the prevention of venous thromboembolism: Systematic reviews of mechanical methods, oral anticoagulation, dextran and regional anaesthesia as thromboprophylaxis. *Health Technol Assess,* 9(49):iii-iv, ix-x, 1-78.

Scurr JH. (2002). Travellers' thrombosis. *J R Soc Health,* 122(1):11-13.

Turpie AG, Bauer KA, Eriksson BI, Lassen MR. (2004). Superiority of fondaparinux over enoxaparin in preventing venous thromboembolism in major orthopedic surgery using different efficacy end points. *Chest,* 126(2):501-508.

Westrich GH, Rana AJ, Terry MA, Taveras NA, Kapoor K, Helfet DL. (2005). Thromboembolic disease prophylaxis in patients with hip fracture: A multimodal approach. *J Orthop Trauma,* 19(4):234-240.

Wille-Jorgensen P, Rasmussen MS, Andersen BR, Borly L. (2003). Heparins and mechanical methods for thromboprophylaxis in colorectal surgery. *Cochrane Database Syst Rev,* (4):CD001217.

DEEP VEIN THROMBOSIS: TREATMENT

Maryanne Crowther, MSN, RN, APNC, CCRN

Definition: Limitation of complications for a patient experiencing an occlusion of the peripheral venous circulation.

NURSING ACTIVITIES

Effective

■ *Use early ambulation for patients with deep vein thrombosis (DVT).* **LOE=I**

 Ambulation as tolerated is recommended for patients with DVT (Buller et al., 2004).

A meta-analysis of DVT patients (N=296) found that early mobilization rather than bed rest neither increased the rate of pulmonary embolism nor increased the complication rate (Trujillo-Santos et al., 2004).

NR = Nursing Research, **MR** = Multidisciplinary Research, **SP** = Standard of Practice, **EO** = Expert Opinion, **LOE** = Level of Evidence

(MR) An RCT of patients (*N*=129) found that ambulation after DVT was safe and did not significantly increase the occurrence of pulmonary embolism compared with those on bed rest (Aschwanden et al., 2001).

(MR) An RCT of patients with proximal DVT (*N*=53) who were receiving low-molecular-weight heparin (LMWH) showed significantly less propagation of thrombus in the walking exercise group than in the bed rest without compression group (Blattler & Partsch, 2003).

(MR) A randomized trial of DVT patients (*N*=146) found no difference in incidence of pulmonary embolism in those treated with ambulation and compression stockings at home versus those treated with 5 days of bed rest in the hospital (Romera et al., 2005).

(MR) An RCT of DVT patients (*N*=53) found that those treated with early ambulation and strong compression had faster pain reduction and resolved edema than those on bed rest without compression (Partsch & Blattler, 2000).

(MR) A descriptive study of patients with DVT (*N*=2650) who were prescribed either bed rest or ambulation found that ambulation did not increase the risk for pulmonary embolism (Trujillo-Santos et al., 2005).

■ *Use elastic compression stockings to prevent post-thrombotic syndrome in patients who have DVT.* **LOE=I**

Note: There is no specific recommendation for timing of elastic compression stocking application, but elastic compression stockings do stimulate fibrinolysis, which suggests that the sooner they are applied, the better. Also, studies by Partsch and Blattler (2000) and Prandoni et al., (2002) randomly assigned patients immediately to elastic compression stocking groups with positive outcomes.

(EO) Use of elastic compression stockings is recommended with a pressure of 30 to 40 mm Hg at the ankle during 2 years after an episode of DVT to prevent post-thrombotic syndrome (Buller et al., 2004).

(MR) A Cochrane systematic review of nonpharmaceutical measures for prevention of post-thrombotic syndrome (*N*=421) found that long-term elastic compression stockings with 20 to 40 mm Hg of compression at the ankle reduced the occurrence of post-thrombotic syndrome after DVT (Kolbach et al., 2004).

(MR) An RCT (*N*=180) demonstrated that prolonged use of below-knee elastic compression stockings for up to 2 years after DVT reduced the risk of post-thrombotic syndrome by half (Prandoni et al., 2004).

■ *Use intermittent compression devices as treatment for patients with post-thrombotic syndrome.* **LOE=I**

(EO) A course of intermittent pneumatic compression for patients with severe edema of the leg due to post-thrombotic syndrome is suggested (Buller et al., 2004).

■ *Administer unfractionated heparin as treatment for patients with DVT as ordered.* **LOE=I**

(EO) Intravenous or subcutaneously administered unfractionated heparin is recommended as one option for short-term treatment of objectively confirmed DVT or for high clinical suspicion of DVT while awaiting the outcome of diagnostic tests (and is the preferred option, particularly for those with severe renal failure) (Buller et al., 2004).

RCT = Randomized Controlled (Clinical) Trial, **NIC** = Nursing Interventions Classification, **NOC** = Nursing Outcomes Classification

■ *Administer low-molecular-weight heparin at home as treatment for patients with DVT as ordered.* LOE=I

(EO) Subcutaneously administered LMWH is recommended as one option for short-term treatment of objectively confirmed DVT as an outpatient if possible or for high clinical suspicion of DVT while awaiting the outcome of diagnostic tests (Buller et al., 2004).

(MR) A Cochrane review comparing LMWH for home versus hospital treatment of patients with DVT ($N=1101$) concluded that home management is cost effective and likely to be preferred by patients (Schraibman et al., 2001).

(MR) A case-control study of DVT patients ($N=100$) found a cost savings of $2578 (Canadian) when using LMWH at an outpatient ambulatory thrombosis clinic rather than unfractionated heparin during inpatient care (Boucher et al., 2003).

(MR) An RCT of DVT patients ($N=298$) found that once-daily subcutaneous enoxaparin in the outpatient setting was as effective and as well tolerated as in-hospital intravenous unfractionated heparin (Chong et al., 2005).

(MR) A controlled study of all eligible presenting patients with DVT ($N=92$) who received home treatment with oral anticoagulants (and LMWH until a therapeutic INR was achieved) demonstrated no pulmonary embolism or major bleeding over 12 weeks of assessment, indicating that most patients did not need to be admitted to hospitals for diagnosis of DVT (Schwarz et al., 2001).

(MR) In a comparison study, patients with DVT receiving outpatient anticoagulation with enoxaparin and warfarin were able to be discharged 2.5 days sooner than those on warfarin monotherapy and had fewer readmissions, at a cost savings of $1151 per patient (Huse et al., 2002).

■ *Administer oral anticoagulation as treatment for patients with DVT as ordered.* LOE=I

(EO) Initiate oral anticoagulation together with either LMWH or unfractionated heparin (discontinuation of heparin when the INR is stable and over 2.0) on the first treatment day; continue for at least 3 months for those with an identifiable risk factor and at least 6 months or indefinitely for those with idiopathic DVT and for those with antiphospholipid antibodies, two or more thrombophilic conditions, or recurrent DVT (Buller et al., 2004).

Possibly Effective

■ *Administer thrombolytic therapy as treatment for selected patients with objectively diagnosed DVT as ordered.* LOE=I

(EO) Intravenous thrombolysis is suggested only for selected patients with DVT, such as those with massive iliofemoral DVT at risk of limb gangrene secondary to venous occlusion (Buller et al., 2004).

(MR) A Cochrane systematic review ($N=668$) found that thrombolysis in addition to anticoagulation for treatment of DVT was effective in removing clot and reducing post-thrombotic syndrome of pain, edema, and skin discoloration (Watson & Armon, 2004).

NR = Nursing Research, **MR** = Multidisciplinary Research, **SP** = Standard of Practice, **EO** = Expert Opinion, **LOE** = Level of Evidence

Not Effective

■ *Administration of nonsteroidal anti-inflammatory agents as initial treatment for patients with DVT.* **LOE=I**

(EO) Use of nonsteroidal anti-inflammatories as initial treatment for patients with DVT is not recommended (Buller et al., 2004).

Possibly Harmful

■ *Bed rest as initial treatment for patients with DVT.* **LOE=IV**

(MR) A retrospective analysis of phlebographic studies comparing early thrombus with its progression several days later demonstrated much greater propagation of thrombus in those on bed rest (26%) than in those who were mobilized between days 0 and 2 (1%) (Schulman, 1985).

OUTCOME MEASUREMENT

TISSUE PERFUSION: PERIPHERAL   (NOC)

Definition: Adequacy of blood flow through the small vessels of the extremities to maintain tissue function.
Tissue Perfusion: Peripheral as evidenced by the following selected NOC indicators:
• Peripheral edema
• Localized extremity pain
(Rate each indicator of **Tissue Perfusion: Peripheral:** 1=severe, 2=substantial, 3=moderate, 4=mild, 5=none) (Moorhead et al., 2004).

REFERENCES

Aschwanden M, Labs KH, Engel H, Schwob A, Jeanneret C, Mueller-Brand J, et al. (2001). Acute deep vein thrombosis: Early mobilization does not increase the frequency of pulmonary embolism. *Thromb Haemost,* 85(1):42-46.

Blattler W, Partsch H. (2003). Leg compression and ambulation is better than bed rest for the treatment of acute deep venous thrombosis. *Int Angiol,* 22(4):393-400.

Boucher M, Rodger M, Johnson JA, Tierney M. (2003). Shifting from inpatient to outpatient treatment of deep vein thrombosis in a tertiary care center: A cost-minimization analysis. *Pharmacotherapy,* 23(3):301-309.

Buller HR, Agnelli G, Hull RD, Hyers TM, Prins MH, Raskob GE. (2004). Antithrombotic therapy for venous thromboembolic disease: The Seventh ACCP Conference on Antithrombotic and Thrombolytic Therapy. *Chest,* 126(3 Suppl):401S-428S.

Chong BH, Brighton TA, Baker RI, Thurlow P, Lee CH; AST DVT Study Group. (2005). Once-daily enoxaparin in the outpatient setting versus unfractionated heparin in hospital for the treatment of symptomatic deep-vein thrombosis. *J Thromb Thrombolysis,* 19(3):173-181.

Huse DM, Cummins G, Taylor DC, Russell MW. (2002). Outpatient treatment of venous thromboembolism with low-molecular-weight heparin: An economic evaluation. *Am J Manag Care,* 8(1 Suppl): S10-S16.

Kolbach DN, Sandbrink MW, Hamulyak K, Neumann HA, Prins MH. (2004). Non-pharmaceutical measures for prevention of post-thrombotic syndrome. *Cochrane Database Syst Rev,* (1):CD004174.

Moorhead M, Johnson M, Maas M (Eds). (2004). *Nursing Outcomes Classification (NOC),* 3rd ed. St. Louis: Mosby.

Partsch H, Blattler W. (2000). Compression and walking versus bed rest in the treatment of proximal deep venous thrombosis with low molecular weight heparin. *J Vasc Surg,* 32(5):861-869.

Prandoni P, Lensing AW, Bernardi E, et al. (2002). The diagnostic value of compression ultrasonography in patients with suspected recurrent deep vein thrombosis, *Thromb Haemost,* 88(3):402-406.

Prandoni P, Lensing AW, Prins MH, Frulla M, Marchiori A, Bernardi E, et al. (2004). Below-knee elastic compression stockings to prevent the post-thrombotic syndrome: A randomized, controlled trial. *Ann Intern Med,* 141(4):249-256.

Romera A, Vila R, Perez-Piqueras A, Marti X, Cairols MA. (2005). Early mobilization in patients with acute deep vein thrombosis: Does it increase the incidence of symptomatic pulmonary embolism? *Phlebology,* 20(3):141, Abstract.

Schraibman IG, Milne AA, Royle EM. (2001). Home versus in-patient treatment for deep vein thrombosis. *Cochrane Database Syst Rev,* (2):CD003076.

Schulman S. (1985). Studies on the medical treatment of deep vein thrombosis. *Acta Med Scand Suppl,* 704:1-68.

Schwarz T, Schmidt B, Hohlein U, Beyer J, Schroder HE, Schellong S. (2001). Eligibility for home treatment of deep vein thrombosis: Prospective study. *BMJ,* 322(7296):1212-1213.

Trujillo-Santos AJ, Martos-Perez F, Perea-Milla E. (2004). Bed rest or early mobilization as treatment of deep vein thrombosis: A systematic review and meta-analysis. *Med Clin (Barc),* 122(17):641-647.

Trujillo-Santos AJ, Perea-Milla E, Jimenez-Puente A, Sanchez-Cantalejo E, del Toro J, Grau E, et al. (2005). Bed rest or ambulation in the initial treatment of patients with acute deep vein thrombosis or pulmonary embolism: Findings from the RIETE registry. *Chest,* 127(5):1631-1636.

Watson LI, Armon MP. (2004). Thrombolysis for acute deep vein thrombosis. *Cochrane Database Syst Rev,* (4):CD002783.

DELIRIUM MANAGEMENT NIC

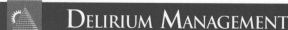

Lenore H. Kurlowicz, PhD, RN, CS, FAAN; Beth Ann Swan, PhD, CRNP, FAAN

NIC Definition: Provision of a safe and therapeutic environment for the patient who is experiencing an acute confusional state (Dochterman & Bulechek, 2004).

NURSING ACTIVITIES

Effective

■ *Assess the patient's risk for delirium, including age 80 or older; presence of preexisting chronic confusion (i.e., dementia or other brain disease/injury); severe illness; two or more chronic health conditions; vision/hearing impairment; polypharmacy (four or more medications); chronic alcohol and/or drug use; dehydration; and history of acute confusion.* **LOE=VI**

MR A descriptive study (*N* = 1285) examined the factors associated with a discharge diagnosis of delirium among hospitalized older adult medical patients. The study revealed the following risk factors: emergency admission, being 80 years of age or older, chronic renal disease, urinary tract infection, abnormal arterial blood gases, low sodium, high creatinine, low albumin, low hematocrit, and proteinuria (Levkoff et al., 1988).

NR = Nursing Research, **MR** = Multidisciplinary Research, **SP** = Standard of Practice, **EO** = Expert Opinion, **LOE** = Level of Evidence

(MR) A prospective cohort study of hip surgery patients (N=225) found delirium in 20% of subjects. Delirious patients were older (80 or older), had impaired hearing and/or vision, had moderate cognitive impairment on admission, more often presented with cerebrovascular or other brain disease, and more often were on psychopharmacological drugs (Duppils & Wikblad, 2000).

(MR) A prospective cohort of elective hip surgery patients (N=105) revealed that postoperative delirium developed in 41% of patients. Risk factors included age older than 80, living in a nursing home prior to admission, mild to severe vision or hearing impairment, prior cognitive impairment, higher comorbidity, depression, and regular use of psychotropic drugs (Galanakis et al., 2001).

(MR) A descriptive study (N=1341) of noncardiac surgery patients, including general surgery, orthopedic surgery, and gynecological surgery, found that risk factors for delirium were age older than 70, abnormal cognitive status examination, poor functional status as measured by the American Society of Anesthesiology Physical Classification I through IV, history of alcohol abuse, and abnormal routine laboratory values (Marcantonio et al., 1994).

(MR) A descriptive study of medical and surgical patients (N=291) with delirium risk factors found that patients who developed delirium during hospitalization had an increased length of stay (LOS). LOS for nondelirious patients was 7.3 days and LOS for delirious patients was 18.8 days (Schor et al., 1992).

(MR) A review of the research literature demonstrated that patients with preexisting dementia who were hospitalized and developed delirium may experience more serious complications and poorer outcomes (Fick et al., 2002).

Additional research: Inouye & Foreman, 2001.

■ *Assess for evidence of other features of delirium as evidenced by the acute onset of the following symptoms that are a change from the patient's baseline mental status: increased lethargy; appears frightened or suspicious of others; illusions/hallucinations (as evidenced by climbing out of bed, disruption of medical therapies, refusing treatments/care, calling out for family); disorientation (most of time); nighttime agitation; new onset of memory problems to decrease the likelihood of adverse events.* **LOE=VI**

(EO) The etiological basis for delirium is multifactorial, including physiological, psychological, sociological, and environmental factors. Delirium is dynamic in that the causes of delirium vary across time and from patient to patient (Foreman et al., 2003).

(MR) A descriptive study of older adult medical patients (N=229) found that 22% of patients developed delirium, and patients who developed delirium experienced longer LOSs, were more likely to be discharged to nursing homes, and died within 6 months of discharge (Francis et al., 1990).

(MR) A quasi-experimental historical cohort study of hip fracture patients (N=214) found that 48% of patients developed delirium, and patients who developed delirium had more pressure ulcers, increased falls, increased urinary retention, and increased LOS (Gustafson et al., 1991).

(MR) A descriptive study of medical, surgical, and terminally ill patients (N=727) found that delirium was a significant predictor of functional decline at hospital discharge and 3 months after discharge (Inouye et al., 1998).

(NR) A quasi-experimental study of older adult medical patients (N=400) found that patients in the intervention group (reorganization of nursing and medical care intervention) experienced less delirium, had a shorter LOS, and had less in-hospital deaths (Lundstrom et al., 2005).

■ *Assess patients for predisposing factors for delirium, including vision impairment, severe illness, dehydration defined as blood urea nitrogen/creatinine ratio exceeding 18, and preexisting cognitive impairment.* **LOE=VI**

(MR) A study with two prospective cohorts of hospitalized medical older adults (N=281) done in tandem established a predictive model for the occurrence of new delirium in hospitalized medical patients based on admission characteristics. Delirium developed in 25% of the development cohort and 17% of the validation cohort, and four factors selected in the final model were vision impairment, severe illness, dehydration, and preexisting cognitive impairment (Inouye et al., 1993).

(NR) A descriptive study of hospitalized medical-surgical older adults (N=20) found that eight of the nine patients with dementia on admission developed delirium during hospitalization. All eight patients with dementia and delirium developed urinary incontinence, five of the eight patients were restrained during hospitalization (none of the delirium-only patients were restrained), and five of the eight patients were readmitted to the hospital within 30 days (none of the delirium-only patients were readmitted) (Fick & Foreman, 2000).

(MR) A review of the research literature (N=14 studies) demonstrated that patients with preexisting dementia who were hospitalized and developed delirium may experience more serious complications and poorer outcomes (Fick et al., 2002).

(NR) A prospective study of hip fracture patients (N=92) examined the predisposing and precipitating factors for delirium that could be recognized by nurses. Delirium developed in 19.6% of patients, and nurses identified that patients who developed delirium were more often dependent in activities of daily living, lived more frequently in a residential home, and suffered more frequently from serious cognitive decline (Schuurmans et al., 2003).

(MR) A prospective cohort study of 36 men undergoing primary coronary artery bypass graft (CABG) surgery revealed that atherosclerosis in the carotid arteries, aorta, and coronary circulation was associated with the development of delirium following CABG surgery (Rudolph et al., 2005).

(MR) A prospective cohort study of patients with an acute stroke (N=218) found that 13% (29) of patients developed delirium. In 9 patients, delirium was secondary to stroke without additional causes, 10 had medical complications, and 10 had multiple potential causes for the delirium (Caeiro et al., 2004).

(MR) A prospective cohort study of patients (N=220) undergoing CABG surgery found that 34% of patients developed delirium. Predisposing factors included increasing age, BUN level, cardiothoracic index, hypertension, and smoking habits (Santos et al., 2004).

■ *Assess patients for precipitating factors for delirium, including use of physical restraints, malnutrition, addition of three or more medications on the previous day, use of an indwelling catheter, and any iatrogenic event.* **LOE=VI**

(MR) A study with two prospective cohorts of hospitalized medical older adults (N=508) done in tandem established a predictive model for the occurrence of new delirium in hospitalized medical patients based on admission characteristics. Delirium developed in 18% of the development cohort and 15% of the validation cohort, and five factors selected in the final model were use of physical restraints, malnutrition, more than three medications added, use of bladder catheter, and any iatrogenic event (Inouye & Charpentier, 1996).

NR = Nursing Research, **MR** = Multidisciplinary Research, **SP** = Standard of Practice, **EO** = Expert Opinion, **LOE** = Level of Evidence

(MR) A prospective cohort study of patients ($N=220$) undergoing CABG surgery found that 34% of patients developed delirium. Precipitating factors included blood replacement during bypass, atrial fibrillation, pneumonia, and blood balance in the postoperative period (Santos et al., 2004).

(MR) A retrospective review of case series data found 20 cases of excited delirium death associated with struggle and restraints (Stratton et al., 2001).

(MR) A descriptive study of hospitalized medical patients ($N=444$) examined the relationship between environmental factors and changes over time in delirium and found development of delirium associated with room changes, presence of medical or physical restraints, absence of a clock or watch, not wearing glasses, and absence of family (McCusker et al., 2001).

(NR) A descriptive study of hip fracture patients ($N=9598$) found that the rate of restraint use for hospitalized hip fracture patients was 31.5% during the 11-year study period. Sixty-eight percent of the patients restrained had delirium (Sullivan-Marx, 2001).

■ *Screen patients with risk factors, predisposing factors, and precipitating factors using the Confusion Assessment Method.* **LOE=VI**

(MR) In a prospective cohort study, elective orthopedic surgery patients ($N=236$) were screened by nurses for delirium using the DSM-III characteristics that form the basis for the Confusion Assessment Method (CAM). Twenty-two percent of the hip replacement patients and 32% of the knee replacement patients developed delirium. Variables related to delirium were age older than 70, bupivacaine with epinephrine, morphine, pain, LOS in the recovery room, and the type of surgery (Contin et al., 2005).

(MR) A prospective cohort study of hip fracture patients ($N=571$) at risk for delirium used screening with the CAM and found that 7% were delirious on admission, 30% became delirious before surgery, 9% were delirious on the day of surgery, and 54% were delirious postoperatively. In attempting to classify the cause as (1) drug-induced delirium, (2) related to infection, (3) fluid-electrolyte disturbance, (4) metabolic disturbance, (5) intracranial process, (6) low perfusion state, (7) alcohol and drug withdrawal, and (8) sensory/environmental delirium, only four were assigned a definite cause: drugs (1); infection (2); or fluid-electrolyte (1) (Brauer et al., 2000).

(NR) In a prospective descriptive study, patients admitted to an acute geriatric ward ($N=258$) were screened by bedside nurses using the CAM. Bedside nurses had trouble with identifying delirium but succeeded in diagnosing correctly the patients without delirium 90% of the time (Lemiengre et al., 2006).

■ *Provide supportive nursing care, including identifying self by name at each contact with the patient and calling the patient by his or her preferred name; using appropriate communication techniques including providing clear and simple explanations; using orientation techniques; providing reassurance to the patient and family; anticipating basic needs such as feeding, toileting, and hydration, and anticipating pain-producing conditions and identifying, evaluating, and treating pain quickly.* **LOE=VI**

(NR) A prospective comparative survey design involving older adult hip fracture patients ($N=88$) found that pain was treated poorly in older adults postoperatively and that age and cognitive impairment strongly influenced the amount of pain medication given the older adults (Feldt & Griffin, 1999).

RCT = Randomized Controlled (Clinical) Trial, **NIC** = Nursing Interventions Classification, **NOC** = Nursing Outcomes Classification

(NR) A pretest/post-test quasi-experimental design tested whether the Elder Care Supportive Interventions Protocol decreased discomfort among hospitalized medical and surgical older adult patients (N=81) with delirium and its associated negative consequences. The intervention group had less discomfort; however, there were no differences in physical functioning, acute confusion, and LOS (Miller et al., 2004).

(NR) A descriptive study of older adult hip surgery patients (N=43) found that 35% developed postoperative delirium; patients with delirium had a very high level of dissatisfaction with sleep. In addition, patients with delirium who had unplanned surgery had the highest pain scores of any group, and patients with delirium who had planned surgery had the lowest measured pain scores of any group (Bowman, 1997).

(NR) A quasi-experimental study of older adult medical patients (N=400) found that patients in the intervention group (reorganization of nursing and medical care intervention) experienced less delirium, had a shorter LOS, and had less in-hospital deaths (Lundstrom et al., 2005).

Additional research: Milisen et al., 2005.

■ *Provide a supportive environment, including minimizing environmental stimulation by reducing lights when not necessary, providing privacy as necessary, keeping activity/noise to a minimum, explaining the need for environmental characteristics to the patient, and organizing care to provide periods of rest and less physical stimuli, as well as avoiding/minimizing the use of restraints/medical immobilization that may increase risk for delirium.*
LOE=V

(MR) A descriptive study of hospitalized medical patients (N=444) examined the relationship between environmental factors and changes over time in delirium and found development of delirium associated with room changes, presence of medical or physical restraints, absence of a clock or watch, not wearing glasses, and absence of family (McCusker et al., 2001).

(NR) An RCT of hip and knee surgery patients (N=66) found that patients who listened to music had fewer episodes of delirium and higher readiness to ambulate scores than those receiving standard postoperative care without music (Ruth & Locsin, 2004).

(NR) A quasi-experimental study, two groups in tandem, of hip fracture patients (N=120) found that patients in the intervention group (a nurse-led interdisciplinary program) experienced delirium of shorter duration (Milisen et al., 2001).

(NR) A review of the research literature found that supportive environmental characteristics were beneficial in reducing delirium (Segatore & Adams, 2001).

■ *Normalize sleep pattern; reorganize care to provide increased amounts of uninterrupted sleep (i.e., consolidate/cluster treatments, medications, vital signs).*
LOE=VI

(NR) A descriptive study of older adult hip surgery patients (N=43) found that 35% developed postoperative delirium; patients with delirium had a very high level of dissatisfaction with sleep (Bowman, 1997).

(MR) A cross-sectional study (N=133) found that patients with sleep apnea were more likely to become delirious (Sandberg et al., 2001).

NR = Nursing Research, **MR** = Multidisciplinary Research, **SP** = Standard of Practice, **EO** = Expert Opinion, **LOE** = Level of Evidence

■ *Clarify use and dosage of existing ordered psychotropic medication. Neuroleptic agents such as haloperidol (Haldol) and risperidone (Risperdal) should be used only in the short term for target symptoms such as hallucinations, paranoid thoughts, or severe agitation (use with caution with older adults). Benzodiazepines are usually the drug of choice for alcohol withdrawal but have the potential to worsen delirium in non–alcohol withdrawal cases.* **LOE=V**

(MR) A review of the research literature (*N*=22 studies) on the association between psychoactive medications and delirium found that these medications contributed to the development of delirium in hospitalized older adults (Gaudreau et al., 2005).

(EO) Expert consensus guidelines for using antipsychotic medications in older adults advise prescribers to be knowledgeable of the possible disease-drug and drug-drug interactions (Alexopoulos et al., 2004).

Additional research: Inouye, 2006.

Possibly Effective

No applicable published research was found in this category.

Not Effective

No applicable published research was found in this category.

Possibly Harmful

No applicable published research was found in this category.

OUTCOME MEASUREMENT

COGNITIVE ORIENTATION   (NOC)

Definition: Ability to identify person, place, and time accurately.

Cognitive Orientation as evidenced by the following selected NOC indicators:
• Identifies self
• Identifies significant other
• Identifies current place
• Identifies significant current events

(Rate each indicator of **Cognitive Orientation:** 1=severely compromised, 2=substantially compromised, 3=moderately compromised, 4=mildly compromised, 5=not compromised) (Moorhead et al., 2004).

REFERENCES

Alexopoulos GS, Streim J, Carpenter D, Docherty JP; Expert Consensus Panel for Using Antipsychotic Drugs in Older Patients. (2004). Using antipsychotic agents in older patients. *J Clin Psychiatry,* 65(Suppl 2):5-99.

Bowman AM. (1997). Sleep satisfaction, perceived pain and acute confusion in elderly clients undergoing orthopaedic procedures. *J Adv Nurs,* 26(3):550-564.

Brauer C, Morrison RS, Silberzweig SB, Siu AL. (2000). The cause of delirium in patients with hip fracture. *Arch Intern Med,* 160(12):1856-1860.

Caeiro L, Ferro JM, Claro MI, Coelho J, Albuquerque R, Figueira ML. (2004). Delirium in acute stroke: A preliminary study of the role of anticholinergic medications. *Eur J Neurol,* 11(10):699-704.

RCT = Randomized Controlled (Clinical) Trial, **NIC** = Nursing Interventions Classification, **NOC** = Nursing Outcomes Classification

Contin AM, Perez-Jara J, Alonso-Contin A, Enguix A, Ramos F. (2005). Postoperative delirium after elective orthopedic surgery. *Int J Geriatr Psychiatry,* 20(6):595-597.

Dochterman JM, Bulechek GM (Eds). (2004). *Nursing Interventions Classification (NIC),* 4th ed. St. Louis: Mosby.

Duppils GS, Wikblad K. (2000). Acute confusional states in patients undergoing hip surgery. A prospective observation study. *Gerontology,* 46(1):36-43.

Feldt K, Griffin P. (1999). Clinical comments—Delirium in hip-fractured elders. *Clin Gerontologist,* 20(2):75-78.

Fick D, Foreman M. (2000). Consequences of not recognizing delirium superimposed on dementia in hospitalized elderly individuals. *J Gerontol Nurs,* 26(1):30-40.

Fick DM, Agostini JV, Inouye SK. (2002). Delirium superimposed on dementia: A systematic review. *J Am Geriatr Soc,* 50(10):1723-1732.

Francis J, Martin D, Kapoor WN. (1990). A prospective study of delirium in hospitalized elderly. *JAMA,* 263(8):1097-1101.

Galanakis P, Bickel H, Gradinger R, Von Gumppenberg S, Forstl H. (2001). Acute confusional state in the elderly following hip surgery: Incidence, risk factors and complications. *Int J Geriatr Psychiatry,* 16(4):349-355.

Gaudreau JD, Gagnon P, Roy MA, Harel F, Tremblay A. (2005). Association between psychoactive medications and delirium in hospitalized patients: A critical review. *Psychosomatics,* 46(4):302-316.

Gustafson Y, Brannstrom B, Berggren D, Ragnarsson JI, Sigaard J, Bucht G, et al. (1991). A geriatric-anesthesiologic program to reduce acute confusional states in elderly patients treated for femoral neck fractures. *J Am Geriatr Soc,* 39(7):655-662.

Inouye SK. (2006). Delirium in older persons. *N Engl J Med,* 354(11):1157-1165.

Inouye SK, Charpentier PA. (1996). Precipitating factors for delirium in hospitalized elderly persons. Predictive model and interrelationship with baseline vulnerability. *JAMA,* 275(11):852-857.

Inouye SK, Foreman MD. (2001). Nurses' recognition of delirium and its symptoms: Comparison of nurse and researcher ratings. *Arch Intern Med,* 161(20):2467-2473.

Inouye SK, Rushing JT, Foreman MD, Palmer RM, Pompei P. (1998). Does delirium contribute to poor hospital outcomes? A three-site epidemiologic study. *J Gen Intern Med,* 13(4):234-242.

Inouye SK, Viscoli CM, Horwitz RI, Hurst LD, Tinetti ME. (1993). A predictive model for delirium in hospitalized elderly medical patients based on admission characteristics. *Ann Intern Med,* 119(6):474-481.

Lemiengre J, Nelis T, Joosten E, Braes T, Foreman M, Gastmans C, et al. (2006). Detection of delirium by bedside nurses using the confusion assessment method. *J Am Geriatr Soc,* 54(4):685-689.

Levkoff SE, Safran C, Cleary PD, Gallop J, Phillips RS. (1988). Identification of factors associated with the diagnosis of delirium in elderly hospitalized patients. *J Am Geriatr Soc,* 36(12):1099-1104.

Lundstrom M, Edlund A, Karlsson S, Brannstrom B, Bucht G, Gustafson Y. (2005). A multifactorial intervention program reduces the duration of delirium, length of hospitalization, and mortality in delirious patients. *J Am Geriatr Soc,* 53(4):622-628.

Marcantonio ER, Goldman L, Mangione CM, Ludwig LE, Muraca B, Haslauer CM, et al. (1994). A clinical prediction rule for delirium after elective noncardiac surgery. *JAMA,* 271(2):134-139.

McCusker J, Cole M, Abrahamowicz M, Han L, Podoba JE, Ramman-Haddad L. (2001). Environmental risk factors for delirium in hospitalized older people. *J Am Geriatr Soc,* 49(10):1327-1334.

Milisen K, Foreman MD, Abraham IL, De Geest S, Godderis J, Vandermeulen E, et al. (2001). A nurse-led interdisciplinary intervention program for delirium in elderly hip-fracture patients. *J Am Geriatr Soc,* 49(5):523-532.

Milisen K, Lemiengre J, Braes T, Foreman MD. (2005). Multicomponent intervention strategies for managing delirium in hospitalized older adults: Systematic review. *J Adv Nurs,* 52(1):79-90.

Miller J, Campbell J, Moore K, Schofield A. (2004). Elder care supportive interventions protocol: Reducing discomfort in confused, hospitalized older adults. *J Gerontol Nurs,* 30(8):10-18.

Moorhead M, Johnson M, Maas M (Eds.). (2004). *Nursing Outcomes Classification (NOC),* 3rd ed. St. Louis: Mosby.

Rudolph JL, Babikian VL, Birjiniuk V, Crittenden MD, Treanor PR, Pochay VE, et al. (2005). Atherosclerosis is associated with delirium after coronary artery bypass graft surgery. *J Am Geriatr Soc,* 53(3):462-466.

Ruth M, Locsin R. (2004). The effect of music listening on acute confusion and delirium in elders undergoing elective hip and knee surgery. *J Clin Nurs,* 13(6B):91-96.

Sandberg O, Franklin KA, Bucht G, Gustafson Y. (2001). Sleep apnea, delirium, depressed mood, cognition, and ADL ability after stroke. *J Am Geriatr Soc,* 49(4):391-397.

Santos FS, Velasco IT, Fraguas R Jr. (2004). Risk factors for delirium in the elderly after coronary artery bypass graft surgery. *Int Psychogeriatr,* 16(2):175-193.

Schor JD, Levkoff SE, Lipsitz LA, Reilly CH, Cleary PD, Rowe JW, et al. (1992). Risk factors for delirium in hospitalized elderly. *JAMA,* 267(6):827-831.

Schuurmans MJ, Duursma SA, Shortridge-Baggett LM, Clevers G, Pel-Littel R. (2003). Elderly patients with a hip fracture: The risk for delirium. *Appl Nurs Res,* 16(2):75-84.

Segatore M, Adams D. (2001). Managing delirium and agitation in elderly hospitalized orthopaedic patients: Part 2—Interventions. *Orthop Nurs,* 20(2):61-73.

Stratton SJ, Rogers C, Brickett K, Gruzinski G. (2001). Factors associated with sudden death of individuals requiring restraint for excited delirium. *Am J Emerg Med,* 19(3):187-191.

Sullivan-Marx EM. (2001). Achieving restraint-free care of acutely confused older adults. *J Gerontol Nurs,* 27(4):56-61.

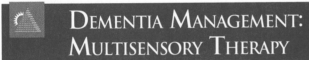

DEMENTIA MANAGEMENT: MULTISENSORY THERAPY

L. Julia Ball, PhD, RN

NIC **Definition:** Provision of a modified environment for the patient who is experiencing a chronic confusional state (Dochterman & Bulechek, 2004).

(This guideline focuses on the use of multisensory stimulation for dementia management.)

NURSING ACTIVITIES

Effective

■ *Use multisensory stimulation in a specially designed multisensory room (snoezelen room) involving the five senses (hearing, sight, smell, taste, and touch) to improve mood and decrease disruptive behaviors for individuals with dementia.* **LOE=II**

MR A random crossover trial studied institutionalized older adults using a specially designed multisensory room (snoezelen room) and traditional activities in a day room ($N=17$). Multisensory stimulation in the specially designed room produced decreased levels of apathy, restlessness, and disturbing behavior in the participants (Lancioni et al., 2002).

MR In an RCT of older noninstitutionalized adults with dementia who attended a day hospital, the experimental group received eight multisensory stimulation sessions ($N=31$) and the control group received traditional recreational therapy. The long-term effects for the experimental group were decreased nonsocial behaviors at home and improved mood compared with the control group. Short-term postsession measures were inconclusive between the groups (Baker et al., 1997).

(MR) In an unblinded RCT across three day care centers for individuals with dementia in Dorset, UK (N=50), inconclusive results were obtained. Individuals assigned to multisensory stimulation and traditional activity groups had an immediate beneficial effect on mood and behavior. However, the effect was carried over to the home setting for the multisensory stimulation group only. After the treatments stopped, the beneficial effects were lost in both groups (Baker et al., 2001).

(NR) In an RCT conducted across three countries (UK, Netherlands, and Sweden) (N=136), it was found that "that" was a repeated word in individuals with dementia; multisensory stimulation was no better than traditional activities for improving behavior, mood, or cognition (Baker et al., 2003).

■ *Create an environment of trust and relaxation facilitated by the presence and nondirective approach of a trained person.* **LOE=VII**

(EO) An essential component of the multisensory room is the one-to-one presence of a trained individual who enables the resident to enjoy the sensory experiences without pressure to achieve any specific goal. The experience in the multisensory room for the individual with dementia must be considered as a recreational activity without requirement for intellectual work of any kind (Ball & Haight, 2005).

■ *Provide a room about the size of a patient's room with specialized equipment that includes, but is not limited to, constantly changing colors in bubble tubes, reflections on the wall from a mirror ball, and fiberoptic sprays or strands; soothing unfamiliar music with interspersed dolphin or whale sounds; diffusers to disperse soothing aromas such as ylang ylang, bergamot, or lavender along with scented lotions for hand massage; and "touchy feely" items to touch and hold such as a soft fuzzy toy, a "cush" ball, or a vibrating cushion. Comfortable seating, a vibrating recliner, and a comfortable wheelchair are essential components of the multisensory room.* **LOE=VII**

(EO) Specialized equipment to stimulate the senses of sight, hearing, smell, and touch are essential components in the multisensory room and enable the resident to enjoy the sensory experiences without pressure to achieve any specific goal (Ball & Haight, 2005).

■ *Use multisensory stimulation without a specially designed room involving the five senses (hearing, sight, smell, taste, and touch) for individuals with dementia.* **LOE=III**

(MR) The effects of multisensory stimulation was investigated in a 6-month controlled study of institutionalized males with dementia who were 80 years or older (N=28). The control group received regularly scheduled activities. The experimental group demonstrated increased levels of energy, motivation, interest in newspapers, smiling, continence, and improved personal cleanliness (Loew & Silverstone, 1971).

(MR) Institutionalized older adults divided into four groups according to behaviors received multisensory stimulation. All groups were observed to have increased enthusiasm for life, improvement of behavior and mood, and decreased wandering, anxiety, and hostility (Bryant, 1991).

(MR) In a loosely controlled descriptive study, institutionalized individuals with advanced Alzheimer's disease (N=15) received multisensory stimulation for 15 minutes for an unspecified period of time. Results indicated that there was an immediate increase in well-being and lowered psychological discomfort (Witucki & Twibell, 1997).

Possibly Effective

■ *Use sensory integration activities with multisensory stimulation instead of traditional recreational therapy.* **LOE=IV**

MR In an RCT (*N*=40), multisensory activities were provided for 45 minutes three times per week for 10 weeks to older institutionalized individuals from three different locations in Canada. No significant change in behavior was observed. However, the authors stated that further research was needed to determine effectiveness of the therapy (Robichaud et al., 1994).

EO The research is inconclusive regarding the effectiveness of multisensory stimulation in a specially designed room (snoezelen room). The literature suggests that sensory deprivation and boredom are at the root of disruptive behavior, apathy, and restlessness (Chitsey et al., 2002; Ball & Haight, 2005). Therefore, multisensory stimulation or appropriate pleasurable activities or therapies conducted in a comfortable environment with a trained individual may be equally effective for mood elevation and reduction of disruptive behavior for people with dementia (MacDonald, 2002).

■ *Provide interventions that may be used without a specially designed multisensory room, such as finger painting; sorting colored buttons; winding yarn; dangling hands in warm water; feeling sponges, balloons, bean bags, and different fabric textures; listening to music and rhythmical sounds and dancing; drinking wine, hot chocolate, hot tea, and coffee, and food tasting; aromatherapy, smelling flowers, lotions and oils, cookie baking (good for working the dough, tasting it, smelling the baking cookies, then eating them); looking at family photographs in a colorful environment with mobiles; and watching slides.* **LOE=VII**

EO Congruent with the philosophy and goal of multisensory stimulation in the multisensory room, multisensory stimulation that is nonintellectually challenging, relaxing, and pleasurable may be employed without a specially designed multisensory room. Researchers have used a myriad of interventions with a trained individual in these studies. The individual designing a multisensory intervention is limited only by the imagination. However, it must be remembered that the key to any intervention is the presence of a trained facilitator who clearly understands the philosophy and goal of multisensory stimulation (Ball & Haight, 2005).

Not Effective

No applicable published research was found in this category.

Possibly Harmful

No applicable published research was found in this category.

RCT = Randomized Controlled (Clinical) Trial, **NIC** = Nursing Interventions Classification, **NOC** = Nursing Outcomes Classification

OUTCOME MEASUREMENT

PERSONAL WELL-BEING (NOC)

Definition: Extent of positive perception of one's health status and life circumstances.
Personal Well-Being as evidenced by the following selected NOC indicators:
- Performance of activities of daily living
- Performance of usual roles
- Psychological health
- Social relationships
- Ability to cope
- Ability to express emotions

(Rate each indicator of **Personal Well-Being:** 1 = not at all satisfied, 2 = somewhat satisfied, 3 = moderately satisfied, 4 = very satisfied, 5 = completely satisfied) (Moorhead et al., 2004).

REFERENCES

Baker R, Bell S, Baker E, Gibson S, Holloway J, Pearce R, et al. (2001). A randomized controlled trial of the effects of multi-sensory stimulation (MSS) for people with dementia. *Br J Clin Psychol,* 40 (Pt 1):81-96.

Baker R, Dowling Z, Wareing LA, Dawson J, Assey J. (1997). Snoezelen: Its long-term and short-term effects on older people with dementia. *Br J Occup Ther,* 60(5):213-218.

Baker R, Holloway J, Holtkamp CC, Larsson A, Hartman LC, Pearce R, et al. (2003). Effects of multisensory stimulation for people with dementia. *J Adv Nurs,* 43(5):465-477.

Ball J, Haight BK. (2005). Creating a multisensory environment for dementia: The goals of a Snoezelen room. *J Gerontol Nurs,* 31(10):4-10.

Bryant W. (1991). Creative group work with confused elderly people. A development of sensory integration therapy. *Br J Occup Ther,* 54(5):187-192.

Chitsey AM, Haight BK, Jones MM. (2002). Snoezelen: A multisensory environmental intervention. *J Gerontol Nurs,* 28(3):41-49.

Dochterman JM, Bulechek GM (Eds). (2004). *Nursing Interventions Classification (NIC),* 4th ed. St. Louis: Mosby.

Doenges ME, Moorehouse MF, Geissler-Murr AC. (2005). *Nursing diagnosis manual.* Philadelphia: FA Davis.

Lancioni GE, Cuvo AJ, O'Reilly MF. (2002). Snoezelen: An overview of research with people with developmental disabilities and dementia. *Disabil Rehabil,* 24(4):175-184.

Loew CA, Silverstone BM. (1971). A program of intensified stimulation and response facilitation for the senile aged. *Gerontologist,* 11(4):341-347.

MacDonald C. (2002). Back to the real sensory world our"care" has taken away. *J Dement Care,* 10(1): 33-36.

Moorhead M, Johnson M, Maas M. (Eds). (2004). *Nursing Outcomes Classification (NOC),* 3rd ed. St. Louis: Mosby.

Robichaud L, Hebert R, Desrosiers J. (1994). Efficacy of a sensory integration program on the behaviors of inpatients with dementia. *Am J Occup Ther,* 48(4):355-360.

Witucki JM, Twibell RS. (1997). The effect of sensory stimulation activities on the psychological well being of patients with advanced Alzheimer's disease. *Am J Alzheimers Dis,* 12(1):10-15.

NR = Nursing Research, **MR** = Multidisciplinary Research, **SP** = Standard of Practice, **EO** = Expert Opinion, **LOE** = Level of Evidence

DIARRHEA MANAGEMENT

Kathleen A. Fitzgerald, PhD, RN

NIC **Definition:** Management and alleviation of diarrhea (Dochterman & Bulechek, 2004).

NURSING ACTIVITIES

Effective

■ **Teach health care providers, patients, and significant others techniques for prevention of diarrheal illnesses using hygiene principles and safe food handling practices. LOE=I**

MR A meta-analysis of 17 studies relating hand washing to the risk of infectious diarrhea in the community was conducted. Interventions to promote hand washing with soap were associated with a decrease of 47% in risk of diarrheal disease (Curtis & Cairncross, 2003).

NR A prospective RCT (N=46) compared the effects of a 2% chlorhexidine gluconate (CHG) antiseptic wash and a 61% ethanol with emollients (ALC) waterless hand rub on skin condition and skin microbiology. The ALC and CHG products were equally effective as skin cleansers; however, the ALC product was associated with improved skin condition and took less time to use (Larson et al., 2001).

MR An observational survey was conducted to compare nosocomial drug-resistant organisms for 3 years before and 3 years after the institution of an alcohol-based hand rub. The incidence of new, nosocomial isolates of methicillin-resistant *Staphylococcus aureus* (MRSA) was decreased by 21%, and vancomycin-resistant *Enterococcus* (VRE) was reduced by 41% after implementation of the alcohol-based hand rub. The incidence of *Clostridium difficile* was unchanged (Gordin et al., 2005). (Please refer to the guideline on Infection Control: Hand Hygiene for more information.)

■ SP *Identify the history and cause of the diarrhea.* **LOE=VI**

EO The approach to and management of acute infectious diarrhea require careful assessment of duration of diarrhea; stool characteristics; frequency of bowel movements; history of foreign travel; ingestion of potentially contaminated food; family, friends, or coworkers with the same symptoms; institutional or day care residence; presence of blood in the stool; immunocompromised status; recent antibiotic administration; accompanying symptoms of dehydration, nausea, vomiting, and fever; and current medication use (Bushen & Guerrant, 2003).

EO Nursing care and assessment of patients with acute diarrhea found in the community as well as those with hospital-acquired infections are recommended as described previously (Walker, 2004).

MR A case study described a comprehensive approach to the diagnosis and treatment of a patient presenting with acute diarrhea (Thielman & Guerrant, 2004).

RCT = Randomized Controlled (Clinical) Trial, **NIC** = Nursing Interventions Classification, **NOC** = Nursing Outcomes Classification

■ (SP) *Note and record the color, volume, frequency, and consistency of stools using objective and quantitative descriptions. Using a descriptive stool instrument is useful in characterizing bowel habits and eliminating variation among patients describing diarrhea.* **LOE=VI**

(MR) A descriptive study was conducted of a population of patients with HIV to develop a self-report measure of diarrhea using pictures representing stool consistencies, specific questions about diarrhea discomfort, complications, number of bowel movements, and consistency of stools. The tool was useful in characterizing bowel habits and eliminating variations among patients in describing diarrhea (Mertz et al., 1995).

■ (SP) *Assess the patient carefully for signs of dehydration.* **LOE=VII**

(NR) A review article described age-related changes, risk factors, assessment, and nursing interventions for dehydration, especially in the aged patient. Factors to assess included irritability, confusion, dizziness (especially when standing up), weakness, thirst, dry skin and membranes, decreased urine output, increased heart rate, and decreased blood pressure. The article contained a dehydration risk appraisal checklist (Mentes, 2006). (Please refer to the guideline on Fluid Management.)

■ *Recommend that patients with acute infectious diarrhea eat foods containing probiotics such as yogurt with active cultures or kefir products.* **LOE=I**

(MR) A Cochrane systematic review assessed the effects of probiotics in infectious diarrhea and concluded that probiotics reduced the risk of diarrhea at 3 days with a mean duration of 30 to 48 hours. Subset analysis was unable to account for the influence of a specific type of probiotic, age of the subjects, or type of diarrheal illness on the results. The analysis concluded that probiotics appeared to be a useful adjunct to rehydration therapy in treating acute infectious diarrhea, but more research is necessary to identify specific probiotic regimens (Allen et al., 2004).

(MR) In a meta-analysis of nine RCTs of the effect of probiotics on infectious diarrhea, the reduction of diarrhea duration and diarrhea frequency were used as the primary outcomes. Results indicated that use of *Lactobacillus* reduced the diarrhea duration by 0.7 day and reduced the diarrhea frequency to 1.6 stools on day 2 of treatment (Van Niel et al., 2002).

(MR) A systematic review of 10 double-blind RCTs was performed to evaluate the effect of probiotics in the treatment or prevention of acute diarrhea in infants and children. The use of probiotics compared with placebo demonstrated a significantly reduced duration of diarrhea, particularly in rotaviral gastroenteritis. The analysis was unable to determine prevention of diarrhea because of insignificant data. *Lactobacillus* GG demonstrated the most consistent effect, although other probiotics were effective (Szajewska & Mrukowicz, 2001).

(MR) A scientific review article described the evidence for the potential and known effects of probiotics in promoting health of the gastrointestinal system, including decreasing diarrhea (Adolfsson et al., 2004).

(MR) A clinical review article found that probiotics were beneficial in various gastrointestinal disorders (Broekaert & Walker, 2006).

NR = Nursing Research, **MR** = Multidisciplinary Research, **SP** = Standard of Practice, **EO** = Expert Opinion, **LOE** = Level of Evidence

Antibiotic-Related Diarrhea

■ *Request that the patient taking antibiotics eat daily foods containing probiotics such as yogurt with active cultures or kefir products. Specific probiotic and dosage have yet to be determined.* **LOE=I**

(MR) A meta-analysis was performed to evaluate the effectiveness of *Saccharomyces boulardii* in preventing antibiotic-associated diarrhea. The results of five RCTs showed that *S. boulardii* was moderately effective in preventing antibiotic-associated diarrhea. The number of patients needing treatment to prevent one case of antibiotic-associated diarrhea was 10 (Szajewska & Mrukowicz, 2005).

(MR) A meta-analysis of nine RCTs investigated the effects of probiotics in prevention of antibiotic-associated diarrhea. The analysis suggested that probiotics (*Saccharomyces boulardii, Lactobacillus*) may be effective in preventing antibiotic-associated diarrhea in children (D'Souza et al., 2002).

■ *Observe for signs and symptoms of diarrhea (e.g., duration of diarrhea, stool characteristics, frequency of bowel movements, and concomitant symptoms of fever, abdominal distention, nausea, or vomiting). Notify the physician of watery diarrhea or an increase in frequency or pitch of bowel sounds indicating the development of colitis.* **LOE=IV**

(MR) A case study approach reviewed the potential complications and treatment of patients with antibiotic-associated diarrhea including ruling out *C. difficile* infection and monitoring for the serious complication of colitis (Bartlett, 2002).

Irritable Bowel Syndrome

■ *Document in detail the patient's description of the stool characteristics, length of time the diarrhea has been present, and presence or lack of concomitant symptoms of abdominal pain, nausea, vomiting, and weight loss.* **LOE=I**

(EO) Patients are diagnosed as having functional diarrhea (also described as irritable bowel syndrome [IBS] with diarrhea) when they have had continuous or recurrent symptoms of the passage of loose or mushy stools without abdominal pain for at least 12 weeks (Thompson et al., 1999).

(MR) Evidence and consensus-based practice guidelines were developed based on systematic literature review of articles that evaluated the performance of diagnostic tests and procedures for IBS and expert opinion. This study identified only 13 published studies that validated symptom criteria (Fass et al., 2001).

Possibly Effective

■ *Ask patients to examine intake of high-fructose corn syrup and fructose sweeteners in relation to onset of diarrhea symptoms. If diarrhea is associated with fructose ingestion, intake should be limited or eliminated.* **LOE=III**

(MR) High-fructose corn syrup or fructose sweeteners from fruit juices can cause gastrointestinal (GI) symptoms of bloating, rumbling, flatulence, and diarrhea at amounts of 25 to 50 g.

RCT = Randomized Controlled (Clinical) Trial, **NIC** = Nursing Interventions Classification, **NOC** = Nursing Outcomes Classification

A 16-oz glass of apple juice frequently contains as much as 30 g of fructose, and 22 oz of soft drink contains approximately 30 to 40 g. In a controlled study, hydrogen breath testing and a symptom scale were used to determine malabsorption of fructose in healthy volunteers. After overnight fasting, 15 healthy volunteers were given 25- and 50-g doses of fructose. Results revealed that half of the subjects demonstrated fructose malabsorption after 25 g and as many 80% after 50 g. Ten of 15 subjects reported GI symptoms, although diarrhea was not as frequently reported as other symptoms (Beyer et al., 2005).

Irritable Bowel Syndrome

■ *Recognize that low to moderate fiber in the diet may control the diarrhea and other symptoms of IBS.* **LOE=II**

(MR) An RCT of the effects of a high-fiber diet on symptoms of IBS was conducted ($N=56$). One group was randomly assigned to receive 10.5 g fiber/day, and a second group received 30.5 g fiber/day. Patients in group 2 consumed about 25 g fiber/day, and group 1 consumed 6 g/day. The difference in fiber intake was not significant. Pain scores, bowel scores, and general symptom scores were not significantly different. Low to moderate fiber intake may be beneficial for patients with IBS, but it is difficult to draw these conclusions because all the patients improved (Aller et al., 2004).

(MR) A descriptive study of 205 IBS patients was conducted to determine whether a low-fiber diet was beneficial in relieving symptoms of IBS. The subjects were instructed on a low (10 g) fiber diet. Patients with diarrhea were instructed on the use of bulking agents only if they became constipated. Postal questionnaires were mailed 4 weeks later with 151 returns. A significant improvement (60% to 100%) was reported by 49% of the patients. Of the patients with diarrhea, 57% reported symptom improvement. The conclusion suggested that low-fiber diets may be an effective treatment for IBS, but further studies are required (Woolner & Kirby, 2000).

(NR) A phenomenological analysis was conducted to describe the perception of women with IBS regarding the relationship of their diet with their symptoms. The women used a trial-and-error method to determine links between food and symptoms but frequently could not pinpoint specific foods that consistently triggered symptoms. The majority felt that there was not a single trigger but frequently a combination of factors (i.e., environment, stress, or food together could trigger symptoms) (Jarrett et al., 2001).

■ *Explain to patients that there is no significant research to support use of herbal remedies at this time for IBS, although some of them may be effective.* **LOE=I**

(MR) A systematic review of alternative therapies for IBS was conducted to determine which therapies had the research data to support recommendations. The therapies with the most support from the literature included Chinese herbal therapy (one RCT), psychological therapy (multiple poorly controlled studies), elimination diets and oral cromolyn (appear equally efficacious in treatment of chronic diarrheal illness), and carbohydrate, lactose, and fructose (may cause more symptoms in the patient with IBS than the normal population) (Spanier et al., 2003).

NR = Nursing Research, **MR** = Multidisciplinary Research, **SP** = Standard of Practice, **EO** = Expert Opinion, **LOE** = Level of Evidence

(MR) A Cochrane review of the effectiveness and safety of herbal medicines in patients with IBS analyzed 75 RCTs. The variety of herbs and poor methodology did not allow a meta-analysis to be performed. The authors concluded that some herbal medicines may improve the symptoms of IBS, but they were unable to draw conclusions about specific herbal preparations (Liu et al., 2006).

Not Effective

■ *Use of water filters to remove bacteria and viruses that can cause diarrhea.*
LOE=II

(MR) An RCT of filtering drinking water comparing the use of an active tap water filter ($N=227$) versus a sham device ($N=229$) over 6 months demonstrated that there was no reduction of diarrheal illnesses or other gastrointestinal illnesses with the use of a filter designed to remove microorganisms (Colford et al., 2005).

Possibly Harmful

No applicable published research was found in this category.

OUTCOME MEASUREMENT

BOWEL ELIMINATION (NOC)

Definition: Formation and evacuation of stool.
Bowel Elimination as evidenced by the following selected NOC indicators:
• Stool soft and formed
• Control of bowel movements
• Comfort of stool passage
(Rate each indicator of **Bowel Elimination:** 1=severely compromised, 2=substantially compromised, 3=moderately compromised, 4=mildly compromised, 5=not compromised) (Moorhead et al., 2004).

REFERENCES

Adolfsson O, Meydani SN, Russell RM. (2004). Yogurt and gut function. *Am J Clin Nutr,* 80(2):245-256.

Allen SJ, Okoko B, Martinez E, Gregorio G, Dans LF. (2004). Probiotics for treating infectious diarrhoea. *Cochrane Database Syst Rev,* (2):CD003048.

Aller R, de Luis DA, Izaola O, la Calle F, del Olmo L, Fernandez L, et al. (2004). Effects of a high-fiber diet on symptoms of irritable bowel syndrome: A randomized clinical trial. *Nutrition,* 20(9):735-737.

Bartlett JG. (2002). Antibiotic-associated diarrhea. *N Engl J Med,* 346(5):334-338.

Beyer PL, Caviar EM, McCallum RW. (2005). Fructose intake at current levels in the United States may cause gastrointestinal distress in normal adults. *J Am Diet Assoc,* 105(10):1559-1566.

Broekaert IJ, Walker WA. (2006). Probiotics as flourishing benefactors for the human body. *Gastroenterol Nurs,* 29(1):26-34.

Bushen OY, Guerrant RL. (2003). Acute infectious diarrhea: Approach and management in the emergency department. *Top Emerg Med,* 25(2):139-149.

Colford JM, Wade TJ, Sandhu SK, Wright CC, Lee S, Shaw S, et al. (2005). A randomized, controlled trial of in-home drinking water intervention to reduce gastrointestinal illness. *Am J Epidemiol,* 161(5):472-482.

RCT = Randomized Controlled (Clinical) Trial, **NIC** = Nursing Interventions Classification, **NOC** = Nursing Outcomes Classification

Curtis V, Cairncross S. (2003). Effect of washing hands with soap on diarrhoea risk in the community: A systematic review. *Lancet Infect Dis,* 3(5):275-281.

Dochterman JM, Bulechek GM (Eds). (2004). *Nursing Interventions Classification (NIC),* 4th ed. St. Louis: Mosby.

D'Souza AL, Rajkumar C, Cooke J, Bulpitt CJ. (2002). Probiotics in prevention of antibiotic associated diarrhoea: Meta-analysis. *BMJ,* 324(7350):1361-1374.

Fass R, Longstreth GF, Pimentel M, Fullerton S, Russak SM, Chiou C, et al. (2001). Evidence- and consensus-based practice guidelines for the diagnosis of irritable bowel syndrome. *Arch Intern Med,* 161(17):2081-2088.

Gordin FM, Schultz ME, Huber RA, Gill JA. (2005). Reduction in nosocomial transmission of drug-resistant bacteria after introduction of an alcohol-based handrub. *Infect Control Hosp Epidemiol,* 26(7):650-653.

Jarrett M, Visser R, Heitkemper M. (2001). Diet triggers symptoms in women with irritable bowel syndrome. *Gastroenterol Nurs,* 24(5):246-252.

Larson EL, Aiello AE, Bastyr J, Lyle C, Stahl J, Cronquist A, et al. (2001). Assessment of two hand hygiene regimens for intensive care unit personnel. *Crit Care Med,* 29(5):944-951.

Liu JP, Liu YX, Wei ML, Grimsgaard S. (2006). Herbal medicines for the treatment of irritable bowel syndrome. *Cochrane Database Syst Rev,* (1):CD004116.

Mentes J. (2006). Oral hydration in older adults: Greater awareness is needed in preventing, recognizing, and treating dehydration. *Am J Nurs,* 106(6):40-49.

Mertz HR, Beck CK, Dixon W, Esquivel MA, Hays RD, Shapiro MF. (1995). Validation of a new measure of diarrhea. *Dig Dis Sci,* 40(9):1873-1882.

Moorhead M, Johnson M, Maas M (Eds). (2004). *Nursing Outcomes Classification (NOC),* 3rd ed. St. Louis: Mosby.

Spanier JA, Howden CW, Jones MP. (2003). A systematic review of alternative therapies in the irritable bowel syndrome. *Arch Intern Med,* 163(3):265-274.

Szajewska H, Mrukowicz J. (2005). Meta-analysis: Non-pathogenic yeast *Saccharomyces boulardii* in the prevention of antibiotic-associated diarrhoea. *Aliment Pharmacol Ther,* 22(5):365-372.

Szajewska H, Mrukowicz JZ. (2001). Probiotics in the treatment and prevention of acute infectious diarrhea in infants and children: A systematic review of published randomized, double-blind, placebo-controlled trials. *J Pediatr Gastroenterol Nutr,* 33(Suppl 2):S17-S25.

Thielman NM, Guerrant RL. (2004). Clinical practice: Acute infectious diarrhea. *N Engl J Med,* 350(1):38-47.

Thompson WG, Longstreth GF, Drossman DA, Heaton KW, Irvine EJ, Muller-Lissner SA. (1999). Functional bowel disorders and functional abdominal pain. *Gut,* 45(Suppl 2):II43-II47.

Van Niel CW, Feudtner C, Garrison MM, Christakis DA. (2002). Lactobacillus therapy for acute infectious diarrhea in children: A meta-analysis. *Pediatrics,* 109(4):678-684.

Walker BW. (2004). Assessing gastrointestinal infections. Common but rarely life-threatening, GI infections have many possible causes. Here's how to gather the clues so your patient gets appropriate care. *Nursing,* 34(5):48-52.

Woolner JT, Kirby GA. (2000). Clinical audit of the effects of low-fibre diet on irritable bowel syndrome. *J Hum Nutr Diet,* 13(4):249-253.

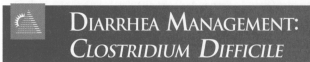

DIARRHEA MANAGEMENT: CLOSTRIDIUM DIFFICILE

Kathleen A. Fitzgerald, PhD, RN

Definition: Prevention, management, and alleviation of diarrhea caused by *C. difficile.*

NURSING ACTIVITIES

Effective

■ *Prevent* C. difficile *transmission by appropriate infection control methods.* **LOE=I**

(EO) A nursing review summary of the most recent developments in patients' care related to *C. difficile* includes contact isolation, soap and water hand washing, use of disposable equipment, and intensive housekeeping utilizing hypochlorite-based products for disinfection (Todd, 2006).

(MR) An extensive and comprehensive review of hand hygiene and evaluation of the agents for scrubs and rubs discussed the importance of environmental and hand contamination in the spread of *C. difficile*. Bacterial spores such as *C. difficile* are not destroyed by alcohol, chlorhexidine, and triclosan products. Even vigorous hand washing is minimally effective. Vegetative cells of *C. difficile* can survive for at least 24 hours on inanimate surfaces and spore survival can be up to 5 months (Kampf & Kramer, 2004).

(EO) Pay close attention to cleaning and disinfecting high-touch surface areas in patients' rooms. Patients with contact precautions should have all disposable patient care items (e.g., blood pressure cuffs) to avoid cross contamination (Sehulster & Chinn, 2003).

(EO) Use contact isolation, wear gloves and gowns to prevent spread of *C. difficile* infections (Garner, 1996).

(MR) In a laboratory study comparing a variety of disinfectants on dried *C. difficile* spores, high-concentration bleach products could inactivate the *C. difficile* spores on hard surfaces in less than 10 minutes (Perez et al., 2005).

(MR) In a descriptive study of an acute-care hospital and long-term care facility, electronic rectal thermometers were found to be cultured with *C. difficile* toxin. All electronic rectal thermometers were replaced with disposable rectal thermometers. During the 6-month post intervention period, the incidence of *C. difficile* diarrhea was reduced from 2.71 per 1000 patient days to 1.76 per 1000 patient days in the acute care facility (Brooks et al., 1992).

Possibly Effective

■ *Administer probiotics to patients with antibiotic-associated diarrhea to prevent the incidence of* C. difficile. **LOE=I**

(MR) A double-blind, placebo-controlled study of 138 patients was conducted to determine whether *Lactobacillus acidophilus* and *Bifidobacterium bifidum* could prevent the development of *C. difficile* in patients with antibiotic-associated diarrhea. The probiotics were combined into a capsule and provided daily to the treatment group. Only 46% of the patients receiving the probiotics were *C. difficile* toxin positive compared with 78% of the placebo group (Plummer et al., 2004).

(MR) A meta-analysis of 25 RCTs was performed to compare the efficacy of probiotics for the prevention of antibiotic-associated diarrhea and the treatment of *C. difficile* diarrhea and colitis. The study concluded that three types of probiotics (*Saccharomyces boulardii, Lactobacillus rhamnosus* GG, and probiotic mixtures) significantly reduced the development of

---

RCT = Randomized Controlled (Clinical) Trial, **NIC** = Nursing Interventions Classification, **NOC** = Nursing Outcomes Classification

antibiotic-associated diarrhea, but only *Saccharomyces boulardii* was effective in treatment of *C. difficile* (McFarland, 2006).

■ *Watch for the presence of watery stools in patients receiving antibiotics, especially third-generation cephalosporin and quinolone drugs.* **LOE=IV**

(MR) In a case-control study of 27 patients diagnosed with nosocomial *C. difficile*, cephalosporin antibiotic use demonstrated significant association with *C. difficile* diarrhea. In addition, patients with prior use of quinolones were five times more likely to develop *C. difficile* diarrhea (Yip et al., 2001).

(MR) A prospective study using a multidisciplinary team approach to minimize the inappropriate use of third-generation cephalosporins was implemented and evaluated over 7 years. There was a 22% decrease in the use of cephalosporins despite an increase in overall patients' acuity. There was a concomitant significant decrease in nosocomial infections caused by *C. difficile* and resistant Enterobacteriaceae (VRE) (Carling et al., 2003).

■ *Obtain a stool culture and sensitivity as ordered during the first 3 days of illness with diarrhea or if the patient is hospitalized. Obtain stool for* **C. difficile** *toxin if the diarrhea persists despite treatment or if it becomes watery in consistency.* **LOE=IV**

(MR) A prospective multicenter case-control study was designed to evaluate whether specific antibiotics caused the development of *C. difficile* in hospitalized patients. Results revealed that no specific antibiotic or combination of antibiotics accounted for the difference in the patients with *C. difficile*–positive stool compared with the control group of patients with diarrhea. However, the patients with *C. difficile*–positive stool were more severely ill as rated on a severity of illness scale (Vesta et al., 2005).

■ *Teach patients that probiotic use may prevent recurrent* **C. difficile** *infections.* **LOE=II**

(MR) A randomized double-blind, placebo-controlled trial was conducted to determine whether *Lactobacillus plantarum* 299v, a probiotic, in combination with metronidazole would be effective in preventing recurrent episodes of *C. difficile*. Participants treated with the probiotic had less recurrence, but because the sample size was small ($N=21$), the results could not be generalized (Wullt et al., 2003).

(MR) An RCT of treatment of *C. difficile* and incidence of recurrence randomly allocated patients to receive low-dose vancomycin, high-dose vancomycin, and metronidazole. The groups were further randomly assigned to receive the antibiotic plus *Saccharomyces boulardii* or placebo. The results were not significant because of the small number of participants in each group; however, the group receiving high-dose vancomycin plus the *S. boulardii* demonstrated a lower incidence of recurrence (Surawicz et al., 2000).

■ *Watch for the presence of watery stools in patients receiving antibiotics, especially third-generation cephalosporin and quinolone drugs.* **LOE=IV**

(MR) In a case-control study of 27 patients diagnosed with nosocomial *C. difficile*, cephalosporin antibiotic use demonstrated significant association with *C. difficile* diarrhea. In addition, patients with prior use of quinolones were five times more likely to develop *C. difficile* diarrhea (Yip et al., 2001).

(MR) A prospective study using a multidisciplinary team approach to minimize the inappropriate use of third-generation cephalosporins was implemented and evaluated over 7 years. There was a 22% decrease in the use of cephalosporins despite an increase in overall patients' acuity. There was a concomitant significant decrease in nosocomial infections caused by *C. difficile* and resistant Enterobacteriaceae (VRE) (Carling et al., 2003).

■ *Recognize that patients receiving proton pump inhibitors to suppress gastric acid secretion may be at a greater risk for developing* C. difficile. **LOE=IV**

(MR) A retrospective case-control review was performed with 170 patients positive for *C. difficile* toxin. The highest risk of developing *C. difficile* (43.2 odds ratio) was found with patients receiving proton pump inhibitors, antibiotics, and chemotherapy agents. Proton pump inhibitors alone had an odds ratio of 2.5 (Cunningham et al., 2003).

Not Effective

■ *Recognize that the spores of* C. difficile *are very difficult to eradicate. They are not destroyed by alcohol hand washing agents; vigorous hand washing is mechanically required to remove them.* **LOE=I**

(EO) Contact isolation, use of disposable equipment, and washing with soap and water to remove spores from hands mechanically are recommended. Bleach products should be used to clean surfaces and disinfect the room when the patient has been discharged (Todd, 2006).

(EO) Alcohol-based hand rubs are not effective against spore-forming bacteria. The physical action of washing hands with soap and water removes spores (Boyce & Pittet, 2002).

(MR) An extensive and comprehensive review of hand hygiene and evaluation of the agents for scrubs and rubs discussed the importance of environmental and hand contamination in the spread of *C. difficile*. Bacterial spores such as *C. difficile* are not destroyed by alcohol, chlorhexidine, and triclosan products. Vigorous hand washing is minimally effective. Vegetative cells of *C. difficile* can survive for at least 24 hours on inanimate surfaces, and spore survival can be up to 5 months (Kampf & Kramer, 2004).

(MR) An observational study done in a 500-bed hospital demonstrated there was not an increased incidence of *C. difficile* infection with increased use of an alcohol-based hand rub (Boyce et al., 2006).

Possibly Harmful

■ *Use of antiperistaltic agents, including narcotics, in patients with severe* C. difficile *infection. These agents may precipitate toxic megacolon.* **LOE=VI**

(EO) Avoid antiperistaltic drugs in patients with severe *C. difficile* infection (Sunenshine & McDonald, 2006).

RCT = Randomized Controlled (Clinical) Trial, **NIC** = Nursing Interventions Classification, **NOC** = Nursing Outcomes Classification

OUTCOME MEASUREMENT

BOWEL ELIMINATION (NOC)

Definition: Formation and evacuation of stool.

Bowel Elimination as evidenced by the following selected NOC indicators:

- Stool soft and formed
- Control of bowel movements
- Comfort of stool passage
- Elimination pattern

(Rate each indicator of **Bowel Elimination:** 1=severely compromised, 2=substantially compromised, 3=moderately compromised, 4=mildly compromised, 5=not compromised) (Moorhead et al., 2004).

REFERENCES

Boyce JM, Ligi C, Kohan C, Dumigan D, Havill NL. (2006). Lack of association between the increased incidence of *Clostridium difficile*-associated disease and the increasing use of alcohol-based hand rubs. *Infect Control Hosp Epidemiol,* 27(5):479-483.

Boyce JM, Pittet D; Healthcare Infection Control Practices Advisory Committee. Society for Healthcare Epidemiology of America. Association for Professionals in Infection Control. Infectious Diseases Society of America. Hand Hygiene Task Force. (2002). Guideline for hand hygiene in health-care settings: Recommendations of the Healthcare Infection Control Practices Advisory Committee and the HICPAC/SHEA/APIC/IDSA Hand Hygiene Task Force. *Infect Control Hosp Epidemiol,* 23(12 Suppl): S3-S40.

Brooks SE, Veal RO, Kramer M, Dore L, Schupf N, Adachi M. (1992). Reduction in the incidence of *Clostridium difficile*-associated diarrhea in an acute care hospital and a skilled nursing facility following replacement of electronic thermometers with single-use disposables. *Infect Control Hosp Epidemiol,* 13(2):98-103.

Carling P, Fung T, Killion A, Barza M. (2003). Favorable impact of a multidisciplinary antibiotic management program conducted during 7 years. *Infect Control Hosp Epidemiol,* 24(9):699-706.

Cunningham R, Dale B, Undy B, Gaunt N. (2003). Proton pump inhibitors as a risk factor for *Clostridium difficile* diarrhoea. *J Hosp Infect,* 54(3):243-245.

Garner JS. (1996). Guideline for isolation precautions in hospitals. The Hospital Infection Control Practices Advisory Committee. *Infect Control Hosp Epidemiol,* 17(1):53-80.

Kampf G, Kramer A. (2004). Epidemiologic background of hand hygiene and evaluation of the most important agents for scrubs and rubs. *Clin Microbiol Rev,* 17(4):863-893.

McFarland LV. (2006). Meta-analysis of probiotics for the prevention of antibiotic associated diarrhea and the treatment of *Clostridium difficile* disease. *Am J Gastroenterol,* 101(4):812-822.

Moorhead M, Johnson M, Maas M (Eds). (2004). *Nursing Outcomes Classification (NOC),* 3rd ed. St. Louis: Mosby.

Perez J, Springthorpe VS, Sattar SA. (2005). Activity of selected oxidizing microbicides against the spores of *Clostridium difficile:* Relevance to environmental control. *Am J Infect Control,* 33(6):320-325.

Plummer S, Weaver MA, Harris JC, Dee P, Hunter J. (2004). *Clostridium difficile* pilot study: Effects of probiotic supplementation on the incidence of *C. difficile* diarrhoea. *Int Microbiol,* 7(1):59-62.

Sehulster L, Chinn RY; CDC; HICPAC. (2003). Guidelines for environmental infection control in health-care facilities. Recommendations of CDC and the Healthcare Infection Control Practices Advisory Committee (HICPAC). *MMWR Recomm Rep,* 52(RR-10):1-42.

Sunenshine RH, McDonald LC. (2006). *Clostridium difficile*-associated disease: New challenges from an established pathogen. *Cleve Clin J Med,* 73(2):187-197.

NR = Nursing Research, **MR** = Multidisciplinary Research, **SP** = Standard of Practice, **EO** = Expert Opinion, **LOE** = Level of Evidence

Surawicz CM, McFarland LV, Greenberg RN, Rubin M, Fekety R, Mulligan ME, et al. (2000). The search for a better treatment for recurrent *Clostridium difficile* disease: Use of high-dose vancomycin combined with *Saccharomyces boulardii*. *Clin Infect Dis*, 31(4):1012-1017.

Todd B. (2006). *Clostridium difficile:* Familiar pathogen, changing epidemiology: A virulent strain has been appearing more often, even in patients not taking antibiotics. *Am J Nurs*, 106(5):33-36.

Vesta KS, Wells PG, Gentry CA, Stipek WJ. (2005). Specific risk factors for *Clostridium difficile*-associated diarrhea: A prospective, multicenter, case control evaluation. *Am J Infect Control*, 33(8):469-472.

Wullt M, Hagslatt ML, Odenholt I. (2003). *Lactobacillus plantarum* 299v for the treatment of recurrent *Clostridium difficile*-associated diarrhoea: A double-blind, placebo-controlled trial. *Scand J Infect Dis*, 35(6-7):365-367.

Yip C, Loeb M, Salama S, Moss L, Olde J. (2001). Quinolone use as a risk factor for nosocomial *Clostridium difficile*-associated diarrhea. *Infect Control Hosp Epidemiol*, 22(9):572-575.

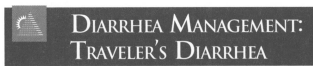

DIARRHEA MANAGEMENT: TRAVELER'S DIARRHEA

Kathleen A. Fitzgerald, PhD, RN

Definition: Management and alleviation of diarrhea associated with travel.

NURSING ACTIVITIES

Effective

■ ⓢⓟ *Teach the patient preventive measures to avoid food- and water-related bacterial diarrheal illnesses while traveling in high-risk areas.* **LOE=VII**

ⓔⓞ Foods and fluids to avoid include foods or beverages from street vendors or any area where less than hygienic conditions may exist, raw or undercooked meat or seafood, raw fruits or vegetables (unless self-peeled), tap water, ice, unpasteurized milk, or dairy products. Bottled water, hot tea and coffee, or beer and wine are generally safe to consume (CDC, 2006).

■ *Recognize that people who travel should generally avoid using prophylactic antibiotics.* **LOE=VII**

ⓔⓞ A review article on drug therapy for prevention of traveler's diarrhea emphasized the problem of the development of organisms resistant to antibiotics (tetracycline and trimethoprim-sulfamethoxazole). The 4-fluoroquinolones were effective in preventing traveler's diarrhea, but because the risk of the development of resistant bacteria outweighs the benefits, routine prescribing for prophylaxis was recommended only for people with chronic gastrointestinal, immunological, endocrine, and hematological disorders (Rendi-Wagner & Kollaritsch, 2002).

ⓜⓡ An RCT of rifaximin, a nonabsorbable antibiotic, was successful in preventing diarrhea caused by *Escherichia coli* in Mexico. Further studies are required to evaluate effectiveness in other bacteria-caused diarrhea (DuPont et al., 2005).

ⓜⓡ A systematic review of the use of bismuth, the active ingredient of Pepto-Bismol, to prevent traveler's diarrhea found only four original, experimental studies. When the data from the four studies were combined, it was determined that bismuth subsalicylate was effective in

---

RCT = Randomized Controlled (Clinical) Trial, **NIC** = Nursing Interventions Classification, **NOC** = Nursing Outcomes Classification

preventing traveler's diarrhea without the cost, side effects, and resistance associated with prophylactic antibiotic use (Rao et al., 2004).

■ Recognize that antibiotic treatment is the recommended therapy for traveler's diarrhea. LOE=I

(MR) A Cochrane review assessed the effects of antibiotics on traveler's diarrhea in relation to the duration of illness, severity of illness, and the adverse effects of antibiotics. A meta-analysis was not performed because of lack of consistency among the studies. The majority of trials utilizing antibiotics reported significant reduction in the duration of the diarrhea, with six trials reporting a greater number of subjects cured by 72 hours. Reports of medication side effects were higher in the treated versus placebo group. The review concluded that antibiotic treatment of traveler's diarrhea was associated with a shorter duration of diarrhea but a higher incidence of side effects (De Bruyn et al., 2000).

Possibly Effective

■ Instruct patients with traveler's diarrhea that the combination of antibiotics and probiotics may reduce the duration of the diarrhea. LOE=I

(MR) A Cochrane review assessed the effects of probiotics in infectious diarrhea. The analysis concluded that probiotics reduced the risk of diarrhea at 3 days with a mean duration of 30 to 48 hours. Subset analysis was unable to account for the influence of a specific type of probiotic, age of the subjects, or type of diarrheal illness on the results. The review concluded that probiotics appeared to be a useful adjunct to rehydration therapy in treating acute infectious diarrhea, but more research is necessary to identify specific probiotic regimens (Allen et al., 2004).

(MR) In a meta-analysis of nine RCT studies of the effect of probiotics on infectious diarrhea, the reduction of diarrhea duration and diarrhea frequency were used as the primary outcomes. Results indicated that use of *Lactobacillus* reduced the diarrhea duration by 0.7 day and reduced the diarrhea frequency to 1.6 stools on day 2 of treatment (Van Niel et al., 2002).

Not Effective

■ Using probiotics (yogurt or other foods containing active normal bacteria) for prevention of traveler's diarrhea. LOE=II

(MR) An RCT of healthy military recruits ($N=502$) demonstrated no significant effect of probiotics on the incidence of diarrhea. Recruits were given yogurt with *Lactobacillus casei* (probiotic) or plain yogurt. The difference in the incidence of diarrhea was not significant (Pereg et al., 2005).

(EO) In a review article, only one small study was located demonstrating probiotics to be effective in preventing traveler's diarrhea. Because of the lack of evidence, probiotics could not be recommended to prevent traveler's diarrhea (Rendi-Wagner & Kollaritsch, 2002).

(MR) In an RCT of 174 travelers, one randomized group served as the control using a placebo and the other interventional group took a nonviable *Lactobacillus acidophilus* twice daily start-

---

NR = Nursing Research, **MR** = Multidisciplinary Research, **SP** = Standard of Practice, **EO** = Expert Opinion, **LOE** = Level of Evidence

ing 1 day before departure and continuing until 3 days after their return. There was no significant difference in the onset of diarrhea and no beneficial effect of treatment with *L. acidophilus* (Briand et al., 2006).

Possibly Harmful

■ *Using antimotility agents if the patient has a fever or bloody diarrhea.* **LOE=VII**

EO Antimotility agents can increase the severity of traveler's diarrhea in these situations by delaying the clearance of the organisms through defecation. Toxic megacolon, sepsis, and disseminated intravascular coagulation have been reported from use of these medications to treat diarrhea (CDC, 2006).

OUTCOME MEASUREMENT

BOWEL ELIMINATION **NOC**

Definition: Formation and evacuation of stool.
Bowel Elimination as evidenced by the following selected NOC indicators:
• Stool soft and formed
• Control of bowel movements
• Comfort of stool passage
(Rate each indicator of **Bowel Elimination:** 1=severely compromised, 2=substantially compromised, 3=moderately compromised, 4=mildly compromised, 5=not compromised) (Moorhead et al., 2004).

REFERENCES

Allen SJ, Okoko B, Martinez E, Gregorio G, Dans LF. (2004). Probiotics for treating infectious diarrhoea. *Cochrane Database Syst Rev*, (2):CD003048.

Briand V, Buffet P, Genty S, Lacombe K, Godineau N, Salomon J, et al. (2006). Absence of efficacy of nonviable *Lactobacillus acidophilus* for the prevention of traveler's diarrhea: A randomized, double-blind, controlled study. *Clin Infect Dis*, 43(9):1170-1175.

Centers for Disease Control and Prevention (CDC). (2006). *Travelers' diarrhea.* Available online: http://www.cdc.gov/. Retrieved on May 10, 2007.

De Bruyn G, Hahn S, Borwick A. (2000). Antibiotic treatment for travellers' diarrhoea. *Cochrane Database Syst Rev*, (3):CD002242.

DuPont HL, Jiang Z, Okhuysen PC, Ericsson CD, de la Cabada FJ, Ke S, et al. (2005). A randomized, double-blind, placebo-controlled trial of rifaximin to prevent travelers' diarrhea. *Ann Intern Med*, 142(10):805-812.

Moorhead M, Johnson M, Maas M (Eds). (2004). *Nursing Outcomes Classification (NOC)*, 3rd ed. St. Louis: Mosby.

Pereg D, Kimhi O, Tirosh A, Orr N, Kayouf R, Lishner M. (2005). The effect of fermented yogurt on the prevention of diarrhea in a healthy adult population. *Am J Infect Control*, 33(2):122-125.

Rao G, Aliwalas MG, Slaymaker E, Brown B. (2004). Bismuth revisited: An effective way to prevent travelers' diarrhea. *J Travel Med*, 11(4):239-241.

RCT = Randomized Controlled (Clinical) Trial, **NIC** = Nursing Interventions Classification, **NOC** = Nursing Outcomes Classification

Rendi-Wagner P, Kollaritsch H. (2002). Drug prophylaxis for travelers' diarrhea. *Clin Infect Dis*, 34(5):628-633.

Van Niel CW, Feudtner C, Garrison MM, Christakis DA. (2002). Lactobacillus therapy for acute infectious diarrhea in children: A meta-analysis. *Pediatrics*, 109(4):678-684.

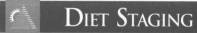 # DIET STAGING

Joseph T. DeRanieri, MSN, RN, CPN, BCECR

NIC **Definition:** Instituting required diet restrictions with subsequent progression of diet as tolerated (Dochterman & Bulechek, 2004).

NURSING ACTIVITIES

Effective

■ **NIC** *Determine presence of bowel sounds.* **LOE=VI**

NR A prospective survey demonstrated that bowel sounds may represent uncoordinated early contractions in the small intestines. A survey was sent to clinicians (*N*=246); bowel sounds were identified by participants as important (Madsen et al., 2005).

■ **NIC** *Determine if the patient is passing flatus.* **LOE=VI**

NR A prospective survey demonstrated that bowel sounds may represent uncoordinated early contractions in the small intestines. A survey was completed (*N*=246); the 15 included physicians ranked flatus as the top clinical parameter to indicate gastrointestinal motility (Madsen et al., 2005).

■ **NIC** *Progress the diet from clear liquid, full liquid, soft, to a regular or special diet as tolerated for adults and children.* **LOE=VII**

MR A multidisciplinary consensus paper reported that stroke patients' progress in diet should be based on the presence or absence of dysphagia. In the postacute phase, patients moved from a pureed to mechanically altered to advanced diet (Rotilio et al., 2004).

EO Nutritional management of patients after bariatric surgery demonstrates the progression of diet in the following order: clear liquid, full liquid, pureed/soft, solid foods (Parkes, 2006).

■ **NIC** *Monitor tolerance to ingestion of ice chips and water.* **LOE=VII**

EO Nutritional management of patients after bariatric surgery supports patients starting with a clear liquid diet (Parkes, 2006).

■ **NIC** **SP** *Institute NPO as needed.* **LOE=VII**

■ **NIC** **SP** *Clamp the NG tube and monitor tolerance as appropriate.* **LOE=VII**

■ **NIC** **SP** *Post the diet restrictions at bedside, on the chart, and in the care plan.* **LOE=VII**

NR = Nursing Research, **MR** = Multidisciplinary Research, **SP** = Standard of Practice, **EO** = Expert Opinion, **LOE** = Level of Evidence

Possibly Effective

No applicable published research was found in this category.

Not Effective

No applicable published research was found in this category.

Possibly Harmful

No applicable published research was found in this category.

OUTCOME MEASUREMENT

NUTRITIONAL STATUS   NOC

Definition: Extent to which nutrients are available to meet metabolic needs.
Nutritional Status as evidenced by the following selected NOC indicators:

- Nutrient intake
- Fluid intake
- Food intake
- Hydration

(Rate each indicator of **Nutritional Status:** 1=severe deviation from normal range, 2=substantial deviation from normal range, 3=moderate deviation from normal range, 4=mild deviation from normal range, 5=no deviation from normal range) (Moorhead et al., 2004).

REFERENCES

Dochterman JM, Bulechek GM (Eds). (2004). *Nursing Interventions Classification (NIC),* 4th ed. St. Louis: Mosby.

Madsen D, Sebolt T, Cullen L, Folkedahl B, Mueller T, Richardson C, et al. (2005). Listening to bowel sounds: An evidence-based practice project: Nurses find that a traditional practice isn't the best indicator of returning gastrointestinal motility in patients who've undergone abdominal surgery. *Am J Nurs,* 105(12):40-49.

Moorhead M, Johnson M, Maas M (Eds). (2004). *Nursing Outcomes Classification (NOC),* 3rd ed. St. Louis: Mosby.

Parkes E. (2006). Nutritional management of patients after bariatric surgery. *Am J Med Sci,* 331(4): 207-213.

Rotilio G, Berni Cananf R, Branca F, Cairella G, Fieschi C, Garbagagnatf F, et al. (2004). Nutritional recommendations for the management of stroke patients. *Rivista Italiana di Nutrizione Paremterale ed Enterale,* 22(4):227-236.

DISCHARGE PLANNING   NIC

Diane E. Holland, PhD, RN

NIC **Definition:** Preparation for moving a patient from one level of care to another within or outside the current health care agency (Dochterman & Bulechek, 2004).

RCT = Randomized Controlled (Clinical) Trial, **NIC** = Nursing Interventions Classification, **NOC** = Nursing Outcomes Classification

NURSING ACTIVITIES

Effective

■ **NIC** *Assist the patient/family/significant others in planning for the supportive environment necessary to provide the patient's posthospital care.* **LOE=II**

(Please refer to the guideline on Environmental Management: Home Preparation.)

■ **NIC** *Arrange for caregiver support, as appropriate.* **LOE=I**

NR A systematic review of family caregiver intervention research identified that social support for caregivers decreased caregiver distress, improved caregiver physical health, and delayed care-receiver nursing home placement (Farran, 2001).

NR A systematic review of stress and coping among caregivers of people with traumatic brain injuries demonstrated that social support contributed to the development of effective coping mechanisms by caregivers (Verhaeghe et al., 2005).

MR An RCT (N=296) of family support over 1 year of caregiving for a person following stroke demonstrated that family support significantly improved quality of life for caregivers (Mant et al., 2005).

■ **NIC** *Coordinate referrals relevant to linkages among health care providers.* **LOE=I**

NR A systematic review demonstrated that access to health and social services resources was problematic for older adults. Referrals by health care providers were a necessary priority in the transitional care of older adults (Naylor, 2002).

NR A systematic review of interventions designed to alleviate caregiver distress in family members of older people with cancer concluded that coordinating care could affect distress (Given & Sherwood, 2006).

MR A systematic review demonstrated that caregivers of people with dementia who did not use support services mainly lacked awareness of the availability of support services (Brodaty et al., 2005).

NR A qualitative exploratory study (N=10) of older adults with cognitive impairment and their caregivers revealed that referrals to and communication with home care service providers were essential (Naylor et al., 2005).

■ **NIC** *Communicate the patient's discharge plans, as appropriate.* **LOE=I**

NR A systematic review of transitional care of older people identified effective communication between health care team members, patients, and family as an essential characteristic of quality discharge planning (Naylor, 2002).

Possibly Effective

■ *Assist the patient/family/significant others in discharge planning.* **LOE=IV**

MR A systematic review of comprehensive discharge planning protocols concluded that evidence from RCTs was not available to support the general adoption of discharge planning protocols or discharge support schemes as means of improving discharge outcomes (Parker et al., 2002).

NR = Nursing Research, **MR** = Multidisciplinary Research, **SP** = Standard of Practice, **EO** = Expert Opinion, **LOE** = Level of Evidence

(MR) A systematic review of discharge planning interventions for older patients with congestive heart failure identified that for most studies the intervention was not explicitly described (Phillips et al., 2004).

(NR) A systematic review of transitional care (including discharge planning) of older adults concluded that evidence about the effects on patients' quality and cost of care was sparse (Naylor, 2002).

■ **NIC** **SP** *Assist the patient/family/significant others to prepare for discharge.* **LOE=VII**

Assist in preparing for discharge by:
• Encouraging self-care, as appropriate.
• Assessing the patient's and primary caregiver's understanding of knowledge or skills required after discharge.
• Identifying patient's teaching needed for postdischarge care.
• Developing a plan that considers the health care and social needs of the patient.
• Documenting the patient's discharge plans on the patient's chart.
• Coordinating efforts of different health care providers in planning for continuity of health care.
• Monitoring readiness for discharge.
• Arranging discharge to the next level of care.

(EO) The preceding interventions are included as part of a nursing standard of practice protocol for discharge planning (Zwicker & Picariello, 2003; Ignatavicius & Workman, 2006; Taylor et al., 2005).

(EO) Assessment of patient's readiness for discharge is important for patient's safety, satisfaction, and outcomes (Weiss et al., 2007).

(EO) Identifying family and others who are willing, able, and available to provide needed postdischarge support is an essential part of nursing case management (Cohen & Cesta, 2005; CMSA, 2002).

OUTCOME MEASUREMENT

DISCHARGE READINESS: SUPPORTED LIVING   **NOC**

Definition: Readiness of a patient to relocate from a health care institution to a lower level of supported living.

Discharge Readiness: Supported Living as evidenced by the following NOC indicators:
• Patient needs consistent with available staff support
• Patient needs consistent with available family support
• Oriented to care at new residence
• Accepts transfer to new residence
• Describes special needs
• Describes short-term plan
• Describes long-term plan
• Describes plan for continuity in care

(Rate each indicator of **Discharge Readiness: Supported Living**: 1=never demonstrated, 2=rarely demonstrated, 3=sometimes demonstrated, 4=often demonstrated, 5=consistently demonstrated) (Moorhead et al., 2004).

Continued

OUTCOME MEASUREMENT—*cont'd*

DISCHARGE READINESS: INDEPENDENT LIVING NOC

Definition: Readiness of a patient to relocate from a health care institution to living independently.

Discharge Readiness: Independent Living as evidenced by the following selected NOC indicators:

- Seeks assistance appropriately
- Uses available social support
- Describes signs and symptoms to health care professional
- Describes prescribed treatments
- Describes risks for complications
- Manages own medications
- Performs activities of daily living (ADLs) independently
- Performs instrumental activities of daily living (IADLs) independently

(Rate each indicator of **Discharge Readiness: Independent Living:** 1 = never demonstrated, 2 = rarely demonstrated, 3 = sometimes demonstrated, 4 = often demonstrated, 5 = consistently demonstrated) (Moorhead et al., 2004).

SELF-DIRECTION OF CARE NOC

Definition: Care recipient actions taken to direct others who assist with or perform physical tasks and personal health care.

Self-Direction of Care as evidenced by the following selected NOC indicators:

- Sets health care goals
- Describes appropriate care
- Obtains resources as necessary
- Instructs others in appropriate care behaviors

(Rate each indicator of **Self-Direction of Care:** 1 = never demonstrated, 2 = rarely demonstrated, 3 = sometimes demonstrated, 4 = often demonstrated, 5 = consistently demonstrated) (Moorhead et al., 2004).

HEALTH-SEEKING BEHAVIOR NOC

Definition: Personal actions to promote optimal wellness, recovery, and rehabilitation.

Health-Seeking Behavior as evidenced by the following selected NOC indicators:

- Seeks assistance from health care professionals when indicated
- Performs ADLs consistent with energy and tolerance
- Performs prescribed health behavior when indicated
- Seeks current health-related information

(Rate each indicator of **Health-Seeking Behavior:** 1 = never demonstrated, 2 = rarely demonstrated, 3 = sometimes demonstrated, 4 = often demonstrated, 5 = consistently demonstrated) (Moorhead et al., 2004).

SAFE HOME ENVIRONMENT NOC

Definition: Physical arrangements to minimize environmental factors that might cause physical harm or injury in the home.

NR = Nursing Research, **MR** = Multidisciplinary Research, **SP** = Standard of Practice, **EO** = Expert Opinion, **LOE** = Level of Evidence

OUTCOME MEASUREMENT—*cont'd*

Safe Home Environment as evidenced by the following selected NOC indicators:
- Placement of handrails
- Smoke detector maintenance
- Provision of assistive devices in accessible location
- Provision of equipment that meets safety standards
- Arrangement of furniture to reduce risks

(Rate each indicator of **Safe Home Environment:** 1 = not adequate, 2 = slightly adequate, 3 = moderately adequate, 4 = substantially adequate, 5 = totally adequate) (Moorhead et al., 2004).

REFERENCES

Brodaty H, Thomson C, Thompson C, Fine M. (2005). Why caregivers of people with dementia and memory loss don't use services. *Int J Geriatr Psychiatry*, 20(6):537-546.

Case Management Society of America (CMSA). (2002). *Standards of Practice for Case Management*, Little Rock, AR: CMSA.

Cohen EL, Cesta TG. (Eds). (2005). *Nursing Case Management*, 4th ed. St Louis: Elsevier.

Dochterman JM, Bulechek GM (Eds). (2004). *Nursing Interventions Classification (NIC)*, 4th ed. St. Louis: Mosby.

Farran CJ. (2001). Family caregiver intervention research: Where have we been? Where are we going? *J Gerontol Nurs*, 27(7):38-45.

Given B, Sherwood PR. (2006). Family care for the older person with cancer. *Semin Oncol Nurs*, 22(1):43-50.

Ignatavicius DD, Workman ML (Eds). (2006). *Medical surgical nursing: Critical thinking for collaborative care*, 5th ed. St. Louis: Saunders.

Mant J, Winner S, Roche J, Wade DT. (2005). Family support for stroke: One year follow up of a randomised controlled trial. *J Neurol Neurosurg Psychiatry*, 76(7):1006-1008.

Moorhead M, Johnson M, Maas M (Eds). (2004). *Nursing Outcomes Classification (NOC)*, 3rd ed. St. Louis, Mosby.

Naylor MD. (2002). Transitional care of older adults. *Annu Rev Nurs Res*, 20:127-147.

Naylor MD, Stephens C, Bowles KH, Bixby MB. (2005). Cognitively impaired older adults: From hospital to home. *Am J Nurs*, 105(2):52-61.

Parker SG, Peet SM, McPherson A, Cannaby AM, Abrams K, Baker R, et al. (2002). A systematic review of discharge arrangements for older people. *Health Technol Assess*, 6(4):1-183.

Phillips CO, Wright SM, Kern DE, Singa RM, Shepperd S, Rubin HR. (2004). Comprehensive discharge planning with postdischarge support for older patients with congestive heart failure: A meta-analysis. *JAMA*, 291(11):1358-1367.

Taylor C, Lillis C, LeMone P (Eds). (2005). *Fundamentals of nursing: The art and science of nursing care*, Philadelphia: Lippincott Williams & Wilkins.

Verhaeghe S, Defloor T, Grypdonck M. (2005). Stress and coping among families of patients with traumatic brain injury: A review of the literature. *J Clin Nurs*, 14(8):1004-1012.

Weiss ME, Piacentine LB, Lokken L, Ancona J, Archer J, Gresser S, et al. (2007). Perceived readiness for hospital discharge in adult medical-surgical patients. *Clin Nurs Spec*, 21(1):31-42.

Zwicker D, Picariello G. (2003). Discharge planning for the older adult. In Mezey M, Fulmer T, Abraham I (Eds): *Geriatric nursing protocols for best practice*, New York: Springer.

RCT = Randomized Controlled (Clinical) Trial, **NIC** = Nursing Interventions Classification, **NOC** = Nursing Outcomes Classification

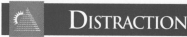

DISTRACTION

Kathleen L. Patusky, PhD, APRN-BC

NIC **Definition:** Purposeful focusing of attention away from undesirable sensations (Dochterman & Bulechek, 2004).

NURSING ACTIVITIES

Effective

■ **NIC** *Instruct the patient on the benefits of stimulating a variety of senses (e.g., through music, counting, television, and reading).* **LOE=II**

NR A four-group controlled study (*N*=80) of massage, verbal coaching, and slow breathing or massage plus verbal coaching and slow breathing versus usual care alone, with patients receiving ocular block injection anesthesia prior to cataract surgery, demonstrated that any of the distraction combinations were superior to usual care in reducing anxiety and discomfort (Simmons et al., 2004).

NR A review of music therapy used with older adults indicated that music could be used for relaxation and distraction (Kramer, 2001).

NR An RCT (*N*=99) of the effect of audio-taped lullabies on children ages 3 to 6 years during routine immunization demonstrated that, although pain perception and physiological measures across five time points (baseline through 2 minutes after immunization) were the same for experimental and control groups, total distress was significantly less for the lullaby group (Megel et al., 1998).

■ **NIC** *Consider distraction techniques as play, activity therapy, reading stories, singing songs, or rhythm activities for children that are novel, appeal to more than one sense, and do not require literacy or thinking ability.* **LOE=II**

NR A three-group controlled study (*N*=105) of 4- to 6-year-old children receiving DPT immunizations was conducted with the distraction interventions of touch, bubble blowing, or standard care. Both the touch and bubble blowing groups showed decreased pain perception compared with the standard care group (Sparks, 2001).

NR A three-group controlled study of preschool children receiving immunizations (*N*=80) and distracted with a party blower or a pinwheel found that children's distress and parental rating of strength needed to hold the child were significantly lower with the party blower. The party blower was more distracting than the pinwheel (Bowen & Dammeyer, 1999).

NR An RCT (*N*=99) of the effect of audio-taped lullabies on children ages 3 to 6 years during routine immunization demonstrated that, although pain perception and physiological measures across five time points (baseline through 2 minutes after immunization) were the same for experimental and control groups, total distress was significantly less for the lullaby group (Megel et al., 1998).

NR = Nursing Research, **MR** = Multidisciplinary Research, **SP** = Standard of Practice, **EO** = Expert Opinion, **LOE** = Level of Evidence

■ **NIC** *Suggest techniques consistent with energy level, ability, age appropriateness, developmental level, and effective use in the past.* **LOE=I**

NR A review of pain management in aging found that nonpharmacological techniques currently in use included cognitive behavioral therapy, guided imagery, and other types of distraction (Hanks-Bell et al., 2004).

NR A systematic review of the literature on clinical guidelines for managing acute pain in older adults demonstrated that relaxation techniques (including the Jacobson jaw relaxation technique), guided imagery, and other distraction techniques could be used to focus attention away from pain. However, patients may not appear to be in pain while distracted—which should be factored into assessment—and physical or mental fatigue may interfere with distraction techniques (Ardery et al., 2003).

NR In a controlled study of 30 adolescents with cancer receiving a lumbar puncture (LP), with 17 using virtual reality (VR) glasses to view a video, there was no difference in pain scores between the two groups. However, the pain scores tended to be lower in the VR group, and the majority of intervention participants reported that the VR experience did help distract them from the LP (Sander Wint et al., 2002).

NR A three-group controlled study (N=105) of 4- to 6-year olds receiving DPT immunizations was conducted with the distraction interventions of touch, bubble blowing, or standard care. Both the touch and bubble blowing groups showed decreased pain perception compared with the standard care group (Sparks, 2001).

NR A three-group controlled study of preschool children receiving immunizations (N=80) and distracted with a party blower or a pinwheel found that children's distress and parental rating of strength needed to hold the child were significantly lower with the party blower. The party blower was more distracting than the pinwheel (Bowen & Dammeyer, 1999).

NR An RCT (N=99) of the effect of audio-taped lullabies on children ages 3 to 6 years during routine immunization demonstrated that, although pain perception and physiological measures across five time points (baseline through 2 minutes after immunization) were the same for experimental and control groups, total distress was significantly less for the lullaby group (Megel et al., 1998).

■ *Use distraction with patients having pain or disability to enhance physical function.* **LOE=I**

MR A Cochrane systematic review found that cognitive therapy and progressive relaxation therapy were more effective than waitlist control in the short-term relief of chronic low back pain. No differences were found between various types of cognitive-behavioral therapy, and long-term results were unknown. The authors could not conclude whether behavioral treatment was superior to active conservative treatment (Ostelo et al., 2005).

MR A Cochrane systematic review found that cognitive-behavioral therapy significantly aided the physical functioning of outpatients with chronic fatigue syndrome (CFS). No evidence was found for effectiveness with milder forms of CFS, with level of disability that prevents attendance at outpatient treatment, or with group cognitive-behavioral therapy. Further studies were recommended (Price & Couper, 2000).

Note: Distraction techniques are used in cognitive-behavioral therapies as a form of coping strategy.

RCT = Randomized Controlled (Clinical) Trial, **NIC** = Nursing Interventions Classification, **NOC** = Nursing Outcomes Classification

■ *Use distraction with adults for perioperative interventions or for medical procedures to decrease pain and/or anxiety.* **LOE=I**

(NR) A systematic review of perioperative procedures found that distraction techniques (music, short stories, relaxation) could decrease preoperative anxiety (Richardson-Tench et al., 2005). **LOE=II**

(NR) A four-group controlled study ($N=80$) of massage, verbal coaching, and slow breathing or massage plus verbal coaching and slow breathing versus usual care alone, with patients receiving ocular block injection anesthesia prior to cataract surgery, demonstrated that any of the distraction combinations were superior to usual care in reducing anxiety and discomfort (Simmons et al., 2004).

(NR) An RCT ($N=96$) of distraction use with adults (a kaleidoscope) during phlebotomy demonstrated that adults using the kaleidoscope experienced lower perceived pain than members of the control group (Cason & Grissom, 1997).

(MR) An RCT ($N=80$) of distraction therapy using nature scenes or sounds versus no distraction therapy with adults undergoing fiberoptic bronchoscopy demonstrated that the intervention, applied before, during, and after the procedure, significantly reduced pain, although anxiety was not reduced. In one adverse event, a patient listening to a tape of nature sounds urinated during the procedure and attributed this to sounds of running water (Diette et al., 2003).

■ *Use distraction with adult cancer patients to reduce nausea and vomiting.* **LOE=I**

(NR) A systematic review of the literature on chemotherapy-related nausea and vomiting demonstrated that distraction techniques could be used as adjuncts to standard antiemetic therapies as a means of optimizing quality of life (Miller & Kearney, 2004).

(NR) An RCT ($N=60$) involving Japanese cancer patients receiving chemotherapy demonstrated that progressive muscle relaxation training reduced nausea and vomiting during the first cycle of chemotherapy. Additional study is needed to determine whether the results hold for subsequent chemotherapy cycles (Arakawa, 1997).

(MR) An RCT of Chinese cancer patients receiving chemotherapy determined that the duration and intensity of nausea were lower in the experimental group (borderline significance), but both experimental and control groups experienced nausea and vomiting with subsequent chemotherapy cycles (Molassiotis, 2000).

(MR) An RCT ($N=60$) of cancer patients examined three interventions (cognitive distraction, relaxation, control) by two psychological states (high anxiety, low anxiety) across five chemotherapy sessions with the following findings: less nausea before and lower systolic BP after chemotherapy with distraction as compared with controls; less nausea before and lower systolic and diastolic BP after chemotherapy with relaxation as compared with controls; and no significant differences between the distraction and relaxation groups on measures (Vasterling et al., 1993).

■ *Use distraction with children as a diversion to reduce distress and pain during immunization.* **LOE=II**

(NR) A three-group controlled study ($N=105$) of 4- to 6-year olds receiving DPT immunizations was conducted with the distraction interventions of touch, bubble blowing, or standard care. Both the touch and bubble blowing groups showed decreased pain perception compared with the standard care group (Sparks, 2001).

(NR) A three-group controlled study of preschool children receiving immunizations ($N=80$) and distracted with a party blower or a pinwheel found that children's distress and parental rating of strength needed to hold the child were significantly lower with the party blower. The party blower was more distracting than the pinwheel (Bowen & Dammeyer, 1999).

(NR) An RCT ($N=99$) of the effect of audio-taped lullabies on children ages 3 to 6 years during routine immunization demonstrated that, although pain perception and physiological measures across five time points (baseline through 2 minutes after immunization) were the same for experimental and control groups, total distress was significantly less for the lullaby group (Megel et al., 1998).

■ *Use distraction with children to reduce physiological pain or anxiety.* **LOE=I**

(NR) A controlled study ($N=76$) of children with musculoskeletal trauma comparing the effect of standard care, ibuprofen, and distraction on pain demonstrated that allowing children to select music or toys as distracters served as an effective adjunct to analgesia, with pain reduction maintained at 60 minutes (Tanabe et al., 2002).

(MR) A Cochrane systematic review found that relaxation and cognitive behavior therapy were effective in decreasing the severity and frequency of headache pain in children and adolescents. Little or no evidence was found for other types of pain or for improving consequences of pain (Eccleston et al., 2003).

■ *Instruct the patient/family member on the benefits of distraction.* **LOE=II**

(MR) An RCT ($N=44$) of parental distraction education for use with chronically ill children receiving IVs demonstrated that the experimental group did use significantly more distraction than the control group. Although there were no differences between the groups in children's distress or pain, there was a trend toward reduced behavioral distress between the preparation phase and the needle insertion phase for the experimental group (Kleiber et al., 2001).

Possibly Effective

■ (NIC) *Encourage the individual to choose the distraction technique(s) desired, such as music, engaging in conversation or telling a detailed account of an event or story, guided imagery, or humor.* **LOE=II**

(NR) A systematic review of perioperative procedures found that distraction techniques (music, short stories, relaxation) could decrease preoperative anxiety (Richardson-Tench et al., 2005).

(NR) A review of pain management in aging found that nonpharmacological techniques currently in use included cognitive-behavioral therapy, guided imagery, and other types of distraction (Hanks-Bell et al., 2004).

(NR) A three-group RCT ($N=58$) of listening to patient-chosen music, listening to patient-chosen books on tape, and usual care with cancer patients undergoing medical procedures (e.g., tissue biopsy, port placement or removal) demonstrated no significant differences between the groups with regard to levels of pain, anxiety, or perceived control. Some patients found both types of distraction to be an annoyance or an interference with attending to the physician, the procedure, and what was happening to them, leading to the conclusion that patients should be given the choice of the use/type of distraction (Kwekkeboom, 2003).

RCT = Randomized Controlled (Clinical) Trial, **NIC** = Nursing Interventions Classification, **NOC** = Nursing Outcomes Classification

(NR) A controlled study ($N=76$) of children with musculoskeletal trauma comparing the effect of standard care, ibuprofen, and distraction on pain demonstrated that allowing children to select music or toys as distracters served as an effective adjunct to analgesia, with pain reduction maintained at 60 minutes (Tanabe et al., 2002).

■ *Use distraction to assist asthma patients with breathing control and improved health.* **LOE=I**

(MR) A Cochrane systematic review found that existing studies were insufficient to indicate that relaxation therapy and cognitive-behavioral therapy were effective treatments for improving health outcomes for adults with asthma. Better designed studies were recommended (Yorke et al., 2006).

(MR) A Cochrane systematic review found that no RCTs were available to evaluate the use of the "Alexander technique," a form of physical therapy that corrects posture and may aid relaxation, in people with chronic, stable asthma. More research was recommended (Dennis, 2000).

■ *Use distraction as an adjunct in programs to achieve a healthy weight.* **LOE=I**

(NR) An evidence-based review in support of an eating disorder program provided anecdotal support for the use of distraction techniques, including milieu activities and "feeling masks," to decrease anxiety among pediatric patients (Breiner, 2003).

(MR) A Cochrane systematic review found that cognitive-behavioral therapy improved weight loss among overweight or obese individuals, although cognitive therapy alone was not effective. Insufficient evidence addressed relaxation therapy and hypnotherapy to offer a conclusion, but available evidence suggested that these therapies might also be useful (Shaw et al., 2005).

(MR) A Cochrane systematic review found that there was insufficient evidence to indicate that behavioral therapies, including relaxation, were useful in treating childhood obesity. Further research was recommended (Summerbell et al., 2003).

■ *Use distraction to assist patients with mental disorders to overcome or become more comfortable with symptoms.* **LOE=I**

(MR) A Cochrane systematic review found that existing studies were insufficient to indicate that meditation therapy was an effective treatment for anxiety. One study showed that transcendental meditation decreased anxiety compared with relaxation therapy and biofeedback, and another study showed no difference between Kundalini yoga and relaxation/mindfulness meditation. Further research was recommended (Krisanaprakornkit et al., 2006).

(MR) A Cochrane systematic review examined studies on the use of distraction techniques with the mental state and hallucinations of schizophrenia. Although no clear effect was found, the authors recommended further trials and better designed studies because even a negligible effect could prove clinically useful (Crawford-Walker et al., 2005).

(MR) A Cochrane systematic review found that existing studies were insufficient to indicate that hypnosis was an effective treatment for the symptoms of schizophrenia. Better designed studies were recommended (Izquierdo & Khan, 2004).

■ *Use distraction with specific disorders to enhance functioning.* **LOE=I**

(MR) A Cochrane systematic review of nonulcer dyspepsia found that existing studies could not confirm the efficacy of psychological interventions, including relaxation therapy, hypnosis, and cognitive-behavioral therapy, as treatments. Better designed trials were recommended (Soo et al., 2005).

(MR) A Cochrane systematic review found no RCTs and no evidence apart from uncontrolled case studies that relaxation techniques were useful in treating vaginismus. Better designed studies with controls were recommended (McGuire & Hawton, 2003).

▪ *Use distraction with adult cancer patients to reduce distress, fatigue, nausea, and vomiting.* **LOE=II**

(NR) A crossover study of 20 women (ages 18 to 55 years) receiving chemotherapy for breast cancer serving as their own controls demonstrated that the use of virtual reality (VR) distraction resulted in reduced symptom distress and fatigue following chemotherapy (Schneider et al., 2004).

(NR) A three-group RCT ($N=58$) of listening to patient-chosen music, listening to patient-chosen books on tape, and usual care with cancer patients undergoing medical procedures (e.g., tissue biopsy, port placement or removal) demonstrated no significant differences between the groups with regard to levels of pain, anxiety, or perceived control. Some patients found both types of distraction to be an annoyance or an interference with attending to the physician, the procedure, and what was happening to them, leading to the conclusion that patients should be given the choice of the use/type of distraction (Kwekkeboom, 2003).

▪ *Use distraction with children for perioperative interventions or for medical procedures to reduce pain and/or anxiety.* **LOE=I**

(NR) An RCT ($N=43$) comparing the effect of parental positioning and age-appropriate child distracters versus standard care on pain, fear, and distress during venipuncture found that, although children in the intervention group did not report lower levels of pain and fear, child life specialist and parental ratings of the child's fear level were significantly lower for the intervention group. Despite the lack of significance for children's responses, the levels of self-reported fear, self-reported pain, and observed distress in the experimental group tended to be lower, prompting the recommendation for further study (Cavender et al., 2004).

(NR) In a controlled study of 30 adolescents with cancer receiving a lumbar puncture (LP), with 17 using VR glasses to view a video, there was no difference in pain scores between the two groups. However, the pain scores tended to be lower in the VR group, and the majority of intervention participants reported that the VR experience did help distract them from the LP (Sander Wint et al., 2002).

(NR) An RCT ($N=384$, at 13 children's hospitals) of distraction (use of illusion kaleidoscope) versus verbal preoccupation and standard care in reducing distress, pain, and fear during venipuncture or IV insertion with children ages 4 to 18 years did not demonstrate a significant difference between the approaches. The authors noted that multiple factors may have influenced results and recommended further study of distraction as an intervention that has been supported anecdotally (Carlson et al., 2000).

(NR) A systematic review and meta-analysis of children's distress behavior and pain during medical procedures found that distraction had a positive effect on distress behavior; the effect on pain varied with age (Kleiber & Harper, 1999).

(MR) An RCT ($N=240$) of nonpharmacological means of pain and anxiety management for children ages 6 to 18 years receiving laceration repair in the emergency department demonstrated that, although age-appropriate distracters did not affect the pain perception in children

RCT = Randomized Controlled (Clinical) Trial, **NIC** = Nursing Interventions Classification, **NOC** = Nursing Outcomes Classification

younger than 10 years, distracters were effective in reducing anxiety for older children and in reducing parents' perception of pain distress in younger children (Sinha et al., 2006).

(MR) An RCT (*N*=40) of using clown doctors to address preoperative anxiety in children ages 5 to 12 years demonstrated that the practice, combined with parental presence, significantly reduced the children's and parents' anxiety during anesthesia induction compared with the control group. However, medical personnel resisted the intervention because they felt it interfered with operating room procedures (Vagnoli et al., 2005).

Use distraction with pediatric or adolescent cancer patients to reduce discomfort. LOE=IV

(NR) In a controlled study of 30 adolescents with cancer receiving an LP, with 17 using VR glasses to view a video, there was no difference in pain scores between the two groups. However, the pain scores tended to be lower in the VR group, and the majority of intervention participants reported that the VR experience did help distract them from the LP (Sander Wint et al., 2002).

(NR) A pilot controlled study (*N*=11) of 10- to 17-year-old chemotherapy patients reported that the use of a VR device as a distracter resulted in a more positive perception of the treatment for 82% of the children, with all participants stating they would like to use the VR for future treatments. Further investigation was recommended (Schneider & Workman, 2000).

Use distraction with older adults for pain management and as a diversion from agitation. LOE=I

(NR) A review of pain management in aging found that nonpharmacological techniques currently in use included cognitive-behavioral therapy, guided imagery, and other types of distraction (Hanks-Bell et al., 2004).

(NR) A systematic review of the literature on clinical guidelines for managing acute pain in older adults demonstrated that relaxation techniques (including the Jacobson jaw relaxation technique), guided imagery, and other distraction techniques could be used to focus attention away from pain. However, patients may not appear to be in pain while distracted—which should be factored into assessment—and physical or mental fatigue may interfere with distraction techniques (Ardery et al., 2003).

(NR) A review of music therapy used with older adults indicated that music can be used for relaxation and distraction (Kramer, 2001).

(MR) A review of treatment strategies for older adults with arthritis indicated that nonpharmacological approaches in use included cognitive therapy, massage, relaxation, and other distraction techniques (Blumstein & Gorevic, 2005).

(MR) A Cochrane systematic review identified one small, methodologically flawed trial that supported the use of aromatherapy for the agitation and neuropsychiatric symptoms of dementia. Large-scale RCTs were recommended before firm conclusions could be offered (Thorgrimsen et al., 2003).

Not Effective

Use of distraction to decrease the seizures of epilepsy. LOE=I

(MR) A Cochrane systematic review of epilepsy found no evidence that relaxation therapy, cognitive-behavioral therapy, EEG, or biofeedback, alone or in combination, had an effect on seizures or quality of life (Ramaratnam et al., 2005).

NR = Nursing Research, **MR** = Multidisciplinary Research, **SP** = Standard of Practice, **EO** = Expert Opinion, **LOE** = Level of Evidence

■ *Use of distraction with children to reduce anxiety during dental treatment.*
LOE=II

(MR) An RCT (*N*=60) of choice-based distraction using a wide variety of CDs with children ages 5 to 12 years receiving routine dental treatment demonstrated that, although dentists were more likely to rate the distraction group as "cooperative," the intervention as assessed by direct coded observation of average disruptive behavior was not sufficient to reduce distress or behavioral problems (Filcheck et al., 2004).

Possibly Harmful

No applicable published research was found in this category.

OUTCOME MEASUREMENT

HEALTH-PROMOTING BEHAVIOR   (NOC)

Definition: Personal actions to sustain or increase wellness.
Health-Promoting Behavior as evidenced by the following selected NOC indicators:
• Uses effective stress reduction behaviors
• Performs healthy behaviors routinely
(Rate each indicator of **Health-Promoting Behavior:** 1=never demonstrated, 2=rarely demonstrated, 3=sometimes demonstrated, 4=often demonstrated, 5=consistently demonstrated) (Moorhead et al., 2004).

REFERENCES

Arakawa S. (1997). Relaxation to reduce nausea, vomiting and anxiety induced by chemotherapy in Japanese patients. *Cancer Nurs,* 20(5):342-349.

Ardery G, Herr KA, Titler MG, Sorofman BA, Schmitt MB. (2003). Assessing and managing acute pain in older adults: A research base to guide practice. *Medsurg Nurs,* 12(1):7-18.

Blumstein H, Gorevic PD. (2005). Rheumatologic illnesses: Treatment strategies for older adults. *Geriatrics,* 60(6):28-35.

Bowen AM, Dammeyer MM. (1999). Reducing children's immunization distress in a primary care setting. *J Pediatr Nurs,* 14(5):296-303.

Breiner S. (2003). An evidence-based eating disorder program. *J Pediatr Nurs,* 18(1):75-80.

Carlson KL, Broome M, Vessey JA. (2000). Using distraction to reduce reported pain, fear, and behavioral distress in children and adolescents: A multisite study. *J Soc Pediatr Nurs,* 5(2):75-85.

Cason CL, Grissom NL. (1997). Ameliorating adults' acute pain during phlebotomy with a distraction intervention. *Appl Nurs Res,* 10(4):168-173.

Cavender K, Goff MD, Hollon EC, Guzzetta CE. (2004). Parents' positioning and distracting children during venipuncture. Effects on children's pain, fear, and distress. *J Holist Nurs,* 22(1):32-56.

Crawford-Walker CJ, King A, Chan S. (2005). Distraction techniques for schizophrenia. *Cochrane Database Syst Rev,* (1):CD004717.

Dennis J. (2000). Alexander technique for chronic asthma. *Cochrane Database Syst Rev,* (2):CD000995.

Diette GB, Lechtzin N, Haponik E, Devrotes A, Rubin HR. (2003). Distraction therapy with nature sights and sounds reduces pain during flexible bronchoscopy. A complementary approach to routine analgesia. *Chest,* 123(3):941-948.

Dochterman JM, Bulechek GM (Eds). (2004). *Nursing Interventions Classification (NIC),* 4th ed. St. Louis: Mosby.

Eccleston C, Yorke L, Morley S, Williams AC, Mastroyannopoulou K. (2003). Psychological therapies for the management of chronic and recurrent pain in children and adolescents. *Cochrane Database Syst Rev*, (1):CD003968.

Filcheck HA, Allen KD, Ogren H, Darby JB, Holstein B, Hupp S. (2004). The use of choice-based distraction to decrease the distress of children at the dentist. *Child Fam Behav Ther*, 26(4):59-68.

Hanks-Bell M, Halvey K, Paice JA. (2004). Pain assessment and management in aging. *Online J Issues Nurs*, 9(3):8.

Izquierdo SA, Khan M. (2004). Hypnosis for schizophrenia. *Cochrane Database Syst Rev*, (3):CD004160.

Kleiber C, Craft-Rosenberg M, Harper DC. (2001). Parents as distraction coaches during i.v. insertion: A randomized study. *J Pain Symptom Manage*, 22(4):851-861.

Kleiber C, Harper DC. (1999). Effects of distraction on children's pain and distress during medical procedures: A meta-analysis. *Nurs Res*, 48(1):44-49.

Kramer MK. (2001). A trio to treasure: The elderly, the nurse, and music. *Geriatr Nurs*, 22(4):191-195.

Krisanaprakornkit T, Krisanaprakornkit W, Piyavhatkul N, Laopaiboon M. (2006). Meditation therapy for anxiety disorders. *Cochrane Database Syst Rev*, (1):CD004998.

Kwekkeboom KL. (2003). Music versus distraction for procedural pain and anxiety in patients with cancer. *Oncol Nurs Forum*, 30(3):433-440.

McGuire H, Hawton K. (2003). Interventions for vaginismus. *Cochrane Database Syst Rev*, (1):CD001760.

Megel ME, Houser CW, Gleaves LS. (1998). Children's responses to immunizations: Lullabies as distraction. *Issues Compr Pediatr Nurs*, 21(3):129-145.

Miller M, Kearney N. (2004). Chemotherapy-related nausea and vomiting—Past reflections, present practice and future management. *Eur J Cancer Care*, 13(1):71-81.

Molassiotis A. (2000). A pilot study of the use of progressive muscle relaxation training in the management of post-chemotherapy nausea and vomiting. *Eur J Cancer Care*, 9(4):230-234.

Moorhead M, Johnson M, Maas M (Eds). (2004). *Nursing Outcomes Classification (NOC)*, 3rd ed. St. Louis: Mosby.

Ostelo RW, van Tulder MW, Vlaeyen JW, Linton SJ, Morley SJ, Assendelft WJ. (2005). Behavioural treatment for chronic low back pain. *Cochrane Database Syst Rev*, (1):CD002014.

Price JR, Couper J. (2000). Cognitive behaviour therapy for chronic fatigue syndrome in adults. *Cochrane Database Syst Rev*, (2):CD001027.

Ramaratnam S, Baker GA, Goldstein LH. (2005). Psychological treatments for epilepsy. *Cochrane Database Syst Rev*, (4):CD002029.

Richardson-Tench M, Pearson A, Birks M. (2005). The changing face of surgery: Using systematic reviews. *Br J Perioper Nurs*, 15(6):240-242, 244-246.

Sander Wint S, Eshelman D, Steele J, Guzzetta CE. (2002). Effects of distraction using virtual reality glasses during lumbar punctures in adolescents with cancer. *Oncol Nurs Forum*, 29(1):E8-E15.

Schneider SM, Prince-Paul M, Allen MJ, Silverman P, Talaba D. (2004). Virtual reality as a distraction intervention for women receiving chemotherapy. *Oncol Nurs Forum*, 31(1):81-88.

Schneider SM, Workman ML. (2000). Virtual reality as a distraction intervention for older children receiving chemotherapy. *Pediatr Nurs*, 26(6):593-597.

Shaw K, O'Rourke P, Del Mar C, Kenardy J. (2005). Psychological interventions for overweight or obesity. *Cochrane Database Syst Rev*, (2):CD003818.

Simmons D, Chabal C, Griffith J, Rausch M, Steele B. (2004). A clinical trial of distraction techniques for pain and anxiety control during cataract surgery. *Insight*, 29(4):13-16.

Sinha M, Christopher NC, Fenn R, Reeves L. (2006). Evaluation of nonpharmacologic methods of pain and anxiety management for laceration repair in the pediatric emergency department. *Pediatrics*, 117(4):1162-1168.

Soo S, Moayyedi P, Deeks J, Delaney B, Lewis M, Forman D. (2005). Psychological interventions for non-ulcer dyspepsia. *Cochrane Database Syst Rev*, (2):CD002301.

Sparks L. (2001). Taking the "ouch" out of injections for children. Using distraction to decrease pain. *MCN Am J Matern Child Nurs*, 26(2):72-78.

Summerbell CD, Ashton V, Campbell KJ, Edmunds L, Kelly S, Waters E. (2003). Interventions for treating obesity in children. *Cochrane Database Syst Rev*, (3):CD001872.

Tanabe P, Ferket K, Thomas R, Paice J, Marcantonio R. (2002). The effect of standard care, ibuprofen, and distraction on pain relief and patient satisfaction in children with musculoskeletal trauma. *J Emerg Nurs*, 28(2):118-125.

Thorgrimsen L, Spector A, Wiles A, Orrell M. (2003). Aroma therapy for dementia. *Cochrane Database Syst Rev,* (3):CD003150.

Vagnoli L, Caprilli S, Robiglio A, Messeri A. (2005). Clown doctors as a treatment for preoperative anxiety in children: A randomized, prospective study. *Pediatrics,* 116(4):e563-e567.

Vasterling J, Jenkins RA, Tope DM, Burish TG. (1993). Cognitive distraction and relaxation training for the control of side effects due to cancer chemotherapy. *J Behav Med,* 16(1):65-80.

Yorke J, Fleming SL, Shuldham CM. (2006). Psychological interventions for adults with asthma. *Cochrane Database Syst Rev,* (1):CD002982.

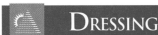 # DRESSING

Cornelia Beck, PhD, RN, FAAN; Valorie M. Shue, BA

NIC   **Definition:** Choosing, putting on, and removing clothes for a person who cannot do this for self (Dochterman & Bulechek, 2004).

NURSING ACTIVITIES

Effective

■ *Refer the patient to occupational therapy.* **LOE=II**

   MR An RCT in Stockholm, Sweden of 100 people recovering from a hip fracture found that early individualized postoperative occupational training that began during the person's hospital stay and included a home visit before discharge sped up the elder's ability to perform activities of daily living (ADLs). Compared with the control group, the intervention group significantly improved in ability to dress themselves (Hagsten et al., 2004).

   MR An RCT of 319 older community dwellers who reported difficulty with one or more ADLs involved home modifications and training in their use: instruction in problem solving, energy conservation, safe performance, and fall recovery techniques and balance and muscle strength training. After 6 months, the treatment group had significantly less difficulty with dressing (Gitlin et al., 2006).

   MR A controlled study involved 50 people who had ischemic stroke and were consecutively admitted to two postacute units in Rome, Italy. One randomly chosen unit added two occupational therapists to the rehabilitation team. The other unit received only physiotherapy. The team constructed individualized plans of treatment that could include strengthening and range-of-motion exercise, musculoskeletal control, trunk and upper extremity positioning, transfer training, postural and gait training, functional and self-care retraining, and adaptive equipment training. Differences between the intervention and control groups were statistically significant for dressing (Landi et al., 2006).

■ *Provide graded assistance.* **LOE=III**

   MR An evidence-based review of controlled studies classified graded assistance (from verbal prompts to physical demonstration, physical guidance, practical physical assistance, and complete physical assistance) as a guideline (recommendation that reflects moderate clinical certainty) for ADLs, including dressing, in people with dementia (Doody et al., 2001).

RCT = Randomized Controlled (Clinical) Trial, **NIC** = Nursing Interventions Classification, **NOC** = Nursing Outcomes Classification

(MR) A controlled study comparing usual care and functional rehabilitation in 17 nursing home residents with dementia found that functional rehabilitation, which included substituting nondirective and directive verbal assists for physical assists, could reduce functional decline during dressing (Rogers et al., 2000).

(MR) A case study showed that certified nursing assistants learned and used a system of least prompts at each step of a task, beginning with less intrusive prompts and gradually proceeding to more intrusive prompts, with three nursing home residents with dementia. The residents' independence in dressing increased (Engelman et al., 2002).

Possibly Effective

■ *Provide nurse and staff education and training.* **LOE=III**

(NR) In a controlled study, nurse educators supported three nursing homes over a 2-year period by helping staff match the correct care practice with residents' capacity for self-care. The rate of resident dressing decline decreased four times more than it did in 10 control facilities that provided usual care (Goldman et al., 2004).

(NR) A controlled study with repeated measures of 40 nursing home residents with dementia found that residents whose caregivers received a comprehensive education program improved level of functioning in morning care (bathing, grooming, dressing, and toileting) (Wells et al., 2000).

■ *Use goal-focused therapy.* **LOE=IV**

(MR) In a controlled study with a pretest/post-test design of 31 patients being treated for neurological, cardiopulmonary, and orthopedic deficits; back injury; and debilitation at a rehabilitation hospital, both groups received physical therapy and occupational therapy. However, participants in the experimental group also received a goal notebook and discussed goals with their therapists daily. The experimental group made significantly greater gains in upper-body dressing than the control group (Gagné & Hoppes, 2003).

Not Effective

No applicable published research was found in this category.

Possibly Harmful

No applicable published research was found in this category.

OUTCOME MEASUREMENT

SELF-CARE: ACTIVITIES OF DAILY LIVING   (NOC)

Definition: Ability to perform the most basic physical tasks and personal care activities independently with or without assistive device.

Self-Care: Activities of Daily Living as evidenced by the following selected NOC indicators:
• Dressing
• Grooming

NR = Nursing Research, **MR** = Multidisciplinary Research, **SP** = Standard of Practice, **EO** = Expert Opinion, **LOE** = Level of Evidence

OUTCOME MEASUREMENT—*cont'd*

(Rate each indicator of **Self-Care: Activities of Daily Living:** 1=severely compromised, 2=substantially compromised, 3=moderately compromised, 4=mildly compromised, 5=not compromised) (Moorhead et al., 2004).

Additional non-NOC indicators:

- Gets clothing from drawer and closet
- Puts clothing on upper body
- Puts clothing on lower body
- Buttons/zips/or fastens clothes as needed
- Puts on socks and shoes
- Removes clothing from upper body
- Removes clothes from lower body

REFERENCES

Dochterman JM, Bulechek GM (Eds). (2004). *Nursing Interventions Classification (NIC),* 4th ed. St. Louis: Mosby.

Doody RS, Stevens JC, Beck C, Dubinsky RM, Kaye JA, Gwyther L, et al. (2001). Practice parameter: Management of dementia (an evidence-based review). Report of the Quality Standards Subcommittee of the American Academy of Neurology. *Neurology,* 56(9):1154-1166.

Engelman KK, Mathews RM, Altus DE. (2002). Restoring dressing independence in persons with Alzheimer's disease: A pilot study. *Am J Alzheimers Dis Other Demen,* 17(1):37-43.

Gagné DE, Hoppes S. (2003). The effects of collaborative goal-focused occupational therapy on self-care skills: A pilot study. *Am J Occup Ther,* 57(2):215-219.

Gitlin LN, Winter L, Dennis MP, Corcoran M, Schinfeld S, Hauck WW. (2006). A randomized trial of a multicomponent home intervention to reduce functional difficulties in older adults. *J Am Geriatr Soc,* 54(5):809-816.

Goldman B, Balgobin S, Bish R, Lee RH, McCue S, Morrison MH, et al. (2004). Nurse educators are key to a best practices implementation program. *Geriatr Nurs,* 25(3):171-174.

Hagsten B, Svensson O, Gardulf A. (2004). Early individualized postoperative occupational therapy training in 100 patients improves ADL after hip fracture. A randomized trial. *Acta Orthop Scand,* 75(2): 177-183.

Landi F, Cesari M, Onder G, Tafani A, Zamboni V, Cocchi A. (2006). Effects of an occupational therapy program on functional outcomes in older stroke patients. *Gerontology,* 52(2):85-91.

Moorhead S, Johnson M, Maas M (Eds). (2004). *Nursing Outcomes Classification (NOC),* 3rd ed. St. Louis: Mosby.

Rogers JC, Holm MB, Burgio LD, Hsu C, Hardin JM, McDowell BJ. (2000). Excess disability during morning care in nursing home residents with dementia. *Int Psychogeriatr,* 12(2):267-282.

Wells DL, Dawson P, Sidani S, Craig D, Pringle D. (2000). Effects of an abilities-focused program on morning care on residents who have dementia and on caregivers. *J Am Geriatr Soc,* 48(4):442-449.

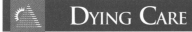 **DYING CARE**

Kathleen Czekanski, PhD, RN, CNE

NIC Definition: Promotion of physical comfort and psychological peace in the final phase of life (Dochterman & Bulecheck, 2004).

NURSING ACTIVITIES

Effective

■ **NIC** *Reduce the demand for cognitive functioning when the patient is ill or fatigued.* **LOE=VII**

EO Assess the patient for interest in participating in activities; allow the patient to rest or sleep during less enjoyable activities to conserve energy (Matzo & Sherman, 2001).

■ *Monitor the patient for psychological changes, such as anxiety, depression, and mood changes.* **LOE=VII**

EO Anxiety is common among patients with advanced disease; there is insufficient evidence about the effectiveness of pharmacotherapy for anxiety in terminally ill patients (Jackson & Lipman, 2004a).

EO The diagnosis and treatment of depression in the terminally ill can improve coping mechanisms for both patients and their families (Block, 2000).

■ **NIC** *Communicate willingness to discuss death. Encourage patient and family to share feelings about death. Facilitate discussion of funeral arrangements.* **LOE=VI**

NR A qualitative study with patients diagnosed with a terminal illness ($N=11$) regarding their discussions with nurses about end-of-life care concluded that patients' participation was highly dependent on professionals' skills in facilitating conversations (Clover et al., 2004).

EO Communicate effectively and compassionately with the patient, family, and health care team members about end-of-life issues (AACN, 2004).

■ **NIC** *Support the patient and family through stages of grief.* **LOE=VII**

EO Grief and bereavement risk assessment is routine and ongoing for the patient and family throughout the illness trajectory (NCPQPC, 2004).

EO Promote patients' self-esteem and dignity by respecting them as individuals with feelings, accomplishments, and acknowledging what they consider as important (Chochinov, 2002).

■ **NIC** *Monitor pain.* **LOE=VI**

MR A descriptive study with terminally ill cancer patients receiving palliative care ($N=120$) regarding the relationship between their level of pain and desire for a hastened death determined that pain had a statistically significant relationship with a desire for a hastened death (Mystakidou et al., 2005).

EO Assess pain thoroughly to determine the quality, intensity, location, and contributing factors (Lewis et al., 2004).

EO The outcome of pain and symptom management is the safe and timely reduction of pain to a level that is acceptable to the patient (NCPQPC, 2004).

■ **NIC** *Minimize discomfort when possible.* **LOE=V**

MR A systematic review demonstrated that breathlessness or dyspnea was a common symptom in people with advanced disease. There was evidence to support the use of oral or parenteral opioids to palliate breathlessness (Jennings et al., 2001).

NR = Nursing Research, **MR** = Multidisciplinary Research, **SP** = Standard of Practice, **EO** = Expert Opinion, **LOE** = Level of Evidence

EO Terminal restlessness occurs in 25% to 88% of dying patients. No single medication was found to be appropriate for treatment; additional trials are needed to determine which protocols are the most effective (Kehl, 2004).

MR A descriptive study of cancer patients (*N*=1296) attending an outpatient radiotherapy program concluded that the most frequently reported symptoms were fatigue, poor sense of well-being, pain, and poor appetite (Bradley et al., 2005).

MR A descriptive study of hospice patients (*N*=74) on the prevalence, causes, and treatment of insomnia determined that insomnia, reported in 52 patients (70%), was most often caused by uncontrolled symptoms such as pain (Hugel et al., 2004).

EO Use scientifically based standardized tools to assess symptoms such as pain, dyspnea, constipation, anxiety, fatigue, nausea/vomiting, and altered cognition experienced by patients at the end of life (AACN, 2004).

EO Treatment of distressing symptoms includes pharmacological, nonpharmacological, and complementary therapies (NCPQPC, 2004).

EO Maximize oxygenation with position changes, supplemental oxygen, maintaining a patent airway, and reducing anxiety or fever (Potter & Perry, 2005).

■ **NIC** *Medicate by an alternate route when swallowing problems develop.*
LOE=VII

EO Crushing medications or burying them in a semisolid food makes swallowing easier (Dahlin & Goldsmith, 2001).

EO Nonessential drugs should be discontinued; the subcutaneous route should be used for essential drugs (Ellershaw & Ward, 2003).

■ **NIC** *Postpone feeding when the patient is fatigued.* **LOE=VII**

EO Smaller meals based on the patient's wishes reduce the burden of eating (Kemp, 2001).

■ **NIC** *Offer fluids and soft foods frequently.* **LOE=VII**

EO Serve smaller portions and bland foods that may be more palatable (Potter & Perry, 2005).

■ **NIC** *Offer culturally appropriate foods.* **LOE=VII**

EO Culturally appropriate or favored foods should be encouraged (Kemp, 2001).

■ **NIC** *Monitor deterioration of physical and/or mental capabilities.* **LOE=V**

MR A systematic review demonstrated that delirium was a common disorder in patients with life-limiting disease and included agitation, confusion, and terminal restlessness. There was insufficient evidence to draw any conclusions about the role of pharmacotherapy in terminally ill patients with delirium. Further research is essential (Jackson & Lipman, 2004b).

MR A prospective assessment of patients with advanced cancer (*N*=104) evaluated the occurrence, precipitating factors, and reversibility of delirium. Delirium was reversible in 50% of the cases with changes in opioid dose, discontinuation of unnecessary psychoactive medications, and hydration (Lawlor et al., 2000).

EO The cancer patient who is in the dying phase becomes bed bound, becomes semicomatose, is able to take only sips of fluid, and is no longer able to take oral drugs (Ellershaw & Ward, 2003).

RCT = Randomized Controlled (Clinical) Trial, **NIC** = Nursing Interventions Classification, **NOC** = Nursing Outcomes Classification

■ **NIC** *Provide frequent rest periods.* **LOE=VII**

⊙ Promote frequent rest periods in a quiet environment; time and pace nursing care activities (Potter & Perry, 2005).

■ **NIC** *Assist with basic care as needed.* **LOE=VII**

⊙ Provide thorough skin and oral care (Potter & Perry, 2005).

⊙ Attend to mouth care, offer sips of water, and moisten mouth and lips (Ellershaw & Ward, 2003).

■ **NIC** *Stay physically close to the frightened patient.* **LOE=VII**

⊙ The nurse's presence can provide comfort and security to a terminally ill patient and can include hand holding, touching, and listening (Lewis et al., 2004).

■ **NIC** *Identify the patient's care priorities.* **LOE=VI**

ⓃⓇ A qualitative study of patients with an advanced cancer diagnosis ($N=7$) regarding preferences for care at the end of life determined that themes included protection of dignity; control of pain and other symptoms; and management of treatment, how time is spent, and impact on family; and control over the dying process (Volker et al., 2004).

ⓂⓇ A qualitative study with dialysis patients ($N=48$), people with HIV infection ($N=40$), and residents of a long-term care facility ($N=38$) assessed their views of end-of-life issues. Participants identified five domains of quality end-of-life care: receiving adequate pain and symptom management, avoiding inappropriate prolongation of dying, achieving a sense of control, relieving burden, and strengthening relationships with loved ones (Singer et al., 1999).

■ **NIC** *Facilitate obtaining spiritual support for the patient and family.* **LOE=VI**

ⓃⓇ A qualitative study with adults receiving palliative care ($N=16$) assessed the meaning of hope. Hope fostering categories included love of family and friends, spirituality, setting goals and maintaining independence, positive relationships with professional careers, humor, personal characteristics, and uplifting memories (Buckley & Herth, 2004).

ⓂⓇ A qualitative study of patients with end-stage heart failure ($N=20$) and patients with inoperable lung cancer ($N=20$) assessed their spiritual needs. Spiritual issues were significant for many patients in their last year of life. Many health care providers lacked the necessary time and skills to uncover and address issues (Murray et al., 2004).

ⓃⓇ A qualitative study with hospice patients ($N=14$) assessed factors associated with decision making at the end of life. Participants described spirituality or faith as factors in coping and decision making (Gauthier, 2005).

■ **NIC** *Respect the patient's and family's specific care requests.* **LOE=VI**

ⓂⓇ A qualitative study with family members ($N=160$) and patients with advanced cancer and chronic end-stage medical conditions ($N=440$) evaluated their perspectives of key elements of quality end-of-life care. Elements rated as extremely important included not being kept alive on life support when there is little hope for recovery (55.7%) and completing things and preparing for life's end with activities such as life review, resolving conflicts, and saying goodbye (43.9%) (Heyland et al., 2006).

NR = Nursing Research, **MR** = Multidisciplinary Research, **SP** = Standard of Practice, **EO** = Expert Opinion, **LOE** = Level of Evidence

(NR) A descriptive study explored the preferences of terminally ill patients with cancer ($N=180$) concerning their place of death. Nearly 90% of subjects preferred to die at home (Tang, 2003).

(EO) The palliative care plan should be based on the identified and expressed values, goals, and needs of the patient and family and is developed with professional guidance and support for decision making (NCPQPC, 2004).

■ **NIC** *Support the family's efforts to remain at the bedside.* **LOE=VII**

(EO) Patient and family wishes regarding the setting for the death should be addressed (NCPQPC, 2004).

■ **NIC** *Include the family in care decisions and activities as desired.* **LOE=IV**

(MR) A cross-sectional, stratified random national survey of seriously ill patients ($N=340$), recently bereaved family members ($N=332$), and MDs and other health care providers ($N=790$) evaluated factors important at the end of life. Items consistently rated as important included pain and symptom management, preparation for death, achieving a sense of completion, decisions about treatment preferences, and being treated as a "whole person" (Steinhauser et al., 2000).

(MR) A qualitative study with family members ($N=461$) of older people who had died from chronic diseases revealed concern about failures in communication and pain control at the end of life (Hanson et al., 1997).

Possibly Effective

■ **NIC** *Minimize discomfort when possible.* **LOE=VI**

(NR) A quasi-experimental study tested the effect of hand massage on hospice patients' comfort ($N=31$). Patients who received hand massage ($N=16$) had increased comfort over time compared with a comparison group; however, results were not significant (Kolcaba et al., 2004).

Not Effective

■ **NIC** *Minimize discomfort when possible.* **LOE=I**

(MR) An RCT investigated the relationship between symptoms and dehydration in patients with malignant disease ($N=82$). No statistically significant association was found between level of hydration and respiratory tract secretions, symptoms of thirst, and dry mouth. Artificial hydration to alleviate these symptoms may be futile (Ellershaw et al., 1995).

■ **NIC** *Facilitate obtaining spiritual support for the patient and family.* **LOE=VI**

(NR) Interviews with adults receiving palliative care ($N=16$) assessed the meaning of hope. Hope-hindering categories included abandonment, isolation, uncontrolled pain, discomfort, and devaluation of personhood (Buckley & Herth, 2004).

Possibly Harmful

No applicable published research was found in this category.

RCT = Randomized Controlled (Clinical) Trial, **NIC** = Nursing Interventions Classification, **NOC** = Nursing Outcomes Classification

OUTCOME MEASUREMENT

DIGNIFIED LIFE CLOSURE   NOC

(Please refer to *Nursing Outcomes Classification* [Moorhead et al., 2004] for the **Dignified Life Closure** outcome.)

REFERENCES

American Association of Colleges of Nursing (AACN). (2004). *Peaceful death: Recommended competencies and curricular guidelines for end-of-life nursing care.* Available online: http://www.aacn.nche.edu/. Retrieved on September 8, 2006.

Block SD. (2000). Assessing and managing depression in the terminally ill patient. ACP-ASIM End-of-Life Care Consensus Panel. American College of Physicians-American Society of Internal Medicine. *Ann Intern Med,* 132(3):209-218.

Bradley N, Davis L, Chow E. (2005). Symptom distress in patients attending an outpatient palliative radiotherapy clinic. *J Pain Symptom Manage,* 30(2):123-131.

Buckley J, Herth K. (2004). Fostering hope in terminally ill patients. *Nurs Stand,* 19(10):33-41.

Chochinov HM. (2002). Perspectives on care at the close of life. Dignity-conserving care—A new model for palliative care: Helping the patient feel valued. *JAMA,* 287(17):2253-2260.

Clover A, Browne J, McErlain P, Vandenberg B. (2004). Patient approaches to clinical conversations in the palliative care setting. *J Adv Nurs,* 48(4):333-341.

Dahlin CM, Goldsmith T. (2001). Dysphagia, dry mouth, and hiccups. In Ferrell BR, Coyle N (Eds). *Textbook of palliative care nursing.* New York: Oxford University Press, pp 122-138.

Dochterman JM, Bulechek GM (Eds). (2004). *Nursing Interventions Classification (NIC),* 4th ed. St. Louis: Mosby.

Ellershaw J, Sutcliffe JM, Saunders CM. (1995). Dehydration and the dying patient. *J Pain Symptom Manage,* 10(3):192-197.

Ellershaw J, Ward C. (2003). Care of the dying patient: The last hours or days of life. *BMJ,* 326(7379):30-34.

Gauthier DM. (2005). Decision making near the end of life. *J Hosp Palliat Nurs,* 7(2):82-90.

Hanson L, Danis M, Garrett J. (1997). What is wrong with end of life care? Opinions of bereaved family members. *J Am Geriatr Soc,* 45(11):1339-1344.

Heyland DK, Dodek P, Rocker G, Groll D, Gafni A, Pichora D, et al. (2006). What matters most in end-of-life care: Perceptions of seriously ill patients and their family members. *CMAJ,* 174(5):627-633.

Hugel H, Ellershaw JF, Cook L, Skinner J, Irvine C. (2004). The prevalence, key causes, and management of insomnia in palliative care patients. *J Pain Symptom Manage,* 27(4):316-321.

Jackson KC, Lipman AG. (2004a). Drug therapy for anxiety in palliative care. *Cochrane Database Syst Rev,* (1):CD004596.

Jackson KC, Lipman AG. (2004b). Drug therapy for delirium in terminally ill patients. *Cochrane Database Syst Rev,* (2):CD004770.

Jennings AL, Davies AN, Higgins JP, Broadley K. (2001). Opioids for the palliation of breathlessness in terminal illness. *Cochrane Database Syst Rev,* (4):CD002066.

Kehl KA. (2004). Treatment of terminal restlessness: A review of the evidence. *J Pain Palliat Care Pharmacother,* 18(1):5-30.

Kemp C. (2001). Anorexia and cachexia. In Ferrell BR, Coyle N (Eds). *Textbook of palliative care nursing.* New York: Oxford University Press, pp. 101-106.

Kolcaba K, Dowd T, Steiner R, Mitzel A. (2004). Efficacy of hand massage for enhancing the comfort of hospice patients. *J Hosp Palliat Nurs,* 6(2):91-102.

Lawlor PG, Gagnon B, Mancini IL, Pereira JL, Hanson J, Suarez-Almazor ME, et al. (2000). Occurrence, causes, and outcome of delirium in patients with advanced cancer: A prospective study. *Arch Intern Med,* 160(6):786-794.

Lewis SM, Heitkemper MM, Dirksen SR. (2004). *Medical-surgical nursing: Assessment and management of clinical problems,* 6th ed. St. Louis: Mosby.

Matzo ML, Sherman DW. (2001). *Palliative care nursing: Quality care to the end of life.* New York, Springer.

Moorhead M., Johnson M., Maas M (Eds). (2004). *Nursing Outcomes Classification (NOC),* 3rd ed. St. Louis: Mosby.

Murray SA, Kendall M, Boyd K, Worth A, Benton TF. (2004). Exploring the spiritual needs of people dying of lung cancer or heart failure: A prospective qualitative interview study of patients and their careers. *Palliat Med,* 18(1):39-45.

Mystakidou K, Parpa E, Katsouda E, Galanos A, Vlahos L. (2005). Pain and desire for hastened death in terminally ill cancer patients. *Cancer Nurs,* 28(4):318-324.

National Consensus Project for Quality Palliative Care (NCPQPC). (2004). *Clinical practice guidelines for quality palliative care.* Available online: http://www.nationalconsensusproject.org. Retrieved on September 8, 2006.

Potter PA, Perry AG. (2005). *Fundamentals of nursing,* 6th ed. St. Louis: Mosby.

Singer P, Martin D, Kelner M. (1999). Quality end-of-life care: Patient's perspectives. *JAMA,* 281(2): 163-168.

Steinhauser KE, Christakis NA, Clipp EC, McNeilly M, McIntyre L, Tulsky JA. (2000). Factors considered important at the end of life by patients, family, physicians, and other care providers. *JAMA,* 284(19):2476-2482.

Tang ST. (2003). When death is imminent: Where terminally ill patients with cancer prefer to die and why. *Cancer Nurs,* 26(3):245-251.

Volker DL, Kahn D, Penticuff JH. (2004). Patient control and end-of-life care part II: The patient perspective. *Oncol Nurs Forum,* 31(5):954-960.

DYSPNEA MANAGEMENT

Virginia L. Carrieri-Kohlman, DNSc, RN, FAAN; DorAnne Donesky-Cuenco, PhD, RN

Definition: Alleviation of dyspnea or a reduction in dyspnea to a level of comfort that is acceptable to the patient. Dyspnea is used interchangeably with the words "shortness of breath" and "breathlessness."

NURSING ACTIVITIES

Effective

■ *Ensure access to fresh air or use a fan directing cold air on the face.* **LOE=II**

(NR) In a descriptive study, use of fresh air or a fan was described as the most effective strategy by 68 patients with shortness of breath across obstructive, restrictive, and vascular pulmonary disease (Janson-Bjerklie et al., 1986).

(MR) In a laboratory observational study, the flow of cool air through the nose reduced breathlessness in eight patients with chronic obstructive pulmonary disease (COPD) (Liss & Grant, 1988).

(MR) In a laboratory case series, flow of warm, humidified air through the mouth via face mask only or with mouthpiece and mask decreased perception of dyspnea in 10 normal volunteers (Simon et al., 1991).

(MR) In an observational laboratory study, cold air directed on the face of 16 healthy volunteers significantly reduced the perception of dyspnea without causing reduction in ventilation (Schwartzstein et al., 1987).

RCT = Randomized Controlled (Clinical) Trial, **NIC** = Nursing Interventions Classification, **NOC** = Nursing Outcomes Classification

■ *Teach the patient to use pursed-lip breathing (PLB).* **LOE=II**

(MR) A crossover design with 12 hypoxemic COPD subjects randomly assigned to either PLB or general relaxation found that PLB significantly improved SaO_2 over baseline whereas relaxation did not (Tiep et al., 1986).

(MR) In an observational study with 22 patients with COPD, volumes of chest wall and compartments (rib cage and abdomen) were assessed using an optoelectronic plethysmograph with dyspnea being assessed using a modified Borg scale. Compared with those spontaneously breathing, participants using PLB exhibited a significant reduction in respiratory rate, dyspnea, and $Paco_2$ with improvement in tidal volume and oxygen saturation (Bianchi et al., 2004).

(MR) Using a crossover design, eight COPD patients wearing a tight-fitting transparent face mask breathed with and without PLB for 8 minutes each at rest and exercise. PLB promoted a slower and deeper breathing pattern and during exercise decreased dyspnea, which was related to the impact of changes in end-expiratory lung volume, and tidal volume on end-respiratory function was variably affected by PLB across patients (Spahija et al., 2005).

(MR) In an observational study of 69 COPD patients who did not spontaneously use PLB, the use of PLB resulted in lower postexercise respiratory rate and a quicker return to preexercise breathlessness after an incremental shuttle walk (Garrod et al., 2005).

■ *Use noninvasive positive-pressure ventilation and continuous positive airway pressure (CPAP, BiPAP) as ordered.* **LOE=II**

(MR) In a crossover study, positive-pressure support used during constant workload exercise in seven patients with COPD improved minute ventilation, decreased inspiratory effort, and improved dyspnea significantly (Maltais et al., 1995).

(MR) In a quasi-experimental study, eight men with disabling breathlessness due to COPD walked on a treadmill with inspiratory pressure support, CPAP, and oxygen in random order on three separate days. Inspiratory pressure support improved median walking distance by 62% compared with the control walk. There was no change in walking distance with either CPAP or oxygen at 2 L/minute. Results showed that inspiratory pressure support could reduce breathlessness and increase exercise tolerance to submaximal treadmill exercise in patients with COPD (Keilty et al., 1994).

(MR) In a prospective RCT, nine outpatients with severe COPD treated with BiPAP for 2 hours a day for 5 days decreased their dyspnea score on the Borg scale from 2 to 0.7 compared with eight controls with COPD who received sham BiPAP (Renston et al., 1994).

(MR) In a crossover design with 10 nonintubated COPD patients in acute respiratory failure, CPAP decreased inspiratory effort and dyspnea and significantly improved pattern of breathing with varying levels of CPAP (Goldberg et al., 1995).

■ *Support the patient to assume the position of choice, including the forward leaning position with arm support.* **LOE=IV**

(EO) A forward leaning position with arm support improves dyspnea because of a favorable diaphragmatic length-tension curve and optimal use of accessory muscles.

(MR) In a quasi-experimental study of 17 patients with COPD, 7 patients who had paradoxical inspiratory motion of the diaphragm while standing had striking relief of dyspnea in the leaning forward position (Sharp et al., 1980).

(MR) In an observational study, the seated leaning forward position was the optimum posture for 40 patients with COPD to generate maximum inspiratory pressures and to obtain greatest

---

NR = Nursing Research, **MR** = Multidisciplinary Research, **SP** = Standard of Practice, **EO** = Expert Opinion, **LOE** = Level of Evidence

subjective relief of dyspnea. No postural effect on inspiratory or expiratory pressures was observed in 140 normal subjects (O'Neill & McCarthy, 1983).

■ *Participate in an 8-week structured pulmonary rehabilitation program.* LOE=I

(MR) An evidenced-based review of more than 20 methodologically well-designed RCTs demonstrated that an 8-week outpatient pulmonary rehabilitation program with education and supervised exercise significantly increased exercise ability and decreased dyspnea during exercise and with activities of daily living (ADLs) compared with controls (Nici et al., 2006).

(MR) A meta-analysis of 14 RCTs showed that a pulmonary rehabilitation program significantly decreased dyspnea with ADLs (Chronic Respiratory Disease Questionnaire) and dyspnea with laboratory exercise, with the treatment effect significantly larger than the minimally important clinical difference and significantly less than the controls. Pulmonary rehabilitation was defined as exercise training (for at least 4 weeks) with or without education, psychological support, or both (Lacasse et al., 2002, 2006).

(MR) In the National Emphysema Treatment Trial, a prospective observational multicenter study ($N=1218$ patients with COPD), dyspnea measured by the modified Borg scale and by the University of California, San Diego, Shortness of Breath Questionnaire significantly improved following rehabilitation (Ries et al., 2005).

■ *Participate in a structured strength or endurance exercise training program.* LOE=I

(MR) In a prospective, unblinded RCT, 40 patients with COPD were randomly assigned to either high-intensity lower extremity endurance training or low-intensity multicomponent calisthenics twice weekly for 8 weeks. Both groups showed significant improvement in exercise variables, dyspnea, functional performance, and health status. Patients in the high-intensity group showed greater increases in treadmill endurance and reductions in exertional dyspnea (Normandin et al., 2002).

(NR) In an RCT, 103 patients with COPD were randomly assigned to a dyspnea self-management program (DSMP) alone with education and home walking, DSMP4 with four supervised exercise sessions, or DSMP24 with 24 supervised sessions. At 2 months, patients in DSMP24 had significantly greater improvements in dyspnea and laboratory exercise performance than those in DSMP (Stulbarg et al., 2002).

(MR) In a case-control study, 30 patients with COPD participated in a 6-week supervised multimodality endurance exercise program; changes in dyspnea and ventilatory measures were compared with 30 matched controls. Supervised exercise training relieved both chronic and acute activity-related breathlessness significantly more than in controls (O'Donnell et al., 1995).

(MR) In an observational study, 151 patients underwent a 12-week exercise program, three times per week for 1 hour, with baseline and follow-up testing. Six-minute walk distance, treadmill time, overhead task completion, dyspnea, and fatigue all improved at the end of the exercise program (Berry et al., 1999).

Possibly Effective

■ *Use humidified low-flow oxygen at various levels at rest and with exercise, depending on individual perception of relief of dyspnea.* LOE=I

(MR) A systematic review of 19 crossover controlled studies found that 14 reported significant relief of dyspnea in patients with COPD using varied flow rates of ambulatory oxygen (2 to 6 L/minute) during exercise (Spathis et al., 2006).

RCT = Randomized Controlled (Clinical) Trial, **NIC** = Nursing Interventions Classification, **NOC** = Nursing Outcomes Classification

MR In a double-blind, randomized crossover trial with 33 patients with lung cancer, supplemental oxygen or air (5 L/minute) was administered via nasal cannula during a 6-minute walk test. No significant differences between treatment groups were observed in dyspnea or 6-minute walk distance (Bruera et al., 2003).

MR In an observational study, eight patients with COPD who had reported less shortness of breath with oxygen at rest had no significant reduction in dyspnea at 0, 2, and 4 L/minute of oxygen (Liss & Grant, 1988).

MR In a single-blind crossover controlled trial with 38 hospice patients reporting dyspnea at rest, dyspnea with either oxygen or room air was significantly reduced from baseline, but there were no significant differences for the mean visual analog scale (VAS) scores between oxygen and air administration (Booth et al., 1996).

MR An observational case study showed significant relief of breathlessness with oxygen in 12 hypoxic COPD patients during rest (Swinburn et al., 1991).

MR An RCT design ($N=1$) was conducted with a 53-year-old female cancer patient who underwent six randomized double-blind crossover trials between oxygen 5 L/minute delivered by mask and air 5 L/minute delivered by mask. The mean VAS for dyspnea was 77 ± 4 during the baseline period compared with 51 ± 7 after air and 40 ± 5 after oxygen (Bruera et al., 1992).

MR Two crossover controlled studies with small samples ($N=20$) found significant relief of dyspnea in patients with interstitial lung disease using varied flow rates of ambulatory oxygen (2 to 6 L/minute) during exercise (Spathis et al., 2006).

MR Fourteen patients with dyspnea related to advanced cancer with six randomized crossover trials with oxygen 5 L/minute and air 5 L/minute demonstrated that dyspnea was significantly more reduced with oxygen (Bruera et al., 1993).

■ *Teach patients relaxation with coaching.* **LOE=III**

NR In an RCT involving the effect of relaxation training, 26 patients with COPD were compared with a control group who were instructed to relax but not given specific instructions. Dyspnea and state anxiety were significantly reduced for the relaxation group during treatment sessions; however, this decrease was not sustained at 4 weeks (Gift et al., 1992).

NR In an RCT, 12 outpatients with COPD practiced relaxation in 4-week sessions combined with daily home practice and 8 patients received usual care. The relaxation significantly decreased dyspnea during the session, but this decrease was not sustained after the sessions (Renfroe, 1988).

■ *Participate in an educational and skills program about pulmonary disease and symptoms.* **LOE=II**

MR Using a quasi-experimental design, patients with COPD in one community ($N=325$) were offered an educational program with assessment and discussion of findings, compared with a second community where patients were only assessed and advised of the findings ($N=213$). Post-test results showed a significant difference in health perception and locus of control but no difference in respiratory symptoms, exercise tolerance, or mental health (Howland et al., 1986).

MR Using an RCT of 89 COPD patients, those who received a limited pulmonary rehabilitation program without exercise training and focused on practice of coping strategies for shortness of breath had significant improvement in only one measure of dyspnea (one out of six)

NR = Nursing Research, **MR** = Multidisciplinary Research, **SP** = Standard of Practice, **EO** = Expert Opinion, **LOE** = Level of Evidence

at one point in time compared with a group who received a health education program (Sassi-Dambron et al., 1995).

(NR) A single-group, observational study of 10 patients with COPD who attended a 6-week nurse-directed self-management program showed no significant change in levels of dyspnea after the program, but self-efficacy for managing dyspnea during activities was improved (Zimmerman et al., 1996).

■ *Participate in a nurse-run clinic.* **LOE=II**

(NR) Patients (*N*=119) with lung cancer participated in a multicenter RCT where they either attended a nursing clinic offering intervention for their breathlessness or received standard treatment for breathlessness and breathing assessments. The intervention combined breathing control, activity pacing, relaxation techniques, and psychosocial support. Breathlessness and distress at best and worst, measured at rest, were found to be decreased significantly more for the intervention group at 8 weeks (Bredin et al., 1999; Corner et al., 1996).

■ *Use in-phase chest wall vibration.* **LOE=II**

(MR) In an observational study of 15 patients with severe COPD, out-of-phase vibration increased dyspnea; however, in-phase vibration (during inspiration) significantly decreased dyspnea (Sibuya et al., 1994).

(MR) In 10 COPD patients with severe dyspnea and hypercapnia, in-phase chest wall vibration significantly reduced dyspnea during hypercapnia but not during exercise (Cristiano & Schwartzstein, 1997).

(MR) In an observational study, in-phase chest wall vibration during exercise in 17 male COPD patients reduced dyspnea and improved respiratory efficiency for all (Fujie et al., 2002).

■ *Suggest use of acupuncture.* **LOE=IV**

(MR) Twenty-four patients with nonmalignant breathlessness received six treatments of acupuncture and transcutaneous electrical nerve stimulation (TENS) in a crossover design. Dyspnea measured daily, before and after each treatment, improved significantly for acupuncture. There was no significant difference between the acupuncture and TENS control groups and no significant differences between treatments (Lewith et al., 2004).

(MR) In a pilot observational study, 20 patients with dyspnea related to lung cancer received one session of acupuncture and had significant decreases in breathlessness and anxiety up to 6 hours after the session with the maximal improvement at 90 minutes (Filshie et al., 1996).

(MR) In an RCT, acupuncture was compared with sham in 24 patients with disabling breathlessness who received "traditional acupuncture points" or sham for 13 sessions over 3 weeks. Groups were matched for gender and severity. Both groups improved their dyspnea at the end of the 6-minute walking distance (6MW); however, the acupuncture group had significantly greater improvement than the placebo group (Jobst et al., 1986).

(MR) In an RCT, 41 patients with chronic obstructive asthma were randomly assigned to 20 acupuncture treatments (*N*=11), self-administered acupressure (*N*=17), or standard care alone (*N*=13) for 8 weeks. There was improvement in dyspnea with all three treatments, with no difference between treatments (Maa et al., 2003).

(MR) With a matched group design, 47 patients with lung or breast cancer and dyspnea received one single session of true or one single session of placebo acupuncture and semipermanent acupuncture "studs" where they applied pressure twice a day. Dyspnea was measured for a

RCT = Randomized Controlled (Clinical) Trial, **NIC** = Nursing Interventions Classification, **NOC** = Nursing Outcomes Classification

week before and after treatments. The acupuncture technique was not superior to placebo for relief of dyspnea (Vickers et al., 2005).

■ *Suggest use of acupressure.* **LOE=II**

(MR) In an RCT, 44 patients with COPD in Taiwan were randomly assigned to true or sham acupressure for five 16-minute sessions per week for 4 weeks. There were significant improvements in dyspnea, anxiety, and fatigue following acupressure compared with control (Wu et al., 2004).

(MR) As an adjunct to pulmonary rehabilitation, 31 patients with COPD received true versus sham acupressure in a 12-week blinded crossover design. There were significant reductions in dyspnea measured by VAS but not with the modified Borg scale (Maa et al., 1997).

(MR) In an RCT, 41 patients with chronic obstructive asthma were randomly assigned to 20 acupuncture treatments ($N=11$), self-administered acupressure ($N=17$), or standard care alone ($N=13$) for 8 weeks. There was improvement in dyspnea with all three treatments, with no difference between treatments (Maa et al., 2003).

■ *Participate in a yoga program.* **LOE=III**

(MR) In an RCT, 11 males with COPD were trained in yoga breathing exercises and 10 postures. A matched group was randomly assigned to receive physiotherapy. Significantly more subjects in the yoga group stated that they had "easier control" of their dyspnea attacks (Tandon, 1978).

(MR) A single group pretest/post-test test design was used to study 15 males with chronic bronchitis who practiced eight body postures and five breathing exercises in the laboratory 30 minutes daily for 1 week and then continued in the home for 3 weeks with reinforcement. There were significant reductions in dyspnea at 4 weeks (Behera, 1998).

■ *Teach the patient to exercise with music for distraction.* **LOE=II**

(MR) In an RCT, 24 patients with COPD were randomly assigned to walk with or without music two to five times per week for 20 to 45 minutes. Subjects who walked with music had significantly less dyspnea during ADLs after 8 weeks. There were no differences between groups in dyspnea at the end of 6MW (Bauldoff et al., 2002).

(MR) In an RCT, 30 subjects with COPD were randomly assigned to no music, moderate tempo music, or fast tempo music during 15 minutes of upper body ergometry training two to three times per week for 4 weeks. Although functional performance improved, there were no differences between groups in dyspnea with ADLs after training (Bauldoff et al., 2005).

(MR) Twenty-four subjects with COPD were instructed to listen to music whenever they felt short of breath. Dyspnea decreased significantly after music sessions, but there was no decrease in dyspnea over time (McBride et al., 1999).

(MR) Using an observational one-group crossover design, 30 subjects with COPD showed no difference in dyspnea or anxiety levels at the end of the 6-minute walk with or without music (Brooks et al., 2003).

■ *Use biofeedback during exercise.* **LOE=III**

(NR) In an RCT, 39 COPD patients were randomly allocated to a 6-week 18-session program of ventilation-feedback combined with cycle exercise, ventilation-feedback only, or exercise only. The ventilation-feedback combined with cycle exercise group had significant improvements in dyspnea and breathing pattern parameters, including minute ventilation, tidal volume, frequency, and expiratory time (Collins et al., 2003).

■ *Use energy conservation techniques.* **LOE=IV**

(MR) Using a quasi-experimental design, 16 male patients with COPD were significantly less dyspneic while using energy conservation techniques during ADLs than when they performed ADLs without energy conservation techniques (Velloso & Jardim, 2006).

■ *Teach controlled breathing; coach the patients to change their breathing pattern to slow, deep breathing with optimal thoracoabdominal movements.* **LOE=IV**

(MR) A review of the literature supports the inclusion of controlled techniques in the relief of dyspnea because of reduced dynamic hyperinflation, increased strength, endurance of respiratory muscles, and optimal pattern of thoracoabdominal motion (Gosselink, 2003).

(MR) In an evidence-based review of the efficacy of diaphragmatic breathing in adults (25 investigations; 424 patients), six studies showed that diaphragmatic breathing was efficacious in improving symptoms. Most studies did not measure symptoms (15), two found no change in symptoms, and two showed a worsening of symptoms. Improvements were most evident in patients with COPD who had elevated respiratory rates, low tidal volumes, and adequate diaphragmatic movement (Cahalin et al., 2005).

Not Effective

■ *Use of guided imagery.* **LOE=II**

(MR) In an RCT with a small sample of 26 patients with COPD, 13 practiced guided imagery for six sessions. As a standard guided imagery script was read, subjects were asked to visualize the scene described and audiotapes were used for practice. Thirteen controls rested quietly. No change in perceived dyspnea was measured during the seventh session (Louie, 2004).

(NR) In a single case design, 19 COPD patients met weekly for 4 weeks for 1 hour of practice with written script. There was no change in dyspnea, although there was improved perceived health-related quality of life (Moody et al., 1993).

■ *Participation in a maintenance exercise program after pulmonary rehabilitation program.* **LOE=II**

(MR) In multiple RCTs on maintenance exercise programs that followed patients longer than 6 months, benefits diminish in about 1 year (Griffiths et al., 2000; Ries et al., 1995; Strijbos et al., 1996; Troosters et al., 2000).

(MR) An RCT evaluated a 12-month maintenance program with weekly telephone contact and monthly supervised exercise sessions ($N=87$) and standard care ($N=85$). There was progressive decline in the improvement of dyspnea with ADL in both groups over 2 years (Ries et al., 2003).

Possibly Harmful

No applicable published research was found in this category.

RCT = Randomized Controlled (Clinical) Trial, **NIC** = Nursing Interventions Classification, **NOC** = Nursing Outcomes Classification

OUTCOME MEASUREMENT

RESPIRATORY STATUS: VENTILATION NOC

Definition: Movement of air in and out of the lungs.

Respiratory Status: Ventilation as evidenced by the following selected NOC indicators:

- Respiratory rate
- Respiratory rhythm
- Ease of breathing
- Tidal volume
- Vital capacity
- Pulmonary function tests

(Rate each indicator of **Respiratory Status: Ventilation:** 1=severely compromised, 2=substantially compromised, 3=moderately compromised, 4=mildly compromised, 5=not compromised) (Moorhead et al., 2004).

REFERENCES

Bauldoff GS, Hoffman LA, Zullo TG, Sciurba FC. (2002). Exercise maintenance following pulmonary rehabilitation: Effect of distractive stimuli. *Chest,* 122(3):948-954.

Bauldoff GS, Rittinger M, Nelson T, Doehrel J, Diaz PT. (2005). Feasibility of distractive auditory stimuli on upper extremity training in persons with chronic obstructive pulmonary disease. *J Cardiopulm Rehabil,* 25(1):50-55.

Behera D. (1998). Yoga therapy in chronic bronchitis. *J Assoc Physicians India,* 46(2):207-208.

Berry MJ, Rejeski WJ, Adair NE, Zaccaro D. (1999). Exercise rehabilitation and chronic obstructive pulmonary disease stage. *Am J Respir Crit Care Med,* 160(4):1248-1253.

Bianchi R, Gigliotti F, Romagnoli I, Lanini B, Castellani C, Grazzini M, et al. (2004). Chest wall kinematics and breathlessness during pursed-lip breathing in patients with COPD. *Chest,* 125(2):459-465.

Booth S, Kelly MJ, Cox NP, Adams L, Guz A. (1996). Does oxygen help dyspnea in patients with cancer? *Am J Respir Crit Care Med,* 153(5):1515-1518.

Bredin M, Corner J, Krishnasamy M, Plant H, Bailey C, A'Hern R. (1999). Multicentre randomised controlled trial of nursing intervention for breathlessness in patients with lung cancer. *BMJ,* 318(7188): 901-904.

Brooks D, Sidani S, Graydon J, McBride S, Hall L, Weinacht K. (2003). Evaluating the effects of music on dyspnea during exercise in individuals with chronic obstructive pulmonary disease: A pilot study. *Rehabil Nurs,* 28(6):192-196.

Bruera E, de Stoutz N, Velasco-Leiva A, Schoeller T, Hanson J. (1993). Effects of oxygen on dyspnoea in hypoxaemic terminal-cancer patients. *Lancet,* 342(8862):13-14.

Bruera E, Schoeller T, MacEachern T. (1992). Symptomatic benefit of supplemental oxygen in hypoxemic patients with terminal cancer: The use of the N of 1 randomized controlled trial. *J Pain Symptom Manage,* 7(6):365-368.

Bruera E, Sweeney C, Willey J, Palmer JL, Strasser F, Morice RC, et al. (2003). A randomized controlled trial of supplemental oxygen versus air in cancer patients with dyspnea. *Palliat Med,* 17(8):659-663.

Cahalin LP, Hernandez ED, Matsuo Y. (2005). Diaphragmatic breathing training: Further investigation needed. *Phys Ther,* 85(4):369-370; author reply 370-373.

Collins E, Fehr L, Bammert C, O'Connell S, Laghi F, Hanson K, et al. (2003). Effect of ventilation-feedback training on endurance and perceived breathlessness during constant work-rate leg-cycle exercise in patients with COPD. *J Rehabil Res Dev,* 40(5 Suppl 2):35-44.

Corner J, Plant H, A'Hern R, Bailey C. (1996). Non-pharmacological intervention for breathlessness in lung cancer. *Palliat Med,* 10(4):299-305.

Cristiano LM, Schwartzstein RM. (1997). Effect of chest wall vibration on dyspnea during hypercapnia and exercise in chronic obstructive pulmonary disease. *Am J Respir Crit Care Med*, 155(5):1552-1559.

Filshie J, Penn K, Ashley S, Davis C. (1996). Acupuncture for the relief of cancer-related breathlessness. *Palliat Med*, 10(2):145-150.

Fujie T, Tojo N, Inase N, Nara N, Homma I, Yoshizawa Y. (2002). Effect of chest wall vibration on dyspnea during exercise in chronic obstructive pulmonary disease. *Respir Physiol Neurobiol*, 130(3): 305-316.

Garrod R, Dallimore K, Cook J, Davies V, Quade K. (2005). An evaluation of the acute impact of pursed lips breathing on walking distance in nonspontaneous pursed lips breathing chronic obstructive pulmonary disease patients. *Chron Respir Dis*, 2(2):67-72.

Gift AG, Moore T, Soeken K. (1992). Relaxation to reduce dyspnea and anxiety in COPD patients. *Nurs Res*, 41(4):242-246.

Goldberg P, Reissmann H, Maltais F, Ranieri M, Gottfried SB. (1995). Efficacy of noninvasive CPAP in COPD with acute respiratory failure. *Eur Respir J*, 8(11):1894-1900.

Gosselink R. (2003). Controlled breathing and dyspnea in patients with chronic obstructive pulmonary disease (COPD). *J Rehabil Res Dev*, 40(5 Suppl 2):25-33.

Griffiths TL, Burr ML, Campbell IA, Lewis-Jenkins V, Mullins J, Shiels K, et al. (2000). Results at 1 year of outpatient multidisciplinary pulmonary rehabilitation: A randomised controlled trial. *Lancet*, 355(9201):362-368.

Howland J, Nelson EC, Barlow PB, McHugo G, Meier FA, Brent P, et al. (1986). Chronic obstructive airway disease. Impact of health education. *Chest*, 90(2):233-238.

Janson-Bjerklie S, Carrieri VK, Hudes M. (1986). The sensations of pulmonary dyspnea. *Nurs Res*, 35(3):154-159.

Jobst K, Chen J, McPherson K, Arrowsmith J, Brown V, Efthimiou J, et al. (1986). Controlled trial of acupuncture for disabling breathlessness. *Lancet*, 2(8521-22):1416-1419.

Keilty SE, Ponte J, Fleming TA, Moxham J. (1994). Effect of inspiratory pressure support on exercise tolerance and breathlessness in patients with severe stable chronic obstructive pulmonary disease. *Thorax*, 49(10):990-994.

Lacasse Y, Brosseau L, Milne S, Martin S, Wong E, Guyatt GH, et al. (2002). Pulmonary rehabilitation for chronic obstructive pulmonary disease. *Cochrane Database Syst Rev*, (3):CD003793.

Lacasse Y, Goldstein R, Lasserson T, Martin S. (2006). Pulmonary rehabilitation for chronic obstructive pulmonary disease. *Cochrane Database Syst Rev*, (4):CD003793.

Lewith GT, Prescott P, Davis CL. (2004). Can a standardized acupuncture technique palliate disabling breathlessness: A single-blind, placebo-controlled crossover study. *Chest*, 125(5):1783-1790.

Liss HP, Grant BJ. (1988). The effect of nasal flow on breathlessness in patients with chronic obstructive pulmonary disease. *Am Rev Respir Dis*, 137(6):1285-1288.

Louie SW. (2004). The effects of guided imagery relaxation in people with COPD. *Occup Ther Int*, 11(3):145-159.

Maa SH, Gauthier D, Turner M. (1997). Acupressure as an adjunct to a pulmonary rehabilitation program. *J Cardiopulm Rehabil*, 17(4):268-276.

Maa SH, Sun M, Hsu KH, Hung TJ, Chen HC, Yu CT, et al. (2003). Effect of acupuncture or acupressure on quality of life of patients with chronic obstructive asthma: A pilot study. *J Altern Complement Med*, 9(5):659-670.

Maltais F, Reissmann H, Gottfried SB. (1995). Pressure support reduces inspiratory effort and dyspnea during exercise in chronic airflow obstruction. *Am J Respir Crit Care Med*, 151(4):1027-1033.

McBride S, Graydon J, Sidani S, Hall L. (1999). The therapeutic use of music for dyspnea and anxiety in patients with COPD who live at home. *J Holist Nurs*, 17(3):229-250.

Moody LE, Fraser M, Yarandi H. (1993). Effects of guided imagery in patients with chronic bronchitis and emphysema. *Clin Nurs Res*, 2(4):478-486.

Moorhead M, Johnson M, Maas M (Eds.) (2004). *Nursing Outcomes Classification (NOC)* (3rd ed). St. Louis: Mosby.

Nici L, Donner C, Wouters E, Zuwallack R, Ambrosino N, Bourbeau J, et al. (2006). American Thoracic Society/European Respiratory Society statement on pulmonary rehabilitation. *Am J Respir Crit Care Med*, 173(12):1390-1413.

Normandin EA, McCusker C, Connors M, Vale F, Gerardi D, ZuWallack RL. (2002). An evaluation of two approaches to exercise conditioning in pulmonary rehabilitation. *Chest,* 121(4):1085-1091.

O'Donnell DE, McGuire M, Samis L, Webb KA. (1995). The impact of exercise reconditioning on breathlessness in severe chronic airflow limitation. *Am J Respir Crit Care Med,* 152(6 Pt 1):2005-2013.

O'Neill S, McCarthy DS. (1983). Postural relief of dyspnoea in severe chronic airflow limitation: Relationship to respiratory muscle strength. *Thorax,* 38(8):595-600.

Renfroe KL. (1988). Effect of progressive relaxation on dyspnea and state anxiety in patients with chronic obstructive pulmonary disease. *Heart Lung,* 17(4):408-413.

Renston JP, DiMarco AF, Supinski GS. (1994). Respiratory muscle rest using nasal BiPAP ventilation in patients with stable severe COPD. *Chest,* 105(4):1053-1060.

Ries AL, Kaplan RM, Limberg TM, Prewitt LM. (1995). Effects of pulmonary rehabilitation on physiologic and psychosocial outcomes in patients with chronic obstructive pulmonary disease. *Ann Intern Med,* 122(11):823-832.

Ries AL, Kaplan RM, Myers R, Prewitt LM. (2003). Maintenance after pulmonary rehabilitation in chronic lung disease: A randomized trial. *Am J Respir Crit Care Med,* 167(6):880-888.

Ries AL, Make BJ, Lee SM, Krasna MJ, Bartels M, Crouch R, et al. (2005). The effects of pulmonary rehabilitation in the national emphysema treatment trial. *Chest,* 128(6):3799-3809.

Sassi-Dambron DE, Eakin EG, Ries AL, Kaplan RM. (1995). Treatment of dyspnea in COPD. A controlled clinical trial of dyspnea management strategies. *Chest,* 107(3):724-729.

Schwartzstein RM, Lahive K, Pope A, Weinberger SE, Weiss JW. (1987). Cold facial stimulation reduces breathlessness induced in normal subjects. *Am Rev Respir Dis,* 136(1):58-61.

Sharp JT, Drutz WS, Moisan T, Foster J, Machnach W. (1980). Postural relief of dyspnea in severe chronic obstructive pulmonary disease. *Am Rev Respir Dis,* 122(2):201-211.

Sibuya M, Yamada M, Kanamaru A, Tanaka K, Suzuki H, Noguchi E, et al. (1994). Effect of chest wall vibration on dyspnea in patients with chronic respiratory disease. *Am J Respir Crit Care Med,* 149(5):1235-1240.

Simon PM, Basner RC, Weinberger SE, Fencl V, Weiss JW, Schwartzstein RM. (1991). Oral mucosal stimulation modulates intensity of breathlessness induced in normal subjects. *Am Rev Respir Dis,* 144(2):419-422.

Spahija J, de Marchie M, Grassino A. (2005). Effects of imposed pursed-lips breathing on respiratory mechanics and dyspnea at rest and during exercise in COPD. *Chest,* 128(2):640-650.

Spathis A, Wade R, Booth S. (2006). Oxygen in the palliation of breathlessness. In S Booth & D Dudgeon (Eds): *Dyspnoea in advanced disease: A guide to clinical management.* New York: Oxford University Press, pp 205-236.

Strijbos JH, Postma DS, van Altena R, Gimeno F, Koeter GH. (1996). Feasibility and effects of a home-care rehabilitation program in patients with chronic obstructive pulmonary disease. *J Cardiopulm Rehabil,* 16(6):386-393.

Stulbarg MS, Carrieri-Kohlman V, Demir-Deviren S, Nguyen HQ, Adams L, Tsang AH, et al. (2002). Exercise training improves outcomes of a dyspnea self-management program. *J Cardiopulm Rehabil,* 22(2):109-121.

Swinburn CR, Mould H, Stone TN, Corris PA, Gibson GJ. (1991). Symptomatic benefit of supplemental oxygen in hypoxemic patients with chronic lung disease. *Am Rev Respir Dis,* 143(5 Pt 1):913-915.

Tandon MK. (1978). Adjunct treatment with yoga in chronic severe airways obstruction. *Thorax,* 33(4):514-517.

Tiep BL, Burns M, Kao D, Madison R, Herrera J. (1986). Pursed lips breathing training using ear oximetry. *Chest,* 90(2):218-221.

Troosters T, Gosselink R, Decramer M. (2000). Short- and long-term effects of outpatient rehabilitation in patients with chronic obstructive pulmonary disease: A randomized trial. *Am J Med,* 109(3): 207-212.

Velloso M, Jardim JR. (2006). Study of energy expenditure during activities of daily living using and not using body position recommended by energy conservation techniques in patients with COPD. *Chest,* 130(1):126-132.

Vickers AJ, Feinstein MB, Deng GE, Cassileth BR. (2005). Acupuncture for dyspnea in advanced cancer: a randomized, placebo-controlled pilot trial. *BMC Palliat Care,* 4:5.

Wu HS, Wu SC, Lin JG, Lin LC. (2004). Effectiveness of acupressure in improving dyspnoea in chronic obstructive pulmonary disease. *J Adv Nurs,* 45(3):252-259.

Zimmerman BW, Brown ST, Bowman JM. (1996). A self-management program for chronic obstructive pulmonary disease: Relationship to dyspnea and self-efficacy. *Rehabil Nurs*, 21(5):253-257.

 # DYSREFLEXIA MANAGEMENT   NIC

Paula R. Sherwood, PhD, RN, CNRN; Elizabeth A. Crago, MSN, RN

NIC Definition: Prevention and elimination of stimuli that cause hyperactive reflexes and inappropriate autonomic responses in a patient with a cervical or high thoracic cord lesion (Dochterman & Bulechek, 2004).

NURSING ACTIVITIES

Effective

No applicable research was found in this category.

Possibly Effective

■ *Identify patients with higher levels of injury and more complete lesions at risk for autonomic dysreflexia (AD), even in the acute phase of recovery.* **LOE=III**

MR In a retrospective descriptive study involving 58 patients with acute spinal cord injury (SCI), onset of AD in the acute recovery phase was associated with cervical versus thoracic lesions (Krassioukov et al., 2003).

MR In a descriptive survey of 330 patients with SCI, having a more complete lesion significantly predicted AD (Widerstrom-Noga et al., 2004).

■ *Identify patients who undergo late surgery (>72 hours after injury) at risk for AD.* **LOE=VI**

MR In a retrospective case series, data for 779 patients with SCI revealed that those who underwent late (>72 hours after injury) spinal stabilization surgery had a higher incidence of AD than those who did not undergo surgery (McKinley et al., 2004).

■ *Use a bowel management program to avoid constipation and bowel obstruction to lower the risk of AD (although "silent" AD may still occur).* **LOE=III**

MR In a prospective descriptive study involving 10 participants with a complete SCI above T6 who underwent a routine bowel program, increases in systolic blood pressure occurred despite the absence of subjective signs of AD (Kirshblum et al., 2002).

MR In a retrospective descriptive study involving patients with acute onset of AD (cervical lesions), fecal impaction and abdominal distention were associated with AD (Krassioukov et al., 2003).

■ *Use a urinary management program to avoid bladder distention to lower the risk of AD.* **LOE=III**

MR In a descriptive survey of 330 patients with SCI, having a full bladder was associated with a higher incidence of AD (Widerstrom-Noga et al., 2004).

RCT = Randomized Controlled (Clinical) Trial, **NIC** = Nursing Interventions Classification, **NOC** = Nursing Outcomes Classification

■ *Assess the patient with SCI regularly for pain and teach adequate pain management techniques.* **LOE=VI**

(MR) In a descriptive survey of 330 patients with SCI, AD was significantly associated with widespread pain and pain worsened by infections (Widerstrom-Noga et al., 2004).

■ *Teach the patient methods for reducing mental stress, such as guided imagery and relaxation.* **LOE=VI**

(MR) In a descriptive survey of 330 patients with SCI, anxiety significantly predicted AD (Widerstrom-Noga et al., 2004).

Not Effective

No applicable published research was found in this category.

Possibly Harmful

■ *Acupuncture for patients with SCI.* **LOE=III**

(MR) In a controlled nonrandomized study involving 15 patients with SCI at or above T8, acupuncture was associated with an acute elevation in systolic blood pressure in three cases (Averill et al., 2000).

■ *Patients undergoing anorectal procedures; treatment with lidocaine may prevent symptoms of AD.* **LOE=II**

(MR) In an RCT, patients with SCI above T6 who received lidocaine anal blocks prior to anorectal procedures had significantly lower mean systolic pressure than patients with saline injections (Cosman & Vu, 2005).

■ *Sexual intercourse in AD patients.* **LOE=VI**

(MR) In a descriptive study involving 315 women with SCI, 11.4% reported AD during sexual activity (Moreno et al., 1995).

(MR) In a review of case studies involving three men with SCI, ejaculation was cited as the trigger for prolonged (>1 week) AD (Elliott & Krassioukov, 2006).

OUTCOME MEASUREMENT

NEUROLOGICAL STATUS: AUTONOMIC   (NOC)

(Please refer to *Nursing Outcomes Classification* [Moorhead et al., 2004] for the **Neurological Status: Autonomic** outcome.)

REFERENCES

Averill A, Cotter AC, Nayak S, Matheis RJ, Shiflett SC. (2000). Blood pressure response to acupuncture in a population at risk for autonomic dysreflexia. *Arch Phys Med Rehabil,* 81(11):1494-1497.

Cosman BC, Vu TT. (2005). Lidocaine anal block limits autonomic dysreflexia during anorectal procedures in spinal cord injury: A randomized, double-blind, placebo-controlled trial. *Dis Colon Rectum,* 48(8):1556-1561.

Dochterman JM, Bulechek GM (Eds). (2004). *Nursing Interventions Classification (NIC),* 4th ed. St. Louis: Mosby.

NR = Nursing Research, **MR** = Multidisciplinary Research, **SP** = Standard of Practice, **EO** = Expert Opinion, **LOE** = Level of Evidence

Elliott S, Krassioukov A. (2006). Malignant autonomic dysreflexia in spinal cord injured men. *Spinal Cord,* 44(6):386-392.

Kirshblum SC, House JG, O'Connor KC. (2002). Silent autonomic dysreflexia during a routine bowel program in persons with traumatic spinal cord injury: A preliminary study. *Arch Phys Med Rehabil,* 83(12):1774-1776.

Krassioukov AV, Furlan JC, Fehlings MG. (2003). Autonomic dysreflexia in acute spinal cord injury: An under-recognized clinical entity. *J Neurotrauma,* 20(8):707-716.

McKinley W, Meade MA, Kirshblum S, Barnard B. (2004). Outcomes of early surgical management versus late or no surgical intervention after acute spinal cord injury. *Arch Phys Med Rehabil,* 85(11):1818-1825.

Moorhead M, Johnson M, Maas M (Eds). (2004). *Nursing Outcomes Classification (NOC),* 3rd ed. St. Louis: Mosby.

Moreno JG, Chancellor MB, Karasick S, King S, Abdill CK, Rivas DA. (1995). Improved quality of life and sexuality with continent urinary diversion in quadriplegic women with umbilical stoma. *Arch Phys Med Rehabil,* 76(8):758-762.

Tsai SJ, Lew HL, Date E, Bih LI. (2002). Treatment of detrusor-sphincter dyssynergia by pudendal nerve block in patients with spinal cord injury. *Arch Phys Med Rehabil,* 83(5):714-717.

Widerstrom-Noga E, Cruz-Almeida Y, Krassioukov A. (2004). Is there a relationship between chronic pain and autonomic dysreflexia in persons with cervical spinal cord injury? *J Neurotrauma,* 21(2):195-204.

DYSRHYTHMIA MANAGEMENT (NIC)

Sharon Wallace, MSN, RN, CCRN

(NIC) **Definition:** Preventing, recognizing, and facilitating treatment of abnormal cardiac rhythms (Dochterman & Bulechek, 2004).

NURSING ACTIVITIES

Effective

■ (NIC) *Ascertain patient and family history of heart disease and dysrhythmias.*
LOE=I

 Findings from a national quantitative study (*N*=1008) of women's awareness of history of cardiovascular disease (CVD), awareness of CVD as a leading cause of death, and knowledge of personal risk and risk to family members indicated that awareness of CVD risk was positively associated with action. Study participants took measures to lower risk in themselves and their families (Mosca et al., 2006).

 In a quantitative study of adults (*N*=193) aged 21 to 55 years, elevated catecholamine levels, epinephrine and norepinephrine, and elevated levels of cortisol were associated with lower socioeconomic status, independent of race, age, gender, and body mass. Elevated levels of catecholamines and cortisol were linked to increased blood pressure, increased heart rate, and abnormal cardiac rhythms, including sudden death (Cohen et al., 2006).

 Modifiable risk factors in men (*N*=3681) and women (*N*=1910) who lived beyond 80 years and 85 years, respectively, were compared with those in men (*N*=1333) and women (*N*=543) who died before 80 years and 85 years of age, respectively. Modifiable risk factors associated with decreased probability of late survival included high pulse pressure and hyperglycemia in men and women. Increased heart rate was linked to decreased probability of late survival in males. Physical activity was associated with increased probability of late survival for men and women (Benetos et al., 2005).

(EO) For women, history and assessment of factors known to increase heart disease risk include blood markers of risk: cholesterol, C-reactive protein, homocysteine, lipoprotein(a), and fibrinogen. Other risk factors include smoking and lack of physical activity. Diet and body weight are assessed to determine risk. Stress and depression should be evaluated as contributing factors along with blood pressure. Finally, a Framingham score to project 10-year risk should be completed (Johnson & Manson, 2005).

(MR) Findings from a systematic review of randomized controlled trials ($N=18$) examining multiple risk factor primary prevention programs suggested that multiple risk factor intervention had no effect on mortality. Reviewers concluded that individual or family counseling and education appeared to be more effective (Ebrahim & Davey Smith, 2000).

(MR) In a descriptive study examining the difference between perceived risk and objective risk for CVD in African-American women ($N=128$), it was found that personal cardiac risk was underestimated despite family history of heart disease (DeSalvo et al., 2005). **LOE=VI**

■ (NIC) *Monitor for and correct oxygen deficits, acid-base imbalances, and electrolyte imbalances, which may precipitate dysrhythmias.* **LOE=V**

(NR) In a systematic review of research regarding vital signs, it was recommended that pulse oximetry be added to the traditional vital signs of temperature, pulse, blood pressure, and respiratory rate because changes in planned management of patients resulted more often from changes in pulse oximetry than from changes in vital signs (Joanna Briggs Institute, 1999).

(NR) In a qualitative study ($N=16$) describing the ways nurses recognize problems in patients, it was found that knowing the patient through repeated assessments, the family, and variation from the typical trajectory enabled nurses to detect subtle changes and distinctions. The skill of early recognition facilitated early intervention and the avoidance of further deterioration in patients' status (Minick & Harvey, 2003). **LOE=VI**

(EO) In one hospital, initiation of a nurse-led rapid response team reduced hospital mortality by 16% and code team activation by 33%, and there was a 55% decrease in codes outside the ICU by providing early intervention (Repasky & Pfeil, 2005).

■ (NIC) (SP) *Apply EKG electrodes and connect to a cardiac monitor.* **LOE=VII**

(EO) Electrocardiographic monitoring in the hospital setting is recommended for class I patients. Class II patients may benefit, but it is not essential. ECG monitoring is not indicated for class III patients (Drew et al., 2004).

■ (NIC) *Monitor EKG changes that increase the risk of dysrhythmia development: prolonged QT interval, frequent premature ventricular contractions, and ectopy close to the T wave.* **LOE=VI**

(EO) Highest priority candidates for QT-interval monitoring include patients with a genetic history; risk for torsades de pointes; QT-prolonging drugs associated with increased dose or overdose; ischemia and infarction; acute decreases in heart rate; and neurological events, hypokalemia, and hypomagnesemia (Drew et al., 2004).

(MR) In a descriptive study of members of two families ($N=12$), an extensive cardiac work-up identified that short QT syndrome was associated with syncope, palpitations, and sudden death. Short QT syndrome, an autosomal dominant inheritance, is thought to be associated with an alteration in the function of ion channels related to repolarization of the myocardium (Gaita et al., 2003).

NR = Nursing Research, **MR** = Multidisciplinary Research, **SP** = Standard of Practice, **EO** = Expert Opinion, **LOE** = Level of Evidence

■ **NIC** **SP** *Facilitate acquisition of a 12-lead EKG as appropriate.* **LOE=VII**

EO Highest priority candidates for ST-segment monitoring include patients with acute coronary syndrome (ACS) and myocardial infarction after thrombolytic therapy, primary angioplasty, and ongoing and recurrent ischemia, infarct extension, transient ischemia, and unstable angina (Drew et al., 2004).

EO Obtain serial 12-lead ECGs in patients with unstable angina/non-ST-segment elevation to increase sensitivity of the ECG for detecting ACS if the initial ECG is nondiagnostic (Gibler et al., 2005).

■ **NIC** **SP** *Determine whether the patient has chest pain or syncope associated with the dysrhythmia.* **LOE=VII**

EO Chest pain assessment includes gathering data about the pain. Traditionally, the PQRST method has been used, which includes provocative and palliative, quality, region, severity, and temporal aspects associated with chest pain (DeVon & Ryan, 2005).

EO Perform risk stratification to screen for ACS in unstable angina, non-ST-segment elevation myocardial infarction, and atypical presentations. Chest pain is not always a central feature of ACS. Patients who present with less typical symptoms include older adults, patients with diabetes and chronic renal failure, and women (Gibler et al., 2005).

EO Multiple studies have shown that atypical symptoms can lead to treatment delays and increased mortality in patients with ACS. Therefore, it is important for nurses, as first contact points within the health care system, to be knowledgeable of typical and atypical symptoms of ACS. Most frequently, women and older adults present with atypical symptoms (Ryan et al., 2005).

■ **NIC** *Assist the patient and family in understanding treatment options.* **LOE=I**

EO Clinical efficacy of β-blockers, contraindications excluded, has been well documented in the management of acute myocardial infarction, secondary prevention after infarction, non-ST-segment elevation ACS, chronic stable ischemic heart disease, heart failure, chronic heart failure, arrhythmias, prevention of sudden cardiac death, aortic dissection, hypertrophic cardiomyopathy, and hypertension (Lopez-Sendon et al., 2004).

MR In a systematic review of randomized controlled trials (N=5) involving a total of 5239 patients with persistent or recurrent atrial fibrillation, it was found that ventricular rate control and anticoagulation may be superior to rhythm control with regard to survival when compared with use of current antidysrhythmic agents (de Denus et al., 2005).

EO ACC/AHA/NASPE practice guidelines for implantation of cardiac pacemakers and antidysrhythmia devices include patients' identification and associated level of evidence (Gregoratos et al., 2002).

■ **NIC** *Teach the patient and family about actions and side effects of prescribed medications.* **LOE=II**

MR In an RTC (N=169) of congestive heart failure patients defined according to Framingham criteria, interventions to improve use of β-blockers by a nurse-facilitator, computerized reminders and patient letters, and provider education (control) were evaluated. Findings showed that nurse-facilitator intervention was more effective at 1-year follow-up (Ansari et al., 2003).

MR In an RTC, patients (N=792) were assigned to usual care and the COACH (Coaching patients On Achieving Cardiovascular Health) program or usual care. The COACH program

RCT = Randomized Controlled (Clinical) Trial, **NIC** = Nursing Interventions Classification, **NOC** = Nursing Outcomes Classification

involved multiple coaching strategies by nurses or dieticians, including prescribing and management of antilipidemic agents, associated with increased patients' compliance. Study findings demonstrated a statistically significant reduction in total cholesterol, body weight, body mass index, and a lesser increase in blood pressure than in the control group. Patients in the COACH group were found to have improved mood, diets, and increased walking exercise time with decreased reports of breathlessness and chest pain (Vale et al., 2003).

(EO) Teaching patients about drug-food interactions should include seasonal or geographic variation related to increased consumption of grapefruit juice. Grapefruit juice is an inhibitor of the cytochrome P450 enzyme system. Drugs used to treat dyslipidemia and CVD can accumulate with grapefruit juice (Karch, 2004).

■ (NIC) *Teach the patient and family measures to decrease the risk of reccurrence of the dysrhythmia(s).* **LOE=I**

(NR) A systematic review of research (*N*=6) related to the effectiveness of nurse-led cardiac clinics for adults with coronary heart disease showed that interventions led to statistically significant differences in lifestyle including diet change, smoking cessation, and adherence to medication. Improvements in general health status and quality of life and reduction in depression and severity of angina were found (Joanna Briggs Institute, 2005).

(MR) A systematic review of randomized controlled trials (*N*=29) of nursing interventions related to smoking cessation indicated the potential benefit of advice/counseling given by nurses to patients and that support from nurses could increase success of quitting. Some degree of evidence existed to suggest a greater effect in hospitalized patients with CVD than in inpatients with other conditions (Rice & Stead, 2004).

(MR) In a systematic review of systematic reviews (*N*=15), it was recommended that all patients be asked if they use tobacco and have their smoking status documented. Screening had been found to be effective as an intervention to lead to smoking cessation (Joanna Briggs Institute, 2001).

(MR) In the Women's Health Initiative Observational Study (*N*=73,743), a prospective study of postmenopausal women 50 to 79 years old, it was found that walking could reduce CVD risk with rates comparable to those for vigorous exercise (Manson et al., 2003).

(MR) In a cross-sectional, descriptive study (*N*=113) of nonsmoking men 30 to 40 years old, it was found that exercise was a significant predictor of low levels of total cholesterol and LDL cholesterol. Obesity and sedentary lifestyle were associated with elevated levels of triglycerides and unfavorable levels of HDL cholesterol (O'Donovan et al., 2005).

Possibly Effective

■ (NIC) *Teach the patient and family how to access the emergency medical system.* **LOE=VI**

(MR) In a descriptive study of men (*N*=38) and women (*N*=9) who were diagnosed with myocardial infarction, it was found that delay time (1.6 hours versus 6.1 hours) decreased significantly if symptoms occurred and a family member was present or if the patient talked to a family member (2.2 hours versus 6.5 hours) after onset of symptoms (Perry et al., 2001).

(MR) In a descriptive study of men (*N*=38) and women (*N*=9) who were diagnosed with myocardial infarction, it was found that delay in seeking treatment was associated with a mismatch between expected symptoms and symptoms experienced, particularly experiencing symptoms less dramatic than expected. Degree of mismatch was a significant correlate of delay (Perry et al., 2001).

NR = Nursing Research, **MR** = Multidisciplinary Research, **SP** = Standard of Practice, **EO** = Expert Opinion, **LOE** = Level of Evidence

■ **NIC** *Teach a family member cardiopulmonary resuscitation (CPR) as appropriate.* **LOE=IV**

MR In a retrospective observational cohort study, all witnessed nontraumatic cardiac arrests in Boston between 1994 and 1998 were evaluated to compare CPR rates of strangers versus known bystanders. Results were statistically significant and indicated that it was more likely that a stranger (45.8%) would perform CPR than a known bystander (15.5%) in a witnessed arrest (Casper et al., 2003).

MR In a prospective study of bystander-witnessed cardiac arrests, all cases of cardiac arrests resuscitated by EMS were recorded. For the patients surviving cardiac arrest ($N=922$), it was found that family members (44%) witnessed the arrest but rarely initiated CPR (11%). Study findings indicated that in the cardiac arrests witnessed by family members, 21% called others before calling EMS (Waalewijn et al., 2001).

MR In a prospective observational study conducted from January 1997 to May 2003 of bystander-witnessed cardiac arrest ($N=868$), it was found that of the bystanders interviewed ($N=684$), 69.6% were family members of the victim and 54.1% had been taught CPR. Reasons for a CPR-trained bystander not to perform CPR included panic (37.5%), perceived inability to perform CPR correctly (9.1%), and perception that they would hurt the patient (1.1%) (Swor et al., 2006).

Not Effective

No applicable published research was found in this category.

Possibly Harmful

No applicable published research was found in this category.

OUTCOME MEASUREMENT

KNOWLEDGE: CARDIAC DISEASE MANAGEMENT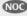

Definition: Extent of understanding conveyed about heart disease and the prevention of complications.

Knowledge: Cardiac Disease Management as evidenced by the following selected NOC indicators:

• Description of usual course of disease process
• Description of symptoms of early disease
• Description of symptoms of worsening disease
• Description of family caregiver's role in treatment plan

(Rate each indicator of **Knowledge: Cardiac Disease Management:** 1=none, 2=limited, 3=moderate, 4=substantial, 5=extensive) (Moorhead et al., 2004).

REFERENCES

Ansari M, Shlipak MG, Heidenreich PA, Van Ostaeyen D, Pohl EC, Browner WS, et al. (2003). Improving guideline adherence: A randomized trial evaluating strategies to increase beta-blocker use in heart failure. *Circulation*, 107(22):2799-2804.

RCT = Randomized Controlled (Clinical) Trial, **NIC** = Nursing Interventions Classification, **NOC** = Nursing Outcomes Classification

Benetos A, Thomas F, Bean KE, Pannier B, Guize L. (2005). Role of modifiable risk factors in life expectancy in the elderly. *J Hypertens,* 23(10):1803-1808.

Casper K, Murphy G, Weinstein C, Brinsfield K. (2003). A comparison of cardiopulmonary resuscitation rates of strangers versus known bystanders. *Prehosp Emerg Care,* 7(3):299-302.

Cohen S, Doyle WJ, Baum A. (2006). Socioeconomic status is associated with stress hormones. *Psychosom Med,* 68(3):414-420.

de Denus S, Sanoski CA, Carlsson J, Opolski G, Spinler SA. (2005). Rate vs rhythm control in patients with atrial fibrillation: A meta-analysis. *Arch Intern Med,* 165(3):258-262.

DeSalvo KB, Gregg J, Kleinpeter M, Pederson BR, Stepter A, Peabody J. (2005). Cardiac risk underestimation in urban, black women. *J Intern Med,* 20(12):1127-1131.

DeVon HA, Ryan CJ. (2005). Chest pain and associated symptoms of acute coronary syndromes. *J Cardiovasc Nurs,* 20(4):232-238.

Dochterman JM, Bulechek GM (Eds). (2004). *Nursing Interventions Classification (NIC),* 4th ed. St. Louis: Mosby.

Drew BJ, Califf RM, Funk M, Kaufman ES, Krucoff MW, Laks MM, et al. (2004). Practice standards for electrocardiographic monitoring in hospital settings: An American Heart Association scientific statement from the Councils on Cardiovascular Nursing, Clinical Cardiology, and Cardiovascular Disease in the Young. *Circulation,* 110(17):2721-2746.

Ebrahim S, Davey Smith G. (2000). Multiple risk factor interventions for primary prevention of coronary heart disease. *Cochrane Database Syst Rev,* (2):CD001561.

Gaita F, Giustetto C, Bianchi F, Wolpert C, Schimpf R, Riccardi R, et al. (2003). Short QT syndrome: A familial cause of sudden death. *Circulation,* 108(8):965-970.

Gibler WB, Cannon CP, Blomkalns AL, Char DM, Drew BJ, Hollander JE, et al. (2005). Practical implementation of the guidelines for unstable angina/non-ST-segment elevation myocardial infarction in the emergency department: A scientific statement from the American Heart Association Council on Clinical Cardiology (Subcommittee on Acute Cardiac Care), Council on Cardiovascular Nursing, and Quality of Care and Outcomes Research Interdisciplinary Working Group, in collaboration with the Society of Chest Pain Centers. *Circulation,* 111(20):2699-2710.

Gregoratos G, Abrams J, Epstein AE, Freedman RA, Hayes DL, Hlatky MA, et al. (2002). ACC/AHA/NASPE 2002 Guideline Update for Implantation of Cardiac Pacemakers and Antiarrhythmia Devices: Summary Article: A report of the American College of Cardiology/American Heart Association Task Force on Practice Guidelines (ACC/AHA/NASPE Committee to Update the 1998 Pacemaker Guidelines). *Circulation,* 106(16):2145-2161.

Joanna Briggs Institute. (1999). Vital signs. *Best Pract,* 3(3):1-6.

Joanna Briggs Institute. (2001). Smoking cessation interventions and strategies. *Best Pract,* 5(3):1-6.

Joanna Briggs Institute. (2005). Nurse-led cardiac clinics for adults with coronary heart disease. *Best Pract,* 9(1):1-6.

Johnson P, Manson J. (2005). How to make sure the beat goes on: Protecting a woman's heart. *Circulation,* 111(4):e28-e33.

Karch AM. (2004). The grapefruit challenge: The juice inhibits a crucial enzyme, with possibly fatal consequences. *Am J Nurs,* 104(12):33-35.

Lopez-Sendon J, Swedberg K, McMurray J, Tamargo J, Maggioni AP, Dargie H, et al. (2004). Expert consensus document on beta-adrenergic receptor blockers. *Eur Heart J,* 25(15):1341-1362.

Manson JE, Greenland P, LaCroix AZ, Stefanick ML, Mouton CP, Oberman A, et al. (2003). What type of exercise prevents cardiovascular disease in postmenopausal women? *N Engl J Med,* 168(3):314-320.

Minick P, Harvey S. (2003). The early recognition of patient problems among medical-surgical nurses. *Medsurg Nurs,* 12(5):291-297.

Moorhead M, Johnson M, Maas M (Eds). (2004). *Nursing Outcomes Classification (NOC),* 3rd ed. St. Louis: Mosby.

Mosca L, Mochari H, Christian A, Berra K, Taubert K, Mills T, et al. (2006). National study of women's awareness, prevention action, and barriers to cardiovascular health. *Circulation,* 113(4):525-534.

O'Donovan G, Owen A, Kearney EM, Jones DW, Nevill AM, Woolf-May K, et al. (2005). Cardiovascular disease risk factors in habitual exercisers, lean sedentary men and abdominally obese men. *Int J Obes,* 29(9):1063-1069.

NR = Nursing Research, **MR** = Multidisciplinary Research, **SP** = Standard of Practice, **EO** = Expert Opinion, **LOE** = Level of Evidence

Perry K, Petrie KJ, Ellis CJ, Horne R, Moss-Morris R. (2001). Symptom expectations and delay in acute myocardial infarction patients. *Heart,* 86(1):91-93.

Repasky TM, Pfeil C. (2005). Experienced critical care nurse-led rapid response team rescues patients on in-patient units. *J Emerg Nurs,* 31(4):376-379.

Rice VH, Stead LF. (2004). Nursing interventions for smoking cessation. *Cochrane Database Syst Rev,* (1): CD001188.

Ryan CJ, DeVon HA, Zerwic JJ. (2005). Typical and atypical symptoms: Diagnosing acute coronary syndromes accurately. *Am J Nurs,* 105(2):34-36.

Swor R, Khan I, Domeier R, Honeycutt L, Chu K, Compton S. (2006). CPR training and CPR performance: Do CPR-trained bystanders perform CPR? *Acad Emerg Med,* 13(6):596-601.

Vale MJ, Jelinek MV, Best JD, Dart AM, Grigg LE, Hare DL, et al. (2003). Coaching patients On Achieving Cardiovascular Health (COACH): A multicenter, randomized trial in patients with coronary heart disease. *Arch Intern Med,* 163(22):2775-2783.

Waalewijn RA, Tijssen JG, Koster RW. (2001). Bystander initiated actions in out-of-hospital cardiopulmonary resuscitation: Results from the Amsterdam resuscitation study. *Resuscitation,* 50(3):273-279.

EDEN THERAPY

Betty J. Ackley, MSN, EdS, RN

Definition: "A model for transforming skilled care facilities from institutions based on a medical model of care into human habitats that promote human growth. This change is accomplished through decentralizing the organizational structure of the facility to empower front-line care delivery staff, and through introduction of plants, animals, gardening, and children into the daily lives of residents" (Hamilton & Tesh, 2002, p. 1).

Eden Therapy is *not* a nursing intervention. It is a concept of care for extended-care facilities that influences how nursing care is delivered. It is included here because many nurses are employed in extended care.

NURSING ACTIVITIES

Effective

No applicable published research was found in this category.

Possibly Effective

■ *Use Eden Therapy to decrease boredom, helplessness, and depression in extended care residents.* **LOE = III**

NR A controlled study of nursing home residents exposed to Eden Therapy versus a control group (*N* = 34) demonstrated decreased boredom and helplessness, but loneliness was not affected (Bergman-Evans, 2004).

NR A controlled study of nursing home residents exposed to Eden Therapy versus a control group (*N* = 60) demonstrated significant differences in helplessness, boredom, and loneliness between the two groups. There were also improvements in the Geriatric Depression Scale (Parsons, 2004).

RCT = Randomized Controlled (Clinical) Trial, **NIC** = Nursing Interventions Classification, **NOC** = Nursing Outcomes Classification

(MR) A case study ($N = 120$) in a nursing home in Switzerland where Eden Therapy was instituted resulted in improved outcomes for residents (less loneliness, helplessness, and boredom) and financial stability (Monkhouse, 2003).

■ *Use Eden Therapy to increase physical and social function.* **LOE = VI**

(MR) A descriptive study ($N = 135$) demonstrated that the change to Eden Therapy helped promote increased function in residents, especially in the physical and social domain. However, there was no change in the minimum data set indicators (Hinman & Heyl, 2002).

■ *Use Eden Therapy to increase family satisfaction with care.* **LOE = III**

In a controlled study ($N = 37$) of families of residents in nursing homes where Eden Therapy was instituted, the satisfaction scores of families obtained from a mailed survey were significantly improved (Rosher & Robinson, 2005).

■ *Provide an on-site training process to begin Eden Therapy that involves a large number of the facility staff.* **LOE = VII**

(EO) Instituting Eden Therapy in facilities was more effective when training was done in the facility with a defined process. Facilities found that after Eden Therapy was instituted, there was a significant decrease in staff turnover, which led to better quality of care. Many facilities found that there was a decreased use of medications such as sleeping pills, antianxiety medications, and antidepressants with the institution of Eden Therapy (Steiner et al., 2004).

■ *Recognize that instituting Eden Therapy may or may not be sufficient to meet the needs of the elderly person. A change in the facility environment may also be necessary.* **LOE = VII**

(EO) The Green House concept grew out of Eden Therapy and includes an environment that promotes quality of care for the elderly (Thomas, 2003). (Note: Dr. William Thomas is the creator of Eden Therapy.)

Not Effective

■ *Using Eden Therapy in a nursing home environment to decrease rates of infection and falls, improve cognition, and decrease cost of care.* **LOE = III**

(MR) A controlled study comparing residents in an Eden Therapy facility versus a controlled facility ($N = 174$) found no major effect of the Eden facility utilizing MDS data on survival of residents, functional status, rate of infection, rate of falls, cognition, cost of care, or nutrition status. The researchers did acknowledge that there were more skilled care residents with lower cognition in the Eden group (Coleman et al., 2002).

Possibly Harmful

No applicable published research was found in this category.

NR = Nursing Research, **MR** = Multidisciplinary Research, **SP** = Standard of Practice, **EO** = Expert Opinion, **LOE** = Level of Evidence

OUTCOME MEASUREMENTS

THE GERIATRIC DEPRESSION SCALE (Yesavage et al., 1982-1983)

THE UCLA LONELINESS SCALE, VERSION 3 (Russell, 1996)

PERSONAL WELL-BEING NOC

Definition: Extent of positive perception of one's health status and life circumstances.

Personal Well-Being as evidenced by the following selected NOC indicators:
- Performance of activities of daily living
- Performance of usual roles
- Psychological health
- Social relationships
- Physical health
- Cognitive function
- Ability to cope
- Ability to relax

(Rate each indicator of **Personal Well-Being:** 1 = not at all satisfied, 2 = somewhat satisfied, 3 = moderately satisfied, 4 = very satisfied, 5 = completely satisfied) (Moorhead et al., 2004).

REFERENCES

Bergman-Evans B. (2004). Beyond the basics: Effects of the Eden Alternative Model on quality of life issues. *J Gerontol Nurs,* 30(6):27-34.

Coleman MT, Looney S, O'Brien J, Ziegler C, Pastorino CA, Turner C. (2002). The Eden Alternative: Findings after 1 year of implementation. *J Gerontol A Biol Sci Med Sci,* 57(7):M422-M427.

Hamilton N, Tesh AS. (2002). The North Carolina Eden Coalition: Facility environmental transformation. *J Gerontol Nurs,* 28(3):35-40.

Hinman MR, Heyl DM. (2002). Influence of the Eden Alternative on the functional status of nursing home residents. *Phys Occup Ther Geriatr,* 20(2):1-20.

Monkhouse C. (2003). Beyond the medication model—the Eden Alternative in practice: A Swiss experience. *J Social Work Long Term Care,* 2(3-4):339-353.

Moorhead M, Johnson M, Maas M (Eds). (2004). *Nursing Outcomes Classification (NOC),* 3rd ed. St. Louis: Mosby.

Parsons ME. (2004). *The impact of the Eden Alternative on quality of life of nursing home residents.* Unpublished doctoral dissertation, University of Nebraska, Nebraska.

Rosher RB, Robinson S. (2005). Impact of the eden alternative on family satisfaction. *J Am Med Dir Assoc,* 6(3):189-193.

Russell DW. (1996). UCLA Loneliness Scale (Version 3): Reliability, validity, and factor structure. *J Pers Assess,* 66(1):20-40.

Steiner JL, Eppelheimer C, De Vries M. (2004). Successful Edenization through education. *Nurs Home Long Term Care Manag,* 53(3):46-49.

Thomas W. (2003). The evolution of Eden. *J Soc Work Long Term Care,* 1(1/2):141-157.

Yesavage JA, Brink TL, Rose TL, Lum O, Huang V, Adey M, et al. (1982-1983). Development and validation of a geriatric depression screening scale: A preliminary report. *J Psychiatr Res,* 17(1):37-49.

RCT = Randomized Controlled (Clinical) Trial, **NIC** = Nursing Interventions Classification, **NOC** = Nursing Outcomes Classification

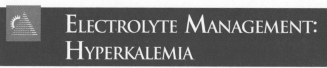

ELECTROLYTE MANAGEMENT: HYPERKALEMIA

 NIC

Elizabeth Speakman, EdD, RN, FANE, CDE

NIC **Definition:** Promotion of potassium balance and prevention of complications resulting from serum potassium levels higher than desired (Dochterman & Bulechek, 2004).

NURSING ACTIVITIES

Effective

■ *Obtain specimen(s) and monitor laboratory values of potassium levels and associated electrolyte imbalances.* **LOE = V**

NR A systematic review documented that serum electrolyte concentrations influenced movement of fluid within and between body compartments. Abnormal electrolytes may reflect fluid or acid-base imbalance or renal, neuromuscular, endocrine, or skeletal dysfunction (Elgart, 2004).

■ **NIC** *Monitor cause(s) of increasing serum potassium levels (e.g., renal failure, excessive intake, and acidosis) as appropriate.* **LOE = I**

NR A systematic review of the literature revealed that the most common cause of hyperkalemia was related to chronic or acute renal failure. In addition, the use of potassium supplements or salt substitutes and the intravenous administration of potassium could contribute to excessive serum potassium. In the case of metabolic acidosis, hyperkalemia is the result of the shift of potassium from intracellular to extracellular space (Burger, 2004).

MR A Cochrane review examined emergency management of hyperkalemia and found that hyperkalemia occurred in outpatients and between 1% and 10% of hospitalized patients because of renal failure, hyperglycemia, or inappropriate use of potassium supplements (Mahoney et al., 2005).

NR A systematic review of the literature noted that hyperkalemia may be the result of excessive parenteral administration of solutions containing potassium, tissue trauma that liberates intracellular potassium, respiratory or metabolic acidosis, or an adrenal cortical insufficiency (Speakman & Weldy, 2002).

■ **NIC** *Administer electrolyte-binding and -excreting resins (e.g., Kayexalate) as prescribed, if appropriate.* **LOE = VII**

NR A systematic review of the literature revealed that sodium polystyrene sulfonate (Kayexalate), a cation-exchange resin, was a common treatment for hyperkalemia with sorbitol, or another osmotic substance, to promote its excretion. Kayexalate can be given orally, through a nasogastric tube, or as a retention enema. As the medication sits in the intestine, sodium moves across the bowel into the blood and potassium moves out of the blood into the intestine. Loose stool removes potassium from the body (Hayes, 2003).

NR = Nursing Research, **MR** = Multidisciplinary Research, **SP** = Standard of Practice, **EO** = Expert Opinion, **LOE** = Level of Evidence

■ **NIC** *Administer prescribed medications to shift potassium into the cell (e.g., 50% dextrose and insulin, sodium bicarbonate, calcium chloride, and calcium gluconate), as appropriate.* **LOE = I**

MR A Cochrane review found that commonly practiced management options (salbutamol, insulin with glucose, dialysis) were effective in treating hyperkalemia (Mahoney et al., 2005).
MR A Cochrane review noted that in animal and human studies IV calcium stabilized membranes and reduced the arrhythmic threshold. The recommendation was that calcium chloride be given in the presence of ECG changes or dysrhythmia (Mahoney et al., 2005).

■ **NIC** *Avoid potassium-sparing medications (e.g., spironolactone [Aldactone] and triamterene [Dyrenium]), as appropriate. Monitor for unintentional potassium intake (e.g., penicillin G potassium or dietary potassium) as appropriate.* **LOE = V**

MR The randomized aldactone evaluation study (RALES) ($N = 44$) demonstrated that a dose of spironolactone larger than 25 to 50 mg a day was an important factor contributing to hyperkalemia (Wrenger et al., 2003).
MR A systematic review of the literature identified that potassium-sparing diuretics impaired the ability of the cortical collecting tubule to secrete potassium (Palmer, 2004).
MR A population-based time-series analysis examined trends in the rate of spironolactone prescriptions and the rate of hospitalization for hyperkalemia in ambulatory patients before and after the publication of RALES. Prescription claims data and hospital admission records were examined for more than 1.3 million adults 66 years of age or older in Ontario, Canada for the years 1994 through 2001. The analysis noted that closer laboratory monitoring and more judicious use of spironolactone may reduce the complication of hyperkalemia-associated morbidity and mortality (Juurlink, et al., 2004).

■ **NIC** *Maintain potassium restrictions.* **LOE = V**

NR A systematic review of the literature noted that the method to treat hyperkalemia depended on the cause and severity of the hyperkalemia. An uncomplicated excess of potassium can be treated by avoiding additional potassium intake either orally or parenterally (Speakman & Weldy, 2002).

■ **NIC** *Monitor for symptoms of inadequate tissue oxygenation (e.g., pallor, cyanosis, and sluggish capillary refill).* **LOE = I**

MR A Cochrane review identified that patients with hyperkalemia may experience weakness, fatigue, distal paresthesias, and respiratory depression (Mahoney et al., 2005).
MR Case-control methodological procedures identified risk factors for hyperkalemia in outpatients prescribed angiotensin-converting enzyme inhibitors during 1992 and 1993 at a Veterans Affairs medical center ($N = 1818$). The study revealed that elevated serum urea nitrogen, elevated creatinine level, and congestive heart failure were strongly and independently associated with hyperkalemia (Reardon & Macpherson, 1998).

■ **NIC** *Monitor renal function (e.g., BUN and Cr levels) if appropriate.* **LOE = V**

NR A systematic review documented that typically volume depletion causes increased urea absorption causing an elevated BUN level disproportionate to the serum creatinine (Elgart, 2004).

RCT = Randomized Controlled (Clinical) Trial, **NIC** = Nursing Interventions Classification, **NOC** = Nursing Outcomes Classification

(MR) A systematic review noted that patients with chronic renal failure who even had a small change in glomerular filtration would experience an elevation in Cr levels (Palmer, 2002).

■ (NIC) *Monitor fluid status, including intake and output, as appropriate.*
LOE = VII

(EO) Patients who demonstrate alterations in their volume status are likely to have electrolyte abnormalities (Elgart, 2004).

■ (NIC) *Monitor for therapeutic effect of diuretic (e.g., increased urine output, decreased CVP/PCWP, and decreased adventitious breath sounds).*
LOE = V

(MR) A systematic review determined that diuretics are drugs that cause a net loss of sodium and water from the body by net action on the kidney. Their primary effect was to decrease the reabsorption of sodium and chloride from the filtrate, increased water loss being secondary to the increased excretion of salt (Haji, 2005).

■ (NIC) *Administer prescribed diuretics, as appropriate.* **LOE = VII**

(EO) Mild hyperkalemia may be treated with a loop diuretic to increase potassium loss from the body or to resolve any acidosis present. Dietary potassium is restricted and medications associated with a high potassium level should be readjusted or stopped. Underlying disorders leading to the high potassium level are treated (Hayes, 2003).

■ (NIC) *Monitor for fluid overload resulting from associated renal failure, as appropriate.* **LOE = V**

(MR) A systematic review revealed that the management of patients with acute renal failure was frequently complicated by pulmonary edema and the effects of both fluid overload and metabolic acidosis (Pierson, 2006).
(MR) A single cohort, longitudinal, prospective study of peritoneal dialysis patients ($N = 28$) investigated the possible role of fluid overload in the development of malnutrition. Fluid status was evaluated by means of repeated bioimpedance analysis, and nutritional status was assessed by means of handgrip strength and subjective global assessment. All patients were observed closely for 9 months. Results revealed that there was a strong association between fluid status and nutritional state (Cheng et al., 2005).

■ (NIC) *Provide food low in potassium (e.g., fruits, beef, gelatin, and olives).*
LOE = VII

(EO) When kidneys are not healthy, patients should limit their potassium-rich foods (NKF, 2002).

■ (NIC) *Instruct patient on appropriate use of salt substitutes, as necessary.*
LOE = IV

(MR) A case study analysis observed a 74-year-old woman who had developed end-stage renal disease because of nephrolithiasis, hypertension, and renal vascular disease and also had

---

NR = Nursing Research, **MR** = Multidisciplinary Research, **SP** = Standard of Practice, **EO** = Expert Opinion, **LOE** = Level of Evidence

chronic obstructive pulmonary disease after 30 years of smoking. In November 2000, chronic intermittent hemodialysis was started three times weekly. The study demonstrated that patients with impaired renal potassium excretion related to renal disease, especially those taking angiotensin-converting enzyme inhibitors, angiotensin II receptor blockers, potassium-sparing diuretics, or NSAIDs, should be warned by their doctors and dieticians about the danger of hyperkalemia. Prescribers of these drugs to such patients should inquire about their use of potassium-containing salt substitutes (Doorenbos & Vermeij, 2003).

■ **NIC** *Monitor potassium levels after diuresis.* **LOE = V**

MR A systematic review identified that the loss of just 1% of total body potassium content would seriously disturb the delicate balance between intracellular and extracellular potassium and would result in profound physiological changes (Cohn et al., 2000).

MR A systematic review identified that a serum potassium level should be monitored frequently throughout diuresis treatment (Kraft et al., 2005).

■ **NIC** *Monitor infused and returned volume of peritoneal dialysate as appropriate.* **LOE = I**

MR A Cochrane review noted two studies that documented that the use of low-potassium and potassium-free dialysate was safe and effective in reducing serum potassium (Mahoney et al., 2005).

MR A systematic review noted that the rate of fluid removal was greatest at the beginning of each exchange and became less effective with time. The volume of fluid filled and drained is carefully recorded to allow close monitoring of fluid balance (Blowey & Alon, 2005).

EO When the dwell time is complete, open the drain clamp and let the dialysate drain by gravity into the drainage bag, taking impurities with it. Observe and document the characteristics and amount of outflow (Hathaway, 2004).

■ **NIC** *Monitor neurological manifestations of hyperkalemia (e.g., muscle weakness, reduced sensation, hyporeflexia, and paresthesias).* **LOE = VII**

EO In hyperkalemia, skeletal muscle weakness may occur, which in turn may lead to flaccid paralysis. Muscle weakness tends to spread from the legs to the trunk and involves respiratory muscles. Hyperkalemia also causes smooth muscle hyperactivity, particularly in the gastrointestinal tract, which can result in nausea, abdominal cramping, and diarrhea, an early sign. Other early warning signs may include restlessness and tingling in the lips and fingers (Hayes, 2003).

■ **NIC** *Monitor cardiac manifestations of hyperkalemia (e.g., decreased cardiac output, heart blocks, peaked T waves, fibrillation, or asystole).* **LOE = I**

MR A Cochrane review documented that patients with hyperkalemia may experience changes in the ECG rhythm (Mahoney et al., 2005).

EO Possible cardiac complications of hyperkalemia include a decreased heart rate, irregular pulse, decreased cardiac output, hypotension, and possibly cardiac arrest. The tall, tented T wave is a prominent ECG characteristic in hyperkalemia. Other ECG changes with worsening hyperkalemia include prolonged PR intervals, loss of P waves, widened QRS complexes, and atrioventricular conduction delays. This condition can also lead to heart block, ventricular dysrhythmias, and asystole. The more serious dysrhythmias become especially dangerous when serum potassium levels reach 7 mEq/L or more (Hayes, 2003).

▪ **NIC** *Instruct the patient and/or family on measures instituted to treat the hyperkalemia.* **LOE = VII**

EO Patients' education is an integral part of the nursing process, and nurses can use this process to assess, plan, implement, and evaluate an effective and individualized patients' education program (Wingard, 2005).

▪ **NIC** *Monitor for rebound hypokalemia (e.g., excessive diuresis, excessive use of cation-exchanging resins).* **LOE = V**

MR A systematic review noted that the goal of hyperkalemia therapy was to antagonize the cardiac effects of potassium to normal while avoiding overcorrection (Kraft et al., 2005).

Possibly Effective

▪ *Obtain specimen(s) and monitor laboratory values of potassium levels and associated electrolyte imbalances.* **LOE = I**

MR A Cochrane review demonstrated that a number of studies did not report absolute values of serum potassium for time points later than baseline or did not report variance in a usable way. Some papers reported change in potassium and standard error of the change rather than the absolute values of potassium (Mahoney et al., 2005).

▪ **NIC** *Monitor for therapeutic effect of diuretics (e.g., increased urine output, decreased CVP/PCWP, and decreased adventitious breath sounds).* **LOE = I**

MR A Cochrane review indicated that no studies were identified that examined the role of increasing urine output (e.g., by fluid resuscitation if appropriate or loop diuretics) to promote potassium excretion (Mahoney et al., 2005).

▪ **NIC** *Administer prescribed diuretics, as appropriate.* **LOE = I**

MR A Cochrane review indicated that no studies were identified that examined the role of increasing urine output (e.g., by fluid resuscitation if appropriate or loop diuretics) to promote potassium excretion (Mahoney et al., 2005).

Not Effective

No applicable published research was found in this category.

Possibly Harmful

No applicable published research was found in this category.

NR = Nursing Research, **MR** = Multidisciplinary Research, **SP** = Standard of Practice, **EO** = Expert Opinion, **LOE** = Level of Evidence

OUTCOME MEASUREMENT

ELECTROLYTE & ACID/BASE BALANCE NOC

Definition: Balance of electrolytes and non-electrolytes in the intracellular and extracellular compartments of the body.

Electrolyte & Acid/Base Balance as evidenced by the following selected NOC indicators:

- Serum potassium
- Apical heart rate
- Apical heart rhythm
- Serum creatinine
- Blood urea nitrogen
- Neuromuscular non-irritability

(Rate each indicator of **Electrolyte & Acid/Base Balance:** 1 = severely compromised, 2 = substantially compromised, 3 = moderately compromised, 4 = mildly compromised, 5 = not compromised) (Moorhead et al., 2004).

REFERENCES

Blowey DL, Alon US. (2005). Dialysis principles for primary health-care providers. *Clin Pediatr,* 44(1):19-27.

Burger CM. (2004). Hyperkalemia. *Am J Nurs,* 104(10):66-70.

Cheng LT, Tang W, Wang T. (2005). Strong association between volume status and nutritional status in peritoneal dialysis patients. *Am J Kidney Dis,* 45(5):891-902.

Cohn JN, Kowey PR, Whelton PK, Prisant LM. (2000). New guidelines for potassium replacement in clinical practice. A contemporary review by the National Council on Potassium in Clinical Practice. *Arch Intern Med,* 160(16):2429-2436.

Dochterman JM, Bulechek GM (Eds). (2004). *Nursing Interventions Classification (NIC),* 4th ed. St. Louis: Mosby.

Doorenbos CJ, Vermeij CG. (2003). Danger of salt substitutes that contain potassium in patients with renal failure. *BMJ,* 326(7379):35-36.

Elgart HN. (2004). Assessment of fluids and electrolytes. *AACN Clin Issues,* 15(4):607-621.

Haji A. (2005). The role of diuretics in the intensive care unit: A review. *Internet J Emerg Intensive Care Med,* 8(2):1-12.

Hathaway L. (2004). Peak technique. Peritoneal dialysis: Filtering out the bad guys. *Nurs Made Incredibly Easy,* 2(5):55-58.

Hayes DD. (2003). When potassium tips the balance. *Nurs Made Incredibly Easy,* 1(2):38-45.

Juurlink DN, Mamdani MM, Lee DS, Kopp A, Austin PC, Laupacis A, et al. (2004). Rates of hyperkalemia after publication of the Randomized Aldactone Evaluation Study. *N Engl J Med,* 351(6):543-551.

Kraft MD, Btaiche IF, Sacks GS, Kudsk KA. (2005). Treatment of electrolyte disorders in adult patients in the intensive care unit. *Am J Health Syst Pharm,* 62(16):1663-1682.

Mahoney BA, Smith WA, Lo DS, Tsoi K, Tonelli M, Clase CM. (2005). Emergency interventions for hyperkalaemia. *Cochrane Database Syst Rev,* (2):CD003235.

Moorhead M, Johnson M, Maas M (Eds). (2004). *Nursing Outcomes Classification (NOC),* 3rd ed. St. Louis: Mosby.

National Kidney Foundation (NKF). (2002). K/DOQI clinical practice guidelines for chronic kidney disease: Evaluation, classification, and stratification. *Am J Kidney Dis,* 39(2 Suppl 1):S1-S266.

Palmer BF. (2002). Renal dysfunction complicating the treatment of hypertension. *N Engl J Med,* 347(16): 1256-1261.

Palmer BF. (2004). Managing hyperkalemia caused by inhibitors of the renin-angiotensin-aldosterone system. *N Engl J Med,* 351(6):585-592.

RCT = Randomized Controlled (Clinical) Trial, **NIC** = Nursing Interventions Classification, **NOC** = Nursing Outcomes Classification

Pierson DJ. (2006). Respiratory considerations in the patient with renal failure. *Respir Care*, 51(4): 413-422.

Reardon LC, Macpherson DS. (1998). Hyperkalemia in outpatients using angiotensin-converting enzyme inhibitors. How much should we worry? *Arch Intern Med*, 158(1):26-32.

Speakman E, Weldy NJ. (2002). *Body fluids & electrolytes*, 8th ed. St. Louis: Mosby.

Wingard R. (2005). Patient education and the nursing process: Meeting the patient's needs. *Nephrol Nurs J*, 32(2):211-214.

Wrenger E, Müller R, Moesenthin M, Welte T, Frölich JC, Neumann KH. (2003). Interaction of spirono-lactone with ACE inhibitors or angiotensin receptor blockers: analysis of 44 cases. *BMJ* 327, (7407) 147-149.

Yelamanchi VP, Molnar J, Ranade V, Somberg JC. (2001). Influence of electrolyte abnormalities on interlead variability of ventricular repolarization times in 12-lead electrocardiography. *Am J Ther*, 8(2):117-122.

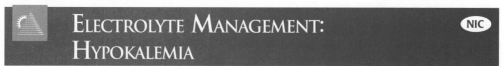

ELECTROLYTE MANAGEMENT: HYPOKALEMIA　　NIC

Elizabeth Speakman, EdD, RN, FANE, CDE

> **NIC**　**Definition:** Promotion of potassium balance and prevention of complications result-ing from serum potassium levels lower than desired (Dochterman & Bulechek, 2004).

NURSING ACTIVITIES

Effective

■ *Obtain specimens for laboratory analysis of potassium levels and associated electrolyte imbalances.* **LOE = V**

NR A systematic review documented that serum electrolyte concentrations influenced move-ment of fluid within and between body compartments. Abnormal electrolytes may reflect fluid or acid-base imbalance or renal, neuromuscular, endocrine, or skeletal dysfunction (Elgart, 2004).

■ *Monitor laboratory values for changes in oxygenation or acid-base balance.* **LOE = II**

MR In a controlled trial (*N* = 636), all patients who experienced severe hypokalemia (serum K⁺ < 3.0 mEq/L) during their hospitalization were enrolled. The study demonstrated that modest improvements in the management of a severe electrolyte disturbance in hospitalized patients could be achieved using a simple computerized alert system that highlighted abnor-mal laboratory values (Paltiel et al., 2003).

NR A systematic review documented that serum electrolyte concentrations influenced move-ment of fluid within and between body compartments. Abnormal electrolytes may reflect fluid or acid-base imbalance or renal, neuromuscular, endocrine, or skeletal dysfunction (Elgart, 2004).

NR A systematic review noted that monitoring laboratory values and performing physical assessments were the infusion nurse's primary role when caring for a patient receiving enteral or parenteral nutrition (Lauts, 2005).

NR = Nursing Research, **MR** = Multidisciplinary Research, **SP** = Standard of Practice, **EO** = Expert Opinion, **LOE** = Level of Evidence

■ **NIC** *Monitor intracellular shifts causing decreasing serum potassium levels (e.g., metabolic alkalosis; dietary, especially carbohydrate, intake; and administration of insulin), as appropriate.* **LOE = V**

MR A systematic review noted that hypokalemia could be the result of intracellular shifts of potassium, increased losses of potassium, or, less commonly, decreased ingestion or administration of potassium (Kraft et al., 2005).

MR An evidence-based review noted that in the absence of an inciting drug, hypokalemia could result from an acute shift of potassium from the extracellular compartment to cells, from inadequate intake, or from abnormal losses. Most commonly, hypokalemia is the result of either abnormal loss through the kidney induced by metabolic alkalosis or loss in the stool induced by diarrhea (Gennari, 1998).

EO Loss of potassium may occur as a result of high sodium intake or excessive administration of bicarbonate or other alkaline substances that stimulate the urinary loss of potassium (Speakman & Weldy, 2002).

■ **NIC** *Monitor renal cause(s) of decreasing serum potassium levels (e.g., diuretics, diuresis, metabolic alkalosis, and potassium-losing nephritis), as appropriate.* **LOE = V**

NR A systematic review of the literature noted that hemodialysis, continuous renal replacement therapy, and peritoneal dialysis could reduce serum potassium levels (Burger, 2004).

EO Diuretics and potassium depletion through the kidneys by osmotic diuresis from high urine glucose can cause a decrease in the body's overall potassium level (Nursing, 2002).

■ **NIC** *Monitor gastrointestinal cause(s) of decreasing serum potassium levels (e.g., diarrhea, fistulas, vomiting, and continuous NG suction), as appropriate.* **LOE = V**

EO Excessive potassium losses may occur with severe gastrointestinal fluid losses from continuous nasogastric suction, lavage, or prolonged vomiting. Diarrhea, intestinal fistulas, laxative abuse, and severe diaphoresis also contribute to potassium loss (Hayes, 2003).

NR A systematic review noted that increased potassium losses that exceed supplementation usually result from renal or gastrointestinal problems such as metabolic alkalosis, diarrhea, high nasogastric tube outputs, and chronic malnutrition (Lyman, 2002).

NR A systematic review documented that hypokalemia was much more common than hyperkalemia among patients receiving parenteral nutrition (Lyman, 2002).

NR A systematic review identified that the metabolic change that occurs with starvation is the shift from carbohydrate metabolism to fat and protein catabolism for energy, resulting in intracellular loss of potassium (Lauts, 2005).

■ **NIC** *Administer prescribed supplemental potassium (PO, NG, or IV) per policy.* **LOE = II**

MR An RCT (*N* = 38) of the use of potassium supplementation versus diet enriched with potassium foods demonstrated that postoperative cardiac patients receiving diuretic therapy could maintain serum potassium levels at clinically adequate concentrations by eating potassium-rich foods (Norris et al., 2004).

NR An evidence-based review noted that oral potassium replacement therapy was preferable if there were bowel sounds, except when life-threatening dysrhythmias existed. However, no

RCT = Randomized Controlled (Clinical) Trial, **NIC** = Nursing Interventions Classification, **NOC** = Nursing Outcomes Classification

empirical evidence was found in support of, or opposition to, the use of potassium protocols. The recommendation was to treat hypokalemia based on the patient's other associated deficiencies and the seriousness of the potassium deficiency (Harrington, 2005).

(MR) A systematic review noted that hypokalemia was treated by administering oral or IV potassium supplements. IV potassium supplementation is reserved for the treatment of severe hypokalemia and symptomatic hypokalemia or when the gastrointestinal tract cannot be used (Kraft et al., 2005).

■ **(NIC)** *Monitor renal functions, EKG, and serum potassium levels during replacement, as appropriate.* **LOE = V**

(NR) An evidenced-based review noted that IV intervention required careful monitoring including hourly urinary output; potassium administered incorrectly could greatly increase the risk of dysrhythmias and cardiac arrest (Burger, 2004).

(MR) A systematic review noted that serum potassium levels should be monitored frequently (1 to 6 hours) in patients with severe hypokalemia, 2 to 8 hours in patients with mild to moderate hypokalemia, and routinely (24 to 48 hours) in asymptomatic patients with hypokalemia that is not severe (Kraft et al., 2005).

■ **(NIC)** *Prevent/reduce irritation from potassium supplement (e.g., administer PO or NG potassium supplements during or after meals to minimize GI irritation, dilute IV potassium adequately, administer IV supplement slowly, and apply topical anesthetic to IV site), as appropriate.* **LOE = V**

(NR) A systematic review noted that the controlled-release microencapsulated tablet appeared to be better tolerated and caused less gastrointestinal erosion than the extended-release wax matrix tablet (Kraft et al., 2005).

(NR) An evidence-based review revealed that potassium supplements could cause stomach irritation and small bowel lesions. Taking smaller oral doses with food or after meals decreased this irritation (Burger, 2004).

■ **(NIC)** *Consider appropriate potassium preparations when supplementing potassium (e.g., chloride-associated hypochloremia; gluconate; acetate; citrate; bicarbonate, decreased chloride levels, and decreased serum potassium; sugar-free, for extracellular increases; or non–sugar free, for intracellular increases), as appropriate.* **LOE = VII**

(NR) An evidenced-based review noted that potassium replacement must always be diluted and delivered using an infusion controller, preferably through a central line to reduce the risk of phlebitis and sclerosis from local irritation (Burger, 2004).

■ **(NIC)** *Administer potassium-sparing diuretics (e.g., spironolactone [Aldactone] or triamterene [Dyrenium]), as appropriate.* **LOE = V**

(MR) An evidenced-based review noted that a more effective way to restore serum potassium to normal concentrations was to use a second diuretic drug that inhibits potassium excretion such as triamterene or spironolactone (Gennari, 1998).

(MR) A systematic review of the literature noted that an alternative therapy of potassium supplementation in correcting or preventing hypokalemia was the use of potassium-sparing diuretics (Kraft et al., 2005).

NR = Nursing Research, **MR** = Multidisciplinary Research, **SP** = Standard of Practice, **EO** = Expert Opinion, **LOE** = Level of Evidence

■ **NIC** *Monitor for digitalis toxicity (e.g., report serum levels above therapeutic range, monitor heart rate and rhythm before administering dose, and monitor for side effects), as appropriate.* **LOE = V**

NR A case study noted that a 55-year-old postoperative patient taking digoxin and furosemide (Lasix) complained of visual changes of halos and spots. The nurse recognized that hypokalemia is the most frequent cause of digitalis toxicity (Burger, 2004).

EO A deficit in potassium enhances the action of digitalis; if digitalis is given to a person with hypokalemia, toxicity is more likely to occur (Speakman & Weldy, 2002).

■ **NIC** *Monitor neurological manifestations of hypokalemia (e.g., muscle weakness, altered level of consciousness, drowsiness, apathy, lethargy, confusion, and depression).* **LOE = I**

MR A prospective cohort study ($N = 5600$) of people age 65 and older who were free of stroke at enrollment revealed that among diuretic users, there was an increased risk for stroke associated with lower serum potassium. Among individuals not taking diuretics, there was an increased risk for stroke associated with low dietary potassium intake. The small number of diuretic users with lower serum potassium and atrial fibrillation had a 10-fold greater risk for stroke than those with higher serum potassium and normal sinus rhythm (Green et al., 2002).

MR A retrospective chart review ($N = 158$) noted that admission hypokalemia was more frequent in patients with head injuries than those without head injuries and that hypokalemic patients on average had lower Glasgow coma scores than those without hypokalemia (Beal et al., 2002).

■ **NIC** *Monitor GI manifestations of hypokalemia (e.g., anorexia, nausea, cramps, constipation, distention, and paralytic ileus). Monitor pulmonary manifestations of hypokalemia (e.g., hypoventilation and respiratory muscle weakness). Monitor renal manifestations of hypokalemia (e.g., acidic urine, reduced urine, osmolality, nocturia, polyuria, and polydipsia). Monitor cardiac manifestations of hypokalemia (e.g., hypotension, broad T-wave, U wave, ectopy, tachycardia, and weak pulse).* **LOE = V**

MR A case study examined ECG changes resulting from an abnormal serum potassium level. The effect of hypokalemia on the cell membrane was to increase the resting membrane potential and increase the duration of the action potential and refractory period (Webster et al., 2002).

MR A systematic review noted that signs and symptoms of hypokalemia included nausea, vomiting, weakness, constipation, paralysis, and respiratory compromise with severe adverse effects of ECG changes, cardiac dysrhythmias, and sudden death (Kraft et al., 2005).

MR An evidence-based review noted that ECG changes were not common with mild to moderate hypokalemia, and it was only when the serum concentration was severe that changes readily appeared (Slovis & Jenkins, 2002).

■ **NIC** *Monitor for symptoms of respiratory failure (e.g., low Pao$_2$ and elevated Paco$_2$ levels and respiratory muscle fatigue).* **LOE = VI**

MR A retrospective chart review ($N = 158$) noted that hypokalemic patients were more likely to need a ventilator; however, no statistical significance was noted when comparing the amount of days the patient was vented with those of the nonhypokalemic patient (Beal et al., 2002).

NR A systematic review noted that as hypokalemia progressed, deep tendon reflexes may be decreased or absent and respiratory muscles could become paralyzed (Nursing, 2002).

RCT = Randomized Controlled (Clinical) Trial, **NIC** = Nursing Interventions Classification, **NOC** = Nursing Outcomes Classification

■ **NIC** *Monitor for rebound hyperkalemia.* **LOE = V**

NR A triangulated study that examined empirical evidence, a comparison of potassium protocols currently used, and an evaluation of the potential benefits and risks of using a potassium protocol in a sample of patients concluded that the use of narrowly defined potassium protocols may lead to overtreatment or incorrect treatment (Harrington, 2005).

NR A systematic review of the literature noted that the oral route potassium supplements were the safest way to increase the patient's potassium; IV potassium supplements could cause rebound hyperkalemia in patients with hypokalemia caused by transcellular potassium shifts (Sweeney, 2005).

MR An evidence-based review identified that although potassium replacement was the cornerstone of therapy for hypokalemia, it was also the most common cause of severe hyperkalemia in patients who were hospitalized (Gennari, 1998).

■ **NIC** *Monitor for excessive diuresis.* **LOE = II**

MR An observational cohort study ($N = 7653$) found an association of mild hypokalemia with increased cardiovascular effects among diuretic-treated hypertensive patients (Cohen et al., 2001).

MR In a controlled study ($N = 36$), elderly clients were evaluated after receiving sodium phosphate for colonic preparation. Hypokalemia and hypocalcemia were noted in 56% and 58% of the patients, respectively. Researchers concluded that sodium phosphate induced serious electrolyte abnormalities in elderly persons (Beloosesky et al., 2003).

MR A systematic review of the literature noted that diuretic use was associated with a 68% increase in in-hospital mortality and a 77% increase in odds of death or nonrecovery of renal function (Haji, 2005).

Possibly Effective

■ *Monitor laboratory values for changes in oxygenation or acid-base balance as appropriate.* **LOE = II**

MR In a controlled trial ($N = 636$), all patients who experienced severe hypokalemia (serum K^+ <3.0 mEq/L) during their hospitalization were enrolled. The authors noted that although completed blood work was successfully tracked using computer-based software, the use of a computerized alert system without a follow-up call may delay the transfer of information (Paltiel et al., 2003).

■ **NIC** *Administer prescribed supplemental potassium (PO, NG, or IV), per policy.* **LOE = V**

NR A triangulated study that examined empirical evidence, a comparison of potassium protocols currently used, and an evaluation of the potential benefits and risks of using a potassium protocol in a sample of patients concluded that there was a wide variation in potassium protocols and no empirical evidence in support of or opposition to these protocols (Harrington, 2005).

MR A systematic review documented that although calculation of the amount of potassium needed to replace the loss that had occurred before the onset of treatment was straightforward, there was no simple formula for calculating the amount needed in patients in whom potassium loss was continuing (Gennari, 1998).

NR = Nursing Research, **MR** = Multidisciplinary Research, **SP** = Standard of Practice, **EO** = Expert Opinion, **LOE** = Level of Evidence

Not Effective

No applicable published research was found in this category.

Possibly Harmful

No applicable published research was found in this category.

OUTCOME MEASUREMENT

ELECTROLYTE & ACID/BASE BALANCE

Definition: Balance of electrolytes and non-electrolytes in the intracellular and extracellular compartments of the body.

Electrolyte & Acid/Base Balance as evidenced by the following selected NOC indicators:

- Serum potassium
- Apical heart rate
- Apical heart rhythm
- Serum creatinine
- Blood urea nitrogen
- Neuromuscular non-irritability

(Rate each indicator of **Electrolyte & Acid/Base Balance:** 1 = severely compromised, 2 = substantially compromised, 3 = moderately compromised, 4 = mildly compromised, 5 = not compromised) (Moorhead et al., 2004.)

REFERENCES

Beal AL, Scheltema KE, Beilman GJ, Deuser WE. (2002). Hypokalemia following trauma. *Shock*, 18(2): 107-110.

Beloosesky Y, Grinblat J, Weiss A, Grosman B, Gafter U, Chagnac A. (2003). Electrolyte disorders following oral sodium phosphate administration for bowel cleansing in elderly patients. *Arch Intern Med*, 163(7):803-808.

Burger CM. (2004). Emergency: Hypokalemia. *Am J Nurs*, 104(11):61-65.

Cohen HW, Madhavan S, Alderman MH. (2001). High and low serum potassium associated with cardiovascular events in diuretic-treated patients. *J Hypertens*, 19(7):1315-1323.

Dochterman JM, Bulechek GM (Eds). (2004). *Nursing Interventions Classification (NIC)*, 4th ed. St. Louis: Mosby.

Elgart, NH. (2004). Assessment of fluids and electrolytes. *AACN Clin Issues*, 15(4): 607-621.

Gennari FJ. (1998). Hypokalemia. *N Engl J Med*, 339(7):451-458.

Green DM, Ropper AH, Kronmal RA, Psaty BM, Burke GL; Cardiovascular Health Study. (2002). Serum potassium level and dietary potassium intake as risk factors for stroke. *Neurology*, 59(3):314-320.

Haji A. (2005). The role of diuretics in the intensive care unit: A review. *Internet J Emerg Intensive Care Med*, 8(2):1-12.

Harrington L. (2005). Potassium protocols: In search of evidence. *Clin Nurs Spec*, 19(3):137-141.

Hayes DD. (2003). When potassium tips the balance. *Nurs Made Incredibly Easy*, 1(2):38-45.

Kraft MD, Btaiche IF, Sacks GS, Kudsk KA. (2005). Treatment of electrolyte disorders in adult patients in the intensive care unit. *Am J Health Syst Pharm*, 62(16):1663-1682.

Lauts NM. (2005). Management of the patient with refeeding syndrome. *J Infus Nurs*, 28(5):337-342.

Lyman B. (2002). Metabolic complications associated with parenteral nutrition. *J Infus Nurs*, 25(1): 36-44.

Moorhead M, Johnson M, Maas M (Eds). (2004). *Nursing Outcomes Classification (NOC)*, 3rd ed. St. Louis: Mosby.

Norris W, Kunzelman K, Bussell S, Rohweder L, Cochran RP. (2004). Potassium supplementation, diet vs pills: A randomized trial in postoperative cardiac surgery patients. *Chest*, 125(2):404-409.

Nursing. (2002). Understanding hypokalemia. *Nursing*, 32(3):65.

Paltiel O, Gordon L, Berg D, Israeli A. (2003). Effect of a computerized alert on the management of hypokalemia in hospitalized patients. *Arch Intern Med*, 163(2):200-204.

Slovis C, Jenkins R. (2002). ABC of clinical electrocardiography: Conditions not primarily affecting the heart. *BMJ*, 324(7349):1320-1323.

Speakman E, Weldy NJ. (2002). *Body fluids & electrolytes*, 8th ed. St. Louis: Mosby.

Sweeney J. (2005). What causes sudden hypokalemia? *Nursing*, 35(4):12.

Webster A, Brady W, Morris F. (2002). Recognising signs of danger: ECG changes resulting from an abnormal serum potassium concentration. *Emerg Med J*, 19(1):74-77.

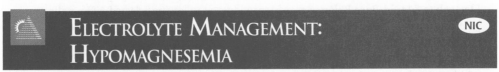

ELECTROLYTE MANAGEMENT: HYPOMAGNESEMIA

NIC

JoAnne Konick-McMahan, RN, MSN, CCRN

NIC **Definition:** Promotion of magnesium balance and prevention of complications resulting from serum magnesium levels lower than desired (Dochterman & Bulechek, 2004).

NURSING ACTIVITIES

Effective

■ *Identify patients at risk for hypomagnesemia (i.e., patients with electrolyte deficiencies, diabetes, alcoholism, on diuretic therapy).* **LOE = VI**

(MR) In a descriptive study (*N* = 1000) quantifying the frequency of hypomagnesemia in relation to other electrolyte abnormalities, hypomagnesemia occurred in 42% of patients with hypokalemia, 29% of patients with hypophosphatemia, 27% of patients with hyponatremia, and 22% of patients with hypocalcemia (Whang et al., 1984).

(MR) A case-control study of patients with type 2 diabetes in an outpatient setting (*N* = 290) found that 49% had hypomagnesemia (ionized serum magnesium less than 0.46 mmol/L) (Corica et al., 2006).

(MR) An RCT of chronic alcoholics (*N* = 49) comparing oral magnesium supplementation versus placebo for 6 weeks found reduction in liver enzymes; correction of sodium, calcium, and potassium levels; and increased muscle strength with magnesium supplementation (Gullestad et al., 1992).

(EO) Loop and thiazide diuretics are associated with loss of magnesium along with water loss (Stark, 2006).

■ *Identify cardiac populations at risk for dysrhythmias of hypomagnesemia, including patients after myocardial infarction, patients after coronary artery bypass grafting, and patients with heart failure.* **LOE = II**

NR = Nursing Research, **MR** = Multidisciplinary Research, **SP** = Standard of Practice, **EO** = Expert Opinion, **LOE** = Level of Evidence

(MR) An RCT (N = 100) of patients after acute myocardial infarction demonstrated that administration of intravenous magnesium in a continuous infusion over a 48-hour period decreased the incidence of dysrhythmia, pump dysfunction, and death (Gyamlani et al., 2000).

(MR) An RCT of patients with heart failure (N = 68) who received magnesium over 12 hours showed a significant decrease in ventricular dysrhythmias. Of note, 38% of patients had hypomagnesemia and 72% had excessive magnesium loss through the kidney (Ceremuzynski et al., 2000).

(MR) A meta-analysis of RCTs of prophylactic magnesium in the setting of cardiothoracic surgery found that magnesium reduced cardiothoracic surgery patients' risk of postoperative atrial fibrillation and length of stay. Lower doses and preoperative initiation provided the best reduction of postoperative atrial fibrillation (Henyan et al., 2005).

■ (NIC) *Monitor for neuromuscular manifestations of hypomagnesemia (e.g., muscle twitching, paresthesias, hyperactive reflexes, positive Babinski reflex, dysphagia, nystagmus, seizures, and tetany).* **LOE = VII**

(EO) Hyperreflexia is one sign of hypomagnesemia. Trousseau and Chvostek signs are both hyperreflexic responses to lack of magnesium (Stark, 2006).

■ *Administer magnesium along with potassium replacements in the setting of hypomagnesemia and hypokalemia.* **LOE = II**

(MR) An RCT (N = 32) in a surgical intensive care unit demonstrated increased circulating magnesium and decreased required potassium replacement with simultaneous infusions of potassium and magnesium versus potassium and placebo (Hamill-Ruth & McGory, 1996).

■ *Use caution when administering magnesium to patients with renal insufficiency or failure.* **LOE = VII**

(EO) Magnesium is excreted by the renal system and may accumulate in the presence of decreased glomerular filtration rate. The dose should be halved and levels checked daily in the acute care setting (Tong & Rude, 2005).

Possibly Effective

No applicable published research was found in this category.

Not Effective

No applicable published research was found in this category.

Possibly Harmful

■ *Use of antacids as magnesium replacement.* **LOE = VII**

(EO) Magnesium-containing antacids have been used to replete magnesium. These antacids cause diarrhea, a cause of magnesium deficiency, and should be used with caution. Safer oral replacement therapies are available and should be used for replacement (Innerarity, 2000).

RCT = Randomized Controlled (Clinical) Trial, **NIC** = Nursing Interventions Classification, **NOC** = Nursing Outcomes Classification

OUTCOME MEASUREMENT

ELECTROLYTE & ACID/BASE BALANCE NOC

Definition: Balance of electrolytes and non-electrolytes in the intracellular and extracellular compartments of the body.

Electrolyte & Acid/Base Balance as evidenced by the following selected NOC indicators:

- Serum magnesium
- Apical heart rate
- Apical heart rhythm
- Cognitive orientation

(Rate each indicator of **Electrolyte & Acid/Base Balance:** 1 = severely compromised, 2 = substantially compromised, 3 = moderately compromised, 4 = mildly compromised, 5 = not compromised) (Moorhead et al., 2004).

REFERENCES

Ceremuzynski L, Gebalska J, Wolk R, Makowska E. (2000). Hypomagnesemia in heart failure with ventricular arrhythmias. Beneficial effects of magnesium supplementation. *J Intern Med,* 247(1):78-86.

Corica F, Corsonello A, Ientile R, Cucinotta D, Di Benedetto A, Perticone F, et al. (2006). Serum ionized magnesium levels in relation to metabolic syndrome in type 2 diabetic patients. *J Am Coll Nutr,* 25(3):210-215.

Dochterman JM, Bulechek GM (Eds). (2004). *Nursing Interventions Classification (NIC),* 4th ed. St. Louis: Mosby.

Gullestad L, Dolva LO, Soyland E, Manger AT, Falch D, Kjekshus J. (1992). Oral magnesium supplementation improves metabolic variables and muscle strength in alcoholics. *Alcohol Clin Exp Res,* 16(5):986-990.

Gyamlani G, Parikh C, Kulkarni AG. (2000). Benefits of magnesium in acute myocardial infarction: Timing is crucial. *Am Heart J,* 139(4):703.

Hamill-Ruth RJ, McGory R. (1996). Magnesium repletion and its effect on potassium homeostasis in critically ill adults: Results of a double-blind, randomized, controlled trial. *Crit Care Med,* 24(1):38-45.

Henyan NN, Gillespie EL, White CM, Kluger J, Coleman CI. (2005). Impact of intravenous magnesium on post-cardiothoracic surgery atrial fibrillation and length of hospital stay: A meta-analysis. *Ann Thorac Surg,* 80(6):2402-2406.

Innerarity S. (2000). Hypomagnesemia in acute and chronic illness. *Crit Care Nurs Q,* 23(2):1-19.

Moorhead M, Johnson M, Maas M (Eds). (2004). *Nursing Outcomes Classification (NOC),* 3rd ed. St. Louis: Mosby.

Stark J. (2006). The renal system. In Alspach JG (Ed) *Core curriculum for critical care nursing.* St. Louis: Saunders, p 601.

Tong GM, Rude RK. (2005). Magnesium deficiency in critical illness. *J Intensive Care Med,* 20(1):3-17.

Whang R, Oei TO, Aikawa JK, Watanabe A, Vannatta J, Fryer A, et al. (1984). Predictors of clinical hypomagnesemia. Hypokalemia, hypophosphatemia, hyponatremia, and hypocalcemia. *Arch Intern Med,* 144(9):1794-1796.

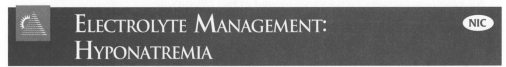

ELECTROLYTE MANAGEMENT: HYPONATREMIA NIC

JoAnne Konick-McMahan, RN, MSN, CCRN

NIC **Definition:** Promotion of sodium balance and prevention of complications resulting from serum sodium levels lower than desired (Dochterman & Bulechek, 2004).

NURSING ACTIVITIES

Effective

- *Identify individuals at risk for hyponatremia with encephalopathy in the acute care setting (i.e., postoperative premenopausal women, patients taking thiazide diuretics).* **LOE = IV**

  (MR) A case-control study of risk factors for encephalopathy ($N = 650$) as well as a cohort study of clinical course among patients with encephalopathy ($N = 674$) revealed that menstruant women were 25 times more likely to have permanent brain damage or die (Ayus et al., 1992).
  (MR) A systematic review ($N = 129$) of cases of severe diuretic-induced hyponatremia reported in the literature from 1962 to 1990 revealed that hyponatremia developed within 14 days in those treated with thiazide diuretics. None occurred in patients treated with furosemide (Sonnenblick et al., 1993).

- **NIC** *Monitor intake and output.* **LOE = VII**

  (NR) A systematic review demonstrated that a fluid intake sheet was the best method of monitoring daily fluid intake (JBI, 2001).

- *Monitor urine color, preferably a morning specimen, using a color chart.* **LOE = V**

  (NR) A systematic review demonstrated the effectiveness of caregiver's or patient's comparison of urine color with a chart as an indicator of fluid balance (Mentes, 2000).

- *Administer hypertonic saline at 1 to 2 mL/kg/hr or per policy for correction of severe, symptomatic hyponatremia. Adjust the rate to raise serum sodium levels by no more than 0.5 mEq/hr for a total of 8 to 12 mEq/L/24 hr.* **LOE = VI**

  (MR) A descriptive study ($N = 56$) of treatment-related complications of severe hyponatremia found no neurological complications among patients corrected slowly (less than 12 mEq/24 hr or less than 0.55 mEq/hr) (Sterns et al., 1994).

- **NIC** **SP** *Avoid excessive administration of hypotonic IV fluids, especially in the presence of syndrome of inappropriate antidiuretic hormone (SIADH) as appropriate. Maintain fluid restriction, as appropriate.* **LOE = VII**

  (EO) This standard of care is based on the rationale that free water is retained in SIADH, leading to dilutional hyponatremia. Reducing the amount of free water decreases serum free water and leads to correction of hyponatremia (Stark, 2006).

- *Withhold diuretics in the presence of hyponatremia related to the use of diuretics.* **LOE = VII**

  (EO) Diuretics, especially thiazide diuretics, are known to lead to hyponatremia, especially in the first 14 days of treatment (Sonnenblick et al., 1993).

- *Minimize the loss of gastrointestinal secretions related to vomiting, diarrhea, and continuous nasogastric suction.* **LOE = VII**

  (EO) Gastrointestinal secretions are sodium rich. Prolonged loss of these secretions without adequate replacement leads to hyponatremia. The use of medications to correct vomiting and diarrhea and prompt removal of nasogastric suction assist in correction of hyponatremia (Johnson & Criddle, 2004).

Possibly Effective

No applicable published research was found in this category.

Not Effective

No applicable published research was found in this category.

Possibly Harmful

No applicable published research was found in this category.

OUTCOME MEASUREMENT

ELECTROLYTE & ACID/BASE BALANCE NOC

Definition: Balance of electrolytes and non-electrolytes in the intracellular and extracellular compartments of the body.

Electrolyte & Acid/Base Balance as evidenced by the following selected NOC indicators:

• Serum sodium
• Urine specific gravity
• Mental alertness
• Cognitive orientation
• Sensation in extremities

(Rate each indicator of **Electrolyte & Acid/Base Balance:** 1 = severely compromised, 2 = substantially compromised, 3 = moderately compromised, 4 = mildly compromised, 5 = not compromised) (Moorhead et al., 2004).

REFERENCES

Ayus JC, Wheeler JM, Arieff AI. (1992). Postoperative hyponatremic encephalopathy in menstruant women. *Ann Intern Med,* 117(11):891-897.

Dochterman JM, Bulechek GM (Eds). (2004). *Nursing Interventions Classification (NIC),* 4th ed. St. Louis: Mosby.

The Joanna Briggs Institute (JBI). (2001). Maintaining oral hydration in older people. *Best Pract,* 5(1):1-6. Available online: http://www.joannabriggs.edu.au. Retrieved November 29, 2006.

Johnson AL, Criddle LM. (2004). Pass the salt: Indications for and implications of using hypertonic saline. *Crit Care Nurse,* 24(5):36-46.

Mentes JC. (2000). *Hydration management: A long-term care nursing intervention to prevent acute confusion and other hydration-linked events.* Doctoral Dissertation, University of Iowa.

Moorhead M, Johnson M, Maas M (Eds). (2004). *Nursing Outcomes Classification (NOC),* 3rd ed. St. Louis: Mosby.

Sonnenblick M, Friedlander Y, Rosin AJ. (1993). Diuretic-induced severe hyponatremia: Review and analysis of 129 reported patients. *Chest,* 103(2):601-606.

Stark J. (2006). The renal system. In Alspach JG (Ed). *Core curriculum for critical care nursing.* St Louis: Saunders.

Sterns RH, Cappuccio JD, Silver SM, Cohen EP. (1994). Neurologic sequelae after treatment of severe hyponatremia: A multicenter perspective. *J Am Soc Nephrol,* 4(8):1522-1530.

NR = Nursing Research, **MR** = Multidisciplinary Research, **SP** = Standard of Practice, **EO** = Expert Opinion, **LOE** = Level of Evidence

ENEMA ADMINISTRATION

Marilee Schmelzer, PhD, RN

NIC **Definition:** Instillation of a substance into the lower gastrointestinal tract (Dochterman & Bulechek, 2004).

NURSING ACTIVITIES

(Note: The large-volume enema technique is described here.)

Effective

No applicable published research was found in this category.

Possibly Effective

■ *Tell the patient exactly what to expect and how to cooperate during the procedure. Provide privacy by closing the door, putting a "do not disturb" sign on the door, and draping the patient so that only the anus is exposed. Reassure the patient that privacy will be maintained.* **LOE = VII**

   (NR) In a qualitative study describing experienced nurses' enema techniques (N=25), the nurses identified strategies to reduce the patients' embarrassment, including providing privacy, draping the area carefully, and being sensitive to the patients' feelings (Schmelzer & Wright, 1996).

■ *Ask the patient to lie in the left lateral Sims position.* **LOE = VII**

   (EO) No studies about the effectiveness of the Sims position were found, but it does place the patient in a position that makes the anus easily visible.

   (NR) In a qualitative study describing experienced nurses' enema techniques (N = 25), all the nurses said that they positioned patients on the left side for an enema, and most said that this was because the anatomy of the colon allowed the enema solution to flow by gravity from the rectum into the sigmoid colon (Schmelzer & Wright, 1996).

   (MR) In a case report of a 52-year-old man with multiple sclerosis whose anterior rectum was perforated by an enema tube, the authors suspected that the perforation occurred because the enema was given while the patient was sitting upright on a commode rather than lying down (May & Reynolds, 1968).

   (MR) An experimental study with healthy young men (N = 10) determined that flexing the hip to 90 degrees or more straightened the angle between the anus and the rectum (Tagart, 1966). Although the researchers did not discuss enemas, one would logically expect that the tube could be inserted more easily when the anal-rectal angle is straightened by knee flexion as occurs in the Sims position.

■ *Visually check the anus for sores, fissures, bleeding, or hemorrhoids, and perform a digital examination with a well-lubricated, gloved finger in order to feel any hemorrhoids or lesions and to determine the tract for inserting the enema catheter.* **LOE = VII**

   (MR) Case studies of three patients with perforations of the rectum found that all three had hemorrhoids, two had experienced pain during insertion of the enema, and the third had a perforation above the dentate line where the rectum is insensitive to pain. The authors concluded that the anus and rectum should have been assessed before giving the enema to identify any preexisting perianal pathology (e.g., hemorrhoids) and that the enema should have been immediately stopped and the physician notified if the patient experienced any difficulties or pain during insertion of the enema tip and delivery of the solution (Saltzstein et al., 1988).

(MR) Case studies of three patients who developed rectal gangrene from phosphate enemas found that all three patients had hemorrhoids, which may have made their rectums more susceptible to perforation by enema tips (Sweeney et al., 1986).

■ *Prepare 1000 to 1500 mL of enema solution as ordered.* **LOE = VII**

(EO) No studies were found comparing the effectiveness of various amounts of enema solution on cleansing ability, but studies have measured the amount of solution that people can take.

(MR) In a controlled study describing the number of tap water enemas needed to obtain clear returns, 123 patients were given 1.75-L enemas, and the researchers wrote that they had learned through experience that few patients tolerated enemas larger than 2 L (Pietilä et al., 1990).

(NR) In a quasi-experimental study comparing the effectiveness of tap water and soapsuds enemas ($N = 25$) in patients scheduled for liver transplantation, patients were able to retain from 400 to 980 mL (mean 890 mL) of enema solution (Schmelzer et al., 2000).

(NR) In a study in which healthy patients were given three enemas (tap water, soapsuds, and polyethylene glycol electrolyte solution [PEG-ES]) a week apart using a repeated measures design ($N = 24$), all but two patients were able to retain 1 L of each enema type. One person took the entire 1-L soapsuds enema but only 381 mL of tap water and 654 mL of PEG-ES, and a second person took only 974 mL of the PEG-ES but the entire liter of the other two solutions (Schmelzer et al., 2004).

(MR) In a study comparing rectal function in healthy volunteers ($N = 32$), patients with chronic constipation ($N = 14$), and patients with incontinence ($N = 16$), all the healthy participants took the entire 1.5-L water enema, the incontinent patients were unable to retain the enema, and the researcher did not comment about the chronically constipated patients' retention (Shafik, 1992).

■ *Warm the enema solution to slightly warmer than body temperature just before administering.* **LOE = VII**

(EO) No studies were found comparing the effectiveness and comfort of enema solutions given at various temperatures, but common sense indicates that a temperature that is close to normal body temperature would be safest. Nursing textbooks traditionally recommend that the enema solution be administered at about 105°F (Harmer & Henderson, 1939, p. 655).

(NR) In a qualitative study describing experienced nurses' enema techniques ($N = 25$), the nurses described warming the temperature of the enema solution so that it is "warm to touch," "body temperature," "lukewarm," "like a baby's bath water," or "room temperature." Two nurses said the temperature should be 105°F, but only one nurse reported using a thermometer (Schmelzer & Wright, 1996).

■ *Make sure that there are no air bubbles in the enema tubing.* **LOE = VII**

(EO) Air is generally considered to have an effect similar to that of intestinal gases; that is, it leads to cramping. People experience abdominal discomfort when air is injected into the rectum during proctoscopy.

NR = Nursing Research, **MR** = Multidisciplinary Research, **SP** = Standard of Practice, **EO** = Expert Opinion, **LOE** = Level of Evidence

■ *Lubricate the end of the enema tube and gently insert the catheter about 5.5 cm (2 to 3 inches) into the rectum to ensure that the tube is beyond the sphincters in the anal canal and to decrease the chance of perforating the rectum.* **LOE = VI**

(EO) No data have been collected regarding the number of perforations compared with the total number of enemas given, but the risk is probably much smaller than with sigmoidoscopy because the tube is inserted a much shorter distance (Richards et al., 2006).

(MR) A descriptive study of Japanese patients ($N = 920$) undergoing barium enema found that the mean length of the rectum was 17.31 cm (7.2 inches) (Sadahiro et al., 1992). The anal canal is about 2 to 3 cm long (Doughty & Jackson, 1993).

(MR) A study that included examination of the gross and histological features of adult ($N = 18$) and infant ($N = 10$) cadaver rectums and radiological examinations of the rectums of healthy volunteers ($N = 50$) found a narrowed junction between the rectum and sigmoid colon and other features suggestive of an anatomical sphincter in this area (Shafik et al., 1999). A sharp curve marks the connection of the rectum to the sigmoid colon; the sigmoid colon's mobility and tortuosity make it particularly challenging for the endoscopist to negotiate (Keljo & Squires, 1998).

■ *Open the clamp on the tubing when the bag is just above the anus and raise it until the solution starts to flow in at a slow, steady rate. Regulate it according to the patient's tolerance. Never raise the bag higher than 18 inches above the anus.* **LOE = III**

(EO) For more than 65 years, textbooks have been instructing nurses to raise the enema bag no higher than 18 inches above the anus (Harmer & Henderson, 1939, p. 657), but the origin of this advice was not determined.

(NR) In a qualitative study describing experienced nurses' enema technique ($N = 25$), all participants said that they raised the enema bag no higher than 18 inches above the rectum (Schmelzer & Wright, 1996).

(NR) During quasi-experimental studies comparing the effectiveness of large-volume enema solutions, researchers found that the enemas flowed in easily and most people were able to retain about a liter of enema solution when the enemas were given slowly and the bag was never raised above 18 inches (Schmelzer et al., 2004).

(MR) An experimental study in which colonic perforations were induced in juvenile pigs ($N = 135$) determined that perforations occurred when barium and water-soluble enemas were given at an average height of 57 inches (143 cm) (Shiels et al., 1993).

(MR) A 3-year retrospective study of all colorectal perforations caused by enemas in a surgical service (serving a population of 400,000 that included about 3500 nursing home patients) revealed 13 cases: 8 with perforations of the sigmoid colon and 5 with perforations of the rectum. Researchers ruled out possible causes other than the enemas but could not determine whether the injury was caused by the enema tip or hydrostatic pressure (Paran et al., 1999).

■ *If the patient complains of cramps or defecation urge, lower the bag to the level of the anus (so that nothing flows in), and instruct the patient to take slow, deep breaths until the cramps or defecation urge disappears.* **LOE = III**

(NR) When this procedure was used in a quasi-experimental study of enema solution effectiveness ($N = 25$), 20 people with chronic liver failure took almost the entire 1000-mL enema and reported little or no discomfort during the enemas (Schmelzer et al., 2000).

RCT = Randomized Controlled (Clinical) Trial, **NIC** = Nursing Interventions Classification, **NOC** = Nursing Outcomes Classification

(NR) When this procedure was used in a study of large-volume enemas in healthy participants ($N = 24$, repeated measures design), the entire 1000 mL of solution was retained by participants during 69 of the 72 enemas (Schmelzer et al., 2004).

(EO) When the enema bag is lowered to the level of the anus to stop the infusion, cramping and the defecation urge decrease, perhaps because the rectal muscle relaxes and fluid passes from the rectum into the sigmoid colon. Also, by lowering the bag rather than using the clamp, excessive pressure within the rectum is relieved as the gas and sometimes fluid can flow back into the bag (Miller, 1975).

■ *Measure the amount of enema solution given and the volume of the enema returns.* **LOE = III**

(NR) A quasi-experimental study, with random assignment to treatment groups and participants "blinded" to solution ($N = 25$), found that 11 of 12 people who received tap water enemas and 6 of 13 people who received soapsuds enemas eliminated a smaller amount (stool plus enema) than was given as an enema (Schmelzer et al., 2000).

(NR) A repeated measures design (double blind, random order of enema delivery) found negative mean outputs (i.e., the amount of solution infused was larger than the size of the returns) for all three enema solutions given to healthy volunteers ($N = 24$) (Schmelzer et al., 2004).

(MR) A case study described a 42-year-old woman who commonly took colonic irrigations and developed hyponatremia from a colonic irrigation with a hypotonic solution (Norlela et al., 2004).

(MR) A case study described a 65-year-old man with C6 quadriplegia who developed confusion and seizures after being given five tap water enemas (1.5 to 3.0 L each over 10 days) (Chertow & Brady, 1994).

Not Effective

No applicable published research was found in this category.

Possibly Harmful

■ *Holding the enema solution as long as possible before defecating.* **LOE = III**

(NR) A repeated measures design (double blind, random order of enema delivery) showed significantly greater loss of surface epithelium on biopsies following soapsuds, distilled water, and PEG-ES enemas ($N = 21$); 50% or more loss of surface epithelium occurred in 17 people following a soapsuds enema, in 12 people following a tap water enema, and in no participants following a PEG-ES enema. The researchers questioned whether surface epithelium loss could be minimized by instructing patients to eliminate the enema immediately rather than waiting 10 minutes as requested during the study (Schmelzer et al., 2004).

■ *Giving three or more tap water enemas until clear.* **LOE = III**

(NR) A quasi-experimental study with random assignment to treatment groups and participants blinded to solution ($N = 25$) found that 11 of 12 people who received tap water enemas and 6 of 13 people who received soapsuds enemas eliminated a smaller amount (stool plus enema) than was given as an enema. The researchers suggested that nurses measure the size of the enema returns to monitor each successive enema's effects on fluid volume and determine whether enemas should continue (Schmelzer et al., 2000).

NR = Nursing Research, **MR** = Multidisciplinary Research, **SP** = Standard of Practice, **EO** = Expert Opinion, **LOE** = Level of Evidence

(NR) A repeated measures design (double blind, random order of enema delivery) found negative mean outputs (i.e., the amount of solution infused was larger than the size of the returns) for all three enema solutions given to healthy volunteers ($N = 24$).

(MR) A case study described a 42-year-old woman who commonly took colonic irrigations and developed hyponatremia from a colonic irrigation with a hypotonic solution (Norlela et al., 2004).

(MR) A case study described a 65-year-old man with C6 quadriplegia who developed confusion and seizures after being given five tap water enemas (1.5 to 3.0 L each over 10 days) (Chertow & Brady, 1994).

(MR) A descriptive study of the number of cleansing enemas needed to obtain clear returns ($N = 123$) determined that 12 people received one or two enemas, 60 received three or four enemas, 35 received five or six enemas, and 16 received more than six enemas. The researchers reported no episodes of water intoxication (Pietilä et al., 1990).

OUTCOME MEASUREMENT

BOWEL ELIMINATION

Definition: Formation and evacuation of stool.

Bowel Elimination as evidenced by the following selected NOC indicators:
- Constipation
- Blood in stool
- Pain with passage of stool

(Rate each indicator of **Bowel Elimination:** 1 = severe, 2 = substantial, 3 = moderate, 4 = mild, 5 = none) (Moorhead et al., 2004).

REFERENCES

Chertow GM, Brady HR. (1994). Hyponatraemia from tap-water enema. *Lancet*, 344(8924):748.

Dochterman JM, Bulechek GM (Eds). (2004). *Nursing Interventions Classification (NIC)*, 4th ed. St. Louis: Mosby.

Doughty DB, Jackson DB. (1993). *Gastrointestinal disorders*. St. Louis: Mosby.

Harmer B, Henderson V. (1939). *Textbook of the principles and practice of nursing*. New York: Macmillan.

Keljo DJ, Squires RH. (1998). Anatomy and anomalies of the small and large intestines. In Feldman M, Scharschmidt BF, Sleisenger MH (Eds). *Sleisenger & Fordtran's gastrointestinal and liver disease*, 6th ed. Philadelphia: Saunders, pp 1419-1436.

May RE, Reynolds KW. (1968). Extraperitoneal perforation of the rectum with a rubber rectal tube. *Br J Clin Pract*, 22(11):491-492.

Miller R. (1975). The cleansing enema. *Radiology*, 117(2):483-485.

Moorhead M, Johnson M, Maas M. (Eds). (2004). *Nursing Outcomes Classification (NOC)*, 3rd ed. St. Louis: Mosby.

Norlela S, Izham C, Khalid BA. (2004). Colonic irrigation-induced hyponatremia. *Malays J Pathol*, 26(2):117-118.

Paran H, Butnaru G, Neufeld D, Magen A, Freund U. (1999). Enema-induced perforation of the rectum in chronically constipated patients. *Dis Colon Rectum*, 42(12):1609-1612.

Pietilä JA, Kinnunen J, Lindén H. (1990). The cleansing enema: How many for a good quality double-contrast enema? *Acta Radiol*, 31(5):489-492.

Richards DG, McMillin DL, Mein EA, Nelson CD. (2006). Colonic irrigations: A review of the historical controversy and the potential for adverse effects. *J Altern Complement Med*, 12(4):389-393.

Sadahiro S, Ohmura T, Yamada Y, Saito T, Taki Y. (1992). Analysis of length and surface area of each segment of the large intestine according to age, sex and physique. *Surg Radiol Anat,* 14(3):251-257.

Saltzstein RJ, Quebbeman E, Melvin JL. (1988). Anorectal injuries incident to enema administration: A recurring avoidable problem. *Am J Phys Med Rehabil,* 67(4):186-188.

Schmelzer M, Case P, Chappell SM, Wright KB. (2000). Colonic cleansing, fluid absorption, and discomfort following tap water and soapsuds enemas. *Appl Nurs Res,* 13(2):83-91.

Schmelzer M, Schiller LR, Meyer R, Rugari SM, Case P. (2004). Safety and effectiveness of large-volume enema solutions. *Appl Nurs Res,* 17(4):265-274.

Schmelzer M, Wright KB. (1996). Enema administration techniques used by experienced registered nurses, *Gastroenterol Nurs* 19(5):171-175.

Shafik A. (1992). The water enema test: A means of assessing rectal function. *Practical Gastroenterol,* 16(9):24J-24P.

Shafik A, Doss S, Asaad S, Ali YA. (1999). Rectosigmoid junction: Anatomical, histological, and radiological studies with special reference to a sphincteric function. *Int J Colorectal Dis,* 14(4-5):237-244.

Shiels WE 2nd, Kirks DR, Keller GL, Ryckman FR, Daugherty CC, Specker BL, et al. (1993). Colonic perforation by air and liquid enemas: Comparison study in young pigs. *AJR Am J Roentgenol,* 160(5):931-935.

Sweeney JL, Hewett P, Riddell P, Hoffmann DC. (1986). Rectal gangrene: A complication of phosphate enema. *Med J Aust,* 144(7):374-375.

Tagart RE. (1966). The anal canal and rectum: Their varying relationship and its effect on anal continence. *Dis Colon Rectum,* 9(6):449-452.

ENERGY MANAGEMENT

Barbara Given, PhD, RN, FAAN; Paula R. Sherwood, PhD, RN, CNRN

> **NIC Definition:** Regulating energy use to treat or prevent fatigue and optimize function (Dochterman & Bulechek, 2004).

NURSING ACTIVITIES

Effective

■ *Identify patients who may benefit from interventions including energy management.* **LOE = I**

 Energy management techniques have been associated with positive outcomes in elderly people with difficulty in activities of daily living (ADLs) (Gitlin et al., 2006) and people with cancer (Barsevick et al., 2004, 2002; Jantarakupt & Porock, 2005), multiple sclerosis (Finlayson, 2005; Lamb et al., 2005; Mathiowetz et al., 2005), HIV (Siegel et al., 2004), and fibromyalgia (Dobkin et al., 2006; Sim & Adams, 2003).

■ *Implement psychoeducational programs for patients that focus on energy management techniques and consist of assessment/observation, problem solving, and periodically reviewing effectiveness of techniques.* **LOE = I**

 A psychoeducational intervention consisting of five contacts by an occupational therapist (OT) and one contact by a physical therapist was associated with less difficulty in instrumental activities of daily living (IADLs) and ADLs, greater self-efficacy, less fear of falling, fewer home hazards, and greater use of adaptive strategies in a randomized controlled trial (RCT) involving 319 adults older than 70 years who reported difficulty with one or more ADLs (Gitlin et al., 2006).

(MR) In an RCT involving 37 people with progressive multiple sclerosis, an 8-week energy conservation course significantly decreased the impact of fatigue on physical, cognitive, and psychosocial health (Vanage et al., 2003).

(MR) In an RCT involving 169 people with multiple sclerosis, a 6-week psychoeducational intervention delivered by OTs was associated with improvements in self-efficacy and vitality and reductions in the impact of fatigue on physical and social health (Mathiowetz et al., 2005).

(NR) In an RCT involving 396 people initiating chemotherapy or radiation therapy for cancer, a 5-week, three-contact energy management intervention delivered by an oncology nurse led to decreased fatigue, although overall functional performance was not affected (Barsevick et al., 2004).

■ *Consider interventions that contain a physical exercise component when appropriate.* **LOE = I**

(NR) In a meta-analysis of 30 studies involving patients undergoing treatment for cancer, exercise interventions were associated with lower levels of fatigue, less severe symptoms, and improved physical function, quality of life, and mood (Conn et al., 2006).

Possibly Effective

■ *Use energy management techniques in people with chronic pain.* **LOE = II**

(MR) In a sample of 156 women with fibromyalgia, a descriptive study found that palliative coping styles such as energy management modified the influence of pain on health status (Dobkin et al., 2006).

(MR) In a descriptive survey of 142 OTs and PTs, energy management/conservation techniques were among the most commonly delivered interventions for people with fibromyalgia (Sim & Adams, 2003).

■ *Consider delivering energy management interventions by telephone.* **LOE = III**

(MR) In a descriptive pilot study involving 29 people with multiple sclerosis, an educational program delivered by telephone by OTs was associated with reductions in fatigue and improvements in pain and general health (Finlayson, 2005).

■ *Consider using self-study modules as part of an intervention to educate people about energy management.* **LOE = IV**

(MR) In a secondary analysis from an RCT involving 92 people with multiple sclerosis, there were no significant differences in outcomes between individuals who attended six sessions of an energy management intervention in person and individuals who missed one or more sessions and received a self-study module (Lamb et al., 2005).

■ *Implement a variety of techniques such as simplifying activities and allowing sufficient time for tasks.* **LOE = III**

(MR) In a descriptive pilot study involving 29 people with multiple sclerosis, the most commonly used energy management strategies were simplifying activities, adjusting priorities,

---

RCT = Randomized Controlled (Clinical) Trial, **NIC** = Nursing Interventions Classification, **NOC** = Nursing Outcomes Classification

changing body position, resting, and planning the day to balance work and rest (Finlayson, 2005).

(NR) In a review of dyspnea management in people with lung cancer, suggested energy management strategies included planning activities and allowing sufficient time for tasks (Jantarakupt & Porock, 2005).

(MR) In a descriptive study involving 108 people without evidence of chronic disease, the use of labor-saving equipment was cited as the most effective strategy in energy conservation for people 30 to 59 years old (Ip et al., 2006).

■ *Provide an intervention with multiple contacts with the caregiver.* **LOE = III**

(NR) In a descriptive study involving 80 people initiating either chemotherapy or radiation therapy for cancer treatment, patients were able to adhere to a three-session psychoeducational program on energy management and also expressed a commitment to continuing the techniques after the intervention was complete (Barsevick et al., 2002).

■ *Evaluate the age of the patient and adapt intervention strategies accordingly.* **LOE = VI**

(MR) In a descriptive study involving people between 30 and 78 years of age without evidence of chronic disease, energy conservation was associated with a reduction in energy expenditure for younger (30 to 59 year old) people versus those 60 years and older (Ip et al., 2006).

Not Effective

■ *Energy conservation techniques for people with multiple sclerosis.* **LOE = I**

(MR) In a systematic review of three studies involving energy management/conservation interventions with people diagnosed with multiple sclerosis, the authors reported insufficient evidence to prescribe energy management interventions in this population because of problems with study designs and small sample sizes (Steultjens et al., 2003).

Possibly Harmful

No applicable published research was found in this category.

OUTCOME MEASUREMENT

ENERGY MANAGEMENT

Definition: Activities are regulated and scheduled to decrease fatigue and optimize physical, social, and mental function.

Energy Management as evidenced by the following indicators:
- Reports acceptable level of fatigue
- Performs ADLs and IADLs
- Verbalizes adaptive strategies to use in performing activities
- Prioritizes activities throughout the day, including rest periods
- Identifies external sources of support for assisting with activities

(Note: This is not a NOC outcome.)

NR = Nursing Research, **MR** = Multidisciplinary Research, **SP** = Standard of Practice, **EO** = Expert Opinion, **LOE** = Level of Evidence

REFERENCES

Barsevick AM, Dudley W, Beck S, Sweeney C, Whitmer K, Nail L. (2004). A randomized clinical trial of energy conservation for patients with cancer-related fatigue. *Cancer,* 100(6):1302-1310.

Barsevick AM, Whitmer K, Sweeney C, Nail LM. (2002). A pilot study examining energy conservation for cancer treatment-related fatigue. *Cancer Nurs,* 25(5):333-341.

Conn VS, Hafdahl AR, Porock DC, McDaniel R, Nielsen PJ. (2006). A meta-analysis of exercise interventions among people treated for cancer. *Support Care Cancer,* 14(7):699-712.

Dobkin PL, De Civita M, Abrahamowicz M, Baron M, Bernatsky S. (2006). Predictors of health status in women with fibromyalgia: A prospective study. *Int J Behav Med,* 13(2):101-108.

Dochterman JM, Bulechek GM (Eds). (2004). *Nursing Interventions Classification (NIC),* 4th ed. St. Louis: Mosby.

Finlayson M. (2005). Pilot study of an energy conservation education program delivered by telephone conference call to people with multiple sclerosis. *Neurorehabilitation,* 20(4):267-277.

Gitlin LN, Winter L, Dennis MP, Corcoran M, Schinfeld S, Hauck WW. (2006). A randomized trial of a multicomponent home intervention to reduce functional difficulties in older adults. *J Am Geriatr Soc,* 54(5):809-816.

Ip WM, Woo J, Yue SY, Kwan M, Sum SM, Kwok T, et al. (2006). Evaluation of the effect of energy conservation techniques in the performance of activity of daily living tasks. *Clin Rehabil,* 20(3):254-261.

Jantarakupt P, Porock D. (2005). Dyspnea management in lung cancer: Applying the evidence from chronic obstructive pulmonary disease. *Oncol Nurs Forum,* 32(4):785-797.

Lamb AL, Finlayson M, Mathiowetz V, Chen HY. (2005). The outcomes of using self-study modules in energy conservation education for people with multiple sclerosis. *Clin Rehabil,* 19(5):475-481.

Mathiowetz VG, Finlayson ML, Matuska KM, Chen HY, Luo P. (2005). Randomized controlled trial of an energy conservation course for persons with multiple sclerosis. *Mult Scler,* 11(5):592-601.

Siegel K, Brown-Bradley CJ, Lekas HM. (2004). Strategies for coping with fatigue among HIV-positive individuals fifty years and older. *AIDS Patient Care STDS,* 18(5):275-288.

Sim J, Adams N. (2003). Therapeutic approaches to fibromyalgia syndrome in the United Kingdom: A survey of occupational therapists and physical therapists. *Eur J Pain,* 7(2):173-180.

Steultjens EM, Dekker J, Bouter LM, Cardol M, Van de Nes JC, Van den Ende CH. (2003). Occupational therapy for multiple sclerosis. *Cochrane Database Syst Rev,* (3):CD003608.

Vanage SM, Gilbertson KK, Mathiowetz V. (2003). Effects of an energy conservation course on fatigue impact for persons with progressive multiple sclerosis. *Am J Occup Ther,* 57(3):315-323.

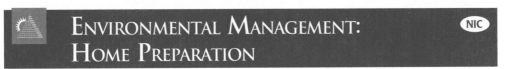

ENVIRONMENTAL MANAGEMENT: HOME PREPARATION   NIC

Diane E. Holland, PhD, RN

NIC Definition: Preparing the home for safe and effective delivery of care (Dochterman & Bulechek, 2004).

NURSING ACTIVITIES

Effective

■ **NIC** *Consult with the patient and caregivers concerning preparation for care delivery at home.* **LOE = V**

NR A systematic review of the literature revealed that there is a need for increased involvement of patients and caregivers in decision making related to transitional care (Naylor, 2002).

RCT = Randomized Controlled (Clinical) Trial, **NIC** = Nursing Interventions Classification, **NOC** = Nursing Outcomes Classification

(NR) A qualitative descriptive study ($N = 24$) to determine elements of a proper hospital discharge for elderly patients revealed that ongoing, open communication with the patient and family was vital for a successful discharge (Bull & Roberts, 2001).

(MR) A qualitative descriptive study ($N = 17$) of the perspectives of people with disabilities on the process of home adaptations revealed that preparation for the adaptation process was key to successful home preparation for care delivery (Picking & Pain, 2003).

■ *Order and ensure the operation and training of the patient and caregivers in the use of any equipment needed.* **LOE = II**

(MR) An RCT ($N = 53$) of an intervention designed to train older adults in the use of bathing devices in the home demonstrated that a higher level of functioning and independence could be achieved by prescribing and training older adults in the use of assistive devices (Chiu & Man, 2004).

■ (NIC) *Provide written materials regarding medications, supplies, and assistive devices as guides for caregivers, as needed.* **LOE = I**

(MR) A Cochrane systematic review recommended the use of both written and verbal information in communicating about care issues with patients and caregivers on discharge from the hospital to the home (Johnson et al., 2003).

Possibly Effective

■ (NIC) *Check the layout of the home and eliminate obstacles.* **LOE = IV**

(MR) A controlled study ($N = 16$) demonstrated that an intervention program to remove environmental barriers in the homes of older adults improved occupational performance of elderly subjects (Stark, 2004).

(MR) A descriptive study ($N = 15$) to determine the validity and reliability of an assessment protocol to enhance the delivery of home modifications identified one domain of "moving around in the house" as important in correctly identifying problems and providing effective recommendations (Sanford et al., 2002).

(MR) A Cochrane systematic review concluded that there was insufficient evidence to determine the effects of interventions to modify environmental home hazards (Lyons et al., 2006).

■ (NIC) *Arrange scheduling of support personnel.* **LOE = VI**

(MR) A descriptive, qualitative study ($N = 65$) of key stakeholders' perceptions of what was important to continuity of home care revealed that clients emphasized consistency of timing of service delivery as an important attribute for providing continuity of home care (Woodward et al., 2004).

■ (NIC) *Confirm date and time of transfer to the home.* **LOE = VI**

(MR) A descriptive survey study ($N = 1183$) of home care personnel's perspectives on successful discharge of elderly patients from the hospital to the home demonstrated that a factor most associated with a successful discharge was timely information about the patient's transfer to home care (Eija & Marja-Leena, 2005).

NR = Nursing Research, **MR** = Multidisciplinary Research, **SP** = Standard of Practice, **EO** = Expert Opinion, **LOE** = Level of Evidence

- ■ **NIC** **SP** *Prepare teaching plans for use in the home to coincide with any earlier teaching already accomplished.* **LOE = VII**

  EO Written material provided to the patient and family members reinforces learning and provides support with the technique after discharge (Ignatavicius & Workman, 2006).

- ■ **NIC** **SP** *Confirm arrangements for transportation to the home with accompanying escort, as needed.* **LOE = VII**

  EO Confirming transportation arrangements is part of standard nursing discharge planning practice (Munden, 2007).

- ■ **NIC** **SP** *Follow up to ensure that plans were feasible and carried out.* **LOE = VII**

  EO Evaluation of outcomes is an important part of a nursing discharge planning standard of practice protocol (Zwicker & Picariello, 2003; Ignatavicius & Workman, 2006).

OUTCOME MEASUREMENT

SAFE HOME ENVIRONMENT **NOC**

Definition: Physical arrangements to minimize environmental factors that might cause physical harm or injury in the home.

Safe Home Environment as evidenced by the following selected NOC indicators:

- Provision of accessible telephone
- Provision of assistive devices in accessible location
- Provision of equipment that meets safety standards

(Rate each indicator of **Safe Home Environment:** 1 = not adequate, 2 = slightly adequate, 3 = moderately adequate, 4 = substantially adequate, 5 = totally adequate) (Moorhead et al., 2004).

DISCHARGE READINESS: SUPPORTED LIVING **NOC**

Definition: Readiness of a patient to relocate from a health care institution to a lower level of supported living.

Discharge Readiness: Supported Living as evidenced by the following selected NOC indicator:

- Patient needs consistent with available family support

(Rate this indicator of **Discharge Readiness: Supported Living:** 1 = never demonstrated, 2 = rarely demonstrated, 3 = sometimes demonstrated, 4 = often demonstrated, 5 = consistently demonstrated) (Moorhead et al., 2004).

DISCHARGE READINESS: INDEPENDENT LIVING **NOC**

Definition: Readiness of a patient to relocate from a health care institution to living independently.

Discharge Readiness: Independent Living as evidenced by the following selected NOC indicators:

Continued

OUTCOME MEASUREMENT—*cont'd*

- Seeks assistance appropriately
- Describes prescribed treatments
- Manages own medications

(Rate each indicator of **Discharge Readiness: Independent Living:** 1 = never demonstrated, 2 = rarely demonstrated, 3 = sometimes demonstrated, 4 = often demonstrated, 5 = consistently demonstrated) (Moorhead et al., 2004).

REFERENCES

Bull MJ, Roberts J. (2001). Components of a proper hospital discharge for elders. *J Adv Nurs,* 35(4):571-581.

Chiu CW, Man DW. (2004). The effect of training older adults with stroke to use home-based assistive devices. *OTJR,* 24(3):113-120.

Dochterman JM, Bulechek GM (Eds). (2004). *Nursing Interventions Classification (NIC),* 4th ed. St. Louis: Mosby.

Eija G, Marja-Leena P. (2005). Home care personnel's perspectives on successful discharge of elderly clients from hospital to home setting. *Scand J Caring Sci,* 19(3):288-295.

Ignatavicius DD, Workman ML (Eds). (2006). *Medical-surgical nursing: Critical thinking for collaborative care,* 5th ed. Philadelphia: Saunders.

Johnson A, Sandford J, Tyndall J. (2003). Written and verbal information versus verbal information only for patients being discharged from acute hospital settings to home. *Cochrane Database Syst Rev,* (4): CD003716.

Lyons RA, John A, Brophy S, Jones SJ, Johansen A, Kemp A, et al. (2006). Modification of the home environment for the reduction of injuries. *Cochrane Database Syst Rev,* (4):CD003600.

Moorhead M, Johnson M, Maas M (Eds). (2004). *Nursing Outcomes Classification (NOC),* 3rd ed. St. Louis, Mosby.

Munden J (Ed). (2007). *Best practices: Evidenced-based nursing procedures,* 2nd ed. Philadelphia: Lippincott Williams & Wilkins.

Naylor MD. (2002). Transitional care for older adults. *Annu Rev Nurs Res,* 20:127-147.

Picking C, Pain H. (2003). Home adaptations: User perspectives on the role of professionals. *Br J Occup Ther,* 66(1):2-8.

Sanford JA, Pynoos J, Tejral A, Browne A. (2002). Development of a comprehensive assessment for delivery of home modifications. *Phys Occup Ther Geriatr,* 20(2):43-55.

Stark S. (2004). Removing environmental barriers in the homes of older adults with disabilities improves occupational performance. *OTJR,* 24(1):32-39.

Woodward CA, Abelson J, Tedford S, Hutchison B. (2004). What is important to continuity in home care? Perspectives of key stakeholders. *Soc Sci Med,* 58(1):177-192.

Zwicker D, Picariello G. (2003). Discharge planning for the older adult. In Mezey M, Fulmer T, Abraham I (Eds). *Geriatric nursing protocols for best practice.* New York: Springer.

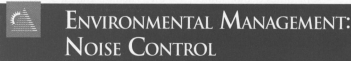

ENVIRONMENTAL MANAGEMENT: NOISE CONTROL

Joyce A. Overman Dube, MS, RN; Melissa M. Barth, MS, RN, CCRN; Cheryl A. Cmiel, RN

Definition: Management of the patient's environment for therapeutic benefit, sensory appeal, and psychological well-being.

NR = Nursing Research, **MR** = Multidisciplinary Research, **SP** = Standard of Practice, **EO** = Expert Opinion, **LOE** = Level of Evidence

NURSING ACTIVITIES

(Note: Many studies related to noise have been performed in non–health care workplaces or specialty practice areas; however, they contribute to knowledge on the effects of noise, the relationship to stress and health, and the implications for the health care environment.)

Effective

■ *Use sleep enhancement protocols or quiet time guidelines.* LOE = III

(NR) A controlled study of critically ill patients in a neurocritical care unit using a pretest/post-test design ($N = 239$) determined that increased sleep frequency (more people slept during quiet time versus nonquiet time) was associated with decreased sound and light levels during the quiet time (Olson et al., 2001).

(MR) A controlled study of critically ill patients ($N = 9$ preimplementation, $N = 8$ postimplementation) in a surgical ICU found a decrease in noise level equivalent, peak noise level, and acoustic alarms. In addition, results demonstrated that lowered mean light disturbance intensity with increased variability of light levels may impair sleep quality (Walder et al., 2000).

(MR) A controlled study of preterm infants ($N = 10$) using a quiet period in the neonatal intensive care unit (NICU) found significant environmental reductions in light intensity, noise levels, alarm events, staff conversation, staff activity, and infant handling. Significant physiological findings of decreased diastolic blood pressure, decreased mean arterial pressure, and decreased infant movements were also found (Slevin et al., 2000).

(NR) A case study designed a five-step process (assess, develop, educate, implement, and evaluate) to develop a quiet hour protocol in a 70-bed special care nursery that resulted in decreased decibel levels sustained 14 months after implementation (Johnson, 2003).

(NR) A case study implemented a quiet time period between two ICUs to promote rest and relaxation by controlling the external environment (measured decibel levels, implemented interventions to reduce noise, and communicated expectations to all visitors and staff). Patient and family satisfaction scores, especially regarding unit noise levels, increased from 50% to 88.9% (Lower et al., 2003).

■ *Use questionnaires or surveys to identify sleep or noise issues.* LOE = II

(NR) An RCT ($N = 60$) assigned participants to a group in which audiotaped critical care unit sounds (e.g., patient monitoring devices, ventilators, staff activities) played throughout the night or to a quiet group where the tape was withheld. A self-rating questionnaire was used to assess sleep subjectively and found that the noise group reported taking longer to fall asleep, spent less time sleeping, woke more frequently, and described their sleep more negatively (Topf et al., 1996).

(NR) A controlled study tested and found the Richards-Cambell Sleep Questionnaire ($N = 70$) to be reliable and valid. This simple screening measure can be used to identify patients who may benefit from sleep-promoting interventions (Richards et al., 2000).

(NR) A secondary analysis of a controlled study ($N = 97$) using the Disturbance Due to Hospital Noise Scale demonstrated that hospital patients' noise-induced stress interacted with other stress to predict poor sleep (Topf & Thompson, 2001).

(MR) A cohort descriptive study ($N = 11$ nurses) in which audiogram, questionnaire, salivary amylase, and heart rate were collected and decibel levels measured sought to determine whether there was a correlation with nursing stress. Higher sound levels were predictive of

---

RCT = Randomized Controlled (Clinical) Trial, **NIC** = Nursing Interventions Classification, **NOC** = Nursing Outcomes Classification

subjective stress and annoyance with average daytime sound levels of 61.2 dB(A) and night-time levels of 58.8 dB(A) (Morrison et al., 2003).

(MR) A descriptive study (N = 150 hospitalized patients, N = 50 healthy controls) used the Pittsburgh Sleep Quality Index and a sociodemographic information form and compared sleep characteristics with sociodemographic and illness variables. Psychiatric patients had worse sleep quality than other types of patients, and health care staff were identified as needing to be educated about sleep and providing intervention when required (Doğan et al., 2005).

■ *Assess the level of noise using a dosimeter to identify sleep or noise issues.* LOE = III

(NR) A mixed method (controlled and descriptive-qualitative) study using pre-post intervention with patients (N = 1479) and staff (N = 3668) found a difference in noise level ratings during three of four times of day, with mornings being most bothersome. Intermittently measured noise levels made health care staff cognizant of noise, and evidence suggests that this highlighted periods of unacceptable noise for patients and staff, requiring investigation of the sources of noise and possible solutions (Overman Dube et al., 2006).

(MR) A descriptive two-part study found excessive noise levels in the main resuscitation area in a level-one emergency department with a time-weighted average of 43 (stand-alone) and 52.9 (following a resident) dB during the study periods, and investigators identified sources of noise that, with modification, may decrease stress in the emergency department (Tijunelis et al., 2005).

(MR) A descriptive study (N = 355) evaluated the relationships between NICU sound, equipment, infant characteristics, and infant responses and found a significant positive relationship between census and sound levels (Byers et al., 2005).

(NR) A descriptive study that looked at the correlation between presence of staff, patients, and visitors in a room with six beds and the impact on ambient noise in a general surgical nursing ward (28 beds) found an increase in noise levels related to the number of staff and, to a lesser degree, the number of patients and visitors present on the ward (Christensen, 2005).

■ *Use ambient background music.* LOE = II

(MR) An RCT (N = 80) study showed decreased propofol (Diprivan) use for patients undergoing urological surgery under spinal anesthesia when music was used in the operating room (Ayoub et al., 2005).

(MR) A controlled multicenter qualitative and quantitative study assessed patients' (N = 325) and staffs' (N = 91) perceptions of composed music played through ceiling speakers to patients in a postanesthesia recovery room and found that staff-perceived noise levels were less during the time music was played and that most patients found the music pleasant (Thorgaard et al., 2005).

(NR) A controlled study (N = 97) showed significant reduction in pain during postanesthesia care unit stay when soothing music and lowering noise levels were used (Shertzer & Keck, 2001).

(NR) A controlled study (N = 40) found that patients had a lower level of noise annoyance during music intervention during two periods when compared with baseline (Byers & Smyth, 1997).

(EO) Establishing a "department of sound" within a hospital setting to oversee noise reduction and the incorporation of therapeutic music to reduce patients' stress and anxiety is recommended (Cabrera & Lee, 2000).

NR = Nursing Research, **MR** = Multidisciplinary Research, **SP** = Standard of Practice, **EO** = Expert Opinion, **LOE** = Level of Evidence

Possibly Effective

Use environmental modification. LOE = III

(MR) A systematic review of the literature on environmental interventions (e.g., noiseless paging system, single-patient rooms, sound-absorbing ceiling tiles and flooring) showed that they effectively reduced noise in the hospital setting and improved patients' sleep (Ulrich & Zimring, 2004).

(MR) A controlled study (N = 69) found lower sound levels and a perceived change to a quieter environment in the experimental patients' room compared with the control patients' room following the implementation of environmental modifications (Walsh-Sukys et al., 2001).

(EO) Detailing environmental considerations for modifying existing laboratory settings, building new settings, and incorporating sound level criteria when making new equipment purchases would be beneficial to control noise levels (Mortland & Mortland, 2002).

(EO) Good nursing is defined as preventing the accidental or intentional awakening of a patient, and unnecessary noise, which may include intermittent, sudden, or sharp noise or noise from conversation outside a patient's room causing the patient to strain to hear it, is described as the "most cruel absence of care" (Nightingale, p. 27, 1860).

Use environmental modification and behavioral modification. LOE = II

(MR) An RCT (N = 267) involving a behavioral intervention program with staff feedback about noise levels in eight nursing homes demonstrated that reduction in noise and light events did not lead to improvement in sleep, suggesting that the intervention did not reduce noise levels enough for sleep. However, it was suggested that combined behavioral and environmental modification may improve sleep (Schnelle et al., 1999).

(NR) A systematic review of the literature using Als's synactive model of neonatal behavioral organization found that behavioral/clinical interventions and environmental changes provided a practical guide and starting point for reducing noise levels and determined that the assessment of noise levels was essential for noise abatement or reduction programs in NICUs (Bremmer et al., 2003).

(EO) A relationship exists between environmental noise and stress and implications for nursing. Suggestions for environmental and behavioral interventions to reduce noise levels include decreasing phone ringer volume, providing headphones or ear plugs, providing music, oiling squeaky equipment, dimming lights, and using conference rooms for conversations (Topf, 2000).

Use staff education and environmental modification. LOE = III

(NR) A controlled longitudinal design study of one bed space described the cumulative effects of environment changes with staff education and showed that a combined approach was more successful in creating a quiet environment than staff education alone (Philbin & Gray, 2002).

(NR) A case study using the PDSA (Plan, Do, Study, Act) process demonstrated decreased decibel levels following staff education and implementation of various environmental noise control interventions (e.g., reduce alarm and voice volume, decrease traffic, close doors, dim lights) with peak noise levels reduced from 113 to 86 dB(A), as well as a reduction in average night shift noise levels (Cmiel et al., 2004).

RCT = Randomized Controlled (Clinical) Trial, **NIC** = Nursing Interventions Classification, **NOC** = Nursing Outcomes Classification

■ *Use staff education and behavioral modification.* **LOE = III**

(MR) A two-phase controlled study that identified noise in two groups (equipment with volume parameters and human behavior) tested a 3-week behavior modification program that involved all medical ICU staff and reduced mean peak sound levels in three of four time blocks in a three-bed room in a medical and a respiratory ICU (Kahn et al., 1998).

(NR) A controlled study ($N = 52$), using pretest/post-test design with an interventional staff education program demonstrated that noise levels could be decreased by increasing staff awareness of the issue (Elander & Hellström, 1995).

(MR) A controlled study in a neuro-ICU examined sleep disturbance and recorded noise levels before ($N = 9$ patients) and after ($N = 14$ patients) a behavioral modification program for all staff and demonstrated a reduction in noise activities associated with implementation of nondisturbance periods in the afternoon and night (Monsén & Edéll-Gustafsson, 2005).

■ *Identify sources of sleep disruptions.* **LOE = II**

(MR) An RCT ($N = 7$ patients and $N = 6$ healthy subjects) with continuous 24-hour polysomnography (PSG) found that noise peaks and patients' care activities accounted for 28% of arousal and awakening from sleep, suggesting that there were other factors in the environment that may contribute to ICU sleep disruption (Gabor et al., 2003).

(MR) A controlled study in which patients ($N = 22$) were monitored with continuous PSG found that the average patients' arousals from environmental noise were 11.5% and awakenings were 17%, which supports the theory that environmental noise is not responsible for the majority of sleep fragmentation, as previous literature suggests (Freedman et al., 2001).

■ *Use hearing protection devices.* **LOE = II**

(MR) A crossover RCT ($N = 81$) demonstrated that use of noise cancellation devices (headphones) reduced subjective assessment of noise by 2 out of 10 on a visual analog scale in adult medical and pediatric intensive care units (Akhtar et al., 2000).

(NR) A descriptive study ($N = 400$) described the use of hearing protection devices and perceptions of noise exposure and hearing loss among construction workers. The study found inadequate use of hearing protection and perceived hearing loss (Lusk et al., 1998).

■ *Provide input into the design process of unit environment to decrease noise.* **LOE = V**

(MR) A descriptive study ($N = 36$) found that sound-absorbing ceiling tiles improved speech intelligibility and reverberation times compared with sound reflective tiles. In addition, staff questionnaires indicated that the afternoon shift experienced lower work demands and less pressure and strain (Blomkvist et al., 2005).

(NR) A case study described the benefits of a healing environment and reviewed the literature related to effects of light, color, noise, and privacy on patients. The authors suggested that a healing environment must be created and was shown to have a positive impact on a patient's recovery, optimizing clinical care/outcomes as well as staff satisfaction, morale, and retention, and fostered repeat business (Altimier, 2004).

(NR) A review of the critical care environment literature provided environmental recommendations for light, color, noise control, sleep promotion, music, aromatherapy, and family/pet visitation (Fontaine et al., 2001).

NR = Nursing Research, **MR** = Multidisciplinary Research, **SP** = Standard of Practice, **EO** = Expert Opinion, **LOE** = Level of Evidence

(EO) Using elements of nature, light, soothing colors, therapeutic sounds, and family interactions enhances the healing process (Stichler, 2001).

■ *Maintain knowledge of current standards related to noise impact on personal health or hearing conservation.* **LOE = V**

(NR) A review of occupational health literature found an inconclusive relationship between increased noise levels and hypertension. Nevertheless, it advocated blood pressure screening as part of a hearing conservation program for workers in environments with exposure to elevated noise levels (Penney & Earl, 2004).

(EO) It is important to understand and maintain the role of occupational and environmental health nurses in ensuring preventive services, including hypertension screening (Lusk, 2001).

Not Effective

No applicable published research was found in this category.

Possibly Harmful

No applicable published research was found in this category.

OUTCOME MEASUREMENT

REST (NOC)

Definition: Quantity and pattern of diminished activity for mental and physical rejuvenation.

Rest as evidenced by the following selected NOC indicators:
• Amount of rest
• Rest pattern
• Rest quality

(Rate each indicator of **Rest:** 1 = extremely compromised, 2 = substantially compromised, 3 = moderately compromised, 4 = mildly compromised, 5 = not compromised) (Moorhead et al., 2004).

REFERENCES

Akhtar S, Weigle CG, Cheng EY, Toohill R, Berens RJ. (2000). Use of active noise cancellation devices in caregivers in the intensive care unit. *Crit Care Med,* 28(4):1157-1160.

Altimier LB. (2004). Healing environments: For patients and providers. *Newborn Infant Nurs Rev,* 4(2):89-92.

Ayoub CM, Rizk LB, Yaacoub CI, Gaal D, Kain ZN. (2005). Music and ambient operating room noise in patients undergoing spinal anesthesia. *Anesth Analg,* 100(5):1316-1319.

Blomkvist V, Eriksen CA, Theorell T, Ulrich R, Rasmanis G. (2005). Acoustics and psychosocial environment in intensive coronary care. *Occup Environ Med,* 62(3):e1.

Bremmer P, Byers JF, Kiehl E. (2003). Noise and the premature infant: Physiological effects and practice implications. *J Obstet Gynecol Neonatal Nurs,* 32(4):447-454.

Byers JF, Lowman LB, Waugh WR. (2005). Neonatal intensive care unit sound levels, environment, and infant responses. *Neonatal Intensive Care,* 18(3):48-53.

Byers JF, Smyth KA. (1997). Effect of a music intervention on noise annoyance, heart rate, and blood pressure in cardiac surgery patients. *Am J Crit Care,* 6(3):183-191.

RCT = Randomized Controlled (Clinical) Trial, **NIC** = Nursing Interventions Classification, **NOC** = Nursing Outcomes Classification

Cabrera IN, Lee MH. (2000). Reducing noise pollution in the hospital setting by establishing a department of sound: A survey of recent research on the effects of noise and music in health care. *Prev Med,* 30(4):339-345.

Christensen M. (2005). Noise levels in a general surgical ward: A descriptive study. *J Clin Nurs,* 14(2): 156-164.

Cmiel CA, Karr DM, Gasser DM, Oliphant LM, Neveau AJ. (2004). Noise control: A nursing team's approach to sleep promotion. *Am J Nurs,* 104(2):40-48.

Doğan O, Ertekin Ş, Doğan S. (2005). Sleep quality in hospitalized patients. *J Clin Nurs,* 14(1):107-113.

Elander G, Hellström G. (1995). Reduction of noise levels in intensive care units for infants: Evaluation of an intervention program. *Heart Lung,* 24(5):376-379.

Fontaine DK, Briggs LP, Pope-Smith B. (2001). Designing humanistic critical care environments. *Crit Care Nurs Q,* 24(3):21-34.

Freedman NS, Gazendam J, Levan L, Pack AI, Schwab RJ. (2001). Abnormal sleep/wake cycles and the effect of environmental noise on sleep disruption in the intensive care unit. *Am J Respir Crit Care Med,* 163(2):451-457.

Gabor JY, Cooper AB, Crombach SA, Lee B, Kadikar N, Bettger HE, et al. (2003). Contribution of the intensive care unit environment to sleep disruption in mechanically ventilated patients and healthy subjects. *Am J Respir Crit Care Med,* 167(5):708-715.

Johnson AN. (2003). Adapting the neonatal intensive care environment to decrease noise. *J Perinat Neonatal Nurs,* 17(4):280-288.

Kahn DM, Cook TE, Carlisle CC, Nelson DL, Kramer NR, Millman RP. (1998). Identification and modification of environmental noise in an ICU setting. *Chest,* 114(2):535-540.

Lower JS, Bonsack C, Guion J. (2003). Peace and quiet. *Nurs Manage,* 34(4):40A-40D.

Lusk SL. (2001). Priorities for preventive services. *AAOHN J,* 49(12):540-541.

Lusk SL, Kerr MJ, Kauffman SA. (1998). Use of hearing protection and perceptions of noise exposure and hearing loss among construction workers. *Am Ind Hyg Assoc J,* 59(7):466-470.

Monsén MG, Edéll-Gustafsson UM. (2005). Noise and sleep disturbance factors before and after implementation of a behavioural modification programme. *Intensive Crit Care Nurs,* 21(4):208-219.

Moorhead M, Johnson M, Maas M (Eds). (2004). *Nursing Outcomes Classification (NOC),* 3rd ed. St. Louis: Mosby.

Morrison WE, Haas EC, Shaffner DH, Garrett ES, Fackler JC. (2003). Noise, stress, and annoyance in a pediatric intensive care unit. *Crit Care Med,* 31(1):113-119.

Mortland KK, Mortland DB. (2002). Seeking a quiet place: Controlling noise in the laboratory. *Clin Leadersh Manag Rev,* 16(4):253-256.

Nightingale F. (1860). *Notes on nursing: What it is, and what it is not.* New York: Appleton and Co.

Olson DM, Borel CO, Laskowitz DT, Moore DT, McConnell ES. (2001). Quiet time: A nursing intervention to promote sleep in neurocritical care units. *Am J Crit Care,* 10(2):74-78.

Overman Dube JA, Barth MM, Cmiel CA, Olson SM, Cutshall SM, Sulla SJ, et al. (2006). *Shh . . . patients healing: From nursing empowerment to innovation.* Presented at the Fifteenth Annual Nursing Research Conference, Mayo Clinic, Rochester, MN, March 8, 2006.

Penney PJ, Earl CE. (2004). Occupational noise and effects on blood pressure: Exploring the relationship of hypertension and noise exposure in workers. *AAOHN J,* 52(11):476-480.

Philbin MK, Gray L. (2002). Changing levels of quiet in an intensive care nursery. *J Perinatol,* 22(6): 455-460.

Richards KC, O'Sullivan PS, Phillips RL. (2000). Measurement of sleep in critically ill patients. *J Nurs Meas,* 8(2):131-144.

Schnelle JF, Alessi CA, Al-Samarrai NR, Fricker RD Jr, Ouslander JG. (1999). The nursing home at night: Effects of an intervention on noise, light, and sleep. *J Am Geriatr Soc,* 47(4):430-438.

Shertzer KE, Keck JF. (2001). Music and the PACU environment. *J Perianesth Nurs,* 16(2):90-102.

Slevin M, Farrington N, Duffy G, Daly L, Murphy JF. (2000). Altering the NICU and measuring infants' responses. *Acta Paediatr,* 89(5):577-581.

Stichler JF. (2001). Creating healing environments in critical care units. *Crit Care Nurs Q,* 24(3):1-20.

Thorgaard P, Ertmann E, Hansen V, Noerregaard A, Hansen V, Spanggaard L. (2005). Designed sound and music environment in postanaesthesia care units–a multicentre study of patients and staff. *Intensive Crit Care Nurs,* 21(4):220-225.

Tijunelis MA, Fitzsullivan E, Henderson SO. (2005). Noise in the ED. *Am J Emerg Med*, 23(3):332-335.

Topf M. (2000). Hospital noise pollution: An environmental stress model to guide research and clinical interventions. *J Adv Nurs*, 31(3):520-528.

Topf M, Bookman M, Arand D. (1996). Effects of critical care unit noise on the subjective quality of sleep. *J Adv Nurs*, 24(3):545-551.

Topf M, Thompson S. (2001). Interactive relationships between hospital patients' noise-induced stress and other stress with sleep. *Heart Lung*, 30(4):237-243.

Ulrich R, Zimring C. (2004). The role of the physical environment in the hospital of the 21st century: A once-in-a-lifetime opportunity. Report to the Center for Health Design for the Designing the 21st Century Hospital Project, 15-17. Available online: http://www.healthdesign.org. Retrieved June 12, 2006.

Walder B, Francioli D, Meyer JJ, Lançon M, Romand JA. (2000). Effects of guidelines implementation in a surgical intensive care unit to control nighttime light and noise levels. *Crit Care Med*, 28(7):2242-2247.

Walsh-Sukys M, Reitenbach A, Hudson-Barr D, DePompei P. (2001). Reducing light and sound in the neonatal intensive care unit: An evaluation of patient safety, staff satisfaction and costs. *J Perinatol*, 21(4):230-235.

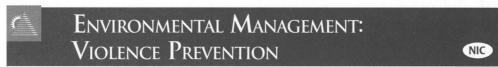

ENVIRONMENTAL MANAGEMENT: VIOLENCE PREVENTION

NIC

Rose E. Constantino, PhD, JD, RN, FAAN, FACFE; Patricia A. Crane, PhD, MSN, RN-C, WHNP

NIC **Definition:** Monitoring and manipulation of the physical environment to decrease the potential for violent behavior directed toward the self, others, or the environment (Dochterman & Bulechek, 2004).

NURSING ACTIVITIES

Effective

■ *Educate young people in violence prevention by focusing on positive alternatives to aggression-based interpersonal problem solving and gender-based role expectations.* **LOE = II**

MR A study with a community-based, random, two-group, two-level growth curve experimental design was used to help 158 teens (14 to 16 years old) develop healthy, nonabusive relationships with dating partners. The intervention group showed a reduced incidence of physical and emotional abuse and reduced symptoms of emotional distress (Wolfe et al., 2003).

MR A study group (*N* = 38) was blindly and randomly sentenced to attend the Turning Point: Rethinking Violence (TPRV) program, a unique, multi-agency, 6-week, 14-hour, court-ordered program that was developed to expose, educate, and remediate first-time violent offenders regarding the real-world consequences of violence. Results showed a statistically significant difference between the study group and the control group (38 participants pulled from a subject pool of first-time offenders who received standard sentencing options), which suggests that the TPRV program could potentially reduce adolescent violence and the subsequent impact on violence care (Scott et al., 2002).

RCT = Randomized Controlled (Clinical) Trial, **NIC** = Nursing Interventions Classification, **NOC** = Nursing Outcomes Classification

(EO) The need for violence prevention among children is great, because even the impact of a child witnessing violence is cumulative, affecting both the mental and physical health as adults and increasing the risk for children to be in violent relationships as adults, thus perpetuating the cycle of violence (Ernst, 2006).

■ (NIC) *Remove potential weapons from the environment (e.g., sharps and ropelike objects). Search the patient and belongings for weapons/potential weapons during inpatient admission procedure as appropriate. Search the environment routinely to maintain it as hazard free. Monitor the safety of items being brought to the environment by visitors. Instruct visitors and other caregivers about relevant patient safety issues. Apply mitts, splints, helmets, or restraints to limit mobility and ability to initiate self-harm as appropriate.* **LOE = VI**

(NR) A case study described restraining a patient with paraplegia along with aggressive and suicidal behaviors who was admitted to the intensive care unit after a suicide attempt by falling from her third story apartment window and proceeding in the intensive care unit to swallow a thermometer cover, a straw, and handfuls of egg crate mattress in an attempt to self-asphyxiate. Multiple nursing strategies were recommended: (1) assess the family's understanding of the use of restraints; (2) request consultation with a psychiatric nurse liaison; (3) record all communication, consultation, and implementation in the patient health record; and (4) consult the ethics committee, legal counsel, and/or a risk manager (Constantino et al., 1997).

(MR) A critical review of 41 published articles about administrative and behavioral interventions directed at addressing workplace violence revealed that only nine of the articles reported results of an evaluation, all of which included interventions that were aimed at preventing assaults between patients and employees, and none of which employed experimental designs. The authors concluded that there was a significant lack of rigorous research that assessed administrative and behavioral measures to address workplace violence (Runyan et al., 2000).

Possibly Effective

■ *Refer young survivors of violence from the emergency department directly to a social services agency.* **LOE = II**

(MR) In this experimental study, the effects of a case management model and an alliance between a health care system's emergency department and a social services agency on the recurrence of violence among youth was examined in 188 victims of interpersonal violence. The treatment group ($N = 96$) that was referred directly from the emergency department to social services agencies showed significant reductions in the recurrence of victimization than the control group ($N = 92$) (Zun et al., 2003).

■ *Provide primary prevention to perpetrators of violence.* **LOE = I**

(MR) A meta-analysis of 22 violence perpetrator intervention studies with a comparison group found that the overall effect on perpetrator intervention was small, with a net effect of only 5%, which was inadequate. Intervention programs for violence perpetrators need more study and longer evaluation periods to determine whether treatment truly has a lasting behavioral modification outcome (Babcock et al., 2004).

NR = Nursing Research, **MR** = Multidisciplinary Research, **SP** = Standard of Practice, **EO** = Expert Opinion, **LOE** = Level of Evidence

Not Effective

No applicable published research was found in this category.

Possibly Harmful

No applicable published research was found in this category.

OUTCOME MEASUREMENT

ABUSE PROTECTION 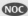

Definition: Protection of self or dependent others from abuse
Abuse Protection as evidenced by the following selected NOC indicators:
- Self-advocacy
- Plan for avoiding abuse
- Implementation of plan to avoid abuse
- Safety of self
- Safety of children
- Facilitation of abuser obtaining counseling

(Rate each above indicator of **Abuse Protection:** 1 = not adequate, 2 = slightly adequate, 3 = moderately adequate, 4 = substantially adequate, 5 = totally adequate) (Moorhead et al., 2004).

AGGRESSION SELF-CONTROL

Definition: Self-restraint of assaultive, combative, or destructive behaviors toward others.
Aggression Self-Control as evidenced by the following selected NOC indicators:
- Identifies when angry
- Identifies when frustrated
- Identifies situations that precipitate hostility
- Identifies when feeling aggressive
- Refrains from verbal outbursts
- Refrains from violating others' personal space
- Refrains from striking others
- Refrains from harming others
- Refrains from harming animals
- Refrains from destroying property
- Uses physical outlets to reduce pent-up energy
- Uses specific techniques to control frustration
- Controls impulses
- Upholds contract to restrain aggressive behaviors
- Maintains self-control without supervision

(Rate each indicator of **Aggression Self-Control:** 1 = never demonstrated, 2 = rarely demonstrated, 3 = sometimes demonstrated, 4 = often demonstrated, 5 = consistently demonstrated) (Moorhead et al., 2004).

REFERENCES

Babcock JC, Green CE, Robie C. (2004). Does batterers' treatment work? A meta-analytic review of domestic violence treatment. *Clin Psychol Rev,* 23(8):1023-1053.

Constantino RE, Boneysteele G, Gesmond SA, Nelson B. (1997). Restraining an aggressive suicidal, paraplegic patient: A look at the ethical and legal issues. *Dimens Crit Care Nurs,* 16(3):144-151.

Dochterman JM, Bulechek GM (Eds). (2004). *Nursing interventions classification (NIC),* 4th ed. St Louis: Mosby.

Ernst AA. (2006). Intimate partner violence: Steps for future generations. *Ann Emerg Med,* 47(2): 200-202.

Moorhead M, Johnson M, Maas M (Eds). (2004). *Nursing outcomes classification (NOC),* 3rd ed. St Louis: Mosby.

Runyan CW, Zakocs RC, Zwerling C. (2000). Administrative and behavioral interventions for workplace violence prevention. *Am J Prev Med,* 18(4 Suppl):116-127.

Scott KK, Tepas JJ, Frykberg E, Taylor PM, Plotkin AJ. (2002). Turning point: Rethinking violence—Evaluation of program efficacy in reducing adolescent violent crime recidivism. *J Trauma,* 53(1): 21-27.

Wolfe DA, Wekerle C, Scott K, Straatman A, Grasley C, Reitzel-Jaffe D. (2003). Dating violence prevention with at-risk youth: A controlled outcome evaluation. *J Consult Clin Psychol,* 71(2): 279-291.

Zun LS, Downey LV, Rosen J. (2003). Violence prevention in the ED: Linkage of the ED to a social service agency. *Am J Emerg Med,* 21(6):454-457.

EXERCISE PROMOTION: MOTIVATIONAL TECHNIQUES

Barbara Resnick, PhD, CRNP, FAAN, FAANP; Sherry H. Pomeroy, PhD, MS, RN

Definition: Facilitation of regular physical activity to maintain or advance to a higher level of fitness and health (Dochterman & Bulechek, 2004).

NURSING ACTIVITIES

Effective

■ *Promote social support from family and friends, which has been associated with long-term exercise adherence in older adults. Examples of social support strategies include peer support (e.g., bringing a friend) and professional educator support (e.g., telephone counseling, computer-based or written information).*
LOE = I

MR An RCT (*N* = 105) testing the impact of a 6-week program that included weekly 2-hour sessions of health education by a peer and physical exercises taught by a physical therapist found that there was an initial improvement at 6 weeks for time spent in exercise activities (Hopman-Rock & Westhoff, 2000).

MR In an RCT (*N* = 66) in which participants were exposed to either a print or print-plus-telephone exercise intervention, participants received an instructional newsletter and use of a pedometer (both groups) and individualized telephone calls (print-plus-telephone group

NR = Nursing Research, **MR** = Multidisciplinary Research, **SP** = Standard of Practice, **EO** = Expert Opinion, **LOE** = Level of Evidence

only) over the 12-week intervention. Both groups showed evidence of increased physical activity (Ball et al., 2005).

(MR) An RCT ($N = 100$) comparing the effects of brief advice with exercise from a clinician supplemented by telephone-based counseling by health educators (extended advice) and with brief advice from a clinician alone (brief advice) found that the extended-advice intervention resulted in greater participation in moderate-intensity physical activity than the brief advice (Pinto et al., 2005).

(MR) A controlled study that evaluated whether 13 diverse local lead agencies could effectively implement a choice-based, telephone-assisted physical activity promotion program for older adults based on intervention models proved efficacious in research settings. Participants received regular telephone calls over a 1-year period from a trained staff member or volunteer support buddy. The intervention resulted in increased physical activity among participants (Hooker et al., 2005).

(MR) A randomized controlled ($2 \times 2 \times 2$) factorial trial ($N = 151$) studying interventions including prescription from general practitioners, counseling by nurses, and exposure to a health education booklet found that only prescription combined with counseling resulted in increased physical activity (Little et al., 2004).

(MR) In a controlled study, matched physician offices were nonrandomly assigned to intervention or control. Healthy, sedentary, adult patients ($N = 255$) were recruited from physician offices. The intervention consisted of brief, behaviorally based counseling by physicians plus a telephone follow-up 2 weeks later. Intervention patients reported increased walking more than controls (Calfas et al., 1996).

(MR) In a controlled study, primary care doctors (117) were randomly allocated to Green Prescription or usual care. A brief activity consultation was provided, followed by telephone support from an exercise specialist. Participants ($N = 270$) exposed to treatment spent more time in physical activity than controls (Kerse et al., 2005).

▪ *Use self-efficacy-based interventions using single or multiple sources (performance of the activity, verbal encouragement, role of self-modeling, and addressing physiological feedback).* LOE = I

(MR) A randomized trial ($N = 240$) testing a self-efficacy-based treatment that involved developing action goals and using barrier-focused mental strategies versus a standard care control group found that the treatment group demonstrated more physical activity at follow-up and better adherence to recommended levels of exercise intensity than did the control group (Sniehotta et al., 2005).

(NR) An RCT ($N = 198$) including minority older adults exposed to a self-efficacy-based motivational and exercise intervention in senior centers (senior self-efficacy program) found that participants in the treatment group spent more time in physical activity than those in the control groups (Resnick et al., 2006).

(NR) An RCT ($N = 208$) testing the impact of the exercise plus program, a self-efficacy-based intervention developed for older women after hip fracture, found that participants exposed to the intervention demonstrated increased time in physical activity at 6 and 12 months after hip fracture (Resnick et al., 2006).

(MR) A randomized trial ($N = 250$) tested the effectiveness of CHANGE (Change Habits by Applying New Goals and Experiences), a lifestyle modification program that was designed to increase exercise maintenance in the year following a cardiac rehabilitation program. The CHANGE intervention (supplemental to usual care) was compared with usual care.

RCT = Randomized Controlled (Clinical) Trial, **NIC** = Nursing Interventions Classification, **NOC** = Nursing Outcomes Classification

Participants in the usual-care group were 76% more likely than those in the CHANGE group to stop exercising during the year after a cardiac rehabilitation program (Moore et al., 2006).

Possibly Effective

■ *Implement stages of change–based interventions. Stages include precontemplation, contemplation, preparation, action, and maintenance (Samuelson, 1998).* **LOE = I**

(MR) An RCT tested a stage-based exercise intervention that was either moderate or vigorous and either home based or center based. After 6 months, all participants exercised at home. The intervention was seen to be effective regardless of location or intensity of exercise. The effectiveness of the stage-based intervention was questionable, because women with less readiness to change were just as likely to adopt or maintain exercise (Cox et al., 2003).

(MR) A randomized study (Increasing Motivation for Physical ACTivity or IMPACT study) promoted adoption and maintenance of physical activity (PA) in sedentary, low-income women participating in federally funded job training programs ($N = 98$). The intervention consisted of 2 months of weekly 1-hour classes, then random assignment to 10 months of behavior change strategies including either home-based telephone counseling for PA plus information and feedback via mailed newsletters (phone + mail counseling condition) or just the mailed newsletters (mail support condition). The combined phone + mail counseling condition resulted in significantly greater increases in estimated total energy expenditure compared with mail alone, providing some support for stage-based interventions.

(MR) Two reviews of the literature found inconsistent evidence that individualized stage-based activity promotion interventions were any more effective than control conditions in promoting long-term adherence to increased levels of physical activity. Possible reasons for this were that these approaches focus too much on stage and not enough on behavior, and they may be too simplified (Adams & White, 2005; Timperio et al., 2004).

■ *Use health contracts.* **LOE = VI**

(MR) In a quasi-experimental study ($N = 25$) in which older adults developed health contracts focused on exercise goals, 20 achieved at least 75% of their exercise goals and 15 had a 100% success rate (Haber & Rhodes, 2004).
(Please refer to the guideline on Patient Contracting.)

Not Effective

■ *Use of a one-time counseling interaction with limited follow-up (i.e., one-time telephone call).* **LOE = I**

(MR) An RCT ($N = 812$) testing Physician-Based Assessment and Counseling for Exercise (PACE) with physicians trained to deliver PACE exercise counseling protocols during a regular medical visit and then provide one reminder telephone call a month later found that a one-time PACE counseling session with minimal reinforcement did not further increase activity (Norris et al., 2000).

■ *Use of a computerized intervention.* **LOE = III**

(MR) A quasi-experimental study recruited 10 primary care practices and worked closely with project staff to develop a practice-specific plan for incorporating the physical activity focused computer-based program into the workflow and office routine. Feasibility was measured by the percentage of patients who used the program during the day of their visit. Only 1 of 10 offices was able to incorporate the program successfully into their office workflow and delivery of routine care (Sciamanna et al., 2004).

Possibly Harmful

No applicable published research was found in this category.

OUTCOME MEASUREMENT

MOTIVATION (NOC)

Definition: Inner urge that moves or prompts an individual to positive action(s).
Motivation as evidenced by the following selected NOC indicators:
• Develops an action plan
• Obtains needed support
• Self-initiates goal-directed behavior
• Completes tasks or activities
• Expresses intent to act
(Rate each indicator of **Motivation:** 1 = never demonstrated, 2 = rarely demonstrated, 3 = sometimes demonstrated, 4 = often demonstrated, 5 = consistently demonstrated) (Moorhead et al., 2004).
Additional non-NOC indicators:
• Self-efficacy expectations related to physical activity/exercise
• Outcome expectations related to physical activity/exercise
• Stage of change related to physical activity/exercise
• Social support for physical activity

REFERENCES

Adams J, White M. (2005). Why don't stage-based activity promotion interventions work? *Health Educ Res,* 20(2):237-243.

Ball K, Salmon J, Leslie E, Owen N, King AC. (2005). Piloting the feasibility and effectiveness of print- and telephone-mediated interventions for promoting the adoption of physical activity in Australian adults. *J Sci Med Sport,* 8(2):134-142.

Calfas KJ, Long BJ, Sallis JF, Wooten WJ, Pratt M, Patrick K. (1996). A controlled trial of physician counseling to promote the adoption of physical activity. *Prev Med,* 25(3):225-233.

Cox KL, Gorely TJ, Puddey IB, Burke V, Beilin LJ. (2003). Exercise behaviour change in 40 to 65-year-old women: The SWEAT Study (Sedentary Women Exercise Adherence Trial). *Br J Health Psychol,* 8(Pt 4): 477-495.

Dochterman JM, Bulechek GM (Eds). (2004). *Nursing Interventions Classification (NIC)*, 4th ed. St. Louis: Mosby.

Haber D, Rhodes D. (2004). Health contract with sedentary older adults. *Gerontologist*, 44(6):827-835.

Hooker SP, Seavey W, Weidmer CE, Harvey DJ, Stewart AL, Gillis DE, et al. (2005). The California active aging community grant program: Translating science into practice to promote physical activity in older adults. *Ann Behav Med*, 29(3):155-165.

Hopman-Rock M, Westhoff MH. (2000). The effects of a health educational and exercise program for older adults with osteoarthritis for the hip or knee. *J Rheumatol*, 27(8):1947-1954.

Kerse N, Elley CR, Robinson E, Arroll B. (2005). Is physical activity counseling effective for older people? A cluster randomized, controlled trial in primary care. *J Am Geriatr Soc*, 53(11):1951-1956.

Little P, Dorward M, Gralton S, et al. (2004). A randomised controlled trial of three pragmatic approaches to initiate increased physical activity in sedentary patients with risk factors for cardiovascular disease, *Br J Gen Pract*, 54(500): 189-195.

Moore SM, Charvat JM, Gordon NH, Pashkow F, Ribisl P, Roberts BL, et al. (2006). Effects of a CHANGE intervention to increase exercise maintenance following cardiac events. *Ann Behav Med*, 31(1):53-62.

Moorhead M, Johnson M, Maas M (Eds). (2004). *Nursing Outcomes Classification (NOC)*, 3rd ed. St. Louis: Mosby.

Norris SL, Grothaus LC, Buchner DM, Pratt M. (2000). Effectiveness of physician-based assessment and counseling for exercise in a staff model HMO. *Prev Med*, 30(6):513-523.

Pinto BM, Goldstein MG, Ashba J, Sciamanna CN, Jette A. (2005). Randomized controlled trial of physical activity counseling for older primary care patients. *Am J Prev Med*, 29(4):247-255.

Resnick B, Vogel A, Luisi D. (2006). Motivating minority older adults to exercise. *Cultur Divers Ethnic Minor Psychol*, 12(1):17-29.

Samuelson, M. (1998). Stages of change: from theory to practice. *The Art of Health Promotion*, 2(5): 1-8.

Sciamanna CN, Marcus BH, Goldstein MG, Lawrence K, Swartz S, Bock B, et al. (2004). Feasibility of incorporating computer-tailored health behaviour communications in primary care settings. *Inform Prim Care*, 12(1):40-48.

Sniehotta FF, Scholz U, Schwarzer R, Fuhrmann B, Kiwus U, Voller H. (2005). Long-term effects of two psychological interventions on physical exercise and self-regulation following coronary rehabilitation. *Int J Behav Med*, 12(4):244-255.

Timperio A, Salmon J, Ball K. (2004). Evidence-based strategies to promote physical activity among children, adolescents and young adults: Review and update. *J Sci Med Sport*, 7(1 Suppl):20-29.

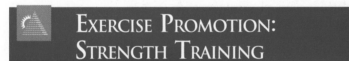

EXERCISE PROMOTION: STRENGTH TRAINING

Barbara Resnick, PhD, CRNP, FAAN, FAANP; Sherry H. Pomeroy, PhD, MS, RN

NIC **Definition:** Facilitating regular resistive muscle training to maintain or increase muscle strength (Dochterman & Bulechek, 2004).

NURSING ACTIVITIES

Effective

■ *Encourage prescriptive resistance exercise of each major muscle group (hips, thighs, legs, back, chest, shoulders, abdomen) using free weights, bands, or machines 2 to 3 nonconsecutive days per week for approximately one set of 8 to*

NR = Nursing Research, **MR** = Multidisciplinary Research, **SP** = Standard of Practice, **EO** = Expert Opinion, **LOE** = Level of Evidence

12 repetitions (range between 3 and 20, e.g., 3 to 5, 8 to 10) performed at a moderate repetition duration (~3 seconds concentric and ~3 seconds eccentric) for accrued health benefits, including reduced risk of osteoporosis, sarcopenia, low back pain, hypertension, and diabetes, and increased ability to perform activities of daily living needed to maintain functional independence throughout the lifespan. Resistance training in individuals with moderate- to high-risk cardiac disease must be closely evaluated for safety and effectiveness and adverse cardiovascular events. **LOE = I**

(EO) Resistance training significantly enhances endurance as well as muscular strength. Benefits of resistance training include development of muscular strength, endurance, and lean body mass and maintenance of basal metabolic rate that can assist in weight control. Most cardiac, frail, and older adults experience substantial benefits from both upper and lower body exercise that includes maintaining independence and preventing falls (Pollock et al., 2000).

(MR) A systematic review of 83 studies found that virtually all the benefits of resistance training could be obtained in 15- to 20-minute training sessions two times per week. Precise controlled movements for each major muscle group without very heavy resistance would result in overall profound effects on the musculoskeletal system. Resistance training combined with steady-state aerobic exercise was recommended as a central component of health promotion (Winett & Carpinelli, 2001).

(MR) A systematic review of 41 studies reported that the benefits of strength training included muscle strength, increased bone and muscle mass, flexibility, dynamic balance, self-confidence, self-esteem, and reduced falls in older adults with functional limitations. The symptoms of arthritis, depression, type 2 diabetes, osteoporosis, heart disease, and sleep disorders were reduced (Seguin & Nelson, 2003).

■ *Use a resistance exercise program in older adults with knee osteoarthritis to improve pain and physical performance and reduce disability.* **LOE = I**

(MR) An RCT, the Fitness and Arthritis in Seniors Trial (FAST), compared the effects of an aerobic training program and a resistance exercise program with a health education control in older adults with symptomatic knee osteoarthritis ($N = 365$). The resistance exercise program was 1 hour in duration with participants performing two sets of 12 repetitions of each major muscle group 3 days per week for 18 months. Participants had consistently modest improvements on measures of functional performance and self-reported disability and pain compared with the control group (Ettinger et al., 1997).

(MR) A systematic review of the effects of strengthening exercise in people with knee osteoarthritis ($N = 11$) showed a positive effect on pain and disability even in settings with relatively limited supervision and low intensity. People with osteoarthritis of the knee should be counseled to engage in strengthening exercises and progress to both open and closed-chain isotonic exercise, such as stair-stepping and squatting exercises (Baker & McAlindon, 2000).

■ *Encourage progressive resistance training following stroke to reduce musculoskeletal impairment.* **LOE = I**

(MR) A systematic review of studies that evaluated the effect of progressive resistance training for people after stroke found that preliminary evidence indicated that such programs reduced

RCT = Randomized Controlled (Clinical) Trial, **NIC** = Nursing Interventions Classification, **NOC** = Nursing Outcomes Classification

musculoskeletal impairment after stroke ($N = 350$ with eight studies meeting criteria for review). Three studies reported improvements in walking and climbing stairs. Few negative effects of strength training after stroke were reported and were very minor (Morris et al., 2004).

(MR) In an RCT, inpatient stroke patients ($N = 64$) were randomly assigned to standard care, functional task practice, or strength-training groups. The strength-training group had upper extremity exercise using eccentric, isometric, or concentric muscle contractions using the available arm and progressing to free weights, therabands, or grip devices 3 days a week on alternate days for 4 to 6 weeks. Strength training significantly improved motor scores (Fugl-Meyer Assessment) and strength (isometric torque), with more improvement in less severe participants (Winstein et al., 2004).

■ *Encourage resistance training as a modality for reducing falls in older adults.*
   LOE = II

(MR) A Cochrane systematic review of 62 clinical trials involving 21,668 participants assessed the effectiveness of various interventions to reduce the number of falls or fallers in older adults. Muscle strengthening and balance training supervised by health professionals at home had a pooled relative risk of 0.80, 95% confidence interval (0.66 to 0.98) (Gillespie et al., 2003).

(MR) Four controlled trials of a home exercise fall prevention program (muscle strengthening and balance retraining exercises) for older adults were pooled and analyzed ($N = 1016$). The number of falls and injuries from falls was reduced by 35%. The program was most effective in reducing injurious falls for participants 80 years and older compared with those aged 65 to 79 (Robertson et al., 2002).

Possibly Effective

■ *Use social cognitive theory–based interventions combined with traditional strength training to improve upper body and lower body strength efficacy gains.*
   LOE = II

(MR) Older adults with knee osteoarthritis were randomly assigned to an aerobic exercise, resistance training, or health education control. Self-efficacy for stair climbing increased in both groups compared with control, and self-efficacy mediated the effect of the treatments on the stair climb, suggesting that control beliefs mediated the effects that exercise programs had on disability (Rejeski et al., 1998).

(MR) An RCT ($N = 38$) tested the addition of a psychological empowerment intervention compared with a traditional strength training program on self-efficacy for upper and lower body strength and desire to lift weight of varying amounts using three sessions per week (two center based and one home based). The study results showed that theoretically based strength training programs to empower older adults may be more motivating than traditional programs (Katula et al., 2006).

Not Effective

No applicable published research was found in this category.

NR = Nursing Research, **MR** = Multidisciplinary Research, **SP** = Standard of Practice, **EO** = Expert Opinion, **LOE** = Level of Evidence

Possibly Harmful

■ *Use of intensive strength training at high resistance loads (>60% 1-RM [repetition maximum]) in individuals with moderate to severe cardiac disease and older adults with low aerobic exercise capacity.* **LOE = I**

(EO) Careful evaluation and initial monitoring of individuals with cardiac disease or severe left ventricular dysfunction and older adults with low aerobic fitness are advised. An aerobic exercise program for 2 to 4 weeks before beginning resistance training is recommended for individuals with low- to moderate-risk cardiac conditions. Resistance training is contraindicated for individuals with unstable angina, uncontrolled hypertension (systolic >160 mm Hg and/or diastolic >100 mm Hg), uncontrolled dysrhythmias or congestive heart failure, severe valvular stenosis or regurgitation, and hypertrophic cardiomyopathy (Pollock et al., 2000).

(MR) A systematic review of the literature regarding exercise testing and safety monitoring for people aged 75 years or older recommended that previously sedentary older people with known cardiovascular disease should "start low and go slow," such as lower extremity resistance training with ankle weights or elastic tubing. Older adults may progress to more intensive strength training, such as weight machines or free weights, if low-intensity exercise is tolerated (Gill et al., 2000).

(MR) In a quasi-experimental study, left ventricular function during 1-RM resistance exercise with individuals with moderate left ventricular function ($N = 15$) resulted in ischemic changes with the highest resistance workloads and larger muscle mass. However, the changes were small in magnitude and did not suggest a reduction in cardiac performance. Individuals with low- to moderate-risk cardiac disease can safely engage in resistance exercise using 10 to 15 repetitions at 20%, 40%, and 60% of 1-RM (Werber-Zion et al., 2004).

OUTCOME MEASUREMENT

PHYSICAL FITNESS (NOC)

Definition: Performance of physical activities with vigor.

Physical Fitness (strength and endurance) as evidenced by the following selected NOC indicators:

- Muscle strength
- Muscle endurance
- Joint flexibility
- Performance of physical activities

(Rate each indicator of **Physical Fitness:** 1 = severely compromised, 2 = substantially compromised, 3 = moderately compromised, 4 = mildly compromised, 5 = not compromised) (Moorhead et al., 2004).

Additional non-NOC indicators:

- 1-RM (repetition maximum) test (ACSM, 2006)
- Push up test and curl-up crunch (ACSM, 2006)
- Timed up and go test (Podsiadlo & Richardson, 1991)
- Chair stand (Rikli & Jones, 1999)
- Arm curl (Rikli & Jones, 1999)

REFERENCES

American College of Sports Medicine (ACSM). (2006). *ACSM's guidelines for exercise testing and prescription,* 7th ed. Philadelphia: Lippincott Williams & Wilkins.

Baker K, McAlindon T. (2000). Exercise for knee osteoarthritis. *Curr Opin Rheumatol,* 12(5):456-463.

Dochterman JM, Bulechek GM (Eds). (2004). *Nursing Interventions Classification (NIC),* 4th ed. St. Louis: Mosby.

Ettinger WH, Burns R, Messier SP, Applegate W, Rejeski WJ, Morgan T, et al. (1997). A randomized trial comparing aerobic exercise and resistance training with a health education program in older adults with knee osteoarthritis: The Fitness Arthritis and Seniors Trial (FAST). *JAMA,* 277(1):25-31.

Gill TM, DiPietro L, Krumholz HM. (2000). Role of exercise stress testing and safety monitoring for older persons starting an exercise program. *JAMA,* 284(3):342-349.

Gillespie LD, Gillespie WJ, Robertson MC, Lamb SE, Cumming RG, Rowe BH. (2003). Interventions for preventing falls in elderly people. *Cochrane Database Syst Rev,* (4):CD000340.

Katula JA, Sipe M, Rejeski WJ, Focht BC. (2006). Strength training in older adults: An empowering intervention. *Med Sci Sports Exerc,* 38(1):106-111.

Moorhead M, Johnson M, Maas M (Eds). (2004). *Nursing Outcomes Classification (NOC),* 3rd ed. St. Louis: Mosby.

Morris SL, Dodd KJ, Morris ME. (2004). Outcomes of progressive resistance strength training following stroke: A systematic review. *Clin Rehabil,* 18(1):27-39.

Podsiadlo D, Richardson S. (1991). The timed "Up and Go": A test of basic functional mobility for frail elderly persons. *J Am Geriatr Soc,* 39(2):142-148.

Pollock ML, Franklin BA, Balady GJ, Chaitman BL, Fleg JL, Fletcher B, et al. (2000). AHA Science Advisory. Resistance exercise in individuals with and without cardiovascular disease: Benefits, rationale, safety, and prescription: An advisory from the Committee on Exercise, Rehabilitation, and Prevention, Council on Clinical Cardiology, American Heart Association; Position paper endorsed by the American College of Sports Medicine. *Circulation,* 101(7):828-833.

Rejeski WJ, Ettinger WH, Morgan T. (1998). Treating disability in knee osteoarthritis with exercise therapy: A central role for self-efficacy and pain. *Arthritis Care Res,* 11(2):94-101.

Rikli RE, Jones CJ. (1999). Development and validation of a functional fitness test for community residing older adults. *J Aging Phys Activity,* 7:129-161.

Robertson MC, Campbell AJ, Gardner MM, Devlin N. (2002). Preventing injuries in older people by preventing falls: A meta-analysis of individual-level data. *J Am Geriatr Soc,* 50(5):905-911.

Seguin R, Nelson M. (2003). The benefits of strength training for older adults. *Am J Prev Med,* 25(3 Suppl 2):141-149.

Werber-Zion G, Goldhammer E, Shaar A, Pollock ML. (2004). Left ventricular function during strength testing and resistance exercise in patients with left ventricular dysfunction. *J Cardiopulm Rehabil,* 24(2):100-109.

Winett RA, Carpinelli RN. (2001). Potential health-related benefits of resistance training. *Prev Med,* 33(5):503-513.

Winstein CJ, Rose DK, Tan SM, Lewthwaite R, Chui HC, Azen SP. (2004). A randomized controlled comparison of upper-extremity rehabilitation strategies in acute stroke: A pilot study of immediate and long-term outcomes. *Arch Phys Med Rehabil,* 85(4):620-628.

 # EXERCISE PROMOTION: STRETCHING

Barbara Resnick, PhD, CRNP, FAAN, FANNP; Sherry H. Pomeroy, PhD, MS, RN

NIC **Definition:** Facilitation of systematic slow-stretch-hold muscle exercises to induce relaxation, to prepare muscles/joints for more vigorous exercise, or to increase or maintain body flexibility (Dochterman & Bulechek, 2004).

NR = Nursing Research, **MR** = Multidisciplinary Research, **SP** = Standard of Practice, **EO** = Expert Opinion, **LOE** = Level of Evidence

NURSING ACTIVITIES

Effective

■ *Encourage prescriptive stretching including repeated feedback-controlled or intelligent stretching.* **LOE = I**

(MR) In a pretest/post-test trial of repeated feedback-controlled and programmed "intelligent" stretching of the ankle plantar and dorsiflexors to treat individuals with spasticity and/or contractures after stroke, participants engaged in stretching of the plantar and dorsiflexors of the ankle three times a week for 45 minutes over a 4-week period. This exercise had a positive influence on the joint properties of the ankle with regard to spasticity and contracture. Stretching may be an effective alternative to passive range of motion, as it can be done alone rather than provided by a trained clinician (Selles et al., 2005).

(MR) A systematic literature review of 28 studies including 1338 participants considered the impact of stretching the hamstrings using a variety of stretching techniques, positions, and durations. All studies reported improvements in range of motion after stretching. Given the type of studies completed, however, it was impossible to determine the most effective hamstring stretching method (Decoster et al., 2005).

(MR) An RCT ($N = 45$) compared the effects of a conventional physical therapy program that involved 20 exercises. The treatment group was exposed to the experimental protocol based on the postural affectation of ankylosing spondylitis and the treatment of the shortened muscle chains in these patients. A total of 15 weekly sessions were provided. The treatment group had greater improvement than the control group in all the clinical measures (Fernandez-de-Las-Penas et al., 2005).

(MR) A systematic review of 43 RCTs in which individually designed stretching was delivered showed that individually designed and supervised programs did better than home programs. High-dose exercise programs versus low-dose programs did better. Overall findings indicated that individually designed programs of stretching exercise delivered with supervision may improve pain and function in chronic nonspecific low back pain (Hayden et al., 2005).

(MR) In a controlled laboratory study ($N = 29$), participants were randomly assigned to a static stretching, ballistic stretching, or control group. On each of 4 consecutive days they completed four maximal range-of-motion stretches of the hamstrings. The results indicated that stretching groups had an increase in range of motion and stretch tolerance after 4 weeks of stretching (LaRoche & Connolly, 2006).

Possibly Effective

■ *Support the utility of stretching for sports injury risk.* **LOE = I**

(MR) In a meta-analysis of a systematic review of randomized trials or cohort studies for interventions that included stretching, 361 studies weighted pooled odds ratios using an intention to treat analysis as well as subgroup analyses. Stretching was not significantly associated with a reduction in total injuries. Consequently, there was not sufficient evidence to endorse or discontinue routine stretching before or after exercise to prevent injury among competitive or recreational athletes (Thacker et al., 2004).

RCT = Randomized Controlled (Clinical) Trial, **NIC** = Nursing Interventions Classification, **NOC** = Nursing Outcomes Classification

MR In a systematic review of RCTs that included stretching prior to exercise in studies from 1966 to 2005, five high-quality studies were evaluated. Three of the studies found that performing warm-up prior to performance significantly reduced the injury risk, and the other two studies found that warm-up was not effective in significantly reducing the number of injuries. Although there was some support for the utility of stretching for risk reduction, there was insufficient evidence to endorse or discontinue routine warm-up prior to sports-related exercise (Fradkin et al., 2006).

Not Effective

■ *Stretching for the relief of leg cramps.* **LOE = I**

NR A two (start exercises) by two (stop quinine) factorial design RCT ($N = 191$) was conducted to compare the impact of stretching versus use of quinine alone or combined with stretching exercises in the treatment of nocturnal leg cramps. Study results indicated that calf-stretching exercises were not effective in reducing the frequency or severity of night cramps (Coppin et al., 2005).

Possibly Harmful

■ *Heavy static stretching exercise of a muscle group prior to any performance requiring maximal muscle strength endurance.* **LOE = I**

NR Two trials were done using a pretest/post-test approach ($N = 52$). The first considered knee-flexion muscle strength endurance with a no-stretching and stretching regimen; the second tested a knee flexion muscle strength endurance exercise at 50% body weight following a no-stretching and a stretching regimen. In both studies, stretching significantly reduced muscle strength endurance. Therefore, stretching should not be recommended prior to any performance requiring maximal muscle strength endurance (Nelson et al., 2005).

(Note: Stretching involves major muscle groups. Stretches should be performed in a "stretch and hold" fashion, not in a "ballistic" or "bouncing" fashion. Clinically relevant muscle groups include hip extensors, knee extensors, ankle plantar flexors, and dorsiflexors, biceps, triceps, shoulders, back extensor, and abdominal muscles.)

OUTCOME MEASUREMENT

FLEXIBILITY

Definition: Normal range of motion; passive and active range of motion in all clinically relevant muscle groups.

Flexibility as evidenced by the following indicators:
• Normal range of motion
• Free of injury
• Free of pain
• Presence of joint stiffness
(Note: This is not a NOC outcome.)

NR = Nursing Research, **MR** = Multidisciplinary Research, **SP** = Standard of Practice, **EO** = Expert Opinion, **LOE** = Level of Evidence

OUTCOME MEASUREMENT—*cont'd*

PHYSICAL FITNESS (NOC)

Definition: Performance of physical activities with vigor.

Physical Fitness as evidenced by the following selected NOC indicators:

- Muscle strength
- Muscle endurance
- Joint flexibility
- Performance of physical activities
- Performance of routine exercise

(Rate each indicator of **Physical Fitness:** 1 = severely compromised, 2 = substantially compromised, 3 = moderately compromised, 4 = mildly compromised, 5 = not compromised) (Moorhead et al., 2004).

REFERENCES

Coppin RJ, Wicke DM, Little PS. (2005). Managing nocturnal leg cramps–calf-stretching exercises and cessation of quinine treatment: A factorial randomised controlled trial. *Br J Gen Pract*, 55(512):186-191.

Decoster LC, Cleland J, Altieri C, Russell P. (2005). The effects of hamstring stretching on range of motion: A systematic literature review. *J Orthop Sports Phys Ther*, 35(6):377-387.

Dochterman JM, Bulechek GM (Eds). (2004). *Nursing Interventions Classification (NIC)*, 4th ed. St. Louis: Mosby.

Fernandez-de-Las-Penas C, Alonso-Blanco C, Morales-Cabezas M, Miangolarra-Page JC. (2005). Two exercise interventions for the management of patients with ankylosing spondylitis: A randomized controlled trial. *Am J Phys Med Rehabil*, 84(6):407-419.

Fradkin AJ, Gabbe BJ, Cameron PA. (2006). Does warming up prevent injury in sport? The evidence from randomised controlled trials. *J Sci Med Sport*, 9(3):214-220.

Hayden JA, van Tulder MW, Tomlinson G. (2005). Systematic review: Strategies for using exercise therapy to improve outcomes in chronic low back pain. *Ann Intern Med*, 142(9):776-785.

LaRoche DP, Connolly DA. (2006). Effects of stretching on passive muscle tension and response to eccentric exercise. *Am J Sports Med*, 34(6):1000-1007.

Moorhead M, Johnson M, Maas M (Eds). (2004). *Nursing Outcomes Classification (NOC)*, 3rd ed. St. Louis: Mosby.

Nelson AG, Kokkonen J, Arnall DA. (2005). Acute muscle stretching inhibits muscle strength endurance performance. *J Strength Cond Res*, 19(2):338-343.

Selles RW, Li X., Lin F, Chung SG, Roth EJ, Zhang LQ. (2005). Feedback-controlled and programmed stretching of the ankle plantarflexors and dorsiflexors in stroke: Effects of a 4-week intervention program. *Arch Phys Med Rehabil*, 86(12):2330-2336.

Thacker SB, Gilchrist J, Stroup DF, Kimsey CD Jr. (2004). The impact of stretching on sports injury risk: A systematic review of the literature. *Med Sci Sports Exerc*, 36(3):371-378.

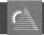 # EXERCISE THERAPY: BALANCE (NIC)

Barbara Resnick, PhD, CRNP, FAAN, FAANP; Sherry H. Pomeroy, PhD, MS, RN

NIC **Definition:** Use of specific activities, postures, and movements to maintain, enhance, or restore balance (Dochterman & Bulechek, 2004).

RCT = Randomized Controlled (Clinical) Trial, **NIC** = Nursing Interventions Classification, **NOC** = Nursing Outcomes Classification

NURSING ACTIVITIES

Effective

■ *Encourage balance training that includes sit-to-stand activities, stepping in all directions, reaching to limits of stability, and activities (e.g., ball throwing) that encourage these activities to improve participation in balance, functional activities, and mobility and to prevent falls or reduce risk for falls. There is insufficient evidence to support a preferred type, duration, or intensity of exercise.*
LOE = I

(MR) The Balance-Strategy Training Programme ($N = 73$), which involved balance exercises with community-dwelling older adults done once a week for 10 weeks, demonstrated improvements in balance, function, and mobility (Nitz & Choy, 2004).

(MR) The FICSIT meta-analysis of seven interventions found that the overall effect of any kind of exercise training was a 10% reduction in fall rates in the subsequent year. Balance training of any type reduced falls by 17% (Province et al., 1995).

(MR) An RCT ($N = 16$) of hemiparetic subjects at least 6 months after stroke showed that an 8-week task-oriented exercise program focusing on balance and mobility exercises resulted in improvements in the center of pressure and displacement under sensory conditions (Bayouk et al., 2006).

(MR) An RCT testing a 6-week enhanced balance training program consisting of a series of repetitive tasks of increasing difficulty specific to functional balance was compared with traditional physical therapy in patients with mobility problems. The intervention showed improved balance in the Berg Balance Scale (Steadman et al., 2003).

(MR) A randomized three-group parallel controlled study ($N = 34$) tested the difference between an exercise program with an emphasis on balance, an exercise group with an emphasis on gait reeducation, and no treatment (control). The study results showed that the balance exercise group showed an improvement in the Functional Balance Scale compared with the other two groups (Shimada et al., 2002).

■ *Use Tai Chi to improve balance with a more efficacious use of mechanisms controlling stepping strategies of the swing leg.* **LOE = I**

(MR) An RCT comparing Tai Chi with brisk walking ($N = 19$) showed that participants exposed to treatment had improved gait and single-leg stance time (Audette et al., 2006).

(MR) An RCT comparing Tai Chi with a stretching exercise program ($N = 256$) and walking found that Tai Chi participants showed improvements in measures of functional balance at the intervention endpoint and significantly reduced their risk of falls (Li et al., 2004).

(MR) A 48-week RCT was provided at 10 matched pairs of congregate living facilities in the Atlanta metropolitan area to 291 women and 20 men. Those in the Tai Chi groups demonstrated a decrease in falls (Wolf et al., 2006).

■ *Use progressive resistive training to improve balance.* **LOE = I**

(MR) A 10-week RCT ($N = 40$) compared a group of community dwelling older adults who participated in a progressive resistance exercise program that included upper and lower extremity exercise for 45 minutes twice a week with those in a flexibility program. Results

NR = Nursing Research, **MR** = Multidisciplinary Research, **SP** = Standard of Practice, **EO** = Expert Opinion, **LOE** = Level of Evidence

demonstrated improvements in balance based on functional reach among those in the resistance exercise group (Barrett & Smerdely, 2002).

MR A 16-week RCT of 64 volunteers (average age 83.5 years) from an independent-living facility were randomly assigned to walking, resistance training, or control groups. Participants in the walking and resistance-training groups engaged in two exercise sessions per week for 16 weeks. Both exercise groups showed significant improvements relative to control groups in upper and lower body strength, shoulder flexibility, and agility and balance exercise (Simons & Andel, 2006).

MR An RCT ($N = 112$) of community-dwelling healthy older adults (69 ± 6 years) compared 8 to 12 weeks of power training at low, medium, and high levels of intensity strength training with a nontraining control group. Participants trained twice weekly (five exercises; three sets of eight rapid concentric/slow eccentric repetitions) using pneumatic resistance machines. The low-intensity power training produced the greatest improvement in balance performance (Orr et al., 2006).

MR In a small randomized trial ($N = 15$), Parkinson's patients were randomly assigned to a combined group (balance and resistance training) and balance group (balance training only). The 10-week high-intensity resistance training (knee extensors and flexors, ankle plantar flexion) and/or balance training under altered visual and somatosensory conditions was done three times a week on nonconsecutive days. Results showed that both groups could balance longer before falling, and this effect persisted for at least 4 weeks (Hirsch et al., 2003).

Possibly Effective

■ *Use cobblestone mat walking to improve balance in older adults.* **LOE = III**

MR An RCT ($N = 108$) of community-dwelling older adults tested the impact of cobblestone mat walking compared with regular walking exercise three times per week for a 16-week period. Functional reach and static standing improved in the treatment group exposed to cobblestone mat walking (Li et al., 2004).

■ *Use dance-based aerobic activities to improve balance and decrease the risk of falls.* **LOE = III**

MR A randomized trial testing the effectiveness of a dance-based aerobic exercise among older community-dwelling women ($N = 20$) showed improved single-leg balance, functional reach, and walking time around two cones (Shigematsu et al., 2002).

MR In a monoinstitutional, randomized, controlled clinical trial, 40 subjects (aged 58 to 68 years) were randomly allocated into two separate groups: the dance group ($N = 20$), which followed a 3-month dance program, and the control group ($N = 20$), which did not engage in physical activities. Results showed a significant improvement in balance in the dance group at the end of the exercise program (Federici et al., 2005).

Not Effective

No applicable published research was found in this category.

Possibly Harmful

No applicable published research was found in this category.

RCT = Randomized Controlled (Clinical) Trial, **NIC** = Nursing Interventions Classification, **NOC** = Nursing Outcomes Classification

OUTCOME MEASUREMENTS

STATIC BALANCE INVENTORY

Summary measure from the Frailty and Injuries: Cooperative Studies of Intervention Techniques (FICSIT) and includes stance with feet together, semitandem stance, tandem stance, and single-leg stance (Rossiter-Fornoff et al., 1995).

BERG BALANCE SCALE (Berg et al., 1995)

FUNCTIONAL REACH

The distance a person can lean forward with the arm flexed to 90 degrees (Duncan et al., 1992).

BALANCE NOC

(Please refer to *Nursing Outcomes Classification* [Moorhead et al., 2004] for the **Balance** outcome.)

REFERENCES

Audette JF, Jin YS, Newcomer R, Stein L, Duncan G, Frontera WR. (2006). Tai Chi versus brisk walking in elderly women. *Age Ageing,* 35(4):388-393.

Barrett CJ, Smerdely P. (2002). A comparison of community-based resistance exercise and flexibility exercise for seniors. *Aust J Physiother,* 48(3):215-219.

Bayouk JF, Boucher JP, Leroux A. (2006). Balance training following stroke: Effects of task-oriented exercises with and without altered sensory input. *Int J Rehabil Res,* 29(1):51-59.

Berg K, Wood-Dauphinee S, Williams JI. (1995). The Balance Scale: Reliability assessment with elderly residents and patients with an acute stroke. *Scand J Rehabil Med,* 27(1):27-36.

Dochterman JM, Bulechek GM (Eds). (2004). *Nursing Interventions Classification (NIC),* 4th ed. St. Louis: Mosby.

Duncan PW, Studenski S, Chandler J, Prescott B. (1992). Functional reach: Predictive validity in a sample of elderly male veterans. *J Gerontol,* 47(3):M93-M98.

Federici A, Bellagamba S, Rocchi MB. (2005). Does dance-based training improve balance in adult and young old subjects? A pilot randomized controlled trial. *Aging Clin Exp Res,* 17(5):385-389.

Hirsch MA, Toole T, Maitland CG, Rider RA. (2003). The effects of balance training and high-intensity resistance training on persons with idiopathic Parkinson's disease. *Arch Phys Med Rehabil,* 84(8): 1109-1117.

Li F, Harmer P, Fisher KJ, McAuley E. (2004). Tai Chi: Improving functional balance and predicting subsequent falls in older persons. *Med Sci Sports Exerc,* 36(12):2046-2052.

Moorhead M, Johnson M, Maas M (Eds). (2004). *Nursing Outcomes Classification (NOC),* 3rd ed. St. Louis, Mosby.

Nitz JC, Choy NL. (2004). The efficacy of a specific balance-strategy training programme for preventing falls among older people: A pilot randomised controlled trial. *Age Ageing,* 33(1):52-58.

Orr R, de Vos NJ, Singh NA, Ross DA, Stavrinos TM, Fiatarone-Singh MA. (2006). Power training improves balance in healthy older adults. *J Gerontol A Biol Sci Med Sci,* 61(1):78-85.

Province MA, Hadley EC, Hornbrook MC, Lipsitz LA, Miller JP, Mulrow CD, et al. (1995). The effects of exercise on falls in elderly patients. A preplanned meta-analysis of the FICSIT Trials. Frailty and Injuries: Cooperative Studies of Intervention Techniques. *JAMA,* 273(17):1341-1347.

Rossiter-Fornoff JE, Wolf SL, Wolfson LI, Buchner DM. (1995). A cross sectional validation study of the FICSIT common data base static balance measures. Frailty and Injuries: Cooperative Studies of Intervention Techniques. *J Gerontol A Biol Sci Med Sci,* 50(6):M291-M297.

Shigematsu R, Chang M, Yabushita N. (2002). Dance-based aerobic exercise may improve indices of falling risk in older women. *Age Aging,* 31(4):261-266.

Shimada H, Uchiyama Y, Kakurai S. (2002). Relationship between lifestyle activities and physical functions in elderly persons utilizing care facilities. *Jpn J Geriatrics,* 39(2):197-203.

Simons R, Andel R. (2006). The effects of resistance training and walking on functional fitness in advanced old age. *J Aging Health,* 18(1):91-105.

Steadman J, Donaldson N, Kalra L. (2003). A randomized controlled trial of an enhanced balance training program to improve mobility and reduce falls in elderly patients. *J Am Geriatr Soc,* 51(6):847-852.

Wolf SL, O'Grady M, Easley KA, Guo Y, Kressig RW, Kutner M. (2006). The influence of intense Tai Chi training on physical performance and hemodynamic outcomes in transitionally frail, older adults. *J Gerontol A Biol Sci Med Sci,* 61(2):184-189.

EXERCISE THERAPY: CARDIORESPIRATORY (AEROBIC)

Barbara Resnick, PhD, CRNP, FAAN, FAANP; Sherry H. Pomeroy, PhD, MS, RN

Definition: Cardiorespiratory (aerobic) exercises in adults to maintain or advance to a higher level of fitness and health.

NURSING ACTIVITIES

Effective

■ *Encourage 30 minutes of moderate intensity physical activity on 5 or more days of the week, continuously or accumulated in 10-minute intervals, to reduce risk for coronary heart disease (CHD), hypertension, stroke, type 2 diabetes mellitus, osteoporosis, obesity, breast and colon cancer, gallbladder disease, anxiety, depression, and all-cause mortality. Physical activity of greater amounts, a longer duration, or more vigorous intensity results in greater health benefits. There is sufficient evidence to support a preferred frequency, duration, and intensity of exercise but insufficient evidence for type of exercise.* **LOE = I**

(MR) A systematic review was followed by an expert multidisciplinary panel that derived a consensus statement based on scientific evidence. The consensus conference report concluded that all Americans should engage in 30 minutes of moderate intensity physical activity on most, preferably all, days of the week at a level appropriate to their capacity, needs, and interests (NIH, 1996), utilizing specific recommendations for healthy adults and older adults (ACSM, 1998).

(MR) A systematic review of the literature concluded that there was sufficient evidence that physical activity produced major health benefits. Independent living of older adults and improved physical function were further benefits of physical activity at the recommended levels. Exercise benefits that occurred in the hours after physical activity (acute effects) had beneficial effects on blood pressure, lipoproteins, and insulin sensitivity. A dose-response relationship existed between physical activity and all-cause mortality rates, total cardiovascular disease, incidence and mortality of CHD, and incidence of type 2 diabetes mellitus (Kesaniemi et al., 2001).

RCT = Randomized Controlled (Clinical) Trial, **NIC** = Nursing Interventions Classification, **NOC** = Nursing Outcomes Classification

(MR) A meta-analysis of 651 participants in 13 studies found that endurance exercise training was efficacious in decreasing resting heart rate in older adults and may provide protective benefits for cardiovascular aging (Huang et al., 2005).

■ Use walking to increase physical activity for health benefits. LOE = II

(NR) A walking intervention study with sedentary older women ($N = 17$) that addressed pain, fear, and fatigue experienced while exercising, combined with exercise cueing and knowledge about exercise, resulted in more exercise, more free-living activity, and stronger self-efficacy expectations (Resnick, 2002).

(NR) A quasi-experimental study of midlife women aged 40 to 65 years ($N = 90$) who participated in a 24-week home-based walking program (four times per week for 30 minutes) showed that 64% of participants adhered to the prescribed walks 6 months after the end of the intervention phase (Wilbur et al., 2005).

(NR) In an RCT study, a home-based walking program for older adults with osteoarthritis of the knee who used arthritis self-management education and a pedometer walking program significantly increased their daily steps walked by 23% and improved muscle strength and walking performance (Talbot et al., 2003).

Possibly Effective

■ Use Tai Chi to improve aerobic capacity and physical functioning. LOE = II

(MR) A meta-analysis of Tai Chi exercise studies ($N = 441$) that measured aerobic capacity ($N = 7$) was conducted to estimate the effect of Tai Chi exercise on aerobic capacity in older adults. The classical Yang style (108 postures) of Tai Chi was most effective with participants who were initially sedentary and when the Tai Chi exercise was performed for at least 1 year (Taylor-Piliae & Froelicher, 2004).

(MR) An RCT with community residents age 65 and older ($N = 94$) tested a Tai Chi intervention over 6 months compared with a waitlist control group. The Tai Chi group had 65% improvement in six functional status measures and in physical functioning such as walking and lifting (Li et al., 2001).

■ Use walking to reduce risk of osteoporosis. LOE = II

(MR) A meta-analysis of walking interventions with participants age 50 years and older ($N = 10$) found that walking alone would not prevent decreases in bone mineral density and that training regimens should incorporate additional modes of exercise to reduce the risk of osteoporosis (Palombaro, 2005).

■ Use physical activity to reduce risk of all-cause dementia. LOE = III

(MR) A prospective study of men and women age 65 years and older ($N = 3375$) reported that engaging in various and different physical activities could protect against future risk of all-cause dementia, Alzheimer's disease, and vascular dementia among people who were apolipoprotein E 4 allele carriers (Podewils et al., 2005). The results suggest that in terms of dementia risk, participation in different physical activities may be as important as frequency, duration, and intensity of physical activity.

Not Effective

No applicable published research was found in this category.

NR = Nursing Research, **MR** = Multidisciplinary Research, **SP** = Standard of Practice, **EO** = Expert Opinion, **LOE** = Level of Evidence

Possibly Harmful

■ *Beginning a vigorous exercise program with diagnosed cardiovascular disease, severe hypertension, fever, and other signs of illness.* **LOE = I**

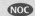 A consensus statement from the American Heart Association recommended that individuals who have diagnosed cardiovascular diseases should begin an exercise program that is low to moderate intensity, such as self-paced walking, and gradually increase exercise intensity, duration, and frequency to recommended levels. Exercise testing may be indicated before individuals with known cardiovascular conditions engage in vigorous exercise (Thompson et al., 2003).

Aerobic exercise is contraindicated in the presence of hypertension greater than 200/100; a heart rate greater than 120; a fever or infection accompanied by muscle aches and pains; and chest pain, dizziness, cramps, acute pain, or shortness of breath (Resnick, 2005).

OUTCOME MEASUREMENT

PHYSICAL FITNESS   NOC

Definition: Performance of physical activities with vigor.

Physical Fitness as evidenced by the following selected NOC indicators:
- Cardiovascular function
- Respiratory function
- Target heart rate
- Resting heart rate
- Aerobic fitness

(Rate each indicator of **Physical Fitness:** 1 = severely compromised, 2 = substantially compromised, 3 = moderately compromised, 4 = mildly compromised, 5 = not compromised) (Moorhead et al., 2004).

REFERENCES

American College of Sports Medicine (ACSM) Position Stand. (1998). The recommended quantity and quality of exercise for developing and maintaining cardiorespiratory and muscular fitness, and flexibility in healthy adults. *Med Sci Sports Exerc*, 30(6):975-991.

Huang G, Shi X, Davis-Brezette JA, Osness WH. (2005). Resting heart rate changes after endurance training in older adults: A meta-analysis. *Med Sci Sports Exerc*, 37(8):1381-1386.

Kesaniemi YK, Danforth E Jr, Jensen MD, Kopelman PG, Lefebvre P, Reeder BA. (2001). Dose-response issues concerning physical activity and health: An evidence-based symposium. *Med Sci Sports Exerc*, 33(6 Suppl):S351-S358.

Li F, Harmer P, McAuley E, Duncan TE, Duncan SC, Chaumeton N, et al. (2001). An evaluation of the effects of Tai Chi exercise on physical function among older persons? A randomized controlled trial. *Ann Behav Med*, 23(2):139-146.

Moorhead M, Johnson M, Maas M (Eds). (2004). *Nursing Outcomes Classification (NOC)*, 3rd ed. St. Louis: Mosby.

National Institutes of Health (NIH). (1996). Physical activity and cardiovascular health. NIH Consensus Development Panel on Physical Activity and Cardiovascular Health. *JAMA*, 276(3):241-246.

Palombaro KM. (2005). Effects of walking-only interventions on bone mineral density at various skeletal sites: A meta-analysis. *J Geriatr Phys Ther*, 28(3):102-107.

RCT = Randomized Controlled (Clinical) Trial, **NIC** = Nursing Interventions Classification, **NOC** = Nursing Outcomes Classification

Podewils LJ, Guallar E, Kuller LH, Fried LP, Lopez OL, Carlson M, et al. (2005). Physical activity, APOE genotype, and dementia risk: Findings from the Cardiovascular Health Cognition Study. *Am J Epidemiol,* 161(7):639-651.

Resnick B. (2002). Testing the effect of the WALC intervention on exercise adherence in older adults. *J Gerontol Nurs,* 28(6):40-49.

Resnick B. (2005). Across the aging continuum: Motivating older adults to exercise. *Adv Nurse Pract,* 13(9):37-40.

Talbot LA, Gaines JM, Huynh TN, Metter EJ. (2003). A home-based pedometer-driven walking program to increase physical activity in older adults with osteoarthritis of the knee: A preliminary study. *J Am Geriatr Soc,* 51(3):387-392.

Taylor-Piliae RE, Froelicher ES. (2004). Effectiveness of Tai Chi exercise in improving aerobic capacity: A meta-analysis. *J Cardiovasc Nurs,* 19(1):48-57.

Thompson PD, Buchner D, Pina IL, Balady GJ, Williams MA, Marcus BH, et al. (2003). Exercise and physical activity in the prevention and treatment of atherosclerotic cardiovascular disease: A statement from the Council on Clinical Cardiology (Subcommittee on Exercise, Rehabilitation, and Prevention) and the Council on Nutrition, Physical Activity, and Metabolism (Subcommittee on Physical Activity). *Circulation,* 107(24):3109-3116.

Wilbur J, Vassalo A, Chandler P, McDevitt J, Miller AM. (2005). Midlife women's adherence to home-based walking during maintenance. *Nurs Res,* 54(1):33-40.

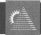 # FALL PREVENTION NIC

Deanna Gray-Miceli, DNSc, APRN, FAANP

NIC **Definition:** Instituting special precautions with patients at risk for injury from falling (Dochterman & Bulechek, 2004).

NURSING ACTIVITIES

Activities included are individually determined and used on a case-by-case basis.

Effective

■ **SP** *Determine the patient's risk for falling, ideally accomplished by use of a scientifically validated and reliable fall risk tool, following admission to a licensed medical care facility, when a change in the patient's medical condition occurs, and/or when a patient is transferred within the facility.* **LOE = VI**

NR A quasi-experimental cohort study examined the effectiveness of a nurse-led fall program in a hospital using the Morse Scale for fall risk identification and found that the program reduced multiple falls (*N* = 198) compared with the usual care (*N* = 211) (Schwendimann et al., 2006).

■ **SP** *Following determination of the patient's risk for falling, develop targeted nursing and multifactorial interventions to reduce risk and manage falls.* **LOE = I**

MR A meta-analysis of 40 clinical trials showed that multifactorial fall risk assessment and management was the most effective intervention to reduce risk of falling in elderly persons (Chang et al., 2004).

MR A systematic review of 62 RCTs of interventions designed to minimize the effect of risk factors for falling in elderly people (*N* = 21,668) concluded that interventions likely to be most beneficial were multidisciplinary and multifactorial (Gillespie et al., 2003).

NR = Nursing Research, **MR** = Multidisciplinary Research, **SP** = Standard of Practice, **EO** = Expert Opinion, **LOE** = Level of Evidence

(NR) A systematic review of RCTs in which the primary intervention was implementing a falls prevention protocol ($N = 156$) found that developing a plan of care or guidelines for interventions to prevent falls in nursing care facilities reduced falls (Torres et al., 2005).

■ (SP) *Following a patient's fall, reassess fall risk (including medications) and perform a comprehensive postfall assessment (including laboratory assays) to determine the cause of the fall and presence of injury. This forms the basis of a care plan to reduce further falls and injury. Refer to a specialist as indicated.* **LOE = VI**

(NR) A descriptive validation study reported reliability and interrater agreement of a 30-item comprehensive postfall assessment tool useful in identifying underlying causes of falls and guiding targeted nursing interventions for older nursing home residents (Gray-Miceli et al., 2006).

(NR) A retrospective review of 220 patients' medical records from an acute care hospital found statistically significant results in confused adults who fell and alkaline phosphatase blood values (O'Hagan & O'Connell, 2005).

(EO) Assessment of laboratory data is recommended as part of the comprehensive postfall evaluation (AGS, 2001; AMDA, 2003).

■ (SP) *Use low-rise beds with locked brakes to reduce serious injury from a bed-related fall.* **LOE = VII**

(EO) The mattress of a low-rise bed is about 14 inches from the floor. This intervention decreases the distance to the floor should a bed fall occur (AMDA, 2003; JHF, 2003; UIGN, 2004).

■ (SP) *Determine the appropriate use of an assistive device; refer as needed to physical therapy.* **LOE = VII**

(EO) Assistive devices help stabilize balance and ambulation (AGS, 2001; AMDA, 2003; JHF, 2003; UIGN, 2004).

■ (SP) *Place the call bell and/or bedside chair or side table in reach of the patient and in locked position. Check the environment including bed and chair brakes, and perform universal safety inspections. Patients' falls occur when reaching for a call bell or leaning on unstable furniture.* **LOE = VI**

(NR) A patients' safety educational program for older adults with chronic illness significantly reduced numbers of patients requiring care for fall-related injuries when they received nursing assessment, education, and postfall evaluation (Bright, 2005).

(NR) A case report of an innovative intervention in acute care to prevent patients' falls included identification of high risk. Communication among staff and patients along with case-specific and universal precautions held promise as an intervention to prevent falls (McCarter-Bayer et al., 2005).

■ *Use assistive devices, hip protectors, and personal alarms as indicated.* **LOE = II**

(MR) A nonexperimental descriptive study of 17 severely disabled and elderly people showed improvement when walking with the WalkAbout (Wolfe et al., 2004).

(MR) In an RCT, older women living at home ($N = 600$) with two or more falls or a fall requiring hospitalization were given hip protectors, which prevented hip fracture compared with controls (Cameron et al., 2003).

RCT = Randomized Controlled (Clinical) Trial, **NIC** = Nursing Interventions Classification, **NOC** = Nursing Outcomes Classification

(MR) A nonrandomized descriptive study using an intervention called NOC WATCH (a non-intrusive personal alarm) found a statistically significant reduction (91%; $p = .02$) in falls among users (Kelly et al., 2002).

■ *Provide urinary incontinence care and exercise opportunities.* **LOE = II**

(NR) A randomized, blinded study with an intervention consisting of low-intensity exercise and incontinent care in nursing home residents ($N = 92$) significantly reduced the number of falls (odds ratio 0.46, $p < .04$) compared with usual care (Messecar, 2003).

(NR) In a cohort study of community-dwelling women ($N = 6049$), a 35% increase in the risk of falls existed with daily urge incontinence compared with a 21% increase in risk of falls with weekly urge incontinence. Also, associated increased risk of falls and nonspinal, nontraumatic fractures occurred (Brown et al., 2000).

■ *Educate on the advantages of wearing flat, supportive footwear.* **LOE = VI**

(MR) A descriptive study ($N = 1371$) of older adults found the use of athletic and canvas shoe wear associated with the lowest risk of falling; fall risk was highest among those not wearing shoes (Koepsell et al., 2004).

■ *Educate on the benefits of taking vitamin D or calcium supplementation, or both.* **LOE = I**

(MR) A systematic review and meta-analysis only of double-blinded RCTs using vitamin D supplementation among ambulatory or institutionalized older adults ($N = 1237$) showed more than a 20% reduction in the risk of falls (Bischoff-Ferrari et al., 2004).

(MR) A randomized controlled, double-blind study using intramuscular vitamin D supplementation among elders ($N = 139$) showed significant improvements in reaction time, balance, and performance but no significant change in number of falls between groups (Dhesi et al., 2004).

(MR) In an RCT ($N = 378$) of community-dwelling older adults, use of alfacalcidol significantly and safely reduced the number of falls, provided participants had a calcium intake of more than 500 mg daily (Dukas et al., 2004).

(MR) A randomized placebo-controlled trial showed that people aged 70 years and older ($N = 5292$) before developing low-trauma fracture who received oral supplementation of calcium and vitamin D alone or in combination failed to differ from controls in all-new fractures, hip fractures, or number of falls (Grant et al., 2005).

■ *Educate on the benefit of supervised exercise programs.* **LOE = II**

(MR) An RCT showed that people ($N = 163$) participating in supervised group exercise and ancillary home exercises had 40% lower rates of falls than controls. Group exercise is valuable for older adults at risk for falls by improving balance (Barnett et al., 2003).

(MR) A controlled, quasi-experimental study in two geriatric hospitals ($N = 134$) examining exercise through qualitative and quantitative measures found that women reporting regular exercise before age 40 had higher quantitative ultrasound measures of strength and fewer falls (Bischoff et al., 2001).

(MR) An RCT involving 65- to 75-year-old women with osteoporosis ($N = 80$) found that the intervention group receiving twice weekly exercise had improvements in dynamic balance and strength and reduced risk for falls compared with controls (Carter et al., 2002).

NR = Nursing Research, **MR** = Multidisciplinary Research, **SP** = Standard of Practice, **EO** = Expert Opinion, **LOE** = Level of Evidence

(MR) In a systematic review of controlled trials ($N = 13$) examining the value of balance and agility training in preventing falls and injuries, six trials demonstrated significant reduction in the rate of falls in the elderly (Davis et al., 2004).

(MR) An RCT showed that exercise (progressive resistance) training and progressive functional training were safe and effective methods of increasing strength and functional performance, with a nonsignificant reduction in fall incidence of 25% during ambulation among older adults ($N = 57$) with a history of injurious falls (Hauer et al., 2001).

■ *Obtain geriatric nurse practitioner (GNP) consultation.* **LOE = VI**

(NR) A descriptive nonexperimental study found that use of consultant GNPs and use of models of clinical care reduced the fall rate by 5.8% in an acute care unit in the hospital (Smyth et al., 2001).

Possibly Effective

No applicable published research was found in this category.

Not Effective

No applicable published research was found in this category.

Possibly Harmful

■ *Use of physical restraints.* **LOE = VI**

(MR) Analysis of incident report data for falls over a 1-year period in a teaching hospital setting showed more serious injuries in older patients who were restrained than not restrained (Tan et al., 2005).

(NR) A retrospective, cross-sectional analysis of 419 patients' falls in an acute care hospital over a 7-year period found that patients in a "nonrational" state at the time of the fall were significantly more likely to have fallen with the bed rails elevated than not, and a patient's death resulted from overelevated bedrails (van Leeuwen et al., 2002).

OUTCOME MEASUREMENT

FALL PREVENTION BEHAVIOR (NOC)

(Please refer to *Nursing Outcomes Classification* [Moorhead et al., 2004] for the **Fall Prevention Behavior** outcome.)

REFERENCES

American Geriatrics Society, British Geriatrics Society, American Academy of Orthopedic Surgeons (AGS/BGS/AAOS). (2001). Guidelines for the prevention of falls in older persons. American Geriatrics Society, British Geriatrics Society, American Academy of Orthopedic Surgeons Panel on Falls Prevention. *J Am Geriatr Soc,* 49(5):664-672.

American Medical Directors Association (AMDA). (2003). *Falls and fall risk.* Columbia, MD: AMDA.

Barnett A, Smith B, Lord SR, Williams M, Baumand A. (2003). Community-based group exercise improves balance and reduces falls in at risk older people: A randomized controlled trial. *Age Ageing,* 32(4):407-414.

RCT = Randomized Controlled (Clinical) Trial, **NIC** = Nursing Interventions Classification, **NOC** = Nursing Outcomes Classification

Bischoff HA, Conzelmann M, Lindemann D, Singer-Lindpaintner L, Stucki G, Vonthein R, et al. (2001). Self-reported exercise before age 40: Influence on quantitative skeletal ultrasound and fall risk in the elderly. *Arch Phys Med Rehabil,* 82(6):801-806.

Bischoff-Ferrari HA, Dawson-Hughes B, Willett WC, Staehelin HB, Bazemore MG, Zee RY, et al. (2004). Effect of vitamin D on falls: A meta-analysis. *JAMA,* 291(16):1999-2006.

Bright L. (2005). Strategies to improve the patient safety outcome indicator: Preventing or reducing falls. *Home Healthc Nurse,* 23(1):29-36.

Brown JS, Vittinghoff E, Wyman JF, Stone KL, Nevitt MC, Ensrud KE, et al. (2000). Urinary incontinence: Does it increase risk of falls and fractures? Study of Osteoporotic Fractures Research Group. *J Am Geriatr Soc,* 48(7):721-725.

Cameron ID, Cumming RG, Kurrle SE, Quine S, Lockwood K, Salkeld G, et al. (2003). A randomized trial of hip protector use by frail older women living in their homes. *Inj Prev,* 9(2):138-141.

Carter ND, Khan KM, McKay HA, Petit MA, Waterman C, Heinonen A, et al. (2002). Community-based exercise program reduces risk factors for falls in 65-to 75-year-old women with osteoperosis: Randomized control trial. *CMAJ,* 167(9):997-1004.

Chang JT, Morton SC, Rubenstein LZ, Mojica WA, Maglione M, Suttorp MJ, et al. (2004). Interventions for the prevention of falls in older adults: Systematic review and meta-analysis of randomized clinical trials. *BMJ,* 328(7441):680.

Davis JC, Donaldson MG, Ashe MC, Khan KM. (2004). The role of balance and agility training in fall reduction: A comprehensive review. *Eura Medicophys,* 40(3):211-221.

Dhesi JK, Jackson SH, Bearne LM, Moniz C, Hurley MV, Swift CG, et al. (2004). Vitamin D supplementation improved neuromuscular function in older people who fall. *Age Ageing,* 33(6):589-595.

Dochterman JM, Bulechek GM (Eds). (2004). *Nursing Interventions Classifications (NIC),* 4th ed. St. Louis: Mosby.

Dukas L, Bischoff HA, Lindpaintner LS, Schacht E, Birkner-Binder D, Damm TN, et al. (2004). Alfacalcidol reduces number of fallers in a community-dwelling elderly population with a minimum calcium intake of more than 500 mg daily. *J Am Geriatr Soc,* 52(2):230-236.

Gillespie LD, Gillespie WJ, Robertson MC, Lamb SE, Cumming RG, Rowe BH. (2003). Interventions for preventing falls in elderly people. *Cochrane Database Syst Rev,* (4):CD000340.

Grant AM, Avenell A, Campbell MK, McDonald AM, MacLennan GS, McPherson GC, et al. (2005). Oral vitamin D3 and calcium for the secondary prevention of low-trauma fractures in elderly people: A randomized placebo-controlled trial. *Lancet,* 365(9471):1621-1628.

Gray-Miceli DL, Strumpf NE, Johnson J, Draganescu M, Ratcliffe SJ. (2006). Psychometric properties of the Post-Fall Index. *Clin Nurs Res,* 15(3):157-176.

Hauer K, Rost B, Rutschle K, Opitz H, Specht N, Bartsch P, et al. (2001). Exercise training for rehabilitation and secondary prevention of falls in geriatric patients with a history of injurious falls. *J Am Geriatr Soc,* 49(1):10-20.

The John A. Hartford Foundation (JHF) Institute for Geriatric Nursing. (2003). Preventing falls in acute care. In: Mezey M, Fulmer T, Abraham I, Zwicker DA (Eds). *Geriatric nursing protocols for best practice,* 2nd ed. New York: Springer, pp 141-64.

Kelly KE, Phillips CL, Cain KC, Polissar NL, Kelly PB. (2002). Evaluation of a nonintrusive monitor to reduce falls in nursing home patients. *J Am Med Dir Assoc,* 3(6):377-382.

Koepsell TD, Wolf ME, Buchner DM, KuKull WA, LaCroix AZ, Tencer AF, et al. (2004). Footwear style and risk of falls in older adults. *J Am Geriatr Soc,* 52(9):1495-1501.

McCarter-Bayer A, Bayer F, Hall K. (2005). Preventing falls in acute care: An innovative approach. *J Gerontol Nurs,* 31(3):25-33.

Messecar D. (2003). An exercise and incontinence intervention did not reduce the incidence or cost of acute conditions in nursing home residents. *Evid Based Nurs,* 6(4):116-117.

Moorhead M, Johnson M, Maas M (Eds). (2004). *Nursing Outcomes Classification (NOC),* 3rd ed. St. Louis: Mosby.

O'Hagan C, O'Connell B. (2005). The relationship between patient blood pathology values and patient falls in an acute-care setting: A retrospective analysis. *Int J Nurs Pract* 11(4):161-168.

Schwendimann R, Milisen K, Buhler H, De Geest S. (2006). Fall prevention in a Swiss acute care hospital setting: Reducing multiple falls. *J Gerontol Nurs,* 32(3):13-22.

Smyth C, Dubin S, Restrepo A, Nueva-Espana H, Capezuti E. (2001). Creating order out of chaos: Models of GNP practice with hospitalized older adults. *Clin Excell Nurse Pract,* 5(2):88-95.

NR = Nursing Research, **MR** = Multidisciplinary Research, **SP** = Standard of Practice, **EO** = Expert Opinion, **LOE** = Level of Evidence

Tan KM, Austin B, Shaughnassy M, Higgins C, McDonald M, Mulkerrin EC, et al. (2005). Falls in acute care hospital and their relationship to restraint use. *Ir J Med Sci*, 174(3):28-31.

Torres EP, Sanchez Castillo PD, Gonzano Rubio M, Martinez Sellares R. (2005). Importance of the continuing education of professionals in the prevention of falls among institutionalized geriatric patients. *Gerokomos*, 16(1):6-17.

University of Iowa Gerontological Nursing Interventions Research Center (UIGN). (2004). *Fall prevention for older adults.* Iowa City (IA): University of Iowa Gerontological Nursing Interventions Research Center, Research Dissemination Core.

van Leeuwen M, Bennett L, West S, Wiles V, Grasso J. (2002). Patient falls from bed and role of bedrails in acute care setting. *Aust J Adv Nurs*, 19(2):8-13.

Wolfe RR, Jordan D, Wolfe ML. (2004). The WalkAbout: A new solution for preventing falls in the elderly and disabled. *Arch Phys Med Rehabil*, 85(12):2067-2069.

 # FAMILY INTEGRITY PROMOTION

Elizabeth R. Van Horn, PhD, RN, CCRN; Donald D. Kautz, PhD, RN, CNRN, CRRN-A

> **NIC** **Definition:** Promotion of family cohesion and unity (Dochterman & Bulechek, 2004).

NURSING ACTIVITIES

Effective

■ **NIC** *Monitor current family relationships.* **LOE = I**

MR A meta-analysis of 70 randomized studies comparing family-centered psychosocial interventions with usual medical care in a variety of patients' illnesses found that depression decreased in family members with interventions that included a relationship focus. However, patients' depression decreased with interventions that included only spouses (Martire et al., 2004).

■ **NIC** *Counsel family members on additional effective coping skills for their own use.* **LOE = I**

MR An RCT of women with recurrent breast cancer and their family caregivers (N = 134 dyads) tested a family-based program of care (FOCUS). In the intervention group, patients reported a significant decrease in negative appraisal of illness and hopelessness, and family members reported a significant decrease in negative appraisal of caregiving from baseline to 3 months. However, no significant effects were sustained at 6 months (Northouse et al., 2005).

MR An RCT of family caregiver and patient dyads (N = 94 dyads) testing a community-based, 14-hour stress and coping program showed that the treatment group had lessened caregiver burden and depression (Hepburn et al., 2001; Ostwald et al., 2003).

MR A descriptive study of family members (N = 123) of patients with brain injury found that higher family coping scores were associated with increased family functioning and decreased psychological distress among family members (Carnes & Quinn, 2005).

RCT = Randomized Controlled (Clinical) Trial, **NIC** = Nursing Interventions Classification, **NOC** = Nursing Outcomes Classification

(MR) A review of 12 RCTs that included a family member in psychosocial interventions for chronic illness revealed that 5 of the studies found positive effects for patients regarding symptoms, stress, and self-efficacy. However, few findings for family member benefits were reported (Martire, 2005).

■ (NIC) *Facilitate open communication among family members.* **LOE = II**

(NR) An RCT of women with recurrent breast cancer and their family caregivers ($N = 134$ dyads) evaluated a family-based program of care (FOCUS); family members in the intervention group demonstrated significantly higher mean scores on satisfaction with family involvement in discussions (Northouse et al., 2002).

(NR) A qualitative study of patients with myocardial infarction or cerebral vascular accident and their family members ($N = 11$) revealed that nurses encouraging family members' sharing of experiences of the illness aided family members in venting emotions, relieving suffering, and promoted increased understanding among family members (Duhamel & Talbot, 2004).

(NR) A qualitative descriptive study of cancer survivors and their family members (123 dyads, $N = 246$) revealed that some families had improved communication after cancer diagnosis and other families preferred not to talk or think about the cancer too much (Mellon, 2002).

(NR) A qualitative study of patients with heart disease and their families ($N = 10$) in which families received four clinical sessions promoting therapeutic conversations revealed improved family understanding of the illness experience; enhanced communication of worries, conflicts, and concerns; and facilitated family support (Tapp, 2001).

(MR) A qualitative study of two cancer patients and their family members ($N = 10$) using family therapy sessions found that facilitating open communication aided families in integrating the cancer experience into their lives. However, families also benefited from occasionally not talking about or addressing the presence of cancer in their lives (Robinson et al., 2005). Additional Research: Logue, 2003; Bohn et al., 2003.

■ (NIC) *Provide for family visitation.* **LOE = III**

(NR) A controlled study of critical care patients and their family members ($N = 40$) revealed that increased visitation significantly improved satisfaction with visitation and also resulted in increased family involvement with patients' care, increased communication with nurses, and decreased family complaints (Roland et al., 2001).

(NR) A descriptive study of 84 family members of ICU patients identified liberal patients' visitation as an important support intervention for family members (De Jong & Beatty, 2000).

(EO) Support of family visitation is desirable to maintain family relationships and promote emotional closeness (Leske, 2002).

■ (NIC) *Provide family members with information about the patient's condition regularly, according to the patient's preference.* **LOE = III**

(NR) A controlled study using a two-group pretest and post-test design tested a needs-based informational session intervention with family members of critical care patients ($N = 66$) in Hong Kong and found that subjects in the intervention group had significantly less anxiety and greater family needs satisfaction than the control group (Chiu et al., 2004).

(NR) A descriptive study of 84 family members of ICU patients revealed that informational support was the nursing intervention rated most important and most frequently used by family members (De Jong & Beatty, 2000).

NR = Nursing Research, **MR** = Multidisciplinary Research, **SP** = Standard of Practice, **EO** = Expert Opinion, **LOE** = Level of Evidence

(EO) Providing information about patients to family members facilitates family decision making and decreased anxiety (Leske, 2002).

■ (NIC) *Provide for care of the patient by family members, as appropriate.*
   LOE = II

(NR) An RCT pilot study of caregivers of a hospitalized elderly family member ($N = 49$) tested a nursing intervention designed to aid family members in providing patients' care and found that patients in the intervention group experienced lower incidences of acute confusion, bowel and bladder incontinence, depression, and hospital readmission at 2 months after discharge. Also, caregivers experienced more role rewards than the comparison group (Li et al., 2003).

(MR) A controlled study using a pre– and post–nursing home placement design of family caregivers of relatives with Alzheimer's or dementia examined caregiver stress and found that after nursing home placement, family visitation and family provision of patients' care were associated with decreased role overload and decreased loss of intimate exchange (Gaugler et al., 2004).

(EO) To reduce the stress response for critically ill patients and their family members, family provision of complementary and alternative therapies to patients including centering, presence, guided imagery, massage, and therapeutic touch are recommended. However, more research is needed on the effects of these activities (Jansen & Schmitt, 2003).

■ (NIC) (SP) *Establish a trusting relationship with family members.* **LOE = VI**

(NR) A qualitative study of patients with myocardial infarction or cerebral vascular accident and their family members ($N = 11$) revealed that establishing a trusting relationship with patients and family members through a humanistic attitude approach facilitated expression of fears and anxieties and created a context for healing (Duhamel & Talbot, 2004).

■ (NIC) (SP) *Provide for family privacy.* **LOE = VII**

(EO) To promote the role of the family advanced practice nurse in long-term care settings, maintenance of family stability and connectedness through preestablished family caregiving activities is recommended, including "drop by" visits, e-mail communication, private dining areas, addressing changing relationships and communication gaps, ongoing communication, and updates about family members (Logue, 2003).

■ (NIC) (SP) *Be a listener for the family members.* **LOE = VII**

(EO) Family support can greatly affect a patient's physical, psychological, and spiritual well-being. Therefore, it is important for the nurse to support family members through active listening to enhance communication of their needs, garnering of support, and increasing their ability to support the patient (O'Brien, 2004).

■ (NIC) (SP) *Determine family understanding of causes of illness.* **LOE = VII**

(EO) Health education can aid in health promotion and disease prevention. Therefore, nurses should determine family understanding of causes of patients' illness through effective and therapeutic communication skills and explain disease etiology and processes in clear terms without use of medical jargon or complex language (O'Brien, 2004).

RCT = Randomized Controlled (Clinical) Trial, **NIC** = Nursing Interventions Classification, **NOC** = Nursing Outcomes Classification

Possibly Effective

■ **NIC** *Identify typical family coping mechanisms.* LOE = VI

NR A qualitative study of patients with myocardial infarction or cerebral vascular accident and their family members ($N = 11$) revealed that the use of interventive questioning helped families identify coping mechanisms and reinforce helpful behaviors that promoted family adaptation to illness (Duhamel & Talbot, 2004).

■ **NIC** *Assist the family with conflict resolution.* LOE = VII

EO Recommendations from the Commissioned Report by the Committee on Health and Behavior: Research, Practice, and Policy include the development of family interventions to minimize hostility, reduce stress associated with disease, and promote conflict management and resolution among family members to improve disease management and health among all family members (Weihs et al., 2002).

■ **NIC** *Facilitate a tone of togetherness within/among the family.* LOE = V

NR A qualitative descriptive study of cancer survivors and their family members (123 dyads, $N = 246$) revealed that family member participation during cancer diagnosis and treatment increased family cohesiveness (Mellon, 2002).

MR A qualitative study of two cancer patients and their family members ($N = 10$) using family therapy sessions suggested that sharing stories and validating family members' unique experiences related to cancer promoted family cohesion and created a shared experience of healing (Robinson et al., 2005).

EO Recommendations from the Commissioned Report by the Committee on Health and Behavior: Research, Practice, and Policy include the development of family interventions that promote family cohesiveness, teamwork, and enhancement of closeness and mutually supportive interactions to improve disease management and health among all family members (Weihs et al., 2002).

MR A qualitative study of patients with diabetes and their spouses ($N = 72$) found that supportive behaviors that promoted working together to manage health, including helping with dietary control, regimen-specific and relationship support, and helpful reminders, were perceived as beneficial by patients (Trief et al., 2003).

EO To promote optimal couple functioning and coping in response to breast cancer, helping couples develop a "we" awareness, increasing awareness of the story each has constructed around the illness, and developing a plan to promote healing together are recommended (Skerrett, 2003).

■ **NIC** *Collaborate with the family in problem solving.* LOE = III

NR A controlled study of family members ($N = 25$) caring for patients recently discharged home after an acute psychiatric admission for depression tested the PLUS intervention (addressing caregiver's personal resources, learning/skill development needs, unanticipated needs, and stress/illness management) versus standard home care and found no significant outcome differences in depression in patients or caregivers. However, when patients made significant functional recovery, the PLUS group caregivers showed less emotional distress (Horton-Deutsch et al., 2002).

NR = Nursing Research, **MR** = Multidisciplinary Research, **SP** = Standard of Practice, **EO** = Expert Opinion, **LOE** = Level of Evidence

MR A descriptive study of anxiety and depression in newly diagnosed adult cancer patients ($N = 48$) and their adult relatives ($N = 99$; total $N = 147$) in Australia revealed that families that were able to act openly, directly express feelings, and effectively solve problems had lower levels of depression, and direct communication of information within the family was associated with lower levels of anxiety in patients (Edwards & Clarke, 2004).

MR A systematic review of empirical intervention research for family members of patients during the recovery phase of an acute cardiac event ($N = 7$ studies), including problem solving, family relationships, role clarification, conflict management, and educational and emotional support interventions, revealed some significant improvements in individual outcomes such as anxiety and self-esteem. However, no significant improvements were found regarding family functioning or other family-related outcomes (Van Horn et al., 2002).

▪ NIC *Encourage the family to maintain positive relationships.* LOE = II

MR An RCT of spouses of 226 male and 70 female ($N = 296$) coronary artery bypass graft patients tested three informational interventions—(1) an optimistically slanted informational tape, (2) a tape emphasizing coping with ups and downs, or (3) standard discharge information—and found that the patients whose spouses viewed the optimistic tape experienced fewer problems requiring physician office visits at 3 and 6 months follow-up (Mahler & Kulik, 2002).

▪ NIC *Refer the family to support groups of other families dealing with similar problems.* LOE = II

MR A controlled study of nine patients with traumatic brain injury (TBI) and their family members ($N = 20$) revealed that a community-based peer support program improved knowledge of TBI, quality of life, general outlook, and coping with depression but had inconsistent impact on social support, happiness, and management of feelings of anger, anxiety, and control (Hibbard et al., 2002).

MR A systematic review of empirical intervention research for family members of patients during the acute phase of an acute cardiac event ($N = 6$ studies) including support groups and educational or orientation sessions found that the majority of studies failed to reduce significantly family member anxiety, stress, or depression. However, qualitative data suggested that some family members benefited from the group sessions (Van Horn et al., 2002).

MR A descriptive survey of family members ($N = 23$) of individuals with mental illness who participated in a church-based support group found great increases in participants' knowledge of mental illness, treatment, etiology, and support services and greatly increased morale (Pickett-Schenk, 2002).

MR An RCT of Chinese family caregivers ($N = 48$) of patients with schizophrenia tested a mutual support group intervention comprising 12 sessions over 3 months and found that subjects in the intervention group experienced lower family burden and greater family function than controls at 1 and 3 months after the intervention (Chien et al., 2004).

▪ NIC *Refer for family therapy, as indicated.* LOE = II

MR An RCT of a five-session counseling intervention that focused on communication techniques was tested with couples ($N = 59$) from the Netherlands in which one member had cancer. The study found that subjects in the intervention group experienced increased feelings of equity or balance in the relationship, higher levels of relationship quality of both partners, and decreased levels of psychological distress in patients (Kuijer et al., 2004).

- ■ **NIC** *Assist the family to resolve feelings of guilt.* **LOE = V**

   EO A world-renowned death and dying clinical nurse specialist recommended that a niece, having recurrent nightmares and anxiety attacks after her aunt committed suicide, speak with a therapist in order to overcome post-traumatic stress disorder, resolve feelings of anger and guilt, and work on her grief (Ufema, 2002).

   MR A qualitative study of family caregivers of demented elders in Sweden ($N = 8$) found that husbands sustained the most anger, worry, weariness, guilt, distress, and isolation related to caregiving burden, especially after symptom onset but before diagnosis. Therefore, the authors recommended preventive interventional home visits (Samuelsson et al., 2001).

   MR A descriptive survey of dementia and palliative care staff ($N = 437$) found that participants identified the most important measures for supporting families as support groups, offering respite care, educating families, relieving family's feeling of guilt, being available, creating a sense of security, and supporting family members after the patient's death (Albinsson & Strang, 2003).

Not Effective

No applicable published research was found in this category.

Possibly Harmful

No applicable published research was found in this category.

OUTCOME MEASUREMENT

FAMILY FUNCTIONING    **NOC**

(Please refer to *Nursing Outcomes Classification* [Moorhead et al., 2004] for the **Family Functioning** outcome.)

REFERENCES

Albinsson L, Strang P. (2003). Differences in supporting families of dementia patients and cancer patients: A palliative perspective. *Palliat Med*, 17(4):359-367.

Bohn U, Wright LM, Moules NJ. (2003). A family systems nursing interview following a myocardial infarction: The power of commendations. *J Fam Nurs*, 9(1):151-165.

Carnes SL, Quinn WH. (2005). Family adaptation to brain injury: Coping and psychological distress. *Fam Syst Health*, 23(2):186-203.

Chien WT, Norman I, Thompson DR. (2004). A randomized controlled trial of a mutual support group for family caregivers of patients with schizophrenia. *Int J Nurs Stud*, 41(6):637-649.

Chiu YL, Chien WT, Lam LW. (2004). Effectiveness of a needs-based education programme for families with a critically ill relative in an intensive care unit. *J Clin Nurs*, 13(5):655-656.

De Jong MJ, Beatty DS. (2000). Family perceptions of support interventions in the intensive care unit. *Dimens Crit Care Nurs*, 19(5):40-47.

Dochterman JM, Bulechek GM (Eds). (2004). *Nursing Interventions Classification (NIC)*, 4th ed. St. Louis: Mosby.

Duhamel F, Talbot LR. (2004). A constructivist evaluation of family systems nursing interventions with families experiencing cardiovascular and cerebrovascular illness. *J Fam Nurs*, 10(1):12-32.

NR = Nursing Research, **MR** = Multidisciplinary Research, **SP** = Standard of Practice, **EO** = Expert Opinion, **LOE** = Level of Evidence

Edwards B, Clarke V. (2004). The psychological impact of a cancer diagnosis on families: The influence of family functioning and patients' illness characteristics on depression and anxiety. *Psychooncology*, 13(8):562-576.

Gaugler JE, Anderson KA, Zarit SH, Pearlin LI. (2004). Family involvement in nursing homes: Effects on stress and well-being. *Aging Ment Health*, 8(1):65-75.

Hepburn KW, Tornatore J, Center B, Ostwald SW. (2001). Dementia family caregiver training: Affecting beliefs about caregiving and caregiver outcomes. *J Am Geriatr Soc*, 49(4):450-457.

Hibbard MR, Cantor J, Charatz H, Rosenthal R, Ashman T, Gundersen N, et al. (2002). Peer support in the community: Initial findings of a mentoring program for individuals with traumatic brain injury and their families. *J Head Trauma Rehabil*, 17(2):112-131.

Horton-Deutsch SL, Farran CJ, Choi EE, Fogg L. (2002). The PLUS intervention: A pilot test with caregivers of depressed older adults. *Arch Psychiatr Nurs*, 16(2):61-71.

Jansen MP, Schmitt NA. (2003). Family-focused interventions. *Crit Care Nurs Clin North Am*, 15(3): 347-354.

Kuijer RG, Buunk BP, De Jong GM, Ybema JF, Sanderman R. (2004). Effects of a brief intervention program for patients with cancer and their partners on feelings of inequity, relationship quality and psychological distress. *Psychooncology*, 13(5):321-334.

Leske JS. (2002). Interventions to decrease family anxiety. *Critical Care Nurse*, 22(6):61-65.

Li H, Melnyk BM, McCann R, Chatcheydang J, Koulouglioti C, Nichols LW, et al. (2003). Creating avenues for relative empowerment (CARE): A pilot test of an intervention to improve outcomes of hospitalized elders and family caregivers. *Res Nurs Health*, 26(4):284-299.

Logue RM. (2003). Maintaining family connectedness in long-term care: An advanced practice approach to family-centered nursing homes. *J Gerontol Nurs*, 29(6):24-31.

Mahler HI, Kulik JA. (2002). Effects of a videotape information intervention for spouses on spouse distress and patient recovery from surgery. *Health Psychol*, 21(5):427-437.

Martire LM. (2005). The "relative" efficacy of involving family in psychosocial interventions for chronic illness: Are there added benefits to patients and family members? *Fam Syst Health*, 23(3):312-328.

Martire LM, Lustig AP, Schulz R, Miller GE, Helgeson VS. (2004). Is it beneficial to involve a family member? A meta-analysis of psychosocial interventions for chronic illness. *Health Psychol*, 23(6): 599-611.

Mellon S. (2002). Comparisons between cancer survivors and family members on meaning of the illness and family quality of life. *Oncol Nurs Forum*, 29(7):1117-1125.

Moorhead S, Johnson M, Maas M (Eds). (2004). *Nursing outcomes classification (NOC)*, 3rd ed. St. Louis: Mosby.

Northouse L, Kershaw T, Mood D, Schafenacker A. (2005). Effects of a family intervention on the quality of life of women with recurrent breast cancer and their family caregivers. *Psychooncology*, 14(6): 478-491.

Northouse LL, Walker J, Schafenacker A, Mood D, Mellon S, Galvin E, et al. (2002). A family-based program of care for women with recurrent breast cancer and their family members. *Oncol Nurs Forum*, 29(10):1411-1419.

O'Brien PG. (2004). Patient and family teaching. In SM Lewis, MM Heitkemper, SR Dirksen (Eds): *Medical-surgical nursing: Assessment and management of clinical problems*. 6th ed, pp. 43-57. St. Louis: Mosby.

Ostwald SK, Hepburn KW, Burns T. (2003). Training family caregivers of patients with dementia: A structured workshop approach. *J Gerontol Nurs*, 29(1):37-44.

Pickett-Schenk SA. (2002). Church-based support groups for African American families coping with mental illness: Outreach and outcomes. *Psychiatr Rehabil J*, 26(2):173-180.

Robinson WD, Carroll JS, Watson WL. (2005). Shared experience building around the family crucible of cancer. *Fam Syst Health*, 23(2):131-147.

Roland P, Russell J, Richards KC, Sullivan SC. (2001). Visitation in critical care: Processes and outcomes of a performance improvement initiative. *J Nurs Care Qual*, 15(2):18-26.

Samuelsson AM, Annerstedt L, Elmstahl S, Samuelsson SM, Grafstrom M. (2001). Burden of responsibility experienced by family caregivers of elderly dementia sufferers. Analyses of strain, feelings and coping strategies. *Scand J Caring Sci*, 15(1):25-33.

Skerrett K. (2003). Couple dialogues with illness: Expanding the "We". *Fam Syst Health*, 21(1):69-80.

Tapp DM. (2001). Conserving the vitality of suffering: Addressing family constraints to illness conversations. *Nurs Inq*, 8(4):254-263.

RCT = Randomized Controlled (Clinical) Trial, **NIC** = Nursing Interventions Classification, **NOC** = Nursing Outcomes Classification

Trief PM, Sandberg J, Greenberg RP, Graff K, Castronova N, Yoon M, et al. (2003). Describing support: A qualitative study of couples living with diabetes. *Fam Syst Health*, 21(1):57-67.

Ufema J. (2002). Insights on death and dying. Suicide: A niece's guilt. *Nursing*, 32(11):68-69.

Van Horn E, Fleury J, Moore S. (2002). Family interventions during the trajectory of recovery from cardiac event: An integrative literature review. *Heart Lung*, 31(3):186-198.

Weihs K, Fisher L, Baird M. (2002). Families, health, and behavior: A section of the commissioned report by the Committee on Health and Behavior: Research, practice, and policy Division of Neuroscience and Behavioral Health and Division of Health Promotion and Disease Prevention Institute of Medicine, National Academy of Sciences. *Fam Syst Health*, 20(1):7-46.

FAMILY INVOLVEMENT PROMOTION

Keith A. Anderson, PhD; Joseph E. Gaugler, PhD

NIC Definition: Facilitating family participation in the emotional and physical care of the patient (Dochterman & Bulechek, 2004).

NURSING ACTIVITIES

Effective

■ *Assess family members' coping styles, abilities, resources, and challenges in response to the health care needs of the patient.* **LOE = II**

EO The Family Management Style framework can be effective for understanding and assessing the coping responses and management styles of family members of children with serious illnesses (Deatrick et al., 2006).

EO The Calgary Family Assessment Model can be an effective instrument for assessing the structural, developmental, and functional attributes of family systems (Wright & Leahey, 2005).

MR A controlled study ($N = 50$ prospective; $N = 72$ retrospective) comparing the interchangeability of the self-reported Family Assessment Device and administered McMaster Structured Interview for Families found that there was general agreement between the measures and that the self-reported measure could effectively serve as a proxy for the "gold standard" of the administered assessment (Barney & Max, 2005).

EO The Friedman Family Assessment Model can be an effective instrument for assessing the structure, functions, and interactions that families have with other social systems, particularly in the community setting (Friedman et al., 2003).

EO The Family System Stressor-Strength Inventory can be an effective instrument for assessing the stressors and coping resources of families (Hanson, 2001).

■ *Facilitate and encourage effective communication between family members and health care providers.* **LOE = II**

EO Multidisciplinary strategies to improve communication (e.g., formal family meetings, ethics consultations) can improve communication between health care professionals, patients, and family members, which in turn can improve quality of care (Boyle et al., 2005).

NR = Nursing Research, **MR** = Multidisciplinary Research, **SP** = Standard of Practice, **EO** = Expert Opinion, **LOE** = Level of Evidence

(NR) A descriptive study ($N = 34$) of a program to include family members in daily work rounds demonstrated that participants felt better informed on patients' condition and plan of care and that communication between the nurses and family members was enhanced (Schiller & Anderson, 2003).

(EO) There is weak evidence that some interventions (i.e., structured group interventions) may lead to increased knowledge and better overall psychological well-being in participants (Scott et al., 2003).

(NR) A descriptive study ($N = 300$) of the Perioperative Clinical Nurse Specialist program in which trained nurses serve as liaisons between surgical teams and family members found that the enhanced communication provided through this program during the perioperative period was highly valued by family members and surgeons (Carmichael & Agre, 2002).

(NR) A descriptive study ($N = 1802$) of a technology-based information and communication intervention (e.g., multimedia programs, videophones) for family caregivers and older adults revealed that participants reported an enhanced sense of control, empowerment in decision making, and greater opportunity for social contact (Magnusson et al., 2002).

■ *Encourage family members to take active roles in the planning and provision of care and facilitate the development of partnerships between family members and health care professionals.* **LOE = II**

(NR) A controlled study ($N = 114$ parent-child dyads) of a developmentally supportive family-centered care program in one neonatal intensive care unit found that inclusion and participation of family members were linked to fewer behavioral stress symptoms and lower medication costs (Byers et al., 2006).

(NR) A controlled study ($N = 185$ family caregivers; $N = 845$ staff members) of a program to enhance the participation of family members with nursing home residents demonstrated that participation in the program was associated with fewer feelings of loss and captivity, greater feelings of satisfaction with care, and enhanced relationships between family caregivers and staff members (Specht et al., 2005). (See also Maas et al., 2001.)

(NR) A descriptive study ($N = 14$ neonatal intensive care units) of visitation policies and efforts to establish and facilitate family-centered care revealed that less restrictive visitation rules, less punitive and restrictive language toward family members, and an enhanced view of parents as participants in care were critical in encouraging active family member participation (Browne et al., 2004).

(MR) An RCT ($N = 932$ family members; $N = 655$ staff members) of a family-staff partnership program in the nursing home setting found that both family members and staff members who participated in the program viewed each more favorably and reported less conflict and better communication (Pillemer et al., 2003).

(NR) An RCT ($N = 144$) of a family-based intervention to improve involvement and coping for family members of women with recurrent breast cancer demonstrated that the program was effective in increasing satisfaction with care and improving communication and information exchange between nurses and family members (Northouse et al., 2002).

■ *Develop, implement, and encourage participation in educational and training programs for family members.* **LOE = I**

(NR) A controlled study ($N = 64$) of an educational intervention conducted in one intensive care unit demonstrated that participation in an individual education program can allay anxiety and meet psychosocial needs of family members (Chien et al., 2006).

RCT = Randomized Controlled (Clinical) Trial, **NIC** = Nursing Interventions Classification, **NOC** = Nursing Outcomes Classification

(MR) An RCT ($N = 32$) of an educational, problem-solving intervention for family members of children with traumatic brain injury revealed that participants in the program reported significantly greater improvement in reducing problematic child behaviors than their counterparts in the control group (Wade et al., 2006).

(NR) An RCT ($N = 100$) of a nurse-led educational intervention for spouses of stroke patients found that spouses who participated fully in the program experienced significant decreases in negative well-being and increases in quality of life over time (Larson et al., 2005).

(NR) An RCT ($N = 163$) of an educational intervention for mothers of critically ill children demonstrated that participation in the program was associated with improved maternal functioning, better emotional coping outcomes, and fewer child adjustment problems (Melnyk et al., 2004).

(NR) A controlled study ($N = 57$) of an educational intervention for parents of children with asthma revealed that participants in the program made significant gains in their perceived knowledge, ability to make decisions, sense of control, and ability to provide care (McCarthy et al., 2002).

■ *Encourage family members to organize and participate in either facilitated or peer-led support groups.* **LOE = I**

(MR) A descriptive study ($N = 41$) of a telephone support group for caregivers of family members with dementia revealed that participants experienced gains in knowledge and skill as well as enhanced emotional and social support (Bank et al., 2006).

(NR) A descriptive study ($N = 114$) of an Internet-based support group program for parents of children with special needs revealed that participants gained insight and social support and reported improvements and greater satisfaction in their caregiver relationship (Baum, 2004).

(NR) An RCT ($N = 48$) of a mutual support group for family caregivers of patients with schizophrenia demonstrated that participation in the support group was associated with decreased levels of caregiver burden and a decrease in the duration of patients' hospitalization as well as increased levels of family functioning (Chien et al., 2004).

(EO) Participation in cancer peer support groups is consistently linked to informational, emotional, and instrumental gains for family members (Campbell et al., 2004).

(NR) An RCT ($N = 60$) of a nurse-led support group for family caregivers of relatives with dementia demonstrated that participation in the support group was associated with less distress and greater improvement in perceived quality of life (Fung & Chien, 2002).

Possibly Effective

■ *Facilitate and encourage family members to organize and participate in facility-based advocacy and decision-making groups (e.g., family advisory boards).* **LOE = V**

(EO) The existence of and participation in family councils may be effective in providing family members with support, education, advocacy opportunities, and avenues for communication (Anderson, 2005).

NR = Nursing Research, **MR** = Multidisciplinary Research, **SP** = Standard of Practice, **EO** = Expert Opinion, **LOE** = Level of Evidence

(MR) A descriptive study of a family advisory board in one heart and kidney unit of a children's hospital revealed that family members and nurses who participated in this multidisciplinary group felt empowered and better informed and understood their roles with greater clarity (Titone et al., 2004).

(EO) Family advisory councils may be effective in enhancing family-centered care (Moore et al., 2003).

■ *Facilitate the presence of family members during emergency procedures and resuscitation activities through proper assessment and preparation.* **LOE = III**

(EO) Consensus recommendations from a national conference on family presence during pediatric resuscitation concluded that family members should be appropriately assessed and, when possible, offered the option of being present during resuscitation (Henderson & Knapp, 2006).

(EO) Family presence during resuscitation has a number of potential benefits and risks for family members, staff, and facilities. However, more research is warranted (Halm, 2005).

(EO) Family members generally want to be present during the final moments of life, and there are benefits to both patients and family members when they are allowed to do so (Moreland, 2005).

(EO) Family members who choose to be present during pediatric resuscitation may benefit as evidenced by decreased anxiety, less subsequent litigation, and less second-guessing of staff efforts (Nibert & Ondrejka, 2005).

■ *Facilitate the presence of family members during induction of anesthesia in children through proper assessment and preparation.* **LOE = III**

(MR) A cohort study ($N = 568$) examining children's anxiety during induction of anesthesia demonstrated that the presence of a calm parent during induction of anesthesia could benefit an anxious child, but the presence of an anxious parent had no benefit (Kain et al., 2006).

(EO) Parental presence may help to alleviate fear and anxiety in children, provided that the parents are properly assessed and prepared (Romino et al., 2005).

(MR) An RCT ($N = 80$) examining stress associated with parental presence during induction of anesthesia demonstrated that parental presence was associated with increased parental heart rate and skin conductance level. However, no increased incidence of electrocardiogram abnormalities was found (Kain et al., 2003).

(NR) An RCT ($N = 80$) examining a video education intervention for parents prior to the induction of anesthesia in children demonstrated that viewing the video was effective in lowering anxiety in parents, which may also have positive effects for the children (Zuwala & Barber, 2001).

OUTCOME MEASUREMENT

FAMILY PARTICIPATION IN PROFESSIONAL CARE   (NOC)

(Please refer to *Nursing Outcomes Classification* [Moorhead et al., 2004] for the **Family Participation in Professional Care** outcome.)

RCT = Randomized Controlled (Clinical) Trial, **NIC** = Nursing Interventions Classification, **NOC** = Nursing Outcomes Classification

REFERENCES

Anderson KA. (2005). Family councils in residential long-term care. In Gaugler JE (Ed). *Promoting family involvement in long-term care settings.* Baltimore, MD: Health Professions Press, pp 25-44.

Bank AL, Arguelles S, Rubert M, Eisdorfer C, Czaja SJ. (2006). The value of telephone support groups among ethnically diverse caregivers of persons with dementia. *Gerontologist,* 46(1):134-138.

Barney MC, Max JE. (2005). The McMaster family assessment device and clinical rating scale: Questionnaire vs interview in childhood traumatic brain injury. *Brain Inj,* 19(10):801-809.

Baum LS. (2004). Internet parent support groups for primary caregivers of a child with special health care needs. *Pediatr Nurs,* 30(5):381-388, 401.

Boyle DK, Miller PA, Forbes-Thompson SA. (2005). Communication and end-of-life care in the intensive care unit: Patient, family, and clinician outcomes. *Crit Care Nurs Q,* 28(4):302-316.

Browne JV, Sanchez E, Langlois A, Smith S. (2004). From visitation policies to family participation guidelines in the NICU: The experience of the Colorado Consortium of Intensive Care Nurseries. *Neonat Paediatr Child Health Nurs,* 7(2):16-23.

Byers JF, Lowman LB, Francis J, Kaigle L, Lutz NH, Waddell T, et al. (2006). A quasi-experimental trial on individualized, developmentally supportive family-centered care. *J Obstet Gynecol Neonatal Nurs,* 35(1):105-115.

Campbell HS, Phaneuf MR, Deane K. (2004). Cancer peer support programs—Do they work? *Patient Educ Couns,* 55(1):3-15.

Carmichael JM, Agre P. (2002). Preferences in surgical waiting area amenities. *AORN J,* 75(6):1077-1083.

Chien W, Chiu YL, Lam L, Ip W. (2006). Effects of a needs-based education programme for family carers with a relative in an intensive care unit: A quasi-experimental study. *Int J Nurs Stud,* 43(1):39-50.

Chien WT, Norman I, Thompson DR. (2004). A randomized controlled trial of a mutual support group for family caregivers of patients with schizophrenia. *Int J Nurs Stud,* 41(6):637-649.

Deatrick JA, Thibodeaux AG, Mooney K, Schmus C, Pollack R, Davey BH. (2006). Family management style framework: A new tool with potential to assess families who have children with brain tumors. *J Pediatr Oncol Nurs,* 23(1):19-27.

Dochterman JM, Bulechek GM (Eds). (2004). *Nursing Interventions Classification (NIC),* 4th ed. St. Louis: Mosby.

Friedman MM, Bowden VR, Jones EG. (2003). *Family nursing: Research, theory, and practice,* 5th ed. Upper Saddle River, NJ: Pearson.

Fung WY, Chien WT. (2002). The effectiveness of a mutual support group for family caregivers of a relative with dementia. *Arch Psychiatr Nurs,* 16(3):134-144.

Halm MA. (2005). Family presence during resuscitation: A critical review of the literature. *Am J Crit Care,* 14(6):494-511.

Hanson SM. (2001). Family nursing assessment and intervention. In Hanson SM, Gedaly-Duff V, Kaakinen JR (Eds). *Family health care nursing: Theory, practice, and research,* 2nd ed. Philadelphia: FA Davis, pp 170-195.

Henderson DP, Knapp JF. (2006). Report of the National Conference on Family Presence during Pediatric Cardiopulmonary Resuscitation and Procedures. *J Emerg Nurs,* 32(1):23-29.

Kain ZN, Caldwell-Andrews AA, Maranets I, Nelson W, Mayes LC. (2006). Predicting which child-parent pair will benefit from parental presence during induction of anesthesia: A decision-making approach. *Anesth Analg,* 102(1):81-84.

Kain ZN, Caldwell-Andrews AA, Mayes LC, Wang SM, Krivutza DM, LoDolce ME. (2003). Parental presence during induction of anesthesia: Physiological effects on parents. *Anesthesiology,* 98(1):58-64.

Larson J, Franzen-Dahlin A, Billing E, Arbin M, Murray V, Wredling R. (2005). The impact of a nurse-led support and education programme for spouses of stroke patients: A randomized controlled trial. *J Clin Nurs,* 14(8):995-1003.

Maas M, Reed D, Specht J, Swanson S, Tripp-Reimer T, Buckwalter K, et al. (2001). Family involvement in care: Negotiated family-staff partnerships in special care units for persons with dementia. In Funk SG, Tomquist EM, Champagne MT, Wiese RA (Eds). *Key aspects of elder care: Managing falls, incontinence, and cognitive impairment.* New York: Springer, pp 330-345.

NR = Nursing Research, **MR** = Multidisciplinary Research, **SP** = Standard of Practice, **EO** = Expert Opinion, **LOE** = Level of Evidence

Magnusson L, Hanson E, Brito L, Berthold H, Chambers M, Daly T. (2002). Supporting family carers through the use of information and communication technology—The EU project ACTION. *Int J Nurs Stud,* 39(4):369-381.

McCarthy MJ, Herbert R, Brimacombe M, Hansen J, Wong D, Zelman M. (2002). Empowering parents through asthma education. *Pediatr Nurs,* 28(5):465-473.

Melnyk BM, Alpert-Gillis L, Feinstein NF, Crean HF, Johnson J, Fairbanks E, et al. (2004). Creating opportunities for parent empowerment: Program effects on the mental health/coping outcomes of critically ill young children and their mothers. *Pediatrics,* 113(6):e597-e607.

Moore KA, Coker K, DuBuisson AB, Swett B, Edwards WH. (2003). Implementing potentially better practices for improving family-centered care in neonatal intensive care units: Successes and challenges. *Pediatrics,* 111(4 Pt 2):e450-e460.

Moorhead S, Johnson M, Maas M (Eds). (2004). *Nursing Outcomes Classification (NOC),* 3rd ed. St. Louis: Mosby.

Moreland P. (2005). Family presence during invasive procedures and resuscitation in the emergency department: A review of the literature. *J Emerg Nurs,* 31(1):58-72.

Nibert L, Ondrejka D. (2005). Family presence during pediatric resuscitation: An integrative review for evidence-based practice. *J Pediatr Nurs,* 20(2):145-147.

Northouse LL, Walker J, Schafenacker A, Mood D, Mellon S, Galvin E, et al. (2002). A family-based program of care for women with recurrent breast cancer and their families. *Oncol Nurs Forum,* 29(10): 1411-1419.

Pillemer K, Suitor JJ, Henderson CR, Meador R, Schultz L, Robison J, et al. (2003). A cooperative communication intervention for nursing home staff and family members of residents. *Gerontologist,* 43(Special No 2):96-106.

Romino SL, Keatley VM, Secrest J, Good K. (2005). Parental presence during anesthesia induction in children. *AORN J,* 81(4):780-792.

Schiller WR, Anderson BF. (2003). Family as a member of the trauma rounds: A strategy for maximized communication. *J Trauma Nurs,* 10(4):93-101.

Scott JT, Prictor MJ, Harmsen M, Broom A, Entwistle V, Sowden A, et al. (2003). Interventions for improving communication with children and adolescents about a family member's cancer. *Cochrane Database Syst Rev,* (4):CD004511.

Specht JK, Reed D, Maas ML. (2005). Family involvement in the care of residents with dementia: An important resource for quality of life and care. In Gaugler JE (Ed). *Promoting family involvement in long-term care settings.* Baltimore, MD: Health Professions Press, pp 163-200.

Titone NJ, Cross R, Sileo M, Martin G. (2004). Taking family-centered care to a higher level on the heart and kidney unit. *Pediatr Nurs,* 30(6):495-497.

Wade SL, Michaud L, Brown TM. (2006). Putting the pieces together: Preliminary efficacy of a family problem-solving intervention for children with traumatic brain injury. *J Head Trauma Rehabil,* 21(1):57-67.

Wright LM, Leahey M. (2005). *Nurses and families: A guide to family assessment and intervention,* 4th ed. Philadelphia: FA Davis.

Zuwala R, Barber KR. (2001). Reducing anxiety in parents before and during pediatric anesthesia induction. *AANA J,* 69(1):21-25.

FAMILY PRESENCE FACILITATION

Cathie E. Guzzetta, PhD, RN, AHN-BC, FAAN; Angela P. Clark, PhD, RN, CNS, FAAN, FAHA; Margo A. Halm, PhD, RN, CCRN, APRN-BC

NIC **Definition:** Facilitation of the family's presence in support of an individual undergoing resuscitation and/or invasive procedures (Dochterman & Bulechek, 2004).

RCT = Randomized Controlled (Clinical) Trial, **NIC** = Nursing Interventions Classification, **NOC** = Nursing Outcomes Classification

NURSING ACTIVITIES

Effective

■ (SP) *Assess the family member's ability to cope emotionally while at the bedside.*
LOE = V

(NR) A descriptive study using quantitative and qualitative methods ($N = 43$ family presence [FP] events) found that family members did not interrupt patients' care during invasive procedures and cardiopulmonary resuscitation (CPR) when they were first assessed for appropriate levels of coping and the absence of combative behaviors, extreme emotional instability, and behaviors consistent with intoxication or an altered mental status (Meyers et al., 2000).

(NR) A process evaluation ($N = 54$ family members) of an FP policy demonstrated that families did not disrupt patients' care during pediatric invasive procedures or CPR when they were first assessed for appropriate levels of coping and the absence of combative behaviors, extreme emotional instability, behaviors consistent with an altered mental status, and suspected child abuse (Mangurten et al., 2005).

(NR) A descriptive study using quantitative and qualitative methods ($N = 64$ FP events) found that families did not interrupt patients' care or the medical team during pediatric invasive procedures and resuscitation interventions when families were assessed for appropriate levels of coping and the absence of combative behaviors, extreme emotional instability, behaviors consistent with an altered mental status, and suspected child abuse (Mangurten et al., 2006).

(EO) A consensus conference of 18 national organizations regarding FP during pediatric procedures and CPR recommended that FP be offered to family members when care to the child will not be interrupted and after assessment for combative and threatening behaviors, extreme emotional volatility, behaviors consistent with intoxication or altered mental status, disagreement among family members, or a threat to the safety of the health care team (Henderson & Knapp, 2006).

(EO) Criteria should be established for assessing families to ensure uninterrupted patients' care (AACN, 2004).

■ *Offer all families the option of FP during CPR and/or invasive procedures.*
LOE = V

(NR) A qualitative study ($N = 9$) of patient's experiences with FP found that patients believed FP was a right and associated with many benefits, including being comforted and receiving help, maintaining patient-family connectedness, and reminding others of the patient's "personhood" (Eichhorn et al., 2001).

(NR) An RCT ($N = 25$) found that all family members who chose to be present ($N = 13$) were satisfied with their decision and experienced no adverse psychological effects from witnessing their relative's CPR (Robinson et al., 1998).

(NR) A descriptive study ($N = 25$) found that almost all relatives (96%) surveyed believed families should have the option to be present, and 80% stated they would have wanted to be present had they been given a choice because they believed such presence would help not only their loved one but also themselves (Meyers et al., 1998).

(NR) In a systematic review of 28 studies (descriptive, RCTs, qualitative), patients, family members, and health care professionals in 18 studies (64%) reported that FP should be offered as an option during CPR, and of the family members who experienced FP, the majority stated that they would do so again because of multiple benefits such as aiding their grieving, providing an opportunity to say goodbye, and seeing that everything possible was done (Halm, 2005).

(EO) The option of FP should be offered to families based on its benefits for both patients and families: feeling comforted and supported, maintaining family bonds, and reminding staff of their human dignity (patients' benefits) and knowing that everything possible was being done, reducing fear and anxiety, feeling supportive to their loved one and staff, and facilitating grief (family benefits) (ENA, 2005).

Additional research: EEC Committee, 2005; Morse & Pooler, 2002.

■ (SP) *Ensure that families receive support while at the bedside; provide opportunities for them to ask questions and see, touch, and speak to the patient; and offer support during and following the event.* **LOE = V**

(NR) In a qualitative study ($N = 9$) exploring patients' experiences with FP during invasive procedures, a family facilitator prepared families by (1) providing information about the patient's status and appearance; (2) escorting families to the bedside, stressing their emotionally supportive role; (3) explaining the experience; and (4) offering psychosocial support (Eichhorn et al., 2001).

(NR) In an RCT ($N = 25$), family members were chaperoned during resuscitation by a nursing, chaplain, or medical staff member who prepared them by providing explanations of the procedures being performed, reassuring them they could leave the room if they wished, and offering them emotional support (Robinson et al.,1998).

(NR) In a qualitative study ($N = 88$), nurse-to-family support was characteristic of patient-family interaction patterns: nurses refrained from interacting with "families who were enduring" compared with people who were very distraught ("family emotionally suffering/patient enduring"); nurses assumed a comforting role to ease distress; and when "patients were failing to endure," nurses gave little explanation, but when "families were learning to endure," nurses coached them to talk to the patient (Morse & Pooler, 2002).

(EO) Family members who choose to be present during resuscitation need to be supported before, during, and after the event (AACN, 2004).

(EO) All providers need to be sensitive to the presence of families during CPR, and one member of the health care team should remain with the family to answer questions, clarify information, and comfort them (EEC Committee, 2005).

Additional research: ENA, 2005; Sacchetti et al., 2005.

■ (SP) *Implement and evaluate an approved evidence-based practice guideline (i.e., policy, procedure, standard of care) for presenting the option of FP during CPR and invasive procedures.* **LOE = V**

(NR) Coinvestigators of a national survey of critical care and emergency nurses ($N = 984$) found that only 5% worked on units with written policies allowing FP. It was recommended that nurses work with their institutions to advocate for written, sanctioned FP guidelines (MacLean et al., 2003).

(EO) A consensus conference of 18 national organizations recommended that FP policies be developed to include the preparation, escort process, and role of the family; guidelines for handling disagreements; methods to provide staff support; and methods to evaluate best

RCT = Randomized Controlled (Clinical) Trial, **NIC** = Nursing Interventions Classification, **NOC** = Nursing Outcomes Classification

practices for FP and long-term outcomes for patients, families, and staff (Henderson & Knapp, 2006).

(EO) All patients' care units should have an approved written practice document for presenting the option of FP during CPR and invasive procedures that includes criteria for assessing family; the role of the family facilitator in supporting families before, during, and after the event; and strategies for handling the development of untoward reactions by family members (AACN, 2004).

(EO) Formal guidelines should be developed to support the option of FP to include principles of facilitating FP, delineation of roles and responsibilities, resources for staff support, and strategies to evaluate patient, family, and provider outcomes (ENA, 2001).

■ (SP) *Educate all health care providers about FP in academic core curricula and hospital orientations.* **LOE = V**

(NR) In an experimental design, a hospital-based FP education program influenced experienced nurses' ($N = 46$) attitudes in intensive care and emergency department settings to give families a choice for FP, with improvements from 11% to 79% after the program (Bassler, 1999).

(EO) Representatives from 18 national organizations recommended that FP education be included in academic core curricula for all providers (physicians, nurses, prehospital care providers, social workers, mental health professionals, security personnel, pastoral care) and also provided in health care settings as part of hospital orientation (Henderson & Knapp, 2006).

(EO) Educational programs for professional staff should include benefits of FP for the patient/family, criteria for assessing families to ensure uninterrupted care of patients, the role of a family facilitator in preparing family members, and contraindications to FP (AACN, 2004).

(EO) Health care organizations should develop and disseminate educational resources for emergency nurses and other staff supporting the option of FP, and continuing education programs should be provided to increase understanding about FP (ENA, 2005).

Possibly Effective

■ *Use a designated staff support person (i.e., nurse, chaplain, social worker, child life specialist) to prepare, support, and guide family members through the bedside FP event.* **LOE = V**

(NR) A descriptive study ($N = 64$ pediatric FP events) found positive benefits for families when they were offered the option of FP by a family facilitator who had received training in a formal FP protocol, including assessing and preparing families for bedside presence and crisis intervention (Mangurten et al., 2006).

(NR) A process evaluation of an evidence-based practice guideline for FP ($N = 65$ families considered for FP) demonstrated that 54 families (83%) were assessed as appropriate candidates, 9 (14%) were deemed inappropriate, 2 (3%) declined, and patients' care was not interrupted when a family facilitator prepared families and guided them through the event (Mangurten et al., 2005).

(NR) A descriptive study ($N = 43$ FP events) found no interruption in patients' care and positive benefits for family members during CPR and invasive procedures when a family facilitator, who had received training in FP, assessed families, prepared and escorted them to the bedside, and guided them through the experience (Meyers et al., 2000).

NR = Nursing Research, **MR** = Multidisciplinary Research, **SP** = Standard of Practice, **EO** = Expert Opinion, **LOE** = Level of Evidence

(MR) A descriptive study (N = 30 FP events) found that patients' care and medical efforts during CPR had not been disrupted or otherwise adversely affected when a designated support person (i.e., a nurse or chaplain) prepared families and guided them through the FP event (Doyle et al., 1987).

(MR) A prospective observational study (N = 37 FP events) of families at the bedside with their children during invasive procedures without a designated support person found two minor interruptions from family members that did not significantly alter patients' care; the only staff present were the emergency department personnel involved in the care of the patient (Sacchetti et al., 2005).

(Note: More research is needed to evaluate the role of the family facilitator because positive outcomes for families and no interruption in patients' care have been documented in studies with and without a designated family support person.)

Additional research: Powers & Rubenstein, 1999; Sacchetti et al., 1996.

Not Effective

No applicable published research was found in this category.

Possibly Harmful

■ *Requiring families, who desire to be at the bedside with their loved one, to wait in the family room.* **LOE = V**

(MR) A prospective study of 74 relatives of 53 people with sudden, unexpected death (most of whom died at home and were treated by emergency medical services) found that relatives who left the room for fear of disturbing the interventions afterward regretted not having given support to their loved ones (Merlevede et al., 2004).

(NR) A descriptive study of family members' (N = 8) experiences with death in the ICU setting found that family members had regrets about missed opportunities to say goodbye to their loved ones (Kirchhoff et al., 2002).

OUTCOME MEASUREMENT

FAMILY SUPPORT DURING TREATMENT (NOC)

Definition: Family presence and emotional support for an individual undergoing treatment.

Family Support During Treatment as evidenced by the following selected NOC indicators:

- Members express desire to support ill member
- Members express feelings and emotions of concern for ill member
- Requests information about patient condition or status
- Seeks social and/or spiritual support for ill member

(Rate each indicator of **Family Support During Treatment:** 1 = never demonstrated, 2 = rarely demonstrated , 3 = sometimes demonstrated, 4 = often demonstrated, 5 = consistently demonstrated) (Moorhead et al., 2004).

Continued

OUTCOME MEASUREMENT—*cont'd*

Additional non-NOC indicators:
• Verbalizes meaning of health crisis
• Maintains appropriate level of coping at the bedside
• Touches, talks to, prays for, helps position, and/or emotionally supports ill family member
• Collaborates with ill family member and/or health care providers in determining care
• Respects care being delivered to ill family member and ensures it is not interrupted by their presence

REFERENCES

American Association of Critical-Care Nurses (AACN). (2004). Practice alert: Family presence during CPR and invasive procedures. *AACN News,* 21(11):4.

Bassler PC. (1999). The impact of education on nurses' beliefs regarding family presence in a resuscitation room. *J Nurses Staff Dev,* 15(3):126-131.

Dochterman JM, Bulechek GM (Eds). (2004). *Nursing Interventions Classification (NIC),* 4th ed. St. Louis: Mosby.

Doyle CJ, Post H, Burney RE, Maino J, Keefe M, Rhee KJ. (1987). Family participation during resuscitation: An option. *Ann Emerg Med,* 16(6):673-675.

EEC Committee, Subcommittees and Task Forces of the American Heart Association (AHA). (2005). 2005 American Heart Association Guidelines for Cardiopulmonary Resuscitation and Emergency Cardiovascular Care. *Circulation,* 112(24 Suppl):IV1-IV203.

Eichhorn DJ, Meyers TA, Guzzetta CE, Clark AP, Klein JD, Taliaferro E, et al. (2001). Family presence during invasive procedures and resuscitation: Hearing the voice of the patient. *Am J Nurs,* 101(5):48-55.

Emergency Nurses Association (ENA). (2001). *Presenting the option of family presence,* 2nd ed. Des Plaines, IL: ENA.

Emergency Nurses Association (ENA). (2005). Position statement: Family presence at the bedside during invasive procedures and cardiopulmonary resuscitation. Available online: http://www.ena.org/. Retrieved on May 25, 2007.

Halm MA. (2005). Family presence during resuscitation: A critical review of the literature. *Am J Crit Care,* 14(6):494-511.

Henderson DP, Knapp JF. (2006). Report of the National Consensus Conference on Family Presence During Pediatric Cardiopulmonary Resuscitation and Procedures. *J Emerg Nurs,* 32(1):23-29.

Kirchhoff K, Walker L, Hutton A, Spuhler V, Cole BV, Clemmer T. (2002). The vortex: Families' experiences with death in the intensive care unit. *Am J Crit Care,* 11(3):200-209.

MacLean SL, Guzzetta CE, White C, Fontaine D, Eichhorn DJ, Meyers TA, et al. (2003). Family presence during cardiopulmonary resuscitation and invasive procedures: Practices of critical care and emergency nurses. *Am J Crit Care,* 12(3):246-257.

Mangurten J, Scott SH, Guzzetta CE, Clark AP, Vinson L, Sperry J, et al. (2006). Effects of family presence during resuscitation and invasive procedures in a pediatric emergency department. *J Emerg Nurs,* 32(3):225-233.

Mangurten JA, Scott SH, Guzzetta CE, Sperry JS, Vinson LA, Hicks BA, et al. (2005). Family presence: Making room. *Am J Nurs,* 105(5):40-48.

Merlevede E, Spooren D, Henderick H, Portzky G, Buylaert W, Jannes C, et al. (2004). Perceptions, needs and mourning reactions of bereaved relatives confronted with a sudden unexpected death. *Resuscitation,* 61(3):341-348.

Meyers T, Eichhorn D, Guzzetta CE. (1998). Do families want to be present during CPR? A retrospective survey. *J Emerg Nurs,* 24(5):400-405.

Meyers TA, Eichhorn DJ, Guzzetta CE, Clark AP, Klein J, Taliaferro E, et al. (2000). Family presence during invasive procedures and resuscitation. *Am J Nurs,* 100(2):32-42.

Moorhead S, Johnson M, Maas M (Eds). (2004). *Nursing Outcomes Classification (NOC)*, 3rd ed. St. Louis: Mosby.

Morse JM, Pooler C. (2002). Patient-family-nurse interactions in the trauma-resuscitation room. *Am J Crit Care*, 11(3):240-249.

Powers KS, Rubenstein JS. (1999). Family presence during invasive procedures in the pediatric intensive care unit: A prospective study. *Arch Pediatr Adolesc Med*, 153(9):955-958.

Robinson SM, Mackenzie-Ross S, Campbell Hewson GL, Egleston CV, Prevost AT. (1998). Psychological effect of witnessed resuscitation on bereaved relatives. *Lancet*, 352(9128):614-617.

Sacchetti A, Lichenstein R, Carraccio CA, Harris RH. (1996). Family member presence during pediatric emergency department procedures. *Pediatr Emerg Care*, 12(4):268-271.

Sacchetti A, Paston C, Carraccio C. (2005). Family members do not disrupt care when present during invasive procedures. *Acad Emerg Med*, 12(5):477-479.

 # FEEDING

Sandra F. Simmons, PhD

NIC Definition: Providing nutritional intake for a patient who is unable to feed self (Dochterman & Bulechek, 2004).

NURSING ACTIVITIES

Effective

■ **SP** *Conduct an observation and/or performance-based assessment to determine a patient's ability to feed self and the type of assistance necessary to enhance self-feeding ability and oral food and fluid consumption.* **LOE=III**

MR A controlled study (*N*=74 nursing home residents) demonstrated that a 2-day (six meals) performance-based assessment wherein trained staff provided one-to-one assistance using a graduated-prompting protocol was effective in determining a resident's ability to self feed and respond to staff assistance as defined by an increase in oral food and fluid consumption (Simmons et al., 2001b).

NR In a descriptive study on a group of cognitively impaired patients (*N*=23 nursing home residents), the Self-Feeding Assessment Tool, which can be used as both a performance and observation-based tool to determine a patient's self-feeding ability (performance based) and received care (observation based), was tested and shown to be effective in identifying feeding problems (Osborn & Marshall, 1993).

NR In a descriptive study with a group of Alzheimer's patients (*N*=30) to measure functional ability during eating, the Eating Behavior Scale, an observation-based assessment tool developed by nurses at the National Institutes of Health, was tested. The tool was shown to be effective in identifying feeding problems and could also be used to assess the effect of an intervention to improve eating ability (Tully et al., 1997).

NR In a descriptive study on a group of Alzheimer's patients (*N*=20), the Feeding Behaviors Inventory, an observation-based assessment tool developed by nurses, was shown to be effective in identifying problem behaviors exhibited by patients at mealtimes, including self-feeding behaviors, staff assistance needed, and time required to eat (Durnbaugh et al., 1996).

RCT = Randomized Controlled (Clinical) Trial, **NIC** = Nursing Interventions Classification, **NOC** = Nursing Outcomes Classification

- (SP) *Provide adequate staff assistance during meals for residents who show an increase in oral intake in response to assistance.* **LOE = III**

(MR) A controlled study (*N* = 74 nursing home residents) showed that 50% of patients with low oral food and fluid consumption during meals ate significantly more when provided with an average of 35+ minutes of one-to-one assistance that enhanced self-feeding ability. Assistance also could be effectively provided in small groups (one staff member to three residents), which required an average of 45 minutes per meal per group (Simmons et al., 2001b).

(MR) A controlled study (*N* = 134 nursing home residents) showed that 46% of residents with low oral food and fluid consumption during meals ate significantly more when provided with an average of 35 minutes of one-to-one assistance. These findings replicated those of a previous study (Simmons & Schnelle, 2004).

(MR) A descriptive study (*N* = 349 nursing home residents) showed that residents who were physically dependent on staff for eating required at least 20 minutes of assistance (Steele et al., 1997).

(MR) A descriptive study with cognitively impaired nursing home residents (*N* = 25) and elderly people residing at home (*N* = 19) showed that caregivers spent an average of 40 minutes per day on feeding assistance (Hu et al., 1986).

(MR) A descriptive study in 32 nursing homes showed that facilities with total staffing (nurse aides plus licensed nurses) above 4.1 total hours per resident per day provided significantly better feeding assistance care as measured by direct observation and resident interview protocols than facilities with total staffing below this level (Schnelle et al., 2004b).

(MR) A descriptive study (*N* = 58 nursing home residents) showed that inadequate nurse aide staffing and inadequate licensed nurse supervision resulted in the following poor feeding assistance care practices for many patients at risk for undernutrition: being fed in bed; improper positioning for eating; food being served at an inappropriate temperature; feeding assistance being rendered in a sporadic, rapid manner even to residents who ate slowly because of swallowing difficulties; and assistance being forced upon residents who could eat independently but who did so slowly (Kayser-Jones & Schell, 1997). (Note: An increase in both nurse aide staffing to provide feeding assistance and licensed nurses for supervision of care delivery has been recommended by multiple groups, including the American Nurses Association [Kayser-Jones & Schell, 1997; Kayser-Jones, 1996; Mondoux, 1998]. A new federal regulation allows nursing homes to hire single-task workers to provide feeding assistance.)

(MR) A descriptive study in seven nursing homes representing three states showed that most of the study homes trained existing nonnursing staff to help residents during meals, and the quality of care provided by these workers was comparable to, if not better than, the care provided by nurse aides. These workers also assisted in other mealtime tasks such as transporting residents to and from the dining room for meals and meal tray delivery and setup (Simmons et al., 2006).

- *Use social stimulation, verbal cueing, and physical guidance to enhance self-feeding ability, oral food and fluid consumption, and quality of life.* **LOE = III**

(MR) A controlled study (*N* = 20) showed that the use of physical touch and verbal cueing provided by nurse aides resulted in a significant increase in oral intake among hospitalized elderly patients with severe cognitive impairment (Lange-Alberts & Shott, 1994).

NR = Nursing Research, **MR** = Multidisciplinary Research, **SP** = Standard of Practice, **EO** = Expert Opinion, **LOE** = Level of Evidence

(MR) A controlled study ($N = 40$ nursing home residents) showed that the use of volunteers during meals to assist with feeding, ensuring that all residents in need of assistance were taken to the dining room for at least one meal per day, and an afternoon group activity that encouraged socialization and hydration were effective in promoting weight gain and quality of life (Musson et al., 1990).

(MR) A controlled study ($N = 74$ nursing home residents) showed that the use of a graduated-prompting protocol that included social stimulation, verbal cueing, and physical guidance enhanced self-feeding ability and oral food and fluid consumption during meals for 50% of patients with oral intake problems (Simmons et al., 2001b).

(MR) A controlled study ($N = 134$ nursing home residents) showed that the use of a graduated-prompting protocol that included social stimulation, verbal cueing, and physical guidance enhanced self-feeding ability and oral food and fluid consumption during meals for 46% of the patients with oral intake problems. These findings replicated those of a previous study (Simmons & Schnelle, 2004).

■ *Offer additional foods and fluids between meals.* LOE = II

(MR) An RCT ($N = 68$ nursing home residents) with patients at risk for poor nutritional status showed that daily provision of additional calories by supplement or snack delivery three times per day for 6 weeks resulted in significant gains in daily caloric intake and weight for both the supplement and snack intervention groups compared with a control group (Turic et al., 1998).

(MR) A controlled study ($N = 134$ nursing home residents) showed that 44% of residents with low oral food and fluid consumption during meals significantly increased their daily caloric intake when offered additional foods and fluids three times per day between meals (Simmons & Schnelle, 2004).

(MR) An RCT ($N = 63$ incontinent nursing home residents) showed that 78% of residents increased their daily fluid intake and improved their hydration status in response to an intervention that included multiple prompts per day to consume fluids between meals, availability of fluid choices, and consistent toileting assistance (Simmons et al., 2001a).

■ (SP) *Monitor daily feeding assistance care provision through standardized direct observation.* LOE = IV

(MR) A descriptive study ($N = 302$ nursing home residents) showed that the adequacy and quality of feeding assistance care provision can be measured by a standardized direct observational protocol (Simmons et al., 2002a).

(MR) A descriptive study in 16 nursing homes showed that nurse aide documentation of feeding assistance care delivery and residents' oral food and fluid consumption were inaccurate in all study homes compared with observations during meals using a standardized protocol. The results of this study underscored the importance of directly observing care delivery as opposed to relying on medical record documentation alone (Schnelle et al., 2004a).

(MR) A controlled study ($N = 48$ nursing home residents) showed that nurse aide staff improved on five care process measures related to the adequacy and quality of feeding assistance care provision when supervisory nurses monitored care provision weekly by a standardized direct observational protocol and provided feedback to direct care staff about their performance

---

RCT = Randomized Controlled (Clinical) Trial, **NIC** = Nursing Interventions Classification, **NOC** = Nursing Outcomes Classification

(Simmons & Schnelle, 2006). Note: The Borun Center for Gerontological Research, University of California, Los Angeles School of Medicine website (www.borun.medsch.ucla.edu) provides standardized direct observational protocols that can be used by supervisory nurses to monitor the adequacy and quality of feeding assistance care provision during meals and the delivery of oral liquid nutritional supplements or other foods and fluids between meals.

■ (SP) *Assess and treat symptoms of depression using a standardized interview protocol.* **LOE = IV**

(EO) Assessment and treatment of depressive symptoms are recommended in the nutritional care practice guidelines to address problems with oral food and fluid consumption and weight loss (Thomas et al., 2000).

(MR) A descriptive study ($N = 156$ nursing home residents) showed that depression was the most common cause of weight loss (Morley & Kraenzle, 1994).

(MR) A cross-sectional study ($N = 396$ nursing home residents) showed that the prevalence of depressive symptoms among patients was significantly higher according to a standardized interview (Geriatric Depression Scale) than prevalence based on medical record information. The treatment and management of depression needed improvement for all patients (Simmons et al., 2004a).

■ (SP) *Assess patients' preferences related to nutritional care using a standardized interview.* **LOE = V**

(MR) A descriptive study ($N = 105$) showed that family members of nursing home residents preferred that noninvasive nutrition interventions, such as improvements in food quality and staff assistance, be attempted before the use of oral liquid supplements or appetite stimulant medications (Simmons et al., 2003).

(MR) A descriptive study ($N = 75$) showed that medical record documentation (minimum data set [MDS]) of residents' oral food and fluid intake and food complaints was inaccurate compared with independent assessments by research staff using standardized direct observation (oral intake) and interview (food complaints) protocols. Specifically, research staff documentation based on direct observation and resident interviews identified a significantly larger number of residents as potentially at risk for undernutrition related to low oral intake (73%) and/or stable complaints about the taste of food (32%) as compared with staff documentation of MDS items K4c (44%) and K4a (0%), respectively, within the same month. A total of 47% of the participants expressed stable complaints about some aspect of the nursing home food service (e.g., variety, appearance, temperature) (Simmons et al., 2002b).

(EO) The FoodEx-LTC is a 44-item questionnaire for cognitively intact to mildly impaired nursing home residents to assess their satisfaction with the food and food service (Crogan et al., 2004; Evans & Crogan, 2005). Note: The Borun Center for Gerontological Research, University of California, Los Angeles School of Medicine website (www.borun.medsch.ucla.edu) provides a standardized, brief seven-item interview to assess nursing home residents' dining location preferences and satisfaction with the food service (refer to the guideline on Weight Gain Assistance). This interview can be conducted with nursing home residents who have mild to moderate cognitive impairment. Criteria for how to select residents appropriate for interview are also provided.

NR = Nursing Research, **MR** = Multidisciplinary Research, **SP** = Standard of Practice, **EO** = Expert Opinion, **LOE** = Level of Evidence

Possibly Effective

■ *Reevaluate the need for restricted and/or modified texture diets for malnourished patients.* **LOE = V**

(MR) A descriptive chart review study (N = 217 nursing home residents) showed that a restricted diet (i.e., altered texture and/or reduced sodium, sugar, or calories) may contribute to malnutrition in nursing home residents (Buckler et al., 1994).

(EO) The liberalization of dietary restrictions may help to increase caloric intake and prevent malnutrition in elderly patients (Aldrich & Massey, 1999).

(MR) A descriptive chart review and observation-based study (N = 212 nursing home residents) showed that many residents may be inappropriately placed or maintained on altered texture diets, and patients needed to be reevaluated for feeding and swallowing skills and the appropriateness of the diet order (Groher & McKaig, 1995).

■ *Ensure that patients at risk for undernutrition and/or in need of staff assistance are taken to the dining room, or other common area, for most meals.* **LOE = V**

(MR) A descriptive study (N = 407 residents) of dementia patients in assisted-living and nursing home facilities showed that over half had low food and fluid intake, and having meals in a public dining area as well as staff monitoring was associated with higher food and fluid intake (Reed et al., 2005).

(MR) A cross-sectional study (N = 761 nursing home residents) showed that nutritional care quality was significantly better according to two of four care process measures when patients ate meals in the dining room compared with their rooms. First, patients rated by staff as requiring assistance to eat were more likely to receive assistance in the dining room than in their rooms. Second, staff medical record documentation of oral food and fluid consumption was more accurate when residents ate in the dining room (Simmons & Levy-Storms, 2005).

■ *Provide oral liquid nutritional supplements between meals to promote adequate nutrient intake.* **LOE = II**

(MR) An RCT (N = 91) of Alzheimer's patients showed that daily supplementation for 3 months resulted in significant gain in daily caloric intake and weight gain among intervention subjects compared with control subjects (Lauque et al., 2004).

(MR) An RCT (N = 68 nursing home residents) of patients at risk for poor nutritional status showed that daily provision of additional calories via supplement or snack delivery three times per day for 6 weeks resulted in significant gains in daily caloric intake and weight for both the supplement and snack intervention groups compared with a control group (Turic et al., 1998).

(MR) A descriptive study (N = 40 nursing home residents) showed that less than 5% received supplements consistent with their orders in daily care practice, and consumption of the supplement was low (Kayser-Jones et al., 1998).

(MR) A descriptive study (N = 132 nursing home residents) showed that less than 10% received supplements consistent with their orders in daily care practice. In addition, supplements were often provided with regularly scheduled meals instead of between meals, and staff provided little to no assistance to encourage consumption (Simmons & Patel, 2006).

RCT = Randomized Controlled (Clinical) Trial, **NIC** = Nursing Interventions Classification, **NOC** = Nursing Outcomes Classification

(MR) A descriptive study ($N = 40$) showed that compliance with oral liquid nutritional supplements among hospitalized and community-dwelling geriatric patients was low because of personal preferences and the palatability of supplements (Lad et al., 2005).

(MR) A descriptive study ($N = 105$) showed that family members of nursing home residents preferred that noninvasive nutrition interventions, such as improvements in food quality and staff assistance, be attempted before the use of oral liquid nutritional supplements or appetite stimulant medications (Simmons et al., 2003).

Not Effective

No applicable published research was found in this category.

Possibly Harmful

■ *Feeding patients in less than 35 minutes who show an increase in oral intake in response to assistance.* **LOE = III**

(MR) A controlled study ($N = 74$ nursing home residents) showed that 50% of patients with low oral food and fluid consumption during meals ate significantly more when provided with an average of 35+ minutes of one-to-one assistance that enhanced self-feeding ability. Assistance could also be effectively provided in small groups (one staff member to three residents), which required an average of 45 minutes per meal per group (Simmons et al., 2001b).

(MR) A controlled study ($N = 134$ nursing home residents) showed that 46% of residents with low oral food and fluid consumption during meals ate significantly more when provided with an average of 35 minutes of one-to-one assistance. These findings replicated those of a previous study (Simmons & Schnelle, 2004).

(MR) A descriptive study ($N = 349$ nursing home residents) showed that residents who were physically dependent on staff for eating required at least 20 minutes of assistance (Steele et al., 1997).

(MR) A descriptive study of cognitively impaired nursing home residents ($N = 25$) and elderly people residing at home ($N = 19$) showed that caregivers spent an average of 40 minutes per day on feeding assistance (Hu et al., 1986).

(MR) A descriptive study of 32 nursing homes showed that facilities with total staffing (nurse aides plus licensed nurses) above 4.1 total hours per resident per day provided significantly better feeding assistance care as measured by direct observation and resident interview protocols than facilities with total staffing below this level (Schnelle et al., 2004b).

(NR) A descriptive study ($N = 58$ nursing home residents) showed that inadequate nurse aide staffing and inadequate licensed nurse supervision resulted in the following poor feeding assistance care practices for many patients at risk for undernutrition: being fed in bed; improper positioning for eating; food being served at an inappropriate temperature; feeding assistance being rendered in a sporadic, rapid manner even to residents who ate slowly because of swallowing difficulties; and assistance being forced upon residents who could eat independently but who did so slowly (Kayser-Jones & Schell, 1997). (Note: An increase in both nurse aide staffing to provide feeding assistance and licensed nurses for supervision of care delivery has been recommended by multiple groups, including the American Nurses Association [Kayser-Jones & Schell, 1997; Kayser-Jones, 1996; Mondoux, 1998].)

(MR) A descriptive study in seven nursing homes representing three states showed that most of the study homes trained existing nonnursing staff to help residents during meals, and the quality of care provided by these workers was comparable to, if not better than, the care provided by nurse aides. These workers also assisted in other mealtime tasks, such as transporting residents to and from the dining room for meals and meal tray delivery and setup (Simmons et al., 2006). (Note: A new federal regulation allows nursing homes to hire single-task workers to provide feeding assistance.)

■ Use of megestrol acetate as an appetite stimulant medication. LOE = II

(MR) An RCT (N = 69 Veterans Administration nursing home residents) of Megace OS, an oral liquid suspension of megestrol acetate, as given daily in an 800-mg dose for 12 weeks with 13 weeks of follow-up, showed that the medication had an effect on improved appetite and well-being, according to patients' self-report, after 12 weeks of treatment and a delayed effect on weight gain during the 13-week follow-up period (Yeh et al., 2000).

(MR) A prospective, controlled study (N = 17 nursing home residents) showed that Megace OS, as given daily in a 400-mg dose for 63 days, had an effect on oral food and fluid intake only when combined with adequate feeding assistance. The medication was not an effective nutritional intervention to increase oral intake under usual nursing home care conditions, which were characterized by inadequate feeding assistance (Simmons et al., 2004b).

(MR) A retrospective chart review study (N = 816 nursing home residents) showed that the incidence of deep venous thrombosis was significantly higher among patients receiving megestrol acetate than in the general population of institutionalized elderly people (Kropsky et al., 2003).

(MR) A descriptive study (N = 105) showed that family members of nursing home residents preferred that noninvasive nutrition interventions, such as improvements in food quality and staff assistance, be attempted before the use of oral liquid nutritional supplements or appetite stimulant medications, such as Megace (Simmons et al., 2003).

■ Use of feeding tubes in dementia patients. LOE = I

(MR) A review article of published literature (years 1966 to 1999) showed no evidence that tube feeding improved clinical outcomes (e.g., survival, aspiration pneumonia, pressure sores) for patients with advanced dementia but much evidence of substantial risks associated with tube feeding (Finucane et al., 1999).

(EO) There may be a financial incentive for nursing homes to place feeding tubes for patients with advanced dementia because of a higher per diem from Medicaid and a reduction in staff time necessary for feeding assistance care provision. The clinical appropriateness of feeding tube placement as a nutritional intervention should be carefully considered in light of these financial and staff resource incentives (Mitchell, 2003; Simmons, 2003).

(MR) A descriptive study of surrogate decision makers (N = 58) for elderly patients showed that, after 5 weeks of use, 84% stated that they would repeat the decision to place a feeding tube for their relative, although almost one third felt the patient would not want the tube. A greater emphasis may need to be placed on the wishes of the patient before placing feeding tubes (McNabney et al., 1994).

(MR) A descriptive study of nursing home residents (N = 379) deemed capable of making decisions showed that 33% would prefer a feeding tube if no longer able to eat because of brain damage. However, 25% changed their minds about wanting a tube when told that physical restraints are sometimes used during the feeding process. Providers need to ensure that decisions to place a feeding tube are based on comprehensive information about care practices and potential risks and benefits (O'Brien et al., 1997).

RCT = Randomized Controlled (Clinical) Trial, **NIC** = Nursing Interventions Classification, **NOC** = Nursing Outcomes Classification

OUTCOME MEASUREMENT

NUTRITIONAL STATUS ⬭NOC

Definition: Extent to which nutrients are available to meet metabolic needs.

Nutritional Status as evidenced by the following selected NOC indicators:

- Food intake
- Fluid intake
- Hydration

(Rate each indicator of **Nutritional Status:** 1 = severe deviation from normal range, 2 = substantial deviation from normal range, 3 = moderate deviation from normal range, 4 = mild deviation from normal range, 5 = no deviation from normal range) (Moorhead et al., 2004)

Additional non-NOC indicators:

- Weight status
- Body mass index
- Medical record documentation of feeding assistance care provision
- Medical record documentation of food and fluid intake
- Medical record documentation of oral supplement intake

REFERENCES

Aldrich JK, Massey LK. (1999). A liberalized geriatric diet fits most dietary prescriptions for long-term-care residents. *J Am Diet Assoc,* 99(4):478-480.

Buckler DA, Kelber ST, Goodwin JS. (1994). The use of dietary restrictions in malnourished nursing home patients. *J Am Geriatr Soc,* 42(10):1100-1102.

Crogan NL, Evans B, Velasquez D. (2004). Measuring nursing home resident satisfaction with food and food service: Initial testing of the FoodEx-LTC. *J Gerontol A Biol Sci Med Sci,* 59(4):370-377.

Dochterman JM, Bulechek GM (Eds). (2004). *Nursing Interventions Classification (NIC),* 4th ed. St. Louis: Mosby.

Durnbaugh T, Haley B, Roberts S. (1996). Assessing problem feeding behaviors in mid-stage Alzheimer's disease. *Geriatr Nurs,* 17(2):63-67.

Evans B, Crogan NL. (2005). Using the FoodEx-LTC to assess institutional food service practices through nursing home residents' perspectives on nutrition care. *J Gerontol A Biol Sci Med Sci,* 60(1):125-128.

Finucane TE, Christmas C, Travis K. (1999). Tube feeding in patients with advanced dementia: A review of the evidence. *JAMA,* 282(14):1365-1370.

Groher ME, McKaig TN. (1995). Dysphagia and dietary levels in skilled nursing facilities. *J Am Geriatr Soc,* 43(5):528-532.

Hu TW, Huang LF, Cartwright WS. (1986). Evaluation of the costs of caring for the senile demented elderly: A pilot study. *Gerontologist,* 26(2):158-163.

Kayser-Jones J. (1996). Mealtime in nursing homes: The importance of individualized care. *J Gerontol Nurs,* 22(3):26-31.

Kayser-Jones J, Schell E. (1997). The effect of staffing on the quality of care at mealtime. *Nurs Outlook,* 45(2):64-72.

Kayser-Jones J, Schell ES, Porter C, Barbaccia JC, Steinbach C, Bird WF, et al. (1998). A prospective study of the use of liquid oral dietary supplements in nursing homes. *J Am Geriatr Soc,* 46(11): 1378-1386.

Kropsky B, Shi Y, Cherniack EP. (2003). Incidence of deep-venous thrombosis in nursing home residents using megestrol acetate. *J Am Med Dir Assoc,* 4(5):255-256.

Lad H, Gott M, Gariballa S. (2005). Elderly patients compliance and elderly patients and health professional's views and attitudes towards prescribed sip-feed supplements. *J Nutr Health Aging,* 9(5):310-314.

Lange-Alberts ME, Shott S. (1994). Nutritional intake. Use of touch and verbal cuing. *J Gerontol Nurs,* 20(2):36-40.

Lauque S, Arnaud-Battandier F, Gillette S, Plaze JM, Andrieu S, Cantet C, et al. (2004). Improvement of weight and fat-free mass with oral nutritional supplementation in patients with Alzheimer's disease at risk of malnutrition: A prospective randomized study. *J Am Geriatr Soc,* 52(10):1702-1707.

McNabney MK, Beers MH, Siebens H. (1994). Surrogate decision-makers' satisfaction with the placement of feeding tubes in elderly patients. *J Am Geriatr Soc,* 42(2):161-168.

Mitchell SL. (2003). Financial incentives for placing feeding tubes in nursing home residents with advanced dementia. *J Am Geriatr Soc,* 51(1):129-131.

Mondoux L. (1998). *Testimony of the American Nurses Association before the National Academy of Sciences Institute of Medicine Committee on Improving Quality in Long Term Care.* Washington, DC.

Moorhead M, Johnson M, Maas M (Eds). (2004). *Nursing Outcomes Classification (NOC),* 3rd ed. St. Louis: Mosby.

Morley JE, Kraenzle D. (1994). Causes of weight loss in a community nursing home. *J Am Geriatr Soc,* 42(6):583-585.

Musson ND, Kincaid J, Ryan P, Glussman B, Varone L, Gamarra N, et al. (1990). Nature, nurture, nutrition: Interdisciplinary programs to address the prevention of malnutrition and dehydration. *Dysphagia,* 5(2):96-101.

O'Brien LA, Siegert EA, Grisso JA, Maislin GM, LaPann K, Evans LK, et al. (1997). Tube feeding preferences among nursing home residents. *J Gen Intern Med,* 12(6):364-371.

Osborn CL, Marshall MJ. (1993). Self-feeding performance in nursing home residents. *J Gerontol Nurs,* 19(3):7-14.

Reed PS, Zimmerman S, Sloane PD, Williams CS, Boustani M. (2005). Characteristics associated with low food and fluid intake in long-term care residents with dementia. *Gerontologist,* 45 Spec No 1(1):74-80.

Schnelle JF, Bates-Jensen BM, Chu L, Simmons SF. (2004a). Accuracy of nursing home medical record information about care-process delivery: Implications for staff management and improvement. *J Am Geriatr Soc,* 52(8):1378-1383.

Schnelle JF, Simmons SF, Harrington C, Cadogan M, Garcia E, M Bates-Jensen B. (2004b). Relationship of nursing home staffing to quality of care. *Health Serv Res,* 39(2):225-250.

Simmons SF. (2003). Should reimbursement rates be increased for feeding assistance in nursing homes? *J Am Med Dir Assoc,* 4(1):52-53.

Simmons SF, Alessi C, Schnelle JF. (2001a). An intervention to increase fluid intake in nursing home residents: Prompting and preference compliance. *J Am Geriatr Soc,* 49(7):926-933.

Simmons SF, Babineau S, Garcia E, Schnelle JF. (2002a). Quality assessment in nursing homes by systematic direct observation: Feeding assistance. *J Gerontol A Biol Sci Med Sci,* 57(10):M665-M671.

Simmons SF, Bertrand R, Shier V, Sweetland R, Moore T, Hurd D, et al. (2006). A preliminary evaluation of the Paid Feeding Assistant regulation: Impact on feeding assistance care process quality in nursing homes. *Gerontologist,* 47(2):184-192.

Simmons SF, Cadogan MP, Cabrera GR, Al-Samarrai NR, Jorge JS, Levy-Storms L, et al. (2004a). The minimum data set depression quality indicator: Does it reflect differences in care processes? *Gerontologist,* 44(4):554-564.

Simmons SF, Lam H, Rao G, Schnelle JF. (2003). Family members' preferences for nutrition interventions to improve nursing home residents' oral food and fluid intake. *J Am Geriatr Soc,* 51(1):69-74.

Simmons SF, Levy-Storms L. (2005). The effect of dining location on nutritional care quality in nursing homes. *J Nutr Health Aging,* 9(6):434-439.

Simmons SF, Lim B, Schnelle JF. (2002b). Accuracy of minimum data set in identifying residents at risk for undernutrition: Oral intake and food complaints. *J Am Med Dir Assoc,* 3(3):140-145.

Simmons SF, Osterweil D, Schnelle JF. (2001b). Improving food intake in nursing home residents with feeding assistance: A staffing analysis. *J Gerontol A Biol Sci Med Sci,* 56(12):M790-M794.

Simmons SF, Patel AV. (2006). Nursing home staff delivery of oral liquid nutritional supplements to residents at risk for unintentional weight loss. *J Am Geriatr Soc,* 54(9):1372-1376.

Simmons SF, Schnelle JF. (2004). Individualized feeding assistance care for nursing home residents: Staffing requirements to implement two interventions. *J Gerontol A Biol Sci Med Sci,* 59(9):M966-M973.

Simmons SF, Schnelle JF. (2006). A continuous quality improvement pilot study: Impact on nutritional care quality. *J Am Med Dir Assoc,* 7(8):480-485.

RCT = Randomized Controlled (Clinical) Trial, **NIC** = Nursing Interventions Classification, **NOC** = Nursing Outcomes Classification

Simmons SF, Walker K, Osterweil D. (2004b). The effect of megestrol acetate on oral food and fluid intake in nursing home residents: A pilot study. *J Am Med Dir Assoc,* 5(1):24-30.

Steele CM, Greenwood C, Ens I, Robertson C, Seidman-Carlson R. (1997). Mealtime difficulties in a home for the aged: Not just dysphagia. *Dysphagia,* 12(1):43-50.

Thomas DR, Ashmen W, Morley JE, Evans WJ. (2000). Nutritional management in long term care: Development of a clinical guideline. Council for Nutritional Strategies in Long-Term Care. *J Gerontol A Biol Sci Med Sci,* 55(12):M725-M734.

Tully MW, Matrakas KL, Muir J, Musallam K. (1997). The Eating Behavior Scale. A simple method of assessing functional ability in patients with Alzheimer's disease. *J Gerontol Nurs,* 23(7):9-15.

Turic A, Gordon KL, Craig LD, Ataya DG, Voss AC. (1998). Nutrition supplementation enables elderly residents of long-term care facilities to meet or exceed RDAs without displacing energy or nutrient intakes from meals. *J Am Diet Assoc,* 98(12):1457-1459.

Yeh SS, Wu SY, Lee TP, Olson JS, Stevens MR, Dixon T, et al. (2000). Improvement in quality-of-life measures and stimulation of weight gain after treatment with megestrol acetate oral suspension in geriatric cachexia: Results of a double-blind, placebo-controlled study. *J Am Geriatr Soc,* 48(5):485-492.

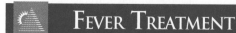 # FEVER TREATMENT

Margaret Griffiths, MSN, RN, CNE

NIC **Definition:** Management of a patient with hyperpyrexia caused by nonenvironmental factors (Dochterman & Bulechek, 2004).

NURSING ACTIVITIES

Effective

■ *Select tympanic or oral temperature measurement devices as appropriate.* **LOE = II**

NR An RCT ($N = 60$) compared tympanic (measured with an infrared thermometer) and oral temperature (measured with a predictive thermistor thermometer) at four times during the perioperative period in adults having major surgery. The tympanic site offered some advantage, but either tympanic or oral readings were satisfactory for routine intermittent monitoring of body temperature during the perioperative period (Erickson & Yount, 1991).

■ *Use a convection cooling device.* **LOE = II**

NR An RCT of ICU patients ($N = 27$) demonstrated that an airflow blanket was more effective than a water-cooling blanket (Loke et al., 2005).

NR An RCT ($N = 20$) found that cooling by convection (airflow blanket) was more effective than cooling by conduction (water-flow blanket) in critically ill adults (Creechan et al., 2001).

MR An RCT ($N = 220$) assigned patients either to cooling blanket therapy plus acetaminophen or to acetaminophen alone. Air blanket therapy resulted in a small increase in the proportion of patients with treatment success (Mayer et al., 2001).

MR An RCT ($N = 37$) found that a system that employed hydrogel-coated water-circulated energy transfer pads applied directly to the trunk and thighs was more effective than the conventional water-circulating cooling blanket (Mayer et al., 2004).

NR = Nursing Research, **MR** = Multidisciplinary Research, **SP** = Standard of Practice, **EO** = Expert Opinion, **LOE** = Level of Evidence

Possibly Effective

■ *Use medications to reduce fever.* **LOE = VII**

(EO) Antipyretic therapy might be justified if the metabolic costs of fever were exceeded by its physiological benefits, if the treatment reduced the metabolic costs or other adverse effects of fever without adversely affecting the course of the febrile illness, or if the side effects of the antipyretic drug regimen were appreciably fewer than its beneficial effects. Insufficient experimental data are available to validate any of these rationales (Greisman & Mackowiak, 2002).

(MR) A systematic review (*N* = 3 studies) found little evidence to support the administration of antipyretics (Hudgings et al., 2004).

■ *Measure and interpret elevated temperatures.* **LOE = VI**

(NR) A descriptive study (*N* = 84) concluded that temperature reading should be interpreted on an individual basis, the same site of measurement should be used, and no adjustment of oral, ear, or axillary temperatures to the rectal site should be made (Sund-Levander et al., 2004).

(EO) Basal body temperatures in frail elderly persons may be lower than the well-established mean value of 37°C or 98.6°F. Lowering the criterion to 100°F (37.8°C) raises the sensitivity to 70% for predicting infection while maintaining excellent specificity at 90%. A single temperature reading of 100°F (37.8°C) is both a sensitive and specific predictor of infection with a positive predictive value of 55% in long-term care facility residents. Other suggested temperature criteria indicative of possible infection in long-term care facility residents are an increase in temperature of at least 2°F (1.1°C) over baseline or an oral temperature of 99°F (37.2°C) or rectal temperature of 99.5°F (37.5°C) on repeated measurements (Bentley et al., 2000).

(MR) In a study of 13 febrile intensive care patients using pulmonary artery catheters with temperature measurement as the standard, temperature was taken with rectal probe, with oral and axillary temperatures obtained with an electronic thermometer, and with tympanic temperatures obtained with an infrared device. Rectal temperature measurements correlated most closely with core temperatures (Schmitz et al., 1995).

(EO) The oral electronic predictive thermometry has higher reliability and a lower standard of error than the infrared ear thermometry (Prentice & Moreland, 1999).

(EO) In the ICU, temperature measurement in the axilla should be discouraged because of its unreliable correlation with core temperature and its poor reproducibility. Temperature is most accurately measured by an intravascular or bladder thermistor, but measurement by electronic probe in the mouth, rectum, or external auditory canal is acceptable in appropriate cases (O'Grady et al., 1998).

■ *Compensate for insensible water loss.* **LOE = VII**

(EO) In a comfortable indoor environment, an extra 600 mL per day of fluid should be supplied to patients with highly elevated body temperature in order to compensate for an increased cutaneous water loss. In tropical or subtropical climates, the extra fluid supply should be substantially increased (Lamke et al., 1980).

RCT = Randomized Controlled (Clinical) Trial, **NIC** = Nursing Interventions Classification, **NOC** = Nursing Outcomes Classification

Not Effective

No applicable published research was found in this category.

Possibly Harmful

■ *Use of infrared thermometers.* **LOE = II**

EO Handheld infrared thermometers are not accurate enough for detecting fever (Ng et al., 2005).

MR A report of a study ($N = 137$) designed to determine the magnitude and frequency of measurement errors with infrared tympanic thermometers in the clinical setting concluded that the variability and inaccuracy of temperatures measured by infrared tympanic thermometers were sufficiently large to suggest that the use of these devices for routine thermometry may be potentially hazardous (Modell et al., 1998).

OUTCOME MEASUREMENT

THERMOREGULATION   **NOC**

Definition: Balance among heat production, heat gain, and heat loss.
Thermoregulation as evidenced by the following selected NOC indicators:
• Increased skin temperature
• Hyperthermia
• Dehydration
(Rate each indicator of **Thermoregulation:** 1 = severe, 2 = substantial, 3 = moderate, 4 = mild, 5 = none) (Moorhead et al., 2004).

REFERENCES

Bentley DW, Bradley S, High K, Schoenbaum S, Taler G, Yoshikawa TT, et al. (2000). Practice guideline for evaluation of fever and infection in long-term care facilities. *Clin Infect Dis,* 31(3):640-653.

Creechan T, Vollman K, Kravutske ME. (2001). Cooling by convection vs cooling by conduction for treatment of fever in critically ill adults. *Am J Crit Care,* 10(1):52-59.

Dochterman JM, Bulechek GM (Eds). (2004). *Nursing Interventions Classification (NIC),* 4th ed. St. Louis: Mosby.

Erickson RS, Yount ST. (1991). Comparison of tympanic and oral temperatures in surgical patients. *Nurs Res,* 40(2):90-93.

Greisman LA, Mackowiak PA. (2002). Fever: Beneficial and detrimental effects of antipyretics. *Curr Opin Infect Dis,* 15(3):241-245.

Hudgings L, Kelsberg G, Safranek S, Neher JO. (2004). Do antipyretics prolong febrile illness? *J Fam Pract,* 53(1):57-58, 61.

Lamke LO, Nilsson G, Reithner L. (1980). The influence of elevated body temperature on skin perspiration. *Acta Chir Scand,* 146(2):81-84.

Loke AY, Chan HC, Chan TM. (2005). Comparing the effectiveness of two types of cooling blankets for febrile patients. *Nurs Crit Care,* 10(5):247-254.

Mayer SA, Commichau C, Scarmeas N, Presciutti M, Bates J, Copeland D. (2001). Clinical trial of an air-circulating cooling blanket for fever control in critically ill neurologic patients. *Neurol,* 56(3):292-298.

Mayer SA, Kowalski RG, Presciutti M, Ostapkovich ND, McGann E, Fitzsimmons BF, et al. (2004). Clinical trial of a novel surface cooling system for fever control in neurocritical patients. *Crit Care Med,* 32(12):2508-2515.

NR = Nursing Research, **MR** = Multidisciplinary Research, **SP** = Standard of Practice, **EO** = Expert Opinion, **LOE** = Level of Evidence

Modell JG, Katholi CR, Kumaramangalam SM, Hudson EC, Graham D. (1998). Unreliability of the infrared tympanic thermometer in clinical practice: a comparative study with oral mercury and oral electronic thermometers. *South Med J,* 91(7):649-654.

Moorhead M, Johnson M, Maas M (Eds). (2004). *Nursing Outcomes Classification (NOC),* 3rd ed. St. Louis: Mosby.

Ng DK, Chan CH, Chan EY, Kwok KL, Chow PY, Lau WF, et al. (2005). A brief report on the normal range of forehead temperature as determined by noncontact, handheld, infrared thermometer. *Am J Infect Control,* 33(4):227-229.

O'Grady NP, Barie PS, Bartlett JG, Bleck T, Garvey G, Jacobi J, et al. (1998). Practice guidelines for evaluating new fever in critically ill adult patients. *Clin Infect Dis,* 26(5):1042-1059.

Prentice D, Moreland J. (1999). A comparison of infrared ear thermometry with electronic predictive thermometry in a geriatric setting. *Geriatr Nurs,* 20(6):314-317.

Schmitz T, Bair N, Falk M, Levine C. (1995). A comparison of five methods of temperature measurement in febrile intensive care patients. *Am J Crit Care,* 4(4):286-292.

Sund-Levander M, Grodzinsky E, Loyd D, Wahren LK. (2004). Errors in body temperature assessment related to individual variation, measuring technique and equipment. *Int J Nurs Pract,* 10(5):216-223.

 # FLUID MANAGEMENT **NIC**

Bonnie J. Wakefield, PhD, RN

NIC **Definition:** Promotion of fluid balance and prevention of complications resulting from abnormal or undesired fluid levels (Dochterman & Bulechek, 2004).

NURSING ACTIVITIES

Effective

■ **SP** *Weigh the patient as indicated by acuity and monitor trends.* **LOE = V**

MR A systematic review demonstrated that measurement of body mass change was a safe technique to assess hydration status, especially for dehydration that occurred over a period of 1 to 4 hours. Less frequent measurement may reflect changes in respiratory water loss or gain/loss of adipose tissue, and thus weight changes may be a less accurate indicator of hydration status (Armstrong, 2005).

EO Weight gain (loss) of 2.2 pounds is equal to fluid gain (loss) of 1 L (Linton & Maebius, 2003).

■ **SP** *Monitor food intake.* **LOE = V**

MR A systematic review demonstrated that water is taken in as food, water content, water produced by food oxidation, and drinking (Ferry, 2005).

NR A systematic review demonstrated that although restrictions on sodium and fluid intake were considered essential in management of heart failure, recommendations were imprecise and not based on evidence (Deaton et al., 2004).

NR A systematic review demonstrated that patients with heart failure were instructed to restrict sodium intake to 2 g per day (Deaton et al., 2004).

RCT = Randomized Controlled (Clinical) Trial, **NIC** = Nursing Interventions Classification, **NOC** = Nursing Outcomes Classification

(NR) A systematic review demonstrated that patients at risk for fluid overload (e.g., heart failure) should be instructed on hidden sodium content in food (Jaarsma et al., 1997).

■ **NIC** (SP) *Monitor vital signs, as appropriate.* **LOE = V**

(MR) A systematic review demonstrated that hypotension and tachycardia, and occasionally fever, were clinical signs of dehydration (Ferry, 2005).

(MR) A systematic review demonstrated that general clinical evaluation and cardiovascular assessment of blood pressure and pulse were objective parameters of dehydration (Weinberg & Minaker, 1995).

(EO) Changes in vital signs can detect changes in fluid balance (Linton & Maebius, 2003).

■ (SP) *Monitor clinical indicators of hydration status: thirst, dry oral mucous membranes, adequacy of pulses, orthostatic blood pressure, breath sounds, edema, neck vein distention, ascites, tongue furrows, and mental status indicators such as anxiety, restlessness, confusion, and lethargy.* **LOE = V**

(MR) A systematic review demonstrated that older adults had a higher osmotic point for thirst sensation and a diminished sensitivity to thirst relative to younger adults (Kenney & Chiu, 2001).

(MR) A quasi-experimental study demonstrated that elderly residents ($N = 12$) in a long-term care setting demonstrated a significant increase in thirst (measured using a visual analogue scale) during dehydration (O'Neill et al., 1997).

(MR) A systematic review demonstrated that thirst sensation usually occurred when total body water loss reached 1% to 2% of body mass (Armstrong, 2005).

(MR) A systematic review demonstrated that dehydration by overnight fluid restriction in both young and older individuals results in impaired alertness. In older individuals it also resulted in slower psychomotor processing speed and impaired memory performance (Ritz & Berrut, 2005).

(MR) A systematic review demonstrated that in adults with suspected blood loss, the most helpful physical findings were either severe postural dizziness (preventing measurement of upright vital signs) or a postural pulse increment of 30 beats per minute or more. The finding of mild postural dizziness had no proven value. In patients with vomiting, diarrhea, or decreased oral intake, the presence of a dry axilla supported the diagnosis of hypovolemia, and moist mucous membranes and a tongue without furrows argued against it. In adults, the capillary refill time and poor skin turgor had no proven diagnostic value (McGee et al., 1999).

■ (SP) *Monitor relevant laboratory results: sodium, serum osmolality, BUN/creatinine ratio, hematocrit, urine osmolality, and urine specific gravity.* **LOE = VI**

(NR) In a cohort study, long-term care residents with delirium ($N = 69$) had significantly higher BUN/creatinine ratios than residents who did not experience delirium ($N = 244$) (Culp et al., 2004).

(NR) In a descriptive study, dehydrated older adults ($N = 89$) admitted to the emergency room had significantly lower systolic and diastolic blood pressure and significantly higher BUN but similar creatinine levels compared with nondehydrated adults ($N = 96$) (Bennett et al., 2004).

NR = Nursing Research, **MR** = Multidisciplinary Research, **SP** = Standard of Practice, **EO** = Expert Opinion, **LOE** = Level of Evidence

(MR) In a large-scale descriptive field study of 230 male and female army soldiers, mild dehydration was associated with elevated urinary specific gravity and creatinine but not hematocrit and serum osmolality. Thus, BUN/creatinine ratio may be a sensitive circulatory index of impending hypohydration (Francesconi et al., 1987).

(MR) A quasi-experimental study of elderly residents (N = 12) in a long-term care setting demonstrated a significant increase in plasma osmolality during dehydration (O'Neill et al., 1997).

■ (SP) *Monitor changes from baseline for laboratory results relevant to fluid balance.* **LOE = V**

(MR) A systematic review demonstrated that because many conditions could contribute to volume depletion, a change from baseline in laboratory values was probably more significant than absolute findings in elderly individuals (Weinberg & Minaker, 1995).

■ (NIC) *Monitor hemodynamic status including CVP, MAP, PAP, and PCWP, if available.* **LOE = I**

(MR) A systematic review demonstrated that arterial cannulation, central venous pressure, and pulmonary artery catheterization provided an accurate measurement of intra-arterial pressure to enable decisions about immediate therapy in critically ill patients (Alspach, 2006; Hollenberg et al., 2004).

■ *Replace fluids through oral rehydration (carbohydrate-electrolyte fluids) or IV therapy, as ordered and appropriate.* **LOE = V**

(MR) In a quasi-experimental study of young healthy men (mean age 22 years) (N = 8), IV and oral fluids were equally effective as rehydration treatments following exercise-induced dehydration (Castellani et al., 1997).

(MR) A systematic review demonstrated that sports drinks were easily absorbed by the stomach and would rapidly correct hypertonic dehydration. Sports drinks were more effective than water in promoting recovery from exercise-induced dehydration in younger individuals (Weinberg & Minaker, 1995).

(MR) A systematic review demonstrated that IV fluids may be used to replace fluids, although this may not be practical outside acute care settings (Weinberg & Minaker, 1995).

■ (SP) *Monitor effects of diuretics.* **LOE = VII**

(EO) Diuretics are indicated in the treatment of conditions associated with fluid overload (e.g., chronic heart failure, hypertension). Monitor for potential adverse or side effects associated with the specific medication (Greenberg, 2000).

■ *Encourage oral intake through systematic prompting, as appropriate.* **LOE = II**

(NR) In a descriptive study, a 5-week hydration program consisting of a beverage cart containing a choice of four beverages and individualized fluid goals in long-term care residents (N = 51) resulted in significant increases in total body water, intracellular body water, and extracellular body water as measured by bioelectric impedance analysis (Robinson & Rosher, 2002).

(NR) In a quasi-experimental study, systematically encouraging oral intake by providing 6 ounces of fluid with each medication administration, instituting fluid rounds morning and

RCT = Randomized Controlled (Clinical) Trial, **NIC** = Nursing Interventions Classification, **NOC** = Nursing Outcomes Classification

evening, and "happy hours" or "tea time" twice a week in the late afternoon reduced hydration-linked events in nursing home residents ($N = 49$) (Mentes & Culp, 2003).

(NR) In a descriptive study, the number of ingestion sessions was positively correlated with water intake adequacy in nursing home residents ($N = 99$) (Gaspar, 1999).

(MR) In an RCT, verbal prompting of cognitively impaired nursing home residents ($N = 63$) during the day significantly increased oral intake (Simmons et al., 2001).

▪ *Encourage oral intake by offering preferred fluids.* LOE = II

(NR) In descriptive study involving long-term care residents ($N = 40$), clinical characteristics (dysphagia, cognitive or functional impairment) and inadequate attention to fluid intake by staff contributed to inadequate fluid intake using three different daily fluid intake standards (Kayser-Jones et al., 1999).

(MR) In a quasi-experimental study, healthy men ($N = 18$) aged 23 to 39 years who were habitual caffeine users did not experience an increase in diuresis when ingesting caffeinated fluids compared with noncaffeinated fluids (water and carbonated citrus drink) (Grandjean et al., 2000).

(MR) In an RCT, verbal prompting during the day and offering a variety of beverages to choose from significantly increased oral intake in less cognitively impaired nursing home residents ($N = 63$) (Simmons et al., 2001).

▪ (NIC) (SP) *Encourage significant other to assist patient with feedings, as appropriate.* LOE = IV

(NR) In a descriptive study of a group of nursing home residents ($N = 13$) who "couldn't drink" (i.e., were physically dependent and incapable of accessing or safely consuming fluids or who had difficulty swallowing), 38% developed dehydration events defined as hospitalization for dehydration, intravenous rehydration, or BUN/creatinine ratio greater than 25:1 (Mentes, 2006).

(NR) In a descriptive study of a group of elderly residents ($N = 57$) on geriatric units, there was a significant inverse relationship between dependence score and mean fluid intake (Armstrong-Esther et al., 1996).

(NR) In a descriptive study, long-term care residents ($N = 40$) who had relatives assist them at mealtimes consumed more fluids than residents without families (Kayser-Jones et al., 1999).

Possibly Effective

▪ (NIC) (SP) *Maintain an accurate intake and output record.* LOE = VI

(NR) In a descriptive study, nurses ($N = 34$) asked to estimate amounts of oral, IV, and simulated body fluids deviated significantly for IV cannula leakage and fluid leakage on bed linens (Daffurn et al., 1994).

(NR) In a descriptive study, an estimated 32% of daily intake and output records ($N = 250$) were estimated to be inaccurate or incomplete; 45% of nurses and 80% of physicians believed the data were not always accurate (Chung et al., 2002).

(NR) In a descriptive study, nurses ($N = 47$) working on geriatric units did not find intake and output records useful because they believed the records were inaccurate (Armstrong-Esther et al., 1996).

(MR) A systematic review demonstrated that intake and output may serve as important collaborating data to other information obtained regarding dehydration (Weinberg & Minaker, 1995).

NR = Nursing Research, **MR** = Multidisciplinary Research, **SP** = Standard of Practice, **EO** = Expert Opinion, **LOE** = Level of Evidence

■ *Monitor urine color.* **LOE = IV**

(NR) In a repeated measures design, significant positive associations were found between urine color, urine specific gravity, and urine osmolality and between urine osmolality and serum sodium and BUN/creatinine ratio in males who were hospitalized ($N = 47$) and residents of a short-term rehabilitation unit (Wakefield et al., 2002).

(NR) In a descriptive correlational design, urine color was significantly correlated with urine specific gravity in 98 frail nursing home residents (Mentes et al., 2006).

(MR) In a quasi-experimental study, urine color, urine osmolality, and urine specific gravity were not significantly correlated with plasma osmolality, plasma sodium, or hematocrit, suggesting that hematological measurements are not as sensitive to mild hypohydration as selected urinary indices. Urine color was strongly correlated with urine specific gravity and urine osmolality (Armstrong et al., 1994).

(MR) In a quasi-experimental study, urine color tracked changes in body water as effectively as (or better than) urine osmolality, urine specific gravity, urine volume, plasma osmolality, plasma sodium, and plasma total protein (Armstrong et al., 1998).

■ *Calculate an appropriate daily fluid intake amount.* **LOE = IV**

(NR) In a cohort study, residents of a long-term care setting with more than 90% compliance with a weight-based fluid intake goal demonstrated significantly higher extracellular fluid volume and lower urine leukocyte counts (Culp et al., 2003).

(MR) In a descriptive study, three standards for calculating recommended fluid intake were tested in nursing home residents ($N = 40$). The standard 100 mL/kg for first 10 kg, 50 mL/kg for next 10 kg, and 15 mL for remaining kg adjusted for extremes in body weight was more reasonable for patients whether they were of normal weight, underweight, or overweight. This standard more closely supports other recommendations of 1500 to 2000 mL fluid intake per day (Chidester & Spangler, 1997).

(MR) In a descriptive study, interviews/examinations of 883 Hispanic and non-Hispanic white men and women (mean age of 74.1 years) were conducted. Seventy-one percent estimated that their usual fluid intake was equal to or exceeded six glasses per day. Significant hypernatremia was not observed in the 227 individuals ingesting less than this; hyponatremia was rare in this population. Encouraging a fluid intake of eight glasses (2 L) per day seemed to serve little useful purpose (Lindeman et al., 2000).

(MR) In an RCT, advice to increase daily fluid intake by 1.5 L had no negative effect in healthy men aged 55 to 75 ($N = 141$). On average, intervention subjects increased daily intake by 1 L, with no significant changes in blood pressure, sodium level, glomerular filtration rate, or quality of life (Spigt et al., 2006).

(MR) A systematic review demonstrated that there was a dearth of research data on estimating daily water requirements for healthy individuals and even less in special populations (e.g., individuals younger than 18, elderly, and pregnant or lactating women) (IOM, 2004).

Not Effective

■ (NIC) *Administer blood products (e.g., platelets and fresh frozen plasma), as appropriate.* **LOE = I**

(MR) In an RCT comparing 4% albumin and normal saline for intravascular fluid resuscitation, patients in both groups had similar outcomes (Finfer et al., 2004).

RCT = Randomized Controlled (Clinical) Trial, **NIC** = Nursing Interventions Classification, **NOC** = Nursing Outcomes Classification

(MR) A systematic review demonstrated that there was no evidence to support the use of albumin over saline for fluid management to reduce mortality in critically ill patients, including those with burns and hypoalbuminemia (Alderson et al., 2004).

(MR) A systematic review demonstrated that there was no evidence that resuscitation with colloids reduced risk of death, compared with crystalloids, in patients with trauma, burns, or following surgery (Roberts et al., 2004).

(MR) A systematic review demonstrated that there was no evidence to support the use of colloids over crystalloids for volume replacement for critically ill patients (Schierhout & Roberts, 1998).

Possibly Harmful

■ (NIC) *Insert a urinary catheter, if appropriate.* **LOE = I**

(MR) A systematic review demonstrated that it was best to avoid use of a catheter if possible and to remove it as soon as possible (Niel-Weise & van den Broek, 2005).

(MR) A systematic review demonstrated that nosocomial urinary tract infection was the most common acquired infection in both hospitals and nursing homes and was usually associated with urinary catheterization (Warren, 2001).

(MR) A systematic review demonstrated that after weighing the risk-benefit ratio, short-term urinary catheterization may be appropriate in critically ill patients requiring accurate measurement of urinary output (Cravens & Zweig, 2000).

OUTCOME MEASUREMENT

FLUID BALANCE (NOC)

Definition: Water balance in the intracellular and extracellular components of the body.
Fluid Balance as evidenced by the following selected NOC indicators:
- Blood pressure
- Radial pulse rate
- Moist mucous membranes
- Central venous pressure
- Mean arterial pressure
- Pulmonary wedge pressure
- Hematocrit
- Urine specific gravity

(Rate each indicator of **Fluid Balance:** 1 = severely compromised, 2 = substantially compromised, 3 = moderately compromised, 4 = mildly compromised, 5 = not compromised) (Moorhead et al., 2004).

Additional non-NOC indicators:
- Fluid intake
- Food intake
- Urine output
- Pulmonary artery pressure
- Serum sodium

OUTCOME MEASUREMENT—*cont'd*

- Serum osmolality
- BUN/creatinine ratio
- Urine color
- Urine osmolality
- Neck vein distention
- Orthostatic blood pressure
- Breath sounds
- Mental status
- Abdominal girth/ascites
- Peripheral edema
- Thirst
- Postural dizziness
- Tongue furrows

REFERENCES

Alderson P, Bunn F, Lefebvre C, Li WP, Li L, Roberts I, et al. (2004). Human albumin solution for resuscitation and volume expansion in critically ill patients. *Cochrane Database Syst Rev,* (4):CD001208.

Alspach JG (Ed). (2006). *Core curriculum for critical care nursing,* 6th ed. St. Louis: Saunders.

Armstrong LE. (2005). Hydration assessment techniques. *Nutr Rev,* 63(6 Pt 2):S40-S54.

Armstrong LE, Maresh CM, Castellani JW, Bergeron MF, Kenefick RW, LaGasse KE, et al. (1994). Urinary indices of hydration status. *Int J Sport Nutr,* 4(3):265-279.

Armstrong LE, Soto JA, Hacker FT Jr, Casa DJ, Kavouras SA, Maresh CM. (1998). Urinary indices during dehydration, exercise, and rehydration. *Int J Sport Nutr,* 8(4):345-355.

Armstrong-Esther CA, Browne KD, Armstrong-Esther DC, Sander L. (1996). The institutionalized elderly: Dry to the bone! *Int J Nurs Stud,* 33(6):619-628.

Bennett JA, Thomas V, Riegel B. (2004). Unrecognized chronic dehydration in older adults: Examining prevalence rate and risk factors. *J Gerontol Nurs,* 30(11):22-28.

Castellani JW, Maresh CM, Armstrong LE, Kenefick RW, Riebe D, Echegaray M, et al. (1997). Intravenous vs. oral rehydration: Effects on subsequent exercise-heat stress. *J Appl Physiol,* 82(3):799-806.

Chidester JC, Spangler AA. (1997). Fluid intake in the institutionalized elderly. *J Am Diet Assoc,* 97(1):23-28.

Chung LH, Chong S, French P. (2002). The efficiency of fluid balance charting: An evidence-based management project. *J Nurs Manag,* 10(2):103-113.

Cravens DD, Zweig S. (2000). Urinary catheter management. *Am Fam Physician,* 61(2):369-376.

Culp K, Mentes J, Wakefield B. (2003). Hydration and acute confusion in long-term care residents. *West J Nurs Res,* 25(3):251-266; discussion 267-273.

Culp KR, Wakefield B, Dyck MJ, Cacchione PZ, DeCrane S, Decker S. (2004). Bioelectrical impedance analysis and other hydration parameters as risk factors for delirium in rural nursing home residents. *J Gerontol A Biol Sci Med Sci,* 59(8):813-817.

Daffurn K, Hillman KM, Bauman A, Lum M, Crispin C, Ince L. (1994). Fluid balance charts: Do they measure up? *Br J Nurs,* 3(16):816-820.

Deaton C, Bennett JA, Riegel B. (2004). State of the science for care of older adults with heart disease. *Nurs Clin North Am,* 39(3):495-528.

Dochterman JM, Bulechek GM (Eds). (2004). *Nursing Interventions Classification (NIC),* 4th ed. St. Louis: Mosby.

Ferry M. (2005). Strategies for ensuring good hydration in the elderly. *Nutr Rev,* 63(6 Pt 2):S22-S29.

Finfer S, Bellomo R, Boyce N, French J, Myburgh J, Norton R, et al. (2004). A comparison of albumin and saline for fluid resuscitation in the intensive care unit. *N Engl J Med,* 350(22):2247-2256.

Francesconi RP, Hubbard RW, Szlyk PC, Schnakenberg D, Carlson D, Leva N, et al. (1987). Urinary and hematologic indexes of hypohydration. *J Appl Physiol,* 62(3):1271-1276.

Gaspar PM. (1999). Water intake of nursing home residents. *J Gerontol Nurs,* 25(4):23-29.

Grandjean AC, Reimers KJ, Bannick KE, Haven MC. (2000). The effect of caffeinated, non-caffeinated, caloric and non-caloric beverages on hydration. *J Am Coll Nutr,* 19(5):591-600.

Greenberg A. (2000). Diuretic complications. *Am J Med Sci,* 319(1):10-24.

Hollenberg SM, Ahrens TS, Annane D, Astiz ME, Chalfin DB, Dasta JF, et al. (2004). Practice parameters for hemodynamic support of sepsis in adult patients: 2004 update. *Crit Care Med,* 32(9):1928-1948.

Institute of Medicine (IOM). (2004). *Dietary reference intakes for water, potassium, sodium, chloride, and sulfate.* Washington DC: The National Academies Press.

Jaarsma T, Abu-Saad HH, Halfens R, Dracup K. (1997). "Maintaining the balance"–nursing care of patients with chronic heart failure. *Int J Nurs Stud,* 34(3):213-221.

Kayser-Jones J, Schell ES, Porter C, Barbaccia JC, Shaw H. (1999). Factors contributing to dehydration in nursing homes: Inadequate staffing and lack of professional supervision. *J Am Geriatr Soc,* 47(10):1187-1194.

Kenney WL, Chiu P. (2001). Influence of age on thirst and fluid intake. *Med Sci Sports Exerc,* 33(9):1524-1532.

Lindeman RD, Romero LJ, Liang HC, Baumgartner RN, Koehler KM, Garry PJ. (2000). Do elderly persons need to be encouraged to drink more fluids? *J Gerontol A Biol Sci Med Sci,* 55(7):M361-M365.

Linton AD, Maebius NK. (2003). *Introduction to medical-surgical nursing,* 3rd ed. Philadelphia: Saunders.

McGee S, Abernethy WB 3rd, Simel DL. (1999). The rational clinical examination. Is this patient hypovolemic? *JAMA,* 281(11):1022-1029.

Mentes JC. (2006). A typology of oral hydration problems exhibited by frail nursing home residents. *J Gerontol Nurs,* 32(1):13-19.

Mentes JC, Culp K. (2003). Reducing hydration-linked events in nursing home residents. *Clin Nurs Res,* 12(3):210-225; discussion 226-228.

Mentes JC, Wakefield B, Culp K. (2006). Use of a urine color chart to monitor hydration status in nursing home residents. *Biol Res Nurs,* 7(3):197-203.

Moorhead M, Johnson M, Maas M (Eds). (2004). *Nursing Outcomes Classification (NOC),* 3rd ed. St. Louis: Mosby.

Niel-Weise BS, van den Broek PJ. (2005). Urinary catheter policies for short-term bladder drainage in adults. *Cochrane Database Syst Rev,* (3):CD004203.

O'Neill PA, Duggan J, Davies I. (1997). Response to dehydration in elderly patients in long-term care. *Aging (Milano),* 9(5):372-377.

Ritz P, Berrut G. (2005). The importance of good hydration for day-to-day health. *Nutr Rev,* 63(6 Pt 2):S6-S13.

Roberts I, Alderson P, Bunn F, Chinnock P, Ker K, Schierhout G. (2004). Colloids versus crystalloids for fluid resuscitation in critically ill patients. *Cochrane Database Syst Rev,* (4):CD000567.

Robinson SB, Rosher RB. (2002). Can a beverage cart help improve hydration? *Geriatr Nurs,* 23(4):208-211.

Schierhout G & Roberts I. (1998). Fluid resuscitation with colloid or crystalloid solutions in critically ill patients: A systematic review of randomised trials. *BMJ,* 316(7136):961-964.

Simmons SF, Alessi C, Schnelle JF. (2001). An intervention to increase fluid intake in nursing home residents: Prompting and preference compliance. *J Am Geriatr Soc,* 49(7):926-933.

Spigt MG, Knottnerus JA, Westerterp KR, Olde Rikkert MG, Schayck CP. (2006). The effects of 6 months of increased water intake on blood sodium, glomerular filtration rate, blood pressure, and quality of life in elderly (aged 55-75) men. *J Am Geriatr Soc,* 54(3):438-443.

Wakefield B, Mentes J, Diggelmann L, Culp K. (2002). Monitoring hydration status in elderly veterans. *West J Nurs Res,* 24(2):132-142.

Warren JW. (2001). Catheter-associated urinary tract infections. *Int J Antimicrob Agents,* 17(4):299-303.

Weinberg AD, Minaker KL. (1995). Dehydration. Evaluation and management in older adults. Council on Scientific Affairs, American Medical Association. *JAMA,* 274(19):1552-1556.

NR = Nursing Research, **MR** = Multidisciplinary Research, **SP** = Standard of Practice, **EO** = Expert Opinion, **LOE** = Level of Evidence

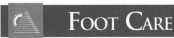

FOOT CARE

Suzanne Lynn Williamson, BSN, RN, CDE

NIC **Definition:** Cleansing and inspecting the feet for the purposes of relaxation, cleanliness, and healthy skin (Dochterman & Bulechek, 2004).

NURSING ACTIVITIES

Effective

■ **NIC** *Inspect skin for irritation, cracking lesions, corns, calluses, deformities or edema, and proper footwear.* **LOE = I**

NR A prospective, randomized, single-center, two-group design ($N = 40$) demonstrated that individualized educational intervention about standard foot care topics improved patients' foot care knowledge and self-efficacy as well as self-care practices. Incorporating interventions such as foot inspection into routine home care services may enhance the quality of care and decrease the incidence of lower extremity complications (Corbett, 2003).

MR An RCT ($N = 530$) demonstrated that education and primary preventive measures provided individually by a podiatrist resulted in a significant improvement in knowledge, foot care practices, and the prevalence of minor foot problems (Hämäläinen et al., 1998).

NR An RCT ($N = 50$) demonstrated that observation and inspection of the feet probably had the greatest value in terms of preventing circulatory complications of the lower extremities (Kruger & Guthrie, 1992).

■ *Cleanse feet in warm, soapy water and dry carefully, especially between toes. After drying, apply lotion as needed.* **LOE = I**

MR A systematic review demonstrated that dry, scaly skin was susceptible to crack or ulcerate providing an entry site for bacteria and that oils or skin creams with lanolin could be used to prevent skin breakdown (Pinzur et al., 2005).

NR A prospective, randomized, single-center, two-group design ($N = 40$) demonstrated that the best preintervention self-care behaviors were reported for washing feet in warm (versus hot or cold) water and applying lotion to dry skin, with 89% of participants stating that they performed these activities (Corbett, 2003).

Possibly Effective

No applicable published research was found in this category.

Not Effective

No applicable published research was found in this category.

RCT = Randomized Controlled (Clinical) Trial, **NIC** = Nursing Interventions Classification, **NOC** = Nursing Outcomes Classification

Possibly Harmful

No applicable published research was found in this category.

OUTCOME MEASUREMENT

TISSUE PERFUSION: PERIPHERAL   NOC

Definition: Adequacy of blood flow through the small vessels of the extremities to maintain tissue function.

Tissue Perfusion: Peripheral as evidenced by the following selected NOC indicators:

• Skin integrity
• Sensation
• Skin color
• Muscle function

(Rate each indicator of **Tissue Perfusion: Peripheral:** 1 = severely compromised, 2 = substantially compromised, 3 = moderately compromised, 4 = mildly compromised, 5 = not compromised) (Moorhead et al., 2004).

REFERENCES

Corbett CF. (2003). A randomized pilot study of improving foot care in home health patients with diabetes. *Diabetes educ*, 29(2):273-282.

Dochterman JM, Bulechek GM (Eds). (2004). *Nursing Interventions Classification (NIC)*, 4th ed. St. Louis: Mosby.

Hämäläinen H, Rönnemaa T, Toikka T, Liukkonen I. (1998). Long-term effects of one year of intensified podiatric activities on foot-care knowledge and self-care habits in patients with diabetes. *Diabetes Educ*, 24(6):734-740.

Kruger S, Guthrie D. (1992). Foot care: Knowledge retention and self-care practices. *Diabetes Educ*, 18(6):487-490.

Moorhead M, Johnson M, Maas M (Eds). (2004). *Nursing Outcomes Classification (NOC)*, 3rd ed. St. Louis: Mosby.

Pinzur MS, Slovenkai MP, Trepman E, Shields NN; Diabetes Committee of the American Orthopaedic Foot and Ankle Society. (2005). Guidelines for diabetic foot care: Recommendations endorsed by the Diabetes Committee of the American Orthopaedic Foot and Ankle Society. *Foot Ankle Int*, 26(1):113-119.

 # GREEN HOUSE CONCEPT

Betty J. Ackley, MSN, EdS, RN

Definition: "A small intentional community for a group of elders and staff. It is a place that focuses on life, and its heart is found in the relationships that flourish there" (The Green House Concept, 2006, p. 1).

The Green House concept takes place in a home that contains 8 to 10 residents. The home is designed to be comfortable and warm, and the presence of medical equipment is minimized. Residents are expected to participate in daily activities in the household as their condition permits. "Its primary purpose is to serve as a place where elders can receive assistance and support with activities of daily living and clinical care, with the assistance and care not becoming the focus of their existence . . . the Green House is intended to de-institutionalize long-term care by eliminating large nursing facilities and creating habilitative, social settings" (The Green House Concept, 2006, p. 1).

The Green House Concept is not a nursing intervention. It is a concept of care for extended care facilities that influences how care is delivered, and it is included here because a large number of nurses are employed in extended care.

On November 7, 2005 the Robert Wood Johnson Foundation announced that they had awarded a $10 million grant to help encourage the adoption of the concept. The goal is to have at least one Green House in every state (Daitz, 2005).

(Note: The Green House is a registered trademark. Any facility desiring to use the term must have an executed license agreement.)

NURSING ACTIVITIES

Effective

No applicable published research was found in this category.

Possibly Effective

■ *Use the Green House concept to decrease boredom, helplessness, and depression in extended care residents.* **LOE = VI**

(MR) A descriptive study ($N = 40$) demonstrated that with the use of the Green House concept including the environment, the results have been positive for residents, family, and staff. Many residents stopped using wheelchairs because they were able to navigate the short distances in the house. Residents and families reported high levels of satisfaction with the privacy afforded by the private rooms. The residents frequently went outdoors, and when indoors they tended to cluster in the hearth room, at the kitchen table, or in the recliners in the living area. Families took advantage of the many areas for visiting and regularly stayed for meals with the residents. Staff turnover and absenteeism decreased. One problem that arose was resistance to implementation of the concept from professional staff, including nurses, which may have been due to lack of sufficient education for the professional staff (Rabig et al., 2006).

(EO) Many elderly people enter nursing homes and become bored, lonely, and lose their human spirit. The Green House Project was designed to help elderly people thrive in a home setting where they have control over their lives, privacy, and supportive relationships. Each person is expected to contribute to the home in any way possible. Care is provided by the Shahbazim, who serves as a homemaker and friend. Nurses provide care only as required, working with the person and the Shahbazim (Thomas, 2004).

Not Effective

No applicable published research was found in this category.

Possibly Harmful

No applicable published research was found in this category.

RCT = Randomized Controlled (Clinical) Trial, **NIC** = Nursing Interventions Classification, **NOC** = Nursing Outcomes Classification

OUTCOME MEASUREMENT

PERSONAL WELL-BEING NOC

Definition: Extent of positive perception of one's health status and life circumstances.
Personal Well-Being as evidenced by the following selected NOC indicators:
- Performance of activities of daily living
- Performance of usual roles
- Psychological health
- Social relationships
- Physical health
- Cognitive function
- Ability to cope
- Ability to relax

(Rate each indicator of **Personal Well-Being:** 1 = not at all satisfied, 2 = somewhat satisfied, 3 = moderately satisfied, 4 = very satisfied, 5 = completely satisfied) (Moorhead et al., 2004).

REFERENCES

Daitz A. (2005). *Developing small community homes as alternatives to nursing homes.* The Robert Wood Johnson Foundation News Release. November 7, 2005. Available online: http://www.ncbdc.org. Retrieved on May 25, 2007.

Moorhead M, Johnson M, Maas M (Eds). (2004). *Nursing Outcomes Classification (NOC),* 3rd ed. St. Louis: Mosby.

NCB Development Corporation. (2006). *The Green House® Concept.* (2006). Available online: http://www.ncbdc.org. Retrieved on May 25, 2007.

Rabig J, Thomas W, Kane RA, Cutler LJ, McAlilly S. (2006). Radical redesign of nursing homes: Applying the green house concept in Tupelo, Mississippi. *Gerontologist,* 46(4):533-539.

Thomas WH. (2004). *What are old people for? How elders will save the world.* Acton, MA: Van Der Wyke and Burnham.

 # GRIEF WORK FACILITATION

Ariella Lang, PhD, RN; Susan Froude, RN, MScN; Andrea Maria Laizner, PhD, RN; Patricia McCarthy, RN, MSc(A); Andrea R. Fleiszer, RN, BN, BSc

NIC **Definition:** Assistance with the resolution of a significant loss (Dochterman & Bulechek, 2004.)

NURSING ACTIVITIES

Effective

No applicable published research was found in this category.

Possibly Effective

■ *Acknowledge and validate the experiences of loss and bereavement. This is central to a caring relationship with bereaved individuals and their families, which may be demonstrated by letting them know their grieving is recognized and understood, supporting opportunities for them to find meaning and make sense of the loss, encouraging the telling of the story including their perceptions related to the death, and showing respect for spiritual and cultural preferences and practices. Be careful not to tell grieving individuals your own experiences with loss and grieving or that the death was for the best.* **LOE = V**

  (NR) A qualitative study ($N = 40$) of bereaved parents (perinatal losses) highlighted the importance of having their feelings acknowledged by health care professionals. This is a significant part of feeling well cared for (Ujda & Bendiksen, 2000).

  (MR) A qualitative study ($N = 20$) of bereaved parents identified that health care providers' demonstrations of compassion and empathy were helpful interventions (Janzen et al., 2003-2004).

  (NR) A qualitative study ($N = 14$ participants from various cultural backgrounds) described the presence of different cultural practices, beliefs, ceremonies, and rituals around the death, reflecting a range of perspectives and reactions (Lobar et al., 2006).

  (MR) A systematic review reported that probably the most important component in all bereavement interventions was the compassionate and empathically attuned caregiver who provided mourners with a healing experience of being understood and supported in their journey of loss (Jordan & Neimeyer, 2003).

■ *Provide anticipatory guidance to individuals and their families to alleviate some of the distress associated with the range and diversity of physical, emotional, and social reactions related to the loss. Explain that strong reactions may surface unexpectedly at different times.* **LOE = V**

  (NR) A qualitative study ($N = 6$ families) showed that the common belief about the need for resolving grief (as measured by absence) was not helpful to the bereaved, but rather grief's presence may contribute to a new relationship with the deceased over time (Moules et al., 2004).

  (NR) A qualitative study ($N = 10$ children) identified needs and issues that were particular to bereaved school-age children and adolescents (Nolbris & Hellstrom, 2005).

  (EO) Individuals grieve in the context of their family, and differences in grieving within the family can contribute to additional pain (Gilbert, 1996).

  (NR) A quasi-experimental study ($N = 70$, $N = 155$ comparison) examined the impact of supportive telephone calls to bereaved individuals following a death. It showed that supportive outreach was correlated with lower grief scores (Kaunonen et al., 2000).

  (NR) A quantitative longitudinal prospective study ($N = 110$ bereaved couples) showed that marital and social supports were important health predictors for men and women individually and as a couple (Lang et al., 2004).

RCT = Randomized Controlled (Clinical) Trial, **NIC** = Nursing Interventions Classification, **NOC** = Nursing Outcomes Classification

■ *Consider the family as the unit of care. The family must be understood in terms of the relationships among its members, not only as a collection of individuals.* **LOE = V**

(NR) A quantitative longitudinal prospective study ($N = 110$ bereaved couples) that tested an explanatory model of health revealed the importance of caring for the marital and family units (Lang et al., 2004).

(EO) When families come together to share the grief experience, distress can be mitigated by the strengthening of relationships among family members (Walsh & McGoldrick, 1991).

(EO) "Grief is a family affair"; family dynamics and structure influence the meanings that family members construe about the loss and about learning to live in the world without the lost one (Nadeau, 2001).

(EO) Acknowledging that a death involves not only the loss of an individual but also a loss of "the family structure as it was" is important (Rycroft & Perlesz, 2001).

■ *Recognize that bereavement care is based on use of therapeutic communication, which is more than words; it attends to genuine presence, active listening, conveying empathy and compassion, as well as appropriate touch.* **LOE = V**

(NR) A mixed-method study ($N = 185$ women) showed that caring-based interventions resulted in "decreased overall emotional disturbance, anger, and depression in the first year after miscarriage" (Swanson, 1999).

(NR) A qualitative study ($N = 57$ interviews) advised that talking about the death event with caregivers following the loss was beneficial for the grieving process of bereaved parents (Saflund et al., 2004).

(NR) A qualitative study ($N = 13$) showed that active listening, understanding the experiences, and communicating empathy were the most important in "what made a difference" for bereaved parents (Caelli et al., 2002).

(NR) A descriptive study ($N = 45$) of bereaved parents evaluating the support they received on the day the child died and since the death reported that staff lacked compassion and were unable to interact effectively and support parents (Davies & Connaughty, 2002).

(EO) Effective communication with bereaved parents requires ongoing dialogue throughout all phases of care. Also, skilled professionals should serve as mentors for their colleagues to ensure the ongoing availability of competent clinicians (Kavanaugh & Paton, 2001).

(EO) Communication with the family and within the family is an important component of bereavement care. Family members use communication as a means of co-constructing a shared reality to help them adapt to changing circumstances (Shapiro, 1994).

(EO) Family members and health care professionals tend to evade talking directly about the death and the presence of grief, motivated by a belief that silence protects against sadness and distress (Wright et al., 1996).

Not Effective

No applicable published research was found in this category.

Possibly Harmful

No applicable published research was found in this category.

NR = Nursing Research, **MR** = Multidisciplinary Research, **SP** = Standard of Practice, **EO** = Expert Opinion, **LOE** = Level of Evidence

Grief may be a lifelong, ever-changing, waxing and waning experience (Moules et al., 2004; Moules, 1998; Stroebe et al., 2001). Nursing care of individuals and families must be approached with receptivity to new understandings of the experience (Becvar, 2001). The bereaved have difficulty recognizing that they may need social support or professional help and are often unable to seek such resources for themselves and their family. Certain situational, personal, and interpersonal factors may have an impact on the risk for poor outcomes (i.e., type of loss—homicides, suicides, trauma, pediatric—or availability of social support).

Nurses can be pivotal in facilitating grief work through caring practices centered around several ways of "being with" and caring for the bereaved (Swanson, 1993). Lang's (2005) supportive bereavement care model, an integrated, evidence-based, theoretical framework, can be used to guide nurses in their practice and research activities related to caring for individuals and their families around a significant loss.

OUTCOME MEASUREMENT

GRIEF RESOLUTION ⬭NOC⬭

(Please refer to *Nursing Outcomes Classification* [Moorhead et al., 2004] for the **Grief Resolution** outcome.)

REFERENCES

Becvar DS. (2001). *In the presence of grief: Helping family members resolve death, dying, and bereavement issues.* New York: Guilford Press.

Caelli K, Downie J, Letendre A. (2002). Parents' experiences of midwife-managed care following the loss of a baby in a previous pregnancy. *J Adv Nurs,* 39(2):127-136.

Davies B, Connaughty S. (2002). Pediatric end-of-life care: Lessons learned from parents. *J Nurs Adm,* 32(1):5-6.

Dochterman JM, Bulechek GM (Eds). (2004). *Nursing Interventions Classification (NIC),* 4th ed. St. Louis: Mosby.

Gilbert KR. (1996). "We've had the same loss, why don't we have the same grief?": Loss and differential grief in families. *Death Stud,* 20 (3):269-283.

Janzen L, Cadell S, Westhues A. (2003-2004). From death notification through the funeral: Bereaved parents' experiences and their advice to professionals. *Omega,* 48(2):149-164.

Jordan JR, Neimeyer RA. (2003). Does grief counseling work? *Death Stud,* 27(9):765-786.

Kaunonen M, Tarkka MT, Laippala P, Paunonen-Ilmonen M. (2000). The impact of supportive telephone call intervention on grief after the death of a family member. *Cancer Nurs,* 23(6):483-491.

Kavanaugh K, Paton JB. (2001). Communicating with parents who experience a perinatal loss. *Illn Crisis Loss,* 9(4):369-380.

Lang A. (2005). Supportive bereavement care model. Paper presented at the VON Canada Annual General Meeting, St. John, NB, November 2005.

Lang A, Goulet C, Amsel R. (2004). Explanatory model of health in bereaved parents post-fetal/infant death. *Int J Nurs Stud,* 41(8):869-880.

Lobar SL, Youngblut JM, Brooten D. (2006). Cross-cultural beliefs, ceremonies, and rituals surrounding death of a loved one. *Pediatr Nurs,* 32(1):44-50.

Moorhead M, Johnson M, Maas M (Eds). (2004). *Nursing Outcomes Classification (NOC),* 3rd ed. St. Louis: Mosby.

Moules NJ. (1998). Legitimizing grief: Challenging beliefs that constrain. *J Fam Nurs,* 4(2):142-166.

Moules NJ, Simonson K, Prins M, Angus P, Bell JM. (2004). Making room for grief: Walking backwards and living forward. *Nurs Inq,* 11(2):99-107.

Nadeau JW. (2001). Family reconstruction of meaning. In Neimeyer RA (Ed). *Meaning reconstruction & the experience of loss*. Washington, DC: American Psychological Association.

Nolbris M, Hellstrom AL. (2005). Siblings' needs and issues when a brother or sister dies of cancer. *J Pediatr Oncol Nurs*, 22(4):227-233.

Rycroft P, Perlesz A. (2001). Speaking the unspeakable: Reclaiming grief and loss in family life. *Aust N Z J Fam Ther*, 22(2):57-65.

Saflund K, Sjogren B, Wredling R. (2004). The role of caregivers after a stillbirth: Views and experiences of parents. *Birth*, 31(2):132-137.

Shapiro ER. (1994). *Grief as a family process: A developmental approach to clinical practice*. New York: Guilford Press.

Stroebe MS, Hansson RO, Stroebe W, Schut H. (2001). Introduction: Concepts and issues in contemporary research on bereavement. In Stroebe MS, Hansson RO, Stroebe W, Schut H (Eds). *Handbook of bereavement research: Consequences, coping, and care*. Washington, DC: American Psychological Association, pp 3-22.

Swanson KM. (1993). Nursing as informed caring for the well-being of others. *Image J Nurs Sch*, 25(4): 352-357.

Swanson KM. (1999). Research-based practice with women who have had miscarriages. *Image J Nurs Sch*, 31(4):339-345.

Ujda RM, Bendiksen R. (2000). Health care provider support and grief after perinatal loss: A qualitative study. *Illn Crisis Loss*, 8(3):265-285.

Walsh F, McGoldrick M. (1991). Loss and the family: A systemic perspective. In Walsh F, McGoldrick M (Eds). *Living beyond loss: Death in the family*. New York: Norton Publishing.

Wright LM, Watson WL, Bell JM. (1996). *Beliefs: The heart of healing in families and illness*. New York: Basic Books.

GUIDED IMAGERY

Christine A. Wynd, PhD, RN, CNAA

NIC **Definition:** Purposeful use of imagination to achieve relaxation and/or direct attention away from undesirable sensations (Dochterman & Bulechek, 2004).

NURSING ACTIVITIES

Effective

■ *Use guided imagery to decrease pain and anxiety in patients experiencing acute or chronic pain.* **LOE = II**

NR A pilot study using a two-group experimental repeated measures design ($N = 13$) demonstrated that guided imagery decreased anxiety and pain in older adult patients receiving joint replacement surgery. Hospital length of stay was also decreased (Antall & Kresevic, 2004).

NR A quasi-experimental study demonstrated less pain but no changes in power in adults ($N = 42$) with chronic pain (Lewandowski, 2004).

MR An RCT studying fibromyalgia patients ($N = 55$) compared the use of pleasant imagery and attention imagery versus routine care and demonstrated that pleasant imagery significantly decreased pain over the study period of 28 days (Fors et al., 2002).

NR = Nursing Research, **MR** = Multidisciplinary Research, **SP** = Standard of Practice, **EO** = Expert Opinion, **LOE** = Level of Evidence

(NR) A pilot, quasi-experimental study ($N = 28$) was conducted with a group of older adults suffering osteoarthritis and demonstrated that the use of guided imagery, along with progressive muscle relaxation, significantly reduced mobility difficulties and pain after 12 days of use (Baird & Sands, 2004).

(NR) A mixed-method design was used to examine how verbal descriptors of pain changed with the use of guided imagery in chronic pain patients ($N = 42$) and showed that those using guided imagery experienced a change in their perception of pain (Lewandowski et al., 2005).

(NR) A systematic literature review of studies involving cancer patients and pain included two imagery studies demonstrating positive results: (1) guided imagery improved pain levels in bone marrow transplant patients ($N = 94$), and (2) guided imagery improved pain levels ($N = 67$) in intermediate to advanced stage cancer patients (Wyatt, 2002).

■ *Use guided imagery with smokers to assist with successful smoking cessation.* **LOE = II**

(NR) An RCT ($N = 71$) using guided health imagery as an intervention for smoking cessation and long-term abstinence demonstrated that after 24 months the intervention group had significantly higher rates of smoking cessation and abstinence (Wynd, 2005).

(NR) An experimental repeated measures design ($N = 84$) was used to compare three groups receiving (1) power imagery, (2) relaxation imagery, or (3) placebo-attention control and demonstrated that both imagery groups had higher cessation rates after the completion of the interventions (Wynd, 1992a).

(NR) Smokers ($N = 76$) who successfully completed a smoking cessation program were invited to participate in a series of relapse prevention sessions. The use of an experimental design demonstrated that guided relaxation imagery versus a placebo-attention control resulted in significantly lowered relapse rates and reduced stress (Wynd, 1992b).

Possibly Effective

■ *Use guided imagery to decrease the need for medications in patients experiencing chronic obstructive pulmonary disease (COPD) and asthma.* **LOE = II**

(MR) An RCT of COPD patients ($N = 26$) who used relaxation tapes versus no tapes demonstrated significant differences in partial percentage of oxygen saturation but no changes in heart rate, temperature, or upper thoracic surface electromyography (Louie, 2004).

(MR) An RCT examining the efficacy of mental imaging to decrease asthma symptoms in patients ($N = 33$) found no significant changes in forced expiratory volume, quality of life, or symptom differences. However, 47% of the mental imaging group participants were able to discontinue their asthma medications (Epstein et al., 2004).

■ *Use guided imagery to improve lung function and decrease anxiety in children with asthma.* **LOE = VI**

(MR) Students with asthma ($N = 4$) who used guided imagery were studied through a nonexperimental descriptive design. Seventy-five percent of the participants experienced improved

RCT = Randomized Controlled (Clinical) Trial, **NIC** = Nursing Interventions Classification, **NOC** = Nursing Outcomes Classification

lung function, 100% of participants experienced a decrease in trait anxiety, 50% of participants had a decrease in state anxiety, and 25% reported improved happiness (Dobson et al.,
2005).

(MR) Students with asthma ($N = 4$) who used guided imagery were studied through a nonexperimental descriptive design. The study demonstrated improved forced expiratory volume
and a decrease in anxiety, and 75% of participants had improved forced expiratory flow rates
(Peck et al., 2003).

■ *Use guided imagery with stroke patients to improve motor function as well as*
relearn trained and untrained tasks. **LOE = II**

(MR) An RCT of subacute stroke patients ($N = 13$) demonstrated that imagery, combined with
standard therapy, resulted in increased scores on the Fugl-Meyer assessment of motor recovery as well as improved scores on the action research arm test over a 6-week period (Page et
al., 2001).

(MR) A prospective RCT of patients suffering a cerebral infarction ($N = 46$) demonstrated that
mental imagery significantly improved relearning in both trained and untrained tasks, leading
to probable retention and generalization of skills and tasks learned in rehabilitation (Liu
et al., 2004a).

(MR) A case study ($N = 2$) using mental imagery in poststroke patients found improved
relearning of tasks and enhancement of patients' day-to-day functioning with an increase in
attention and sequential processing functions but no change in other cognitive or motor
functions (Liu et al., 2004b).

■ *Use guided imagery in patients with cancer as an adjunct to traditional pain*
medication and to improve quality of life. **LOE = II**

(NR) A one-group, pretest/post-test design demonstrated that patients ($N = 62$) with cancer
pain experienced decreased pain intensity after imagery utilization and that previous
positive experiences with imagery were significant predictors of enhanced pain tolerance
(Kwekkeboom et al., 2003).

(NR) In an RCT ($N = 56$), there were no significant differences among four treatment groups
(progressive muscle training, guided imagery training, combined progressive muscle training
and guided imagery training, and control group) on a measure of anxiety. However, there
were significant reductions in depression and increased quality of life for all three treatment
groups (Sloman, 2002).

(MR) A systematic review of the literature demonstrated that guided imagery may be helpful
as an adjuvant therapy (psychosupportive) for cancer patients (Roffe et al., 2005).

(NR) A secondary data analysis from an RCT ($N = 34$) found that patients who used guided
imagery experienced a significant decrease in pain and distress after intervention, but there
were no significant differences between those who used analgesic medications alone and those
who added nonpharmacological interventions (Kwekkeboom, 2001).

(MR) Breast cancer patients ($N = 60$) participated in progressive muscle relaxation and guided
imagery through an RCT. Findings demonstrated reductions in anticipatory nausea and
vomiting and postchemotherapy nausea and vomiting as well as higher quality-of-life scores
(Yoo et al., 2005).

NR = Nursing Research, **MR** = Multidisciplinary Research, **SP** = Standard of Practice, **EO** = Expert Opinion, **LOE** = Level of Evidence

■ *Use guided imagery for improving immune system responses. (Results are inconclusive, although positive effects on mood and well-being are demonstrated.)* **LOE = VI**

(MR) A systematic review of three studies investigating imagery, hypnosis, and relaxation training with immune system activity demonstrated that relaxation and guided imagery improved mood, anxiety, and depression and enhanced immune function in terms of fewer viral infections (Gruzelier, 2002).

(MR) In a case study, one woman with severe dermatomyositis associated with stress used transcendental meditation and visual imagery that resulted in her recovery without use of corticosteroids. The cumulative beneficial influences of imagery and meditation outweighed the negative impact of stress (Collins & Dunn, 2005).

■ *Use guided imagery with invasive procedures to improve patients' satisfaction, mood, and anxiety.* **LOE = II**

(NR) A short review of the literature investigated various nursing interventions (music, massage, therapeutic touch, and guided imagery) and highlighted that these activities could decrease anxiety in patients undergoing cardiac catheterization (McCaffrey & Taylor, 2005).

(MR) A case-control study ($N = 23$) investigating music therapy and relaxation imagery in bone marrow transplant patients found that pain and nausea decreased in the treatment group. There was also a decrease in time to engraftment (Sahler et al., 2003).

(MR) An RCT of patients undergoing conventional colorectal resections ($N = 60$) who were randomly assigned to three groups (guided imagery, progressive muscle relaxation, and control) demonstrated patients' satisfaction with the imagery and relaxation interventions but showed no significant changes in postoperative pain and medication use (Haase et al., 2005).

(NR) An RCT ($N = 150$) comparing five groups (stress management, imagery, touch therapy, remote intercessory prayer, and control) demonstrated that touch therapy, imagery, and stress management all decreased worry/mood and were feasible for use in a critical care unit (Seskevich et al., 2004).

Not Effective

No applicable published research was found in this category.

Possibly Harmful

No applicable published research was found in this category.

Note: Guided imagery is a cost-effective intervention used with minimal risk and demonstrates many positive outcomes when individuals are receptive to participating in the activity. Frequently, studies report small sample sizes with a variety of populations and different diagnoses. Methods of guided imagery delivery vary widely in terms of time, focus, scripts, and the addition of music. Most imagery research is conducted with Caucasians, and more women than men participate in the exercises. Cultural, religious, and gender differences require further investigation.

RCT = Randomized Controlled (Clinical) Trial, **NIC** = Nursing Interventions Classification, **NOC** = Nursing Outcomes Classification

OUTCOME MEASUREMENT

COMFORT LEVEL NOC

Definition: Extent of positive perception of physical and psychological ease.

Comfort Level as evidenced by the following selected NOC indicators:
- Physical well-being
- Symptom control
- Pain control

(Rate each indicator of **Comfort Level:** 1 = not at all satisfied, 2 = somewhat satisfied, 3 = moderately satisfied, 4 = very satisfied, 5 = completely satisfied) (Moorhead et al., 2004).

HEALTH PROMOTING BEHAVIOR NOC

Definition: Personal actions to sustain or increase wellness.

Health Promoting Behavior as evidenced by the following selected NOC indicators:
- Uses effective stress reduction behaviors
- Performs healthy behaviors routinely
- Avoids tobacco use

(Rate each indicator of **Health Promoting Behavior:** 1 = never demonstrated, 2 = rarely demonstrated, 3 = sometimes demonstrated, 4 = often demonstrated, 5 = consistently demonstrated) (Moorhead et al., 2004).

REFERENCES

Antall GF, Kresevic D. (2004). The use of guided imagery to manage pain in an elderly orthopaedic population. *Orthop Nurs*, 23(5):335-340.

Baird CL, Sands L. (2004). A pilot study of the effectiveness of guided imagery with progressive muscle relaxation to reduce chronic pain and mobility difficulties of osteoarthritis. *Pain Manag Nurs*, 5(3): 97-104.

Collins MP, Dunn LF. (2005). The effects of meditation and visual imagery on an immune system disorder: Dermatomyositis. *J Altern Complement Med*, 11(2):275-284.

Dobson RL, Bray MA, Kehle TJ. (2005). Relaxation and guided imagery as an intervention for children with asthma: A replication. *Psychol Sch*, 42(7):707-720.

Dochterman JM, Bulechek GM (Eds). (2004). *Nursing Interventions Classification (NIC)*, 4th ed. St. Louis: Mosby.

Epstein GN, Halper JP, Barrett EA, Birdsall C, McGee M, Baron KP, et al. (2004). A pilot study of mind-body changes in adults with asthma who practice mental imagery. *Altern Ther Health Med*, 10(4):66-71.

Fors EA, Sexton H, Gotestam KG. (2002). The effect of guided imagery and amitriptyline on daily fibromyalgia pain: A prospective, randomized, controlled trial. *J Psychiatr Res*, 36(3):179-187.

Gruzelier JH. (2002). A review of the impact of hypnosis, relaxation, guided imagery and individual differences on aspects of immunity and health. *Stress*, 5(2):147-163.

Haase O, Schwenk W, Hermann C, Muller JM. (2005). Guided imagery and relaxation in conventional colorectal resections: A randomized, controlled, partially blinded trial. *Dis Colon Rectum*, 48(10): 1955-1963.

Kwekkeboom KL. (2001). Pain management strategies used by patients with breast and gynecologic cancer with postoperative pain. *Cancer Nurs*, 24(5):378-386.

Kwekkeboom KL, Kneip J, Pearson L. (2003). A pilot study to predict success with guided imagery for cancer pain. *Pain Manag Nurs*, 4(3):112-123.

Lewandowski W, Good M, Draucker CB. (2005). Changes in the meaning of pain with the use of guided imagery. *Pain Manag Nurs*, 6(2):58-67.

NR = Nursing Research, **MR** = Multidisciplinary Research, **SP** = Standard of Practice, **EO** = Expert Opinion, **LOE** = Level of Evidence

Lewandowski WA. (2004). Patterning of pain and power with guided imagery. *Nurs Sci Q,* 17(3):233-241.

Liu KP, Chan CC, Lee TM, Hui-Chan CW. (2004a). Mental imagery for promoting relearning for people after stroke: A randomized controlled trial. *Arch Phys Med Rehabil,* 85(9):1403-1408.

Liu KP, Chan CC, Lee TM, Hui-Chan CW. (2004b). Mental imagery for relearning of people after brain injury. *Brain Inj,* 18(11):1163-1172.

Louie SW. (2004). The effects of guided imagery relaxation in people with COPD. *Occup Ther Int,* 11(3):145-159.

McCaffrey R, Taylor N. (2005). Effective anxiety treatment prior to diagnostic cardiac catheterization. *Holist Nurs Pract,* 19(2):70-73.

Moorhead M, Johnson M, Maas M (Eds). (2004). *Nursing Outcomes Classification (NOC),* 3rd ed. St. Louis: Mosby.

Page SJ, Levine P, Sisto S, Johnston MV. (2001). A randomized efficacy and feasibility study of imagery in acute stroke. *Clin Rehabil,* 15(3):233-240.

Peck HL, Bray MA, Kehle TJ. (2003). Relaxation and guided imagery: A school-based intervention for children with asthma. *Psychol Sch,* 40(6):657-675.

Roffe L, Schmidt K, Ernst E. (2005). A systematic review of guided imagery as an adjuvant cancer therapy. *Psychooncology,* 14(8):607-617.

Sahler OJ, Hunter BC, Liesveld JL. (2003). The effect of using music therapy with relaxation imagery in the management of patients undergoing bone marrow transplantation: A pilot feasibility study. *Altern Ther Health Med,* 9(6):70-74.

Seskevich JE, Crater SW, Lane JD, Krucof MW. (2004). Beneficial effects of noetic therapies on mood before percutaneous intervention for unstable coronary syndromes. *Nurs Res,* 53(2):116-121.

Sloman R. (2002). Relaxation and imagery for anxiety and depression control in community patients with advanced cancer. *Cancer Nurs,* 25(6):432-435.

Wyatt G. (2002). Complementary therapies. *Cancer Pract,* 10(Suppl 1):S70-S73.

Wynd CA. (1992a). Personal power imagery and relaxation techniques used in smoking cessation programs. *Am J Health Promot,* 6(3):184-189.

Wynd CA. (1992b). Relaxation imagery used for stress reduction in the prevention of smoking relapse. *J Adv Nurs,* 17(3):294-302.

Wynd CA. (2005). Guided health imagery for smoking cessation and long-term abstinence. *J Nurs Scholarsh,* 37(3):245-250.

Yoo HJ, Ahn SH, Kim SB, Kim WK, Han OS. (2005). Efficacy of progressive muscle relaxation training and guided imagery in reducing chemotherapy side effects in patients with breast cancer and in improving their quality of life. *Support Care Cancer,* 13(10):826-833.

 # HALLUCINATION MANAGEMENT   NIC

Susan Brust, MSN, CNS, APNP

> NIC **Definition:** Promoting the safety, comfort, and reality orientation of a patient experiencing hallucinations (Dochterman & Bulechek, 2004).

NURSING ACTIVITIES

Effective

■ **NIC** *Provide antipsychotic and antianxiety medications on a routine and PRN basis.* **LOE = I**

 A systematic review of available data suggested that new-generation antipsychotics have the potential to reduce relapse rates (Leucht et al., 2003).

RCT = Randomized Controlled (Clinical) Trial, **NIC** = Nursing Interventions Classification, **NOC** = Nursing Outcomes Classification

(MR) A systematic review suggested that medications in the conventional neuroleptic, atypical antipsychotic, cholinesterase inhibitor, and serotonergic classes meliorate psychosis and behavioral symptoms in patients with Alzheimer's disease, although the evidence is not conclusive for many medications (Sultzer, 2004).

(MR) A systematic review found that medication treatment for depression with psychosis using a combination of an antidepressant and an antipsychotic may not be more effective than an antidepressant alone. However, combination therapy may be more effective than an antipsychotic alone (Wijkstra et al., 2005).

■ *Provide PRN antianxiety medications as a first-line basis before PRN antipsychotic medications.* **LOE = I**

(NR) A systematic review of the evidence indicated that traditional antipsychotics and benzodiazepines were equally effective in managing acute agitation and other psychotic symptoms. It has been recommended that benzodiazepines should be the first line of action because they do not cause the serious side effects that are common with traditional antipsychotics (Usher & Luck 2004).

(NR) A descriptive study demonstrated a high incidence of PRN psychotropic medication administration compared with similar studies and an excessive reliance on the use of typical antipsychotics over benzodiazepines. This practice is not supported by contemporary literature (Usher et al., 2001).

■ (NIC) *Monitor the patient for medication side effects and desired therapeutic effects.* **LOE = I**

(MR) An RCT ($N = 1460$) confirmed the established relationship between the presence of tardive dyskinesia and age and duration of treatment with antipsychotics (Miller et al., 2005).

(MR) A systematic review demonstrated that neuroleptic-induced akathisia (NIA) was a relatively common side effect of neuroleptics in which patients complained of a subjective sense of restlessness, usually referable to the legs, and had characteristic motor movements. Recognition and treatment of NIA are essential (Adler et al., 1989).

(NR) A descriptive study proposed that the side effects of psychotropic medications made adherence to treatment regimens difficult for many patients (Sin & Gamble, 2003).

■ (NIC) *Establish a trusting interpersonal relationship with the patient.* **LOE = II**

(NR) A systematic review demonstrated that therapeutic interpersonal interactions with patients were an essential competency for advanced practice psychiatric–mental health nurses and should be upheld, promoted, and implemented to improve outcomes (Silverstein, 2006).

(NR) A case study ($N = 6$) revealed that the relationship of patient and nurse was therapeutic, but the degree of positive change from the relationship was difficult to measure (Scanlon, 2006).

(MR) An RCT ($N = 2437$) demonstrated that discrepancies between patients' and practitioners' beliefs about care were an important determinant of trust and satisfaction, and involving patients in the selection of their primary care provider could have an independent positive effect (Krupat et al., 2004).

NR = Nursing Research, **MR** = Multidisciplinary Research, **SP** = Standard of Practice, **EO** = Expert Opinion, **LOE** = Level of Evidence

■ **NIC** *Avoid arguing with the patient about the validity of the hallucinations.* **LOE = VII**

EO "As the dementia becomes more severe, the person may become convinced that what they are hearing or seeing is real. They can find this very frightening. Try to let them know that, although you are not sharing their experience, you understand how very distressing it is for them. Distracting the person may help. There is absolutely no point in arguing about whether or not the things that they are seeing are real" (ASDCR, 2000).

■ **NIC** *Provide medication teaching to the patient and significant others.* **LOE = II**

MR An RCT involving patients with schizophrenia ($N = 1493$) at 57 U.S. sites randomly assigned participants to receive olanzapine, perphenazine, quetiapine, or risperidone for up to 18 months. Ziprasidone was included after its approval by the Food and Drug Administration. The primary aim was to delineate differences in the overall effectiveness of these five treatments. A majority of patients in each group discontinued their assigned treatment owing to inefficacy or intolerable side effects or for other reasons related to the antipsychotic medication (Lieberman et al., 2005).

NR A descriptive study of mental health nurses ($N = 48$) with active patients' caseloads involved completion of a comprehensive questionnaire assessing a number of variables related to medications, including whom the participants felt was primarily responsible for monitoring the side effects of medication, their knowledge skills and confidence in dealing with medication adherence, and their prior education and training in medication adherence strategies. Lack of patients' insight was endorsed as the strongest influence on patients' nonadherence. Over 84% of nurses indicated that they did not have any prior education or training in medication adherence strategies (Coombs et al., 2003).

■ **NIC** *Provide illness teaching to patient/significant others if hallucinations are illness based (e.g., delirium, schizophrenia, and depression).* **LOE = II**

MR An RCT ($N = 236$) suggested that a relatively brief intervention of eight psychoeducational sessions with systematic family involvement in simultaneous groups could considerably improve the treatment of schizophrenia (Pitschel-Walz et al., 2006).

MR An RCT compared effects of an 18-month hallucination-focused integrative treatment (HIT) with routine treatment in schizophrenic patients who persistently heard voices ($N = 63$) on outcomes of subjective burden and psychopathology. Using an intent-to-treat analysis, patients were assessed at baseline, 9, and 18 months with sex, age, education, and illness (hallucination) duration used as covariates. The experimental group experienced significant improvements in hallucinations, distress, and negative content of voices, and these gains were maintained over time, suggesting that HIT was an effective treatment strategy with long-lasting effects for treatment-refractory voice hallucinations (Jenner et al., 2006).

■ *Provide group and/or individual cognitive-behavioral therapy (CBT).* **LOE = I**

MR A 2-year RCT ($N = 121$) demonstrated that cognitive enhancement therapy versus enriched supportive therapy improved cognitive deficits and related behaviors of patients with stable schizophrenia when sufficient exposure to relevant rehabilitation was provided (Hogarty et al., 2004).

MR A systematic review demonstrated that cognitive therapy was an important adjunct to standard treatments of schizophrenia (Rector & Beck, 2002).

RCT = Randomized Controlled (Clinical) Trial, **NIC** = Nursing Interventions Classification, **NOC** = Nursing Outcomes Classification

MR An RCT ($N = 90$) showed that group CBT did improve social functioning, but unless therapy was provided by experienced CBT therapists, hallucinations were not reduced (Wykes et al., 2005).

MR A controlled study ($N = 45$) evaluated CBT with coping training in 45 patients with schizophrenia or a related disorder. Follow-up 2 and 4 years later showed that coping training could improve overall symptomatology including auditory hallucinations and quality of life even over longer periods of time, but a status of persistent disablement indicated a continuing need for mental health care (Hogarty et al., 2004).

■ NIC *Point out, if asked, that you are not experiencing the same stimuli.* **LOE = VII**

EO "As the dementia becomes more severe, the person may become convinced that what they are hearing or seeing is real. They can find this very frightening. Try to let them know that, although you are not sharing their experience, you understand how very distressing it is for them. Distracting the person may help. There is absolutely no point in arguing about whether or not the things that they are seeing are real" (ASDCR, 2000).

Possibly Effective

■ NIC *Provide the patient with opportunities to discuss hallucinations.* **LOE = VI**

NR A case study ($N = 20$) suggested that nurses' responses to auditory hallucinations could be conceptualized by patients as facilitators, barriers, and attributions (Coffey et al., 2004).

NR A case study ($N = 1$) described a patient who was increasingly accepting of his voices and established a clear sense of himself as someone who heard voices after a voices group helped him come to terms with his experience (Corren & Lucas, 2004).

MR A qualitative study found that a hearing-voice group was well received by participants who found sharing their experiences helpful (Conway, 2004).

MR A case study ($N = 2$) demonstrated that the use of narratives or life stories was effective in leading to recovery (Lysaker & Buck, 2006).

■ NIC *Educate family and significant others about ways to deal with the patient who is experiencing hallucinations.* **LOE = III**

MR A descriptive study ($N = 15$) demonstrated that families of patients with psychosis had high levels of engagement and satisfaction with family services (Stanbridge et al., 2003).

NR A controlled study ($N = 154$) demonstrated that psychological distress was significantly lower among caregivers who were older, full-time workers and who experienced lower objective and subjective burdens. Caregivers who had perceived more support from friends and had more contacts with their relatives' primary mental health providers demonstrated significantly higher psychological distress (Provencher et al., 2003). Note: Those who received more support actually experienced more psychological distress.

EO In psychosis with Alzheimer's disease, nonpharmacological interventions should be tried first, including educating families about things to avoid that make behaviors worse or trigger behaviors (Katz & Grossberg, 2005).

■ NIC *Monitor and regulate the level of activity and stimulation in the environment.* **LOE = IV**

MR A controlled study ($N = 35$) found that schizophrenic inpatients treated on a more structured and less stimulating unit showed greater improvement in Brief Psychiatric Rating

NR = Nursing Research, **MR** = Multidisciplinary Research, **SP** = Standard of Practice, **EO** = Expert Opinion, **LOE** = Level of Evidence

Scale ratings during the first 2 days of hospitalization compared with the open-ward group (Cohen & Khan, 1990).

■ **NIC** **SP** *Maintain a consistent routine.* **LOE = VII**

EO In psychosis with Alzheimer's disease, nonpharmacological interventions should be tried first, including the use of consistent routine (Katz & Grossberg, 2005).

■ **NIC** **SP** *Monitor hallucinations for presence of content that is violent or self-harmful.* **LOE = V**

MR A systematic review determined that command hallucinations were not sufficient to produce action in isolation and that a psychological process was involved (Braham et al., 2004). **MR** A qualitative study ($N = 100$) determined that the presence of command auditory hallucinations for suicide (CAHS) did not directly predict suicide attempts. However, individuals who were already at risk for suicidal behavior (e.g., past attempters) may be at increased risk for a suicide attempt when experiencing CAHS (Harkavy-Friedman et al., 2003).

■ **NIC** *Encourage the patient to develop control/responsibility over their own behavior, if ability allows.* **LOE = V**

EO The most important intervention in helping patients manage voices is to help them learn what they can do and/or what circumstances make the voices better or worse (Saenger, 2004). **NR** A systematic review emphasized the need to explore patients' efforts at controlling hallucinations as a foundation for promoting patients' self-monitoring and self-regulation of hallucinatory experiences (Williams, 1989). **MR** A qualitative study ($N = 62$) indicated that many patients monitor symptoms that they associate with changes in their illness and alter their behavior on the basis of their symptoms by self-treatment (McCandless-Glimcher et al., 1986).

■ *Teach patients self-management strategies.* **LOE = III**

NR A descriptive study ($N = 200$) researched 36 self-management strategies for auditory hallucinations. The most commonly used management category was behavioral change, the most common strategy was ignoring auditory hallucinations, and the most common resource was self-learning (Tsai & Ku, 2005). **NR** A controlled study ($N = 62$) showed statistically significant improvement at the end of a 10-week class designed to teach behavioral management strategies in persistent auditory hallucinations (Buccheri et al., 2004).

Not Effective

No applicable published research was found in this category.

Possibly Harmful

■ **NIC** **SP** *Provide for safety and comfort of the patient and others when the patient is unable to control behavior (e.g., limit setting, area restriction, physical restraint, and seclusion).* **LOE = V**

NR A descriptive study ($N = 60$ nursing staff, $N = 29$ patients) suggested that nurses believed seclusion to be very necessary, not very punitive, and a highly therapeutic practice that assisted

RCT = Randomized Controlled (Clinical) Trial, **NIC** = Nursing Interventions Classification, **NOC** = Nursing Outcomes Classification

patients to calm down and feel better. Patients, on the other hand, believed that seclusion was used frequently for minor disturbances and as a means of staff exerting power and control. Patients also believed that seclusion resulted in them feeling punished and had little therapeutic value (Meehan et al., 2004).

(NR) A qualitative study suggested that seclusion was far from a therapeutic experience for the patient and that nurses should consider their own behaviors and intentions when initiating seclusion (Trimmer, 2005).

(NR) A qualitative study ($N = 6$) suggested that the experience of seclusion served as an intensification of already existing feelings of exclusion, rejection, abandonment, and isolation. It was not the act of seclusion that affected patients' negative perception and negative emotional experience but rather the lack of nurse-patient contact during the seclusion experience. When patients coped by regressing, acting out, or taking on a more compliant stance, they appeared to be motivated by a need to connect with staff (Holmes et al., 2004).

Note: Although seclusion is a current standard of practice for violent behavior, more research is needed on the effectiveness of seclusion as an intervention for auditory hallucinations and its effect on the patient in helping or delaying recovery because research suggests that patients find it punitive.

OUTCOME MEASUREMENT

DISTORTED THOUGHT SELF-CONTROL (NOC)

(Please refer to *Nursing Outcomes Classification* [Moorhead et al., 2004] for the **Distorted Thought Self-Control** outcome.)

REFERENCES

Adler LA, Angrist B, Reiter S, Rotrosen J. (1989). Neuroleptic-induced akathisia: A review. *Psychopharmacology,* 97(1):1-11.

Alzheimer's Society of Dementia Care and Research (ASDCR). (2000). *Caring for someone with dementia: Hallucinations and delusions.* Alzheimer's Society Advice Sheet. Available online: http://www.alzheimers. org.uk. Retrieved on June 1, 2006.

Braham LG, Trower P, Birchwood M. (2004). Acting on command hallucinations and dangerous behavior: A critique of the major findings in the last decade. *Clin Psychol Rev,* 24(5):513-528.

Buccheri R, Trygstad L, Dowling G, Hopkins R, White K, Griffin JJ, et al. (2004). Long-term effects of teaching behavioral strategies for managing persistent auditory hallucinations in schizophrenia. *J Psychosoc Nurs Ment Health Serv,* 42(1):18-27.

Coffey M, Higgon J, Kinnear J. (2004). 'Therapy as well as the tablets': An exploratory study of service users' views of community mental health nurses' (CMHNs) responses to hearing voices. *J Psychiatr Ment Health Nurs,* 11(4):435-444.

Cohen S, Khan A. (1990). Antipsychotic effect of milieu in the acute treatment of schizophrenia. *Gen Hosp Psychiatry,* 12(4):248-251.

Conway T. (2004). Hearing voices: An experience of group work in a medium secure psychiatric hospital. *Practice,* 16(2):137-145.

Coombs T, Deane FP, Lambert G, Griffiths R. (2003). What influences patients' medication adherence? Mental health nurse perspectives and a need for education and training. *Int J Ment Health Nurs,* 12(2):148-152.

Corren D, Lucas D. (2004). Hearing voices—and proud of it: Dan Corren and Dorte Lucas explain how a hearing voices group helped a client to come to terms with his experience. *Ment Health Pract*, 7(7):16.

Dochterman JM, Bulechek GM (Eds). (2004). *Nursing Interventions Classification (NIC)*, 4th ed. St. Louis: Mosby.

Harkavy-Friedman JM, Kimhy D, Nelson EA, Venarde DF, Malaspina D, Mann JJ. (2003). Suicide attempts in schizophrenia: The role of command auditory hallucinations for suicide. *J Clin Psychiatry*, 64(8):871-874.

Hogarty GE, Flesher S, Ulrich R, Carter M, Greenwald D, Pogue-Geile M, et al. (2004). Cognitive enhancement therapy for schizophrenia: Effects of a 2-year randomized trial on cognition and behavior. *Arch Gen Psychiatry*, 61(9):866-876.

Holmes D, Kennedy SL, Perron A. (2004). The mentally ill and social exclusion: A critical examination of the use of seclusion from the patient's perspective. *Issues Ment Health Nurs*, 25(6):559-578.

Jenner JA, Nienhuis FJ, van de Willige G, Wiersma D. (2006). "Hitting" voices of schizophrenia patients may lastingly reduce persistent auditory hallucinations and their burden: 18-month outcome of a randomized controlled trial. *Can J Psychiatry*, 51(3):169-177.

Katz I, Grossberg GT. (2005). Psychosis in Alzheimer's disease. (Archived web conference.) June 29, 2005. Available online: http://www.medscape.com. Retrieved on May 10, 2006.

Krupat E, Hsu J, Irish J, Schmittdiel JA, Selby J. (2004). Matching patients and practitioners based on beliefs about care: Results of a randomized controlled trial. *Am J Manag Care*, 10(11 Pt 1):814-822.

Leucht S, Barnes TR, Kissling W, Engel RR, Correll C, Kane JM. (2003). Relapse prevention in schizophrenia with new-generation antipsychotics: A systematic review and exploratory meta-analysis of randomized, controlled trials. *Am J Psychiatry*, 160(7):1209-1222.

Lieberman JA, Stroup TS, McEvoy JP, Swartz MS, Rosenheck RA, Perkins DO, et al. (2005). Effectiveness of antipsychotic drugs in patients with chronic schizophrenia. *N Engl J Med*, 353(12):1209-1223.

Lysaker P, Buck K. (2006). Moving toward recovery within clients' personal narratives: Directions for a recovery-focused therapy. *J Psychosoc Nurs Ment Health Serv*, 44(1):28-35.

McCandless-Glimcher L, McKnight S, Hamera E, Smith BL, Peterson KA, Plumlee AA. (1986). Use of symptoms by schizophrenics to monitor and regulate their illness. *Hosp Community Psychiatry*, 37(9):929-933.

Meehan T, Bergen H, Fjeldsoe K. (2004). Staff and patient perceptions of seclusion: Has anything changed? *J Adv Nurs*, 47(1):33-38.

Miller DD, McEvoy JP, Davis SM, Caroff SN, Saltz BL, Chakos MH, et al. (2005). Clinical correlates of tardive dyskinesia in schizophrenia: Baseline data from the CATIE schizophrenia trial. *Schizophr Res*, 2005, 80(1):33-43.

Moorhead M, Johnson M, Maas M (Eds). (2004). *Nursing Outcomes Classification (NOC)*, 3rd ed. St. Louis: Mosby.

Pitschel-Walz G, Bauml J, Bender W, Engel RR, Wagner M, Kissling W. (2006). Psychoeducation and compliance in the treatment of schizophrenia: Results of the Munich Psychosis Information Project Study. *J Clin Psychiatry*, 67(3):443-452.

Provencher HL, Perreault M, St Onge M, Rousseau M. (2003). Predictors of psychological distress in family caregivers of persons with psychiatric disabilities. *J Psychiatr Ment Health Nurs*, 10(5):592-607.

Rector NA, Beck AT. (2002). A clinical review of cognitive therapy for schizophrenia. *Curr Psychiatry Rep*, 4(4):284-292.

Saenger E. (2004). Treatment-resistant schizophrenia: An expert interview with Ralph Hoffman, MN. *Medscape Psychiatry and Mental Health*, 9(2). Available online: http://www.medscape.com. Retrieved on May 10, 2006.

Scanlon A. (2006). Psychiatric nurses' perceptions of the constituents of the therapeutic relationship: A grounded theory study. *J Psychiatr Ment Health Nurs*, 13(3):319-329.

Silverstein CM. (2006). Therapeutic interpersonal interactions: The sacrificial lamb? *Perspect Psychiatr Care*, 42(1):33-41.

Sin J, Gamble C. (2003). Managing side-effects to the optimum: Valuing a client's experience. *J Psychiatr Ment Health Nurs*, 10(2):147-153.

Stanbridge RI, Burbach FR, Lucas AS, Carter K. (2003). A study of families' satisfaction with a family interventions in psychosis service in Somerset. *J Fam Ther*, 25(2):181.

RCT = Randomized Controlled (Clinical) Trial, **NIC** = Nursing Interventions Classification, **NOC** = Nursing Outcomes Classification

Sultzer DL. (2004). Psychosis and antipsychotic medications in Alzheimer's disease: Clinical management and research perspectives. *Dement Geriatr Cogn Disord,* 17(1-2):78-90.

Trimmer W. (2005). Does seclusion result in a calmer patient? *Whitireia Nurs J,* 12:9-13.

Tsai YF, Ku YC. (2005). Self-care symptom management strategies for auditory hallucinations among inpatients with schizophrenia at a Veterans' Hospital in Taiwan. *Arch Psychiatr Nurs,* 19(4):194-199.

Usher K, Lindsay D, Sellen J. (2001). Mental health nurses' PRN psychotropic medication administration practices. *J Psychiatr Ment Health Nurs,* 8(5):383-390.

Usher K, Luck L. (2004). Psychotropic PRN: A model for best practice management of acute psychotic behavioural disturbance in inpatient psychiatric settings. *Int J Ment Health Nurs,* 13(1):18-21.

Wijkstra J, Lijmer J, Balk F, Geddes J, Nolen WA. (2005). Pharmacological treatment for psychotic depression. *Cochrane Database Syst Rev,* (4):CD004044.

Williams CA. (1989). Perspectives on the hallucinatory process. *Issues Ment Health Nurs,* 10(2):99-119.

Wykes T, Hayward P, Thomas N, Green N, Surguladze S, Fannon D, et al. (2005). What are the effects of group cognitive behaviour therapy for voices? A randomised control trial. *Schizophr Res,* 77(2-3):201-210.

HAND MASSAGE

Katharine Kolcaba, PhD, RN-C; Annette R. Mitzel, MSN, RN, LMT, CNS

Definition: Stimulating the skin and underlying tissues of each hand with varying strokes and degrees of digital pressure to produce relaxation and/or connectedness.

NURSING ACTIVITIES

Effective

■ *Greet the patient and establish a therapeutic rapport. Place the patient in a comfortable position with the forearm and hand easily accessible to the therapist. Explain the procedure to the patient, that both hands will be massaged equally unless contraindicated. Clarify any questions or concerns.* **LOE = II**

(EO) Presence and a therapeutic relationship prior to implementing hand massage make the massage more effective. A therapeutic relationship is part of the holistic experience (Dossey et al., 1995).

(NR) An RCT of 31 hospice patients randomly allocated into treatment and comparison groups concluded that a thorough introduction was nonthreatening and communication and caring (verbal and nonverbal) were enhanced because the focus was on the whole person (Kolcaba et al., 2004).

(EO) When the nurse puts the patient at ease, the effectiveness of the intervention is enhanced (Mitzel-Wilkinson, 2000).

■ *Use an antibacterial moist, prepackaged towelette to cleanse hands prior to physical contact.* **LOE = II**

(NR) An RCT of 31 alert hospice patients randomly allocated into treatment and comparison groups demonstrated that cleaning hands with a towelette was refreshing, cooling, and provided confidence that nosocomial infection was prevented (Kolcaba et al., 2004).

NR = Nursing Research, **MR** = Multidisciplinary Research, **SP** = Standard of Practice, **EO** = Expert Opinion, **LOE** = Level of Evidence

■ *Hold the patient's hand between the therapist's hands to establish contact. Request that the patient report any sensations that are not comfortable as the hand is massaged.* **LOE = II**

(NR) An RCT of 31 alert hospice patients randomly allocated into treatment and comparison groups demonstrated that individual contact connected the caregiver to the care recipient in a profound way (Kolcaba et al., 2004).

(EO) The nurse's use of self as a therapeutic instrument and putting the patient at ease influence the effectiveness of the intervention (Kolcaba, 2003).

■ *Place the patient's forearm and hand in a palm-up position with the thumb abducted.* **LOE = VII**

(EO) This position facilitates kneading of the specific body region (Andrade, 2001).

■ *Apply lubricant to the palm and dorsal surfaces of the patient's hand.* **LOE = II**

(NR) An RCT of 31 hospice patients randomly allocated into treatment and comparison groups demonstrated that warmed lubricant facilitated easy sliding movements on fragile skin (Kolcaba et al., 2004).

■ *Begin stroking, gliding over the skin without moving deep muscle masses. The direction of stroking is up the midline of the palm around the base of the thumb to the wrist. Stroke in the same direction several times.* **LOE = VII**

(EO) Basic sliding effleurage is performed on the palms and fingers of the patient's hands. Thumbs can be used in small places such as the metacarpals. This enhances venous return and may provide a passive stretch (Tappen & Benjamin, 1998).

(NR) An RCT of 31 hospice patients randomly allocated into treatment and comparison groups demonstrated that movement from distal to proximal surfaces improved circulation and increased patients' comfort (Kolcaba et al., 2004).

■ *Observe the patient's response and inquire about the patient's comfort.* **LOE = II**

(NR) An RCT of 31 hospice patients randomly allocated into treatment and comparison groups revealed that a small percentage of patients (2 of 31 participants) were unreceptive or uncomfortable with hand massage. Hand massage cannot be assumed to be a comfortable intervention for everyone (Kolcaba et al., 2004).

■ *Across the surface of the palm, apply friction, which is a massage stroke that permits deeper work with the tissue involving small circular movements with the tips of the fingers, thumb, or the heel of the nurse's hand.* **LOE = VII**

(EO) Friction addresses small areas at a time and adds specificity to the massage by affecting targeted structures such as a muscle or tendon (Tappen & Benjamin, 1998).

■ *Moving to the fingers, apply friction to each digit in a "pilling" action with each digit being massaged individually and on all surfaces (side, top, and bottom).* **LOE = II**

(NR) An RCT of 31 hospice patients randomly allocated into treatment and comparison groups demonstrated that applying friction to each digit enhanced relaxation and further promoted connectedness (Kolcaba et al., 2004).

RCT = Randomized Controlled (Clinical) Trial, **NIC** = Nursing Interventions Classification, **NOC** = Nursing Outcomes Classification

■ *Lightly stroke the entire palmar surface with long motions toward the heart, slowing strokes to move to the patient's other hand.* **LOE = II**

(NR) An RCT of 31 hospice patients randomly allocated into treatment and comparison groups revealed that gentle transition to the other hand facilitated the opportunity for meaningful conversation (Kolcaba et al., 2004).

■ *Reposition, and repeat the massage on the other hand.* **LOE = II**

(NR) An RCT of 31 hospice patients randomly allocated into treatment and comparison groups revealed that symmetry was important for a sense of completeness and balance (Kolcaba et al., 2004).

Possibly Effective

■ *If culturally appropriate, use face-to-face positioning with eye contact.* **LOE = VII**

(EO) Clinicians must seek to "see through the eyes of the other," demonstrating commitment to understanding and compassion and returning the focus toward what is important to the patient (Thompson, 2006).

■ *Warm a small amount of lubricant (nonfragrant, hypoallergenic) in the nurse's hands if the patient is not too warm already. If the patient expresses feeling warm or hot or the room is warm, cool lubricant may be more refreshing.* **LOE = II**

(NR) An RCT of 31 alert hospice patients randomly allocated into treatment and comparison groups revealed that patients had unique preferences regarding temperature of the lotion and would express these preferences to the person giving the massage (Kolcaba et al., 2004).

■ *Support the dorsal surface of the patient's hand with the nurse's hands, maintaining the physical connection between patient and nurse throughout the procedure.* **LOE = II**

(EO) Physical connection demonstrates consistency by showing respect and caring (Thompson, 2006).

■ *If the patient affirms the method and pressure, repeat as often as desired.* **LOE = II**

(NR) An RCT of 31 alert hospice patients randomly allocated into treatment and comparison groups revealed that patients gave verbal and nonverbal indicators of pleasure and comfort with each step of the procedure (Kolcaba et al., 2004).

■ *In fleshy areas, begin kneading in a two-handed movement, attempting to move muscle mass gently by pressing and rolling the tissue under the nurse's hands. Across the surface of the palm, concurrently apply friction in a massage stroke that permits deeper work with the tissue involving small circular movements with the tips of the fingers, thumb, or the heel of the nurse's hand.* **LOE = II**

(NR) An RCT of 31 alert hospice patients randomly allocated into treatment and comparison groups showed that this step was effective for increasing relaxation, but the sample size was small (Kolcaba et al., 2004).

NR = Nursing Research, **MR** = Multidisciplinary Research, **SP** = Standard of Practice, **EO** = Expert Opinion, **LOE** = Level of Evidence

EO These two strokes when done together on the hand increase local circulation, assist venous return, and evoke muscular relaxation (Tappen & Benjamin, 1998).

■ *Reposition the hand so that the dorsal surface (back of the hand) is up.* **LOE = II**

NR An RCT of 31 alert hospice patients randomly allocated into treatment and comparison groups revealed that a resting hand position was the most comfortable for the patient (Kolcaba et al., 2004).

■ *Vary the duration of the procedure on one hand according to the patient's comfort level (approximately 5 to 10 minutes for each hand).* **LOE = II**

NR An RCT of 31 alert hospice patients randomly allocated into treatment and comparison groups showed that the duration of the actual procedure depended on signs and verbal cues from the patient (Kolcaba et al., 2004).

■ *Use aromatherapy with massage.* **LOE = II**

NR An RCT ($N = 103$) of cancer patients in a palliative care setting demonstrated that both whole body massage and aromatherapy improved outcomes, but improvements between the intervention group and control group were not significantly different (Wilkinson et al., 1999).

■ *Teach hand massage to family members, visitors, and auxiliary personnel.* **LOE = II**

NR In an RCT of 31 alert hospice patients randomly allocated into treatment and comparison groups, nonprofessional people learned and enjoyed doing hand massage for their loved one. The simplicity of the massage procedure and the acceptability of personal variation of the method made teaching others uncomplicated (Kolcaba et al., 2004).

Not Effective

■ *Use of tapotement, which is repeated tapping, cupping, and hacking (with the sides of the hands).* **LOE = VII**

EO Tapotement is a finishing stroke for broad body parts. The strokes of tapotement are not suitable for the small surface of the hands (Tappen & Benjamin, 1998).

Possibly Harmful

■ *Use of friction over inflamed joints, fragile skin, obvious tumors, or bruises.* **LOE = II**

NR In an RCT ($N = 31$) of hospice patients who were randomly allocated into treatment (receiving hand massage twice weekly for 3 weeks) or comparison groups (receiving hand massage once at the study's end), findings demonstrated that friction over areas of concern led to possible damage (Kolcaba et al., 2004).

■ *Kneading nonfleshy areas.* **LOE = VII**

EO Kneading is a movement for fleshy areas only and may cause discomfort if performed on other areas (Tappen & Benjamin, 1998).

RCT = Randomized Controlled (Clinical) Trial, **NIC** = Nursing Interventions Classification, **NOC** = Nursing Outcomes Classification

■ *Repositioning to reach dorsal and palmar surfaces when the patient manifests pain or discomfort.* **LOE = II**

NR In an RCT ($N = 31$) of hospice patients who were randomly allocated into treatment (receiving hand massage twice weekly for 3 weeks) or comparison groups (receiving hand massage once at the study's end), findings indicated that repositioning of hands decreased pain and discomfort (Kolcaba et al., 2004).

■ *Using direct and firm pressure on the center of the palm (this is an acupressure point).* **LOE = II**

NR In an RCT ($N = 31$) of hospice patients who were randomly allocated into treatment (receiving hand massage twice weekly for 3 weeks) or comparison groups (receiving hand massage once at the study's end), researchers stated that direct and firm pressure on the center of the palm was contraindicated (Kolcaba et al., 2004).

OUTCOME MEASUREMENT

COMFORT LEVEL    NOC

Definition: Extent of positive perception of physical and psychological ease
Comfort Level as evidenced by the following selected NOC indicators:
• Physical well-being
• Psychological well-being
(Rate each indicator of **Comfort Level:** 1 = not at all satisfied, 2 = somewhat satisfied, 3 = moderately satisfied, 4 = very satisfied, 5 = completely satisfied) (Moorhead et al., 2004)

TOTAL COMFORT

Total comfort as evidenced by a pain and/or comfort scale per institutional policy to demonstrate increased comfort or decreased pain
   Rate the patient's total comfort from 0 to 10, with 10 being as comfortable as possible. This is similar to rating of pain and is easy and familiar for patients. (Kolcaba, 2003)

PERSONAL WELL-BEING   NOC

Definition: Extent of positive perception of one's health status and life circumstances.
Personal Well-Being as evidenced by the following selected NOC indicators:
• Ability to cope
• Ability to relax
• Level of happiness
(Rate each indicator of **Personal Well-Being:** 1 = not at all satisfied, 2 = somewhat satisfied, 3 = moderately satisfied, 4 = very satisfied, 5 = completely satisfied) (Moorhead et al., 2004).

COMMUNICATION   NOC

Definition: Reception, interpretation, and expression of spoken, written, and nonverbal messages.

NR = Nursing Research, **MR** = Multidisciplinary Research, **SP** = Standard of Practice, **EO** = Expert Opinion, **LOE** = Level of Evidence

OUTCOME MEASUREMENT—*cont'd*

Communication as evidenced by the following selected NOC indicators:
- Use of spoken language
- Use of nonverbal language
- Acknowledgment of messages received
- Accurate interpretation of messages received
- Exchanges messages accurately with others

(Rate each indicator of **Communication:** 1 = severely compromised, 2 = substantially compromised, 3 = moderately compromised, 4 = mildly compromised, 5 = not compromised) (Moorhead et al., 2004).

REFERENCES

Andrade C. (2001). *Outcome based massage.* Philadelphia: Lippincott Williams & Wilkins.

Dossey B, Montgomery K, Guzzetta C, Kolkmeier L. (1995). *Holistic nursing: A handbook for practice,* 2nd ed. Gaithersburg, MD: Aspen.

Kolcaba K. (2003). Comfort theory and practice. New York: Springer.

Kolcaba K, Dowd T, Steiner R, Mitzel A. (2004). Efficacy of hand massage for enhancing the comfort of hospice patients. *J Hosp Palliat Nurs,* 6(2):91-102.

Mitzel-Wilkinson A. (2000). Massage therapy as a nursing practice. *Holist Nurs Pract,* 14(2):48-56.

Moorhead M, Johnson M, Maas M (Eds). (2004). *Nursing Outcomes Classification (NOC),* 3rd ed. St. Louis: Mosby.

Tappen F, Benjamin PJ. (1998). *Tappen's handbook of healing massage techniques,* 3rd ed. Stamford, CT: Appleton & Lange.

Thompson D. (2006). *Hands heal: Communication, documentation, and insurance billing for manual therapists,* 3rd ed. Philadelphia: Lippincott Williams & Wilkins.

Wilkinson S, Aldridge J, Salmon I, Cain E, Wilson B. (1999). An evaluation of aromatherapy massage in palliative care. *Palliat Med,* 13(5):409-417.

HEALING TOUCH

Diane Wind Wardell, PhD, RN-C, AHN-BC

Definition: Healing Touch is a "biofield therapy that is an energy based approach to health and healing" (Mentgen, 2003). It uses a variety of hands-on techniques that facilitate balance for the physical, emotional, mental, and spiritual well-being. It is taught as a nursing continuing education program throughout the world.

NURSING ACTIVITIES

Effective

■ *Provide Healing Touch to improve quality of life.* **LOE = II**

(MR) An RCT using "blinding" of participants to treatment was conducted with 62 women receiving radiation therapy for gynecological or breast cancer. Participants received either a mock treatment (control group) or noncontact Healing Touch. The Healing Touch group demonstrated statistically significant gains in total score and also physical functioning, pain reduction, and vitality compared with the control group on the quality-of-life instrument, the SF-36 from the Medical Outcomes Study at the Rand Corporation. The Healing Touch group had improvements in all nine of the domains compared with the control (Cook et al., 2004).

NR A review of studies found indications of benefit in the area of quality of life using Healing Touch (Wardell & Weymouth, 2004).

Possibly Effective

■ *Provide Healing Touch to promote personal well-being, defined as the extent of positive perception of one's health status and life circumstances (Wardell & Weymouth, 2004).* LOE = II

MR A randomized, prospective, two-period crossover intervention study was conducted with 230 participants recruited and 164 completing the study to measure the effects of therapeutic massage (MT) and Healing Touch on pain, nausea, fatigue, and anxiety of chemotherapy patients in comparison with caring presence (P) or standard cancer treatment alone. Classic crossover analysis yielded significant immediate and overall effects for both MT and Healing Touch in reducing blood pressure and heart rate in comparison with P and significantly reducing level of pain in comparison with P. MT and Healing Touch also reduced mood disturbance during the intervention periods. Fatigue was less in the Healing Touch period (Kinney et al., 2002).

MR In a randomized-by-group (visit $N = 13$, massage $N = 13$, and Healing Touch $N = 10$) controlled study, the effects on anxiety, depression, caregiver burden, and fatigue were evaluated in caregivers of patients undergoing stem cell transplants. Using the Beck Anxiety Inventory, the Center for Epidemiologic Studies Depression Scale, the Subjective Burden Scale, and the Multidimensional Fatigue Inventory, findings indicated in the Healing Touch group scores for anxiety, depression, and subjective burden decreased but did not reach significance. The fatigue scores in the Healing Touch group increased. A poststudy survey of 9 of the 10 participants in the Healing Touch group found that most reported a time for self-focus and decreased worry, and 2 reported a decrease in pain symptoms (Rexilius et al., 2002).

MR In an RCT, 55 participants were randomly assigned to standard care or Healing Touch groups to determine their effects on the quality of life among people at the end stage of life. The outcomes measured were quality of life, physical symptoms, and spiritual meaning using the Missoula Vitas instrument. Although there were no significant differences between Healing Touch and standard hospice care, the Healing Touch group did improve on interpersonal, well-being, and function scores over time as compared with worsening in the control group (Ziembroski et al., 2003).

NR In a phenomenologic-hermeneutic study, Healing Touch sessions with cancer participants revealed a distinct pattern of interactions that included caring for each other; connecting to each other and themselves; opening into trust, receptibility, and intuition; cocreating; and being-one-with that created a sense of bonding or being as one with each other. A change in consciousness allowed participants to see themselves as whole, being unified with themselves (body-emotion-mind-spirit), and having a sense of well-being (Christiano, 1997). Findings were similar in two other phenomenological studies of women receiving Healing Touch during therapy for breast cancer (Kopecki, 2001; Mooreland, 1998).

NR = Nursing Research, **MR** = Multidisciplinary Research, **SP** = Standard of Practice, **EO** = Expert Opinion, **LOE** = Level of Evidence

(MR) Three clinical trials plan to demonstrate improved quality of life with Healing Touch, and one will explore physiological mechanisms of action. However, there are no published findings to date from these studies (HTI, 2005).

■ *Use the HEALTH tool to obtain a thorough, holistic history from a patient, determine the meaning the patient holds for each aspect of that history, document and assess the outcome of all energetic healing treatments done, and determine the concerns, plans, and goals for care on the part of the patient as well as the practitioner.* **LOE = I**

(NR) The HEALTH tool (Healing Energy and Life Through Holism) was developed to encompass who the practitioner is, who the patient is, what techniques are used in what order, and what the environment is like. It is a modular, holistic assessment tool that reflects the physical, emotional-mental, social, and spiritual human being; the Healing Touch process; and the environment. No reliability or validity is available (Hutchison, 1997).

■ *Provide Healing Touch for pain relief; the areas are the subset of pain, immune status, pre- and post-therapeutic interventions outcome, mood/stress, and the elderly.* **LOE = II/III**

(NR) A quasi-experimental design study was conducted on the effects of Healing Touch on chronic nonmalignant abdominal pain using interview data with 23 participants experiencing lingering (4 months to 9 years) postsurgical abdominal pain (Slater, 1996). The groups were a placebo interview, treatment by a naïve healer, and treatment by an experienced Healing Touch practitioner. There was a decrease in pain using the McGill-Melzack Pain Questionnaire in both the naïve and experienced healer groups. Recipients' responses indicated relaxation and some pain relief, with the most dramatic and long-lasting pain relief occurring after treatment by the experienced providers (Benor, 2001).

(MR) A quasi-experimental controlled study with 20 participants receiving either Healing Touch or chiropractic treatment was used to determine the efficacy of Healing Touch for chronic low back pain. Groups were equivalent on pain, range of motion, orthopedic tests, and quality of life. Using a *t*-test, both Healing Touch and chiropractic groups were found to have significantly decreased pain, improved range of motion, and improved orthopedic measurements. The chiropractic group had improvement in quality of life (Weymouth & Sandberg-Lewis, 2000).

(NR) In a retrospective descriptive study on chronic pain in response to the specific Healing Touch technique trauma release, 10 seminar participants demonstrated variations in pain. At least 1 month following the Healing Touch trauma release, the responses included complete absence of pain ($N = 4$), decrease in pain ($N = 2$), an initial decrease and then return ($N = 2$), and no change ($N = 2$). None experienced an increase in pain (Wardell, 2000).

(NR) A single-blind three-group design including control, mock treatment, and Healing Touch treatment groups found no changes in pain using a numerical pain rating scale of 1 to 10 or in medication usage in a study of 48 postoperative participants with total knee replacements. Using a goniometer, there was a 30.6% average increase in joint mobility with Healing Touch and 27.0% with mock treatment compared with the control group (Cordes et al., 2002).

(MR) A pilot study using a nonrandomized two-group design of Healing Touch and progressive muscle relaxation with 12 veterans experiencing chronic neuropathic pain suggested that Healing Touch might have some effect on altering the pain experience. There was a large

RCT = Randomized Controlled (Clinical) Trial, **NIC** = Nursing Interventions Classification, **NOC** = Nursing Outcomes Classification

variation within the groups and a significant difference in the Healing Touch group on the Composite of Interference on the Brief Pain Inventory. The mean score of the fatigue subscale of the Profile of Moods decreased in the Healing Touch group and in the subscale of confusion. In both of these subscales, the control group remained stable. The Diener Satisfaction with Life Scale showed nonsignificant increased well-being in the Healing Touch group, whereas the control group remained stable (Wardell et al., 2006).

NR A quasi-experimental one-group pretest/post-test design study of 138 inpatients with varying pain syndromes who received a single Healing Touch session demonstrated a change in pain scores and anxiety. There was a change in pre- to post-treatment pain from 5.94 to a mean of 3.64 on a scale of 1 to 10. The mean level of anxiety significantly decreased from pretreatment to after treatment (Welcher & Kish, 2001).

MR In a case study report of five participants with fibromyalgia, there were varied responses to Healing Touch treatments. Preexperiment pain ratings on a scale of 0 to 9 ranged from 3.4 to 5.7, and postexperiment ratings ranged from 1.2 to 5.5. Three participants reported changes that included decreased stress, spiritual uplifting, and improved mobility and mental clarity (Diener, 2001).

■ *Use the Healing Touch Comfort Questionnaire (HTCQ) to assess the effectiveness of treatment.* **LOE = I**

MR The HTCQ is based on the middle range theory of Kolcaba's Comfort Theory. Personal well-being and comfort are similar types of constructs; comfort is an immediate holistic outcome of treatment and can be used to measure the benefits of treatment for any Healing Touch therapy. The HTCQ was specifically designed for HT, a Likert-type questionnaire with six options. Internal consistency and reliability were established with a Cronbach alpha = .94 with 56 recipients (Dowd et al., 2006).

■ *Provide Healing Touch to enhance immune function.* **LOE = III**

MR In an RCT using a repeated measures design in which 22 healthy individuals received no treatment, treatment with standard Healing Touch, or treatment with Healing Touch plus music, immunological effects were found. The results indicated a significant interaction effect of the treatment series on secretory immunoglobulin (sIgA) and the practitioner training level with a nearly four times average positive change for the people with the more highly trained practitioner. Stress rating (on a scale of 1 to 10) indicated a significant reduction after treatment for both Healing Touch and Healing Touch plus music. Pain relief was reported by 55% of respondents experiencing pain (Wilkinson et al., 2002).

MR A quasi-experimental repeated measures design with HIV-infected individuals investigated the clinical effectiveness of Healing Touch for increasing sIgA in saliva and quality of life with 15 participants. Twenty-seven percent met the criteria for positive response, one on the sIgA measure and three on quality of life as measured by the Functional Assessment of HIV Infections. All positive responders were HIV symptomatic and showed evidence of change over the treatment series as compared with change over a single Healing Touch treatment. Healing Touch could not be isolated as solely responsible for the positive changes, which may have been affected by therapeutic alliance factors (Wilkinson, 2002).

■ *Provide Healing Touch to improve mood and decrease stress.* **LOE = II**

MR In an RCT, 150 cardiac patients were evaluated for the effects of noetic therapies (stress management, prayer, imagery, and Healing Touch therapy) on mood immediately before cardiac intervention. Mood was assessed before and after treatment using a visual analogue scale (VAS) of eight scales: four positive mood descriptors of happy, hopeful, calm, and satisfied; three negative mood descriptors (worried, sad, upset); and one unpleasant physical sensation (shortness of breath). Analysis showed that stress management, imagery, and Healing Touch all produced reductions in reported worry as compared with standard therapy and prayer. Healing Touch significantly decreased worry and increased satisfaction. The Healing Touch group also showed a nonsignificant decrease in upsetness, sadness, and shortness of breath (Seskevich et al., 2004).

(NR) A mixed-methodology RCT reviewed the effect of providing Healing Touch to 51 undergraduate students. There was no effect of Healing Touch on the coping ability, self-esteem, and general health of first-year students, but there were significant effects for the third-year students in less transient stress, less chronic stress, and coping by committing more effort than those in the control group (Taylor, 2001).

(NR) A qualitative study using a grounded theory case study approach explored the experiential process of Healing Touch for 15 people with moderate depression verified by the Beck Depression Inventory (BDI). All of the participants demonstrated a reduced score (27 to 10 points) in the BDI at the completion of the research. The grounded theory analysis identified four stages for people with moderate depression participating in Healing Touch sessions. The first two stages partially addressed the basic psychosocial problems of disconnection from self, others, and the world. The final two stages completed the process of emerging from depression and reconnection with self, others, and the world (Van Aken, 2004).

■ *Provide Healing Touch for pre- and post-therapeutic interventions.* **LOE = II**

(MR) An RCT investigating the effects of healing interventions of noetic therapies (stress management, prayer, imagery, and Healing Touch therapy) before angioplasty in 150 patients on complication rates found that there was a 25% to 30% absolute reduction in adverse periprocedural outcomes in those treated with any noetic therapy. The lowest number of events was in the off-site prayer group, and absolute mortality at 6 months was also lowest in this group (Krucoff et al., 2001).

(MR) A multicenter RCT involving 748 cardiac patients was conducted to determine the effects of two noetic therapies (prayer and a combination of music, imagery, and Healing Touch [MIT]) compared with standard care. There was no significant difference for the primary composite endpoints (adverse events in hospital and 6-month readmission or death) in any treatment comparison. For the prespecified secondary endpoints, mortality at 6 months was lower with MIT therapy than with no MIT therapy. The MIT therapy group also had significantly less preprocedural distress (Krucoff et al., 2005).

(NR) In an RCT involving 148 patients who received either Healing Touch or readings from the Big Book during treatment in an early stage of recovery from alcoholism, patients receiving Healing Touch had some significant changes on selected measures compared with control. There was a greater reduction in heart rate and on the VAS scales, indicating that the Healing Touch group was happier, more satisfied, and had a greater reduction in pain than the control group. Healing Touch reduced some areas of stress in the early stages of recovery in patients admitted for alcoholism treatment (Dubrey, 2006).

(NR) The effect of Healing Touch on recovery from abdominal hysterectomy in 60 women randomly assigned to Healing Touch, back massage, or standard care was evaluated. Pre- and postoperative evaluation of the amount of narcotic analgesic self-administered; the frequency of bowel program treatments; medication usage; vital signs; and lung, gastrointestinal, urinary, and motor function was performed. The analysis of covariance (ANCOVA) indicated that the Healing Touch patients had a significantly higher level of recovery than the two controls on lung, gastrointestinal, and activity status. Reductions of blood pressures and pulse rate were statistically significant for the Healing Touch group. The amounts of narcotic analgesia and bowel treatments were less for the Healing Touch patients than for the back massage and control patients but did not reach significance (Silva, 1996).

(NR) A single case study reported a successful intervention to facilitate natural conception with Healing Touch for an elderly primipara with a diagnosis of infertility of unknown origin (Kissinger & Kaczmarek, 2006).

▨ *Provide Healing Touch for the elderly with behavioral issues and pain.* LOE = III

(NR) A blinded-to-reviewer, controlled pilot study of people with dementia experiencing high levels of agitation on the Cohen-Mansfield Agitation Inventory showed significant lowering of these levels with a Healing Touch intervention. The results indicated that the Healing Touch group ($N = 6$) showed a significant decrease in agitation levels during the intervention period. Psychotropic medication use was also noted to have decreased, and the participants verbalized the calming effects of Healing Touch (Wang & Hermann, 2006).

(NR) A quasi-experimental study with a nonrandomized controlled group evaluated the use of Healing Touch and Therapeutic Touch in 26 elderly people residing in a long-term care setting over 6 months. The Healing Touch group had 22 people with a median age of 81.9 years. Pre- and postassessment were done on pain using a VAS scale of 0 to 10 in color; self-report of tension, worry, happiness, and nervousness using a four-point rating system for each emotion; and pulse and respiration. All were significant in an ANCOVA (Forbes et al., 2006).

(NR) A nonrandomized controlled quasi-experimental pilot study involving 12 nursing home residents with Alzheimer's disease evaluated Healing Touch effects on functional behavior using the 10-item Functional Behavior Profile (Ostuni & Pietro, 2001). Results indicated significant improvement in behavior scores across all 10 behavioral items for the Healing Touch group (appetite, sleep, freedom from pain, orientation, compliance with daily routine, socialization, emotional stability, nonverbal responses, freedom from jargon, and conversational communication). There was no improvement in the control group with decline in behavior scores. The composure scores (freedom from agitation, extreme restlessness, catastrophic outbursts) improved significantly, as did the physical comfort (freedom from complaints) for the Healing Touch group but not for the control group.

▨ *Provide Healing Touch to enhance spiritual health, which is defined as connectedness with self, others, higher power, all life, nature, and the universe, that transcends and empowers the self.* LOE = III

(NR) A descriptive study of 477 nurses and nonnurses as students in Healing Touch classes found a significant difference between upper level classes and the lower levels on the Spiritual Perspective Scale. There was also a difference on the Questionnaire on Spiritual and Religious Attitudes between levels of instruction completed. This suggested that there was a heightened sense of spiritual awareness in those in the higher levels of the program (Wardell, 2001).

(NR) Further qualitative analysis of the aforementioned study resulted in a taxonomy of spiritual experiences from the participants ($N = 327$), who recalled their most significant spiritual event. Within three structural domains of circumstance, manifestation, and interpretation, a variety of experiences were reported that indicated the structure of a spiritual experience (Wardell & Engebretson, 2006).

NR = Nursing Research, **MR** = Multidisciplinary Research, **SP** = Standard of Practice, **EO** = Expert Opinion, **LOE** = Level of Evidence

NR A mixed-method study including qualitative analysis of 10 interviews with certified Healing Touch practitioners and quantitative data through a questionnaire completed by 87 practitioners demonstrated the transformational aspects of the work. Spiritual aspects of conducting healing sessions were included. Quantitative data analysis showed the practitioners found the highest efficacy for stress and anxiety reduction, promoting relaxation and relieving pain, promoting and maintaining wellness, accelerating healing, promoting personal and spiritual growth, and easing the dying process (Weymouth, 2002).

NR A phenomenologic-hermeneutic study of cancer participants receiving Healing Touch sessions revealed a distinct pattern of interactions that included caring for each other; connecting to each other and themselves; opening into trust, receptibility, and intuition; cocreating, and being-one-with that created a sense of bonding or being as one with each other (Christiano, 1997). These four themes were further abstracted to meta-themes sensation and perception. A change in consciousness allowed participants to see themselves as whole, being unified with themselves (body-emotion-mind-spirit), and having a sense of well-being. Similar findings were also found in a phenomenological study of six women receiving Healing Touch during chemotherapy for breast cancer (Mooreland, 1998).

NR The qualitative analysis of the experience of three women receiving Healing Touch during breast cancer survivorship resulted in the essence of the Healing Touch experience being one of connection with others. This led to a strengthened self that created a new state of enhanced physical, emotional, and spiritual well-being (Kopecki, 2001).

Not Effective

No applicable published research was found in this category.

Possibly Harmful

■ *Abruptly stopping Healing Touch.* **LOE = VI**

NR One study (unpublished) identified harm when Healing Touch was abruptly terminated for 14 elderly residents of a long-term care facility. During active treatment, all participants (an average of nine sessions per resident) reported noted improvement with decreased pain and functional ability. After the treatments were abruptly discontinued, some of the participants noted severe exacerbation of pain, decreased functional ability, sleep disturbance, and change in emotional status (Peck et al., 2001).

OUTCOME MEASUREMENT

PERSONAL WELL-BEING

Definition: Extent of positive perception of one's health status and life circumstances.
Personal Well-Being as evidenced by the following selected NOC indicators:
- Psychological health
- Spiritual life
- Ability to relax
- Level of happiness

(Rate each indicator of **Personal Well-Being:** 1 = not all satisfied, 2 = somewhat satisfied, 3 = moderately satisfied, 4 = very satisfied, 5 = completely satisfied) (Moorhead et al., 2004).

REFERENCES

Benor D. (2001). *Spiritual healing: Scientific validation of a healing revolution*. Southfield, MI: Vision Publications.

Christiano C. (1997). The lived experience of healing touch with cancer patients. Florida International University in Miami, Master's Thesis.

Cook CA, Guerrerio JF, Slater VE. (2004). Healing touch and quality of life in women receiving radiation treatment for cancer: A randomized controlled trial. *Altern Ther Health Med,* 10(3):34-41.

Cordes P, Proffitt C, Roth J. (2002). *The effect of Healing Touch therapy on the pain and joint mobility experienced by patients with total knee replacements*. Healing Touch Research Survey, June 2002. Lakewood, CO: Healing Touch International.

Diener D. (2001). A pilot study of the effect of chakra connection and magnetic unruffle on perception of pain in people with fibromyalgia. *Healing Touch Newslett Res Ed,* 01(3):7-8.

Dowd T, Kolcaba K, Steiner R. (2006). Development of the healing touch comfort questionnaire. *Holist Nurs Pract,* 20(3):122-129.

Dubrey R. (2006). The role of healing touch in the treatment of persons in recovery from alcoholism. *Couns,* in press.

Forbes MA, Gelhaart C, Schmid MM. (2006). The effect of healing touch on pain and mood in institutionalized elders. In review.

Healing Touch International (HTI). (2005). *Research survey,* 7th ed. Lakewood, CO: Healing Touch International.

Hutchinson C. (1997). *The HEALTH tool (Healing Energy and Life Through Holism)*. Healing Touch Newsletter. Lakewood, CO.

Kinney ME, Wilcox C, Post-White J, Lerner IJ, Berntsen J. (2002). The effect of therapeutic massage and healing touch on cancer patients. [Abstract]. Healing Touch International 6th Annual Conference, Denver, CO.

Kissinger J, Kaczmarek L. (2006). Healing touch and fertility: A case report. *J Perinat Educ,* 15(2):13-20.

Kopecki D. (2001). The lived experience of women with breast cancer. The Sage Colleges, Master's Thesis.

Krucoff MW, Crater S, Gallup D, Blankenship J, Cuffe M, Guarneri M, et al. (2005). Music, imagery, touch, and prayer as adjuncts to interventional cardiac care: The Monitoring and Actualization of Noetic Trainings (MANTRA) II randomised study. *Lancet,* 366(9481):211-217.

Krucoff MW, Crater SW, Green CL, Maas AC, Seskevich JE, Lane JD, et al. (2001). Integrative noetic therapies as adjuncts to percutaneous intervention during unstable coronary syndromes: Monitoring and Actualization of Noetic Training (MANTRA) feasibility pilot. *Am Heart J,* 142(5):760-769.

Mentgen J. (2003). *Healing Touch level 1 syllabus*. Lakewood, CO: Colorado Center for Healing Touch.

Mooreland K. (1998). The lived experience of receiving the chakra connection of women with breast cancer who are receiving chemotherapy: A phenomenological study. *Healing Touch Newslett,* 8(3):3, 5.

Moorhead M, Johnson M, Maas M (Eds). (2004). *Nursing Outcomes Classification (NOC),* 3rd ed. St. Louis: Mosby.

Ostuni E, Pietro MJ. (2001). Effects of healing touch on nursing home residents in later stages of Alzheimer disease. [Abstract]. Healing Touch International 5th Annual Conference, Denver, CO. January.

Peck S, Wypyzynski J, Hauser D. (2001). A descriptive study of outcomes with the use of healing touch in elders and adults with chronic illness. Unpublished manuscript.

Rexilius SJ, Mundt C, Erickson Megel M, Agrawal S. (2002). Therapeutic effects of massage therapy and healing touch on caregivers of patients undergoing autologous hematopoietic stem cell transplant. *Oncol Nurs Forum,* 29(3):E35-E44.

Seskevich JE, Crater SW, Lane JD, Krucof MW. (2004). Beneficial effects of noetic therapies on mood before percutaneous intervention for unstable coronary syndromes. *Nurs Res,* 53(2):116-121.

Silva MA. (1996). The effects of relaxation touch on the recovery level of postanesthesia abdominal hysterectomy patients. [Abstract]. *Altern Ther Health Med,* (2)4.

Slater V. (1996). Safety, elements, and effects of healing touch on chronic non-malignant abdominal pain. Unpublished doctoral dissertation, University of Tennessee, College of Nursing. Knoxville, TN.

Taylor B. (2001). The effects of Healing Touch on the coping ability, self esteem and general health of undergraduate nursing students. *Complement Ther Nurs Midwifery,* 7(1):34-42.

NR = Nursing Research, **MR** = Multidisciplinary Research, **SP** = Standard of Practice, **EO** = Expert Opinion, **LOE** = Level of Evidence

Van Aken R. (2004). The experiential process of healing touch for people with moderate depression. Unpublished doctoral dissertation. School of Nursing and Health Care Practices, Southern Cross University, Australia.

Wang KL, Hermann C. (2006). Pilot study to test the effectiveness of Healing Touch on agitation in people with dementia. *Geriatr Nurs*, 27(1):34-40.

Wardell DW. (2000). The trauma release technique: How it is taught and experienced in Healing Touch. *Altern Complement Ther*, 6(1):20-27.

Wardell DW. (2001). Spirituality of healing touch participants. *J Holist Nurs*, 19(1):71-86.

Wardell DW, Engebretson J. (2006). Taxonomy of spiritual experiences. *J Religion Health*, 45(2):215-233.

Wardell DW, Rintala D, Duan Z, Tan G. (2006). A pilot study of healing touch and progressive relaxation for chronic neuropathic pain in persons with spinal cord injury. *J Holist Nurs*, 24(4):231-240.

Wardell DW, Weymouth KF. (2004). Review of studies of healing touch. *J Nurs Scholarsh*, 36(2):147-154.

Welcher B, Kish J. (2001). Reducing pain and anxiety through Healing Touch. *Healing Touch Newslett*, 01(3):19.

Weymouth K. (2002). Healing from a personal perspective: Interviews with certified healing touch practitioners. Unpublished doctoral dissertation, Saybrook Graduate School and Research Center, San Francisco, California.

Weymouth K, Sandberg-Lewis S. (2000). Comparing the efficacy of Healing Touch and chiropractic adjustment in treating chronic low back pain: A pilot study. *Healing Touch Newslett*, 00(3):7-8.

Wilkinson D. (2002). The clinical effectiveness of healing touch on HIV-infected individuals. Unpublished dissertation. Tennessee State University, Nashville, TN.

Wilkinson D, Knox P, Chatman J, Johnson T, Barbour N, Myles Y, et al. (2002). The clinical effectiveness of healing touch. *J Altern Complement Med*, 8(1):33-47.

Ziembroski J, Gilbert N, Bossarte R, Guldberg M. (2003). Healing touch and hospice care: Examining outcomes at the end of life. *Altern Complement Ther*, 9(3):146-151.

HEALTH EDUCATION   NIC

Kathaleen C. Bloom, PhD, CNM; Barbara J. Olinzock, EdD, MSN, RN

NIC   Definition: Developing and providing instruction and learning experiences to facilitate voluntary adaptation of behavior conducive to health in individuals, families, groups, or communities (Dochterman & Bulechek, 2004).

NURSING ACTIVITIES

Effective

■ **NIC** *Determine personal context and social-cultural history of the individual, family, or community health behavior.* **LOE = I**

NR An RCT involving 60 patients with multiple risk factors showed that the use of a targeted health interview plus individual motivational counseling based on personal goals for stroke risk reduction was more successful in the initiation of risk reduction behaviors than a targeted health interview only or a targeted health interview plus brief scripted advice (Miller & Spilker, 2003).

MR An RCT ($N = 733$) investigating mammography adherence found that the use of in-person or telephone tailored messages based on a woman's personal beliefs about breast cancer risks and benefits of mammography was more effective than either a standard reminder postcard regarding mammography or a nontailored mammography recommendation from the primary care physician (Champion et al., 2003).

(MR) An RCT ($N = 150$) of a breast cancer risk counseling intervention designed for lesbian and bisexual women found that the intervention resulted in reduction in breast cancer anxieties and increased breast screening 24 months after intervention (Bowen et al., 2006).

(NR) A systematic review of 52 empirical articles concluded that social, environmental, and cultural factors affected the willingness and ability of racial and ethnic minority men to participate in health screening and health promotion activities (Dallas & Burton, 2004).

(NR) A systematic review of 292 research articles found lack of knowledge as well as attitudes, beliefs, and fears to be associated with lower instances of cervical and breast cancer screening among immigrant women (Aroian, 2001).

(MR) A systematic review of studies investigating factors influencing breast and cervical cancer screening behavior in Hispanic women found that written educational materials and media-based public health campaigns were effective in providing information to Hispanics if they were culturally sensitive and written in Spanish at a grade 6 reading level (Austin et al., 2002).

■ (NIC) *Develop educational materials written at a reading level appropriate to the target audience.* **LOE = I**

(MR) A systematic review of 44 studies investigating the relationship between literacy levels, utilization of health care services, and health care outcomes found that low literacy was associated with low health knowledge and less use of preventive health services (Berkman et al., 2004; Dewalt et al., 2004).

(MR) A systematic review of 20 studies using interventions to improve health outcomes for low-literacy patients found that the use of simplified educational materials generally had a positive effect on knowledge and comprehension (Berkman et al., 2004; Pignone et al., 2005).

(MR) An RCT involving 255 individuals found that a quick look at a few photographs was sufficient to improve the ability to recognize a melanoma and concluded that education by photographs should replace or augment standard "ABCD" messages for self-detection of melanoma (Girardi et al., 2006).

(NR) An RCT ($N = 37$ low-income mothers) testing the use of easy-to-read versus standard immunization information sheets found that simplification of the information in and of itself was not sufficient to increase knowledge (Wilson et al., 2006).

■ (NIC) *Use group presentations to provide support and lessen threat to learners experiencing similar problems or concerns, as appropriate.* **LOE = I**

(MR) A Cochrane review of 31 RCTs revealed that individual and group counseling along with advice from a health professional and nicotine replacement were effective in inducing smoking cessation (Moher et al., 2005).

(MR) A meta-analysis of 43 RCTs investigating interventions to increase physical activity among elderly people revealed that group-delivered interventions were most likely to have an effect on increasing physical activity in older adults (Conn et al., 2002).

(MR) An RCT with 286 low-income minority mothers testing a community-based parent education program that included home visits, group sessions, and standard social services throughout the first year of life found that infants of mothers in the intervention group entered well-baby care earlier, had more frequent well-child visits, and were more likely to be adherent to immunization schedules (El-Mohandes et al., 2003).

(NR) A demonstration project ($N = 124$) using a group-based prenatal care model emphasizing assessment, education, and support was found to have an effect on health care compliance, satisfaction with care, and improvement in rates of premature and low-birth-weight infants (Grady & Bloom, 2004).

■ *Involve the learner in mutual goal-setting.* **LOE = I**

(MR) A systematic review of research related to risk factor intervention for physical activity, diet, smoking, obesity, and risky alcohol use found that assessment of patients' needs with subsequent tailoring of behavioral interventions that include self-monitoring, collaborative goal-setting, and active problem solving was associated with appropriate single and multiple risk factor reduction (Goldstein et al., 2004).

(MR) A systematic review of research related to the effect of behavioral counseling interventions on health outcomes found that shared decision making was associated with an increased sense of personal control, promoted choices that were patient centered, and was less likely to cause resistance. This shared decision making is enhanced by asking questions such as "How important is it to you . . .?" (Whitlock et al., 2002).

(NR) An RCT ($N = 90$) evaluating the effect of a nurse-led intervention to improve women's cardiovascular risk factors found that involving women in reflection on and appropriate changes in personal smoking, nutrition, and exercise patterns resulted in increased aerobic exercise activity and decreased smoking (Anderson et al., 2006).

■ **(NIC)** *Use a variety of strategies and intervention points in the educational program.* **LOE = I**

(MR) A systematic review of research related to risk factor intervention found that the use of multiple modalities was associated with appropriate risk factor reduction (Goldstein et al., 2004).

(MR) In an RCT ($N = 337$), a 4-week educational program combining lecture, engagement in self-assessment workbook activities, shopping trips, and cooking demonstrations was found to have a positive effect on health knowledge and on changes in dietary choices, exercise, resting heart rate, cholesterol level, and percent body fat (Aldana et al., 2005).

(MR) In an RCT ($N = 467$ patients with hypercholesterolemia), an intervention consisting of three nurse-led individual diet counseling sessions (including the use of illustrated goal sheets, educational pamphlets, and a cookbook), referral services, and reinforcement telephone calls and newsletters increased self-reported dietary intake and weight loss but resulted in no difference in cholesterol levels (Ammerman et al., 2003).

(MR) In an RCT of overweight individuals, 91 participants were randomly assigned to a 6-month weight loss program delivered totally via Internet sites or a structured program using Internet sites plus 24 weekly behavioral lessons via e-mail, weekly online self-monitoring submissions, therapist feedback, and an online bulletin board. Participants in the structured program with weekly contact and individualized feedback lost significantly more weight and experienced greater decreases in waist circumference measurements (Tate et al., 2001).

(MR) In an RCT with 251 postmenopausal women in which all participants answered a questionnaire on breast self-examination (BSE) behavior and health beliefs, half were also shown a 15-minute video on BSE. Although self-reported BSE increased significantly in both groups, women in the video group performed BSE more frequently (Janda et al., 2002).

RCT = Randomized Controlled (Clinical) Trial, **NIC** = Nursing Interventions Classification, **NOC** = Nursing Outcomes Classification

■ *Develop structured educational interventions with multiple contact points.*
LOE = I

(NR) A meta-analysis of seven studies of weight loss intervention for children found that the most effective interventions involved longer periods of participation and consistent, structured interventions (Snethen et al., 2006).

(MR) A systematic review of research related to risk factor intervention found that behavioral interventions that include multiple follow-up contacts were associated with appropriate single and multiple risk factor reduction (Goldstein et al., 2004).

(NR) In an RCT ($N = 168$) investigating the effectiveness of a nursing inpatient smoking cessation program in individuals with cardiovascular disease, a 1-hour inpatient counseling session with six telephone follow-up calls in the first 2 months after discharge resulted in a 6-month abstinence rate of 40.1, whereas the abstinence rate for inpatient counseling alone was 30.2% and for usual care was 20% (Chouinard & Robichaud-Ekstrand, 2005).

(MR) An RCT with 286 low-income minority mothers testing the effects of a community-based parent education program on health care utilization in the first year of life found that mothers who had more frequent contact were the most likely to have followed age-appropriate immunization schedules for their infants (El-Mohandes et al., 2003).

■ *Develop and use tailored interventions.* **LOE = I**

(MR) In a Cochrane review of 17 trials evaluating educational materials for smoking cessation, the use of materials tailored to the individual had a stronger effect than either the use of standard materials or no intervention (Lancaster & Stead, 2005).

(MR) A systematic review of 30 RCTs examining the use of computer-tailored interventions to change physical activity and/or dietary habits revealed a positive effect on dietary practices, especially related to reduction of fat intake (Kroeze et al., 2006).

(MR) An RCT ($N = 213$) comparing the use of standardized and tailored educational brochures for parents regarding prevention of child injury revealed that those who received the tailored information reported adoption of more care and home safety behaviors (Nansel et al., 2002).

(MR) An RCT involving 1247 patients who had recently undergone a polypectomy investigated the use of a telephone-delivered intervention plus tailored materials focusing on the six primary behavioral risk factors for colorectal cancer. The study found that this intervention generated a significantly greater reduction in multiple risk factors (Emmons et al., 2005).

(MR) In a cohort study, 146 smokers who received an individually tailored nicotine dependence intervention, 29% (95% C.I. 22% to 37%) were abstinent at 6-month follow-up (Fernander et al., 2006).

■ *Develop collaborative multidisciplinary partnerships.* **LOE = I**

(MR) A Cochrane review of 62 trials of interventions designed to affect risk factors for falling among community-dwelling elders concluded that multidisciplinary and multifactorial interventions were likely to be effective (Gillespie et al., 2003).

(MR) A systematic review of research related to risk factor interventions for physical activity, diet, smoking, obesity, and risky alcohol use found that the use of multidisciplinary teams and nurse-led programs was associated with multiple risk factor reduction (Goldstein et al., 2004).

NR = Nursing Research, **MR** = Multidisciplinary Research, **SP** = Standard of Practice, **EO** = Expert Opinion, **LOE** = Level of Evidence

(MR) A systematic review of research related to the effect of behavioral counseling interventions on health outcomes found that involving a variety of staff and using diverse, complementary intervention methods improved the effectiveness of the interventions (Whitlock et al., 2002).

(NR) A case report of the evaluation of a 9-year community-based, nurse-managed health promotion and chronic disease care management program for community-residing older adults found that these seniors reported better general health, performance of roles, and social functioning as well as fewer physician visits and hospital days per year than the general population (Nūnez et al., 2003).

Possibly Effective

■ *Use technology-based interventions.* **LOE = I**

(MR) In a systematic review of 26 trials, the authors stated that there was not enough evidence to conclude that computer-based patients' education led to better health outcomes (Wofford et al., 2005).

(MR) An RCT ($N = 211$) of a computer-based decision aid about genetic testing for breast cancer susceptibility found that an interactive computer program was more effective in increasing knowledge about breast cancer risk in women at low risk for breast cancer and had the potential to stand alone as an educational intervention for low-risk (but not high-risk) women (Green et al., 2004).

(MR) In an RCT ($N = 91$) involving overweight individuals, participants in a structured program using Internet educational sites plus weekly behavioral lessons via e-mail, weekly online self-monitoring submissions, therapist feedback, and an online bulletin board lost significantly more weight and experienced greater decreases in waist circumference measurements than individuals who were given URLs for weight control websites (Tate et al., 2001).

(MR) An RCT ($N = 511$) found that mailed computer-tailored health messages accompanied by computer-tailored telephone counseling had a positive impact on physical activity (Jacobs et al., 2004).

(MR) An RCT ($N = 91$) investigating the use of computer software to promote physical activity concluded that computer systems that engage participants in repeated interactions are more effective than noninteractive systems and that the addition of emotional and relational elements such as social dialog, empathetic feedback, and humor increased satisfaction with and desire to continue use of the software (Bickmore et al., 2005).

■ *Use incentives or rewards.* **LOE = I**

(MR) A Cochrane review of 64 trials revealed that the use of rewards plus social support (found in two trials) had the greatest effect on reduction of smoking (Lumley et al., 2004).

(MR) A Cochrane review of 15 RCTs found no evidence of higher smoking cessation rates for incentive groups beyond 6 months assessment and no clear evidence that participants who committed their own money did better than those who did not or that different types of incentives were more or less effective (Hey & Perera, 2005).

(MR) In a controlled trial pilot study ($N = 53$) of the use of vouchers during pregnancy and for 12 postpartum weeks to promote smoking abstinence, abstinence rates were high in the initial postpartum period and remained high for as long as 24 postpartum weeks (Higgins et al., 2004).

RCT = Randomized Controlled (Clinical) Trial, **NIC** = Nursing Interventions Classification, **NOC** = Nursing Outcomes Classification

(MR) In an RCT involving 179 veterans, the use of incentives for smoking cessation resulted in significantly higher rates of smoking cessation program enrollment and completion and short-term quit rates (75 days) but not quit rates at 6 months (Volpp et al., 2006).

◼ *Use telephone follow-up.* LOE = I

(MR) An RCT (N = 754) found that tailored written feedback regarding dietary fat and fiber followed by a brief telephone intervention and mailed educational booklets was effective in changing fat and fiber intake in a group of rural residents (Fries et al., 2005).

(MR) In an RCT (N = 952), proactive telephone counseling was shown to be a useful strategy to promote smoking cessation among the parents of young children (Abdullah et al., 2005).

(MR) In an RCT (N = 1911) of an educational and counseling program to increase screening mammography among women 65 years and older, simple written materials about breast cancer screening for older women were followed up 4 months later by telephone contact in which the women who had not yet scheduled a mammogram were offered counseling to address issues and concerns. The simply written information was slightly beneficial; the addition of the telephone consultation showed no benefit (Michielutte et al., 2005).

(MR) An RCT (N = 399) compared walking behaviors in a group who received multiple mailings of a print brochure about the benefits of walking and a group who received the same mailings plus three telephone calls and found that walking increased significantly in both groups, which indicated that the addition of the telephone calls did not provide any additive effect (Humpel et al., 2004).

Not Effective

◼ *Use of self-help materials.* LOE = I

(MR) A Cochrane review of 33 trials involving self-help materials used for smoking cessation failed to find a positive effect of adding self-help materials to either one-on-one counseling or nicotine replacement (Lancaster & Stead, 2005).

(MR) In an RCT (N = 952) comparing printed self-help materials plus three sessions of telephone-based smoking cessation counseling with the use of printed self-help materials only, the addition of telephone counseling yielded twice the 7-day point prevalence quit rate at 6-month follow-up (Abdullah et al., 2005).

Possibly Harmful

No applicable published research was found in this category.

OUTCOME MEASUREMENT

HEALTH PROMOTING BEHAVIOR (NOC)

Definition: Personal actions to sustain or increase wellness.
Health Promoting Behavior as evidenced by the following selected NOC indicators:
- Uses risk avoidance behaviors
- Monitors personal behavior for risks

NR = Nursing Research, **MR** = Multidisciplinary Research, **SP** = Standard of Practice, **EO** = Expert Opinion, **LOE** = Level of Evidence

OUTCOME MEASUREMENT—*cont'd*

- Seeks balance among exercise, work, leisure, rest, and nutrition
- Uses effective stress reduction behaviors
- Performs healthy behaviors routinely

(Rate each indicator of **Health Promoting Behavior:** 1 = never demonstrated, 2 = rarely demonstrated, 3 = sometimes demonstrated, 4 = often demonstrated, 5 = consistently demonstrated) (Moorhead et al., 2004).

HEALTH SEEKING BEHAVIOR 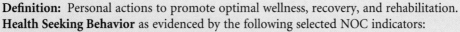 NOC

Definition: Personal actions to promote optimal wellness, recovery, and rehabilitation.
Health Seeking Behavior as evidenced by the following selected NOC indicators:
- Performs self-screening when indicated
- Seeks assistance from health professionals when indicated
- Adheres to self-developed strategies to eliminate unhealthy behavior
- Seeks current health-related information
- Performs prescribed health behavior when indicated

(Rate each indicator of **Health Seeking Behavior:** 1 = never demonstrated, 2 = rarely demonstrated, 3 = sometimes demonstrated, 4 = often demonstrated, 5 = consistently demonstrated) (Moorhead et al., 2004).

ADHERENCE BEHAVIOR NOC

Definition: Self-initiated actions to promote wellness, recovery, and rehabilitation.
Adherence Behavior as evidenced by the following selected NOC indicators:
- Seeks health-related information from a variety of sources
- Weighs risks/benefits of health behavior
- Uses strategies to eliminate unhealthy behavior
- Performs self-screening
- Performs self-monitoring of health status

(Rate each indicator of **Adherence Behavior:** 1 = never demonstrated, 2 = rarely demonstrated, 3 = sometimes demonstrated, 4 = often demonstrated, 5 = consistently demonstrated) (Moorhead et al., 2004).

REFERENCES

Abdullah AS, Mak YW, Loke AY, Lam TH. (2005). Smoking cessation intervention in parents of young children: A randomised controlled trial. *Addiction,* 100(11):1731-1740.

Aldana SG, Greenlaw RL, Diehl HA, Salberg A, Merrill RM, Ohmine S, et al. (2005). Effects of an intensive diet and physical activity modification program on the health risks of adults. *J Am Diet Assoc,* 105(3):371-381.

Ammerman AS, Keyserling TC, Atwood JR, Hosking JD, Zayed H, Krasny C. (2003). A randomized controlled trial of a public health nurse directed treatment program for rural patients with high blood cholesterol. *Prev Med,* 36(3):340-351.

Anderson D, Mizzari K, Kain V, Webster J. (2006). The effects of a multimodal intervention trial to promote lifestyle factors associated with the prevention of cardiovascular disease in menopausal and postmenopausal Australian women. *Health Care Women Int,* 27(3):238-253.

Aroian KJ. (2001). Immigrant women and their health. *Annu Rev Nurs Res,* 19:179-226.

Austin LT, Ahmad F, McNally MJ, Stewart DE. (2002). Breast and cervical cancer screening in Hispanic women: A literature review using the health belief model. *Womens Health Issues,* 12(3):122-128.

Berkman ND, Dewalt DA, Pignone MP, Sheridan SL, Lohr KN, Lux L, et al. (2004). Literacy and health outcomes. *Evid Rep Technol Assess (Summ),* 87:1-8.

Bickmore T, Gruber A, Picard R. (2005). Establishing the computer-patient working alliance in automated health behavior change interventions. *Patient Educ Couns,* 59(1):21-30.

Bowen DJ, Powers D, Greenlee H. (2006). Effects of breast cancer risk counseling for sexual minority women. *Health Care Women Int,* 27(1):59-74.

Champion V, Maraj M, Hui S, Perkins AJ, Tierney W, Menon U, et al. (2003). Comparison of tailored interventions to increase mammography screening in nonadherent older women. *Prev Med,* 36(2): 150-158.

Chouinard MC, Robichaud-Ekstrand S. (2005). The effectiveness of a nursing inpatient smoking cessation program in individuals with cardiovascular disease. *Nurs Res,* 54(4):243-254.

Conn VS, Valentine JC, Cooper HM. (2002). Interventions to increase physical activity among aging adults: A meta-analysis. *Ann Behav Med,* 24(3):190-200.

Dallas C, Burton L. (2004). Health disparities among men from racial and ethnic minority populations. *Annu Rev Nurs Res,* 22:77-100.

Dewalt DA, Berkman ND, Sheridan S, Lohr KN, Pignone MP. (2004). Literacy and health outcomes: A systematic review of the literature. *J Gen Intern Med,* 19(12):1228-1239.

Dochterman JM, Bulechek GM (Eds). (2004). *Nursing Interventions Classification (NIC),* 4th ed. St. Louis: Mosby.

El-Mohandes AA, Katz KS, El-Khorazaty MN, McNeely-Johnson D, Sharps PW, Jarrett MH, et al. (2003). The effect of a parenting education program on the use of preventive pediatric health care services among low-income, minority mothers: A randomized, controlled study. *Pediatrics,* 111(6 Pt 1): 1324-1332.

Emmons KM, McBride CM, Puleo E, Pollak KI, Clipp E, Kuntz K, et al. (2005). Project PREVENT: A randomized trial to reduce multiple behavioral risk factors for colon cancer. *Cancer Epidemiol Biomarkers Prev,* 14(6):1453-1459.

Fernander AF, Patten CA, Schroeder DR, Stevens SR, Croghan IT, Offord KP, et al. (2006). Characteristics of six-month tobacco use outcomes of black patients seeking smoking cessation intervention. *J Health Care Poor Underserved,* 17(2):413-424.

Fries E, Edinboro P, McClish D, Manion L, Bowen D, Beresford SA, et al. (2005). Randomized trial of a low-intensity dietary intervention in rural residents: The Rural Physician Cancer Prevention Project. *Am J Prev Med,* 28(2):162-168.

Gillespie LD, Gillespie WJ, Robertson MC, Lamb SE, Cumming RG, Rowe BH. (2003). Interventions for preventing falls in elderly people. *Cochrane Database Syst Rev,* (4):CD000340.

Girardi S, Gaudy C, Gouvernet J, Teston J, Richard MA, Grob J. (2006). Superiority of a cognitive education with photographs over ABCD criteria in the education of the general population to the early detection of melanoma: A randomized study. *Int J Cancer,* 118(9):2276-2280.

Goldstein MG, Whitlock EP, DePue J; Planning Committee of the Addressing Multiple Behavioral Risk Factors in Primary Care Project. (2004). Multiple behavioral risk factor interventions in primary care: Summary of research evidence. *Am J Prev Med,* 27(2 Suppl):61-79.

Grady MA, Bloom KC. (2004). Pregnancy outcomes of adolescents enrolled in a CenteringPregnancy program. *J Midwifery Womens Health,* 49(5):412-420.

Green MJ, Peterson SK, Baker MW, Harper GR, Friedman LC, Rubinstein WS, et al. (2004). Effect of a computer-based decision aid of knowledge, perceptions, and intentions about genetic testing for breast cancer susceptibility: A randomized controlled trial. *JAMA,* 292(4):442-452.

Hey K, Perera R. (2005). Competitions and incentives for smoking cessation. *Cochrane Database Syst Rev,* (2):CD004307.

Higgins ST, Heil SH, Solomon LJ, Bernstein IM, Lussier JP, Abel RL, et al. (2004). A pilot study on voucher-based incentives to promote abstinence from cigarette smoking during pregnancy and postpartum. *Nicotine Tob Res,* 6(6):1015-1020.

Humpel N, Marshall AL, Iverson D, Leslie E, Owen N. (2004). Trial of print and telephone delivered interventions to influence walking. *Prev Med,* 39(3):635-641.

Jacobs AD, Ammerman AS, Ennett ST, Campbell MK, Tawney KW, Aytur SA, et al. (2004). Effects of a tailored follow-up intervention on health behaviors, beliefs, and attitudes. *J Womens Health,* 13(5): 557-568.

Janda M, Stanek C, Newman B, Obermair A, Trimmel M. (2002). Impact of videotaped information on frequency and confidence of breast self-examination. *Breast Cancer Res Treat,* 73(1):37-43.

Kroeze W, Werkman A, Brug J. (2006). A systematic review of randomized trials on the effectiveness of computer-tailored education on physical activity and dietary behaviors. *Ann Behav Med,* 31(3): 205-223.

Lancaster T, Stead LF. (2005). Self-help interventions for smoking cessation. *Cochrane Database Syst Rev,* (3):CD001118.

Lumley J, Oliver SS, Chamberlain C, Oakley L. (2004). Interventions for promoting smoking cessation during pregnancy. *Cochrane Database Syst Rev,* (4):CD001055.

Michielutte R, Sharp PC, Foley KL, Cunningham LE, Spangler JG, Paskett ED, et al. (2005). Intervention to increase screening mammography among women 65 and older. *Health Educ Res,* 20(2):149-162.

Miller ET, Spilker J. (2003). Readiness to change and brief educational interventions: Successful strategies to reduce stroke risk. *J Neurosci Nurs,* 35(4):215-222.

Moher M, Hey K, Lancaster T. (2005). Workplace interventions for smoking cessation. *Cochrane Database Syst Rev,* (3):CD003440.

Moorhead M, Johnson M, Maas M (Eds). (2004). *Nursing Outcomes Classification (NOC),* 3rd ed. St. Louis: Mosby.

Nansel TR, Weaver N, Donlin M, Jacobsen H, Kreuter MW, Simons-Morton B. (2002). Baby, be safe: The effect of tailored communications for pediatric injury prevention provided in a primary care setting. *Patient Educ Couns,* 46(3):175-190.

Núñez DE, Armbruster C, Phillips WT, Gale BJ. (2003). Community-based senior health promotion program using a collaborative practice model: The Escalante Health Partnerships. *Public Health Nurs,* 20(1):25-32.

Pignone M, DeWalt DA, Sheridan S, Berkman N, Lohr KN. (2005). Interventions to improve health outcomes for patients with low literacy: A systematic review. *J Gen Intern Med,* 19:1228-1239.

Snethen JA, Broome ME, Cashin SE. (2006). Effective weight loss for overweight children: A meta-analysis of intervention studies. *J Pediatr Nurs,* 21(1):45-56.

Tate DF, Wing RR, Winett RA. (2001). Using Internet technology to deliver a behavioral weight loss program. *JAMA,* 285(9):1172-1177.

Volpp KG, Gurmankin Levy A, Asch DA, Berlin JA, Murphy JJ, Gomez A, et al. (2006). A randomized controlled trial of financial incentives for smoking cessation. *Cancer Epidemiol Biomarkers Prev,* 15(1):12-18.

Whitlock EP, Orleans CT, Pender N, Allan J. (2002). Evaluating primary care behavioral counseling interventions: An evidence-based approach. *Am J Prev Med,* 22(4):267-284.

Wilson FL, Brown DL, Stephens-Ferris M. (2006). Can easy-to-read immunization information increase knowledge in urban low-income mothers? *J Pediatr Nurs,* 21(1):4-12.

Wofford JL, Smith ED, Miller DP. (2005). The multimedia computer for office-based patient education: A systematic review. *Patient Educ Couns,* 59(2):148-157.

HEAT/COLD APPLICATION

Deborah Couture, PT, DPT, MS, OCS

NIC **Definition:** Stimulation of the skin and underlying tissues with heat or cold for the purpose of decreasing pain, muscle spasms, or inflammation (Dochterman & Bulechek, 2004).

RCT = Randomized Controlled (Clinical) Trial, **NIC** = Nursing Interventions Classification, **NOC** = Nursing Outcomes Classification

NURSING ACTIVITIES

Effective

■ *Use the intermittent treatment protocol of an ice pack (melting ice in a standard ice pack) for reducing pain.* **LOE = I**

(MR) A randomized controlled double-blind study ($N = 99$) of subjects with mild/moderate acute ankle sprains indicated that those treated with an intermittent treatment protocol of cryotherapy (melting ice water at 0°C in a standard ice pack) had significantly less ankle pain on activity than those using a standard 20-minute protocol (Bleakley et al., 2006).

(MR) A double-blind RCT ($N = 40$) of patients undergoing inguinal hernia repair indicated that localized cooling with ice packs was a safe and effective method for providing pain relief following hernia repair based on significant differences in visual analogue scores between treatment and control groups (Koc et al., 2006).

(NR) An RCT ($N = 25$) found that application of cold promoted relief of pricking pain artificially produced by electrical stimulation and reduced skin blood flow and skin conductance levels, and application of heat caused a significant increase in pain sensation and enhancement of blood flow and skin conductance levels (Saeki, 2002).

(MR) An RCT ($N = 19$) concluded that patients with acute gout treated with ice had significantly greater reduction in pain than the control group (Schlesinger et al., 2002).

■ *Use ice packs for reducing skin surface temperature and intra-articular temperature. The duration of application to reduce temperatures adequately is directly dependent on the thickness of adipose tissue.* **LOE = II**

(MR) A repeated measures design ($N = 50$) comparing the skin surface temperature during the application of four cryotherapy modalities concluded that ice packs and a mixture of water and alcohol were significantly more efficient in reducing skin surface temperature than a gel pack or package of frozen peas (Kanlayanaphotporn & Janwantanakul, 2005).

(MR) A case series with no control group ($N = 30$) examined the intra-articular temperature of the knee after application of an ice pack on the knee following arthroscopic knee surgery. The study concluded that external application of ice is an effective and sure method to diminish the intra-articular temperature of the knee (Sanchez-Inchausti et al., 2005).

(MR) A prospective within-subject controlled trial found that, although both methods were effective, application of ice reduced intra-articular temperature of the knee more than a cryotherapy device but was associated with higher pain scores, suggesting that intra-articular temperatures below a certain threshold were associated with increased perceived pain (Warren et al., 2004).

(MR) A four-group between-group comparison with an independent (skinfold thickness) and a dependent variable (time required to decrease intramuscular temperature 7°C from baseline) found a direct relationship between adipose tissue and cooling time (Otte et al., 2002).

(MR) A clinical trial, repeated measure ($N = 16$), concluded that cold pack therapy applied for 20 minutes produced a significant reduction in temperature in cutaneous and subcutaneous superficial tissues without directly changing the temperature of tissues at or more than 2.0 cm below the skin, and the temperature gradient of both layers of tissue reversed after treatment, indicating that deep tissue was one of the sources of heat used to rewarm the cooled superficial surfaces (Enwemeka et al., 2002).

NR = Nursing Research, **MR** = Multidisciplinary Research, **SP** = Standard of Practice, **EO** = Expert Opinion, **LOE** = Level of Evidence

Additional research: Chesterton et al., 2002; MacAuley, 2001; Martin et al., 2001; Myrer et al., 2001.

■ *Use a continuous cryotherapy device/cryotherapy apparatus/cold compressive dressing (Cryo/Cuff) for reducing intra-articular temperature and pain. The use of thick dressings, however, may impair the cooling effects.* **LOE = I**

(MR) A prospective RCT ($N = 61$) found no significant difference in morphine consumption between patients receiving cold compressive dressings (Cryo/Cuff) and patients receiving epidural anesthesia in the postoperative management of unicondylar knee arthroplasty; it was concluded that the Cryo/Cuff was an effective, risk-free alternative to epidural anesthesia to reduce pain after knee arthroplasty (Holmstrom & Hardin, 2005).

(MR) A systematic review/meta-analysis indicated that use of a cryotherapy apparatus was associated with significantly lower postoperative pain but did not significantly affect postoperative drainage or range of motion (Raynor et al., 2005).

(MR) An RCT ($N = 61$) found that wool and crepe dressings significantly impaired the cooling effects of cryotherapy applied with Cryo/Cuff and autochill, whereas thin adhesive dressings did not (Ibrahim et al., 2005).

(MR) A prospective within-subject controlled trial found that, although both methods were effective, the application of ice reduced intra-articular temperature of the knee more than a cryotherapy device but was associated with higher pain scores (Warren et al., 2004).

(MR) An RCT ($N = 69$) demonstrated that the use of a continuous cryotherapy delivery system reduced the amount of pain and discomfort perceived by patients who underwent arthroscopic or open surgical procedures on the shoulder (Singh et al., 2001).

■ *Use a paraffin wax bath for short-term symptomatic relief for arthritic hands.* **LOE = I**

(MR) A controlled trial ($N = 40$) of patients with rheumatoid arthritis and healthy controls demonstrated a significant increase in skin microcirculation, skin temperature, and core temperature when 30 minutes of local thermotherapy was applied using infrared light, paraffin, or peat. Microcirculation was more intense when paraffin was used (Berliner & Maurer, 2004).

(MR) A controlled trial ($N = 17$) of patients with scleroderma found that hand exercises in combination with a paraffin bath seemed to improve mobility, perceived stiffness, and skin elasticity to a greater extent than treatment with exercises alone (Sandqvist et al., 2004).

(MR) A Cochrane review of thermotherapy for treatment of rheumatoid arthritis concluded that paraffin wax baths combined with exercise could be recommended for beneficial short-term effects for arthritic hands (Robinson et al., 2002).

Possibly Effective

■ *Use a hot pack application to increase tissue temperature and blood flow.* **LOE = II**

(MR) An RCT ($N = 46$) found no difference between the use of dry heat versus moist heat in the tissue temperature rise and thermal transfer through orofacial tissues, although a small number of participants preferred moist heat (Poindexter et al., 2002).

RCT = Randomized Controlled (Clinical) Trial, **NIC** = Nursing Interventions Classification, **NOC** = Nursing Outcomes Classification

■ *Use a hot pack application combined with exercise for treatment of acute and subacute low back pain.* **LOE = I**

(MR) A systematic review found moderate evidence in a small number of trials that heat wrap therapy provided a small short-term reduction in pain and disability in a population with a mix of acute and subacute low back pain. The addition of exercise further reduced pain and improved function (French et al., 2006).

(MR) An RCT ($N = 100$) evaluating the efficacy of combining continuous low-level heat wrap therapy with exercise on the functional ability of patients with acute low back pain concluded that combining heat wrap therapy with exercise improved functional outcomes compared with either intervention alone and that either intervention alone was more effective than control (Mayer et al., 2005).

■ *Use a cooling garment in the treatment of multiple sclerosis (MS).* **LOE = II**

(MR) An RCT ($N = 60$) found that active cooling with a cooling garment for 60 minutes at 7°C improved muscle strength, fatigue, and postural stability in patients with MS. Active cooling was associated with mean leukocyte nitric oxide production of 41%, which could be relevant because it blocks conduction in demyelinated axons (Beenekker et al., 2001).

■ *Use a 10-minute ice massage for pain relief.* **LOE = IV**

(MR) A controlled clinical trial ($N = 16$) indicated that a 10-minute ice massage was an effective procedure for achieving analgesia (Bugaj, 1975).

■ *Use a warm sitz bath to decrease anal sphincter pressures.* **LOE = IV**

(MR) A study of control subjects ($N = 40$) with no anorectal complaints found no significant difference between anal pressures at rest or during voluntary contraction before and after a hot perineal bath (Pinho et al., 1993).

(MR) A controlled trial ($N = 46$) measuring rectal and interstitial sphincter temperature, rectal and rectal neck pressure, and EMG activity of both external and internal sphincters before and after participants sat in warm water baths at 40°, 45°, and 50°C for 10 minutes found that rectal neck pressures and internal sphincter EMG activity dropped significantly while in the bath but gradually returned to pretest levels 25 to 70 minutes after (Shafik, 1993b).

(MR) A controlled trial ($N = 57$) of patients with anorectal complaints and healthy volunteers found that immersion of the anus in warm water (40°C) for 5 minutes significantly decreased resting anal canal pressure over time in all participants and was likely to benefit patients after anorectal operations and those with anorectal pain (Dodi et al., 1986).

■ *Use a warm sitz bath to induce urination.* **LOE = IV**

(MR) A controlled trial ($N = 51$) using 30 healthy volunteers and 21 patients with urinary retention found that spontaneous micturition occurred in 19 of 21 patients with urinary retention when they sat in a warm sitz bath. Sitz baths were tested at temperatures of 40°, 45°, and 50°C (Shafik, 1993a).

■ *Use a warm bath to increase blood flow.* **LOE = II**

(NR) An RCT ($N = 6$) investigating the effect of a warm foot bath on increasing the distal (foot)-proximal (abdominal) skin temperature gradient (DPG) indicated that 40° and 41°C foot bathing could increase the DPG and may be an effective method of affecting whole body skin blood flow and triggering heat dissipation (Liao et al., 2005).

(MR) An RCT ($N = 24$) with repeated measurements of blood flow concluded that although contrast therapy produced fluctuations in blood flow, the warm water therapy (40°C) resulted in significant changes in blood flow compared with the control and contrast conditions. Cold-water therapy (13°C) did not produce significantly decreased blood flow when compared with the controlled condition (Fiscus et al., 2005).

Not Effective

■ *Use of hot packs for increasing tissue extensibility and flexibility.* **LOE = II**

(MR) An RCT ($N = 24$) comparing the effects of deep heating with short-wave diathermy, superficial heating with hydrocollator packs, and no heating on tissue extensibility of the calf muscles in the absence of stretching found that superficial heating was more effective than no heating, but the results were not statistically significant (Robertson et al., 2005).

(MR) An RCT ($N = 27$) found results that supported previous findings that moist heat application did not significantly affect muscle flexibility (Sawyer et al., 2003).

(MR) An RCT ($N = 97$) of patients with limited range of motion in dorsiflexion found no significant difference in improvements in extensibility of the plantar flexors between the group that performed static stretching with superficial moist heat application and the group that performed static stretching without heat (Knight et al., 2001).

(MR) An RCT ($N = 30$) indicated that significant benefits to increase hamstring flexibility could be gained by using moist heat packs in comparison with static stretching (Funk et al., 2001).

■ *Using hot or cold pack application for treatment of rheumatoid arthritis.* **LOE = I**

(MR) A Cochrane review of thermotherapy for treatment of rheumatoid arthritis found that there was no significant effect of hot and ice pack applications, cryotherapy, and faradic baths on objective measures of disease activity including joint swelling, pain, medication intake, range of motion, grip strength, and hand function compared with a control group or active therapy group (Robinson et al., 2002).

■ *Using frozen gel packs to reduce skin surface temperature.* **LOE = II**

(MR) An RCT ($N = 20$) comparing the localized skin cooling effects of a flexible frozen gel pack, a package of frozen peas, and control found that the application of a frozen pea package produced sufficient cooling of skin to produce analgesia, decrease nerve conduction velocity, or decrease metabolic enzyme activity, but flexible frozen gel packs did not cool skin sufficiently (Chesterton et al., 2002).

■ *Using cold pack applications to treat low back pain.* **LOE = I**

(MR) A systematic review found insufficient evidence to evaluate the effects of cold for low back pain (French et al., 2006).

■ *Using cold pack application as a supplement to exercise to treat tendinopathy.* **LOE = II**

(MR) An RCT ($N = 40$) investigating the use of ice as a supplement to an exercise program for treatment of lateral elbow tendinopathy found that eccentric strengthening and static stretching reduced pain in patients whether or not ice was included (Manias & Stasinopoulos, 2006).

RCT = Randomized Controlled (Clinical) Trial, **NIC** = Nursing Interventions Classification, **NOC** = Nursing Outcomes Classification

■ *Using ice massage for reducing exercise-induced muscle damage.* **LOE = II**

(MR) An RCT (*N* = 12) found no significant difference between people treated with ice massage and a placebo group in reducing the indirect markers associated with exercise-induced muscle damage or enhancing recovery of muscle function (Howatson et al., 2005).

(MR) An RCT (*N* = 9) found that ice massage reduced the appearance of plasma creatine kinase but had no other effect on signs and symptoms associated with exercise-induced muscle damage (Howatson & van Someren, 2003).

Possibly Harmful

■ *Using ice packs below certain critical temperatures.* **LOE = V**

(MR) A prospective within-subject controlled trial found that, although both methods were effective, the application of ice to reduce intra-articular temperature of the knee was more effective than a cryotherapy device but was associated with higher pain scores, suggesting that intra-articular temperatures below a certain threshold were associated with increased perceived pain (Warren et al., 2004).

(MR) A review of the literature found that motor performance was affected by temperature with a critical temperature around 18°C at which muscle performance decreased and that the critical temperature of cold with inflammation and edema increasing was below 15°C (Meeusen & Lievens, 1986).

■ *Performing exercise following the use of ice packs on the lower extremity.* **LOE = V**

(MR) A controlled clinical trial (*N* = 30) found that the application of an ice bag to the shoulder for 30 minutes did not impair shoulder joint position sense (Dover & Powers, 2004).

(MR) A clinical trial (*N* = 20) found that the application of a cooling pad at 4°C for 15 minutes made the knee joint stiffer and lessened sensitivity of position sense. This should be taken into account for therapeutic programs that involve exercise immediately after a cooling period (Uchio et al., 2003).

(MR) A systematic review of the literature found that reflex activity and motor function were impaired following ice treatment; thus, patients may be more susceptible to injury after ice treatments (MacAuley, 2001).

(MR) A review of the literature found that motor performance was affected by temperature, with a critical temperature around 18°C, at which muscle performance decreased, and that the critical temperature of cold with inflammation and edema increasing was below 15°C (Meeusen & Lievens, 1986).

OUTCOME MEASUREMENT

PAIN LEVEL (NOC)

Definition: Severity of observed or reported pain.
Pain Level as evidenced by the following NOC indicators:
• Reported pain
• Length of pain episodes
• Moaning and crying

OUTCOME MEASUREMENT—*cont'd*

- Facial expressions of pain
- Restlessness
- Pacing
- Narrowed focus
- Muscle tension
- Loss of appetite

(Rate each indicator of **Pain Level:** 1 = severe, 2 = substantial, 3 = moderate, 4 = mild, 5 = none) (Moorhead et al., 2004).

REFERENCES

Beenekker EA, Oparina TI, Hartgring A, Teelken A, Arutjunyan AV, De Keyser J. (2001). Cooling garment treatment in MS: Clinical improvement and decrease in leukocyte NO production. *Neurology,* 57(5):892-894.

Berliner MN, Maurer AI. (2004). Effect of different methods of thermotherapy on skin microcirculation. *Am J Phys Med Rehabil,* 83(4):292-297.

Bleakley CM, McDonough SM, MacAuley DC, Bjordal J. (2006). Cryotherapy for acute ankle sprains: A randomised controlled study of two different icing protocols. *Br J Sports Med,* 40(8):700-705.

Bugaj R. (1975). The cooling, analgesic, and rewarming effects of ice massage on localized skin. *Phys Ther,* 55(1):11-19.

Chesterton LS, Foster NE, Ross L. (2002). Skin temperature response to cryotherapy. *Arch Phys Med Rehabil,* 83(4):543-549.

Dochterman JM, Bulechek GM (Eds). (2004). *Nursing Interventions Classification (NIC),* 4th ed. St. Louis: Mosby.

Dodi G, Bogoni F, Infantino A, Pianon P, Mortellaro LM, Lise M. (1986). Hot or cold in anal pain? A study of the changes in internal anal sphincter pressure profiles. *Dis Colon Rectum,* 29(4):248-251.

Dover G, Powers ME. (2004). Cryotherapy does not impair shoulder joint position sense. *Arch Phys Med Rehabil,* 85(8):1241-1246.

Enwemeka CS, Allen C, Avila P, Bina J, Konrade J, Munns S. (2002). Soft tissue thermodynamics before, during, and after cold pack therapy. *Med Sci Sports Exerc,* 34(1):45-50.

Fiscus KA, Kaminski TW, Powers ME. (2005). Changes in lower-leg blood flow during warm-, cold-, and contrast water therapy. *Arch Phys Med Rehabil,* 86(7):1404-1410.

French SD, Cameron M, Walker BF, Reggars JW, Esterman AJ. (2006). A Cochrane review of superficial heat or cold for low back pain. *Spine,* 31(9):998-1006.

Funk D, Swank AM, Adams KJ, Treolo D. (2001). Efficacy of moist heat pack application over static stretching on hamstring flexibility. *J Strength Cond Res,* 15(1):123-126.

Hill PD. (1989). Effects of heat and cold on the perineum after episiotomy/laceration. *J Obstet Gynecol Neonatal Nurs,* 18(2):124-129.

Holmstrom A, Hardin BC. (2005). Cryo/Cuff compared to epidural anesthesia after knee unicompartmental arthroplasty: A prospective, randomized and controlled study of 60 patients with a 6-week follow-up. *J Arthroplasty,* 20(3):316-321.

Howatson G, Gaze D, van Someren KA. (2005). The efficacy of ice massage in the treatment of exercise-induced muscle damage. *Scand J Med Sci Sports,* 15(6):416-422.

Howatson G, van Someren KA. (2003). Ice massage. Effects on exercised-induced muscle damage. *J Sports Med Phys Fitness,* 43(4):500-505.

Ibrahim T, Ong SM, Saint Clair Taylor GJ. (2005). The effects of different dressings on the skin temperature of the knee during cryotherapy. *Knee,* 12(1):21-23.

Kanlayanaphotporn R, Janwantanakul P. (2005). Comparison of skin surface temperature during the application of various cryotherapy modalities. *Arch Phys Med Rehabil,* 86(7):1411-1415.

RCT = Randomized Controlled (Clinical) Trial, **NIC** = Nursing Interventions Classification, **NOC** = Nursing Outcomes Classification

Knight CA, Rutledge CR, Cox ME, Acosta M, Hall SJ. (2001). Effect of superficial heat, deep heat, and active exercise warm-up on the extensibility of the plantar flexors. *Phys Ther,* 81(6):1206-1214.

Koc M, Tez M, Yoldas O, Dizen H, Gocmen E. (2006). Cooling for the reduction of postoperative pain: Prospective randomized study. *Hernia,* 10(2):184-186.

Liao WC, Landis CA, Lentz MJ, Chiu MJ. (2005). Effect of foot bathing on distal-proximal skin temperature gradient in elders. *Int J Nurs Stud,* 42(7):717-722.

MacAuley DC. (2001). Ice therapy: How good is the evidence? *Int J Sports Med,* 22(5):379-384.

Manias P, Stasinopoulos D. (2006). A controlled clinical pilot trial to study the effectiveness of ice as a supplement to the exercise programme for the management of lateral elbow tendinopathy. *Br J Sports Med,* 40(1):81-85.

Martin SS, Spindler KP, Tarter JW, Detwiler K, Petersen HA. (2001). Cryotherapy: An effective modality for decreasing intraarticular temperature after knee arthroscopy. *Am J Sports Med,* 29(3):288-291.

Mayer JM, Ralph L, Look M, Erasala GN, Verna JL, Matheson LN, et al. (2005). Treating acute low back pain with continuous low-level heat wrap therapy and/or exercise: A randomized controlled trial. *Spine J,* 5(4):395-403.

Meeusen R, Lievens P. (1986). The use of cryotherapy in sports injuries. *Sports Med,* 3(6):398-414.

Moorhead M, Johnson M, Maas M (Eds). (2004). *Nursing Outcomes Classification (NOC),* 3rd ed. St. Louis: Mosby.

Myrer WJ, Myrer KA, Measom GJ, Fellingham GW, Evers SL. (2001). Muscle temperature is affected by overlying adipose when cryotherapy is administered. *J Athl Train,* 36(1):32-36.

Otte JW, Merrick MA, Ingersoll CD, Cordova ML. (2002). Subcutaneous adipose tissue thickness alters cooling time during cryotherapy. *Arch Phys Med Rehabil,* 83(11):1501-1505.

Pinho M, Correa JC, Furtado A, Ramos JR. (1993). Do hot baths promote anal sphincter relaxation? *Dis Colon Rectum,* 36(3):273-274.

Poindexter RH, Wright EF, Murchison DF. (2002). Comparison of moist and dry heat penetration through orofacial tissues. *Cranio,* 20(1):28-33.

Raynor MC, Pietrobon R, Guller U, Higgins LD. (2005). Cryotherapy after ACL reconstruction: A meta-analysis. *J Knee Surg,* 18(2):123-129.

Robertson VJ, Ward AR, Jung P. (2005). The effect of heat on tissue extensibility: A comparison of deep and superficial heating. *Arch Phys Med Rehabil,* 86(4):819-825.

Robinson V, Brosseau L, Casimiro L, Judd M, Shea B, Wells G, et al. (2002). Thermotherapy for treating rheumatoid arthritis. *Cochrane Database Syst Rev,* (2):CD002826.

Saeki Y. (2002). Effect of local application of cold or heat for relief of pricking pain. *Nurs Health Sci,* 4(3):97-105.

Sanchez-Inchausti G, Vaquero-Martin J, Vidal-Fernandez C. (2005). Effect of arthroscopy and continuous cryotherapy on the intra-articular temperature of the knee. *Arthroscopy,* 21(5):552-556.

Sandqvist G, Akesson A, Eklund M. (2004). Evaluation of paraffin bath treatment in patients with systemic sclerosis. *Disabil Rehabil,* 26(16):981-987.

Sawyer PC, Uhl TL, Mattacola CG, Johnson DL, Yates JW. (2003). Effects of moist heat on hamstring flexibility and muscle temperature. *J Strength Cond Res,* 17(2):285-290.

Schlesinger N, Detry MA, Holland BK, Baker DG, Beutler AM, Rull M, et al. (2002). Local ice therapy during bouts of acute gouty arthritis. *J Rheumatol,* 29(2):331-334.

Shafik A. (1993a) Role of warm water bath in inducing micturition in postoperative urinary retention after anorectal operation. *Urol Int,* 50(4):213-217.

Shafik A. (1993b) Role of warm-water bath in anorectal conditions. The "thermosphincteric reflex." *J Clin Gastroenterol,* 16(4):304-308.

Singh H, Osbahr DC, Holovacs TF, Cawley PW, Speer KP. (2001). The efficacy of continuous cryotherapy on the postoperative shoulder: A prospective, randomized investigation. *J Shoulder Elbow Surg,* 10(6):522-525.

Uchio Y, Ochi M, Fujihara A, Adachi N, Iwasa J, Sakai Y. (2003). Cryotherapy influences joint laxity and position sense of the healthy knee joint. *Arch Phys Med Rehabil,* 84(1):131-135.

Warren TA, McCarty EC, Richardson AL, Michener T, Spindler KP. (2004). Intra-articular knee temperature changes: Ice versus cryotherapy device. *Am J Sports Med,* 32(2):441-445.

HEMORRHAGE CONTROL

Ruth M. Kleinpell, PhD, RN, FAAN, FAANP, FCCM; Thomas Ahrens, DNSc, RN, FAAN

NIC **Definition:** Reduction or elimination of rapid and excessive blood loss (Dochterman & Bulechek, 2004).

NURSING ACTIVITIES

Effective

■ **SP** *Control bleeding loss in hemorrhage by applying manual pressure over the bleeding or the potential bleeding area if possible or applying a pressure dressing as indicated.* **LOE = VII**

EO Emergency and critical care treatment guidelines indicate that initial resuscitation requires rapid restoration of the circulating blood volume along with interventions to control ongoing losses. The initial management of the patient with impending shock requires attention to the "ABCs" of resuscitation: assurance of an airway (A), adequate ventilation (breathing, B), and establishment of an adequate blood volume to support the circulation (C). Control of hemorrhage requires immediate attention (Maier, 2005). Current Advanced Trauma Life Support guidelines call for the replacement of each milliliter of lost blood with three times the amount of isotonic crystalloid while giving careful attention to the physiological response of the patient (Kauvar & Wade, 2005; Alam, 2006; Maier, 2005).

■ **SP** *Assess for signs of shock including changes in vital signs, presence of postural hypotension, presence of anxiety, and new onset of confusion.* **LOE = VII**

EO Emergency and critical care treatment guidelines outline that mild hypovolemia (≤20% of the blood volume) can result in mild tachycardia but relatively few other signs. With moderate hypovolemia (20% to 40% of the blood volume), increasing tachycardia, postural hypotension, and anxiety may be seen. If hypovolemia is severe (≥40% of the blood volume), the classic signs of shock appear with hypotension, marked tachycardia, oliguria, and agitation or confusion. The transition from mild to severe hypovolemic shock can be insidious or extremely rapid (Maier, 2005; Kolecki & Menckhoff, 2006).

EO Consensus definitions outlining sepsis and septic shock identify that the clinical signs of sepsis and septic shock include the systemic inflammatory response syndrome. Two or more of the following conditions can indicate sepsis: temperature >38°C or <36°C, heart rate >90 beats/min, respiratory rate >20 breaths/min or $Paco_2 < 32$ mm Hg (<4.3 kPa), WBC > 12,000 cells/mm³, <4000 cells/mm³, or >10% immature (band) forms. Additional signs and symptoms include chills, hypotension, decreased skin perfusion, decreased urine output, significant edema or positive fluid balance (>20 mL/kg over 24 hours), decreased capillary refill or mottling, hyperglycemia (plasma glucose >120 mg/dL) in the absence of diabetes, and unexplained change in mental status (Levy et al., 2003).

RCT = Randomized Controlled (Clinical) Trial, **NIC** = Nursing Interventions Classification, **NOC** = Nursing Outcomes Classification

■ ⒮ *Note hemoglobin/hematocrit level before and after blood loss, as indicated; if the Hgb is less than 7 mg/dL, administer blood product as ordered.* **LOE = I**

ⓂⓇ Recommendations from a systematic literature review state that red blood cell transfusion should occur in sepsis and septic shock when hemoglobin decreases to less than 7.0 g/dL to target a hemoglobin of 7.0 to 9.0 g/dL (Dellinger et al., 2004).

ⒺⓄ Hypertonic saline is a promising initial resuscitation option, and it has been demonstrated to be more effective at restoring the extravascular volume, cardiac output, and organ perfusion than large-volume resuscitation with Ringer's lactate (Deitch & Dayal, 2006; Kramer, 2003; Kreimeier & Messmer, 2002).

ⒺⓄ The use of recombinant factor VIIa for adjunctive hemorrhage control in trauma and surgical patients has demonstrated benefit in controlling bleeding (Benharash et al., 2005).

■ *Use a rapid response team (RRT) for the early detection of shock.* **LOE = I**

ⓂⓇ RRTs or medical emergency teams provide a team approach to shock to evaluate and treat immediately patients with alterations in vital signs or neurological deterioration. In several prospective clinical trials, the use of RRTs demonstrated decreases in incidence of in-hospital cardiac arrest, bed occupancy of cardiac arrest survivors, and overall in-hospital mortality (Bellomo et al., 2003, 2004; Buist et al., 2002).

ⓂⓇ Consensus guidelines on the use of RRTs recommend that hospitals implement a system that detects urgent unmet medical needs and responds to them rapidly and reliably (DeVita et al., 2006).

■ ⒮ *Use protocols to target early identification and treatment of hemorrhage and onset of shock.* **LOE = IV**

ⓂⓇ In a historical control single-site study, the use of a hospital-wide comprehensive shock program was associated with decreased mortality rates and better outcomes (discharge to home or rehabilitation center). Shock protocols were implemented by nurses to provide early recognition of shock and initiation of indicated therapies, including goal-directed resuscitation protocols (Sebat et al., 2005).

■ *Use early goal-directed therapy.* **LOE = I**

ⓂⓇ Shock is the clinical syndrome that results from inadequate tissue perfusion. Regardless of the cause, the hypoperfusion-induced imbalance between the delivery of oxygen and the uptake of oxygen leads to cellular dysfunction. Rapid infusion of volume resuscitation through large-bore intravenous lines is indicated for initial resuscitation in shock. A randomized clinical trial of emergency room focused resuscitation using goal-directed therapy that targeted optimizing perfusion through the use of fluid resuscitation, transfusion of packed red blood cells to achieve a hematocrit ≥30%, and/or administration of dobutamine infusion (up to a maximum of 20 µg/kg/min) was used to achieve perfusion goals that demonstrated significant improvement in survival (Rivers et al., 2001).

NR = Nursing Research, **MR** = Multidisciplinary Research, **SP** = Standard of Practice, **EO** = Expert Opinion, **LOE** = Level of Evidence

Possibly Effective

■ *If the patient displays signs of shock, consider elevating both legs.* **LOE = VII**

(EO) Elevating both legs can be the optimal method of restoring blood volume to the core of the body. Using the classic Trendelenburg position may increase work of breathing and risk for aspiration (Maier, 2005).

■ *Use blood substitutes to restore blood volume.* **LOE = V**

(MR) A synthesis review of hemoglobin-based O_2 carriers revealed that despite numerous clinical trials, predominantly in animal models, no consensus could be reached on the clinical application of blood substitutes. The critical properties of hemoglobin solutions with regard to oxygen affinity, viscosity, and oncotic pressure need to be studied further (Winslow, 2003).

Not Effective

■ *Use of colloids compared with crystalloids for resuscitation.* **LOE = I**

(MR) Three systematic reviews have demonstrated no differences with fluid resuscitation with colloid or crystalloid solutions in critically ill patients (Schierhout & Roberts, 1998; Choi et al., 1999; Finfer et al., 2004).

Possibly Harmful

No applicable published research was found in this category.

OUTCOME MEASUREMENT

CIRCULATION STATUS

Definition: Unobstructed, unidirectional blood flow at an appropriate pressure through large vessels of the systemic and pulmonary circuits.

Circulation Status as evidenced by the following selected NOC indicators:

- Systolic blood pressure
- Diastolic blood pressure
- Pulse pressure
- Mean blood pressure
- Central venous pressure
- Pulmonary wedge pressure
- Pao$_2$
- Paco$_2$
- Oxygen saturation
- Arterial-venous oxygen difference
- Cognitive status
- Skin temperature

Continued

OUTCOME MEASUREMENT—*cont'd*

- Skin color
- Urinary output

(Rate each indicator of **Circulation Status:** 1 = severely compromised, 2 = substantially compromised, 3 = moderately compromised, 4 = mildly compromised, 5 = not compromised) (Moorhead et al., 2004).

REFERENCES

Alam HB. (2006). An update on fluid resuscitation. *Scand J Surg,* 95(3):136-145.

Bellomo R, Goldsmith D, Uchino S, Buckmaster J, Hart GK, Opdam H, et al. (2003). A prospective before-and-after trial of a medical emergency team. *Med J Aust,* 179(6):283-287.

Bellomo R, Goldsmith D, Uchino S, Buckmaster J, Hart G, Opdam H, et al. (2004). Prospective controlled trial of effect of medical emergency team on postoperative morbidity and mortality rates. *Crit Care Med,* 32(4):916-921.

Benharash P, Bongard F, Putnam B. (2005). Use of recombinant factor VIIa for adjunctive hemorrhage control in trauma and surgical patients. *Am Surg,* 71(9):776-780.

Buist MD, Moore GE, Bernard SA, Waxman BP, Anderson JN, Nguyen TV. (2002). Effects of a medical emergency team on reduction of incidence of and mortality from unexpected cardiac arrests in hospital: Preliminary study. *BMJ,* 324(7334):387-390.

Choi PT, Yip G, Quinonez LG, Cook DJ (1999). Crystalloids vs. colloids in fluid resuscitation: A systematic review. *Crit Care Med,* 27(1):200-210.

Deitch EA, Dayal SD. (2006). Intensive care unit management of the trauma patient. *Crit Care Med,* 34(9):2294-2301.

Dellinger RP, Carlet JM, Masur H, Gerlach H, Calandra T, Cohen J, et al. (2004). Surviving Sepsis Campaign guidelines for management of severe sepsis and septic shock. *Crit Care Med,* 32(3):858-873.

DeVita MA, Bellomo R, Hillman K, Kellum J, Rotondi A, Teres D, et al. (2006). Findings of the first consensus conference on medical emergency teams. *Crit Care Med,* 34(9):2463-2478.

Dochterman JM, Bulechek GM (Eds). (2004). *Nursing Interventions Classification (NIC),* 4th ed. St. Louis: Mosby.

Finfer S, Bellomo R, Boyce N, French J, Myburgh J, Norton R, et al. (2004). A comparison of albumin and saline for fluid resuscitation in the intensive care unit, *N Engl J Med,* 350(22):2247-2256.

Kauvar DS, Wade CE. (2005). The epidemiology and modern management of traumatic hemorrhage: US and international perspectives. *Crit Care,* 9 Suppl 5:S1-S9.

Kolecki P, Menckhoff CR. (2006). Shock, hypovolemic. *eMedicine.* Available online: http://www.emedicine.com. Retrieved on May 27, 2007.

Kramer GC. (2003). Hypertonic resuscitation: Physiologic mechanisms and recommendations for trauma care. *J Trauma,* 54(5 Suppl):S89-S99.

Kreimeier U, Messmer K. (2002). Small-volume resuscitation: From experimental evidence to clinical routine. Advantages and disadvantages of hypertonic solutions. *Acta Anaesthesiol Scand,* 46(6): 625-638.

Levy MM, Fink MP, Marshall JC, Abraham E, Angus D, Cook D, et al. (2003). 2001 SCCM/ESICM/ACCP/ATS/SIS International Sepsis Definitions Conference. *Crit Care Med,* 31(4):1250-1256.

Maier RV. (2005). Approach to the patient with shock. In Kasper DL, Braunwald, E, Fauci, AS, et al (Eds): *Harrison's principles of internal medicine,* 16th ed. New York: McGraw Hill.

Moorhead M, Johnson M, Maas M (Eds). (2004). *Nursing Outcomes Classification (NOC),* 3rd ed. St. Louis: Mosby.

Rivers E, Nguyen B, Havstad S, Ressler J, Muzzin A, Knoblich B, et al. (2001). Early goal-directed therapy in the treatment of severe sepsis and septic shock. *N Engl J Med,* 345(19):1368-1377.

Schierhout G, Roberts I. (1998). Fluid resuscitation with colloid or crystalloid solutions in critically ill patients: A systematic review of randomised trials, *BMJ* 316(7136):961-964.

NR = Nursing Research, **MR** = Multidisciplinary Research, **SP** = Standard of Practice, **EO** = Expert Opinion, **LOE** = Level of Evidence

Sebat F, Johnson D, Musthafa AA, Watnik M, Moore S, Henry K, et al. (2005). A multidisciplinary community hospital program for early and rapid resuscitation of shock in nontrauma patients. *Chest*, 127(5):1729-1743.

Winslow RM. (2003). Current status of blood substitute research: Towards a new paradigm. *J Intern Med*, 253(5):508-517.

HIV PREVENTION

Thomas James Loveless, MSN, CRNP

Definition: Reduction in the transmission and acquisition of HIV infection through a variety of strategies, activities, interventions, and services (CDC, 1998).

NURSING ACTIVITIES

Effective

■ *Maintain universal precautions consistently for all patients.* **LOE = VII**

(EO) Considered the "gold standard" and remaining as the cornerstone of protecting health care workers, universal precautions were implemented by the CDC in 1986 and updated in 1996 and 2005 (Panlilio et al., 2005).

(EO) Occupational transmission of HIV to health care workers has been documented when health care workers are exposed to blood and visibly bloody fluids (Bell, 1997).

(MR) In prospective studies of health care providers, the risks of an occupational transmission of HIV subsequent to a percutaneous exposure to HIV-infected blood has been documented to be approximately 0.3% (95% confidence interval [CI] = 0.2% to 0.5%) and after a mucous membrane exposure, approximately 0.09% (95% CI = 0.006% to 0.5%) (Bell, 1997).

(MR) A prospective review indicated that the risks of transmission after exposure to fluids or tissues other than HIV-infected products have not been quantified but are probably considerably lower than the risks after blood exposure (Henderson et al., 1990).

■ *Evaluate the need for postexposure prophylaxis immediately after an exposure.* **LOE = VII**

(EO) Postexposure prophylaxis (PEP) should be initiated as soon as possible, usually within 1 to 2 hours (Gerberding, 1999) if warranted. Careful consideration needs to be given regarding the source patient as well as the heath care worker. Full evaluation may require consultation with an infectious disease specialist. The median time from exposure to treatment in 432 health care workers with HIV exposure from October 1996 until December 1998 was 1.8 hours (Bartlett & Gallant, 2005-2006). Initiation of PEP should not exceed 36 hours.

(MR) A logistic-regression analysis of 33 case patients and 665 controls showed that the significant risk factors for seroconversion were deep injury, injury with an instrument that showed obvious patient's blood, an injury subsequent to the source patient's artery or vein being punctured, or exposure to the blood of a patient who soon succumbed to AIDS complications (Cardo et al., 1997).

RCT = Randomized Controlled (Clinical) Trial, **NIC** = Nursing Interventions Classification, **NOC** = Nursing Outcomes Classification

(EO) Consideration for PEP, while in consultation with an infectious disease specialist, should evaluate the extent of the injury (the depth of penetration and the size of the inoculum), the absence or presence of obvious blood from the source patient on the inflicting instrument, whether or not the blood from the source patient is directly a result of arterial or venous puncture (hollow bore needles that were in an artery or vein are likely to contain more inoculum and have a greater capacity to transmit infectious blood), and the overall state of health of the source patient. Discuss with the health care provider the risk versus benefits of initiating PEP (Do et al., 2003).

■ *Immediately complete thorough hand washing if an exposure to blood or bloody fluids has occurred.* **LOE = VII**

(EO) Immediate hand washing after blood or body fluid exposure is recommended to prevent HIV transmission (CDC, 1998).

■ *Do not recap or purposely bend or break needles, remove needles from disposable syringes, or otherwise manipulate needles by hand.* **LOE = VII**

(EO) Although certain procedures remain intrinsically riskier than others, the modern-day use of engineered safety devices to prevent percutaneous needle sticks should not be modified or maneuvered (CDC, 1998; Panlilio et al., 2005).

(EO) After needles are used, all should immediately be placed in a puncture-resistant container for disposal (CDC, 1998; Panlilio et al., 2005).

Possibly Effective

■ *Health care workers with open draining or exudative lesions should refrain from all direct care of patients and from handling patient-care equipment until the condition resolves.* **LOE = VII**

(EO) Exposed skin that is chapped, abraded, or afflicted with dermatitis increases the likelihood of a bidirectional transmission of blood-borne pathogens (CDC, 1998).

■ *Wear gloves while performing venipuncture and other vascular procedures; for touching blood or other bloody fluids, mucous membranes, or nonintact skin of patients; or when hand contamination with blood may occur (e.g., with phlebotomy or the uncooperative patient).* **LOE = VII**

(EO) Gloves should reduce the incidence of blood contamination of hands during phlebotomy, *but they cannot prevent penetrating injuries caused by needles or other sharp instruments* (CDC, 1998).

■ *Wear masks and eyewear routinely during procedures that are likely to generate droplets of blood to prevent mucocutaneous exposure.* **LOE = VII**

(EO) Masks and eyewear should reduce the incidence of blood contamination of mucous membranes of the mouth, eye, and nose while performing procedures that may generate droplets of blood or body fluids requiring precautions (CDC, 1998; Panlilio et al., 2005; Larson, 1988, 1999).

NR = Nursing Research, **MR** = Multidisciplinary Research, **SP** = Standard of Practice, **EO** = Expert Opinion, **LOE** = Level of Evidence

Not Effective

No applicable published research was found in this category.

Possibly Harmful

No applicable published research was found in this category.

OUTCOME MEASUREMENT

KNOWLEDGE: HEALTH BEHAVIOR NOC

Definition: Extent of understanding conveyed about the promotion and protection of health.

Knowledge: Health Behavior as evidenced by the following selected NOC indicators:

• Description of measures to avoid exposure to environmental hazards
• Description of measures to prevent transmission of infectious disease

(Rate each indicator of **Knowledge: Health Behavior:** 1 = none, 2 = limited, 3 = moderate, 4 = substantial, 5 = extensive) (Moorhead et al., 2004).

REFERENCES

Bartlett JG, Gallant JE. (2005-2006). *Medical Management of HIV Infection: 2005-2006 Edition.* Baltimore, MD: Johns Hopkins Medicine, Health Publishing Business Group.

Bell DM. (1997). Occupational risk of human immunodeficiency virus infection in health-care workers: An overview. *Am J Med,* 102(5B):9-15.

Cardo DM, Culver DH, Ciesielski CA, Srivastava PU, Marcus R, Abiteboul DJ, et al. (1997). A case-control study of HIV seroconversion in health care workers after percutaneous exposure. *N Engl J Med,* 337(21):1485-1490.

Centers for Disease Control and Prevention (CDC). (1998). Public Health Service guidelines for the management of healthcare worker exposures to HIV and recommendations for postexposure prophylaxis. *MMWR Recomm Rep,* 47(RR-7):1-33.

Do AN, Ciesielski CA, Metler RP, Hammett TA, Li J, Flemming PL. (2003). Occupationally acquired human immunodeficiency virus (HIV) infection: National case surveillance data during 20 years of the HIV epidemic in the United States. *Infect Control Hosp Epidemiol,* 24(2):86-96.

Gerberding JL. (1999). Management of occupational exposures to blood-borne viruses. In Sande MA, Volberding PA. *The medical management of AIDS,* 6th ed. Philadelphia: WB Saunders.

Henderson DK, Fahey BJ, Willy M, Schmitt JM, Carey K, Koziol DE, Lane HC, Fedio J, Saah AJ. (1990). Risk for occupational transmission of human immunodeficiency virus type 1 (HIV-1) associated with clinical exposures. A prospective evaluation. *Ann Intern Med,* 113(10):740-746.

Larson E. (1988). A causal link between handwashing and risk of infection? Examination of the evidence. *Infect Control,* 9(1):28-36.

Larson E. (1999). Skin hygiene and infection prevention: More of the same or different approaches? *Clin Infect Dis,* 29(5):1287-1294.

Moorhead M, Johnson M, Maas M (Eds). (2004). *Nursing Outcomes Classification (NOC),* 3rd ed. St. Louis: Mosby.

Panlilio AL, Cardo DM, Grohskopf LA, Heneine W, Ross CS; U.S. Public Health Service. (2005). Updated U.S. Public Health Service guidelines for the management of occupational exposures to HIV and recommendations for postexposure prophylaxis. *MMWR Recomm Rep,* 54(RR-9):1-17.

HOME MAINTENANCE ASSISTANCE (NIC)

Diane E. Holland, PhD, RN

(NIC) **Definition:** Helping the patient/family to maintain the home as a clean, safe, and pleasant place to live (Dochterman & Bulechek, 2004).

NURSING ACTIVITIES

Effective

■ (NIC) *Determine the patient's home maintenance requirements.* **LOE = I**

(MR) A systematic review of the impact of interventions to improve housing (including rehousing, refurbishment, and energy efficiency measures) on measures of mental or physical health, episodes of illness, and use of health services concluded that the lack of evidence linking housing and health may be attributed to methodological difficulties and political obstacles (Thomson et al., 2001).

(MR) A systematic review demonstrated that a home safety assessment provided the most knowledge in identification and correction of hazards known to promote falls (Ritzel et al., 2001).

(NR) A systematic review identified the development of a plan for additional information and programmatic resources regarding home improvements as strategic in understanding how living arrangements may be a risk factor for patients (Hays, 2002).

(MR) An RCT ($N = 60$) of home assessments by an occupational therapist and an ergotherapist demonstrated that the autonomy of older patients at risk of falling could be preserved (Pardessus et al., 2002).

(NR) A descriptive study ($N = 20,000$) demonstrated that home maintenance is a risk factor for unintentional injuries occurring within the homes of older adults (Fletcher & Hirdes, 2005).

■ (NIC) *Involve the patient/family in deciding home maintenance requirements.* **LOE = I**

(MR) A systematic review indicated the importance of including family members and the patient where possible in the decision-making process regarding home environmental interventions (Gitlin, 2001).

■ (NIC) *Assist family members to develop realistic expectations of themselves in the performance of their roles.* **LOE = I**

(MR) A meta-analysis of the literature indicated that interventions for caregivers of people with dementia had a beneficial effect on caregiver knowledge, psychological distress, and burden (Brodaty et al., 2003).

■ (NIC) *Help the family use a social support network.* **LOE = I**

(NR) A systematic review identified that social support for caregivers decreased caregiver distress, improved caregiver physical health, and delayed care receiver nursing home placement (Farran, 2001).

NR = Nursing Research, **MR** = Multidisciplinary Research, **SP** = Standard of Practice, **EO** = Expert Opinion, **LOE** = Level of Evidence

(NR) A systematic review demonstrated that social support contributed to the development of effective coping mechanisms by caregivers (Verhaeghe et al., 2005).

(MR) An RCT ($N = 296$) of family support for 1 year following caregiving for a person with stroke demonstrated that family support significantly improved quality of life for caregivers (Mant et al., 2005).

(MR) An RCT ($N = 232$) of caregiver training for people with stroke demonstrated that poor family support identified caregivers at risk of adverse outcomes (McCullagh et al., 2005). Additional research: Savard et al., 2006; Plews et al., 2005; Friedman et al., 2005; Upton & Reed, 2006.

■ **(NIC)** *Provide information on how to make the home environment safe and clean.* **LOE = I**

(MR) A systematic review demonstrated that using bleach, antibacterial soaps, and proper food handling procedures can prevent infections in the home (Britton, 2003).

(MR) A systematic review demonstrated that successful strategies for reducing microbial risks in the home included adequate cleaning practices and appropriate use of cleaning and disinfection products (Kagan et al., 2002).

■ **(NIC)** *Advise the alleviation of all offensive odors.* **LOE = VI**

(MR) An observational study ($N = 3241$) found that odors were related to asthma symptoms and current cough (Engvall et al., 2001).

■ **(NIC)** *Suggest services for pest control, as needed.* **LOE = II**

(MR) An RCT ($N = 49$) demonstrated that reducing cockroach counts in homes significantly reduced allergen concentrations in the kitchen (McConnell et al., 2003).

(MR) An RCT ($N = 100$) showed that cockroach extermination in homes with asthmatic children decreased levels of particulate matter and daytime symptoms (Eggleston et al., 2005).

■ **(NIC)** *Facilitate cleaning of dirty laundry.* **LOE = I**

(MR) A systematic review demonstrated that washing bedding regularly reduced house dust mite and animal allergens (Eggleston, 2005).

(MR) An RCT ($N = 104$) of allergen avoidance (including washing bedding once a week in hot water) demonstrated a significant decrease in acute care visits for children with mite allergy (Carter et al., 2001).

■ **(NIC)** *Coordinate the use of community resources.* **LOE = I**

(NR) A systematic review demonstrated that access to health and social services resources was problematic for older adults. Referrals by health care providers are a necessary priority in the transitional care of older adults (Naylor, 2002).

(NR) A systematic review of interventions designed to alleviate caregiver distress in family members of older people with cancer concluded that coordinating care may alleviate distress (Given & Sherwood, 2006).

(MR) A systematic review demonstrated that caregivers of people with dementia who did not use support services mainly lacked awareness of the availability of support services (Brodaty et al., 2005).

RCT = Randomized Controlled (Clinical) Trial, **NIC** = Nursing Interventions Classification, **NOC** = Nursing Outcomes Classification

Possibly Effective

■ **NIC** *Provide information on respite care, as needed.* **LOE = II**

MR A Cochrane systematic review of medical day hospital care for the elderly versus other forms of care concluded that medical day hospital care appeared to be more effective than no intervention but no more effective than other respite interventions (Forster et al., 2000).
MR A Cochrane systematic review of respite care for people with dementia and their caregivers concluded that current evidence did not demonstrate any benefits or adverse effects for people with dementia or their caregivers (Lee & Cameron, 2004).
NR A systematic review demonstrated that a barrier to the use of respite services was a lack of information on the part of the caregiver (Aoun et al., 2005).

■ **NIC** *Suggest necessary structural alterations to make the home accessible.* **LOE = V**

MR A longitudinal observational study of community-dwelling adults ($N = 131$) recommended assessment of accessibility, usability, and dependence in activities of daily living for efficient planning and evaluation of housing adaptations (Fange & Iwarrsson, 2003).
MR A descriptive survey study ($N = 252$) demonstrated that the presence of any home modification was associated with fewer falls with injury in people who used wheelchairs at home (Berg et al., 2002).
MR A mixed-methods study ($N = 19$) demonstrated that usability of the home environment of stroke survivors was enhanced if attention was paid to both the inside and the outside housing environments (Reid, 2004).

■ **NIC** *Provide information on how to make the home environment safe and clean.* **LOE = I**

MR A Cochrane systematic review found that there was insufficient evidence that interventions to modify the home physical environment affected the likelihood of sustaining an injury in the home (Lyons et al., 2006).
MR A systematic review demonstrated that although simply advising people to "take care" and make changes to the home environment was not effective, environmental factors played a role in many falls (Rand Report, 2002).
MR A systematic review and meta-analysis recommended an assessment of risk factors for falls and modifying home environmental hazards (AGS et al., 2001).
Additional research: Clemson et al., 2004; Gitlin et al., 2001; Hogan et al., 2001; Huang & Acton, 2004; Lightbody et al., 2002; Nikolaus & Bach, 2003; Ward et al., 2004; Stevens et al., 2001.

■ *Discuss the cost of needed alterations and repair and available resources.* **LOE = VI**

MR A descriptive study ($N = 82$) identifying home adaptations for older home-dwelling people demonstrated that costs correlated with the degree of mobility disability, yet they were recouped within the average life expectancy through decreased use of formal care services (Lansley et al., 2004).
MR A pilot study ($N = 70$) addressing a multihazard, multimethod intervention for home repair demonstrated that a comprehensive approach to home remediation could be effective and cost efficient (Klitzman et al., 2005).

NR = Nursing Research, **MR** = Multidisciplinary Research, **SP** = Standard of Practice, **EO** = Expert Opinion, **LOE** = Level of Evidence

Not Effective

■ *Suggesting services for home alterations, repair, or maintenance.* **LOE = VII**

(EO) Although simply advising people to "take care" and make changes to the home environment is not effective, it remains an essential element in identifying safety hazards (Rand Report, 2002).

Possibly Harmful

No applicable published research was found in this category.

OUTCOME MEASUREMENT

SAFE HOME ENVIRONMENT (NOC)

Definition: Physical arrangements to minimize environmental factors that might cause physical harm or injury in the home.
Safe Home Environment as evidenced by the following selected NOC indicators:
• Placement of handrails
• Smoke detector maintenance
• Provision of assistive devices in accessible location
• Provision of equipment that meets safety standards
• Arrangement of furniture to reduce risks
(Rate each indicator of **Safe Home Environment**: 1 = not adequate, 2 = slightly adequate, 3 = moderately adequate, 4 = substantially adequate, 5 = totally adequate) (Moorhead et al., 2004).

DISCHARGE READINESS: SUPPORTED LIVING (NOC)

Definition: Readiness of a patient to relocate from a health care institution to a lower level of supported living.
Discharge Readiness: Supported Living as evidenced by the following selected NOC indicators:
• Patient needs consistent with available family support
• Describes special needs
• Describes short-term plan
• Describes long-term plan
• Describes plan for continuity in care
(Rate each indicator of **Discharge Readiness: Supported Living**: 1 = never demonstrated, 2 = rarely demonstrated, 3 = sometimes demonstrated, 4 = often demonstrated, 5 = consistently demonstrated) (Moorhead et al., 2004).

DISCHARGE READINESS: INDEPENDENT LIVING (NOC)

Definition: Readiness of a patient to relocate from a health care institution to living independently.

Continued

OUTCOME MEASUREMENT—*cont'd*

Discharge Readiness: Independent Living as evidenced by the following selected NOC indicators:
- Seeks assistance appropriately
- Uses available social support

(Rate each indicator of **Discharge Readiness: Independent Living**: 1 = never demonstrated, 2 = rarely demonstrated, 3 = sometimes demonstrated, 4 = often demonstrated, 5 = consistently demonstrated) (Moorhead et al., 2004).

REFERENCES

American Geriatrics Society (AGS), British Geriatrics Society (BGS) & American Academy of Orthopaedic Surgeons (AAOS) Panel on Falls Prevention. (2001). Guideline for the prevention of falls in older persons. *J Am Geriatr Soc,* 49(5):664-672.

Aoun SM, Kristjanson LJ, Currow DC, Hudson PL. (2005). Caregiving for the terminally ill: At what cost? *Palliat Med,* 19(7):551-555.

Berg K, Hines M, Allen S. (2002). Wheelchair users at home: Few home modifications and many injurious falls. *Am J Public Health,* 92(1):48.

Britton LA. (2003). Microbiological threats to health in the home. *Clin Lab Sci,* 16(1):10-15.

Brodaty H, Green A, Koschera A. (2003). Meta-analysis of psychosocial interventions for caregivers of people with dementia. *J Am Geriatr Soc,* 51(5):657-664.

Brodaty H, Thomson C, Thompson C, Fine M. (2005). Why caregivers of people with dementia and memory loss don't use services. *Int J Geriatr Psychiatry,* 20(6):537-546.

Carter MC, Perzanowski MS, Raymond A, Platts-Mills TA. (2001). Home intervention in the treatment of asthma among inner-city children. *J Allergy Clin Immunol,* 108(5):732-737.

Clemson L, Cumming RG, Kendig H, Swann M, Heard R, Taylor K. (2004). The effectiveness of a community-based program for reducing the incidence of falls in the elderly: A randomized trial. *J Am Geriatr Soc,* 52(9):1487-1494.

Dochterman JM, Bulechek GM (Eds). (2004). *Nursing Interventions Classification (NIC),* 4th ed. St. Louis: Mosby.

Eggleston PA. (2005). Improving indoor environments: Reducing allergen exposures. *J Allergy Clin Immunol,* 116(1):122-126.

Eggleston PA, Butz A, Rand C, Curtin-Brosnan J, Kanchanaraksa S, Swartz L, et al. (2005). Home environmental intervention in inner-city asthma: A randomized controlled clinical trial. *Ann Allergy Asthma Immunol,* 95(6):518-524.

Engvall K, Norrby C, Norback D. (2001). Asthma symptoms in relation to building dampness and odour in older multifamily houses in Stockholm. *Int J Tuberc Lung Dis,* 5(5):468-477.

Fange A, Iwarrsson S. (2003). Accessibility and usability in housing: Construct validity and implications for research and practice. *Disabil Rehabil,* 25(23):1316-1325.

Farran CJ. (2001). Family caregiver intervention research: Where have we been? Where are we going? *J Gerontol Nurs,* 27(7):38-45.

Fletcher PC, Hirdes JP. (2005). Risk factor for accidental injuries within senior citizens' homes: Analysis of the Canadian Survey on Ageing and Independence. *J Gerontol Nurs,* 31(2):49-57.

Forster A, Young J, Langhorne P. (2000). Medical day hospital care for the elderly versus alternative forms of care. *Cochrane Database Syst Rev,* (2):CD001730.

Friedman LC, Brown AE, Romero C, Dulay MF, Peterson LE, Wehrman P, et al. (2005). Depressed mood and social support as predictors of quality of life in women receiving home health care. *Qual Life Res,* 14(8):1925-1929.

Gitlin LN. (2001). Effectiveness of home environmental interventions for individuals with dementia and family caregivers. *Home Health Care Consultant,* 8(9):22-26.

Gitlin LN, Corcoran M, Winter L, Boyce A, Hauck WW. (2001). A randomized, controlled trial of a home environmental intervention: Effect on efficacy and upset in caregivers and on daily function of persons with dementia. *Gerontologist,* 41(1):4-14.

Given B, Sherwood PR. (2006). Family care for the older person with cancer. *Semin Oncol Nurs,* 22(1): 43-50.

Hays JC. (2002). Living arrangements and health status in later life: A review of recent literature. *Public Health Nurs,* 19(2):136-151.

Hogan DB, MacDonald FA, Betts J, Bricker S, Ebly EM, Delarue B, et al. (2001). A randomized controlled trial of a community-based consultation service to prevent falls. *CMAJ,* 165(5):537-543.

Huang TT, Acton GJ. (2004). Effectiveness of home visit falls prevention strategy for Taiwanese community-dwelling elders: Randomized trial. *Public Health Nurs,* 21(3):247-256.

Kagan LJ, Aiello AE, Larson E. (2002). The role of the home environment in the transmission of infectious diseases. *J Community Health,* 27(4):247-267.

Klitzman S, Caravanos J, Belanoff C, Rothenberg L. (2005). A multihazard, multistrategy approach to home remediation: Results of a pilot study. *Environ Res,* 99(3):294-306.

Lansley P, McCreadie C, Tinker A. (2004). Can adapting the homes of older people and providing assistive technology pay its way? *Age Ageing,* 33(6):571-576.

Lee H, Cameron M. (2004). Respite care for people with dementia and their carers. *Cochrane Database Syst Rev,* (2):CD004396.

Lightbody E, Watkins C, Leathley M, Sharma A, Lye M. (2002). Evaluation of a nurse-led falls prevention programme versus usual care: A randomized controlled trial. *Age Ageing,* 31(3):203-210.

Lyons RA, John A, Brophy S, Jones SJ, Johansen A, Kemp A, et al. (2006). Modification of the home environment for the reduction of injuries. *Cochrane Database Syst Rev,* (4):CD003600.

Mant J, Winner S, Roche J, Wade DT. (2005). Family support for stroke: One year follow up of a randomised controlled trial. *J Neurol Neurosurg Psychiatry,* 76(7):1006-1008.

McConnell R, Jones C, Milam J, Gonzalez P, Berhane K, Clement L, et al. (2003). Cockroach counts and house dust allergen concentrations after professional cockroach control and cleaning. *Ann Allergy Asthma Immunol,* 91(6):546-552.

McCullagh E, Brigstocke G, Donaldson N, Kalra L. (2005). Determinants of caregiving burden and quality of life in caregivers of stroke patients. *Stroke,* 36(10):2181-2186.

Moorhead M, Johnson M, Maas M (Eds). (2004). *Nursing Outcomes Classification (NOC),* 3rd ed. St. Louis, Mosby.

Naylor MD. (2002). Transitional care of older adults. *Annu Rev Nurs Res,* 20:127-147.

Nikolaus T, Bach M. (2003). Preventing falls in community-dwelling frail older people using a home intervention team (HIT): Results from the randomized Falls-HIT trial. *J Am Geriatr Soc,* 51(3):300-305.

Pardessus V, Puisieux F, Di Pompeo C, Gaudefroy C, Thevenon A, Dewailly P. (2002). Benefits of home visits for falls and autonomy in the elderly: A randomized trial study. *Am J Phys Med Rehabil,* 81(4):247-252.

Plews C, Bryar R, Closs J. (2005). Clients' perceptions of support received from health visitors during home visits. *J Clin Nurs,* 14(7):789-797.

Rand Report. (2002). *Evidence report and evidence-based recommendations: Falls prevention interventions in the Medicare population* (No. Contract number 500-98-0281): Southern California Evidence-Based Practice Center.

Reid D. (2004). Accessibility and usability of the physical housing environment of seniors with stroke. *Int J Rehabil Res,* 27(3):203-208.

Ritzel DO, Beasley D, Flynn J, Liefer M. (2001). Injuries to elderly women in the home environment: A research review. *Int Electronic J Health Educ,* 4:64-66.

Savard J, Leduc N, Lebel P, Beland F, Bergman H. (2006). Caregiver satisfaction with support services: Influence of different types of services. *J Aging Health,* 18(1):3-27.

Stevens M, Holman CD, Bennett N, de Klerk N. (2001). Preventing falls in older people: Outcome evaluation of a randomized controlled trial. *J Am Geriatr Soc,* 49(11):1448-1455.

Tanner EK. (2003). Assessing home safety in homebound older adults. *Geriatr Nurs,* 24(4):250-256.

RCT = Randomized Controlled (Clinical) Trial, **NIC** = Nursing Interventions Classification, **NOC** = Nursing Outcomes Classification

Thomson H, Petticrew M, Morrison D. (2001). Health effects of housing improvement: Systematic review of intervention studies. *BMJ*, 323(7306):187-190.

Upton N, Reed V. (2006). The influence of social support on caregiver coping. *Int J Psychiatr Nurs Res*, 11(2):1256-1267.

Verhaeghe S, Defloor T, Grypdonck M. (2005). Stress and coping among families of patients with traumatic brain injury: A review of the literature. *J Clin Nurs*, 14(8):1004-1012.

Ward CD, Turpin G, Dewey ME, Fleming S, Hurwitz B, Ratib S, et al. (2004). Education for people with progressive neurological conditions can have negative effects: Evidence from a randomized controlled trial. *Clin Rehabil*, 18(7):717-725.

HOPE INSPIRATION

Wendy Duggleby, DSN, RN, AOCN

NIC **Definition:** Facilitation of the development of a positive outlook in a given situation (Dochterman & Bulechek, 2004).

NURSING ACTIVITIES

Effective

No applicable published research was found in this category.

Possibly Effective

■ *Utilize the Living with Hope program; view a "Living with Hope" video and choose one of the following hope activities.* **LOE = II**

Write or ask someone to help you write one or more letters to someone:
- Choose people you want to write a letter to.
- Ask someone to help you write the letter or letters.
- You can give the letter to someone if you wish, but you don't have to.

Begin a hope collection:
- You can collect anything you want that gives you hope; these may include poems, writings, pictures, drawings, photographs, music, and stories.
- Place your collection in a special binder or box.

Begin an "About Me" collection (tell your life as a story):
- In your story, tell about your ups and downs beginning as young as you can remember.
- You can tell your story in any way you like. Some examples may be collecting cards, pictures, or writing a journal.
- You can put your story in a scrapbook, or you can audiotape or videotape your story so that others can learn about you.

NR An RCT ($N = 58$) of older terminally ill cancer patients comparing two groups, (1) Living with Hope program and (2) control group who received standard care, demonstrated a significant increase in hope and quality-of-life scores in the treatment group compared with the control (Duggleby et al., 2006, 2007).

NR = Nursing Research, **MR** = Multidisciplinary Research, **SP** = Standard of Practice, **EO** = Expert Opinion, **LOE** = Level of Evidence

■ *Utilize the Hope Intervention program (eight 2-hour group meetings over 8 weeks), which includes building a sense of community, search for hope, connecting with others, expanding the boundaries, building the hopeful veneer, and reflecting and evaluating (Herth, 2000).* **LOE = II**

(NR) An RCT ($N = 115$) of patients with recurrent cancer comparing three groups, (1) Hope Intervention program, (2) informational control, and (3) control (standard care), demonstrated significant increases in hope and quality-of-life scores for the treatment group compared with the other groups (Herth, 2000).

■ *Use humor.* **LOE = III**

(MR) A controlled clinical trial ($N = 180$) in which participants were assigned to view a humor video or a nonhumor video demonstrated a significant increase in hope following the humorous video compared with those in the control group (Vilaythong et al., 2003).

(NR) Participants in a qualitative study of terminally ill cancer patients ($N = 10$) suggested that humor and laughter fostered their hope by distraction from their concerns (Duggleby & Wright, 2004).

■ *Find meaning and purpose in life through life review and telling stories of experiences.* **LOE = IV**

(NR) Participants in a qualitative study of stroke survivors ($N = 9$) described how life review and telling of their experiences fostered their hope (Bays, 2001).

(NR) Participants in a grounded theory qualitative study of terminally ill cancer patients ($N = 10$) identified life review as a way to foster their hope by helping them find meaning and purpose in life (Duggleby & Wright, 2005).

(NR) Participants in a phenomenological qualitative study of terminally ill cancer patients ($N = 11$) described summarizing their life as a way to foster their hope (Benzein et al., 2001).

■ *Set personal short-term goals.* **LOE = IV**

(NR) Participants in a qualitative study of terminally ill cancer patients ($N = 10$) identified setting realistic short-term goals as a way to foster their hope (Duggleby & Wright, 2004).

(NR) Participants in a phenomenological qualitative study of healthy adults ($N = 24$) suggested that the activity of setting goals fostered their hope (Benzein et al., 2000).

(NR) Participants in a qualitative study of chronic renal dialysis patients ($N = 14$) described how setting of short-term goals fostered their hope (Weil, 2000).

■ *Encourage supportive relationships with family, friends, and health care professionals.* **LOE = IV**

(MR) A correlational study of cancer patients ($N = 113$) indicated that patients with a high level of social support felt a decreased sense of hopelessness (Gil & Gilbar, 2001).

(NR) Participants in a mixed-method study of family caregivers of terminally ill patients (quantitative $N = 51$, qualitative $N = 10$) suggested that positive supportive relationships with others fostered their hope (Borneman et al., 2002).

RCT = Randomized Controlled (Clinical) Trial, **NIC** = Nursing Interventions Classification, **NOC** = Nursing Outcomes Classification

NR Participants in a grounded theory quality study of family caregivers of terminally ill cancer patients ($N = 10$) identified supportive positive relationships with family, friends, and health care professionals as fostering their hope (Holtslander et al., 2005).

NR Participants in a qualitative study of terminally ill cancer patients ($N = 10$) identified supportive positive relationships with family and friends as fostering their hope (Duggleby & Wright, 2004).

Not Effective

■ *Use of exercise.* **LOE = II**

NR An RCT of lung cancer patients ($N = 104$) assigned to a preoperative exercise group or a nonexercise group demonstrated no significant differences in hope scores between groups (Wall, 2000).

Possibly Harmful

■ *Poor communication with health care professionals and lack of information regarding diagnosis and treatment.* **LOE = IV**

NR Participants in a phenomenological qualitative study of terminally ill cancer patients ($N = 11$) showed that poor communication and lack of information decreased their hope (Benzein et al., 2001).

NR Participants in a grounded theory qualitative study of family caregivers of terminally ill cancer patients ($N = 10$) described how poor communication and lack of information hindered their hope (Holtslander et al., 2005).

NR Participants in a qualitative study of terminally ill cancer patients ($N = 10$) suggested that lack of information about prognosis and treatment decreased their hope (Duggleby & Wright, 2004).

OUTCOME MEASUREMENT

HOPE NOC

Definition: Optimism that is personally satisfying and life-supporting.
Hope as evidenced by the following selected NOC indicators:
• Expresses expectation of a positive future
• Expresses meaning in life
• Sets goals
• Expresses optimism
• Expresses belief in others
• Expresses inner peace
• Expresses sense of self-control
(Rate each indicator of **Hope:** 1 = never demonstrated, 2 = rarely demonstrated, 3 = sometimes demonstrated, 4 = often demonstrated, 5 = consistently demonstrated) (Moorhead et al., 2004).

NR = Nursing Research, **MR** = Multidisciplinary Research, **SP** = Standard of Practice, **EO** = Expert Opinion, **LOE** = Level of Evidence

REFERENCES

Bays CL. (2001). Older adults' descriptions of hope after a stroke. *Rehabil Nurs,* 26(1):18-20, 23-27.

Benzein E, Norberg A, Saveman B. (2001). The meaning of the lived experience of hope in patients with cancer in palliative home care. *Palliat Med,* 15(2):117-126.

Benzein EG, Saveman B, Norberg A. (2000). The meaning of hope in healthy, nonreligious Swedes. *West J Nurs Res,* 22(3):303-319.

Borneman T, Stahl C, Ferrell BR, Smith D. (2002). The concept of hope in family caregivers of cancer patients at home. *J Hospice Palliat Nurs,* 4(1):21-33.

Dochterman JM, Bulechek GM (Eds). (2004). *Nursing Interventions Classification (NIC),* 4th ed. St. Louis: Mosby.

Duggleby W, Degner L, Williams A, Wright K, Cooper D, Popkin D, et al. (2006). Mixed method evaluation of a Living with Hope program for older terminally ill cancer patients. *Oncol Nurs Forum,* 33(2): 409.

Duggleby W, Degner L, Williams A, Wright K, Cooper D, Popkin D, et al. (2007). Living with hope: Initial evaluation of a psychosocial hope intervention for older palliative home care patients. *J Pain Symptom Manage,* 33(3):247-257.

Duggleby W, Wright K. (2004). Elderly palliative care cancer patients' descriptions of hope-fostering strategies. *Int J Palliat Nurs,* 10(7):352-359.

Duggleby W, Wright K. (2005). Transforming hope: How elderly palliative patients live with hope. *Can J Nurs Res,* 37(2):70-84.

Gil S, Gilbar O. (2001). Hopelessness among cancer patients. *J Pyschosocial Oncol,* 19(1):21-33.

Herth K. (2000). Enhancing hope in people with a first recurrence of cancer. *J Adv Nurs,* 32(6):1431-1441.

Holtslander LF, Duggleby W, Williams AM, Wright KE. (2005). The experience of hope for informal caregivers of palliative patients. *J Palliat Care,* 21(4):285-291.

Moorhead M, Johnson M, Maas M (Eds). (2004). *Nursing outcomes classification (NOC),* 3rd ed. St. Louis: Mosby.

Vilaythong AP, Arnau RC, Rosen DH. (2003). Humor and hope: Can humor increase hope? *Int J Humor Res,* 16(1):79-89.

Wall LM. (2000). Changes in hope and power in lung cancer patients who exercise. *Nurs Sci Q,* 13(3):234-242.

Weil CM. (2000). Exploring hope in patients with end stage renal disease on chronic hemodialysis. *Nephrol Nurs J,* 27(2):219-224.

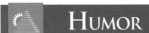 # HUMOR

Mary P. Bennett, PhD, FNP, APRN

NIC **Definition:** Facilitating the patient to perceive, appreciate, and express what is funny, amusing, or ludicrous in order to establish relationships, relieve tension, release anger, facilitate learning, or cope with painful feelings (Dochterman & Bulechek, 2004).

NURSING ACTIVITIES

Effective

No applicable published research was found in this category.

Possibly Effective

Enhanced Immune Function

RCT = Randomized Controlled (Clinical) Trial, **NIC** = Nursing Interventions Classification, **NOC** = Nursing Outcomes Classification

■ *Use humor to decrease proinflammatory cytokines in rheumatoid arthritis patients.* **LOE = III**

(MR) In a controlled clinical trial (*N* = 64) of 41 rheumatoid arthritis (RA) patients and 23 healthy individuals, proinflammatory cytokines were measured before and after a humor stimulus. Levels of interleukin 6 (IL-6) and IL-4 (inflammatory factors) decreased significantly in the RA group but not in the control group (Matsuzaki et al., 2006).

■ *Watch a comical video to create a pleasant feeling that enhances free radical–scavenging capacity in human whole saliva.* **LOE = III**

(MR) In a controlled clinical trial (*N* = 27), free radical–scavenging capacity (FRSC) in saliva was measured in participants before, during, and after viewing a comical video. The FRSC values obtained after watching the video were significantly higher than those before watching it, and those who reported a pleasant feeling following the video had higher FRSC values than those who did not (Atsumi et al., 2004).

■ *Use humor to decrease stress and improve immune function.* **LOE = II**

(NR) An RCT (*N* = 32) measured baseline stress and natural killer cell activity in participants who were randomly assigned to two groups: (1) humor movie and (2) nonhumor movie. The results demonstrated a significant reduction in self-reported stress following the intervention in those viewing the humor movie. There was also significantly improved natural killer cell activity in people viewing the humor movie who laughed, and this improvement in immune function was significantly correlated with the participants' response (measured using a humor response scale) (Bennett et al., 2003). (Note: Only people who laughed out loud had significant improvement in immune function.)

■ *Watch a humorous video to enhance immune function.* **LOE = III**

(MR) A controlled clinical trial (*N* = 52) of healthy men was used to test the effect of a 1-hour humor video on various measures of immune function. Significant increases in natural killer cell functioning, levels of immunoglobins, and active cytotoxic T cells were found (Berk et al., 2001).

■ *Watch a humorous video to decrease the response to allergens in people with atopic dermatitis.* **LOE = III**

(MR) A controlled clinical trial (*N* = 26) tested the effect of an 87-minute humor video on skin wheal response to dust mite allergens in people with known allergies to dust mites. Wheal responses were significantly reduced after viewing the video, and this reduction in size was maintained for 2 hours but not for 4 hours. Wheal responses were not significantly affected by viewing a nonhumorous video (Kimata, 2001).

Enhanced Coping

■ *Use humor to decrease state anxiety.* **LOE = II**

(MR) In two separate controlled clinical trials (*N* = 20 and *N* = 39), the effect of humor was compared with the effects of other interventions on state anxiety in healthy women. Participants were exposed to four treatments in a counterbalanced order (aerobic exercise,

NR = Nursing Research, **MR** = Multidisciplinary Research, **SP** = Standard of Practice, **EO** = Expert Opinion, **LOE** = Level of Evidence

humorous video, new-age music, and sitting quietly). State anxiety was measured before and after each treatment. Negative affect decreased in all conditions except sitting quietly, with the humor intervention being the most effective (Szabo et al., 2005; Szabo, 2003).

■ **Watch a humorous video to decrease allergic wheal response during stressful situations. LOE = II**

(MR) A controlled clinical trial ($N = 52$) of patients with atopic dermatitis tested the effect of viewing a humorous video versus a nonhumorous video on allergic wheal responses during an experimental stressor. Those who viewed the humorous video had decreased wheal response during the stressful situation compared with those who viewed the nonhumorous video (Kimata, 2004b).

■ **Use humor to increase hope. LOE = III**

(MR) A controlled clinical trial ($N = 180$) was used to test the effect of viewing a humorous video versus a nonhumorous video on scores on the Snyder State Hope Scale. Participants were assigned to either a humorous video or a neutral video, with pretest/post-test measurement of hope. There was a significant increase in hope following the humorous video compared with those in the control group (Vilaythong et al., 2003).

■ **Use humor as systematic desensitization to reduce the fear of spiders. LOE = II**

(MR) A controlled clinical trial ($N = 40$) was used to test the effect of humor desensitization in people fearful of spiders. Participants were randomly assigned to one of three groups: systematic desensitization, humor desensitization, and untreated control. Participants in both treatment groups had greater reduction in fear than the controls, and humor desensitization worked as well as traditional desensitization therapy but not significantly better (Ventis et al., 2001).

■ **Watch a humorous video to decrease stress hormones. LOE = II**

(MR) A controlled clinical trial ($N = 10$) of healthy male subjects tested the effect of a 1-hour humorous video on various neuroendocrine measures of stress. Participants were assigned to two groups: (1) humor movie and (2) non-humor movie. Significant reductions in cortisol, dopac (the major serum neuronal catabolite of dopamine), epinephrine, and growth hormone were noted in those who were in the laughter group (Berk et al., 1989).

Therapeutic Relationships

■ **Use humor to develop therapeutic relationships in palliative care. LOE = VI**

(NR) A qualitative ethnographic design ($N = 15$) of patients in palliative care was used to determine the role of humor in the development of authentic person-to person connectedness concluded that humor was a powerful asset in hospice/palliative care (Dean & Gregory, 2005).

■ **Use humor to develop therapeutic relationships in men with testicular cancer. LOE = VI**

(MR) A qualitative design ($N = 45$) was used to determine the role of humor in people with testicular cancer. Men used humor to challenge assumptions about the disease, manage feelings, hide embarrassment, and share a sense of solidarity with others. Jokes helped decrease tension and increase a feeling of being treated as normal. However, men also acknowledged that humor could be hurtful if used in the wrong way, such as jokes that brought humiliation or stigma. The authors concluded that clinicians should use judgment in the use of humor and look for leads from the patient to individualize the use of humor (Chapple & Ziebland, 2004).

■ *Use humor to develop therapeutic relationships with aphasic clients.* LOE = VI

(MR) An ethnographic qualitative design (*N* = 8) was used to examine the role of humor in therapy for people with aphasia. Humor was used to manage the interpersonal interactions between the therapist and patient and to smooth the therapy process. Humor was judged to be a helpful tool to decrease patients' embarrassment and to obtain patients' cooperation with the therapy process. However, the interactions observed indicated that most of the humor was initiated by the therapist, and the authors recommended that greater humor equality between patient and therapist should be considered (Simmons-Mackie & Schultz, 2003).

■ *Use humor as therapy in hospitalized schizophrenic patients.* LOE = III

(MR) A controlled clinical trial (*N* = 34) of hospitalized schizophrenic patients was used to test the effect of viewing movies over a 3-month span. People in the experimental group viewed humorous videos, while those in the control group viewed different kinds of movies. People in the experimental group had significant reductions in measures of verbal hostility and anxiety/depression. There were also perceptions of increased staff support. However, the authors concluded that the results could have been mediated by the incidental exposure of the staff to the humorous movies (Gelkopf et al., 1993).

■ *Use humor to enhance cohesiveness in group therapy.* LOE = III

(MR) A controlled clinical trial (*N* = 28) involving female subjects was used to test the effect of a humorous activity and a nonhumorous group activity. Participants in the humor groups rated their activity higher on factors of evaluation, action, and cohesion (Banning & Nelson, 1987).

Decrease Pain

■ *Use humor to reduce pain perception.* LOE = II

(MR) A controlled study (*N* = 56) compared three groups randomly assigned to different tasks while viewing a humorous video: (1) to get into a cheerful mood without smiling or laughing, (2) to smile and laugh extensively, and (3) to produce a humorous commentary to the video. Pain tolerance was measured before, immediately after, and 20 minutes after the intervention using the cold pressor test. Pain tolerance increased for participants in all three groups following the humor intervention and remained high for 20 minutes (Zweyer et al., 2004).

(MR) A factorial design was used to test the effect of a video (humorous versus serious) and perceived control (choice versus no choice) and expectation (positive versus none) on requests for pain medications in postsurgical orthopedic patients. Participants (*N* = 78) were randomly assigned to one of eight possible conditions. Results indicated that humor increased requests for minor medication when combined with expectations to reduce pain but increased use of heavy analgesics when patients were denied choice over the humor stimulus (Rotton & Shats, 1996).

(MR) A controlled study (*N* = 200) compared nine groups randomly assigned to different types (humorous, neutral, holocaust) and lengths (15, 30, and 45 minutes) of videos. Pain tolerance was tested at baseline, immediately following the video, and 30 minutes later using the cold pressor test. Participants viewing the humorous video had increased pain tolerance following the video. However, those viewing the longer videos also had increased pain tolerance independent of the video content (Weisenberg et al., 1995, 1998).

(MR) A controlled study ($N = 13$) comparing two groups (humorous movies and nonhumorous movies) demonstrated that there was a reduction in subjective reports of pain and use of pain medications and improvement in affect in a group of elderly residents in a long-term care facility who viewed the humorous movies (Adams & McGuire, 1986).

■ *Use humor to reduce pain and inflammation in people with rheumatoid arthritis.* **LOE = III**

(MR) A controlled study ($N = 57$) compared healthy people with RA patients in a pretest/posttest design. All participants were exposed to a 1-hour rakugo (traditional Japanese comic story). Mood increased significantly in both groups following the humor intervention. Pain decreased for patients with RA, along with cortisol and IL-6 levels. Gamma interferon levels decreased significantly for people in both groups. The results indicated that humor could decrease pain levels and physiological measures of inflammation in people with RA (Yoshino et al., 1996).

Enhanced Learning/Memory

■ *Use humor to enhance memory.* **LOE = VI**

(MR) Two studies were reported that examined the effect of various levels of humor in advertising on participants' memory ($N = 303$ and $N = 187$). The results indicated that memory of the advertisement content was improved by moderate levels of humor compared with both high and low levels of humor. However, the second study showed that if the humor could be made more relevant to the advertising claims, higher levels of humor increased memory of the advertisement claims. The authors concluded that humor encouraged the formation of humor memory links, making the learned material easier to recall (Krishnan & Chakravarti, 2003).

■ *Use humor to enhance online teaching.* **LOE = II**

(MR) Students ($N = 44$) were randomly assigned to one of two online learning sections of a general psychology course (standard online course versus humor-enhanced course). Results indicated that humor significantly increased students' interest and participation but did not significantly improve overall course performance compared with those in the standard course (LoSchiavo & Shatz, 2005).

Improve Cardiopulmonary Function

■ *Use humor to enhance arterial blood flow.* **LOE = II**

(MR) Using a crossover design, 20 participants viewed both a humorous movie and scenes from a war movie. Ultrasound measures of blood flow and dilation of the brachial artery were obtained in all participants before and after both videos. The results indicated artery dilation with increased blood flow during the humorous video, whereas the war movie caused vasoconstriction and decreased blood flow. Overall, the authors reported a 22% increase in blood flow during the humorous video compared with a 35% decrease in blood flow during the war video (Miller et al., 2006).

RCT = Randomized Controlled (Clinical) Trial, **NIC** = Nursing Interventions Classification, **NOC** = Nursing Outcomes Classification

■ *Use humor to improve bronchial asthma.* **LOE = II**

(MR) In an RCT of 20 patients with bronchial asthma and 20 healthy participants, baseline bronchial response to methacholine was measured. Participants were randomly assigned to (1) a humorous movie and (2) a nonhumorous movie. Two weeks later, the alternative film was watched. Immediately after viewing both videos, bronchial response to methacholine challenge was measured. Viewing a humorous video significantly reduced bronchial responsiveness to methacholine in people with bronchial asthma (Kimata, 2004a). (Note: There was no significant change in healthy participants. Also, studies concerning the use of humor in asthmatics can be found in the "Possibly Harmful" section.)

■ *Use humor to improve pulmonary function.* **LOE = III**

(MR) A controlled clinical trial ($N = 11$) involving people with chronic obstructive pulmonary diseases measured pulmonary function and chest wall movement in participants during fits of laughter induced by a humorous video. All fits of laughter led to a significant drop in functional residual capacity (FRC), when air was forcefully expelled from the lungs during laughter (Filippelli et al., 2001). As people with obstructive lung diseases have increased FRC because of an inability for air trapping, laughter may have a role in treating people with chronic obstructive pulmonary disease.

■ *Use humor to improve cardiovascular function.* **LOE = III**

(NR) A controlled clinical trial ($N = 8$) of college-age subjects measured cardiac output in participants at 5-minute intervals before, during, and after viewing a humorous video. During laughter, there were significant increases in cardiac output and decreases in total peripheral resistance. After laughter, there was a significant decrease in oxygen consumption (Boone et al., 2000).

Not Effective

■ *Use of humor to affect health outcomes.* **LOE = I**

(MR) Results from a 3-year longitudinal study of Finnish police officers ($N = 87$) demonstrated that measures of sense of humor (self and peer ratings) did not predict any of the measured outcomes of physical health over a 3-year period. Rather, higher sense of humor scores were associated with a greater body mass, increased smoking, and a greater risk of cardiovascular disease (Kerkkänen et al., 2004).

(MR) Results from a population-based study in Norway ($N = 65,333$) determined that sense of humor, as measured on the Sense of Humor Questionnaire, did not significantly correlate with any of the health outcomes measured. Sense of humor was correlated with overall health satisfaction. The authors concluded that "overall, these data, comprising the largest study of humor and health ever undertaken, provide very little evidence for a direct relationship between sense of humor and physical health parameters" (Svebak et al., 2004).

■ *Use of laughter therapy to decrease anxiety.* **LOE = II**

(NR) Using a quasi-experimental design, nursing students ($N = 93$) were randomly assigned to one of three groups. The experimental group received 8 weeks of autogenic training, the attention control group received 8 weeks of laughter therapy, and the time control group received no intervention. State anxiety, burnout scores, blood pressure, and pulse rates were measured at baseline, at the end of the 8-week treatment period, and at 5, 8, and 11 months following the treatment period. Results indicated a statistically greater reduction of state and trait anxiety, blood pressure, and pulse rates in the autogenic group than in the humor or the nontreatment control group following the 8-week intervention. There was no effect on burnout, and there were no significant differences between the groups at later measurement points (Kanji et al., 2006).

▪ Use of humor to decrease pain perception. LOE = III

MR Using a quasi-experimental design, participants ($N = 44$; 24 females and 20 males) were assigned to three interventions in counterbalanced order: (1) mathematical distraction, (2) humor audiotape, and (3) preferred music (provided by participants). Tolerance time was measured using the cold pressor test, pain intensity was measured on a visual analogue scale, and perceived control was also measured. Preferred music significantly increased tolerance compared with the mathematical distraction group and significantly increased perceived control compared with the humor group. There were no significant differences in pain intensity ratings between groups (Mitchell et al., 2006).

MR A 2×2 factorial study was conducted to determine the effect of expectation on the response to humor. Participants ($N = 134$) were assigned to either a humorous video or a relaxation video. In addition, participants were given instructions that led them to believe that the video would either increase or decrease their pain sensitivity. Pain tolerance was tested immediately before and after the video using a blood pressure cuff. Both videos increased pain tolerance, and this effect was increased when the subjects were led to believe that the intervention would work. The authors raised the question that the benefits of humor may be related to expectations of a benefit (Mahony et al., 2001).

MR A controlled study was conducted to determine the effect of humor versus distraction on pain tolerance. Participants were assigned to one of three groups: (1) humorous video, (2) documentary video, and (3) no-video control. Pain tolerance was tested by the cold pressor test during the videos or the control period. Although participants in the humor group estimated that the humor video was more effective at improving their pain tolerance, only those who rated the film as funny tolerated more pain. Overall, participants in the humor group did not have significantly different pain tolerance compared with those viewing the documentary (Nevo et al., 1993).

EO Well-designed large-scale clinical trials of the use of humor have yet to be conducted. More rigorous research is needed before definitive conclusions can be reached about the effects of humor on various outcome measures (Bennett & Lengacher, 2006; Martin, 2001).

Possibly Harmful

▪ Use of humor to relax subjects while measuring blood pressure. LOE = II

NR Using a quasi-experimental design, normotensive volunteers ($N = 16$) had their blood pressure measured at baseline and during three episodes of laughter while viewing a humorous video. There was a significant rise in systolic blood pressure during laughter. The authors concluded that the use of humor during blood pressure measurement could cause falsely elevated readings (McMahon et al., 2005).

▪ Use of humor in people with asthma. LOE = VI

MR In a cross-sectional survey ($N = 826$) and diary ($N = 21$) study of children who presented to the emergency room of a children's hospital with acute asthma, 31.9% of those completing

RCT = Randomized Controlled (Clinical) Trial, **NIC** = Nursing Interventions Classification, **NOC** = Nursing Outcomes Classification

the diary study reported incidents of mirth-triggered asthma. According to the diary data, there were 18 events of mirth-triggered asthma while watching humorous videos, and these events led to mean decreased peak flow readings at 2 and 10 minutes following the naturally occurring stimulus (65% and 76% of baseline, respectively). In the cross-sectional arm designed to determine factors related to mirth-triggered asthma, those who were older needed more doses of bronchodilators, had more wheezing, and had more night symptoms, and those who reported exercise-induced symptoms were also more likely to report mirth-triggered asthma. Cough was the primary symptom and usually occurred within 2 minutes of the mirth. The authors concluded that mirth-triggered asthma was an indicator of poor asthma control (Liangas et al., 2003).

(MR) In a second cross-sectional survey study surveying 105 asthma patients for triggers of asthma, 41.9% reported laughter-induced asthma (Liangas et al., 2004).

■ *Maladaptive use of humor coping.* **LOE = VII**

(MR) A correlational study investigated the hypothesis that sense of humor had a multi-dimensional aspect, with both adaptive and maladaptive components. Participants ($N = 137$) completed measures of eight different components of sense of humor as well as measures of self-esteem, depression, anxiety, and self-competency. Adaptive sense of humor was associated with greater self-esteem, lower depression and anxiety levels, and more positive self-competency judgments. In contrast, the maladaptive components of humor that were self-focused (e.g., self-defeating and belabored humor) were associated with poorer self-esteem, greater depression and anxiety, and poorer judgments of self-competence (Kuiper & Nicholl, 2004).

OUTCOME MEASUREMENT

IMMUNE STATUS (NOC)

Definition: Natural and acquired appropriately targeted resistance to internal and external antigens.
Immune Status as evidenced by the following selected NOC indicators:
• Skin integrity
• Antibody titers
• Differential white blood count
• T4-cell level
• T8-cell level
(Rate each indicator of **Immune Status:** 1 = severely compromised, 2 = substantially compromised, 3 = moderately compromised, 4 = mildly compromised, 5 = not compromised) (Moorhead et al., 2004).

COPING (NOC)

Definition: Personal actions to manage stressors that tax an individual's resources.
Coping as evidenced by the following selected NOC indicators:
• Identifies multiple coping strategies
• Uses effective coping strategies
• Reports decrease in physical symptoms of stress

OUTCOME MEASUREMENT—*cont'd*

(Rate each indicator of **Coping:** 1 = never demonstrated, 2 = rarely demonstrated, 3 = sometimes demonstrated, 4 = often demonstrated, 5 = consistently demonstrated) (Moorhead et al., 2004).

COMFORT LEVEL NOC

Definition: Extent of positive perception of physical and psychological ease.
Comfort Level as evidenced by the following selected NOC indicators:
- Physical well-being
- Symptom control
- Social relationships
- Pain control

(Rate each indicator of **Comfort Level:** 1 = not at all satisfied, 2 = somewhat satisfied, 3 = moderately satisfied, 4 = very satisfied, 5 = completely satisfied) (Moorhead et al., 2004).

MEMORY NOC

Definition: Ability to cognitively retrieve and report previously stored information.
Memory as evidenced by the following NOC indicators:
- Recalls immediate information accurately
- Recalls recent information accurately
- Recalls remote information accurately

(Rate each indicator of **Memory:** 1 = severely compromised, 2 = substantially compromised, 3 = moderately compromised, 4 = mildly compromised, 5 = not compromised) (Moorhead et al., 2004).

REFERENCES

Adams E, McGuire F. (1986). Is laughter the best medicine? A study of the effects of humor on perceived pain and affect. *Act Adapt Aging,* 8(3-4):157-175.

Atsumi T, Fujisawa S, Nakabayashi Y, Kawarai T, Yasui T, Tonosaki K. (2004). Pleasant feeling from watching a comical video enhances free radical-scavenging capacity in human whole saliva. *J Psychosom Res,* 56(3):377-379.

Banning MR, Nelson DL. (1987). The effects of activity-elicited humor and group structure on group cohesion and affective responses. *Am J Occup Ther,* 41(8):510-514.

Bennett MP, Lengacher CA. (2006). Humor and laughter may influence health. I. History and background. *Evid Based Complement Alternat Med,* 3(1):61-63.

Bennett MP, Zeller JM, Rosenberg L, McCann J. (2003). The effect of mirthful laughter on stress and natural killer cell activity. *Altern Ther Health Med,* 9(2):38-45.

Berk LS, Felten DL, Tan SA, Bittman BB, Westengard J. (2001). Modulation of neuroimmune parameters during the eustress of humor-associated mirthful laughter. *Altern Ther Health Med,* 7(2):62-72, 74-76.

Berk LS, Tan SA, Fry WF, Napier BJ, Lee JW, Hubbard RW, et al. (1989). Neuroendocrine and stress hormone changes during mirthful laughter. *Am J Med Sci,* 298(6):390-396.

Boone T, Hansen S, Erlandson A. (2000). Cardiovascular responses to laughter: A pilot project. *Appl Nurs Res,* 13(4):204-208.

Chapple A, Ziebland S. (2004). The role of humor for men with testicular cancer. *Qual Health Res,* 14(8):1123-1139.

Dean RA, Gregory DM. (2005). More than trivial: Strategies for using humor in palliative care. *Cancer Nurs,* 28(4):292-300.

Dochterman JM, Bulechek G (Eds). (2004). *Nursing Interventions Classification (NIC)*, 4th ed. St. Louis: Mosby.

Filippelli M, Pellegrino R, Iandelli I, Misuri G, Rodarte JR, Duranti R, et al. (2001). Respiratory dynamics during laughter. *J Appl Physiol*, 90(4):1441-1446.

Gelkopf M, Kreitler S, Sigal M. (1993). Laughter in a psychiatric ward. Somatic, emotional, social, and clinical influences on schizophrenic patients. *J Nerv Ment Dis*, 181(5):283-289.

Kanji N, White A, Ernst E. (2006). Autogenic training to reduce anxiety in nursing students: Randomized controlled trial. *J Adv Nurs*, 53(6):729-735.

Kerkkänen P, Kuiper NA, Martin RA. (2004). Sense of humor, physical health, and well-being at work: A three-year longitudinal study of Finnish police officers. *Humor*, 17(1-2):21-35.

Kimata H. (2001). Effect of humor on allergen-induced wheal reactions. *JAMA*, 285(6):738.

Kimata H. (2004a). Effect of viewing a humorous vs. nonhumorous film on bronchial responsiveness in patients with bronchial asthma. *Physiol Behav*, 81(4):681-684.

Kimata H. (2004b). Laughter counteracts enhancement of plasma neurotrophin levels and allergic skin wheal responses by mobile phone-mediated stress. *Behav Med*, 29(4):149-152.

Krishnan HS, Chakravarti D. (2003). A process analysis of the effects of humorous advertising executions on brand claims memory. *J Consum Psychol*, 13(3):230-245.

Kuiper NA, Nicholl S. (2004). Thoughts of feeling better? Sense of humor and physical health. *Humor*, 17(1-2):37-66.

Liangas G, Morton JR, Henry RL. (2003). Mirth-triggered asthma: Is laughter really the best medicine? *Pediatr Pulmonol*, 36(2):107-112.

Liangas G, Yates DH, Wu D, Henry RL, Thomas PS. (2004). Laughter-associated asthma. *J Asthma*, 41(2):217-221.

LoSchiavo F, Shatz M. (2005). Enhancing online instruction with humor. *Teach Psychol*, 32(4):246-248.

Mahony DL, Burroughs WJ, Hieatt AC. (2001). The effects of laughter on discomfort thresholds: Does expectation become reality? *J Gen Psychol*, 128(2):217-226.

Martin RA. (2001). Humor, laughter, and physical health: Methodological issues and research findings. *Psychol Bull*, 127(4):504-519.

Matsuzaki T, Nakajima A, Ishigami S, Tanno M, Yoshino S. (2006). Mirthful laughter differentially affects serum pro- and anti-inflammatory cytokine levels depending on the level of disease activity in patients with rheumatoid arthritis. *Rheumatology*, 45(2):182-186.

McMahon C, Mahmud A, Feely J. (2005). Taking blood pressure—no laughing matter! *Blood Press Monit*, 10(2):109-110.

Miller M, Mangano C, Park Y, Goel R, Plotnick GD, Vogel RA. (2006). Impact of cinematic viewing on endothelial function. *Heart*, 92(2):261-262.

Mitchell LA, MacDonald RA, Brodie EE. (2006). A comparison of the effects of preferred music, arithmetic and humour on cold pressor pain. *Eur J Pain*, 10(4):343-351.

Moorhead M, Johnson M, Maas M (Eds). (2004). *Nursing Outcomes Classification (NOC)*, 3rd ed. St. Louis: Mosby.

Nevo O, Keinan G, Teshimovsky-Arditi M. (1993). Humor and pain tolerance. *Humor*, 6(1):71-88.

Rotton J, Shats M. (1996). Effects of state humor, expectancies, and choice on postsurgical mood and self-medication: A field experiment. *J Appl Soc Psychol*, 26(20):1775-1794.

Simmons-Mackie N, Schultz M. (2003). The role of humour in therapy for aphasia. *Aphasiology*, 17(8):751-766.

Svebak S, Martin RA, Holmen J. (2004). The prevalence of sense of humor in a large, unselected county population in Norway: Relations with age, sex, and some health indicators. *Humor*, 17(1-2):121-134.

Szabo A. (2003). The acute effects of humor and exercise on mood and anxiety. *J Leisure Res*, 35(2):152-162.

Szabo A, Ainsworth SE, Danks PK. (2005). Experimental comparison of the psychological benefits of aerobic exercise, humor, and music. *Humor*, 18(3):235-246.

Ventis WL, Higbee G, Murdock SA. (2001). Using humor in systematic desensitization to reduce fear. *J Gen Psychol*, 128(2):214-253.

Vilaythong AP, Arnau RC, Rosen DH, Mascaro N. (2003). Humor and hope: Can humor increase hope? *Humor*, 16(1):79-89.

Weisenberg M, Raz T, Hener T. (1998). The influence of film-induced mood on pain perception. *Pain*, 76(3):365-375.

Weisenberg M, Tepper I, Schwarzwald J. (1995). Humor as a cognitive technique for increasing pain tolerance. *Pain,* 63(2):207-212.

Yoshino S, Fujimori J, Kohda M. (1996). Effect of mirthful laughter on neuroendocrine and immune systems in patients with rheumatoid arthritis. *J Rheumatol,* 23(4):793-794.

Zweyer K, Velker B, Ruch W. (2004). Do cheerfulness, exhilaration, and humor production moderate pain tolerance? A FACS study. *Humor,* 17(1-2):85-119.

 # HYPOTHERMIA TREATMENT NIC

Deborah Pool, MS, RN, CCRN

> **NIC** **Definition:** Rewarming and surveillance of a patient whose core body temperature is below 35°C (Dochterman & Bulechek, 2004).

NURSING ACTIVITIES

Effective

■ ⒮ *Continuously monitor core temperature (via tympanic membrane, bladder, esophageal, or pulmonary artery) with a low recording thermometer.*
LOE = IV

⒠ Oral and axillary thermometers measure 0.6°C to 0.7°C less than core temperatures (Neno, 2005).

⒠ Conventional thermometers may not accurately record temperatures lower than 35°C (Neno, 2005; McCullough & Arora, 2004).

⒨ In a crossover study ($N = 3$), it was demonstrated that rectal temperature lagged considerably behind aural or esophageal temperatures, suggesting that all body compartments were not warmed evenly and rectal temperatures may not reflect the core temperature (Vanggaard et al., 1999).

■ **NIC** ⒮ *Monitor vital signs, as appropriate.* **LOE = IV**

⒠ Hemodynamic status is altered secondary to vasoconstriction and myocardial depression (Kelly, 2005; Biem et al., 2003).

■ ⒮ *Place on a continuous cardiac monitor and assess for dysrhythmias, particularly ventricular fibrillation.* **LOE = IV**

⒨ Multiple case reports demonstrated that ventricular fibrillation may be precipitated by vigorous movement of hypothermia victims (ECC Committee, 2005; Thomas & Cahill, 2000).

■ **NIC** ⒮ *Monitor for electrolyte imbalance. Monitor for acid-base imbalance.*
LOE = VII

⒠ Vasoconstriction and decreased cardiac output result in decreased oxygenation and altered cellular perfusion, which may result in metabolic derangements, altered electrolyte balance, and acidosis (Kelly, 2005; Neno, 2005; Biem et al., 2003).

RCT = Randomized Controlled (Clinical) Trial, **NIC** = Nursing Interventions Classification, **NOC** = Nursing Outcomes Classification

■ **NIC** **SP** *Administer heated oxygen, as appropriate. Institute active external rewarming measures (e.g., application of hot water bottles and placement on a heating blanket), as appropriate.* **LOE = II**

MR A crossover study ($N = 8$) of health volunteers cooled to 33°C demonstrated that the use of resistive heat blankets doubled rewarming rates compared with reflective foil blankets (Greif et al., 2000).

NR In a quasi-experimental study ($N = 298$), three prewarmed cotton blankets, head covering with a reflective blanket, and forced warm air inflatable blankets were equally effective in maintaining body temperature in normothermic trauma patients (Cohen et al., 2002).

MR A crossover study ($N = 9$) of healthy volunteers evaluated on two randomly ordered study days, comparing a circulating water garment with a forced air cover, demonstrated that the heated water garment raised body temperatures more quickly than the forced air cover, largely because of posterior heating (Taguchi et al., 2004).

MR An RCT ($N = 24$) study of patients undergoing intra-abdominal surgery demonstrated that forced air and resistive heating mechanisms were equally effective in maintaining intra-operative core temperatures (Negishi et al., 2003).

■ **SP** *For severe hypothermia (temperature <30°C), institute internal rewarming methods as ordered (e.g., warmed IV fluids and blood products, peritoneal lavage, hemodialysis, cardiopulmonary bypass).* **LOE = III**

MR Long-term outcomes for patients suffering from severe accidental hypothermia who were resuscitated with cardiopulmonary bypass ($N = 32$) demonstrated that cardiopulmonary bypass in young, otherwise healthy adults was likely to result in optimal neurological recovery (Walpoth et al., 1997).

MR In a comparison study ($N = 38$), healthy volunteers were subjected to several methods of rewarming following immersion in cold (10° ± 1°C) water. The most effective method of rewarming was found to be immersion in warm water (38°C) with concurrent hydromassage and ambient air temperature of 65° ± 5°C (Losik & Afanas'eva, 2004).

MR Case reports of patients ($N = 15$) treated with forced air rewarming demonstrated that patients who suffered accidental hypothermia without cardiopulmonary arrest were likely to be resuscitated using forced air rewarming (Kornberger et al., 1999).

MR A prospective randomized unblended trial ($N = 30$) demonstrated that increased core temperature was achieved more quickly with warmed, humidified oxygen in the postanesthesia care unit than in patients receiving oxygen at ambient room temperature (Frank et al., 2000).

■ **SP** *Monitor the patient for "afterdrop" and signs of rewarming shock.* **LOE = IV**

EO As normothermia is achieved, patients may have a reduction in cardiac output related to vasodilation and sequestering of fluid in the periphery (Sommers & Bolton, 2006; Neno, 2005; ECC Committee, 2005; Biem et al., 2003).

Possibly Effective

■ **NIC** *Give the patient warm oral fluids, if alert and able to swallow.* **LOE = VII**

EO Patients who are able to swallow warmed fluids without risk of aspiration may have an increase in body temperature related to warming of the gastrointestinal tract (Neno, 2005).

NR = Nursing Research, **MR** = Multidisciplinary Research, **SP** = Standard of Practice, **EO** = Expert Opinion, **LOE** = Level of Evidence

■ **NIC** *Cover the patient with warm blankets as appropriate.* **LOE = III**

NR In a randomized crossover study ($N = 8$), it was demonstrated that using a blanket, radiant warmer, or forced air device resulted in equal increases in body temperature and that the patient's own body heat production was the most likely factor determining temperature change (Williams et al., 2005).

Not Effective

■ *Use of a water-filled blanket or negative pressure rewarming device to improve body temperature.* **LOE = II**

MR In an RCT ($N = 60$) comparing the use of a negative pressure device with conventional methods of rewarming, patients in the postanesthesia recovery unit demonstrated no advantage in using this device (Smith et al., 1999).

MR In an intraoperative study ($N = 24$) of patients undergoing abdominal surgery, participants were randomly assigned to warming with a full-length water-filled mattress, a lower body forced air blower, or a resistive heating blanket. It was demonstrated that the water-filled mattress was much less effective than the other methods to support body temperature (Negishi et al., 2003).

■ *Measuring temperature using axillary placement of a thermometer.* **LOE = III**

NR A comparative controlled study ($N = 60$) measuring body temperature as a pulmonary artery blood temperature versus an axilla temperature using a chemical thermometer and a tympanic membrane temperature demonstrated that both the tympanic and axillary temperatures were not well correlated with the pulmonary artery temperature (Fullbrook, 1997).

NR A comparative controlled study measuring the temperature of critically ill patients with an infrared ear thermometer versus an axillary mercury-in-glass thermometer ($N = 50$) demonstrated that the tympanic thermometer provided more reliable measurements than the axillary temperature (Leon et al., 2005).

NR A comparative controlled study measuring the temperature of adults ($N = 84$) with oral, tympanic, axillary, and rectal methods demonstrated the greatest variation with tympanic measurements, then axillary temperatures, compared with the standard of the rectal temperature (Thomas et al., 2004).

Possibly Harmful

■ **SP** *Administering intramuscular or subcutaneous medications while the patient remains hypothermic.* **LOE = VII**

EO Hypothermic patients are peripherally vasoconstricted, which decreases absorption. As the patient becomes normothermic, vasodilation occurs and a "bolus" effect of medications may result (ECC Committee, 2005; Good et al., 2006).

RCT = Randomized Controlled (Clinical) Trial, **NIC** = Nursing Interventions Classification, **NOC** = Nursing Outcomes Classification

OUTCOME MEASUREMENT

THERMOREGULATION (NOC)

Definition: Balance among heat production, heat gain, and heat loss.

Thermoregulation as evidenced by the following selected NOC indicators:

- Shivering when cold
- Apical heart rate
- Radial pulse rate
- Respiratory rate
- Reported thermal comfort

(Rate each indicator of **Thermoregulation:** 1 = severely compromised, 2 = substantially compromised, 3 = moderately compromised, 4 = mildly compromised, 5 = not compromised) (Moorhead et al., 2004).

REFERENCES

Biem J, Koehncke N, Classen D, Dosman J. (2003). Out of the cold: Management of hypothermia and frostbite. *CMAJ,* 168(3):305-311.

Cohen S, Hayes JS, Tordella T, Puente I. (2002). Thermal efficiency of prewarmed cotton, reflective, and forced-warm-air inflatable blankets in trauma patients. *Int J Trauma Nurs,* 8(1):4-8.

Dochterman JM, Bulechek GM (Eds). (2004). *Nursing Interventions Classification (NIC)*, 4th ed. St. Louis: Mosby.

ECC Committee, Subcommittees and Task Forces of the American Heart Association (AHA). (2005). 2005 American Heart Association Guidelines for Cardiopulmonary Resuscitation and Emergency Cardiovascular Care. Part 2: Ethical Issues. *Circulation,* 112 (24 Suppl):IV6-IV11.

Frank SM, Hesel TW, El-Rahmany HK, Tran KM, Bamford OS. (2000). Warmed humidified inspired oxygen accelerates postoperative warming. *J Clin Anesth,* 12(4):283-287.

Fulbrook P. (1997). Core body temperature measurement: A comparison of axilla, tympanic membrane and pulmonary artery blood temperature. *Intensive Crit Care Nurs,* 13(5):266-272.

Good KK, Verble JA, Secrest J, Norwood BR. (2006). Postoperative hypothermia—The chilling consequences. *AORN J,* 83(5):1055-1066.

Greif R, Rajek A, Laciny S, Bastanmehr H, Sessler DI. (2000). Resistive heating is more effective than metal-foil insulation in an experimental model of accidental hypothermia: A randomized, controlled trial. *Ann Emerg Med,* 35(4):337-345.

Kelly EM. (2005). External warming/cooling devices. In Weigand D, Carlson K (Eds). *AACN procedure manual for critical care.* St. Louis: Elsevier.

Kornberger E, Schwarz B, Lindner KH, Mair P. (1999). Forced air surface rewarming in patients with severe accidental hypothermia. *Resuscitation,* 41(2):105-111.

Leon C, Rodriguez A, Fernandez A, Flores L. (2005). Infrared ear thermometry in the critically ill patient. *J Crit Care,* 20(1):106-110.

Losik TK, Afanas'eva RF. (2004). Comparative evaluation of different methods for normalizing heat state of persons exposed to cold water. *Med Tr Prom Ekol,* 5:12-17.

McCullough L, Arora S. (2004). Diagnosis and treatment of hypothermia. *Am Fam Physician,* 70(12):2325-2332.

Moorhead M, Johnson M, Maas M (Eds). (2004). *Nursing Outcomes Classification (NOC)*, 3rd ed. St. Louis: Mosby.

Negishi C, Hasegawa K, Mukai S, Nakagawa F, Ozaki M, Sessler DI. (2003). Resistive-heating and forced-air warming are comparably effective. *Anesth Analg,* 96(6):1683-1687.

Neno R. (2005). Hypothermia: Assessment, treatment and prevention. *Nurs Stand,* 19(20):47-52.

Smith CE, Parand A, Pinchak AC, Hagen JF, Hancock DE. (1999). The failure of negative pressure rewarming (Thermostat) to accelerate recovery from mild hypothermia in postoperative surgical patients. *Anesth Analg*, 89(6):1541-1545.

Sommers MS, Bolton PJ. (2006). Multisystem. In JG Alspach (Ed): *Core curriculum for critical care nursing*, 6th ed. St. Louis: Saunders, pp 809-826.

Taguchi A, Ratnaraj J, Kabon B, Sharma N, Lenhardt R, Sessler DI, et al. (2004). Effects of a circulating-water garment and forced-air warming on body heat content and core temperature. *Anesthesiology*, 100(5):1058-1064.

Thomas KA, Burr R, Wang SY, Lentz MJ, Shaver J. (2004). Axillary and thoracic skin temperatures poorly comparable to core body temperature circadian rhythm: Results from 2 adult populations. *Biol Res Nurs*, 5(3):187-194.

Thomas R, Cahill CJ. (2000). Successful defibrillation in profound hypothermia (core body temperature 25.6 degrees C). *Resuscitation*, 47(3):317-320.

Vanggaard L, Eyolfson D, Xu X, Weseen G, Giesbrecht GG. (1999). Immersion of distal arms and legs in warm water (AVA rewarming) effectively rewarms mildly hypothermic humans. *Aviat Space Environ Med*, 70(11):1081-1088.

Walpoth BH, Walpoth-Aslan BN, Mattle HP, Radanov BP, Schroth G, Schaeffler L, et al. (1997). Outcome of survivors of accidental deep hypothermia and circulator arrest treated with extracorporeal blood warming. *N Engl J Med*, 337(21):1500-1505.

Williams AB, Salmon A, Graham P, Galler D, Payton MJ, Bradley M. (2005). Rewarming of healthy volunteers after induced mild hypothermia: A healthy volunteer study. *Emerg Med J*, 22(3):182-184.

INCISION SITE CARE

Maria Marinelli, BSN, CNOR, RNFA

NIC **Definition:** Cleansing, monitoring, and promotion of healing in a wound that is closed with sutures, clips, or staples (Dochterman & Bulechek, 2004).

NURSING ACTIVITIES

Effective

■ *For an incision that has been closed primarily, protect with a sterile dressing for 24 to 48 hours postoperatively.* **LOE = I**

EO Covering a surgical wound for 24 to 48 hours protects the nonepithelialized tissue. "The guideline provides recommendations concerning reduction of the risk for surgical site infections (SSI). Each recommendation is categorized on the basis of existing scientific data, theoretical rationale, and applicability" (CDC, 1996 p. 117). The CDC's National Nosocomial Infections Surveillance system conducted a 10-year survey (1986 to 1996) of 593,344 patients undergoing surgical procedures and determined that SSIs were the most common nosocomial infection (CDC, 1999).

■ *Wash hands before and after dressing changes and any contact with the surgical site.* **LOE = I**

EO Washing the hands before and after dressing changes is strongly recommended and is supported by some experimental, clinical, or epidemiological studies and strong theoretical rationale (CDC, 1999).

RCT = Randomized Controlled (Clinical) Trial, **NIC** = Nursing Interventions Classification, **NOC** = Nursing Outcomes Classification

(MR) An RCT ($N = 100$) studied hand washing by health care workers before and after the physical examination of patients in the health care setting. All participants who did not perform proper hand washing protocol were carriers of potential pathogenic bacteria (Nogueras et al., 2001).

(SP) *Perform surgical hand antisepsis according to established guidelines.* **LOE = VII**

(EO) When performing surgical hand antisepsis using antimicrobial soap, scrub hands and forearms the length of time recommended by the manufacturer. Long scrub times are not necessary. When using an alcohol-based surgical hand scrub product, follow the manufacturer's advice and prewash hands and forearms with a nonantimicrobial soap and dry hands and forearms completely. Also, allow the alcohol-based product to dry thoroughly before donning sterile gloves (Boyce et al., 2002).

When an incision dressing must be changed, use sterile technique. **LOE = I**

(EO) Sterile technique for incision dressing changes is recommended and supported by suggestive clinical or epidemiological studies or theoretical rationale (CDC, 1999).

Educate the patient and family regarding proper incision care, symptoms of SSI, and the need to report such symptoms. **LOE = I**

(EO) The education provided by the nurse is supported by clinical or epidemiological studies or theoretical rationale (CDC, 1999).

Educate the patient and family to protect the wound closed with a topical skin adhesive (2-octyl cyanoacrylate) by keeping the wound dry and using a dressing. **LOE = I**

(MR) A Cochrane systematic review found that surgeons may consider the use of tissue adhesives as an alternative to sutures or adhesive tape for the closure of surgical incisions in the operating room. Areas of high tension such as the elbow and knee have not been studied, however. Traditional closure by sutures, staples, and adhesive tapes has been modernized with the use of tissue adhesives in surgery (Coulthard et al., 2004).

(NIC) *Inspect the incision site for redness, swelling, or signs of dehiscence or evisceration.* **LOE = VII**

(EO) "Surgical literature suggests that direct observation of surgical sites is the most accurate method to detect SSI, although sensitive data are lacking and mostly generated by indirect case-finding methods" (CDC, 1999, p. 116).

(NIC) *Monitor the healing process in the incision site.* **LOE = I**

(EO) "At least two studies have shown that most SSIs become evident within 21 days after operation" (CDC, 1999, p. 116). Therefore, constant monitoring of the incision site is a standard of practice in surgical care.

(MR) In a prospective single-cohort descriptive study ($N = 1772$), there was a definite reduction in clean wound infection rates postoperatively when a nurse, as a trained observer, was allowed to assess, collect, and analyze data. Daily visits with early identification and scoring using a previously validated wound assessment scoring tool minimized the subjective evaluation (Reilly et al., 2001).

NR = Nursing Research, **MR** = Multidisciplinary Research, **SP** = Standard of Practice, **EO** = Expert Opinion, **LOE** = Level of Evidence

Possibly Effective

■ *Use warm air enhanced by ultraviolet light and do not rub hands together while drying hands.* **LOE = II**

> **NR** An RCT ($N = 90$) concluded that holding hands stationary and not rubbing them together was desirable for removing bacteria. Using ultraviolet light reinforced the bacteria removal during warm air drying. Paper towels were useful for removing bacteria from fingertips but not palms and fingers (Yamamoto et al., 2005).

■ **NIC** *Change the dressing at appropriate intervals.* **LOE = IV**

> **MR** In an RCT of postoperative patients ($N = 100$), 50 patients received a wound dressing after 48 hours and 50 did not. There was no significant difference in wound infection outcomes, indicating that wound dressings were not necessary after 48 hours (Meylan & Tschantz, 2001).

> **MR** A Cochrane systematic review concluded that there was insufficient evidence to determine the necessity for specific dressings, topical agents, or frequency of dressing changes to use in the practice setting for wounds healing by secondary intention (Vermeulen et al., 2004).

■ *Use foam or gauze for a postoperative dressing.* **LOE = I**

> **MR** A Cochrane systematic review found that there was no clear evidence of a difference between gauze and foam dressings in terms of healing. However, patients with a foam dressing experienced less pain and fewer nursing visits postoperatively (Vermeulen et al., 2004).

Not Effective

No applicable published research was found in this category.

Possibly Harmful

No applicable published research was found in this category.

OUTCOME MEASUREMENT

KNOWLEDGE: INFECTION CONTROL   **NOC**

Definition: Extent of understanding conveyed about prevention and control of infection.

Knowledge: Infection Control as evidenced by the following selected NOC indicators:
- Description of practices that reduce transmission
- Description of signs and symptoms
- Description of monitoring procedures

(Rate each indicator of **Knowledge: Infection Control:** 1 = none, 2 = limited, 3 = moderate, 4 = substantial, 5 = extensive) (Moorhead et al., 2004).

RCT = Randomized Controlled (Clinical) Trial, **NIC** = Nursing Interventions Classification, **NOC** = Nursing Outcomes Classification

REFERENCES

Boyce JM, Pittet D; Healthcare Infection Control Practices Advisory Committee; HIPAC/SHEA/APIC/IDSA Hand Hygiene Task Force. (2002). Guideline for Hand Hygiene in Health-Care Settings: Recommendations of the Healthcare Infection Control Practices Advisory Committee and the HICPAC/SHEA/APIC/IDSA Hand Hygiene Task Force. *MMWR Recomm Rep,* 51(RR-16):1-45.

Centers for Disease Control (CDC). (1999). *Guideline for prevention of surgical site infection.* Atlanta: Centers for Disease Control and Prevention Hospital Infection Control Practices Advisory Committee.

Coulthard P, Worthington H, Esposito M, Elst M, Waes OJ. (2004). Tissue adhesives for closure of surgical incisions. *Cochrane Database Syst Rev,* (2):CD004287.

Dochterman JM, Bulechek GM (Eds). (2004). *Nursing Interventions Classification (NIC),* 4th ed. St. Louis: Mosby.

Meylan G, Tschantz P. (2001). Surgical wounds with or without dressing: Prospective comparative study. *Ann Chir,* 126(5):459-462.

Moorhead M, Johnson M, Maas M (Eds). (2004). *Nursing Outcomes Classification (NOC),* 3rd ed. St. Louis: Mosby.

Nogueras M, Marinsalta N, Roussell M, Notario R. (2001). Importance of hand germ contamination in health-care workers as possible carriers of nosocomial infections. *Rev Inst Med Trop Sao Paulo,* 43(3):149-152.

Reilly JS, Baird D, Hill R. (2001). The importance of definitions and methods in surgical wound infection audit. *J Hosp Infect,* 47(1):64-66.

Vermeulen H, Ubbink D, Goossens A, de Vos R, Legemate D. (2004). Dressings and topical agents for surgical wounds healing by secondary intention. *Cochrane Database Syst Rev,* (2):CD003554.

Yamamoto Y, Ugai K, Takahashi Y. (2005). Efficiency of hand drying for removing bacteria from washed hands: Comparison of paper towel drying with warm air drying. *Infect Control Hosp Epidemiol,* 26(3):316-320.

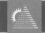 ## INFECTION CONTROL   NIC

Thomas James Loveless, MSN, CRNP

NIC **Definition:** Minimizing the acquisition and transmission of infectious agents (Dochterman & Bulechek, 2004).

NURSING ACTIVITIES

Direct and Nondirect Patient Contact

Effective

■ **NIC** *Institute universal precautions.* **LOE = VII**

   EO Considered the "gold standard" and remaining as the cornerstone of protecting health care workers, universal precautions were implemented by the CDC in 1986 and updated in 1996 (Garner, 1996; Panlilio et al., 2005).

■ **SP** *Perform hand washing and maintain hand care.* **LOE = VII**

   EO According to the CDC and its review of the seminal work of Semmelweis and Holmes in the early 19th century, hand washing has been accepted as one of the most important mechanisms to prevent the spread of infectious agents in health care workers (Boyce et al., 2002).

NR = Nursing Research, **MR** = Multidisciplinary Research, **SP** = Standard of Practice, **EO** = Expert Opinion, **LOE** = Level of Evidence

(EO) Hand washing remains the single most effective method to prevent, control, and reduce infections. Hand washing is a mantra of infection control and is one of the basic fundamental underlying principles of nursing (Bjerke, 2004).

(EO) Always wash hands after touching blood, body fluids, secretions, and contaminated items, regardless of wearing gloves (Boyce et al., 2002).

(EO) Immediate hand washing should be thoroughly completed if an exposure to blood or bloody fluids has occurred (Garner, 1996).

(EO) Wash hands immediately after removing gloves and in between each and every contact with patients (Garner, 1996).

(EO) Use of a nonantibacterial soap is sufficient for routine hand washing (Garner, 1996). When using soap and water, wash hands vigorously for at least 15 seconds, avoiding excessively hot water as this may cause dermatitis. Washing with plain soap and water for 15 seconds reduces bacterial counts on the skin by 0.6 to 1.1 $\log^{10}$, whereas washing for 30 seconds reduces counts by 1.8 to 2.8 $\log^{10}$. Transient flora, which colonizes the superficial layers of the skin, is more amenable to removal by routine hand washing (Kampf & Kramer, 2004).

(EO) Use of an antibacterial soap or a waterless antiseptic agent is needed after caring for any patient with known multidrug-resistant pathogens (e.g., methicillin-resistant *Staphylococcus aureus*) (Boyce et al., 2002). Alcohol-based hand rubs significantly reduce the number of microorganisms (Boyce et al., 2002).

■ (SP) *Put on a gown as appropriate.* **LOE = VII**

(EO) A nonsterile gown is adequate to protect skin and soiling of clothing. Remove soiled gowns as soon as possible and discard according to appropriate biohazard precautions (Garner, 1996).

■ (SP) *Put on masks and eyewear as appropriate.* **LOE = VII**

(EO) Masks and eyewear should be worn routinely during direct contact for procedures that are likely to generate droplets of blood to prevent mucocutaneous exposure.

(EO) Masks and eyewear should reduce the incidence of blood contamination of mucous membranes of the mouth, eyes, and nose while performing procedures that may generate droplets of blood or body fluids requiring precautions (Garner, 1996; Larson, 1988, 1999).

Possibly Effective

■ (NIC) *Wear gloves as mandated by universal precaution policy.* **LOE = VII**

(EO) Gloves do not provide complete protection against hand contamination. Bacterial flora colonizing patients may be recovered from the hands of up to 30% of health care workers who wear gloves during contact with patients (Olsen et al., 1993; Tenorio et al., 2001).

(EO) Clean, nonsterile gloves are adequate protection for routine care of patients. Gloves are required for contact with mucous membranes and nonintact skin. Changing of gloves is required, even while performing sequential, individual tasks on the same patient (Garner, 1996) and particularly when going from contaminated sites to noncontaminated sites (Boyce et al., 2002). Wearing gloves *does not* eliminate the need for consistent hand washing.

(EO) Glove wearing by health care workers is recommended for two main reasons: (1) to prevent microorganisms that may be infecting, commensally carried, or transiently present on health care workers' hands from being transmitted to patients and from one patient to another and (2) to reduce the risk of health care workers acquiring infections from patients (Boyce

RCT = Randomized Controlled (Clinical) Trial, **NIC** = Nursing Interventions Classification, **NOC** = Nursing Outcomes Classification

et al., 2002). The effectiveness of gloves in preventing contamination of health care workers' hands has been reported in several clinical studies (Pittet et al., 1999; Tenorio et al., 2001).

■ *Avoid wearing artificial nails and nail polish.* **LOE = VII**

(EO) The issue of artificial nails and cosmetic polish remains unresolved regarding transmission of infections. The CDC recommends that health care workers avoid wearing artificial nails and keep natural nails less than one quarter of an inch long if they care for patients at risk for acquiring infections (e.g., chemotherapy patient, transplant patient) (Boyce et al., 2002).

(EO) Subungual areas of the hand harbor high concentrations of bacteria, frequently coagulase-negative staphylococci, gram-negative rods, and yeast. Despite thorough hand washing, studies have reported the harboring of substantial bacteria in the subungual space (Gross et al., 1979; Pottinger et al., 1989; McNeil et al., 2001). It is still unclear whether artificial nails contribute definitively to the transmission of infection, and additional studies are warranted. Moreover, the length of the nails remains in debate, but it is reported that the majority of bacterial growth occurs along the proximal 1 mm of the nail bed adjacent to subungual skin (Wynd et al., 1994; Pottinger et al., 1989).

Not Effective

No applicable published research was found in this category.

Possibly Harmful

No applicable published research was found in this category.

Droplet Contact

Effective

■ (NIC) (SP) *Institute universal precautions.* **LOE = VII**

(EO) Standard precautions are the minimal requirement for patients with illness from pathogens known to be transmitted through droplets (Panlilio et al., 2005).

(EO) Patients' placement requires a private room. If no private room is available, avoid discordant placement. Patients with known or suspected microorganisms that are transmitted by droplets should be placed in a room with a patient who also has the same infection.

(EO) If cohorting is not possible, maintain separation of at least 3 feet between patients (Panlilio et al., 2005).

(EO) Special air handling is not required and room doors may remain open (Panlilio et al., 2005).

(EO) Wearing a mask as defined by standard precautions applies while caring for the patient with an infection known to spread by droplets (Panlilio et al., 2005).

(EO) If transport of the source patient is not avoidable, mask the patient to decrease the patient's ability to disperse droplets.

Possibly Effective

No applicable published research was found in this category.

Not Effective

No applicable published research was found in this category.

NR = Nursing Research, **MR** = Multidisciplinary Research, **SP** = Standard of Practice, **EO** = Expert Opinion, **LOE** = Level of Evidence

Possibly Harmful

No applicable published research was found in this category.

Airborne Precautions

Effective

- ■ **NIC** **SP** *Institute universal precautions.* **LOE = VII**

    EO Standard precautions are the minimal requirement for patients with illness from pathogens known to be transmitted through airborne transmission (Panlilio et al., 2005).

- ■ **SP** *In addition to universal precautions, respiratory protection is warranted.* **LOE = VII**

    EO Wearing respiratory protection (N95 respirator) when entering a room of a patient with known infectious pulmonary tuberculosis, measles (rubeola), or varicella (chicken pox) must be done and strictly adhered to (Panlilio et al., 2005).

    EO Patients' placement requires a private room with negative air pressure; a minimum of 6 to 12 air exchanges per hour is mandated. Air discharge to the outdoors is required or high-efficiency filtration before the air is circulated internally (Panlilio et al., 2005). The room door *must* remain closed.

    EO Patients' cohorting is required. When cohorting is not possible, absolute consultation with infectious diseases is warranted (Panlilio et al., 2005).

    EO Patients' transport outside the room should be kept to an absolute minimum. If transport is required, the source patient must be masked; a surgical mask is sufficient (Panlilio et al., 2005).

Possibly Effective

No applicable published research was found in this category.

Not Effective

No applicable published research was found in this category.

Possibly Harmful

No applicable published research was found in this category.

OUTCOME MEASUREMENT

KNOWLEDGE: INFECTION CONTROL   **NOC**

Definition: Extent of understanding conveyed about prevention and control of infection.

Knowledge: Infection Control as evidenced by the following selected NOC indicators:

- Description of practices that reduce transmission
- Description of signs and symptoms
- Description of monitoring procedures

(Rate each indicator of **Knowledge: Infection Control:** 1 = none, 2 = limited, 3 = moderate, 4 = substantial, 5 = extensive) (Moorhead et al., 2004).

RCT = Randomized Controlled (Clinical) Trial, **NIC** = Nursing Interventions Classification, **NOC** = Nursing Outcomes Classification

REFERENCES

Bjerke NB. (2004). The evolution: Handwashing to hand hygiene guidance. *Crit Care Nurs Q*, 27(3): 295-307.

Bolyard EA, Tablan OC, Williams WW, Pearson ML, et al. (1998). Guideline for infection control in health care personnel—CDC personnel health guideline. *Am J Infect Control*, 26(3):289-354.

Boyce JM, Pittet D; Healthcare Infection Control Practices Advisory Committee; HICPAC/SHEA/APIC/ IDSA Hand Hygiene Task Force. (2002). Guideline for hand hygiene in health-care settings. Recommendations of the Healthcare Infection Control Practices Advisory Committee and the HICPAC/SHEA/ APIC/IDSA Hand Hygiene Task Force. Society for Healthcare Epidemiology of America/Association for Professionals in Infection Control/Infectious Diseases Society of America. *MMWR Recomm Rep*, 51(RR-16):1-45.

Dochterman JM, Bulechek GM (Eds). (2004). *Nursing Interventions Classification (NIC)*, 4th ed. St. Louis: Mosby.

Garner JS. (1996). Guideline for isolation precautions in hospitals. The Hospital Infection Control Practices Advisory Committee. *Infect Control Hosp Epidemiol*, 17(1):53-80.

Gross A, Cutright DE, A'Alessandro SM. (1979). Efects of surgical scrub on microbial population under the fingernails. *Am J Surg*, 138(3), 463-467.

Kampf G, Kramer A. (2004). Epidemiologic background of hand hygiene and evaluation of the most important agents for scrubs and rubs. *Clin Microbiol Rev*, 17(4):863-893.

Larson E. (1988). A causal link between handwashing and risk of infection? Examination of the evidence. *Infect Control*, 9(1):28-36.

Larson E. (1999). Skin hygiene and infection prevention: More of the same or different approaches? *Clin Infect Dis*, 29(5):1287-1294.

McNeil SA, Foster CL, Hedderwick SA, Kauffman CA. (2001). Effects of hand cleansing with antimicrobal soap or alcohol-based gel on microbial colonization of artificial fingernails worn by health care workers. *Clin Infect Dis*, 32(3):367-372.

Moorhead M, Johnson M, Maas M (Eds). (2004). *Nursing Outcomes Classification (NOC)*, 3rd ed. St. Louis: Mosby.

Olsen RJ, Lynch P, Coyle MB, Cummings J, Bokete T, Stamm WE. (1993). Examination gloves as barriers to hand contamination in clinical practice. *JAMA* 270:350.

Panlilio AL, Cardo DM, Grohskopf LA, Heneine W, Ross CS; U.S. Public Health Service. (2005). Updated U.S. Public Health Service guidelines for the management of occupational exposures to HIV and recommendations for postexposure prophylaxis. *MMWR Recomm Rep*, 54(RR-9):1-17.

Pittet D, Dharan S, Touveneau S, Sauvan V, Perneger TV. (1999). Bacterial contamination of the hands of hospital staff during routine patient care. *Arch Intern Med*, 159(8):821-826.

Pottinger J, Burns S, Manske C. (1989). Bacterial carriage by artificial versus natural nails. *Am J Infect Control*, 17(6):340-344.

Tenorio AR, Badri SM, Sahgal NB, Hota B, Matushek M, Hayden MK, et al. (2001). Effectiveness of gloves in the prevention of hand carriage of vancomycin-resistant enterococcus species of health care workers after patient care. *Clin Infect Dis*, 32(5):826-829.

Wynd CA, Samstag DE, Lapp AM. (1994). Bacterial carriages on the fingernails of OR nurses. *AORN J*, 60(5):796, 799-805.

INFECTION CONTROL: HAND HYGIENE

Jeannie P. Cimiotti, DNS, RN

NIC **Definition:** Minimizing the acquisition and transmission of infectious agents (Dochterman & Bulechek, 2004).

NR = Nursing Research, **MR** = Multidisciplinary Research, **SP** = Standard of Practice, **EO** = Expert Opinion, **LOE** = Level of Evidence

NURSING ACTIVITIES

Effective

■ **NIC** *Wash hands before and after each patient care activity.* **LOE = I**

EO Perform hand hygiene before and after each contact with a patient (Boyce et al., 2002).

NR A systematic review of the literature demonstrated a relationship between skin hygiene and infection and that hand washing affected skin integrity (Larson, 2001).

NR A systematic review of the literature demonstrated that health care worker hand hygiene was linked to the transmission of infection (Larson, 1999).

■ *Use a waterless alcohol-based hand rub for routine hand hygiene.* **LOE = I**

MR An RCT of health care workers ($N = 50$) that evaluated the efficacy of two hand hygiene products, an unmedicated soap and an alcohol-based hand rub, demonstrated a decrease in microbial hand contamination associated with use of an alcohol-based hand rub (Kac et al., 2005).

MR A controlled study that examined health care–associated drug-resistant organisms in a large urban, tertiary care medical center, before and after the implementation (3 years for each phase) of an alcohol-based hand rub, demonstrated a decrease in health care–associated drug-resistant bacteria with the use of alcohol-based hand rub (Gordin et al., 2005).

MR A controlled study that examined rates of late-onset sepsis in very low birth weight infants in a neonatal intensive care unit before and after implementation ($N = 161$ and $N = 176$, respectively) of an alcohol-based hand rub demonstrated that a decrease in sepsis was associated with the use of alcohol-based hand rub (Ng et al., 2004).

MR A controlled study examined infection rates in an acute care orthopedic surgery unit before and after implementation (6 months and 10 months, respectively) of an alcohol-based hand rub and demonstrated a decrease in the rate of infection (urinary tract and surgical site) associated with the use of alcohol-based hand rub (Hilburn et al., 2003).

EO Use an alcohol-based hand rub for routine hand hygiene when hands are not visibly soiled. Apply the product to the palm of one hand and rub hands together, covering all surfaces of the hands and fingers until completely dry (Boyce et al., 2002).

■ *Use a nonantibacterial soap or an antibacterial soap for hand hygiene. (Note: Soap should be used only if hands are visibly soiled or contaminated with body fluids.)* **LOE = I**

EO Alcohol-based hand rubs are not appropriate for use when hands are visibly dirty, contaminated with proteinaceous material, or soiled with blood or other body fluids. Soiled hands should be cleaned by using a nonantibacterial or antibacterial soap applied to hands wet with water, and hands should be rubbed vigorously for at least 15 seconds, covering all surfaces of the hands and fingers (Boyce et al., 2002).

RCT = Randomized Controlled (Clinical) Trial, **NIC** = Nursing Interventions Classification, **NOC** = Nursing Outcomes Classification

Possibly Effective

■ *Remove hand jewelry (e.g., rings) to enhance hand hygiene and prevent infection.* **LOE = I**

(MR) A Cochrane review demonstrated that there was insufficient evidence and no RCTs to determine adequately if there was an association between surgical team members wearing finger rings and surgical site infections (Arrowsmith et al., 2001).

(MR) A systematic review of the literature and original data demonstrated that wearing hand jewelry affected the efficacy of hand hygiene (Sickbert-Bennett et al., 2004).

(NR) A case-control study of health care workers with and without rings ($N = 50$ both groups) demonstrated that after hand hygiene, there was a greater reduction in the number of bacterial colonies on the hands of health care workers who did not wear rings (Salisbury et al., 1997).

Not Effective

■ *Using alcohol-based hand rub for hand hygiene when a patient is infected with a spore-forming bacterium (i.e.,* Clostridium difficile, anthrax bacillus*).* **LOE = I**

(MR) An RCT to evaluate several hand hygiene agents against *Bacillus atrophaeus,* a surrogate for *B. anthracis,* demonstrated that a waterless alcohol-based hand rub was not effective in removing spores from six healthy adult volunteers (Weber et al., 2003).

(EO) Alcohol-based hand rubs are not effective against spore-forming bacteria; the physical action of washing hands with soap and water removes spores (Boyce et al., 2002).

Possibly Harmful

■ *Presence of artificial fingernails.* **LOE = IV**

(MR) A case-control study of infants ($N = 19$ cases, $N = 54$ controls) in a neonatal intensive care unit demonstrated that exposure to one nurse with artificial fingernails was associated with cases of extended-spectrum beta-lactamase–producing *Klebsiella pneumoniae* (Gupta et al., 2004).

(MR) A case-control study of health care workers with ($N = 21$ cases) and without ($N = 20$ controls) artificial fingernails performing hand hygiene with antimicrobial soap or an alcohol-based hand rub demonstrated that health care workers with artificial fingernails had more pathogens isolated from their hands than controls (McNeil et al., 2001).

(MR) A cohort study of infants ($N = 33$) infected with *Pseudomonas aeruginosa* in a 40-bed neonatal intensive care unit and a step-down nursery examined microbial samples from the hands of all health care workers who had contact with infants ($N = 166$) and demonstrated that exposure to a health care worker with artificial fingernails was associated with a risk of infection (Foca et al., 2000).

■ *Using personal lotions or hand creams.* **LOE = IV**

(MR) A case-control study of in vitro preparations ($N = 35$ cases and $N = 80$ controls) inoculated from five vancomycin-resistant *Enterococcus faecium* clinical isolates revealed that the use of Vaseline Intensive Care lotion inhibited the antiseptic action of chlorhexidine gluconate (Frantz et al., 1997).

NR = Nursing Research, **MR** = Multidisciplinary Research, **SP** = Standard of Practice, **EO** = Expert Opinion, **LOE** = Level of Evidence

■ *Using alcohol-based hand hygiene products when hands are not completely dry, especially before touching electrical equipment.* **LOE = VI**

(MR) A report on the flammability of alcohol-based products stated that an emergency medical technician was the victim of a flash fire when he lit a cigarette after performing hand hygiene with an alcohol-based hand rub (Greene, 2003).

(MR) A case study reported that a health care worker was the victim of a flash fire after using an alcohol-based hand rub and removing a 100% polyester isolation gown that had built up static electricity, then touching a metal door before the alcohol evaporated from her hands (Bryant et al., 2002).

■ *Using hand hygiene products that may lead to irritant or allergic contact dermatitis.* **LOE = VI**

(MR) A descriptive study of neonatal intensive care nurses ($N = 58$) reported that nurses ($N = 7$) exhibited signs of mild to severe contact dermatitis after using an alcohol-based hand rub (Cimiotti et al., 2003).

(MR) A descriptive study of dermatitis in health care workers ($N = 360$) demonstrated that contact dermatitis was classified as occupational in a majority of the cases and that health care workers exhibiting occupational contact dermatitis were significantly more likely to be nurses (Nettis et al., 2002).

OUTCOME MEASUREMENT

KNOWLEDGE: INFECTION CONTROL   (NOC)

Definition: Extent of understanding conveyed about prevention and control of infection.

Knowledge: Infection Control as evidenced by the following selected NOC indicators:
- Description of mode of transmission
- Description of factors contributing to transmission
- Description of practices that reduce transmission

(Rate each indicator of **Knowledge: Infection Control:** 1 = none, 2 = limited, 3 = moderate, 4 = substantial, 5 = extensive) (Moorhead et al., 2004).

REFERENCES

Arrowsmith VA, Maunder JA, Sargent RJ, Taylor R. (2001). Removal of nail polish and finger rings to prevent surgical infection. *Cochrane Database Syst Rev*, (4):CD003325.

Boyce JM, Pittet D; Healthcare Infection Control Practices Advisory Committee. Society for Healthcare Epidemiology of America. Association for Professionals in Infection Control. Infectious Diseases Society of America. Hand Hygiene Task Force. (2002). Guideline for Hand Hygiene in Health-Care Settings: Recommendations of the Healthcare Infection Control Practices Advisory Committee and the HICPAC/SHEA/APIC/IDSA Hand Hygiene Task Force. *Infect Control Hosp Epidemiol*, 23(12 Suppl): S3-S40.

RCT = Randomized Controlled (Clinical) Trial, **NIC** = Nursing Interventions Classification, **NOC** = Nursing Outcomes Classification

Bryant KA, Pearce J, Stover B. (2002). Flash fire associated with the use of alcohol-based antiseptic agent. *Am J Infect Control*, 30(4):256-257.

Cimiotti JP, Marmur ES, Nesin M, Hamlin-Cook P, Larson EL. (2003). Adverse reactions associated with an alcohol-based hand antiseptic among nurses in a neonatal intensive care unit. *Am J Infect Control*, 31(1):43-48.

Dochterman JM, Bulechek GM (Eds). (2004). *Nursing Interventions Classification (NIC)*, 4th ed. St Louis: Mosby.

Foca M, Jakob K, Whittier S, Della Latta P, Factor S, Rubenstein D, et al. (2000). Endemic *Pseudomonas aeruginosa* infection in a neonatal intensive care unit. *N Engl J Med*, 343(10):695-700.

Frantz SW, Haines KA, Azar CG, Ward JI, Homan SM, Roberts RB. (1997). Chlorhexidine gluconate (CHG) activity against clinical isolates of vancomycin-resistant *Enterococcus faecium* (VREF) and the effects of moisturizing agents on CHG residue accumulation on the skin. *J Hosp Infect*, 37(2):157-164.

Gordin FM, Schultz ME, Huber RA, Gill JA. (2005). Reduction in nosocomial transmission of drug-resistant bacteria after introduction of an alcohol-based handrub. *Infect Control Hosp Epidemiol*, 26(7):650-653.

Greene J. (2003). Igniting interest. Hand-rub dispenser locations undergo scrutiny. *Mater Manag Health Care*, 12(3):32-34.

Gupta A, Della-Latta P, Todd B, San Gabriel P, Haas J, Wu F, et al. (2004). Outbreak of extended-spectrum beta-lactamase-producing *Klebsiella pneumoniae* in a neonatal intensive care unit linked to artificial nails. *Infect Control Hosp Epidemiol*, 25(3):210-215.

Hilburn J, Hammond BS, Fendler EJ, Groziak PA. (2003). Use of alcohol hand sanitizer as an infection control strategy in an acute care facility. *Am J Infect Control*, 31(2):109-116.

Kac G, Podglajen I, Gueneret M, Vaupre S, Bissery A, Meyer G. (2005). Microbiological evaluation of two hand hygiene procedures achieved by healthcare workers during routine patient care: A randomized study. *J Hosp Infect*, 60(1):32-39.

Larson E. (1999). Skin hygiene and infection prevention: More of the same or different approaches? *Clin Infect Dis*, 29(5):1287-1294.

Larson E. (2001). Hygiene of the skin: When is clean too clean? *Emerg Infect Dis*, 7(2):225-230.

McNeil SA, Foster CL, Hedderwick SA, Kauffman CA. (2001). Effect of hand cleansing with antimicrobial soap or alcohol-based gel on microbial colonization of artificial fingernails worn by health care workers. *Clin Infect Dis*, 32(3):367-372.

Moorhead M, Johnson M, Mass M (Eds). (2004). *Nursing Outcomes Classification (NOC)*, 3rd ed. St Louis: Mosby.

Nettis E, Colanardi MC, Soccio AL, Ferrannini A, Tursi A. (2002). Occupational irritant and allergic contact dermatitis among healthcare workers. *Contact Dermatitis*, 46(2):101-107.

Ng PC, Wong HL, Lyon DJ, So KW, Liu F, Lam RK, et al. (2004). Combined use of alcohol hand rub and gloves reduces the incidence of late onset infection in very low birthweight infants. *Arch Dis Child Fetal Neonatal Ed*, 89(4):F336-F340.

Salisbury DM, Hutfilz P, Treen LM, Bollin GE, Gautam S. (1997). The effect of rings on microbial load of health care workers' hands. *Am J Infect Control*, 25(1):24-27.

Sickbert-Bennett EE, Weber DJ, Gergen-Teague MF, Rutala WA. (2004). The effects of test variables on the efficacy of hand hygiene agents. *Am J Infect Control*, 32(2):69-83.

Weber DJ, Sickbert-Bennett E, Gergen MF, Rutala WA. (2003). Efficacy of selected hand hygiene agents used to remove *Bacillus atrophaeus* (a surrogate of *Bacillus anthracis*) from contaminated hands. *JAMA*, 289(10):1274-1277.

INFECTION PROTECTION   NIC

Thomas James Loveless, MSN, CRNP

NIC   **Definition:** Prevention and early detection of infection in a patient at risk (Dochterman & Bulechek, 2004).

NR = Nursing Research, **MR** = Multidisciplinary Research, **SP** = Standard of Practice, **EO** = Expert Opinion, **LOE** = Level of Evidence

NURSING ACTIVITIES

Effective

■ *Monitor for fever.* **LOE = VII**

    EO A temperature greater than 100°F (37.2°C) is both a sensitive and specific predictor of infection (Bentley et al., 2000). Maintain a general approach to the evaluation of fever. Other suggestive criteria of infection include an increase in temperature of at least 2°F (1.1°C) over baseline on repeated measurements. Fever is defined as a single oral temperature of ≥38°C (100.4°F) for ≥1 hour (Hughes et al., 2002). Fever, combined with neutropenia (defined as a neutrophil count <500 cell/mm^3 or a count of <1000 cells/mm^3 with a predicted decrease to <500 cells/mm^3) reflects susceptibility to infection (Hughes et al., 2002).

■ *Monitor for subtle clinical manifestations of infection.* **LOE = VII**

    EO The clinical clues to infection vary among patients and may be affected by several components: age, comorbidities, setting, operative history, and functional ability. In the geriatric setting, infection may manifest itself as a change in mental status, may be very subtle, and may show rapid decline. Monitor for increased confusion, incontinence, falling, deteriorating mobility, or failure to cooperate (Bentley et al., 2000).

■ *Monitor for physical signs of infection.* **LOE = VII**

    EO Residents of a long-term care facility who demonstrated tachypnea (respiratory rate ≥25 breaths/min) subsequently had a diagnosis of pneumonia. The respiratory rate had a sensitivity of 90% and a specificity of 95% for pneumonia diagnosis (Bentley et al., 2000).

■ *Monitor for pulse oximetry.* **LOE = VII**

    EO Oxygen saturation less than 90% is indicative of pneumonia. Consider chest radiography (Bentley et al., 2000).

■ *Monitor for dehydration.* **LOE = VII**

    EO Dehydration in the febrile patient can indicate underlying infection. Serology including electrolyte surveillance is critical for the evaluation of infection. Often an elevated ratio of blood urea nitrogen to serum creatinine, or both, reflects underlying infection. Other laboratory tests should include blood cell count, urinalysis, and urine culture (Bentley et al., 2000).

■ **SP** *Maintain universal precautions consistently for* all *patients.* **LOE = VII**

    EO To minimize the acquisition and transmission of infectious agents within the hospital setting, the following standard precautions are considered the minimal precautions that all nurses should incorporate in the care of their patients: prevention of needlestick injury (and other sharps) and use of protective barriers such as gloves, gowns, aprons, mask, or protective equipment with the intent to prevent exposure to potentially infectious materials. Standard precautions synthesize the primary features of universal precautions (Garner, 1996); universal precautions were designed to reduce the risk of transmission of bloodborne pathogens. In addition, the body substance isolation precaution was designed to reduce transmission of

RCT = Randomized Controlled (Clinical) Trial, **NIC** = Nursing Interventions Classification, **NOC** = Nursing Outcomes Classification

pathogens from moist body surfaces. Standardized precautions apply to all patients in all settings (Garner, 1996).

■ ⓈⓅ *Practice hand washing and hand care.* **LOE = VII**

Ⓔ According to the CDC and its review of the seminal work of Semmelweis and Holmes in the early 19th century, hand washing has been accepted as one of the most important mechanisms to prevent the spread of infectious agents in health care workers (Boyce et al., 2002).

Ⓔ Hand washing remains the single most effective method to prevent, control, and reduce infections. Hand washing is a mantra of infection control and is one of the basic, fundamental underlying principles of nursing (Bjerke, 2004).

Ⓔ Always wash hands after touching blood, body fluids, secretions, and contaminated items regardless of wearing gloves (Boyce et al., 2002).

Ⓔ Immediate hand washing should be thoroughly completed if an exposure to blood or bloody fluids has occurred (CDC, 1996).

Ⓔ Wash hands immediately after removing gloves and in between each and every contact with patients (CDC, 1996).

Ⓔ Use of a nonantibacterial soap is sufficient for routine hand washing (CDC, 1996). When using soap and water, wash hands vigorously for at least 15 seconds, avoiding excessively hot water because this may cause dermatitis. Washing with plain soap and water for 15 seconds reduces bacterial counts on the skin by 0.6 to 1.1 $\log^{10}$, whereas washing for 30 seconds reduces counts by 1.8 to 2.8 $\log^{10}$. Transient flora, which colonizes the superficial layers of the skin, is more amenable to removal by routine hand washing (Kampf & Kramer, 2004).

Ⓔ Use of an antibacterial soap or a waterless antiseptic agent is needed after caring for any patient with known multidrug-resistant pathogens (e.g., methicillin-resistant *Staphylococcus aureus*). Alcohol-based hand rubs significantly reduce the number of microorganisms (Boyce et al., 2002).

■ ⓈⓅ *Wear a gown.* **LOE = VII**

Ⓔ A nonsterile gown is adequate to protect skin and soiling of clothing. Remove soiled gowns as soon as possible, and discard following appropriate biohazard precautions (CDC, 1996).

■ ⓈⓅ *Wear mask and eyewear.* **LOE = VII**

Ⓔ The CDC reported that mask and eyewear should reduce the incidence of blood contamination of mucous membranes of the mouth, eye, and nose while performing procedures that may generate droplets of blood or body fluids requiring precautions (CDC, 1996; Larson, 1988, 1999).

Droplet Contact

■ ⓈⓅ *Maintain universal precautions consistently for all patients.* **LOE = VII**

Ⓔ Standard precautions are the minimal requirement for patients with illness from pathogens known to be transmitted through droplets (Panlilio et al., 2005).

Ⓔ Patients' placement requires a private room. If no private room is available, avoid discordant placement. Patients with known or suspected microorganisms that are transmitted via

NR = Nursing Research, **MR** = Multidisciplinary Research, **SP** = Standard of Practice, **EO** = Expert Opinion, **LOE** = Level of Evidence

droplets should be placed in a room with a patient who also has the same infection (CDC, 1996).

⊙ If cohorting (sharing a room with a patient infected with the same microorganism) is not possible, maintain separation of at least 3 feet between patients (Panlilio et al., 2005).

⊙ Special air handling is not required, and room doors may remain open (Panlilio et al., 2005).

⊙ Wearing a mask as defined by standard precautions applies while caring for the patient with an infection known to be spread by droplets (Panlilio et al., 2005).

⊙ If transport of the source patient is not avoidable, mask the patient to decrease the patient's ability to disperse droplets (Panlilio et al., 2005).

Airborne Precautions

■ ⊙ *Maintain universal precautions consistently for all patients.* **LOE = VII**

⊙ Standard precautions are the minimal requirement for patients with illnesses from pathogens known to be transmitted through airborne transmission (Panlilio et al., 2005).

■ ⊙ *In addition to universal precautions, respiratory protection is warranted.* **LOE = VII**

⊙ Wearing respiratory protection (N95 respirator) when entering a room of a patient with known infectious pulmonary tuberculosis, measles (rubeola), or varicella (chicken pox) must be strictly adhered to (Panlilio et al., 2005).

⊙ Patients' placement requires a private room with negative air pressure; a minimum of 6 to 12 air exchanges per hour is mandated. Air discharge to the outdoors is required or high-efficiency filtration before the air is circulated internally (Panlilio et al., 2005). The room door *must* remain closed.

⊙ Patients' cohorting is required. When cohorting is not possible, absolute consultation with infectious diseases is warranted (Panlilio et al., 2005).

⊙ Patients' transport outside of the room should be kept to the absolute minimum. If transport is required, the source patient must be masked; a surgical mask is sufficient (Panlilio et al., 2005).

Possibly Effective

■ *Wear gloves.* **LOE = VII**

⊙ Gloves do not provide complete protection against hand contamination. Bacterial flora colonizing in patients may be recovered from the hands of up to 30% of health care workers who wear gloves during contact with patients (Olsen et al., 1993; Tenorio et al., 2001).

⊙ Clean, nonsterile gloves are adequate protection for routine care of patients. Gloves are required for contact with mucous membranes and nonintact skin. Changing of gloves is required, even while performing sequential individual tasks on the same patient (CDC, 1996) and particularly when going from contaminated sites to noncontaminated sites (Boyce et al., 2002). Wearing gloves does not eliminate the need for consistent hand washing.

⊙ Glove wearing by health care workers is recommended for two main reasons: (1) to prevent microorganisms that may be infectious, commensally carried, or transiently present on health care workers' hands from being transmitted to patients and from one patient to another and (2) to reduce the risk of health care workers acquiring infections from patients (Boyce

RCT = Randomized Controlled (Clinical) Trial, **NIC** = Nursing Interventions Classification, **NOC** = Nursing Outcomes Classification

et al., 2002). The effectiveness of gloves in preventing contamination of health care workers' hands has been reported in several clinical studies (Pittet et al., 1999; Tenorio et al., 2001).

Not Effective

■ *Wearing artificial nails and nail polish.* **LOE = V**

(EO) The issue of artificial nails and cosmetic polish remains unresolved regarding transmission of infections. The CDC recommends that health care workers avoid wearing artificial nails and keep natural nails less than one quarter of an inch long if they care for patients at risk for acquiring infections (e.g., chemotherapy patients, transplant patients) (Boyce et al., 2002).

(EO) Subungual areas of the hand harbor high concentrations of bacteria, frequently coagulase-negative staphylococci, gram-negative rods, and yeast. Despite thorough hand washing, studies have reported the harboring of substantial bacteria in the subungual space (Gross et al., 1979; Pottinger et al., 1989; McNeil et al., 2001). It is still unclear whether artificial nails contribute definitively to the transmission of infection, and additional studies are warranted. Moreover, the length of the nails remains in debate, but it is reported that the majority of bacterial growth occurs along the proximal 1 mm of the nail bed adjacent to subungual skin (Wynd et al., 1994; Pottinger et al., 1989).

Possibly Harmful

No applicable published research was found in this category.

OUTCOME MEASUREMENT

KNOWLEDGE: INFECTION CONTROL   (NOC)

Definition: Extent of understanding conveyed about prevention and control of infection.

Knowledge: Infection Control as evidenced by the following selected NOC indicators:
• Description of practices that reduce transmission
• Description of signs and symptoms
• Description of monitoring procedures
(Rate each indicator of **Knowledge: Infection Control:** 1 = none, 2 = limited, 3 = moderate, 4 = substantial, 5 = extensive) (Moorhead et al., 2004).

REFERENCES

Bentley DW, Bradley S, High K, Schoenbaum S, Taler G, Yoshikawa TT, et al. (2000). Practice guideline for evaluation of fever and infection in long-term care facilities. *Clin Infect Dis,* 31(3):640-653.

Bjerke NB. (2004). The evolution: Handwashing to hand hygiene guidance. *Crit Care Nurs Q,* 27(3): 295-307.

Boyce JM, Pittet D; Healthcare Infection Control Practices Advisory Committee; HICPAC/SHEA/APIC/IDSA Hand Hygiene Task Force. (2002). Guideline for Hand Hygiene in Health-Care Settings. Recommendations of the Healthcare Infection Control Practices Advisory Committee and the HICPAC/SHEA/APIC/IDSA Hand Hygiene Task Force. Society for Healthcare Epidemiology of America/Association for Professionals in Infection Control/Infectious Diseases Society of America. *MMWR Recomm Rep,* 51(RR-16):1-45.

Centers for Disease Control and Prevention (CDC), Department of Health and Human Services, Fact Sheet. (1996). *Universal Precautions for Prevention of Transmission of HIV and Other Bloodborne Infections.* Available online: http://www.cdc.gov/ncidod/dhqp/bp_universal_precautions.html. Retrieved on July 7, 2007.

Dochterman JM, Bulechek GM (Eds). (2004). *Nursing Interventions Classification (NIC),* 4th ed. St. Louis: Mosby.

Garner JS. (1996). Guideline for isolation precautions in hospitals. The Hospital Infection Control Practices Advisory Committee. *Infect Control Hosp Epidemiol,* 17(1):53-80.

Gross A, Cutright DE, A'Alessandro SM. (1979). Efects of surgical scrub on microbial population under the fingernails. *Am J Surg,* 138(3), 463-467.

Hughes WT, Armstrong D, Bodey GP, Bow EJ, Brown AE, Calandra T, et al. (2002). 2002 guidelines for the use of antimicrobial agents in neutropenic patients with cancer. *Clin Infect Dis,* 34(6):730-751.

Kampf G, Kramer A. (2004). Epidemiologic background of hand hygiene and evaluation of the most important agents for scrubs and rubs. *Clin Microbiol Rev,* 17(4):863-893.

Larson E. (1988). A causal link between handwashing and risk of infection? Examination of the evidence. *Infect Control,* 9(1):28-36.

Larson E. (1999). Skin hygiene and infection prevention: More of the same or different approaches? *Clin Infect Dis,* 29(5):1287-1294.

McNeil SA, Foster CL, Hedderwick SA, Kauffman CA. (2001). Effects of hand cleansing with antimicrobial soap or alcohol-based gel on microbial colonization of artificial fingernails worn by health care workers. *Clin Infect Dis,* 32(3):367-372.

Moorhead M, Johnson M, Maas M (Eds). (2004). *Nursing Outcomes Classification (NOC),* 3rd ed. St. Louis: Mosby.

Olsen RJ, Lynch P, Coyle MB, Cummings J, Bokete T, Stamm WE. (1993). Examination gloves as barriers to hand contamination in clinical practice. *JAMA* 270:350.

Panlilio AL, Cardo DM, Grohskopf LA, Heneine W, Ross CS; US Public Health Service. (2005). Updated U.S. Public Health Service guidelines for the management of occupational exposures to HIV and recommendations for postexposure prophylaxis. *MMWR Recomm Rep,* 54(RR-9):1-17.

Pittet D, Dharan S, Touveneau S, Sauvan V, Perneger TV. (1999). Bacterial contamination of the hands of hospital staff during routine patient care. *Arch Intern Med,* 159(8):821-826.

Pottinger J, Burns S, Manske C. (1989). Bacterial carriage by artificial versus natural nails. *Am J Infect Control,* 17(6):340-344.

Tenorio AR, Badri SM, Sahgal NB, Hota B, Matushek M, Hayden MK, et al. (2001). Effectiveness of gloves in the prevention of hand carriage of vancomycin-resistant enterococcus species by health care workers after patient care. *Clin Infect Dis,* 32(5):826-829.

Wynd CA, Samstag DE, Lapp AM. (1994). Bacterial carriages on the fingernails of OR nurses. *AORN J,* 60(5):796, 799-805.

 # INTRAVENOUS INSERTION

Lisa Gorski, MS, APRN-BC, CRNI, FAAN

NIC **Definition:** Insertion of a needle into a peripheral vein for the purpose of administering fluids, blood, or medications (Dochterman & Bulechek, 2004).

NURSING ACTIVITIES

Effective

■ *Use a specialized IV team to place and monitor peripheral IV catheters to reduce the risk of complications and costs.* **LOE = II**

(MR) A randomized, prospective controlled trial found that patients whose peripheral IV catheters were started by and maintained by a dedicated IV team of nurses had significantly

RCT = Randomized Controlled (Clinical) Trial, **NIC** = Nursing Interventions Classification, **NOC** = Nursing Outcomes Classification

less local and bacteremic complications than patients with those started by medical house staff and maintained by floor nurses (Soifer et al., 1998).

(NR) A correlational descriptive study ($N = 413$) examining extending peripheral IV catheter dwell time from 72 to 144 hours found that if nonirritating medications were administered and a dedicated team of IV specialists inserted and evaluated the catheters, catheter dwell time may be extended beyond 72 hours (Catney et al., 2001).

(NR) A descriptive study ($N = 339$) examining the effects of nurse, patient, IV type, and IV insertion on IV outcome found that nurses who were older, more experienced, and certified in a specialty area had significantly more successful IV insertions than less experienced and skilled nurses (Jacobson & Winslow, 2005).

(EO) Specialized "IV teams" have shown unequivocal effectiveness in reducing the incidence of catheter-related infections and associated complications and costs (O'Grady et al., 2002).

■ *Wash hands using conventional antiseptic soap and water or with waterless alcohol-based gels or foams before and after inserting peripheral IV catheters to reduce the risk of intravenous device–related infections.* **LOE = I**

(Please refer to the guideline on Infection Control: Handwashing.)

(EO) Maintain aseptic technique while performing all IV therapy–related procedures to reduce the risk of catheter-related bloodstream infections (BSIs) (O'Grady et al., 2002).

■ (NIC) *Maintain strict aseptic technique.* **LOE = I**

(Please refer to the Infection Control guideline.)

(EO) Maintain aseptic technique while performing all IV therapy–related procedures to reduce the risk of catheter-related BSIs (O'Grady et al., 2002).

■ *Use a 2% chlorhexidine-based preparation for disinfection of the intended venipuncture site to reduce the risk of infection.* **LOE = I**

(MR) A meta-analysis of studies ($N = 8$ studies involving 4143 catheters, of which 1361 were peripheral IV catheters) comparing chlorhexidine gluconate with povidone iodine solutions for catheter site care found that the incidence of bloodstream infections was significantly reduced when chlorhexidine gluconate was used (Chaiyakunapruk et al., 2002).

(EO) The U.S. Food and Drug Administration (FDA) has approved a 2% tincture of chlorhexidine preparation for skin antisepsis before insertion of intravascular catheters (O'Grady et al., 2002).

■ (SP) *Use veins on the dorsal and ventral surface of the upper extremities for adults.* **LOE = VII**

(EO) Lower extremity veins are associated with increased risk for embolism and thrombophlebitis (INS, 2006).

■ (SP) *Initiate site selection in the distal areas of the upper extremities with subsequent cannulation proximal to the previous site.* **LOE = VII**

(EO) When the new peripheral IV insertion site is located above the previous site, avoid infusing medications or solutions through the potentially damaged site where the old IV was placed (INS, 2006).

NR = Nursing Research, **MR** = Multidisciplinary Research, **SP** = Standard of Practice, **EO** = Expert Opinion, **LOE** = Level of Evidence

■ ⓢⓟ *No more than two attempts by any one nurse should be made to place a peripheral IV catheter.* **LOE = VII**

ⒺⓄ This avoids multiple unsuccessful attempts that would cause unnecessary trauma to the patient and potentially limit future vascular access (INS, 2006).

■ ⓢⓟ *Use a catheter of the smallest size and shortest length appropriate for the fluid to be infused.* **LOE = VII**

ⒺⓄ Smaller peripheral IV catheters allow increased blood flow around the catheter within the vein, potentially decreasing the risk for phlebitis (INS, 2006).

■ *Use a local intradermal anesthetic or topical anesthetic cream to decrease pain associated with IV insertion.* **LOE = I**

ⓃⓇ A meta-analysis of 20 studies analyzing the effectiveness of a topical anesthetic (2.5% lidocaine and 2.5% prilocaine mixture, EMLA cream) concluded that use of EMLA significantly decreased venipuncture and IV insertion pain in 85% of the population (Fetzer, 2002).

ⓃⓇ A randomized double-blinded study involving surgical adult patients ($N = 47$) that compared the use of intradermal injections of either lidocaine hydrochloride 1% with sodium bicarbonate or sodium chloride 0.9% with benzyl alcohol demonstrated that there was no significant difference between the anesthetic effects; both were effective in reducing pain and were safe (Brown, 2004).

ⓃⓇ A quasi-experimental study involving surgical adult patients ($N = 30$) that compared use of intradermal injection of lidocaine, EMLA cream, and the "Numby Stuff" system (local anesthetic Iontocaine with use of mild electrical current to deliver the medication through the skin) found the Numby Stuff superior to the other methods in decreasing IV insertion pain (Miller et al., 2001).

ⓃⓇ A descriptive study involving adult medical-surgical patients ($N = 180$) was designed to determine patients' preferences regarding the use of intradermal lidocaine before peripheral IV insertions. Significant findings included the fact that subjects who had any type of experience with lidocaine would prefer to have it used for future IV insertions and that the pain associated with lidocaine injection was less than the pain associated with IV insertion (Brown, 2003).

ⓃⓇ A randomized double-blinded study involving adult inpatients on medical units ($N = 33$) that compared use of subcutaneous injection of buffered lidocaine hydrochloride 1%, sodium chloride 0.9% with benzyl alcohol, and no treatment found a significantly improved pain rating associated with use of lidocaine hydrochloride 1% and no significant difference between no treatment and use of sodium chloride with benzyl alcohol (Hattula et al., 2002).

■ ⓢⓟ *Replace peripheral IV catheters every 96 hours or longer with the infusion of nonirritating medications and when a specialized IV team inserts and evaluates the catheters.* **LOE = III**

ⓃⓇ A correlational descriptive study ($N = 413$) examining extending peripheral IV catheter dwell time from 72 to 144 hours found there was no significant increase in phlebitis or infiltration as the days progressed. However, drug irritation, catheter size, and personnel

RCT = Randomized Controlled (Clinical) Trial, **NIC** = Nursing Interventions Classification, **NOC** = Nursing Outcomes Classification

inserting the catheter were significant predictors of phlebitis or infiltration. When nonirritating medications were administered and a dedicated team of IV specialists inserted and evaluated the catheters, catheter dwell time could be extended beyond 72 hours (Catney et al., 2001).

(MR) A prospective descriptive study ($N = 2503$) found that the rate of phlebitis for peripheral IV catheters at 96 hours was not significantly different from that at 72 hours; peripheral IV catheters were inserted and monitored daily by nurses on the IV team (Lai, 1998).

(MR) A prospective descriptive study ($N = 412$) found that extended dwell time did not lead to significantly higher rates of phlebitis; catheters were inserted by an IV team whenever possible (Cornely et al., 2002).

■ *Use a manufactured catheter securement device to extend peripheral IV dwell time and reduce risk of peripheral IV-related complications.* **LOE = II**

(MR) A systematic review of prospective or prospective randomized studies that compared tape and suture versus other methods of securing peripheral IV catheters or peripherally inserted central catheters was performed. Three prospective studies of peripheral IV catheters ($N = 429$) that compared tape plus a transparent dressing with a manufactured catheter securement device demonstrated a reduction in overall complications up to 69%, reduction in catheter dislodgement by up to 95%, and dwell times prolonged by up to 61% (Frey & Schears, 2006).

(NR) A prospective, quasi-experimental study ($N = 659$) that compared the effects of three peripheral IV catheter securement methods (nonsterile tape, the HubGuard, and StatLock) on the outcome of peripheral IV catheter survival to 96 hours found that the StatLock device resulted in significantly longer dwell times (Smith, 2006).

Possibly Effective

No applicable published research was found in this category.

Not Effective

No applicable published research was found in this category.

Possibly Harmful

■ *Using veins of the lower extremities.* **LOE = VII**

(EO) There is increased risk of embolism and thrombophlebitis when a peripheral IV is placed in the lower extremities (INS, 2006).

■ *Using veins in the palm side of the wrist.* **LOE = VII**

(EO) The radial nerve is located near the vein and can cause excessive pain during insertion and during the insertion period of the IV catheter and could potentially cause nerve damage.

■ *Placing the peripheral IV catheter in an area of flexion.* **LOE = VII**

(EO) There is increased risk of catheter dislodgement and complications such as phlebitis related to excessive movement of the catheter within the vein (INS, 2006).

NR = Nursing Research, **MR** = Multidisciplinary Research, **SP** = Standard of Practice, **EO** = Expert Opinion, **LOE** = Level of Evidence

■ *Placing the peripheral IV catheter in the arm of a patient who has undergone breast surgery requiring axillary node dissection or who has an existing fistula.*
LOE = VII

(EO) Altered venous and lymphatic circulation can cause or exacerbate edema or increase risk for infection (INS, 2006).

OUTCOME MEASUREMENT

PERIPHERAL VASCULAR ACCESS

Definition: Establishment of an access to the bloodstream through a peripheral vein.
Peripheral Vascular Access as evidenced by the following indicators:
• Intravenous catheter securely anchored
• Insertion site free of edema
• Insertion site free of redness
• Patient states site is comfortable
(Note: This is not a NOC outcome.)

REFERENCES

Brown D. (2004). Local anesthesia for vein cannulation: A comparison of two solutions. *J Infus Nurs*, 27(2):85-88.

Brown J. (2003). Using lidocaine for peripheral IV insertions: Patients' preferences and pain experiences. *Medsurg Nurs*, 12(2):95-100.

Catney MR, Hillis S, Wakefield B, Simpson L, Domino L, Keller S, et al. (2001). Relationship between peripheral intravenous catheter dwell time and the development of phlebitis and infiltration. *J Infus Nurs*, 24(5):332-341.

Chaiyakunapruk N, Veenstra DL, Lipsky BA, Saint S. (2002). Chlorhexidine compared with povidone iodine solution for vascular site care: A meta-analysis. *Ann Intern Med*, 136(11):792-801.

Cornely OA, Bethe U, Pauls R, Waldschmidt D. (2002). Peripheral Teflon catheters: Factors determining incidence of phlebitis and duration of cannulation. *Infect Control Hosp Epidemiol*, 23(5):249-253.

Dochterman JM, Bulechek GM (Eds). (2004). *Nursing Interventions Classification (NIC)*, 4th ed. St. Louis: Mosby.

Fetzer SJ. (2002). Reducing venipuncture and intravenous insertion pain with eutectic mixture of local anesthetic: A meta-analysis. *Nurs Res*, 51(2):119-124.

Frey AM, Schears GJ. (2006). Why are we stuck on tape and suture? A review of catheter securement devices. *J Infus Nurs*, 29(1):34-38.

Hattula JL, McGovern EK, Neumann TL. (2002). Comparison of intravenous cannulation injectable pre-anesthetics in an adult medical inpatient population. *App Nurs Res*, 15(3):189-193.

Infusion Nurses Society (INS). (2006). Infusion nursing standards of practice. *J Infus Nurs*, 29(1 Suppl): S1-S92.

Jacobson AF, Winslow EH. (2005). Variables influencing intravenous catheter insertion difficulty and failure: An analysis of 339 intravenous catheter insertions. *Heart Lung*, 34(5):345-359.

Lai KK. (1998). Safety of prolonging peripheral cannula and IV tubing use from 72 hours to 96 hours. *Am J Infect Control*, 26(1):66-70.

Miller KA, Balakrishnan G, Eichbauer G, Betley K. (2001). 1% lidocaine injection, EMLA cream, or "Numby Stuff" for topical analgesia associated with peripheral intravenous cannulation. *AANA J*, 69(3):185-187.

O'Grady NP, Alexander M, Dellinger EP, Gerberding JL, Heard SO, Maki DG, et al. (2002). Guidelines for the prevention of intravascular catheter-related infections. Centers for Disease Control and Prevention. *MMWR Recomm Rep*, 51(RR-10):1-29.

RCT = Randomized Controlled (Clinical) Trial, **NIC** = Nursing Interventions Classification, **NOC** = Nursing Outcomes Classification

Smith B. (2006). Peripheral intravenous catheter dwell times: A comparison of 3 securement methods for implementation of a 96-hour scheduled change protocol. *J Infus Nurs*, 29(1):14-17.

Soifer NE, Borzak S, Edlin BR, Weinstein RA. (1998). Prevention of peripheral venous catheter complications with an intravenous therapy team: A randomized controlled trial. *Arch Intern Med*, 158(5): 473-477.

 # INTRAVENOUS THERAPY

Lisa A. Gorski, MS, APRN-BC, CRNI, FAAN

NIC **Definition:** Administration and monitoring of intravenous fluids and medications (Dochterman & Bulechek, 2004).

NURSING ACTIVITIES

Effective

■ *Wash hands using conventional antiseptic soap and water or waterless alcohol-based gels or foams before and after administering IV therapy to reduce the risk of IV device–related infections.* **LOE = I**

(Please refer to the guideline on Infection Control: Hand Hygiene.)

■ **NIC** *Maintain strict aseptic technique.* **LOE = I**

(Please refer to the guideline on Infection Control.)

■ *Use a specialized IV team to administer and monitor IV therapy to reduce the risk of complications and cost of care.* **LOE = II**

MR A randomized, prospective controlled trial found that patients whose peripheral IV catheters were started by and maintained by a dedicated IV team of nurses had significantly less local and bacteremic complications than patients with those started by medical house staff and maintained by floor nurses (Soifer et al., 1998).

NR A correlational descriptive study ($N = 413$) examining the relationship between extending peripheral IV catheter dwell time from 72 to 144 hours found that if nonirritating medications were administered and a dedicated team of IV specialists inserted and evaluated the catheters, catheter dwell time may be extended beyond 72 hours (Catney et al., 2001).

MR A significant reduction in the rate of hospital-acquired BSIs was demonstrated after the introduction of a dedicated IV team (Meier et al., 1998).

EO Specialized IV teams have shown unequivocal effectiveness in reducing the incidence of catheter-related infections and associated complications and costs (CDC, 2003).

■ **SP** *Administer irritating IV fluids or medications, parenteral nutrition, and continuous vesicant drug infusions through a centrally placed catheter to reduce the risk of phlebitis and damage to peripheral veins.* **LOE = VII**

EO Therapies not appropriate for peripheral short catheters include continuous vesicant therapy, parenteral nutrition, infusates with a pH less than 5 or greater than 9, and infusates with an osmolarity greater than 600 mOsm/L (INS, 2006).

NR = Nursing Research, **MR** = Multidisciplinary Research, **SP** = Standard of Practice, **EO** = Expert Opinion, **LOE** = Level of Evidence

(NR) A correlational descriptive study ($N = 413$) examining extending peripheral IV catheter dwell time from 72 to 144 hours found that if nonirritating medications were administered and a dedicated team of IV specialists inserted and evaluated the catheters, catheter dwell time may be extended beyond 72 hours (Catney et al., 2001).

■ (SP) ***Remove and replace a peripheral IV catheter when it has been placed in an emergency situation as soon as possible and no longer than 48 hours after placement.*** **LOE = VII**

(EO) Removing and replacing a peripheral IV catheter as soon as possible is recommended because of the risk of compromised aseptic technique during insertion (INS, 2006).

■ (SP) ***Disinfect the needleless connector (injection/access cap) using 70% alcohol, 2% chlorhexidine in alcohol, or povidone iodine immediately before use to minimize contamination and decrease the risk of catheter-related BSIs.***
LOE = IV

(MR) An in vitro study compared two needleless access devices with a needle access device by inoculating each device with *Enterococcus faecium* and then accessing each device either without disinfection or with 70% alcohol disinfection. There was no statistically significant difference in the rate of fluid contamination between the two types of devices; failure to disinfect the device prior to access increased the risk for contamination (Arduino et al., 1997).

(MR) A protocol for collecting, processing, and examining needleless connectors found that 63% of needleless connectors ($N = 24$) collected from patients with long-term central venous catheters in a bone marrow transplant center contained biofilms composed of coagulase-negative staphylococci (Donlan et al., 2001).

(MR) A randomized study of cardiac surgical patients with central venous catheters ($N = 77$) found that the use of needleless connectors was associated with significantly less microbial contamination than standard caps. Disinfection with chlorhexidine/alcohol or povidone iodine was more effective than isopropyl alcohol (Casey et al., 2003).

(MR) A retrospective cohort study was completed to determine whether an increase in BSIs in patients with central venous catheters was associated with implementing a needleless device. A significant increase in BSIs occurred after implementation of the device and was associated with nurses' lack of knowledge regarding care practices for the device (Cookson et al., 1998).

(EO) Cleanse the injection or access port with an approved disinfectant immediately prior to use (INS, 2006).

(EO) Minimize contamination risk by wiping the access port with an appropriate antiseptic and accessing the port only with sterile devices (O'Grady et al., 2002).

■ (SP) ***Use single-dose flush solution containers/syringes (saline/heparin) to reduce the risk of infection.*** **LOE = IV**

(MR) Case reports of patient-to-patient transmission of viral illnesses were associated with poor infection control practices. Single-dose vials, ampules, and prefilled syringes were recommended (CDC, 2003).

(MR) A retrospective cohort study was conducted among 41 hospitalized patients; three of four patients who received saline flushes from a multidose saline vial had acute hepatitis C virus (HCV) infection, whereas none of the nine patients who did not receive saline flushes had HCV infection ($P = .01$). No other significant exposures was identified (Krause et al., 2003).

RCT = Randomized Controlled (Clinical) Trial, **NIC** = Nursing Interventions Classification, **NOC** = Nursing Outcomes Classification

(MR) A prevalence study in a large hospital was performed to investigate practices and contamination of multiple-use vials. Risky practices included opened vials with opening dates marked on only on 50% of vials, 13% present on units beyond expiration dates, and lack of proper storage. One vial was contaminated with *Staphylococcus epidermidis* (Mattner & Gastmeier, 2004).

(MR) In an observational study, syringes filled by nursing staff using routine floor procedures were collected and studied. The contents of 14 of 168 syringes collected had microbial contamination with the source appearing to be hand contact (Calop et al., 2000).

(MR) A preliminary study demonstrated microbial contamination of 8 of 100 clinician-prepared saline syringes including contaminated syringe tips and needles ($N = 2$). A further 4% of syringe tips/transportation caps and 3% of needles yielded positive cultures ($N = 100$). A subsequent comparative study found contamination in nurse-prepared syringe solutions and inadequate or inconsistent aseptic technique. Prefilled syringes showed no contamination and showed cost savings (Worthington et al., 2001).

(EO) Single-use flushing systems should be used (INS, 2006).

■ *Use computerized "smart" infusion pumps* to reduce the risk for error when administering high-risk IV medications (e.g., heparin, insulin, morphine, potassium, propofol).* **LOE = II**

(MR) A prospective randomized study ($N = 744$) compared infusion pump use between intervention (pump on) periods and control periods (pump off) in cardiac surgical patients. It was found that the decision support software in a computerized pump intercepted many potentially harmful errors before reaching the patient, including unsafe drug dilutions, inappropriate bolus technique, and initiating drugs without physician orders (Rothschild et al., 2005).

(EO) Dose error reduction systems should be considered in the selection and use of electronic infusion pumps (INS, 2006).

■ (SP) *Identify the patient and assess for the appropriate dose, route, and rate of infusion and for potential incompatibilities between infusates before initiating the IV infusion.* **LOE = VII**

(EO) This is standard practice for care of the patient with an intravenous infusion (INS, 2006).

■ (SP) *Double-check the infusion solution, dosage, and rate with a second health care provider (nurse, pharmacist) when high-risk medications are administered.* **LOE = VIII**

(EO) Intravenous high-risk medications include amiodarone, heparin, low-molecular-weight heparin, lidocaine, nesiritide, nitroprusside, potassium, and sodium chloride (in concentrations >0.9%). Strategies to decrease risk of errors include limiting access to medications, automated alert systems, and automating or double checking the solution, dosage, and rate (ISMP, 2004b).

■ (SP) *Trace the IV catheter from the point of origin every time an infusion container or device is changed and when a patient is transferred from one setting to another (e.g., intensive care unit to medical unit, medical unit to*

---

* Administration set is defined to include the IV tubing and any add-on devices such as extension sets and the needleless connector.

NR = Nursing Research, **MR** = Multidisciplinary Research, **SP** = Standard of Practice, **EO** = Expert Opinion, **LOE** = Level of Evidence

home care) to reduce the risk of accidental connection of an infusion to the wrong type of catheter. **LOE = VII**

(EO) Tubing misconnections have resulted in significant adverse events including patients' deaths. Examples include erroneously connecting IV infusions to epidural catheters or feeding tubes or vice versa (The Joint Commission, 2006; ISMP, 2004a).

■ *Change IV administration sets* for primary and continuous infusions every 96 hours unless contaminated or administering lipids, blood, or blood products.* **LOE = I**

(MR) A systematic review of all randomized or systematically allocated controlled trials that addressed IV administration set frequency and included outcome measures of infusate colonization, infusate-related BSIs, catheter colonization, catheter-related BSIs, and mortality found good evidence that changing the administration set every 72 hours to every 96 hours did not increase the risk for infusate-related BSIs and fair evidence that it did not increase the risk of catheter-related BSIs. There were insufficient data to make recommendations for parenteral nutrition, particularly lipid-containing parenteral nutrition solutions (Gillies et al., 2004).

(EO) Replace administration sets no more frequently than every 72 hours *unless* administering blood, blood products, or lipid emulsions (O'Grady et al., 2002).

(EO) Change primary and secondary continuous administration sets no more frequently than every 72 hours and immediately upon suspected contamination or when the integrity of the product or system has been compromised (INS, 2006).

■ (SP) *Administer IV medications in the home setting when the infusion therapy is appropriate for home care, when planning with attention to appropriateness of patient's condition is assessed, and when the patient or caregiver is able to participate in learning about infusion therapy administration.* **LOE = IV**

(EO) Infusion therapies administered in the home setting include antimicrobial drugs, total parenteral nutrition, some chemotherapy drugs, analgesics, cardiac drugs including dobutamine and milrinone, and intravenous immunoglobulin therapy (Gorski, 2005a, b).

(EO) Factors to address when moving a patient to home infusion therapy include assessment of the patient's clinical stability and tolerance of the intended home infusion medication(s) without significant or unmanageable side effects, willingness and ability to participate in the home care plan, adequacy of the home environment (cleanliness, refrigeration), and reimbursement (Gorski, 2005a).

(NR) In a controlled study, the use of standardized instruction handouts and a skills checklist was shown to decrease teaching time and the number of home visits (Grimes-Holsinger, 2002).

(NR) A grounded theory study ($N = 7$) examined characteristics of the education process from the caregiver's point of view that led to competence in learning home infusion therapy. Defining factors were divided into themes that occurred during the teaching-learning process (Cox & Westbrook, 2005).

---

* Administration set is defined to include the IV tubing and any add-on devices such as extension sets and the needleless connector.

RCT = Randomized Controlled (Clinical) Trial, **NIC** = Nursing Interventions Classification, **NOC** = Nursing Outcomes Classification

(EO) A model was designed to incorporate all the factors to be considered in home infusion therapy administration to aid nurses in comprehensive patient's assessment, planning patient's and caregiver's education, and assisting patients in completing a course of home infusion therapy (Dobson, 2001).

(EO) Patients' education should address adverse reactions, side effects, risks and benefits, and self-care practices and should include validation of understanding and ability to perform infusion-related procedures safely (INS, 2006).

■ (SP) *Assess and monitor the patient and the infusion access device for adverse reactions and complications of infusion therapy, including infection at the catheter site, catheter-related BSIs, signs of catheter malfunction (occlusion), peripheral IV infiltration, phlebitis, and infusion-related adverse reactions or side effects.* **LOE = VII**

(EO) This is safe, appropriate care for the patient receiving IV therapy (Josephson, 2004).

Possibly Effective

■ *Change IV administration sets every 7 days when an antiseptic-coated central venous catheter has been placed or in patients with low-risk infusions (e.g., non–blood product, non-TPN, non–interleukin 2).* **LOE = II**

(NR) A randomized study comparing IV administration set changes on day 4 (approximately 72 hours) or not at all in ICU-placed short-term antiseptic-coated central venous catheters ($N = 414$) found no significant difference in catheter colonization or catheter-related bacteremia (Rickard et al., 2004).

(MR) In an RCT, patients with cancer requiring infusion therapy were randomly assigned to IV tubing changes every 3 days ($N = 280$) or within 4 to 7 days ($N = 232$). There was no significant difference in microbial colonization of the tubing and no incidence of BSIs when high-risk patients (those receiving parenteral nutrition, interleukin 2, or blood transfusions) were excluded (Raad et al., 2001).

(NR) An in vitro randomized study comparing administration sets set at varying rates for 7 days found that there was no deterioration in the administration sets in relation to condition and accuracy of infusion delivery (Rickard et al., 2002).

■ *Use an antiseptic barrier cap over the needleless device to reduce the risk of catheter-related BSIs.* **LOE = II**

(MR) An in vitro study evaluated bacterial contamination of three different types of needleless caps cleaned with the conventional 3- to 5-second disinfection with 70% alcohol compared with the use of an antiseptic barrier cap (containing 2% chlorhexidine in 70% alcohol) left in place for 10 minutes followed by removal and allowing the needleless cap septum to dry. Sixty-seven percent of alcohol-disinfected caps showed transmission of microorganisms and only 1.6% of barrier caps showed any transmission. This technology should be studied in a clinical trial (Menyhay & Maki, 2006).

(MR) A prospective randomized multicenter study in which surgical ICU patients with non-tunneled central venous catheters for 6 or more days ($N = 230$) were randomly assigned to

---

NR = Nursing Research, **MR** = Multidisciplinary Research, **SP** = Standard of Practice, **EO** = Expert Opinion, **LOE** = Level of Evidence

either a standard Luer-Lock cap or a hub with a 3% iodinated alcohol chamber found a significant decrease in culture-positive catheter hubs and catheter-related BSI in the antiseptic hub chamber group (Leon et al., 2003).

Not Effective

No applicable published research was found in this category.

Possibly Harmful

No applicable published research was found in this category.

OUTCOME MEASUREMENT

FREE OF BLOODSTREAM INFECTION

Definition: Free of localized or generalized signs of infection.

Free of Bloodstream Infection as evidenced by the following indicators:

- IV site condition
- Skin around IV insertion
- Swelling around IV site
- Swelling in involved extremity
- Drainage around IV site
- WBC count
- Temperature

(Note: This is not a NOC outcome.)

REFERENCES

Arduino MJ, Bland LA, Danzig LE, McAllister SK, Aguero SM. (1997). Microbiologic evaluation of needleless and needle-access devices. *Am J Infect Control,* 25(5):377-380.

Calop J, Bosson JL, Croize J, Laurent PE. (2000). Maintenance of peripheral and central IV infusion devices by 0.9% sodium chloride with or without heparin as a potential source of catheter microbial contamination. *J Hosp Infect,* 46(2):161-162.

Casey AL, Worthington T, Lambert PA, Quinn D, Faroqui MH, Elliot TS. (2003). A randomized, prospective clinical trial to assess the potential infection risk associated with the PosiFlow needleless connector. *J Hosp Infect,* 54(4):288-293.

Catney MR, Hillis S, Wakefield B, Simpson L, Domino L, Keller S, et al. (2001). Relationship between peripheral intravenous catheter dwell time and the development of phlebitis and infiltration. *J Infus Nurs,* 24(5):332-341.

Centers for Disease Control and Prevention (CDC). (2003). Transmission of hepatitis B and C viruses in outpatient settings: New York, Oklahoma, and Nebraska, 2000-2002. *MMWR,* 52(38):901-906.

Cookson ST, Ihrig M, O'Mara EM, Denny M, Volk H, Banerjee SN, et al. (1998). Increased BSI rates in surgical patients associated with variation from recommended use and care following implementation of a needleless device. *Infect Control Hosp Epidemiol,* 19(1):23-27.

Cox JA, Westbrook LJ. (2005). Home infusion therapy: Essential characteristics of a successful education process: A grounded theory study. *J Infus Nurs,* 28(2):99-105.

Dobson PM. (2001). A model for home infusion therapy initiation and maintenance. *J Infus Nurs,* 24(6):385-394.

Dochterman JM, Bulechek GM (Eds). (2004). *Nursing Interventions Classification (NIC),* 4th ed. St. Louis: Mosby.

RCT = Randomized Controlled (Clinical) Trial, **NIC** = Nursing Interventions Classification, **NOC** = Nursing Outcomes Classification

Donlan RM, Murga R, Bell M, Toscano CM, Carr JH, Novicki TJ, et al. (2001). Protocol for detection of biofilms on needleless connectors attached to central venous catheters. *J Clin Microbiol*, 39(2): 750-753.

Gillies D, O'Riordan L, Wallen M, Rankin K, Morrison A, Nagy S. (2004). Timing of intravenous administration set changes: A systematic review. *Infect Control Hosp Epidemiol*, 25(3):240-250.

Gorski LA. (2005a). Hospital to home care: Discharge planning for the patient requiring home infusion therapy. *Top Adv Pract Nurs*, 5(3). Available online: www.medscape.com. Retrieved on June 4, 2007.

Gorski LA. (2005b). *Pocket guide to home infusion therapy*. Sudbury, MA: Jones & Bartlett.

Grimes-Holsinger V. (2002). Comparing the effect of a skills checklist on teaching time required to achieve independence in administration of infusion medications. *J Infus Nurs*, 25(2):109-120.

Infusion Nurses Society (INS). (2006). Infusion nursing standards of practice. *J Infus Nurs*, 29(1 Suppl): S1-S92.

Institute for Safe Medication Practices (ISMP). (2004a). Problems persist with life threatening tubing misconnections. ISMP Medication Safety Alert (June 17). Available online: http://www.ismp.org/. Retrieved on June 4, 2007.

Institute for Safe Medication Practices (ISMP). (2004b). ISMP's list of high alert medications. Available online: http://www.ismp.org/. Retrieved on June 4, 2007.

The Joint Commission. (2006). Tubing misconnections—A persistent and potentially deadly occurrence. *Sentinel Event Alert*, (36):1-3.

Josephson DL. (2004). *Intravenous infusion therapy for nurses*, 2nd ed. New York: Thomson/Delmar Learning.

Krause G, Trepka M, Whisenhunt R, Katz D, Nainan O, Wiersma ST, Hopkins RS. (2003). Nosocomial transmission of hepatitis C virus associated with the use of multidose saline vials. *Infect Control Hosp Epidemiol*, 24(2):122-127.

Leon C, Alvarez-Lerma F, Ruiz-Santana S, Gonzalez V, de la Torre MV, Sierra R, et al. (2003). Antiseptic chamber-containing hub reduces central venous catheter related infection: A prospective, randomized study. *Crit Care Med*, 31(5):1318-1324.

Mattner F, Gastmeier P. (2004). Bacterial contaminations of multiple dose vials: A prevalence study. *Am J Infect Control*, 32(1):12-16.

Meier PA, Fredrickson M, Catney M, Nettleman MD. (1998). Impact of a dedicated intravenous team on nosocomial bloodstream infection rates. *Am J Infect Control*, 26(4):388-392.

Menyhay SZ, Maki DG. (2006). Disinfection of needleless catheter connectors and access ports with alcohol may not prevent microbial entry: The promise of a novel antiseptic barrier cap. *Infect Control Hosp Epidemiol*, 27(1):23-27.

O'Grady NP, Alexander M, Dellinger EP, Gerberding JL, Heard SO, Maki DG, et al. (2002). Guidelines for the prevention of intravascular catheter-related infections. Centers for Disease Control and Prevention. *MMWR Recomm Rep*, 51(RR-10):1-29.

Raad I, Hanna HA, Awad A, Alrahwan A, Bivins C, Khan A, et al. (2001). Optimal frequency of changing intravenous administration sets: Is it safe to prolong use beyond 72 hours? *Infect Control Hosp Epidemiol*, 22(3):136-139.

Rickard CM, Lipman J, Courtney M, Siversen R, Daley P. (2004). Routine changing of intravenous administration sets does not reduce colonization or infection in central venous catheters. *Infect Control Hosp Epidemiol*, 25(8):650-655.

Rickard CM, Wallis SC, Courtney M, Lipman J, Daley PJ. (2002). Intravascular administration sets are accurate and in appropriate condition after 7 days of continuous use: An in vitro study. *J Adv Nurs*, 37(4):330-337.

Rothschild JM, Keohane CA, Cook EF, et al. (2005). A controlled trial of smart infusion pumps to improve medication safety in critically ill patients. *Crit Care Med*, 33(3):533-540.

Soifer NE, Borzak S, Edlin BR, Weinstein R. (1998). Prevention of peripheral venous catheter complications with an intravenous therapy team: A randomized controlled trial. *Arch Intern Med*, 158(5): 473-477.

Worthington T, Tebbs S, Moss H, Bevan V, Kilburn J, Elliott TS. (2001). Are contaminated flush solutions an overlooked source for catheter related sepsis? *J Hosp Infect*, 49(1):81-83.

LATEX PRECAUTIONS

Leslie H. Nicoll, PhD, MBA, RN-BC

NIC **Definition:** Reducing the risk of a systemic reaction to latex (Dochterman & Bulechek, 2004).

NURSING ACTIVITIES

Effective

▪ **NIC** *Question patient or appropriate other about history of systemic reactions to natural rubber latex (e.g., facial or scleral edema, tearing eyes, urticaria, rhinitis, and wheezing).* **LOE = I**

MR A case-control study ($N = 161$) showed that patients with spina bifida represented the highest risk group of patients for developing natural rubber latex (NRL) hypersensitivity (Buck et al., 2000).

EO Latex allergy in children is most commonly identified in patients who have undergone multiple operations for neural tube defects or genitourinary anomalies (Waseem et al., 2006).

MR A meta-analysis found that health care workers had an increased risk of sensitization and allergic symptoms to latex (Bousquet et al., 2006).

MR A descriptive study ($N = 1300$) confirmed that atopy is an important risk for the development of latex allergy (Proietti et al., 2005).

MR A systematic review showed a high prevalence of latex sensitization and allergy among health care workers, atopic individuals, and children who had undergone multiple surgical operations (spina bifida, congenital anomalies) (Bayrou, 2006).

▪ *If a patient is identified at risk, treat the patient as though an NRL allergy exists.* **LOE = I**

MR A follow-up case study ($N = 17$) found that strict compliance with latex avoidance instructions was essential both inside and outside the hospital. Greater emphasis should be placed on reducing latex exposure in the home and school environments, as such contact could maintain positive immunoglobulin E (IgE) antibody levels (Dieguez Pastor et al., 2006).

MR A systematic review found that anaphylaxis from NRL allergy was a medical emergency and must be treated as such. Latex is a potent allergen, and a type I anaphylactic reaction may be immediate in sensitized individuals. Acute treatment must be carried out in a latex-free environment (Hepner & Castells, 2003).

MR A descriptive study found that even if a person had not experienced an NRL reaction, it could be documented that he or she had been sensitized and should be treated as if an NRL allergy was present (Edlich et al., 2003).

EO The adoption of the following institutional policies designed to prevent new cases of NRL allergy and maximize safety is recommended: (1) NRL gloves should be used only as mandated by accepted standard precautions; (2) only nonpowdered, nonsterile NRL gloves should

RCT = Randomized Controlled (Clinical) Trial, **NIC** = Nursing Interventions Classification, **NOC** = Nursing Outcomes Classification

be used; and (3) nonpowdered, sterile NRL gloves are preferred for use. Low-protein powdered, sterile gloves may be used but only in conjunction with an ongoing assessment for development of allergic reactions (Charous et al., 2002).

■ *If a patient is identified as at risk, consider a skin prick test with NRL extracts to identify IgE-mediated immunity.* **LOE = I**

(MR) A systematic review found that skin prick tests with well-characterized latex extracts were highly sensitive and specific predictors of latex-specific IgE antibodies (Ownby, 2003).

Possibly Effective

■ *If a patient is identified as at risk, reduce latex exposure of the patient.* **LOE = I**

(MR) A systematic review found that anaphylaxis from NRL allergy was a medical emergency and must be treated as such. Latex is a potent allergen, and a type I anaphylactic reaction may be immediate in sensitized individuals. Acute treatment must be carried out in a latex-free environment (Hepner & Castells, 2003).

(MR) A descriptive study stated that safe and readily available immunotherapy for NRL allergy was currently lacking (Brehler & Kutting, 2001; Sutherland et al., 2002).

Not Effective

No applicable published research was found in this category.

Possibly Harmful

No applicable published research was found in this category.

OUTCOME MEASUREMENT

ALLERGIC RESPONSE: LOCALIZED (NOC)

(Please refer to *Nursing Outcomes Classification* [Moorhead et al., 2004] for the **Allergic Response: Localized** outcome.)

REFERENCES

Bayrou O. (2006). Latex allergy. *Rev Prat,* 56(3):289-295.

Bousquet J, Flahault A, Vandenplas O, Ameille J, Duron JJ, Pecquet C, et al. (2006). Natural rubber latex allergy among health care workers: A systematic review of the evidence. *J Allergy Clin Immunol,* 118(2):447-454.

Brehler R, Kutting B. (2001). Natural rubber latex allergy: A problem of interdisciplinary concern in medicine. *Arch Intern Med,* 161(8):1057-1064.

Buck D, Michael T, Wahn U, Niggemann B. (2000). Ventricular shunts and the prevalence of sensitization and clinically relevant allergy to latex in patients with spina bifida. *Pediatr Allergy Immunol,* 11(2):111-115.

Charous BL, Blanco C, Tarlo S, Hamilton RG, Baur X, Beezhold D, et al. (2002). Natural rubber latex allergy after 12 years: Recommendations and perspectives. *J Allergy Clin Immunol,* 109(1):31-34.

Dieguez Pastor MC, Anton Girones M, Blanco R, Pulido Z, Muriel A, de la Hoz Caballer B. (2006). Latex allergy in children: A follow-up study. *Allergol Immunopathol,* 34(1):17-22.

NR = Nursing Research, **MR** = Multidisciplinary Research, **SP** = Standard of Practice, **EO** = Expert Opinion, **LOE** = Level of Evidence

Dochterman JM, Bulechek GM (Eds). (2004). *Nursing Interventions Classification (NIC)*, 4th ed. St. Louis: Mosby.

Edlich RF, Woodard CR, Hill LG, Heather CL. (2003). Latex allergy: A life-threatening epidemic for scientists, healthcare personnel, and their patients. *J Long Term Eff Med Implants*, 13(1):11-19.

Hepner DL, Castells MC. (2003). Latex allergy: An update. *Anesth Analg*, 96(4):1219-1229.

Moorhead M, Johnson M, Maas M (Eds). (2004). *Nursing Outcomes Classification (NOC)*, 3rd ed. St. Louis: Mosby.

Ownby DR. (2003). Strategies for distinguishing asymptomatic latex sensitization from true occupational allergy or asthma. *Ann Allergy Asthma Immunol*, 90(5 Suppl 2):42-46.

Proietti L, Gueli G, La Rocca G, Bonanno G, Vasta N, Bella R, et al. (2005). [Latex allergy prevalence and atopy in 1300 health care workers]. *Recenti Prog Med*, 96(10):478-482.

Sutherland MF, Suphioglu C, Rolland JM, O'Hehir RE. (2002). Latex allergy: Towards immunotherapy for health care workers. *Clin Exp Allergy*, 32(5):667-673.

Waseem M, Ganti S, Hipp A. (2006). Latex-induced anaphylactic reaction in a child with spina bifida. *Pediatr Emerg Care*, 22(6):441-442.

LEARNING FACILITATION   (NIC)

Barbara J. Olinzock, EdD, MSN, RN; Kathaleen C. Bloom, PhD, CNM

NIC **Definition:** Promoting the ability to process and comprehend information (Dochterman & Bulechek, 2004).

NURSING ACTIVITIES

Effective

■ *Use approaches to support patient's choice.* **LOE = I**

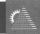 A Cochrane review of 14 publications and 11 studies determined that there was evidence that patients' education for adults with type 2 diabetes using group programs based upon empowerment, patients' participation, and adult learning principles was effective in improving glycemic control (Deakin et al., 2005).

 A Cochrane review of nine RCTs concluded that preoperative education intervention delivered up to 6 weeks prior to surgery over and above routine care had no added effect on knowledge but had a small effect on preoperative anxiety, suggesting that teachings tailored to patients' preferences according to those who are most in need of support may be most beneficial (McDonald et al., 2004).

MR A systematic review of published studies on psychoeducational interventions with pediatric cancer patients found that information content needed to be negotiated with the patient and family to determine its acceptability (Bradlyn et al., 2003).

MR In an RCT (*N* = 700) testing a patient-centered educational intervention to support patients' choice and self-management, patients receiving the intervention had significant improvement in quality of life and confidence in coping ability, greater satisfaction, and a reduction in the need for health care resources (Kennedy et al., 2004).

RCT = Randomized Controlled (Clinical) Trial, **NIC** = Nursing Interventions Classification, **NOC** = Nursing Outcomes Classification

■ *Use multifaceted approaches.* **LOE = I**

(MR) A Cochrane review of 59 RCTs examining educational interventions to improve hypertension control found insufficient evidence to support education alone but concluded that multifaceted efforts with rigorous identification, follow-up, and treatment with antihypertension medication resulted in significant reductions in blood pressure and cardiovascular mortality and morbidity (Fahey et al., 2006).

(MR) A Cochrane review of 36 trials comparing self-care management of asthma with usual care determined that self-management education that included information about a written action plan, self-monitoring, and regular medical review was beneficial for adults with asthma (Gibson et al., 2003).

(MR) A systematic review and meta-analysis of 15 studies comparing patient-centered behavioral interventions including counseling, self-monitoring, and structured training courses found insufficient evidence to support the use of self-monitoring or training courses alone without counseling (Boulware et al., 2001).

(MR) A descriptive systematic review of 12 meta-analyses on the effects of patients' education on chronic disease found that the effects were generally small and of short duration and concluded that collaborative, multidisciplinary patients' education is more likely to be beneficial (Cooper et al., 2001).

■ (NIC) *Provide information appropriate to the developmental level.* **LOE = I**

(MR) A systematic review of published studies on psychoeducational interventions with pediatric cancer patients concluded that individualized and interactive interventions negotiated with the patient and family were the most beneficial (Bradlyn et al., 2003).

(MR) A Cochrane review of 14 publications and 11 studies determined that patients' education for adults with type 2 diabetes using group programs based upon empowerment, patients' participation, and adult learning principles was effective in improving glycemic control (Deakin et al., 2005).

(MR) An RCT ($N = 95$) of an 8-week home-based asthma education program that used written materials tailored for low-literacy adults and children found better caregiver quality of life and improved asthma control at 12 month follow-up for younger children 1 to 3 years of age but not for children 4 to 6 years of age (Brown et al., 2002).

■ *Provide information to support self-efficacy, self-regulation, and self-management.* **LOE = I**

(MR) A Cochrane review of 32 studies examining the effects of self-management education for children with asthma found improved physiological outcomes and self-efficacy as well as reduced school absenteeism and use of health care resources (Wolf et al., 2003).

(MR) A Cochrane review of 15 randomized trials examining the options for self-management education for adults with asthma found that optimal control could be achieved through either self-care management or medical review but that reducing self-management education reduced its effectiveness (Powell & Gibson, 2003).

(NR) An RCT ($N = 237$ cancer patients) on the effects of an 18-week intervention providing information about problem solving and decision making in the management of cancer-related

NR = Nursing Research, **MR** = Multidisciplinary Research, **SP** = Standard of Practice, **EO** = Expert Opinion, **LOE** = Level of Evidence

symptoms found significant improvement in symptom limitations, especially among younger patients (Doorenbos et al., 2005).

(MR) An RCT ($N = 32$ families) examining the use of a problem-solving approach for families of school-age children with traumatic brain injury found that assisting family members to focus on problem identification, learn new coping strategies, and implement plans for managing injury-related stresses reduced the child's symptom internalization, anxiety, depression, and withdrawal (Wade et al., 2006).

(MR) An RCT ($N = 700$) on the impact of a patient-oriented, self-help guidebook and patient-centered consultation on disease management and satisfaction in patients with inflammatory bowel disease found a significant boost in enablement immediately after their introduction to the intervention. Findings from qualitative analysis of patients' and physicians' interviews ascertained that the guidebook did facilitate confidence in self-care management for patients (Kennedy et al., 2004).

■ (NIC) *Adjust the instruction to the patient's level of knowledge and understanding.* LOE = I

(MR) In a systematic review of 29 studies examining the effects of a wide variety of delivery approaches (including written, audio, video, and computer methods), knowledge outcomes and to some extent function and morbidity were improved when materials or methods were designed with literacy in mind. Patients with both higher and lower literacy skills benefited with the use of well-tailored materials (Berkman et al., 2004).

(NR) An RCT ($N = 36$) on the use of a simplified education program focusing on a single component of an educational program for rural patients with heart failure found significant benefits in knowledge and self-care outcomes (Caldwell et al., 2005).

(MR) An RCT ($N = 294$) researching a multifaceted nurse intervention protocol consisting of materials adapted to the literacy and information needs of patients with hypertension resulted in a significant benefit in patient's self-confidence in hypertensive control (Bosworth et al., 2005).

(MR) In a single-group pre- and postintervention pilot study ($N = 25$) of a disease management program designed for low literacy, patients with heart failure experienced improved self-care behavior (DeWalt et al., 2004).

(NR) In a descriptive, correlational design ($N = 65$), readability of materials used to educate older African American patients on anticoagulant therapy was assessed as being four grades above the reading level of the patients and not culturally sensitive to the population (Wilson et al., 2003).

■ *Use methods that are culturally sensitive and support patients' customs, values, and lifestyle.* LOE = I

(MR) In an RCT ($N = 200$) on the effectiveness of a culturally sensitive, symptom-focused, educational intervention using interactive storytelling, shared experiences, and mutual goal setting for elder rural African American women with type 2 diabetes, results showed significant improvement in self-care practices and quality of life as well as decreased distress from symptoms (Keyserling et al., 2002).

(NR) A single-group pre- and post-pilot study ($N = 40$) on the use of a culturally tailored diabetes management program developed for Chinese Americans demonstrated significant improvements in weight, blood pressure, mean hemoglobin A_{1c}, and diabetes quality of life (Wang & Chan, 2005).

RCT = Randomized Controlled (Clinical) Trial, **NIC** = Nursing Interventions Classification, **NOC** = Nursing Outcomes Classification

(NR) In an RCT ($N = 216$) that provided culturally appropriate educational interventions for Mexican Americans with diabetes through the use of preferred language, cultural dietary preferences, family and social involvement, and discussion of cultural health beliefs, significant improvement in diabetes knowledge and self-care behavior resulted (Brown et al., 2007).

(MR) An RCT ($N = 203$) testing a peer mentoring approach to end-of-life decision making with dialysis patients found significant benefit among African Americans (but not white patients) on completion of and comfort in talking about advanced directives, as well as subjective well-being and anxiety, and concluded that peer mentoring and relationship building may be very effective in certain cultural groups where there is more emphasis on oral communication (Perry et al., 2005).

■ Arrange family and peer support, as appropriate. LOE = I

(NR) A systematic review of eight intervention studies critiquing the effectiveness of mass media and public health campaigns to minimize delays in seeking treatment of acute myocardial infarction (AMI) concluded that promoting dialogue between previous AMI patients and high-risk patients, addressing problems of denial, and emphasizing symptom evaluation, problem solving, and decision making were beneficial (Caldwell & Miaskowski, 2002).

(MR) An RCT ($N = 82$) on the effects of a partner-guided protocol that included integrated education and training of patients and partners in cognitive and behavioral coping skills for providing end-of-life pain management for cancer patients found significant improvement in self-efficacy and caregiver strain (Keefe et al., 2005).

(NR) An RCT ($N = 32$ families) on the use of a family-partner education and counseling intervention to manage dietary sodium restriction found a significant difference in urinary sodium levels 3 months after the intervention (Dunbar et al., 2005).

(MR) In an RCT ($N = 203$) on a peer mentoring approach to end-of-life decision making with dialysis patients, significant benefit among African American patients on completion of and comfort in talking about advanced directives as well as subjective well-being and anxiety was noted (Perry et al., 2005).

■ Use the telephone to reinforce information, as appropriate. LOE = I

(NR) An RCT testing a multifaceted nurse-coaching intervention consisting of five individualized sessions and two follow-up telephone calls over 6 months using educational, behavioral, and affective strategies determined that there were improvements in self-management and psychosocial outcomes for women with type 2 diabetes (Whittemore et al., 2004).

(NR) In an RCT ($N = 84$), decreased physical symptoms and anxiety and improved self-care management resulted with the use of an 8-weekly structured telephone education intervention delivered by an expert cardiovascular nurse for first-time patients immediately after an implantable cardioverter defibrillator (Dougherty et al., 2004).

(MR) In an RCT ($N = 272$) evaluating the effectiveness of diabetic education using automated telephone calls and nurse telephone follow-up, improvements in glycemic control and patients' satisfaction proved significant (Piette et al., 2001).

(MR) A quasi-experimental single-group pretest and post-test study ($N = 42$ patients with type 2 diabetes) on the effects of a 12-week educational intervention using cellular phone and Internet interactions found a significant decrease in fasting plasma glucose and 2-hour

NR = Nursing Research, MR = Multidisciplinary Research, SP = Standard of Practice, EO = Expert Opinion, LOE = Level of Evidence

postprandial blood sugar levels and an increase in patients' satisfaction (Kim et al., 2005).

■ *Provide home-based outreach education, as appropriate.* **LOE = I**

(MR) An RCT (*N* = 221) examining the effects of a home-based educational intervention targeted at symptom identification for inner-city families with children ages 2 to 8 years with persistent asthma found that the program was effective in improving symptom identification and overall medication management (Butz et al., 2005) but not asthma severity or health care use (Butz et al., 2005).

(MR) In an RCT (*N* = 62) examining the effects on family functioning of an education and counseling intervention delivered promptly after discharge that included an information packet and three follow-up home visits from a social worker, the effects on outcomes were positive (Clark et al., 2003).

(NR) An RCT (*N* = 176) of the use of posthospitalization outreach from a nurse for stroke survivors and their family/caregivers found that families in the intervention group had significant improvement in psychosocial outcomes, less social isolation, reduced physical dependence, and reduced caregiver strain (Burton & Gibbon, 2005).

(NR) An RCT (*N* = 180) on the effects of an early home recovery information intervention 1 month after coronary artery bypass surgery versus usual discharge protocol information found physical benefits for women and psychological effects of vigor and fatigue for men in the intervention group (Moore & Dolansky, 2001).

Possibly Effective

■ *Use computer and web-based methods as appropriate.* **LOE = I**

(MR) A Cochrane review of 24 RCTs on the use of interactive health applications for people with chronic disease found positive benefits including increased knowledge, social support, and self-efficacy but cautioned that little is known about possible disparities between advantaged and disadvantaged populations and computer use by these populations (Murray et al., 2005).

(MR) In a meta-analysis of 22 research articles on the impact of web-based versus non-web-based interventions to promote knowledge sharing, education, and understanding of the condition for those with chronic illness, web-based interventions contributed to greater behavioral changes and increased knowledge, participation, and social support (Wantland et al., 2004).

(MR) In an RCT (*N* = 244) evaluating a low-literacy diabetes education computer multimedia intervention, improved recognition of susceptibility to diabetes complications was determined to be significant but no difference in glycemic control resulted. There was less use of the computer by elderly and low-health-literacy individuals in both intervention and control groups (Gerber et al., 2005).

(MR) In an RCT (*N* = 75) on a computer-based information tool to support the process of shared decision making for patients with chronic pain, significant improvement in the understanding of the illness and treatment options resulted (Hochehnert et al., 2006).

(MR) An RCT (*N* = 95) of an 8-week home-based asthma education program with written materials tailored for low-literacy adults and children reported better caregiver quality of life and improved asthma control at 12-month follow-up for younger children 1 to 3 years of age but not for children 4 to 6 years of age (Brown et al., 2002).

RCT = Randomized Controlled (Clinical) Trial, **NIC** = Nursing Interventions Classification, **NOC** = Nursing Outcomes Classification

■ **NIC** *Provide adequate time for mastery of content, as appropriate.* **LOE = I**

MR In a Cochrane review of group-based education programs, group-based education proved to have positive effects on glycemic control, diabetes knowledge, self-management, and the need for diabetes medication at 4- to 6-month and 12-month follow-ups with sustained effects up to 2 years with additional follow-up (Deakin et al., 2005).

MR A Cochrane review of 62 studies comparing the effectiveness of clinical pathways as a multidisciplinary intervention with an educational component for stroke patients determined that there was insufficient evidence to support the use of clinical pathways over standard care in a rehabilitation setting and that clinical pathways actually may worsen quality of life for stroke patients. A standardized, time-limited pathway may not be sufficient to affect outcomes (Kwan & Sandercock, 2004).

MR In an RCT ($N = 319$) using a structured 5-day initial diabetes education program with 1-day reeducation follow-up sessions at 1- and 2-year contact points, significant improvements in glycemic control as well as quality of life and feelings of well-being resulted (Tankova et al., 2004).

NR An RCT ($N = 216$) comparing an extended dose (time) of community education (24 hours) versus a compressed dose (16 hours) for self-management of diabetes among Mexican American individuals found that, although both interventions were culturally appropriate, the extended dose resulted in greater metabolic control (Brown et al., 2007).

MR A systematic review examining the impact of arthritis patients' education found little evidence of sustained results of patients' education over time (Schrieber & Colley, 2004).

MR In a descriptive systematic review of 12 meta-analyses on the effects of patients' education on chronic disease, the effects of patients' education were small and of short duration (Cooper et al., 2001).

Not Effective

■ *Using written educational materials as the source of information.* **LOE = I**

MR A Cochrane review of two trials comparing a combination of written and verbal information versus written information alone for patients being discharged from acute care found that a combination of written and verbal information was beneficial for knowledge comprehension and patients' satisfaction (Johnson et al., 2003).

MR An RCT ($N = 59$) assessing the effect of adding educational booklets on inflammatory bowel disease to usual care found that the addition of these booklets focusing on the disease, management, and quality-of-life issues did not improve and actually worsened health-related quality of life (Borgaonkar et al., 2002).

MR An RCT ($N = 60$) comparing the effects of three educational interventions including individualized verbal instruction, educational classes, and written materials found written information to be ineffective (Urek et al., 2005).

MR An RCT ($N = 109$) evaluating the effects of three types of commercially produced written information as an adjunct to routine hospital information concluded that the use of commercially prepared materials supplementing hospital information demonstrated promise if used in combination with routine hospital information, especially for patients who may be "vigilant copers" (Sheard & Garrud, 2006).

NR = Nursing Research, **MR** = Multidisciplinary Research, **SP** = Standard of Practice, **EO** = Expert Opinion, **LOE** = Level of Evidence

OUTCOME MEASUREMENT:

KNOWLEDGE: TREATMENT REGIMEN NOC

Definition: Extent of understanding conveyed about a specific treatment regimen.

Knowledge: Treatment Regimen as evidenced by the following selected NOC indicators:
- Description of specific disease process
- Description of rationale for treatment regimen
- Description of self-care responsibilities for ongoing treatment
- Description of self-monitoring techniques
- Description of expected effects of treatment

(Rate each indicator of **Knowledge: Treatment Regimen:** 1 = none, 2 = limited, 3 = moderate, 4 = substantial, 5 = extensive) (Moorhead et al., 2004).

REFERENCES

Berkman ND, Dewalt DA, Pignone MP, Sheridan SL, Lohr KN, Lux L, et al. (2004). Literacy and health outcomes. *Evid Rep Technol Assess (Summ)*, 87:1-8.

Borgaonkar MR, Townson G, Donnelly M, Irvine EJ. (2002). Providing disease-related information worsens health-related quality of life in inflammatory bowel disease. *Inflamm Bowel Dis*, 8(4): 264-269.

Bosworth HB, Olsen MK, Gentry P, Orr M, Dudley T, McCant F, et al. (2005). Nurse administered telephone intervention for blood pressure control: A patient-tailored multifactorial intervention. *Patient Educ Couns*, 57(1):5-14.

Boulware LE, Daumit GL, Frick KD, Minkovitz CS, Lawrence RS, Powe NR. (2001). An evidence-based review of patient-centered behavioral interventions for hypertension. *Am J Prev Med*, 21(3):221-232.

Bradlyn AS, Beale IL, Kato PM. (2003). Psychoeducational interventions with pediatric cancer patients: Part I: Patient information and knowledge. *J Child Fam Stud*, 12(3):257-277.

Brown JV, Bakeman R, Celano MP, Demi AS, Kobrynski L, Wilson SR. (2002). Home-based asthma education of low-income children and their families. *J Pediatr Psych*, 27(8):677-688.

Brown SA, Blozis SA, Kouzekanani K, Garcia AA, Winchell M, Hanis CL. (2007). Health beliefs of Mexican Americans with type 2 diabetes: The Starr County Border Health Initiative. *Diabetes Educ*, 33(2):300-308.

Burton C, Gibbon B. (2005). Expanding the role of the stroke nurse: A pragmatic clinical trial. *J Adv Nurs*, 52(6):640-650.

Butz AM, Syron L, Johnson B, Spaulding J, Walker M, Bollinger ME. (2005). Home-based asthma self-management education for inner city children. *Public Health Nurs*, 22(3):189-199.

Caldwell MA, Miaskowski C. (2002). Mass media interventions to reduce help-seeking delay in people with symptoms of acute myocardial infarction: Time for a new approach? *Patient Educ Couns*, 46(1): 1-9.

Caldwell MA, Peters KJ, Dracup KA. (2005). A simplified education program improves knowledge, self-care behavior, and disease severity in heart failure patients in rural settings. *Am Heart J*, 150(5): 983.

Clark MS, Rubenach S, Winsor A. (2003). A randomized controlled trial of an education and counseling intervention for families after stroke. *Clin Rehabil*, 17(7):703-712.

Cooper H, Booth K, Fear S, Gill G. (2001). Chronic disease patient education: Lessons from meta-analyses. *Patient Educ Couns*, 44(2):107-117.

Deakin T, McShane CE, Cade JE, Williams RD. (2005). Group based training for self-management strategies in people with type 2 diabetes mellitus. *Cochrane Database Syst Rev*, (2):CD003417.

DeWalt DA, Pignone M, Malone R, Rawls C, Kosnar MC, George G, et al. (2004). Development and pilot testing of a disease management program for low literacy patients with heart failure. *Patient Educ Couns*, 55(1):78-86.

Dochterman JM, Bulechek GM (Eds). (2004). *Nursing Interventions Classification (NIC)*, 4th ed. St. Louis: Mosby.

Doorenbos A, Given B, Given C, Verbitsky N, Cimprich B, McCorkle R. (2005). Reducing symptom limitations: A cognitive behavioral intervention randomized trial. *Psychooncology*, 14(7):574-584.

Dougherty CM, Lewis FM, Thompson EA, Baer JD, Kim W. (2004). Short-term efficacy of a telephone intervention by expert nurses after an implantable cardioverter defibrillator. *Pacing Clin Electrophysiol*, 27(12):1594-1602.

Dunbar SB, Clark PC, Deaton C, Smith AL, De AK, O'Brien MC. (2005). Family education and support interventions in heart failure: A pilot study. *Nurs Res*, 54(3):158-166.

Fahey T, Schroeder K, Ebrahim S. (2006). Interventions to improve control of blood pressure in patients with hypertension. *Cochrane Database Syst Rev*, (2):CD005182.

Gerber BS, Brodsky IG, Lawless KA, Smolin LI, Arozullah AM, Smith EV, et al. (2005). Implementation and evaluation of a low-literacy diabetes education computer multimedia application. *Diabetes Care*, 28(7):1574-1580.

Gibson PG, Powell H, Coughlan J, Wilson AJ, Abramson M, Haywood P, et al. (2003). Self-management education and regular practitioner review for adults with asthma. *Cochrane Database Syst Rev*, (1): CD001117.

Hochlehnert A, Richter A, Bludau HB, Bieber C, Blumenstiel K, et al. (2006). A computer-based information-tool for chronic pain patients. Computerized information to support the process of shared decision-making. *Patient Educ Couns*, 61(1):92-98.

Johnson A, Sandford J, Tyndall J. (2003). Written and verbal information versus verbal information only for patients being discharged from acute hospital settings to home. *Cochrane Database Syst Rev*, (4): CD003716.

Keefe FJ, Ahles TA, Sutton L, Dalton J, Baucom D, Pope MS, et al. (2005). Partner-guided cancer pain management at the end of life: A preliminary study. *J Pain Symptom Manage*, 29(3):263-273.

Kennedy AP, Nelson E, Reeves D, Richardson G, Roberts C, Robinson A, et al. (2004). A randomised controlled trial to assess the effectiveness and cost of a patient orientated self management approach to chronic inflammatory bowel disease. *Gut*, 53(11):1639-1645.

Keyserling TC, Samuel-Hodge CD, Ammerman AS, Ainsworth BE, Henriquez-Roldan CF, Elasy TA, et al. (2002). A randomized trial of an intervention to improve self-care behaviors of African-American women with type 2 diabetes: Impact on physical activity. *Diabetes Care*, 25(9):1576-1583.

Kim HS, Yoo YS, Shim HS. (2005). Effects of an Internet-based intervention on plasma glucose levels in patients with type 2 diabetes. *J Nurs Care Qual*, 20(4):335-340.

Kwan J, Sandercock P. (2004). In-hospital care pathways for stroke. *Cochrane Database Syst Rev*, (4): CD002924.

McDonald A, Hetrick S, Green S. (2004). Pre-operative education for knee or hip replacement. Cochrane Database Syst Rev, (1):CD003526.

Moore SM, Dolansky MA. (2001). Randomized trial of a home recovery intervention following coronary artery bypass surgery. *Res Nurs Health*, 24(2):93-104.

Moorhead M, Johnson M, Maas M (Eds). (2004). *Nursing Outcomes Classification (NOC)*, 3rd ed. St. Louis: Mosby.

Murray E, Burns J, See TS, Lai R, Nazareth I. (2005). Interactive Health Communication Applications for people with chronic disease. *Cochrane Database Syst Rev*, (4):CD004274.

Perry E, Swartz J, Brown S, Smith D, Kelly G, Swartz R. (2005). Peer mentoring: A culturally sensitive approach to end-of-life planning for long-term dialysis patients. *Am J Kidney Dis*, 46(1):111-119.

Piette JD, Weinberger M, Kraemer FB, McPhee SJ. (2001). Impact of automated calls with nurse follow-up on diabetes treatment outcomes in a Department of Veterans Affairs Health Care System: a randomized controlled trial. *Diabetes Care*, 24(2):202-208.

Powell H, Gibson PG. (2003). Options for self-management education for adults with asthma. *Cochrane Database Syst Rev*, (1):CD004107.

Schrieber L, Colley M. (2004). Patient education. *Best Pract Res Clin Rheumatol*, 18(4):465-476.

Sheard C & Garrud P. (2006). Evaluation of generic patient information: Effects on health outcomes, knowledge and satisfaction. *Patient Educ Couns*, 61(1):43-47.

Tankova T, Dakovska G, Koev D. (2004). Education and quality of life in diabetic patients. *Patient Educ Couns*, 53(3):285-290.

NR = Nursing Research, **MR** = Multidisciplinary Research, **SP** = Standard of Practice, **EO** = Expert Opinion, **LOE** = Level of Evidence

Urek MC, Tudoric N, Plavec D, Urek R, Koprivc-Milenovic T, Stojic M. (2005). Effect of educational programs on asthma control and quality of life in adult asthma patients. *Patient Educ Couns,* 58(1):47-54.

Wade SL, Michaud L, Brown TM. (2006). Putting the pieces together: Preliminary efficacy of a family problem-solving intervention for children with traumatic brain injury. *J Head Trauma Rehabil,* 21(1):57-67.

Wang C, Chan S. (2005). Culturally tailored diabetes education program for Chinese Americans: A pilot study. *Nurs Res,* 54(4):347-353.

Wantland DJ, Portillo CJ, Holzemer WL, Slaughter R, McGhee EM. (2004). The effectiveness of Web-based vs. non-Web based interventions: A meta-analysis of behavioral change outcomes. *J Med Internet Res,* 6(4):e40.

Whittemore R, Melkus GD, Sullivan A, Grey M. (2004). A nurse-coaching intervention for women with type 2 diabetes. *Diabetes Educ,* 30(5):795-804.

Wilson FL, Racine E, Tekieli V, Williams B. (2003). Literacy, readability and cultural barriers: Critical factors to consider when educating older African Americans about anticoagulation therapy. *J Clin Nurs,* 12(2):275-282.

Wolf FM, Guevara JP, Grum CM, Clark NM, Cates CJ. (2003). Educational interventions for asthma in children. *Cochrane Database Syst Rev,* (1):CD000326.

LEARNING READINESS ENHANCEMENT   NIC

Barbara J. Olinzock, EdD, MSN, RN; Kathaleen C. Bloom, PhD, CNM

NIC **Definition:** Improving the ability and willingness to receive information (Dochterman & Bulechek, 2004).

NURSING ACTIVITIES

Effective

■ *Use instructional strategies based upon readiness models.* **LOE = I**

NR An integrated literature review and meta-analysis (*N* = 1044) of preoperative education for orthopedic patients concluded that for the most part preoperative teaching demonstrated some value in increasing knowledge, but the direction of the effects on reduction of anxiety, pain, and other outcomes was unknown from existing research. The investigation of empowerment models and those enabling patients to gain mastery of their own resources and situation is recommended for future study (Johansson et al., 2005).

MR An RCT (*N* = 1029) based an intensive 3-month telephone and mail follow-up of individuals with diabetes incorporating readiness strategies on the transtheoretical model of change and determined the readiness strategies to be effective in shifting participants in the intervention group to action stages (Jones et al., 2006).

MR An RCT (*N* = 119) used a readiness-to-learn model and self-regulatory intervention to improve asthma management among urban Latino and African American families and found significant improvements in self-care management and health outcomes (Bonner et al., 2002).

NR A qualitative descriptive study (*N* = 30) on learning readiness for self-direction of care identified five stages of learning readiness (dependent, involved, engagement, self-initiation, and self-direction) for patients with spinal cord injury in rehabilitation with five corresponding nursing roles (authority, guide, motivator, mentor, and consultant) and was organized into a rehabilitation learning readiness assessment model and guide (Olinzock, 2004).

■ **NIC** *Assist the patient to develop confidence in ability, as appropriate.* **LOE = I**

MR A Cochrane review of 32 studies on the effects of self-management education for children with asthma found improved physiological outcomes and self-efficacy as well as reduced school absenteeism and use of health care resources (Wolf et al., 2003).

MR In an RCT ($N = 32$ families) on the use of a problem-solving approach for families of school-age children with traumatic brain injury, assisting family members with problem identification, learning new coping strategies, and implementing plans for managing injury-related stresses was found to reduce the child's symptom internalization, anxiety, depression, and withdrawal (Wade et al., 2006).

MR An RCT ($N = 700$) on the study of a patient-oriented, self-help guidebook and patient-centered consultation on disease management and satisfaction in patients with inflammatory bowel disease determined a significant boost in enablement immediately after their introduction to the intervention. Findings from qualitative analysis of interviews with patients and physicians ascertained that the guidebook facilitated confidence in self-care management for patients (Kennedy et al., 2004).

■ *Use strategies to encourage and sustain patients' motivation and engagement.* **LOE = I**

MR An RCT ($N = 101$) evaluating the effectiveness of an educational multimedia program comprising a CD-ROM program for children (ages 7 to 14 years) and an educational book compared with a group using the booklet alone found that an interactive program for children resulted in better outcomes (McPherson et al., 2006).

NR In a literature review of 23 studies of the early discharge of cardiac patients, the use of motivational and disease management interventions demonstrated promise for improved adherence and lifestyle change (Beswick et al., 2005).

MR An RCT ($N = 200$) used interactive storytelling, shared experiences, and mutual goal setting techniques to engage and educate elder rural African American women about type 2 diabetes and reported significant improvements in self-care practices, improved quality of life, and decreased reports of distress from symptoms for the intervention group (Keyserling et al., 2002).

MR An RCT ($N = 76$) testing the use of a CD-ROM computer-assisted education program for urban low-income children with asthma (9 to13 years of age) found greater self-efficacy and intrinsic motivational benefits of the CD-ROM program (Shegog et al., 2001).

■ *Offer ongoing psychosocial and affective support.* **LOE = I**

NR An RCT ($N = 176$) on the impact of the expanded role of the stroke nurse to promote outreach education after discharge from the hospital for stroke survivors and their family/caregivers found that families in the intervention group demonstrated improved psychosocial outcomes, less social isolation, reduced physical dependence, and reduced caregiver strain than the control group (Burton & Gibbon, 2005).

NR An RCT testing a multifaceted nurse-coaching intervention consisting of five individualized sessions and two follow-up telephone calls over 6 months using behavioral and affective strategies determined that there were improvements in self-management and psychosocial outcomes for women with type 2 diabetes (Whittemore et al., 2004).

NR = Nursing Research, **MR** = Multidisciplinary Research, **SP** = Standard of Practice, **EO** = Expert Opinion, **LOE** = Level of Evidence

(NR) An RCT ($N = 84$) on the use of an 8-weekly structured telephone education intervention delivered by an expert cardiovascular nurse for first-time patients immediately after an implantable cardioverter defibrillator procedure found benefit for physical symptoms, anxiety, and self-care management (Dougherty et al., 2004).

■ (NIC) *Enlist participation of the family/significant others, as appropriate.* **LOE = I**

(NR) An RCT ($N = 61$ dyads) on the use of a family-focused intervention for patients with heart failure to support self-determination and self-management of dietary sodium restriction and enhance communication and support demonstrated significant benefits of the family-focused intervention on urine sodium (Dunbar et al., 2005).

(MR) An RCT ($N = 32$ families) testing the use of a family-centered problem-solving intervention in families with children who experienced a traumatic brain injury found significant benefits improving child functioning (Wade et al., 2006).

Possibly Effective

■ *Use strategies to encourage verbalization of concerns.* **LOE = I**

(MR) An RCT ($N = 232$) comparing an activation intervention to prompt patients with diabetes to ask their provider questions regarding concerns about their diabetes versus a group receiving a passive education video found that the activation intervention group was significantly more likely to be actively involved in the consultation with their provider than the group receiving the passive intervention and was more likely to have improved glycemic control (Williams et al., 2005).

(MR) In an RCT ($N = 321$) testing the effectiveness of a question-prompt intervention given to cancer patients to increase patients' participation in medical consultations, patients who received the question-prompt sheet were more likely to ask questions about the likely course and outcome of the disease, risk of relapse, and chance of cure (Brown et al., 2001).

(MR) An RCT ($N = 105$) testing the long-term efficacy of an FAQ checklist as an intervention with cardiac patients preparing for a medical check-up found value in the use of the aid to reduce anxiety initially but also found that its usefulness over time decreased. The study concluded that it was not a stimulating method to use for preparing patients (Bolman et al., 2005).

(MR) An RCT ($N = 160$) evaluating the use of low-literacy reminder cards with high-risk cardiac patients in the community found that using reminder cards to encourage patients to discuss risk factors with their primary physician did not improve blood pressure, lipid levels, and glycosylated hemoglobin in the intervention group (Echeverry et al., 2005).

Not Effective/Possibly Harmful

■ *Monitoring the use of educational strategies that promote patients'*
understanding and preferences. **LOE = I**

(NR) A meta-analysis of 25 intervention studies concluded that the effects of psychoeducational interventions such as relaxation techniques, cognitive-behavioral strategies, and information on analgesic relief measures for cancer patients, although promising, needed further research because of methodological issues. However, the investigators recommended that nurses should consider continued use of psychoeducational interventions only as an adjunct

RCT = Randomized Controlled (Clinical) Trial, **NIC** = Nursing Interventions Classification, **NOC** = Nursing Outcomes Classification

for pain analgesia and that psychoeducational interventions should fit with patients' preferences (Devine, 2003).

MR   A systematic review of published studies on psychoeducational interventions with pediatric cancer patients concluded that not all information content may be acceptable to families and that information content needed to be negotiated with the patient and family. Information transfer that is highly individualized and interactive was recommended (Bradlyn et al., 2003).

MR   An RCT ($N = 80$) on the effects of a visual CD-ROM in combination with an information leaflet in preparation for breast reduction surgery found that patients' anxiety prior to surgery and knowledge retention were significantly improved over a control group receiving the information leaflet only. However, the investigators recommended that patients be given choices about the type of educational intervention they desire and cautioned about the possibility of too much extra information as anxiety producing for some patients (Danino et al., 2005).

MR   An RCT ($N = 85$) studying the effects of a detailed information drug leaflet on anesthesia determined that although there were no significant changes in anxiety between the intervention group and control group, the majority of patients preferred not to receive such detailed information (Oldman et al., 2004).

MR   An RCT ($N = 225$) comparing two methods of delivering preoperative education (leaflets versus a trained nurse interview from the pain team) about patient-controlled analgesia (PCA) prior to major surgery found that there were no significant differences in anxiety and pain between the intervention group and the control group. Those receiving a preoperative oral interview resulted in no benefits and reported being more confused about self-managing their PCA postoperatively than those receiving a detailed leaflet. The variability in how patients interpret information orally was offered as a possible interpretation of results (Chumbley et al., 2004).

OUTCOME MEASUREMENT

MOTIVATION   NOC

Definition: Inner urge that moves or prompts an individual to positive action(s).
Motivation as evidenced by the following selected NOC indicators:
• Self-initiates goal-directed behavior
• Maintains positive self-esteem
• Expresses belief in ability to perform action
• Obtains needed support
(Rate each indicator of **Motivation:** 1 = never demonstrated, 2 = rarely demonstrated, 3 = sometimes demonstrated, 4 = often demonstrated, 5 = consistently demonstrated) (Moorhead et al., 2004).

SELF-DIRECTION OF CARE   NOC

Definition: Care recipient actions taken to direct others who assist with or perform physical tasks and personal health care.
Self-Direction of Care as evidenced by the following selected NOC indicators:

NR = Nursing Research, **MR** = Multidisciplinary Research, **SP** = Standard of Practice, **EO** = Expert Opinion, **LOE** = Level of Evidence

OUTCOME MEASUREMENT—*cont'd*

- Sets health care goals
- Instructs others in appropriate care behaviors
- Expresses confidence in problem solving
- Instructs others in appropriate health maintenance activities

(Rate each indicator of **Self-Direction of Care:** 1 = never demonstrated, 2 = rarely demonstrated, 3 = sometimes demonstrated, 4 = often demonstrated, 5 = consistently demonstrated) (Moorhead et al., 2004).

REFERENCES

Beswick AD, Rees K, West RR, Taylor FC, Burke M, Griebsch I, et al. (2005). Improving uptake and adherence in cardiac rehabilitation: Literature review. *J Adv Nurs,* 49(5):538-555.

Bolman C, Brug J, Bar F, Martinali J, van den Borne B. (2005). Long-term efficacy of a checklist to improve patient education in cardiology. *Patient Educ Couns,* 56(2):240-248.

Bonner S, Zimmerman BJ, Evans D, Irigoyen M, Resnick D, Mellins RB. (2002). An individualized intervention to improve asthma management among urban Latino and African-American families. *J Asthma,* 39(2):167-179.

Bradlyn AS, Beale IL, Kato PM. (2003). Psychoeducational interventions with pediatric cancer patients: Part I: Patient information and knowledge. *J Child Fam Stud,* 12(3):257-277.

Brown RF, Butow PN, Dunn SM, Tattersall MH. (2001). Promoting patient participation and shortening cancer consultations: A randomised trial. *Br J Cancer,* 85(9):1273-1279.

Burton C, Gibbon R. (2005). Expanding the role of the stroke nurse: A pragmatic clinical trial. *J Adv Nurs,* 52(6):640-650.

Chumbley GM, Ward L, Hall GM, Salmon P. (2004). Pre-operative information and patient-controlled analgesia: Much ado about nothing. *Anaesthesia,* 59(4):354-358.

Danino AM, Chahraoui K, Frachebois L, Jebrane A, Moutel G, Herve C, et al. (2005). Effects of an informational CD-ROM on anxiety and knowledge before aesthetic surgery: A randomised trial. *Br J Plast Surg,* 58(3):379-383.

Devine EC. (2003). Meta-analysis of the effect of psychoeducational interventions on pain in adults with cancer. *Oncol Nurs Forum,* 30(1):75-89.

Dochterman JM, Bulechek GM (Eds). (2004). *Nursing Interventions Classification (NIC),* 4th ed. St. Louis: Mosby.

Dougherty CM, Lewis FM, Thompson EA, Baer JD, Kim W. (2004). Short-term efficacy of a telephone intervention by expert nurses after an implantable cardioverter defibrillator. *Pacing Clin Electrophysiol,* 27(12):1594-1602.

Dunbar SB, Clark PC, Deaton C, Smith AL, De AK, O'Brien MC. (2005). Family education and support interventions in heart failure: A pilot study. *Nurs Res,* 54(3):158-166.

Echeverry D, Dike M, Jovanovic L, Wollitzer AO, Westphal S, Mudaliar S, et al. (2005). Efforts to improve subsequent treatment of cardiovascular risk factors in older patients with diabetes hospitalized for a cardiac event. *Am J Manag Care,* 11(12):758-764.

Johansson K, Nuutila L, Virtanen H, Katajisto J, Salantera S. (2005). Preoperative education for orthopaedic patients: Systematic review. *J Adv Nurs,* 50(2):212-223.

Jones RB, Pearson J, Cawsey AJ, Bental D, Barrett A, White J, et al. (2006). Effect of different forms of information produced for cancer patients on their use of the information, social support, and anxiety: Randomised trial. *BMJ,* 332(7547):942-948.

Kennedy AP, Nelson E, Reeves D, Richardson G, Roberts C, Robinson A, et al. (2004). A randomised controlled trial to assess the effectiveness and cost of a patient orientated self management approach to chronic inflammatory bowel disease. *Gut,* 53(11):1639-1645.

Keyserling TC, Samuel-Hodge CD, Ammerman AS, Ainsworth BE, Henriquez-Roldan CF, Elasy TA, et al. (2002). A randomized trial of an intervention to improve self-care behaviors of African-American women with type 2 diabetes: Impact on physical activity. *Diabetes Care,* 25(9):1576-1583.

McPherson AC, Glazebrook C, Forster D, James C, Smyth A. (2006). A randomized, controlled trial of an interactive educational computer package for children with asthma. *Pediatrics,* 117(4):1046-1054.

Moorhead M, Johnson M, Maas M (Eds). (2004). *Nursing Outcomes Classification (NOC),* 3rd ed. St. Louis: Mosby.

Oldman M, Moore D, Collins S. (2004). Drug patient information leaflets in anaesthesia: Effect on anxiety and patient satisfaction. *Br J Anaesth,* 92(6):854-858.

Olinzock BJ. (2004). A model for assessing learning readiness for self-direction of care in individuals with spinal cord injuries: A qualitative study. *SCI Nurs,* 21(2):69-74.

Shegog R, Bartholomew LK, Parcel GS, Sockrider MM, Masse L, Abramson SL. (2001). Impact of a computer-assisted education program on factors related to asthma self-management behavior. *J Am Med Inform Assoc,* 8(1):49-61.

Wade SL, Michaud L, Brown TM. (2006). Putting the pieces together: Preliminary efficacy of a family problem-solving intervention for children with traumatic brain injury. *J Head Trauma Rehabil,* 21(1):57-67.

Whittemore R, Melkus GD, Sullivan A, Grey M. (2004). A nurse-coaching intervention for women with type 2 diabetes. *Diabetes Educ,* 30(5):795-804.

Williams GC, McGregor H, Zeldman A, Freedman ZR, Deci EL, Elder D. (2005). Promoting glycemic control through diabetes self management: Evaluating a patient activation intervention. *Patient Educ Couns,* 56(1):28-34.

Wolf FM, Guevara JP, Grum CM, Clark NM, Cates CJ. (2003). Educational interventions for asthma in children. *Cochrane Database Syst Rev,* (1):CD000326.

MASSAGE

Katharine Kolcaba, PhD, RN-C; Annette R. Mitzel, MSN, RN, LMT, CNS

NIC **Definition:** Stimulation of the skin and underlying tissues with varying degrees of hand pressure to decrease pain, produce relaxation, and/or improve circulation (Dochterman & Bulechek, 2004).

NURSING ACTIVITIES

Effective

■ *Assess the patient's needs, desires, preferences, and realistic outcomes for the massage.* **LOE = VII**

EO Perform a comprehensive assessment before a massage to address the patient's needs, desires, and preferences in order to establish outcomes (Andrade & Clifford, 2001).

EO Presence and a therapeutic relationship prior to implementing massage make the massage more effective. A therapeutic relationship is part of the holistic experience (Dossey, 1995).

EO A thorough patient's history and benefits of massage should be discussed before the massage is administered in order to address individualized expectations (Bray, 1999).

■ **NIC** *Screen for contraindications, such as decreased platelets, decreased skin integrity, deep vein thrombosis, and hypersensitivity to touch.* **LOE = VII**

EO Screening for contraindications of massage must be done before a massage is performed in order to avoid these areas of concern during the massage (Andrade & Clifford, 2001).

NR = Nursing Research, **MR** = Multidisciplinary Research, **SP** = Standard of Practice, **EO** = Expert Opinion, **LOE** = Level of Evidence

■ **NIC** *Determine the patient's degree of psychological comfort with touch.*
  LOE = V

EO The patient must be comfortable with touch in order to receive the full benefit of the massage (Andrade & Clifford, 2001).

EO Clinicians must seek to "see through the eyes of the other" demonstrating commitment to understanding and compassion and returning the focus toward what is important to the patient (Thompson, 2006).

■ **NIC** *Select the area or areas of the body to be massaged.* **LOE = VII**

EO Selecting areas for massage and preparing equipment, supplies, and appropriate positioning prepare the patient for the massage (Fritz, 2004).

■ **NIC** *Prepare a warm, comfortable environment without distractions.*
  LOE = VII

EO It is important to prepare the environment and have a minimum of distractions for full benefits of the massage (Fritz, 2004). This ensures the peacefulness and appropriateness of the environment for the patient, contributing to the holistic experience.

■ **NIC** *Place the patient in a position that facilitates massage.* **LOE = VII**

EO Position the patient in a position that is comfortable to enhance the benefits of massage (Fritz, 2004).

■ **NIC** *Apply moist heat before massage or during massage to other areas of the body, as indicated.* **LOE = VII**

EO Moist heat may be helpful to enhance the benefits of massage (Fritz, 2004).

■ **NIC** *Drape to expose only the area to be massaged, as needed.* **LOE = VII**

EO Draping is important for the patient's comfort and modesty (Fritz, 2004).

■ **NIC** *Massage using continuous, even, and rhythmical movements.* **LOE = II**

EO Continuous and rhythmical movements facilitate beneficial massage (Okvat et al., 2002).

■ **NIC** *Massage the hands and feet if other areas are inconvenient or if more comfortable for the patient.* **LOE = VII**

EO As an alternative, the hands and feet may be massaged instead if the patient is not comfortable with a full body massage (Fritz, 2004).

■ **NIC** *Establish a period of time for massage that achieves the desired response.*
  LOE = VII

EO The therapist should determine the length of the massage of different parts of the body based on intuition and experience in order to accomplish the desired outcome (Andrade & Clifford, 2001).

RCT = Randomized Controlled (Clinical) Trial, **NIC** = Nursing Interventions Classification, **NOC** = Nursing Outcomes Classification

■ **NIC** *Adapt massage area, technique, and pressure to the patient's perception of comfort and purpose of massage.* **LOE = VII**

EO Sensitivity to touch varies with each individual. Adjusting the pressure exerted in the massage increases effectiveness and comfort (Fritz, 2004).

■ **NIC** *Encourage the patient to deep breathe and relax during massage.* **LOE = VII**

EO Deep breathing stimulates a parasympathetic response and subsequent relaxation (Fritz, 2004).

■ **NIC** *Encourage the patient to concentrate on the good feelings of the massage.* **LOE = VII**

EO Positive reinforcement of the pleasurable sensations from massage enhances the patient's experience (Fritz, 2004).

■ *Avoid massage over areas with open lesions, bruises, tender skin, shunts, or access ports.* **LOE = V**

EO Lesions, bruises, and tender areas on the skin are contraindications for massage because further injury may be caused (Fritz, 2004).

■ **NIC** *Instruct the patient at completion of massage to rest until ready and then to move slowly.* **LOE = V**

EO Rest and gentle activities are recommended after massage to prolong the benefits of the massage. Fluids are encouraged to maintain hydration (Fritz, 2004).

■ **NIC** *Use massage alone or in conjunction with other measures, as appropriate.* **LOE = V**

EO Music and aromatic fragrance can be added as desired by the patient to enhance the massage experience (Fritz, 2004).

■ **NIC** *Evaluate and document the response to massage.* **LOE = VII**

EO Evaluation of the patient's response is based upon observation and active listening. Documentation is important for safety and continuity of care (Thompson, 2006).

Possibly Effective

■ **NIC** *Use warm lotion, oil, or dry powder to reduce friction (no lotion or oils on head or scalp), assessing for any sensitivity or contraindications.* **LOE = VII**

EO Warmed lotion is often preferred, but not always necessary, for reducing friction. Do not apply lotion, powder, or oils to the head or scalp (Fritz, 2004).

■ *Use aromatherapy with massage.* **LOE = II**

NR In an RCT ($N = 103$) of cancer patients in a palliative care setting, patients in the massage-without-aromatherapy group as well as the aromatherapy group experienced improved out-

---

NR = Nursing Research, **MR** = Multidisciplinary Research, **SP** = Standard of Practice, **EO** = Expert Opinion, **LOE** = Level of Evidence

comes. However, improvements between the two groups were not statistically significant (Wilkinson et al., 1999).

Not Effective

No applicable published research was found in this category.

Possibly Harmful

■ *Use of friction over inflamed joints, fragile skin, obvious tumors, or bruises.* **LOE = II**

NR In an RCT (*N* = 31) of hospice patients who were randomly assigned to treatment (receiving hand massage twice weekly for 3 weeks) or comparison groups (receiving hand massage once at the study's end), findings demonstrated that friction over areas of concern led to possible damage (Kolcaba et al., 2004).

■ *Kneading nonfleshy areas.* **LOE = VII**

EO Kneading is a movement for fleshy areas only and may cause discomfort if performed on other areas (Tappen & Benjamin, 1998).

■ *Repositioning to access dorsal and palmar surfaces when the patient manifests pain or discomfort.* **LOE = II**

NR In an RCT (*N* = 31) of hospice patients who were randomly assigned to treatment (receiving hand massage twice weekly for 3 weeks) or comparison groups (receiving hand massage once at the study's end), findings indicated that repositioning of hands decreased pain and discomfort (Kolcaba et al., 2004).

■ *Using direct and firm pressure on the center of the palm (this is an acupressure point).* **LOE = II**

NR In an RCT (*N* = 31) of hospice patients who were randomly assigned to treatment (receiving hand massage twice weekly for 3 weeks) or comparison groups (receiving hand massage once at the study's end), researchers stated that direct and firm pressure on the center of the palm was contraindicated (Kolcaba et al., 2004).

OUTCOME MEASUREMENT

COMFORT LEVEL NOC

Definition: Extent of positive perception of physical and psychological ease.
Comfort Level as evidenced by the following selected NOC indicators:
• Physical well-being
• Psychological well-being
(Rate each indicator of **Comfort Level:** 1 = not at all satisfied, 2 = somewhat satisfied, 3 = moderately satisfied, 4 = very satisfied, 5 = completely satisfied) (Moorhead et al., 2004).

Continued

RCT = Randomized Controlled (Clinical) Trial, **NIC** = Nursing Interventions Classification, **NOC** = Nursing Outcomes Classification

OUTCOME MEASUREMENT—*cont'd*

TOTAL COMFORT

Total Comfort as evidenced by a pain and/or comfort scale per institutional policy to demonstrate increased comfort or decreased pain

Rate the patient's **Total Comfort** from 0 to 10, with 10 being as comfortable as possible. This is similar to rating of pain and is easy and familiar for patients (Kolcaba, 2003).

PERSONAL WELL-BEING   NOC

Definition: Extent of positive perception of one's health status and life circumstances.
Personal Well-Being as evidenced by the following selected NOC indicators:
• Ability to cope
• Ability to relax
• Level of happiness
(Rate each indicator of **Personal Well-Being:** 1 = not at all satisfied, 2 = somewhat satisfied, 3 = moderately satisfied, 4 = very satisfied, 5 = completely satisfied) (Moorhead et al., 2004).

REFERENCES

Andrade C, Clifford P. (2001). *Outcome based massage.* Philadelphia: Lippincott Williams & Wilkins.
Bray R. (1999). Massage: Exploring the benefits. *Elder Care,* 11(5):15-16.
Dochterman JM, Bulechek GM (Eds). (2004). *Nursing Interventions Classification (NIC),* 4th ed. St. Louis: Mosby.
Dossey L. (1995). How should alternative therapies be evaluated: an examination of fundamentals. *Altern Ther Health Med,* 1(2):6-9.
Fritz S. (2004). *Fundamentals of therapeutic massage,* 3rd ed. St. Louis: Mosby.
Kolcaba K. (2003). *Comfort theory and practice.* New York: Springer.
Kolcaba K, Dowd T, Steiner R, Mitzel A. (2004). Efficacy of hand massage for enhancing the comfort of hospice patients. *J Hosp Palliat Nurs,* 6(2):91-102.
Moorhead M, Johnson M, Maas M (Eds). (2004). *Nursing Outcomes Classification (NOC),* 3rd ed. St. Louis: Mosby.
Okvat HA, Oz MC, Ting W, Namerow PB. (2002). Massage therapy for patients undergoing cardiac catheterization. *Altern Ther Health Med,* 8(3):68-70, 72, 74-75.
Tappen F, Benjamin PJ. (1998). *Tappen's handbook of healing massage techniques,* 3rd ed. Connecticut: Appleton & Lange.
Thompson D. (2006). *Hands heal: Communication, documentation, and insurance billing for manual therapists,* 3rd ed. Philadelphia: Lippincott Williams & Wilkins.
Wilkinson S, Aldridge J, Salmon I, Cain E, Wilson B. (1999). An evaluation of aromatherapy massage in palliative care. *Palliat Med,* 13(5):409-417.

 # MEDICATION ADMINISTRATION

Kathleen G. Burke, PhD, RN; Kristie B. Asimos, MSN, CRNP

NIC **Definition:** Preparing, giving, and evaluating the effectiveness of prescription and nonprescription drugs (Dochterman & Bulechek, 2004).

NR = Nursing Research, **MR** = Multidisciplinary Research, **SP** = Standard of Practice, **EO** = Expert Opinion, **LOE** = Level of Evidence

NURSING ACTIVITIES

Effective

■ *Document, verify, and reconcile all medications with the patient, family member, or other health care personnel, especially during transition times.* **LOE = VI**

> (MR) A baseline chart review of 33 ICU discharge charts demonstrated 94% of discharge medication orders changed because of errors. The highest risk of medication errors occurred during transition times, 46% to 56%, including transfers within the hospital and between hospital and home (Pronovost et al., 2003).

> (MR) A longitudinal study of an electronic medication reconciliation process demonstrated a reduction in transfer error rate to zero by the 24th week ($N = 33$) (Pronovost et al., 2003).

> (MR) In a 7-month chart review following the implementation of a medication reconciliation process on admission, during transfer, and at discharge from the hospital in an acute care setting, the medication discrepancy rate was reduced from 213 errors per 100 admissions to 42 errors per 100 admissions (Rozich & Resar, 2001; Rozich et al., 2004).

■ *Document and verify all medication orders with appropriate health care members, as well as question the accuracy and appropriateness of medication orders.* **LOE = VI**

> (EO) The second most common cause of medication error is failure to document and verify medication orders; this failure was responsible for 20% of errors in 2001, 29.4% in 2002, and 18.3% in 2003 (Lewis, 2005).

> (EO) Absent, confusing, or intimating communication accounted for 17.7% of harmful errors in 2002, and 13% in 2003 (Lewis, 2005).

> (EO) The most commonly cited factors associated with medication errors are lack of knowledge or application of knowledge, use of wrong drug name, incorrect drug route, incorrect dosage calculations (Institute of Medicine, 2000), and distractions and interruptions (Cohen et al., 1998).

■ *Reduce interruptions during medication administration.* **LOE = VI**

> (EO) Distractions, inattention, and rushing through medication administration or from patient to patient are associated with increases in errors during the process of administering medications (Hughes & Edgerton, 2005).

> (EO) Interruptions while preparing and administering medications are primary contributors to medication errors (Pape, 2001).

■ *Follow the seven rights of medication administration: right drug, right dose, right preparation, right route, right time, right patient, right documentation.* **LOE = V**

> (EO) Following the seven rights provides a line of defense in preventing adverse drug events (Hughes & Ortiz, 2005).

> (EO) Seventy-five percent of medication errors involve four types of errors: an omission, an order involving an improper dose, a prescribing error, and administration of a drug that was not prescribed. Twenty-one percent of the 235,159 errors reported involved the following types of errors: wrong time, extra dose, wrong patient, wrong drug preparation, wrong dosage,

RCT = Randomized Controlled (Clinical) Trial, **NIC** = Nursing Interventions Classification, **NOC** = Nursing Outcomes Classification

wrong route, wrong administration technique, expired product, and deteriorated product (Lewis, 2005).

■ *Eliminate (reduce) barriers to safe medication administration.* **LOE = VII**

EO A State of the Science Panel on Safe Medication Administration concluded that there were seven significant barriers to safe medication administration: (1) lack of a "just culture of safety," (2) lack of interdisciplinary collaboration and communication, (3) nurses' working environment not supporting safety, (4) voices of front-line nurses missing in decision making and system design, (5) difficulties in translating research into practice, (6) policy not driven by evidence, and (7) insufficient funding for research. Strategies to address those barriers were suggested (Burke et al., 2005).

EO Make sure near misses and errors are quickly reported and reports are disseminated to promote a "just culture of safety" (Burke et al., 2005).

EO Eliminate the use of abbreviations and acronyms by providing patients with "smart cards," cards containing extensive data including their medications and history (Burke et al., 2005).

EO Educate nurses, physicians, and pharmacists together to create interdisciplinary peer review teams for collaborative learning from errors (Burke et al., 2005).

EO Educate health care providers to speak a common language and use agreed-upon definitions to promote interdisciplinary collaboration and communication (Burke et al., 2005).

EO Allow staff nurses time to participate in safety initiatives and create staffing patterns that allow flexibility in responding to unanticipated changes in patients' acuity and volume, thus providing a nurse work environment that supports safety (Burke et al., 2005).

■ *Disseminate information about causes and prevention of medication administration errors.* **LOE = V**

EO Medication errors are the most common type of patient-related error and involve serious consequences; disseminating information reduces their incidence of occurrence (Bates et al., 1995, 1997).

■ *Identify factors contributing to risk of medication administration error and educate health care providers about these risks.* **LOE = VI**

EO One in every three adverse drug events occurs when nurses are administering medications to patients; identifying factors contributing to the errors will reduce the incidence of such errors (Bates et al., 1995; Burke et al., 2005).

EO Nurses and pharmacists are responsible for medication errors involving administration in 26% to 34% of adverse drug error instances (Hughes & Ortiz, 2005).

EO The most commonly cited factors associated with medication errors are lack of knowledge or application of knowledge; use of wrong drug name, dose, or abbreviation; incorrect dosage calculations; and distractions and interruptions (Cohen et al., 1998; Institute of Medicine, 2000).

EO Certain drugs are considered high-alert drugs because of the association with an increase in the number of, or higher risk of, harmful adverse drug events; such drugs include adrenal corticosteroids, analgesics, antibiotics, antihistamines, antineoplastics, asthma medications, bronchodilators, cardiac medications, electrolytes, vitamins and minerals, insulin, opioids, and sedatives (Hughes & Edgerton, 2005).

NR = Nursing Research, **MR** = Multidisciplinary Research, **SP** = Standard of Practice, **EO** = Expert Opinion, **LOE** = Level of Evidence

(MR) A retrospective review of 30,195 charts found that antibiotics and chemotherapy drugs were the medications most involved in adverse medication events (Pape, 2001).

(MR) A cohort study of Medicare enrollees ($N = 30,397$) found that the most frequent classes of drugs associated with adverse drug events were cardiovascular agents, antibiotics, diuretics, nonopioid analgesics, and anticoagulants (Gurwitz et al., 2003).

Possibly Effective

No applicable published research was found in this category.

Not Effective

No applicable published research was found in this category.

Possibly Harmful

No applicable published research was found in this category.

OUTCOME MEASUREMENT

MEDICATION RESPONSE (NOC)

Definition: Therapeutic and adverse effects of prescribed medication.

Medication Response as evidenced by the following selected NOC indicators:

• Adverse effects
• Allergic reaction
• Drug interaction
• Drug intolerance

(Rate each indicator of **Medication Response:** 1 = severe, 2 = substantial, 3 = moderate, 4 = mild, 5 = none) (Moorhead et al., 2004).

REFERENCES

Bates DW, Cullen DJ, Laird N, Petersen LA, Small SD, Servi D, et al. (1995). Incidence of adverse drug events and potential adverse drug events: Implications for prevention. ADE Prevention Study Group. *JAMA*, 274(1):29-34.

Bates DW, Spell N, Cullen DJ, Burdick E, Laird N, Petersen LA, et al. (1997). The costs of adverse drug events in hospitalized patients. Adverse Drug Events Prevention Study Group. *JAMA*, 277(4): 307-311.

Burke KG, Mason DJ, Alexander M, Barnsteiner JH, Rich VL. (2005). Making medication administration safe: Report challenges nurses to lead the way. *Am J Nurs*, 105(3 Suppl):2-3.

Cohen MR, Proulx SM, Crawford SY. (1998). Survey of hospital systems and common serious medication errors. *J Healthc Risk Manage*, 18(1):16-27.

Dochterman JM, Bulechek GM (Eds). (2004). *Nursing Interventions Classification (NIC)*, 4th ed. St. Louis: Mosby.

Gurwitz JH, Field TS, Harrold LR, Rothschild J, Debellis K, Seger AC, et al. (2003). Incidence and preventability of adverse drug events among older persons in the ambulatory setting. *JAMA*, 289(9): 1107-1116.

Hughes RG, Edgerton EA. (2005). Reducing pediatric medication errors: Children are especially at risk for medication errors. *Am J Nurs*, 105(5):79-85.

Hughes RG, Ortiz E. (2005). Medication errors: Why they happen, and how they can be prevented. *Am J Nurs*, 105(3):14-24.

Institute of Medicine. (2000). *To err is human: Building a safer health system.* Washington, DC: National Academies Press.

Lewis L. (2005). Discussion and recommendations: Safe medication administration: An invitational symposium recommends ways of addressing obstacles. *Am J Nurs,* 105(3 Suppl):42-47.

Moorhead M, Johnson M, Maas M (Eds). (2004). *Nursing Outcomes Classification (NOC),* 3rd ed. St. Louis, Mosby.

Pape TM. (2001). Searching for the final answer: Factors contributing to medication administration errors. *J Contin Educ Nurs,* 32(4):152-160.

Pronovost P, Weast B, Schwarz M, Wyskiel RM, Prow D, Milanovich SN, et al. (2003). Medication reconciliation: A practical tool to reduce the risk of medication errors. *J Crit Care,* 18(4):201-205.

Rozich JD, Howard RJ, Justeson JM, Macken PD, Lindsay ME, Resar RK. (2004). Standardization as a mechanism to improve safety in health care. *Jt Comm J Qual Saf,* 30(1):5-14.

Rozich JD, Resar RK. (2001). Medication safety: One organization's approach to the challenge. *J Clin Outcomes Manage,* 8(10):27-34.

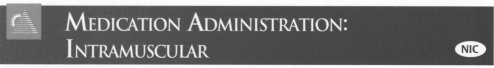

MEDICATION ADMINISTRATION: INTRAMUSCULAR

NIC

Karen A. Papastrat, MSN, RN

NIC **Definition:** Preparing and giving medications via the intramuscular route (Dochterman & Bulechek, 2004).

NURSING ACTIVITIES

Effective

■ *Use the ventrogluteal (VG) over the dorsogluteal (DG) site when administering intramuscular (IM) injections.* **LOE = I**

NR Integrative literature reviews and meta-analyses found that the VG site was safe, used bone landmarks to locate the site, had a greater thickness of the gluteal muscle than the DG site, and was free of large blood vessels and nerves (Greenway, 2004; Small, 2004; Zelman, 1961).

NR An integrative review of the literature resulted in an evidence-based practice guideline for administration of IM injections. The VG site was appropriate for larger volumes; the literature varied with recommendations of 2 to 5 mL (Nicoll & Hesby, 2002).

EO The VG site also provides the most consistent layer of adipose tissue, less than 3.75 cm (Beyea & Nicoll, 1995; Greenway, 2004). This minimizes the risk of not reaching the target muscle in obese people or those with large body mass indexes (BMIs).

EO The VG site can be reached from the prone, supine, or side-lying position. The site is located in the superior lateral aspect of the gluteal muscles. The nurse locates the site by placing the heel of the hand over the greater trochanter; the index finger points to the anterior superior iliac crest, forms a "V" with the middle finger, and the injection site is within the V (Potter & Perry, 2006; Craven & Hirnle, 2006).

EO The VG site is the preferred site for medications that are irritating to subcutaneous tissues, are more viscous, or are of greater volume as much as 5 mL (Perry & Potter, 2006; Harkreader & Hogan, 2004).

NR = Nursing Research, **MR** = Multidisciplinary Research, **SP** = Standard of Practice, **EO** = Expert Opinion, **LOE** = Level of Evidence

▓ *Use the Z-track technique with all intramuscular injections to decrease the leaking of medications into the subcutaneous tissue, thereby lessening pain and complications at the site and promoting absorption from the muscle site.* **LOE = V**

(NR) Systematic reviews of the literature consistently and vigorously supported the use of this technique. The Z-track method has been shown to reduce pain, minimize skin irritation, and prevent leakage into the subcutaneous tissue by creating a zigzag tract that traps the medication in the muscle (Beyea & Nicoll, 1995; Keen, 1986; Nicoll & Hesby, 2002; Newton et al., 1992; Pullen, 2005).

(EO) Fundamental nursing textbooks recommend Z-track technique to be used with deep IM injections to minimize leakage of medications into subcutaneous tissue (Craven & Hirnle, 2006; Harkreader & Hogan, 2004; Perry & Potter, 2006).

Possibly Effective

▓ *Use a filter needle when drawing injectable solutions from an ampule or vial and to change the needle before the injection.* **LOE = V**

(EO) Using a filter needle for drawing up all medications from the ampule or vial is recommended to eliminate medication errors and patients' complaints (Nicoll & Hesby, 2002).

(MR) An integrative review and meta-analyses concluded that needles should be changed to prevent foreign object transmission and to decrease irritation from medication clinging to the outside shaft of the needle (Rodger & King, 2000).

(EO) There is evidence that filter needles have prevented glass from being drawn into a syringe and should be used with glass ampules (Falchuk et al., 1985; Sabon et al., 1989).

(EO) Suggestions to minimize risk of complications when not using a filter needle include the following: insert needle in rubber-topped vial bevel up to prevent coring, withdraw medication from the vial holding the container down and do not withdraw the last drops of medication (McConnell, 1982), and wipe off any medication drips on the needle with a sterile gauze pad (Newton et al., 1992).

▓ *Prior to injection, aspirate by pulling back on the plunger of a syringe to ensure that medication is not injected directly into a blood vessel.* **LOE = III**

(EO) There are no research data documented to support the need for this procedure (Atkinson et al., 2002; CDC, 2006).

(EO) Multiple nursing textbooks recommend the aspiration technique (Craven & Hirnle, 2006; Harkreader & Hogan, 2004; Potter & Perry, 2006).

(NR) An integrative research review cited reports in the literature of intra-arterial or intravenous injection of medication and thus recommended the continued use of this technique (Nicoll & Hesby, 2002).

Not Effective

No applicable published research was found in this category.

RCT = Randomized Controlled (Clinical) Trial, **NIC** = Nursing Interventions Classification, **NOC** = Nursing Outcomes Classification

Possibly Harmful

■ *Using the dorsogluteal site.* **LOE = I**

(NR) Integrative literature reviews and meta-analyses of sciatic nerve injury found that injury to the sciatic nerve was associated with the use of the DG site (Small, 2004).

(EO) Some nursing textbooks recommend against the use of the DG site and no longer include instruction on this site (Perry & Potter, 2006; Potter & Perry, 2006).

(EO) Although other textbooks continue to provide instructions in marking and using the site, they warn against or indicate that this is not a preferred site because of potential injury and complications and/or indicate the VG as the preferred site (Craven & Hirnle, 2006; Harkreader & Hogan, 2004).

■ *Using standard intramuscular needles (1 inch, 25 mm; 1.37 inches, 35 mm; 1.5 inches, 38 mm).* **LOE = II**

(MR) In a retrospective study, 100 patients had CT scans of the pelvis following VG and DG injections. At the VG site, the depth of the adipose tissue ranged from 2.5 to 62.6 mm, and at the DG site the depth ranged from 7.5 to 59.8 mm. Because of the depth of the fat, significant numbers of patients failed to receive an IM injection (Nisbet, 2006).

(EO) Research revealed important reasons for injecting vaccine into the muscle that include (1) decreased immune response of hepatitis B, rabies, and influenza vaccines; (2) the injected antigen takes longer to reach the circulation; (3) antigens remaining in subcutaneous fat may be denatured by enzymes; (4) inadvertent subcutaneous injections can cause abscesses and granulomas (Zuckerman, 2000).

(MR) A prospective study of 220 health care workers concluded that when giving IM injections in the deltoid: (1) for men 59 to 118 kg, a 25-mm (1-inch) needle would penetrate the muscle; (2) for women less than 60 kg, a 16-mm (5/8-inch) needle would penetrate the muscle; (3) for women 60 to 90 kg, a 25-mm needle would be needed; and (4) for women greater than 90 kg, a 38-mm (1.5-inch) needle would be required (Poland et al., 1997).

(MR) In an ultrasound study of 250 elderly patients (≥65 years), it was found that BMI and deltoid subcutaneous thickness were significantly correlated but that females with the same BMI had significantly thicker subcutaneous layers and thinner muscle layers. The minimal needle length required for an IM injection at a 90-degree angle in all BMI males and women with BMI less than 35 was a 25-mm (1-inch) needle. For women with BMI greater than 35, a 32-mm (1.25-inch) needle was required. It was found that females had significantly greater subcutaneous layer thickness and significantly less muscle layer thickness than males (Cook et al., 2006).

(EO) Recommendations for IM injection in the deltoid muscle for adults are a 90-degree angle, 1- to 1.5-inch needle, and 22 to 25 gauge (CDC, 2006).

Additional research: Grabinski et al., 1983; Hodges, 2005; Lindsay et al., 1985; Vukovich et al., 1975; Cohen et al., 1972.

■ *Adding an air bubble to an intramuscular injection; an air bubble should be used only with specific manufacturer's recommendation.* **LOE = VI**

(MR) Adding an air bubble can affect the dosage of a medication in a syringe by 5% to 100%, possibly resulting in delivery of dangerous overdosages (Chaplin et al., 1985; Zenk, 1993). The same is true when using a Carpuject device.

NR = Nursing Research, **MR** = Multidisciplinary Research, **SP** = Standard of Practice, **EO** = Expert Opinion, **LOE** = Level of Evidence

OUTCOME MEASUREMENT

MEDICATION RESPONSE (NOC)

Definition: Therapeutic and adverse effects of prescribed medication.
Medication Response as evidenced by the following selected NOC indicators:
- Adverse effects
- Allergic reaction
- Drug interaction
- Drug intolerance

(Rate each indicator of **Medication Response:** 1 = severe, 2 = substantial, 3 = moderate, 4 = mild, 5 = none) (Moorhead et al., 2004).

REFERENCES

Atkinson WL, Pickering LK, Schwartz B, Weniger BG, Iskander JK, Watson JC, et al. (2002). General recommendations on immunization: Recommendations of the Advisory Committee on Immunization Practices (ACIP) and the American Academy of Family Physicians (AAFP). *MMWR Recomm Rep,* 51(RR-2):1-35.

Beyea SC, Nicoll LH. (1995). Administration of medications via the intramuscular route: An integrative review of the literature and research-based protocol for the procedure. *Appl Nurs Res,* 8(1):23-33.

Centers for Disease Control and Prevention (CDC). (2006). *Epidemiology and prevention of vaccine preventable diseases,* 9th ed. Atkinson W, Hamborsky J, McIntyre L, Wolfe S (Eds). Washington DC: Public Health Foundation.

Chaplin G, Shull H, Welk PC 3rd. (1985). How safe is the air-bubble technique for I.M. injections? Not very, say these experts. *Nursing,* 15(9):59.

Cohen LS, Rosenthal JE, Horner DW Jr, Atkins JM, Matthews OA, Sarnoff SJ. (1972). Plasma levels of lidocaine after intramuscular administration. *Am J Cardiol,* 29(4):520-523.

Cook IF, Williamson M, Pond D. (2006). Definition of needle length required for intramuscular deltoid injection in elderly adults: An ultrasonographic study. *Vaccine,* 24(7):937-940.

Craven RF, Hirnle CJ. (2006). *Fundamentals of nursing: Human health and function,* 5th ed. New York: Lippincott.

Dochterman JM, Bulechek GM (Eds). (2004). *Nursing Interventions Classification (NIC),* 4th ed. St. Louis: Mosby.

Falchuk KH, Peterson L, McNeil BJ. (1985). Microparticulate-induced phlebitis: Its prevention by in-line filtration. *N Engl J Med,* 312(2):78-82.

Grabinski PY, Kaiko RF, Rogers AG, Houde RW. (1983). Plasma levels and analgesia following deltoid and gluteal injections of methadone and morphine. *J Clin Pharmacol,* 23(1):48-55.

Greenway K. (2004). Using the ventrogluteal site for intramuscular injection. *Nurs Stand,* 18(25):39-42.

Harkreader H, Hogan MA. (2004). *Fundamentals of nursing,* 2nd ed. St. Louis: Mosby.

Hodges D. (2005). Big butts a barrier to medication. *Medical Post.* Available online: http://www.medical-post.com. Retrieved on September 2, 2006.

Keen MF. (1986). Comparison of intramuscular injection techniques to reduce site discomfort and lesions. *Nurs Res,* 35(4):207-210.

Lindsay KL, Herbert DA, Gitnick GL. (1985). Hepatitis B vaccine: Low postvaccination immunity in hospital personnel given gluteal injections. *Hepatology,* 5(6):1088-1090.

McConnell EA. (1982). The subtle art of really good injections. *RN,* 45(2):24-35.

Moorhead M, Johnson M, Maas M (Eds). (2004). *Nursing Outcomes Classification (NOC),* 3rd ed. St. Louis: Mosby.

Newton M, Newton DW, Fudin J. (1992). Reviewing the "big three" injection routes. *Nursing,* 22(2):34-41.

Nicoll LH, Hesby A. (2002). Intramuscular injection: An integrative research review and guideline for evidence-based practice. *Appl Nurs Res*, 15(3):149-162.

Nisbet AC. (2006). Intramuscular gluteal injections in the increasingly obese population: Retrospective study. *BMJ*, 332(7542):637-638.

Perry AG, Potter P. (2006). *Clinical skills and techniques*, 6th ed. St. Louis: Mosby.

Poland GA, Borrud A, Jacobson RM, McDermott K, Wollan PC, Brakke D, et al. (1997). Determination of deltoid fat pad thickness: Implications for needle length in adult immunization. *JAMA*, 277(21):1709-1711.

Potter P, Perry AG. (2006). *Fundamentals of nursing*, 6th ed. St. Louis: Mosby.

Pullen RL Jr. (2005). Administering medication by the Z-track method. *Nursing*, 35(7):24.

Rodger MA, King L. (2000). Drawing up and administering intramuscular injections: A review of the literature. *J Adv Nurs*, 31(3):574-582.

Sabon RL Jr, Cheng EY, Stommel KA, Hennen CR. (1989). Glass particle contamination: Influence of aspiration methods and ampule types. *Anesthesiology*, 70(5):859-862.

Small SP. (2004). Preventing sciatic nerve injury from intramuscular injections: Literature review. *J Adv Nurs*, 47(3):287-296.

Vukovich RA, Brannick LJ, Sugerman AA, Neiss ES. (1975). Sex differences in the intramuscular absorption and bioavailability of cephradine. *Clin Pharmacol Ther*, 18(2):215-220.

Zelman S. (1961). Notes on techniques of intramuscular injection: The avoidance of needless pain and morbidity. *Am J Med Sci*, 241:563-574.

Zenk KE. (1993). Beware of overdose. *Nursing*, 23(3):28-29.

Zuckerman JN. (2000). The importance of injecting vaccines into the muscle. Different patients need different needle sizes. *BMJ*, 321(7271):1237-1238.

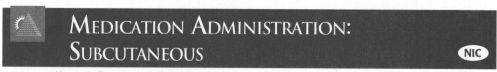

MEDICATION ADMINISTRATION: SUBCUTANEOUS

NIC

Karen A. Papastrat, MSN, RN

NIC **Definition:** Preparing and giving medications via the subcutaneous route (Dochterman & Bulechek, 2004).

NURSING ACTIVITIES

Heparin and Subcutaneous Injection

Effective

■ *Use a 3-mL syringe versus a 1-mL syringe to reduce the size of bruising at the injection site.* **LOE = I**

MR A systematic literature review and meta-analysis supported the use of a 3-mL syringe to reduce bruising (Annersten & Willman, 2005).

NR A quasi-experimental study of 30 patients (58 injections) in a large, urban hospital compared two syringe sizes (3 and 1 mL) and found significant decreases in mean size of bruises. The increase in surface area in the 3-mL syringe decreased the force required to inject the medication by two thirds.

NR An integrative review of research identified the use of a 3-mL syringe as a practice implication to reduce bruising (Beyea & Nicoll, 1999).

NR = Nursing Research, **MR** = Multidisciplinary Research, **SP** = Standard of Practice, **EO** = Expert Opinion, **LOE** = Level of Evidence

Possibly Effective

■ *Use a smaller volume of heparin to decrease bruising.* **LOE = VI**

(MR) A single cohort study with a convenience sample ($N = 29$) reported a high incidence of bruising, as high as 90%, from subcutaneous heparin injection (Hadley et al., 1996).

(MR) A single cohort study with a convenience sample ($N = 29$) comparing heparin concentrations of 5000 units/0.5 mL and 5000 units/0.25 mL found that a smaller volume 0.25 mL of 5000 units of heparin subcutaneously resulted in a smaller bruise size (Hadley et al., 1996).

■ *Slowly inject heparin over 30 seconds to reduce significantly bruising and pain at the injection site.* **LOE = VI**

(NR) A quasi-experimental study with 30 participants analyzing 68 visual analogue scale pain scores and 136 bruise sizes over a 7-month period demonstrated that an injection technique using a 27.5-gauge, 5/8-inch needle injected over 30 seconds versus over 10 seconds significantly reduced bruising at 48 and 60 hours after injection ($P = .0145$ at 48 hours and $P = .0056$ at 60 hours). Site pain intensity was reduced by 50% when administering subcutaneous heparin over 30 seconds versus 10 seconds (Chan, 2001).

■ *Use a finer gauge needle–28 gauge versus 25 gauge–to reduce pain at the injection site.* **LOE = VI**

(MR) A single cohort study ($N = 73$) comparing 28-gauge, $\frac{1}{2}$-inch needles and 25-gauge, $\frac{5}{8}$-inch needles (TB) found that using a finer gauge needle reduced pain but did not significantly affect the size of bruising (Coley et al., 1987).

Not Effective

■ *Changing the needle before the administration of subcutaneous heparin, aspiration for blood return before injection, and pressure on the site following injection.* **LOE = V**

(NR) An experimental study ($N = 161$) of the effect of four different subcutaneous injection techniques found no significance in bruising using this method (McGowan & Wood, 1990).

(NR) A quantitative study using a small convenience sample ($N = 31$) for heparin injections in a large, urban hospital compared whether bruising was decreased by changing needles before the administration of heparin. There was no significant difference (Klingman, 2000).

Additional research: Beyea & Nicoll, 1996; Hadley et al., 1996.

Possibly Harmful

■ *Applying ice to the injection site before and after subcutaneous heparin injection.* **LOE = V**

(NR) A review of the literature indicated that although applying ice before and after subcutaneous injection resulted in less pain, bruising was found to be significantly larger (Ross & Soltes, 1995; Kuzu & Ucar, 2001).

RCT = Randomized Controlled (Clinical) Trial, **NIC** = Nursing Interventions Classification, **NOC** = Nursing Outcomes Classification

Insulin and Subcutaneous Injection

Effective

■ *Administer insulin injections into the subcutaneous fat tissues to provide the most reliable and consistent absorption of insulin.* **LOE = I**

(MR) A meta-analysis supported the subcutaneous injection of insulin (Frid & Linde, 1993; Pemberton & Holman, 1989; Strauss et al., 2002).

■ *Rotate within each site, and use the same anatomical site at the same time each day to have the most consistent absorptive effect.* **LOE = V**

(NR) A systematic review of the literature indicated that absorption rates vary from site to site; it is now generally accepted that the same anatomical site should be used at the same time every day for a more consistent, predictive, absorptive effect (King, 2003; Fleming, 1999).

(EO) Absorption is most rapid from the abdomen and slowest from the buttocks (Wood et al., 2002).

(EO) Rotating within one anatomical site (using an intrarotation technique, separating by 1 to 2 inches each injection site) should be used to avoid lipohypertrophies (King, 2003; Shin & Kim, 2006).

(EO) Rotate injections within one site, and stress consistency within a rotation plan (ADA, 2004; Lumber, 2004).

Possibly Effective

■ *Use needles shorter than 12.5 mm (5, 6, 8 mm), especially in children and thin adults, to prevent inadvertent intramuscular injection.* **LOE = VI**

(EO) The average skin thickness as measured by ultrasound and MRI images has shown that the epidermis and dermis above the subcutaneous fat layer vary between 1.5 and 3 mm. This is true in both obese and thin individuals (NovoCare News, 2000; Pemberton & Holman, 1989).

■ *Adults using a standard size, subcutaneous length needle should inject at 90 degrees using a "pinch-up" technique, holding the skinfold until the needle has been withdrawn from the skin. However, shorter, thinner needles are a clear advantage for all uses as they create less resistance, are easier to inject, and result in less discomfort.* **LOE = V**

(NR) A systematic literature review of 38 studies regarding subcutaneous injection technique concluded that the size of injection needle should be adjusted to the amount of subcutaneous tissue on an individual basis (Annersten & Willman, 2005).

(EO) The pinch-up technique is thought to result in a more diffuse deposit of insulin, thought to promote absorption by increasing distribution of medication, and may prevent accidental injection into the muscle (Becton Dickinson, 2006; Strauss et al., 1999).

(MR) In a multicenter, open-label, randomized two-period, crossover trial that compared needle length and glycemic control for 62 obese and nonobese patents, it was found that 12.7

and 6 mm produced comparable hemoglobin A_{1c}; 89% of patients preferred the shorter needle length (Schwartz et al., 2004).

(FO) Regardless of body weight, body mass index, age, and body type, the epidermal layer does not significantly vary, so shorter 5- to 6-mm needles with gauges of 29 to 31 can be safely recommended for everyone (King, 2003).

■ *Use the insulin pen to administer a more accurate dose using an 8-mm or shorter needle and for improved patients' compliance.* **LOE = II**

(MR) A review of the research literature supported the accuracy in dosing using the insulin pen (Graff & McClanahan, 1998).

(MR) A review of the research literature demonstrated the insulin pen's advantages in maintaining glycemic control, the increased acceptance by pen users, convenience, ease of use, safety, and efficacy (Bohannon, 1999).

(FO) The pen is preferred over traditional subcutaneous injections by patients for the following reasons: convenience, decreased pain, increased control, and decreasing the fear of injections (Fleming, 2000).

(MR) A multicenter survey with 1310 participants found increased patients' compliance with the insulin pen (Graff & McClanahan, 1998).

(FO) Pen use has a faster flow of insulin during delivery and less dribbling from pen tip to completion of the injection. It is recommended that the needle of the pen remain for 6 to 10 seconds after injection (King, 2003; Becton Dickinson, 2006).

Not Effective

■ *Aspiration prior to administration of subcutaneous insulin injection to indicate correct needle placement.* **LOE = V**

(NR) A quasi-experimental study of 204 injections yielded no blood return; however, based on skinfold measurements, some of those injections were documented as being administered into the muscle (Peragallo-Dittko, 1995).

(FO) The American Diabetes Association, along with insulin syringe manufacturers, no longer supports aspiration with insulin injections (ADA, 2004; Becton Dickinson, 2006).

Possibly Harmful

■ *Sharing of syringe, and needle reuse by the same individual.* **LOE = III**

(FO) The risk of transmission of HIV and hepatitis when needles are shared by individuals is well documented (ADA, 2004).

(MR) A pan-European epidemiological study with 1002 patients concluded that needle reuse, even more than once, created a 31% increase in lipohypertrophy. To avoid pain, bruising, and lipohypertrophies, needles should not be reused (Straus, 2002; King, 2003).

Note: The ADA's position statement on insulin administration recognizes the possible need to reuse needles by the same patient and the risks involved but fails to condemn this as unsafe practice. Their recommendation is that if the needle is "noticeably dull or deformed or if it has come in contact with any surface other than skin" it should be discarded (ADA, 2004).

RCT = Randomized Controlled (Clinical) Trial, **NIC** = Nursing Interventions Classification, **NOC** = Nursing Outcomes Classification

OUTCOME MEASUREMENT

MEDICATION RESPONSE NOC

Definition: Therapeutic and adverse effects of prescribed medication.

Medication Response as evidenced by the following selected NOC indicators:

- Adverse effects
- Allergic reaction
- Drug interaction
- Drug intolerance

(Rate each indicator of **Medication Response:** 1 = severe, 2 = substantial, 3 = moderate, 4 = mild, 5 = none) (Moorhead et al., 2004).

REFERENCES

American Diabetes Association (ADA). (2004). Insulin administration. *Diabetes Care*, 27(Suppl 1): S106-S109.

Annersten M, Willman A. (2005). Performing subcutaneous injections: A literature review. *Worldviews Evid Based Nurs*, 2(3):122-130.

Becton Dickinson. (2006). Getting started: Drawing and injecting insulin. Available online: http://www.bddiabetes.com. Retrieved on September 30, 2006.

Beyea SC, Nicoll LH. (1996). Back to basics. Administering i.m. injections the right way. *Am J Nurs*, 96(1):34-35.

Beyea SC, Nicoll LH. (1999). Using data to support decision making. *AORN J*, 70(5):912-913.

Bohannon NJ. (1999). Insulin delivery using pen devices. Simple-to-use tools may help young and old alike. *Postgrad Med*, 106(5):57-68.

Chan H. (2001). Effects of injection duration on site-pain intensity and bruising associated with subcutaneous heparin. *J Adv Nurs*, 35(6):882-892.

Coley RM, Butler CD, Beck BI, Mullane JP. (1987). Effect of needle size on pain and hematoma formation with subcutaneous injection of heparin sodium. *Clin Pharm*, 6(9):725-727.

Dochterman JM, Bulechek GM (Eds). (2004). *Nursing Interventions Classification (NIC)*, 4th ed. St. Louis: Mosby.

Fleming DR. (1999). Challenging traditional insulin injection practices. *Am J Nurs*, 99(2):72-74.

Fleming DR. (2000). Mightier than the syringe. *Am J Nurs*, 100(11):44-48.

Frid A, Linde B. (1993). Clinically important differences in insulin absorption from abdomen in IDDM. *Diabetes Res Clin Pract*, 21(2-3):137-141.

Graff MR, McClanahan MA. (1998). Assessment by patients with diabetes mellitus of two insulin pen delivery systems versus a vial and syringe. *Clin Ther*, 20(3):486-496.

Hadley SA, Chang M, Rogers K. (1996). Effect of syringe size on bruising following subcutaneous heparin injection. *Am J Crit Care*, 5(4):271-276.

King L. (2003). Subcutaneous insulin injection technique. *Nurs Stand*, 17(34):45-52.

Klingman L. (2000). Effects of changing needles prior to administering heparin subcutaneously. *Heart Lung*, 29(1):70-75.

Kuzu N, Ucar H. (2001). The effect of cold on the occurrence of bruising, haematoma and pain at the injection site in subcutaneous low molecular weight heparin. *Int J Nurs Stud*, 38(1):51-59.

Lumber T. (2004). Tips for site rotation. When it comes to insulin, where you inject is just as important as how much and when. *Diabetes Forecast*, 57(7):68-70.

McConnell EA. (2000). Administering subcutaneous heparin. *Nursing*, 30(6):17.

McGowan S, Wood A. (1990). Administering heparin subcutaneously: An evaluation of techniques used and bruising at the injection site. *Aust J Adv Nurs*, 7(2):30-39.

Moorhead M, Johnson M, Maas M (Eds). (2004). *Nursing Outcomes Classification (NOC)*, 3rd ed. St. Louis: Mosby.

NovoCare News. (2000). NovoFine: Very fine needles indeed. Ideal length for needles. *Diabetes Today,* 4(3):2.

Pemberton E, Holman R. (1989). Optimal needle length for subcutaneous injection. *Diabetic Medicine,* 6(Suppl 2):9.

Peragallo-Dittko V. (1995). Aspiration of the subcutaneous insulin injection: Clinical evaluation of needle size and amount of subcutaneous fat. *Diabetes Educ,* 21(4):291-296.

Ross S, Soltes D. (1995). Heparin and hematoma: Does ice make a difference? *J Adv Nurs,* 21(3):434-439.

Schwartz S, Hassman D, Shelmet J, Sievers R, Weinstein R, Liang J, et al. (2004). A multicenter, open-label, randomized, two-period crossover trial comparing glycemic control, satisfaction, and preference achieved with a 31 gauge × 6 mm needle versus a 29 gauge × 12.7 mm needle in obese patients with diabetes mellitus. *Clin Ther,* 26(10):1663-1678.

Shin H, Kim MJ. (2006). Subcutaneous tissue thickness in children with type 1 diabetes mellitus. *J Adv Nurs,* 54(1):29-34.

Strauss K. (2002). An unexpected hazard of insulin injection. *Prac Diabetes Int,* 19(2):63.

Strauss K, Hannet I, McGonigle J, Parkes JL, Ginsberg B, Jamal R, et al. (1999). Ultra-short (5 mm) insulin needles: Trial results and clinical recommendations. *Pract Diabetes Int,* 16(7):218-222.

Strauss K, De Gols H, Hannet I, Partanen T, Frid A. (2002). A pan-European epidemiologic study of insulin injection technique in patients with diabetes. *Pract Diabetes Int,* 19(3):71-76.

Wood L, Wilbourne J, Kyne-Grzebalski D. (2002). Administration of insulin by injection. *Pract Diabetes Int,* 19(2 Suppl):S1-S4.

 # MEMORY TRAINING

Graham J. McDougall, Jr., PhD, RN, APRN-BC, FAAN

NIC   Definition: Facilitation of memory (Dochterman & Bulechek, 2004).

Interventions to improve cognitive and memory function are usually prescribed based on the level of cognitive function of the individual: impaired or nonimpaired. These interventions are designed to improve episodic memory function that is the storage of information about when events happened and the relationship between those events.

NURSING ACTIVITIES

Effective

■ *Refer the patient to an effective and comprehensive memory training program for older adults, which often includes the four components of stress inoculation, health promotion, memory self-efficacy, and memory strategy training.*
LOE = I

MR A meta-analytic review of healthy community-dwelling elderly participants indicated that memory training improved memory performance (objective) with large effect sizes and improved subjective memory functioning (attitudes and beliefs) with smaller effects compared with controls. Treatment gains were negatively affected as the participants increased in age and as the sessions decreased in length from an optimum 90 minutes (Floyd & Scogin, 1997).

MR A meta-analysis found that memory training resulted in significant increases in memory function in healthy subjects aged 60 or older compared with controls. Treatment gains were negatively affected as the participants increased in age and as the sessions decreased in length from an optimum 90 minutes (Verhaeghen et al., 1992).

(NR) An eight-session classroom-based memory intervention pre-post quasi-experimental study ($N = 78$) yielded significant gains in memory performance, memory self-efficacy, and use of memory strategies among a group of healthy octogenarians living in a retirement community (McDougall, 2002).

(MR) Participants ($N = 2832$) of an RCT were assigned to three group interventions targeted at the outcome of verbal episodic memory. The outcomes were favorable for 87% of speed, 74% of reasoning, and 26% of memory-trained groups, resulting in training effects that were of a magnitude equivalent to the amount of decline expected in elderly people without dementia (Ball et al., 2002).

Possibly Effective

■ *Promote classroom-based psychosocial intervention teaching memory strategies to older adults with brief classroom interventions and for older adults with multiple chronic conditions.* LOE = III

(NR) In a controlled study performed on community-dwelling older adults, a 2-week, four-session ($1\frac{1}{2}$ hours per class) intervention ($N = 74$) significantly improved both metamemory and memory performance in the treatment group. The dose of the intervention was not strong enough because participants had little opportunity to practice in class (enactive mastery experiences). Thus, participants had enough exposure to memory techniques to see that the techniques could work but not enough practice to observe actual changes in their memory in everyday situations (Dellefield & McDougall, 1996).

(NR) A classroom-based memory intervention quasi-experimental study with nursing home residents ($N = 30$) was moderately beneficial. There was a significant difference in immediate story recall and memory self-efficacy. Treatment benefits were reduced by the low level of attendance and depression and cognitive impairment of the individuals (McDougall, 2001).

(MR) In a Cochrane systematic review, memory impairment associated with strokes, there is insufficient evidence to determine whether memory training is effective (Majid et al., 2000).

■ *Promote cognitive rehabilitation following stroke to assist with memory, alertness, and sustained attention.* LOE = II

(MR) Help the family develop a memory aid booklet or wallet that contains pictures and labels from the patient's life, or develop a video that includes familiar pictures with narration. The evidence base for memory strategy training improvement was insufficient to refute or support the conclusions because one trial was available ($N = 12$), whereas the attention-focused studies consisted of two trials ($N = 56$) with the results of one trial supporting improvement in alertness and attention (Lincoln et al., 2000a, b; Majid et al., 2000).

Not Effective

■ *Teaching mnemonics to elders.* LOE = III

(EO) Because mnemonic strategies are often seen as useful only for classical episodic memory tasks, older adults may have problems and difficulty in transferring the use of these strategies

---

NR = Nursing Research, **MR** = Multidisciplinary Research, **SP** = Standard of Practice, **EO** = Expert Opinion, **LOE** = Level of Evidence

to their everyday lives. Simply teaching mnemonics to elders has no relationship to their everyday memory performance (McDougall, 1999; McDougall et al., 2006).

MR In a comparison study between younger adults and older adults, older adults often encountered greater difficulty transferring mnemonic strategies into their daily lives when mnemonics are the major emphasis of a unifactorial memory training program (e.g., teaching only one or two mnemonic strategies) (Brooks et al., 1993).

MR Octogenarian survivors of a longitudinal aging study ($N = 96$) participated in four sessions of mnemonic skills training, which minimally enhanced their episodic memory performance (Singer et al., 2003).

Possibly Harmful

▪ *Participating in a comprehensive memory training program when anxiety, depression, and mild cognitive impairment (MCI) are manifest and untreated.* **LOE=VII**

EO A psychosocial intervention (memory training program) may have a negative impact on an individual's beliefs and confidence and negatively influence memory performance (McDougall et al., 2006).

EO Memory complaints may be the earliest manifestation of MCI. An MCI diagnosis includes the five criteria of cognitive complaints: not normal for the age of the individual, no dementia, cognitive decline, memory impairment, and essentially normal functional activities (McDougall et al., 2006; Winblad et al., 2004).

OUTCOME MEASUREMENT

ATTITUDES ABOUT MEMORY FUNCTION

The Metamemory in Adulthood questionnaire is a reliable and nonthreatening assessment for nonimpaired individuals and has been validated to be effective (Dixon et al., 1988; McDougall, 1999). Metamemory, the memory components of knowledge, beliefs, and affect instrument, consists of seven subscales measuring strategy, task, capacity, change, anxiety, achievement, and locus.

MEMORY PERFORMANCE

The Rivermead Everyday Behavioral Memory Test (RBMT) is designed to reflect everyday memory performance and serves as the memory performance measure. The standard profile score (SPS) of the RBMT (with clinical cut points to diagnosis memory impairment) is used as a measure of memory impairment. The components include remembering of a name (first and surname), a hidden belonging, an appointment, picture recognition, a brief news article (immediate and delayed), face recognition, a new route (immediate), a new route (delayed), a message, orientation, and date. The SPS has a possible range from 0 to 24 and is sometimes interpreted with regard to cutoff points for four groups of memory function: normal (22 to 24), poor (17 to 21), moderately impaired (10 to 16), and severely impaired memory (0 to 9).

MEMORY   **NOC**

Definition: Ability to cognitively retrieve and report previously stored information.

Continued

OUTCOME MEASUREMENT—*cont'd*

Memory as evidenced by the following NOC indicators:
- Recalls immediate information accurately
- Recalls recent information accurately
- Recalls remote information accurately

(Rate each indicator of **Memory:** 1 = severely compromised, 2 = substantially compromised, 3 = moderately compromised, 4 = mildly compromised, 5 = not compromised) (Moorhead et al., 2004).

REFERENCES

Ball K, Berch DB, Helmers KF, Jobe JB, Leveck MD, Marsiske M, et al. (2002). Effects of cognitive training interventions with older adults: A randomized controlled trial. *JAMA,* 288(18):2271-2281.

Brooks JO 3rd, Friedman L, Yesavage JA. (1993). A study of the problems older adults encounter when using a mnemonic technique. *Int Psychogeriatr,* 5(1):57-65.

Dellefield KS, McDougall GJ. (1996). Increasing metamemory in older adults. *Nurs Res,* 45(5): 284-290.

Dixon RA, Hultsch DF, Hertzog C. (1988). The Metamemory in Adulthood (MIA) questionnaire. *Psychopharmacol Bull,* 24(4):671-688.

Dochterman JM, Bulechek GM (Eds). (2004). *Nursing Interventions Classification (NIC),* 4th ed. St. Louis: Mosby.

Floyd M, Scogin F. (1997). Effects of memory training on the subjective memory functioning and mental health of older adults: A meta-analysis. *Psychol Aging,* 12(1):150-161.

Lincoln NB, Majid MJ, Weyman N. (2000a). Cognitive rehabilitation for attention deficits following stroke. *Cochrane Database Syst Rev,* (4):CD002842.

Lincoln NB, Majid MJ, Weyman N. (2000b). Cognitive rehabilitation for memory deficits following stroke. *Cochrane Database Syst Rev,* (3):CD002293.

Majid MJ, Lincoln NB, Weyman N. (2000). Cognitive rehabilitation for memory deficits following stroke. Cochrane Database Syst Rev, (3):CD002293.

McDougall GJ. (2001). Rehabilitation of memory and memory self-efficacy in cognitively impaired nursing home residents. *Clin Geron,* 23(3/4):127.

McDougall GJ. (2002). Memory improvement in octogenarians. *Appl Nurs Res,* 15(1):2-10.

McDougall GJ Jr. (1999). Cognitive interventions among older adults. *Annu Rev Nurs Res,* 17:219-240.

McDougall GJ Jr, Becker H, Arheart KL. (2006). Older adults in the SeniorWISE study at risk for mild cognitive impairment. *Arch Psychiatr Nurs,* 20(3):126-134.

Moorhead M, Johnson M, Maas M (Eds). (2004). *Nursing Outcomes Classification (NOC),* 3rd ed. St. Louis: Mosby.

Singer T, Lindenberger U, Baltes PB. (2003). Plasticity of memory for new learning in very old age: A story of major loss? *Psychol Aging,* 18(2):306-317.

Verhaeghen P, Marcoen A, Goossens L. (1992). Improving memory performance in the aged through mnemonic training: A meta-analytic study. *Psychol Aging,* 7(2):242-251.

Winblad B, Palmer K, Kivipelto M, Jelic V, Fratiglioni L, Wahlund LO, et al. (2004). Mild cognitive impairment—Beyond controversies, towards a consensus: Report of the International Working Group on Mild Cognitive Impairment. *J Intern Med,* 256(3):240-246.

 # MUSIC THERAPY

Jill M. Winters, PhD, RN

NIC **Definition:** Using music to help achieve a specific change in behavior, feeling, or physiology (Dochterman & Bulechek, 2004).

NR = Nursing Research, **MR** = Multidisciplinary Research, **SP** = Standard of Practice, **EO** = Expert Opinion, **LOE** = Level of Evidence

NURSING ACTIVITIES

Effective

■ *Identify the specific change in patients with anxiety that is desired after music sessions.* **LOE = I**

(NR) An RCT ($N = 64$) demonstrated lower anxiety scores in women who listened to at least 30 minutes of relaxing music and who underwent cesarean birth experiences compared with the control group who did not listen to music (Chang & Chen, 2005).

(NR) A three-group (music, silent headphones, control) RCT ($N = 180$) demonstrated significant reductions in anxiety in the experimental group who listened to 30 minutes of preferred music compared with the placebo and control groups in preoperative day surgery patients (Cooke et al., 2005).

(MR) An RCT ($N = 28$) demonstrated a significant reduction in anxiety on days 1 and 2 for women who were residing in a women's shelter who had experienced domestic violence and who listened to self-selected 20-minute recordings of relaxing music paired with progressive muscle relaxation compared with their counterparts who did not listen to music (Hernandez-Ruiz, 2005).

(NR) An RCT ($N = 86$) demonstrated lower anxiety scores in the experimental group ($N = 50$) that listened to music for 20 minutes twice daily following cardiac surgery compared with their counterparts in the control group ($N = 30$) who rested quietly in bed without music (Sendelbach et al., 2006).

(NR) A six-group (music a.m.; music a.m. and p.m.; music a.m. and noc; music a.m., p.m., and noc; quiet rest; control) RCT ($N = 180$) demonstrated that 20-minute relaxing music sessions through headphones offered twice (morning and afternoon or morning and evening) or three times per day (morning, afternoon, and evening) were more effective in reducing anxiety than music once per day, quiet rest, or treatment as usual in people who had experienced acute myocardial infarction (AMI) (Winters, 2005).

■ *Identify the specific change in patients with pain/discomfort that is desired after music sessions.* **LOE = I**

(NR) A four-group (relaxation, music, relaxation and music, control) RCT ($N = 311$) demonstrated that all three treatment groups had significantly less postintervention pain than controls during ambulation and rest on postoperative days 1 and 2 following gynecologic surgery. The group provided with both relaxation and music had significantly less postintervention pain than those with all three conditions on postoperative day 2 only. When music alone was compared with relaxation alone, the music group had less pain and the relaxation group had less distress, both on day 2 only (Good et al., 2002).

(NR) A three-group (sedative music, scheduled rest, control) RCT ($N = 61$) demonstrated reduced pain in participants who experienced either 30-minute music or scheduled rest sessions compared with the treatment-as-usual group in patients during chair rest after open-heart surgery (Voss et al., 2004).

(NR) A four-group (music, relaxation, combined music and relaxation, control) RCT ($N = 167$) evaluated pain levels in abdominal surgical patients at rest, during ambulation, and after ambulation on postoperative days 1 and 2. Pain was lower in all intervention groups than the

RCT = Randomized Controlled (Clinical) Trial, **NIC** = Nursing Interventions Classification, **NOC** = Nursing Outcomes Classification

control group at rest and at three of the six ambulation measurement points. There were no differences noted after ambulation (Good et al., 2005).

(MR) In a review of 51 studies involving 1867 participants exposed to music and 1796 controls, the studies ($N = 31$) that evaluated use of music for acute postoperative pain revealed pain intensity that was 0.5 unit lower on a scale of 0 to 10 than noted in unexposed participants. Small reductions in opioid consumption were also noted in eight studies (Cepeda et al., 2006).

(NR) A three-group (investigator-selected music, participant-selected music, control) RCT ($N = 60$) demonstrated reduced pain in both music groups compared with the control group in individuals with chronic, nonmalignant pain (Siedliecki & Good, 2006).

■ (NIC) *Assist the individual in assuming a comfortable position.* **LOE = II**

(NR) An RCT ($N = 60$) demonstrated desired outcomes in older adults who listened to music and were assisted into a comfortable position (Lai & Good, 2005).

(NR) A six-group (music a.m.; music a.m. and p.m.; music a.m. and noc; music a.m., p.m., and noc; quiet rest; control) RCT ($N = 180$) demonstrated desired outcomes in AMI patients who listened to music after participants in all six groups were assisted into comfortable positions (Winters, 2005).

■ (NIC) *Limit extraneous stimuli (e.g., lights, sounds, visitors, telephone calls) during the listening experience.* **LOE = II**

(NR) A controlled study ($N = 17$) demonstrated desired outcomes following music sessions in postoperative patients after turning off television, radio, and phone; asking visitors to leave; and placing a sign on the door to keep visitors from entering the room (Aragon et al., 2002).

(NR) A six-group (music a.m.; music a.m. and p.m.; music a.m. and noc; music a.m., p.m., and noc; quiet rest; control) RCT ($N = 180$) demonstrated desired outcomes following music sessions after limiting extraneous stimuli by lowering lights, unplugging the telephone, turning the television off, asking visitors to step out, closing the door, and standing outside the room to ensure that participants would not be disturbed (Winters, 2005).

■ (NIC) *Ensure that the volume is adequate but not too high.* **LOE = II**

(NR) A three-group (sedative music, scheduled rest, control) RCT ($N = 61$) demonstrated desired outcomes when participants were encouraged to adjust the music volume to a comfortable level (Voss et al., 2004).

(NR) A randomized six-group (music a.m.; music a.m. and p.m.; music a.m. and noc; music a.m., p.m., and noc; quiet rest; control) RCT ($N = 180$) demonstrated desired outcomes after music sessions when participants were encouraged to adjust the music volume to a comfortable level (Winters, 2005).

■ (NIC) *Facilitate the individual's active participation (e.g., playing an instrument or singing) if this is desired and feasible within the setting.* **LOE = III**

(MR) A controlled study ($N = 26$) demonstrated improvements in emotional status/psychological well-being in both songwriting and lyric analysis groups in people undergoing treatment for chemical dependency (Jones, 2005).

NR = Nursing Research, **MR** = Multidisciplinary Research, **SP** = Standard of Practice, **EO** = Expert Opinion, **LOE** = Level of Evidence

■ **NIC** *Choose particular music selections representative of the individual's preferences.* **LOE = I**

NR A three-group (sedative music, scheduled rest, control) RCT ($N = 61$) demonstrated desired outcomes in participants who listened to self-selected music during chair rest after open-heart surgery (Voss et al., 2004).

NR A three-group (music, silent headphones, control) RCT ($N = 180$) demonstrated desired outcomes in the experimental group who listened to 30 minutes of preferred music compared with the placebo and control groups in preoperative day surgery patients (Cooke et al., 2005).

NR An RCT ($N = 60$) demonstrated desired outcomes in older adults who were asked to choose from six 45-minute music recordings (Lai & Good, 2005).

NR A three-group (investigator-selected music, self-selected music, control) RCT ($N = 60$) demonstrated desired outcomes in participants who listened to both investigator-selected and self-selected music groups (Siedliecki & Good, 2006).

NR A six-group (music a.m.; music a.m. and p.m.; music a.m. and noc; music a.m., p.m., and noc; quiet rest; control) RCT ($N = 180$) demonstrated desired outcomes in participants who were encouraged to select from a list of seventeen 20-minute recordings representing a wide array of musical genres (Winters, 2005).

■ **NIC** *Provide headphones, as indicated.* **LOE = I**

NR A three-group (sedative music, scheduled rest, control) RCT ($N = 61$) demonstrated desired outcomes in participants who listened to self-selected music through headphones during chair rest after open-heart surgery (Voss et al., 2004).

NR A four-group RCT ($N = 167$) demonstrated desired outcomes in participants who listened to music through headphones (Good et al., 2005).

NR A three-group (investigator-selected music, self-selected music, control) RCT ($N = 60$) demonstrated desired outcomes in participants who listened to music through headphones (Siedliecki & Good, 2006).

NR A six-group (music a.m.; music a.m. and p.m.; music a.m. and noc; music a.m., p.m., and noc; quiet rest; control) RCT ($N = 180$) demonstrated desired outcomes when music was delivered through headphones (Winters, 2005).

■ **NIC** *Avoid turning music on and leaving it on for long periods.* **LOE = I**

NR A three-group (sedative music, scheduled rest, control) RCT ($N = 61$) demonstrated desired outcomes in participants who listened to 30 minutes of self-selected music through headphones during chair rest after open-heart surgery (Voss et al., 2004).

NR A three-group (music, silent headphones, control) RCT ($N = 180$) demonstrated desired outcomes in participants provided a 30-minute session of preferred music (Cooke et al., 2005).

NR An RCT ($N = 60$) demonstrated desired outcomes in older adults who listened to 45-minute music recordings (Lai & Good, 2005).

NR A six-group (music a.m.; music a.m. and p.m.; music a.m. and noc; music a.m., p.m., and noc; quiet rest; control) RCT ($N = 180$) demonstrated desired outcomes when participants were provided with a 20-minute music listening experience (Winters, 2005).

RCT = Randomized Controlled (Clinical) Trial, **NIC** = Nursing Interventions Classification, **NOC** = Nursing Outcomes Classification

Possibly Effective

■ *Identify the specific change in patients with depression that is desired after the music session.* **LOE = II**

> NR A three-group (investigator-selected music, self-selected music, control) RCT ($N = 60$) demonstrated reduced depression in both music groups compared with the control group in individuals with chronic, nonmalignant pain (Siedliecki & Good, 2006).

■ *Identify the specific change in heart rate that is desired after the music session.* **LOE = II**

> NR A six-group (music a.m.; music a.m. and p.m.; music a.m. and noc; music a.m., p.m., and noc; quiet rest; control) RCT ($N = 180$) demonstrated in people who had experienced AMI that 20-minute relaxing music sessions via headphones offered twice (morning and afternoon or morning and evening) or three times per day (morning, afternoon, and evening) were more effective in reducing heart rate than music once per day, quiet rest, or treatment as usual (Winters, 2005).

■ *Identify the specific change in heart rate variability (HRV) that is desired after the music session.* **LOE = II**

> NR A six-group (music a.m.; music a.m. and p.m.; music a.m. and noc; music a.m., p.m., and noc; quiet rest; control) RCT ($N = 180$) demonstrated that 20-minute relaxing music sessions through headphones offered twice (morning and afternoon or morning and evening) or three times per day (morning, afternoon, and evening) were more effective in increasing HRV than music once per day, quiet rest, or treatment as usual in people who had experienced AMI (Winters, 2005).

■ *Identify the specific change in myocardial oxygen (MVO₂) consumption that is desired after the music session.* **LOE = II**

> NR A six-group (music a.m.; music a.m. and p.m.; music a.m. and noc; music a.m., p.m., and noc; quiet rest; control) RCT ($N = 180$) demonstrated that 20-minute relaxing music sessions through headphones offered twice (morning and afternoon or morning and evening) or three times per day (morning, afternoon, and evening) were more effective in reducing MVO_2 consumption than music once per day, quiet rest, or treatment as usual in people who had experienced AMI (Winters, 2005).

■ *Identify the specific change in respiratory rate (RR) that is desired after the music session.* **LOE = II**

> NR A six-group (music a.m.; music a.m. and p.m.; music a.m. and noc; music a.m., p.m., and noc; quiet rest; control) RCT ($N = 180$) demonstrated that 20-minute relaxing music sessions through headphones offered twice (morning and afternoon or morning and evening) or three times per day (morning, afternoon, and evening) were more effective in reducing RR than music once per day, quiet rest, or treatment as usual in people who had experienced AMI (Winters, 2005).

NR = Nursing Research, **MR** = Multidisciplinary Research, **SP** = Standard of Practice, **EO** = Expert Opinion, **LOE** = Level of Evidence

■ *Identify the specific change in systolic blood pressure (SBP) that is desired after the music session.* **LOE = II**

(NR) A controlled study ($N = 17$) demonstrated that postoperative thoracic surgical patients who listened to a single 20-minute live harp music session experienced reduced SBP (Aragon et al., 2002).

(NR) A six-group (music a.m., music a.m. and p.m., music a.m. and noc, music a.m., p.m., and noc, quiet rest, control) RCT ($N = 180$) demonstrated that 20-minute relaxing music sessions via headphones offered twice (morning and afternoon or morning and evening) or three times per day (morning, afternoon, and evening) were more effective in reducing SBP than music once per day, quiet rest, or treatment as usual (Winters, 2005).

■ *Identify the specific change in oxygen saturation (SPO$_2$) that is desired after the music session.* **LOE = III**

(NR) A controlled study ($N = 17$) demonstrated that postoperative thoracic surgical patients who listened to a single 20-minute live harp music session experienced increased SPO$_2$ (Aragon et al., 2002).

■ *Identify the specific change in quality of life (QOL) that is desired after the music session.* **LOE = II**

(MR) An RCT ($N = 80$) demonstrated that the experimental group that received routine hospice services and clinical music therapy had higher QOL (measured by the Hospice Quality of Life–Revised instrument) over time than their counterparts in the control group who were matched with respect to gender and age. Furthermore, QOL improved over time for the experimental group but a reduction in QOL was observed in the control group (Hilliard, 2003).

■ *Identify the specific change in psychological well-being that is desired after the music session.* **LOE = III**

(MR) A controlled study ($N = 26$) demonstrated improvements in emotional status/psychological well-being in both the songwriting and lyric analysis groups in people undergoing treatment for chemical dependency (Jones, 2005).

■ *Identify the specific change in sleep that is desired after the music session.* **LOE = II**

(MR) An RCT ($N = 28$) demonstrated a significant improvement in sleep quality for women who were residing in a women's shelter who had experienced domestic violence and who listened to self-selected 20-minute recordings of relaxing music paired with progressive muscle relaxation compared with their counterparts who did not listen to music (Hernandez-Ruiz, 2005).

(NR) An RCT ($N = 60$) demonstrated improved sleep quality, longer sleep duration, greater sleep efficiency, shorter sleep latency, less sleep disturbance, and less daytime dysfunction in older adults who listened to sedative music at bedtime for 3 weeks compared with their counterparts who did not (Lai & Good, 2005).

RCT = Randomized Controlled (Clinical) Trial, **NIC** = Nursing Interventions Classification, **NOC** = Nursing Outcomes Classification

- **NIC** *Determine the individual's interest in music.* **LOE = II**

 NR A six-group (music a.m.; music a.m. and p.m.; music a.m. and noc; music a.m., p.m., and noc; quiet rest; control) RCT (N = 180) inquired about music listening practices prior to music experiences and demonstrated desired outcomes (Winters, 2005).

- **NIC** *Identify the individual's musical preferences.* **LOE = II**

 NR An RCT (N = 60) demonstrated desired outcomes in older adults who were asked about their musical preference before music sessions (Lai & Good, 2005).

 NR A six-group (music a.m.; music a.m. and p.m.; music a.m. and noc; music a.m., p.m., and noc; quiet rest; control) RCT (N = 180) demonstrated desired outcomes in patients recovering from myocardial infarction when participants were queried about musical preference before music sessions (Winters, 2005).

- **NIC** *Inform the individual as to the purpose of the music experience.* **LOE = II**

 NR A three-group (sedative music, scheduled rest, control) RCT (N = 61) demonstrated desired outcomes when participants were told about the purpose of the music experience (Voss et al., 2004).

 NR A six-group (music a.m.; music a.m. and p.m.; music a.m. and noc; music a.m., p.m., and noc; quiet rest; control) RCT (N = 180) demonstrated desired outcomes when participants were told about the purpose of the music experience (Winters, 2005).

Not Effective

- **NIC** *Make music tapes/compact discs and equipment available to the individual.* **LOE = II**

 MR An RCT (N = 20) found no differences in pain perception between the experimental group that listened to music of their choosing for at least 45 minutes with music made available for use as desired during the 4 hours following minor foot surgery and their counterparts in the control group (Macdonald et al., 2003).

 MR An RCT (N = 58) found no group-by-time interaction effect on pain perception at rest or with movement or on use of morphine via a PCA pump. Comparisons were made between baseline, operative day, and first and second postoperative day measures for the experimental group that listened to 2 to 6 hours of music of their choosing on the day of surgery and their counterparts in the control group (Macdonald et al., 2003).

Possibly Harmful

No applicable published research was found in this category.

OUTCOME MEASUREMENT

ANXIETY LEVEL **NOC**

Definition: Severity of manifested apprehension, tension, or uneasiness arising from an unidentifiable source.

Anxiety Level as evidenced by the following selected NOC indicators:

NR = Nursing Research, **MR** = Multidisciplinary Research, **SP** = Standard of Practice, **EO** = Expert Opinion, **LOE** = Level of Evidence

OUTCOME MEASUREMENT—*cont'd*

- Restlessness
- Distress
- Uneasiness
- Muscle tension
- Irritability
- Indecisiveness
- Difficulty concentrating
- Verbalized apprehension
- Verbalized anxiety
- Exaggerated concern about life events
- Increased blood pressure
- Increased pulse rate
- Sleep pattern disturbance

(Rate each indicator of **Anxiety Level:** 1 = severe, 2 = substantial, 3 = moderate, 4 = mild, 5 = none) (Moorhead et al., 2004).

SLEEP NOC

Definition: Natural periodic suspension of consciousness during which the body is restored.

Sleep as evidenced by the following selected NOC indicators:
- Hours of sleep (at least 5 hr per 24 hr*)
- Sleep pattern
- Sleep quality
- Sleep efficiency (ratio of sleep time/total time trying)
- Sleeps through the night consistently
- Feels rejuvenated after sleep
- Wakeful at appropriate times

(Rate each indicator of **Sleep:** 1 = severely compromised, 2 = substantially compromised, 3 = moderately compromised, 4 = mildly compromised, 5 = not compromised) (Moorhead et al., 2004).

---

* Appropriate for adults

REFERENCES

Aragon D, Farris C, Byers JF. (2002). The effects of harp music in vascular and thoracic surgical patients. *Altern Ther Health Med*, 8(5):52-54, 56-60.

Cepeda MS, Carr DB, Lau J, Alvarez H. (2006). Music for pain relief. *Cochrane Database Syst Rev*, (2): CD004843.

Chang SC, Chen CH. (2005). Effects of music therapy on women's physiologic measures, anxiety, and satisfaction during cesarean delivery. *Res Nurs Health*, 28(6):453-461.

Cooke M, Chaboyer W, Schluter P, Hiratos M. (2005). The effect of music on preoperative anxiety in day surgery. *J Adv Nurs*, 52(1):47-55.

Dochterman JM, Bulechek GM (Eds). (2004). *Nursing Interventions Classification (NIC)*, 4th ed. St. Louis: Mosby.

RCT = Randomized Controlled (Clinical) Trial, **NIC** = Nursing Interventions Classification, **NOC** = Nursing Outcomes Classification

Good M, Anderson GC, Ahn S, Cong X, Stanton-Hicks M. (2005). Relaxation and music reduce pain following intestinal surgery. *Res Nurs Health,* 28(3):240-251.

Good M, Anderson GC, Stanton-Hicks M, Grass JA, Makii M. (2002). Relaxation and music reduce pain after gynecologic surgery. *Pain Manag Nurs,* 3(2):61-70.

Hernandez-Ruiz E. (2005). Effect of music therapy on the anxiety levels and sleep patterns of abused women in shelters. *J Music Ther,* 42(2):140-158.

Hilliard RE. (2003). The effects of music therapy on the quality and length of life of people diagnosed with terminal cancer. *J Music Ther,* 40(2):113-137.

Jones JD. (2005). A comparison of songwriting and lyric analysis techniques to evoke emotional change in a single session with people who are chemically dependent. *J Music Ther,* 42(2):94-110.

Lai HL, Good M. (2005). Music improves sleep quality in older adults. *J Adv Nurs,* 49(3):234-244.

Macdonald AR, Mitchell LA, Dillon T, Serpell MG, Davies JB, Ashley EA. (2003). An empirical investigation of the anxiolytic and pain reducing effects of music. *Psychol Music,* 31(2):187-203.

Moorhead M, Johnson M, Maas M (Eds). (2004). *Nursing Outcomes Classification (NOC),* 3rd ed. St. Louis: Mosby.

Sendelbach SE, Halm MA, Doran KA, Miller EH, Gaillard P. (2006). Effects of music therapy on physiological and psychological outcomes for patients undergoing cardiac surgery. *J Cardiovasc Nurs,* 21(3):194-200.

Siedliecki SL, Good M. (2006). Effect of music on power, pain, depression and disability. *J Adv Nurs,* 54(5):553-562.

Voss JA, Good M, Yates B, Baun MM, Thompson A, Hertzog M. (2004). Sedative music reduces anxiety and pain during chair rest after open-heart surgery. *Pain,* 112(1-2):197-203.

Winters J. (2005). Effects of timing and frequency of relaxing music interventions during acute recovery from acute myocardial infarction. *Am J Crit Care,* 14(3):254-255.

 # MUTUAL GOAL-SETTING NIC

Catherine E. Lein, MS, APRN, FNP-BC; Celia E. Wills, PhD, RN;
Kathleen Gaskill Bappert, BSN, RN, MS

NIC **Definition:** Collaborating with the patient to identify and prioritize care goals, then developing a plan for achieving those goals (Dochterman & Bulechek, 2004).

NURSING ACTIVITIES

Effective

■ SP *Involve patients (mutuality) in care planning, identifying expected outcomes, and evaluating outcomes.* **LOE = VII**

EO Involving patients in care and outcomes planning is beneficial for the patient (ANA, 2004).

■ *Assist patients to identify personal values, set goals, and prioritize goals in order to improve clinical outcomes and quality of life.* **LOE = II**

NR A controlled study of mutual goal setting versus nurse-determined goals for adult male patients ($N = 27$) hospitalized with a diagnosis requiring key lifestyle changes demonstrated that the mutual goal setting group had better goal attainment than the nurse-determined goals group (Czar, 1987).

NR = Nursing Research, **MR** = Multidisciplinary Research, **SP** = Standard of Practice, **EO** = Expert Opinion, **LOE** = Level of Evidence

NR An RCT of mutual goal setting, behavior modification, and mutual goal setting in combination with behavior modification showed that mutual goal setting combined with behavior modification was best for improving self-care in elderly nursing home residents ($N = 79$) (Blair, 1995).

MR An RCT of goal setting in myocardial infarction patients ($N = 180$) who set personal goals resulted in improved quality of well-being and increasing goal attainment over time (Oldridge et al., 1999).

MR An evidence-based review of research on engaging health care users to improve care quality concluded that collaborative care interventions (involving mutual goal setting) resulted in improved health outcomes for chronic disease management (Hibbard, 2003).

NR An RCT of mutual goal setting with heart failure patients ($N = 88$) in home health care resulted in improvements in mental health and quality of life outcomes (Scott et al., 2004).

MR An RCT of patient-centered primary care (involving mutual goal setting) with adult-age patients with medically unexplained symptoms ($N = 200$) resulted in improved mental health, satisfaction, and reduced physical disability and controlled substance use (Smith et al., 2006).

■ *Use goal attainment scaling (GAS) for improving goals identification, achievement, and clinical outcomes.* **LOE = II**

NR An RCT of mutual goal setting and other interventions with moderately intellectually impaired patients ($N = 15$) with behavior problems (using GAS) demonstrated improvement in self-care behaviors (Mate-Kole et al., 1999).

NR An RCT of a wellness intervention for women with multiple sclerosis ($N = 113$) showed that setting incremental goals (with GAS) helped the women to identify and meet their individualized wellness goals and improve mental health and pain scores (Stuifbergen et al., 2003a, b).

MR An RCT of individualized treatment goals for rural frail elderly patients ($N = 265$) using GAS demonstrated clinically important changes in functioning (Rockwood et al., 2003).

Possibly Effective

No applicable published research was found in this category.

Not Effective

No applicable published research was found in this category.

Possibly Harmful:

No applicable published research was found in this category.

OUTCOME MEASUREMENT

PARTICIPATION IN HEALTH CARE DECISIONS

Definition: Personal involvement in selecting and evaluating health care options to achieve desired outcome.

Participation in Health Care Decisions as evidenced by the following selected NOC indicators:

Continued

RCT = Randomized Controlled (Clinical) Trial, **NIC** = Nursing Interventions Classification, **NOC** = Nursing Outcomes Classification

OUTCOME MEASUREMENT—*cont'd*

- Seeks relevant information
- Specifies health outcome preferences
- Identifies barriers to desired outcome achievement
- States intent to act on decision
- Identifies available support for achieving desired outcomes
- Seeks services to meet desired outcomes
- Negotiates for care preferences
- Evaluates satisfaction with health care outcomes

(Rate each indicator of **Participation in Health Care Decisions:** 1 = never demonstrated, 2 = rarely demonstrated, 3 = sometimes demonstrated, 4 = often demonstrated, 5 = consistently demonstrated) (Moorhead et al., 2004).

GOAL ATTAINMENT SCALING (GAS) METHODOLOGY

(Becker et al., 2000; Garwick, 1976; Kiresuk et al., 1994).

REFERENCES

American Nurses Association (ANA). (2004). *Nursing: Scope & standards of practice.* Washington, DC: ANA.

Becker H, Stuifbergen A, Rogers S, Timmerman G. (2000). Goal attainment scaling to measure individual change in intervention studies. *Nurs Res,* 49(3):176-180.

Blair CE. (1995). Combining behavior management and mutual goal setting to reduce physical dependency in nursing home residents. *Nurs Res,* 44(3):160-165.

Czar M. (1987). Two methods of goal setting in middle-aged adults facing critical life changes. *Clin Nurse Spec,* 1(4):171-177.

Dochterman JM, Bulechek GM (Eds). (2004). *Nursing Interventions Classification (NIC),* 4th ed. St. Louis: Mosby.

Garwick G. (1976). The rudiments of goal attainment scaling. In Brintnall J, Garwick G (Eds). *Applications of goal attainment scaling.* Minneapolis, MN: Program Evaluation Resource Center.

Hibbard JH. (2003). Engaging health care consumers to improve the quality of care. *Med Care,* 41(1 Suppl): I61-I70.

Kiresuk T, Smith A, Cardillo J. (1994). *Goal attainment scaling.* Hillsdale, NJ: Erlbaum Associates.

Mate-Kole CC, Danquah SA, Twum M, Danquah AO. (1999). Outcomes of a nonaversive behavior intervention in intellectually impaired individuals using goal attainment scaling. *Nurs Res,* 48(4):220-225.

Moorhead M, Johnson M, Maas M (Eds). (2004). *Nursing Outcomes Classification (NOC),* 3rd ed. St. Louis: Mosby.

Oldridge N, Guyatt G, Crowe J, Feeny D, Jones N. (1999). Goal attainment in a randomized controlled trial of rehabilitation after myocardial infarction. *J Cardiopulm Rehabil,* 19(1):29-34.

Rockwood K, Howlett S, Stadnyk K, Carver D, Powell C, Stolee P. (2003). Responsiveness of goal attainment scaling in a randomized controlled trial of comprehensive geriatric assessment. *J Clin Epidemiol,* 56(8):736-743.

Scott LD, Setter-Kline K, Britton AS. (2004). The effects of nursing interventions to enhance mental health and quality of life among individuals with heart failure. *Appl Nurs Res,* 17(4):248-256.

Smith RC, Lyles JS, Gardiner JC, Sirbu C, Hodges A, Collins C, et al. (2006). Primary care clinicians treat patients with medically unexplained symptoms: A randomized controlled trial. *J Gen Intern Med,* 21(7):671-677.

Stuifbergen AK, Becker H, Blozis S, Timmerman G, Kullberg V. (2003a). A randomized clinical trial of a wellness intervention for women with multiple sclerosis. *Arch Phys Med Rehabil,* 84(4):467-476.

NR = Nursing Research, **MR** = Multidisciplinary Research, **SP** = Standard of Practice, **EO** = Expert Opinion, **LOE** = Level of Evidence

Stuifbergen AK, Becker H, Timmerman GM, Kullberg V. (2003b). The use of individualized goal setting to facilitate behavior change in women with multiple sclerosis. *J Neurosci Nurs*, 35(2):94-99, 106.

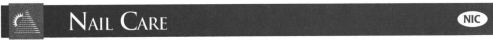

NAIL CARE   NIC

Janet L. Bryant, MSN, RN, CNS, CWCN, COCN; Teresa J. Kelechi, PhD, RN

NIC Definition: Promotion of clean, neat, attractive nails and prevention of skin lesions related to improper care of nails (Dochterman & Bulechek, 2004).

NURSING ACTIVITIES

Effective

■ **SP** *Refer to an appropriate specialist for toenail care for complex conditions including diabetes, peripheral vascular disease, neurological disorders, fungal infections, use of steroids or anticoagulants, and other serious foot disorders.* **LOE = VII**

Diabetes, Peripheral Vascular Disease, Neurological Disorders

EO Periodic professional foot care serves a fundamental role in diabetic preventive care (Harkless et al., 2001).

EO Patients with diabetes and previous foot lesions, especially amputations, require preventive foot care and lifelong surveillance, preferably by a foot care specialist (ADA, 1999).

EO The key to amputation prevention in diabetic patients is early recognition and regular foot screenings from a podiatrist or physician (APMA, 2006).

Fungal Infections

MR A Cochrane systematic review found that fungal infections (onychomycosis) are a common complaint and do not resolve spontaneously. They can be treated either orally or with topical agents; oral treatments are more commonly prescribed for onychomycosis and appear to have the benefit of shorter treatment times and better cure rates than topical preparations (Bell-Syer et al., 2004).

EO People with a toenail infection should be referred to a medical professional for assessment and treatment (Woodrow et al., 2005).

Regular Use of Steroids or Anticoagulants

EO Patients with immunological compromise are susceptible to both bacterial and fungal infections (Harkless et al., 2001).

EO Seniors experience many reasons for the inability to cut their nails, including poor vision, poststroke, cardiac disease, difficulty breathing, and fear that cuts can lead to bleeding, ulceration, infection, and possible amputation (Popoola et al., 2005).

Corns, Calluses, Ingrown Toenails

EO Podiatrists prioritize people with complex needs, such as those taking oral, intra-muscular, or intravenous steroids and those taking regular anticoagulants (Woodrow et al., 2005).

RCT = Randomized Controlled (Clinical) Trial, **NIC** = Nursing Interventions Classification, **NOC** = Nursing Outcomes Classification

(EO) Corns and calluses are caused by friction and pressure when the bony parts of the feet rub against shoes. Over-the-counter medicines contain acids that destroy tissue but do not treat the cause. Seek the advice and treatment of a foot specialist (NIA, 2006).

(EO) Excessive callus acts to elevate pressure, which confirms the importance of professional callus care, especially in the patient at risk for neuropathic ulceration (Cavanaugh et al., 2001).

(MR) A Cochrane systematic review stated that in most cases basic foot care and footwear advice was probably adequate to relieve symptoms of an ingrown toenail, but surgery was the best treatment option to remove permanently either the whole nail or just the troublesome portion of the nail (Rounding & Bloomfield, 2005).

(EO) Conservative management for nondiabetic patients with ingrown toenails includes brief warm water soaks, topical or oral antibiotic therapy, proper nail trimming, and elevation of the corner of the nail with a cotton wick. A more serious ingrown toenail, especially in patients with diabetes, may require surgical intervention (Zuber & Pfenninger, 1995).

Elderly Patients with Sensory Deficits

(EO) Seniors experience many reasons for the inability to cut their nails, including poor vision, poststroke, cardiac disease, difficulty breathing, and fear that cuts can lead to bleeding, ulceration, infection, and possible amputation (Popoola et al., 2005).

■ (SP) *Use mild soap and lukewarm water for washing feet daily.* **LOE = VII**

(EO) Use mild soap in small amounts and a moisturizing cream or lotion on the legs and feet every day (NIA, 2006).

(EO) People who are mobile should wash their feet with mild soap and water daily and pat dry thoroughly with particular attention to the area between the toes (Kelechi & Lukacs, 1994).

■ (SP) *Apply moisturizer to the feet and area around the nails daily but not between the toes.* **LOE = VII**

(EO) To increase skin moisture, apply a lactic acid or urea-based lotion or cream to the feet immediately after bathing. Do not apply lotion in the toe web area because it can macerate, becoming a prime target for infection (Bryant & Beinlich, 1999).

(EO) Applying moisturizing lotion on the feet after bathing can alleviate dry skin (U.S. Food and Drug Administration, 2006).

■ (SP) *Use toenail clippers to trim toenails.* **LOE = VII**

(EO) Nail clippers should be used to trim toenails, maintaining a straight edge (Pattillo, 2004).

(EO) If toenails are fairly thin, nail nippers (clippers) may be used to take small bites of the nail, starting at the outside edge and working in toward the center (Bryant, 1995).

■ (SP) *Trim toenails straight across and not too short.* **LOE = VII**

(EO) Toenails should be trimmed straight across, not too short, and never down into the nail groove (Meadows, 2006; Christensen et al., 1991).

NR = Nursing Research, **MR** = Multidisciplinary Research, **SP** = Standard of Practice, **EO** = Expert Opinion, **LOE** = Level of Evidence

■ **SP** *Use an emery board to maintain toenails between scheduled trimming.*
LOE = VII

EO All sharp or jagged edges or snags of toenails can be smoothed with a file or emery board (Haas & Ahroni, 2001; APMA, 2006).

■ **SP** *Assess nail status and risk for injury.* **LOE = VII**

EO A comprehensive nursing assessment should include status of skin and nails and self-care status (Doughty, 2001).

EO A thorough foot assessment is necessary before the nurse proceeds with nail and foot care. A foot screening tool assists the clinician in performing a consistent, detailed examination (Bryant, 1995).

■ **SP** *Use lamb's wool to separate overlapping toes.* **LOE = VII**

EO Lamb's wool or a small 2 × 2 gauze may be wound between the toes to separate overlapping or contacting toes to help prevent maceration (Haas & Ahroni, 2001; Bryant & Beinlich, 1999).

Possibly Effective

No applicable published research was found in this category.

Not Effective

No applicable published research was found in this category.

Possibly Harmful

■ *Use of a cuticle stick to push back cuticles.* **LOE = VII**

EO Cuticles require special attention; if necessary, gently push them back with a towel or washcloth to avoid injury (Kelechi & Lukacs, 1994).

■ *Use of foot soaks to make nails more conducive to clipping.* **LOE = VII**

EO Soaking is discouraged because excessive soaking can either dry out or macerate the skin (Bryant & Beinlich, 1999; Haas & Ahroni, 2001; Levin, 1993).

OUTCOME MEASUREMENT

NAIL CARE

Definition: Maintaining nails in healthy condition with appropriate grooming.
Nail Care as evidenced by the following indicators:
- Cares for nails
- Nails kept short, clean, and groomed
- Nails free of infection
(Note: This is not a NOC outcome.)

RCT = Randomized Controlled (Clinical) Trial, **NIC** = Nursing Interventions Classification, **NOC** = Nursing Outcomes Classification

REFERENCES

American Diabetes Association (ADA). (1999). Consensus development conference on diabetic foot wound care. *Diabetes Care,* 22(8):1354-1360.

American Podiatric Medical Association (APMA). (2006). *Diabetes: Your podiatric physician talks about diabetes. Information from the American Podiatric Medical Association.* Available online: www.apma.org. Retrieved on June 4, 2007.

Bell-Syer S, Porthouse J, Bigby M. (2004). Oral treatments for toenail onychomycosis. *Cochrane Database Syst Rev,* (2):CD004766.

Bryant JL. (1995). Preventive foot care program: A nursing perspective. *Ostomy Wound Manage,* 41(4):28-30, 32-34.

Bryant JL, Beinlich NR. (1999). Foot care: Focus on the elderly. *Orthop Nurs,* 18(6):53-60.

Cavanaugh P, Ulbrecht J, Caputo G. (2001). The biomechanics of the foot in diabetes mellitus. In Bowker J, Pfeifer M (Eds). *Levin and O'Neal's the diabetic foot,* 6th ed. St. Louis: Mosby, pp 125-196.

Christensen MH, Funnell MM, Ehrlich MR, Fellows EP, Floyd JC. (1991). How to care for the diabetic foot. *Am J Nurs,* 3(3):50-56.

Dochterman JM, Bulechek GM (Eds). (2004). *Nursing Interventions Classification (NIC),* 4th ed. St. Louis: Mosby.

Doughty D. (2001). Role of the wound care nurse. In Bowker J, Pfeifer M (Eds). *Levin and O'Neal's the diabetic foot,* 6th ed. St. Louis: Mosby, pp 676-681.

Haas L, Ahroni J. (2001). Lower limb self-management education. In Bowker J, Pfeifer M (Eds). *Levin and O'Neal's the diabetic foot,* 6th ed. St. Louis: Mosby, pp 665-675.

Harkless L, Satterfield K, Dennis K. (2001). Role of the podiatrist. In Bowker J, Pfeifer M (Eds). *Levin and O'Neal's the diabetic foot,* 6th ed. St. Louis: Mosby, pp 682-699.

Kelechi T, Lukacs K. (1994). Basic foot care: A self-instructional manual. Center for the Study of Aging, Medical University of South Carolina. Charleston, SC.

Levin M. (1993). Pathogenesis and management of diabetic foot lesions. In Levin M, O'Neal L, Bowker J (Eds). *The diabetic foot,* 5th ed. St. Louis: Mosby, pp 17-60.

Meadows M. (2006). Taking care of your feet. *FDA Consum,* 40(2):16-24.

National Institute on Aging (NIA). (2006). *AgePage: Foot Care.* Available online: http://www.nia publications.org. Retrieved on June 4, 2007.

Pattillo MM. (2004). Therapeutic and healing foot care: A healthy feet clinic for older adults. *J Gerontol Nurs,* 30(12):25-32.

Popoola MM, Jenkins L, Griffin O. (2005). Caring for the foot mobile: Holistic foot and nail management. *Holist Nurs Pract,* 19(5):222-227.

Rounding C, Bloomfield S. (2005). Surgical treatments for ingrowing toenails. *Cochrane Database Syst Rev,* (2):CD001541.

U.S. Food and Drug Administration (2006). *Taking Care of Your Feet.* Available online: http://www.fda. gov/fdac/features/2006/206_feet.html. Accessed on June 4, 2007.

Woodrow P, Dickson N, Wright P. (2005). Foot care for non-diabetic older people. *Nurs Older People,* 17(8):31-32.

Zuber TJ, Pfenninger JL. (1995). Management of ingrown toenails. *Am Fam Physician,* 52(1):181-190.

NASOGASTRIC INTUBATION

Kathleen A. Fitzgerald, PhD, RN

Definition: Insertion of a tube through the nares into the pharynx, the esophagus, and down into the stomach for feeding or removal of gastric secretions.

NR = Nursing Research, **MR** = Multidisciplinary Research, **SP** = Standard of Practice, **EO** = Expert Opinion, **LOE** = Level of Evidence

NURSING ACTIVITIES

Effective

■ ⑤ *Prepare patients for the procedure by providing information about the sensations they will experience.* **LOE = VI**

⑥ In a qualitative experiment with hospitalized patients (*N* = 48) undergoing upper endoscopy, four treatment groups (behavioral instruction, sensory information, combination, and control) received information about the procedure in order to reduce emotional reactions and improve cooperative behaviors during the procedure. Outcome measures included amount of diazepam used, heart rate, gagging, and time to effect passage of the tube. The sensory information group received information about the specific sensations they would experience during the procedure. There were significant differences between this group and the other three groups with a decrease in use of diazepam, decrease in gagging, and stable heart rate. There was no effect on the length of time for tube passage (Johnson & Leventhal, 1974).

■ ⑤ *Provide a calm environment and use simple directions describing the patient's experiences and behaviors necessary to facilitate insertion of the nasogastric (NG) tube.* **LOE = VI**

⑥ A qualitative study of the comfort strategies used by emergency room nurses when inserting NG tubes (32 subjects with 49 attempts [*N* = 49]) showed that successful attempts at NG insertion involved a combination or blend of highly technical and affective styles. Strategies used by the nurses while inserting NG tubes included reassuring touch, comforting talk, and keeping things calm. Comforting talk was characterized as melodic and rhythmic, patterned and repetitive. Terms used in the description of the discomfort of the procedure were moderate versus extreme (e.g., uncomfortable instead of terrible). Movement was unhurried and efficient, establishing a calm environment. The goal of these strategies was to keep the patient focused on the task at hand—swallowing the tube (Penrod et al., 1999).

⑥ Videotapes in the previous study were reviewed using a code book of nursing behaviors categorized into four nursing approaches: technical, affective, blended, and mixed. The technical approach placed priority on the technical aspects of tube placement such as curling the tip, warming the tube, and determining the length and little on patients' comfort. The affective approach focused on minimizing the patient's discomfort and considered the technical aspects only when handling the tube. The blended approach focused on the procedure while acknowledging the patient's sensations and forewarning the patient of impending discomfort. The mixed approach was coded when two people were performing the procedure and manifested different approaches. The technical approach took more time to insert the tube than did the blended approach. The blended approach appeared to be the most effective and efficient (Morse et al., 2000).

■ ⑤ *Measure the tube length for placement using the updated Hanson method.* **LOE = VI**

⑥ An observational study using 99 adult cadavers and five normal volunteers demonstrated the nose-to-ear-to-xiphoid (NEX) measurement to be inaccurate. A formula was designed based on the actual measurements ([NEX − 50 cm]/2) + 50 cm. This formula resulted in the tube placement 1 to 10 cm in the stomach 91% of the time (Hanson, 1979).

RCT = Randomized Controlled (Clinical) Trial, **NIC** = Nursing Interventions Classification, **NOC** = Nursing Outcomes Classification

NR A cross-sectional study of adult subjects undergoing esophageal motility studies ($N = 76$) developed a clinical prediction rule or method for predicting gastric tube insertion from the nares to the lower esophageal sphincter (LES) in adults, predicted a placement distance to locate the tube into the stomach, and compared it with the NEX method and Hanson method. The location of the LES was verifiable by the esophageal motility study. Twenty-four variables were used in the prediction calculations and 20 external measurements obtained. The final formula included the patient's gender, weight, and nose-to-umbilicus measurement while lying flat, and a nomogram was created to facilitate use of the complex formula. The final formula had higher predicted accuracy than the NEX and Hanson methods; Hanson's method with some recommended updates for current tube types was validated as accurate by the formula (Ellett et al., 2005).

EO Measurement of the NEX has been the standard practice but has not been verified by research. This procedure more likely measures the length to the LES than the gastric body and should be used with caution with tubes that have multiple openings at the tip (e.g., most feeding tubes) (Ellett et al., 2005).

■ *Provide for patient's comfort during the insertion process by using lidocaine spray alone or in combination with lidocaine gel as ordered.* **LOE = II**

MR In a double-blind, placebo-controlled, randomized trial of adult patients ($N = 70$), 29 patients received nebulized lidocaine and 21 received nebulized normal saline. Patients rated their discomfort on a 100-mm visual analogue scale (0 = no discomfort, 100 = severe discomfort), and the difficulty of insertion was rated on a five-point Likert scale. The results indicated a mean score of 37.7 mm for those receiving lidocaine and 59.3 mm for those receiving normal saline. There was no difference in the difficulty in tube passage identified by nurses, and patients who received lidocaine had more complications including epistaxis and dyspnea, with chest tightness in one patient (Cullen et al., 2004).

MR In a double-blind, double-dummy, randomized triple crossover design involving healthy volunteers ($N = 30$), each patient had three NG tubes placed acting as the patient's own control for the three study medications: lidocaine gel, lidocaine spray, and atomized cocaine. A visual analogue scale (0 to 100) was used for pain and global discomfort. Patients who were asked to identify which study medication they preferred rated all the medications as equally effective in pain control. The lidocaine gel was identified as significantly better for overall discomfort scores. Patients preferred the lidocaine gel (Ducharme & Matheson, 2003).

MR In a randomized, double-blind, placebo-controlled trial with adult patients ($N = 40$) in the emergency room, randomly assigned patients ($N = 20$) received atomized lidocaine or normal saline in their oropharynx. All patients received lidocaine gel intranasally during the insertion. Using a visual analogue scale (0 = least possible pain, 100 = worst possible pain) immediately after securing the tube, mean pain scores for the lidocaine group were statistically and clinically significantly lower than for the placebo group (Wolfe et al., 2000).

■ SP *Obtain an x-ray film to confirm correct placement of a blindly inserted small-bore enteral tube or a large-bore tube before beginning feedings or administering medications.* **LOE = VII**

MR A descriptive review of complications associated with bedside placement of feeding tubes noted that most institutions required feeding tube placement confirmed by chest x-ray films to avoid complications of inadvertent bronchial, pleural, or lung placement. The author also

NR = Nursing Research, **MR** = Multidisciplinary Research, **SP** = Standard of Practice, **EO** = Expert Opinion, **LOE** = Level of Evidence

noted that many institutions now require radiographic confirmation that NG tube ports are in the stomach (as opposed to the esophagus) prior to the administration of bowel preparation solutions, medications, or feedings, to prevent inadvertent aspiration of these materials (Baskin, 2006).

(EO) Because of the possibility of tube malposition in the tracheobronchial tree, radiographic confirmation of the position of the feeding tube tip is recommended (ASPEN, 2002).

(EO) X-ray confirmation of correct placement of any NG tube to be used for feeding or medication administration remains the "gold standard" (Metheny, 2006, 2007).

▪ (SP) *Provide oral care at least every 2 to 4 hours or as needed per day to prevent overgrowth of oropharyngeal bacteria. Patients who are NPO or tube fed should have oral hygiene offered or performed as frequently as patients with endotracheal intubation.* **LOE = VII**

(MR) In a comparative review of three groups of patients in six nursing and skilled nursing facilities, group 1 ($N = 78$) received NG tube feedings, group 2 ($N = 57$) received percutaneous inserted gastrostomy tube feedings, and group 3 ($N = 80$) were orally fed patients and considered the control group. Cultures of the oropharynx were taken in the morning hours before breakfast and before the performance of oral care. There was a significantly higher rate of pathogenic bacteria (i.e., gram-negative bacilli isolated from the oropharynx) of both tube-fed groups versus those who were able to eat. *Pseudomonas aeruginosa* was found only in the oropharynx in the NG tube-fed patients. *Klebsiella* and *Proteus* were cultured from all patients but were most prevalent in those receiving tube feedings (Leibovitz et al., 2003).

(EO) Bacteria grow rapidly in the mouth of patients who do not eat; these patients are missing the process of eating to wash down contaminated oral secretions into the stomach (Logsdon, 2004).

(EO) A summary article discussed the bacterial colonization of the oropharynx that occurs in patients with endotracheal tubes that may result in aspiration pneumonia. Feeding or other NG tubes are also risk factors for aspiration. An oral hygiene protocol was instituted in a community hospital based on evidence in the literature and was described to have decreased the incidence of aspiration pneumonia in the ICU. The protocol emphasized removing dental plaque with brushing of the teeth and use of an antiseptic oral rinse every 2 to 4 hours (Schleder, 2003).

▪ (SP) *Secure the tube to the nose, avoiding pressure on the nare and movement of the tube; change the tape or device holding the nasogastric or nasoenteric tube in place daily. Check the mark or length of the external portion of the tube to make sure that the tube is the same length as when inserted before retaping.* **LOE = VII**

(MR) A case study reported that improper taping of the tube to the nose may result in excessive pulling or pressure on the nare with subsequent necrosis requiring cosmetic surgical repair (Lai et al., 2001).

Possibly Effective

▪ *Measure the pH of the aspirate to determine gastric placement.* **LOE = VI**

(EO) The pH in the stomach is generally in the range of 1 to 5, versus the lung secretions and intestinal aspirate, which usually have a pH of 7 or higher (Metheny & Titler, 2001).

RCT = Randomized Controlled (Clinical) Trial, **NIC** = Nursing Interventions Classification, **NOC** = Nursing Outcomes Classification

(NR) An observational study of patients with an NG tube or nasointestinal tube ($N = 605$ patients, 794 aspirates) demonstrated that pH testing could differentiate gastric placement from intestinal placement, and four tubes inadvertently inserted into the respiratory tract all had values greater than 6.5 (Metheny et al., 1993).

(NR) A summary article on the use of pH meter testing to determine feeding tube placement indicated that 85% of gastric tube aspirates had a pH reading of 6 or less. When the sample was examined for the use of acid-inhibiting medications, it was determined that pH measured greater than 6 in 18% of the patients. Eighty-seven percent of the intestinal aspirates had a pH greater than 6. Results indicated that using pH meters was an alternative method in determining the placement of NG or nasoenteric tubes (Metheny et al., 1994a). (Note: This study was conducted prior to the use of proton pump inhibitors.)

(NR) In a descriptive study of the efficacy of using pH testing to confirm placement of NG tubes, 29% of the patients with NG tubes did not have an accurate pH in determining placement because the patient was receiving H_2 blockers and proton pump inhibitors, which produced false readings; some brands of pH strips were inaccurate or their results were misinterpreted by staff (Taylor & Clemente, 2005).

■ Observe the aspirate. LOE = VII

(NR) In a controlled study, staff nurses were shown photographs of a sample of 106 aspirates from feeding tubes and asked to predict tube position. Their ability to identify 50 gastric aspirates and 50 intestinal aspirates improved significantly after reading a list of suggested characteristics of feeding tube aspirates. Gastric aspirates were most likely to be green (cloudy), off-white or tan (cloudy), bloody or brown (cloudy), or colorless (clear). Intestinal aspirates were most likely to be yellow or bile stained (usually clear but sometimes cloudy). Pleural aspirates were likely to be light yellow in color, clear, and perhaps blood-tinged. Tracheobronchial aspirates primarily contained mucus and were more likely to be opaque and off-white or tan in color (Metheny et al., 1994b).

(EO) Aspirate from the stomach is usually green, brown, clear, and colorless with mucus, whereas aspirate from the lungs is off-white to tan mucus or bloody from trauma. If the tube is in the esophagus, it is generally very difficult to obtain any aspirate (Metheny & Titler, 2001).

■ Measure the external length of the tube and record. LOE = VII

(EO) Once the placement of the feeding tube has been confirmed by x-ray, it is helpful to have a measurement of the external length of the tube. The area of the tube exiting the nare should be marked on the tube. The Salem sump tubes have markings already on the tube, which should be recorded and checked daily or prior to use for medications or feeding. This original distance can be used as the standard distance that should remain to help detect dislodgement of the tube (Metheny et al., 2005).

Not Effective

■ Using the auscultation method to differentiate between respiratory and gastric placement of a nasogastric feeding tube or gastric versus esophagus placement of a nasogastric tube. LOE = VI

(NR) A descriptive study of 85 acutely ill patients and 123 taped auscultations was conducted to determine whether air insufflated through feeding tubes ending in the esophagus, stomach,

---

NR = Nursing Research, **MR** = Multidisciplinary Research, **SP** = Standard of Practice, **EO** = Expert Opinion, **LOE** = Level of Evidence

duodenum, and proximal jejunum would produce different pitch and volume of sounds. Expert raters listened to the sounds and recorded their impressions. X-ray films were taken to verify the feeding tube tip placement. Overall results revealed correct classifications of the tapes 34.4% of the time, indicating that air insufflation was an inaccurate procedure to use to verify feeding tube placement (Metheny et al., 1990).

(EO) There have been multiple case reports of small-bore feeding tubes being inserted into the lung following use of the auscultation method to check placement. This has also happened with large-bore feeding tubes. The auscultatory method can also fail to detect when a tube's ports are situated in the esophagus as opposed to the stomach (Metheny, 2006).

Possibly Harmful

■ *Inserting a nasogastric tube in patients with a severe craniofacial or basilar skull fracture or transsphenoidal surgical procedure.* **LOE = VII**

(EO) Do not place NG tubes when these conditions are present; there have been multiple case reports of an NG tube being inserted into the brain. Because it is possible for even an orally placed tube to enter the brain under these conditions, laryngoscopic or fluoroscopic guidance may be needed to ensure safe placement (Metheny 2006; Baskaya, 1999; Genu et al., 2004; Rahimi-Movaghar et al., 2005; Ferreras et al., 2000).

OUTCOME MEASUREMENT

NASOGASTRIC INTUBATION

Definition: Nasogastric tube inserted into the stomach for feeding or decompression of the stomach without complications.

Nasogastric Intubation as evidenced by the following indicators:
- X-ray confirmation of stomach placement
- pH of gastric secretions below 6
- Appearance of the gastric contents
- Patient's comfort
- Normal lung sounds

(Note: This is not a NOC outcome.)

REFERENCES

ASPEN Board of Directors and the Clinical Guidelines Task Force. (2002). Guidelines for the use of parenteral and enteral nutrition in adult and pediatric patients. Section VIII: Access for administration of nutritional support. *JPEN*, 26(1 Suppl):33SA-35SA.

Baskaya MK. (1999). Inadvertent intracranial placement of a nasogastric tube in patients with head injuries. *Surg Neurol*, 52(4):426-427.

Baskin WN. (2006). Acute complications associated with bedside placement of feeding tubes. *Nutr Clin Pract*, 21(1):40-55.

Cullen L, Taylor D, Taylor S, Chu K. (2004). Nebulized lidocaine decreases the discomfort of nasogastric tube insertion: A randomized, double-blind trial. *Ann Emerg Med*, 44(2):131-137.

Ducharme J, Matheson K. (2003). What is the best topical anesthetic for nasogastric insertion? A comparison of lidocaine gel, lidocaine spray, and atomized cocaine. *J Emerg Nurs*, 29(5):427-430.

RCT = Randomized Controlled (Clinical) Trial, **NIC** = Nursing Interventions Classification, **NOC** = Nursing Outcomes Classification

Ellett ML, Beckstrand J, Flueckiger J, Perkins SM, Johnson CS. (2005). Predicting the insertion distance for placing gastric tubes. *Clin Nurs Res*, 14(1):11-27.

Ferreras J, Junquera LM, Garcia-Consuegra L. (2000). Intracranial placement of a nasogastric tube after severe craniofacial trauma. *Oral Surg Oral Med Oral Pathol Oral Radiol Endod*, 90(5):564-566.

Genu PR, de Oliveira DM, Vasconcellos RJ, Noqueira RV, Vasconcellos BC. (2004). Inadvertent intracranial placement of a nasogastric tube in a patient with severe craniofacial trauma: A case report. *J Oral Maxillofac Surg*, 62(11):1435-1438.

Hanson RL. (1979). Predictive criteria for length of nasogastric tube insertion for tube feeding. *JPEN*, 3(3):160-163.

Johnson JE, Leventhal H. (1974). Effects of accurate expectations and behavioral instructions on reactions during a noxious medical examination. *J Pers Soc Psychol*, 29(5):710-718.

Lai PB, Pang PC, Chan SK, Lau WY. (2001). Necrosis of the nasal ala after improper taping of a nasogastric tube. *Int J Clin Pract*, 55(2):145.

Leibovitz A, Plotnikov G, Habot B, Rosenberg M, Segal R. (2003). Pathogenic colonization of oral flora in frail elderly patients fed by nasogastric tube or percutaneous enterogastric tube. *J Gerontol A Biol Sci Med Sci*, 58(1):52-55

Logsdon BK. (2004). Preventing aspiration pneumonia in at-risk residents. *Nurs Homes Long Term Care Manag*, 53(8):60-62.

Metheny NA. (2006). Preventing respiratory complications of tube feedings: Evidence-based practice. *Am J Crit Care*, 15(4):360-369.

Metheny NA. (2007). Letters to the Editor. Confirmation of nasogastric tube placement. *Am J Crit Care*, 16(1):19.

Metheny NA, Clouse RE, Clark JM, Reed L, Wehrle MA, Wiersema L. (1994a). pH testing of feeding-tube aspirates to determine placement. *Nutr Clin Pract* 9(5):185-190.

Metheny N, McSweeney M, Wehrle MA, Wiersema L. (1990). Effectiveness of the auscultatory method in predicting feeding tube location. *Nurs Res*, 39(5):262-267.

Metheny N, Reed L, Berglund B, Wehrle MA. (1994b). Visual characteristics of aspirates from feeding tubes as a method for predicting tube location. *Nurs Res*, 43(5):282-287.

Metheny N, Reed R, Wiersema L, McSweeney M, Wehrle MA, Clark J. (1993). Effectiveness of pH measurements in predicting feeding tube placement: An update. *Nurs Res*, 42(6):324-331.

Metheny NA, Schnelker R, McGinnis J, Zimmerman G, Duke C, Merritt B, et al. (2005). Indicators of tubesite during feedings. *J Neurosci Nurs*, 37(6):320-325.

Metheny NA, Titler MG. (2001). Assessing placement of feeding tubes, *Am J Nurs*, 101(5):36-45.

Morse JM, Penrod J, Kassab C, Dellasega C. (2000). Evaluating the efficiency and effectiveness of approaches to nasogastric tube insertion during trauma care. *Am J Crit Care*, 9(5):325-333.

Penrod J, Morse JM, Wilson S. (1999). Comforting strategies used during nasogastric tube insertion. *J Clin Nurs*, 8(1):31-38.

Rahimi-Movaghar V, Boroojeny SB, Moghtaderi A, Keshmirian B. (2005). Intracranial placement of a nasogastric tube. A lesson to be re-learnt? *Acta Neurochir*, 147(5):573-574.

Schleder BJ. (2003). Taking charge of hospital-acquired pneumonia *Nurse Pract*. 29(3):50-53.

Taylor SJ, Clemente R. (2005). Confirmation of nasogastric tube position by pH testing. *J Hum Nutr Diet*, 18(5):371-375.

Wolfe TR, Fosnocht DE, Linscott MS. (2000). Atomized lidocaine as topical anesthesia for nasogastric tube placement: A randomized, double-blind, placebo-controlled trial. *Ann Emerg Med*, 35(5):421-425.

 # NAUSEA MANAGEMENT: CANCER

Suzanne L. Dibble, DNSc, RN; Janelle M. Tipton, MSN, RN, AOCN

Definition: Prevention and alleviation of nausea associated with cancer, including cancer treatment.

NR = Nursing Research, **MR** = Multidisciplinary Research, **SP** = Standard of Practice, **EO** = Expert Opinion, **LOE** = Level of Evidence

Anticipatory nausea is nausea that occurs before patients receive their next chemotherapy treatment. It is a conditioned response and can occur after a negative past experience with chemotherapy. Prevention is key, especially early in therapy. *Acute nausea* usually occurs within a few minutes to several hours after chemotherapy administration and often resolves within the first 24 hours. *Delayed nausea* usually occurs more than 24 hours after chemotherapy administration, often peaking 48 to 72 hours after chemotherapy, and can last over a week (NCCN, 2006).

NURSING ACTIVITIES

Effective

■ *Use manual acupressure at P6 to reduce the amount and intensity of nausea.*
   LOE = I

   (NR) An RCT ($N = 160$) demonstrated that use of acupressure at P6 was more effective than placebo acupressure or no intervention in treating delayed chemotherapy-induced nausea (Dibble et al., 2006).

   (NR) An RCT ($N = 17$) demonstrated that use of acupressure at P6 was more effective than no intervention in treating acute and delayed chemotherapy-induced nausea (Dibble et al., 2000).

   (NR) An RCT ($N = 40$) demonstrated that use of acupressure at P6 was more effective than no intervention in treating acute and delayed chemotherapy-induced nausea; nausea was less frequent, less severe, and of shorter duration in the intervention group (Shin et al., 2004).

   (MR) A systematic review pooled the results of 11 clinical trials ($N = 1247$) and determined that acupressure reduced mean acute nausea severity (Ezzo et al., 2005, 2006).

■ *Use guided imagery and progressive muscle relaxation to reduce nausea.*
   LOE = I

   (MR) A meta-analysis of 15 studies ($N = 742$) determined that relaxation training significantly reduced the incidence of nausea (Luebbert et al., 2001).

   (MR) An RCT ($N = 60$) assessing the effectiveness of progressive muscle relaxation training and guided imagery demonstrated significantly less anticipatory and postchemotherapy nausea than in the control group (Yoo et al., 2005).

   (MR) In an RCT ($N = 71$) of Chinese women with breast cancer, 25 minutes of progressive muscle relaxation with 5 minutes of guided imagery was superior to standard antiemetic treatment alone in managing acute and delayed nausea (Molassiotis et al., 2002).

■ *Use psychoeducational support and information to help reduce nausea associated with chemotherapy.* **LOE = I**

   (NR) In a randomized controlled study ($N = 70$), women with breast cancer listened to informational audiotapes on self-care behaviors related to chemotherapy. The occurrence and intensity of nausea were reduced, and the experimental group used more self-care behaviors (Williams & Schreier, 2004).

   (MR) A meta-analysis of 116 intervention studies ($N = 5326$) indicated that psychoeducational and psychosocial care had beneficial effects for nausea in cancer (Devine & Westlake, 1995).

RCT = Randomized Controlled (Clinical) Trial, **NIC** = Nursing Interventions Classification, **NOC** = Nursing Outcomes Classification

■ *Give effective antiemetic drugs to prevent nausea, when possible.* **LOE = I**

(MR) For highly and moderately emetogenic chemotherapy regimens, a 5-HT$_3$ receptor antagonist and a corticosteroid in addition to a neurokinin-1 receptor antagonist are recommended for acute and delayed nausea and vomiting. A benzodiazepine is used effectively for anticipatory nausea and vomiting. Pharmacological interventions for nausea and vomiting are recommended based on the type of nausea and/or vomiting and the emetogenicity of the chemotherapy. The National Comprehensive Cancer Network, Antiemesis Practice Guidelines (2006) and the Results of the 2004 Perugia International Antiemesis Consensus Conference (2006), meta-analyses, and systematic reviews support the use of the various classes of antiemetic agents (NCCN, 2006; Roila et al., 2006).

Possibly Effective

■ *Use a properly placed acustimulation device such as a ReliefBand to assist with treating nausea.* **LOE = II**

(MR) In a randomized, double-blind, placebo-controlled parallel-subjects trial with a follow-up crossover trial ($N = 42$ gynecological cancer patients), the severity of nausea was significantly reduced when patients were using the ReliefBand during days 2 to 4 (Pearl et al., 1999).

(MR) In an RCT using a three-level crossover design ($N = 27$) comparing three groups—(1) acustimulation P6, (2) sham acustimulation, and (3) no intervention—no statistically significant differences in average severity of nausea between the groups was demonstrated. However, the data showed a trend that acustimulation compared with no acustimulation reduced the severity of delayed nausea. In addition, patients took fewer antinausea pills during the active-acustimulation cycle of this experiment compared with the no-acustimulation phase (Roscoe et al., 2002).

(MR) In a randomized double-blind study ($N = 49$) of an active ReliefBand versus an inactive device, there was a significant reduction of nausea severity in those wearing the active device (Treish et al., 2003).

(MR) In an RCT ($N = 729$) comparing three groups—(1) acustimulation P6, (2) acupressure band, and (3) no intervention—no statistically significant differences in delayed nausea between the groups was demonstrated. However, the data showed that the acupressure band group had significantly less nausea on the treatment day (Roscoe et al., 2003).

(MR) A systematic review pooling the results of 11 clinical trials ($N = 1247$) determined that there was no benefit to using the ReliefBand (Ezzo et al., 2005, 2006).

■ *Use a properly placed acupressure device such as a Sea-Band to assist with treating nausea.* **LOE = II**

(MR) In an RCT ($N = 86$) comparing three groups of women undergoing chemotherapy for breast cancer—(1) acupressure bands at P6, (2) acustimulation at P6, and (3) no intervention—the proportion of patients reporting severe nausea was significantly less in the acupressure band group compared with the no-intervention group (Roscoe et al., 2006).

(MR) In an RCT ($N = 729$) comparing three groups—(1) acustimulation at P6, (2) acupressure band, and (3) no intervention—no statistically significant differences in delayed nausea between the groups were demonstrated. However, the data showed that the acupressure band

NR = Nursing Research, **MR** = Multidisciplinary Research, **SP** = Standard of Practice, **EO** = Expert Opinion, **LOE** = Level of Evidence

group had significantly less nausea on the treatment day than the no-intervention group (Roscoe et al., 2003).

■ *Use the herb ginger (Zingiber officinale) to assist with treating nausea.* **LOE = II**

(NR) In a randomized double-blind study ($N = 41$), participants received either ginger or a placebo after the administration of prochlorperazine (Compazine). The ginger group had greater symptomatic relief (Pace, 1987).

(MR) A randomized double-blind crossover study ($N = 48$ gynecologic cancer patients) compared 1 g/day ginger root powder versus placebo for acute nausea and the same ginger dose compared with metoclopramide for delayed nausea. For acute nausea, there was no significant improvement with the addition of ginger. For delayed nausea, there was no significant difference in efficacy between metoclopramide and ginger (Manusirivithaya et al., 2004).

(MR) In a controlled laboratory study on rats, following cisplatin administration, significant inhibition of gastric emptying occurred, which was partially reversed by pretreatment with ginger extract and ginger juice (Sharma & Gupta, 1998).

(MR) In a controlled laboratory study on dogs, following cisplatin administration, significant inhibition of gastric emptying occurred, which was partially reversed by pretreatment with ginger extract and ginger juice (Sharma et al., 1997).

Not Effective

■ *Using virtual reality intervention for reducing symptom distress through the use of distraction in patients receiving chemotherapy.* **LOE = II**

(NR) A study using a crossover design ($N = 20$) utilized virtual reality as a distraction intervention for women receiving chemotherapy. Symptom distress scores, including the incidence of nausea, were significantly lower immediately following the intervention. When symptoms were measured 48 hours after chemotherapy, the results were not statistically significant but trended toward a reduction in symptom distress, including nausea (Schneider et al., 2004).

(NR) A randomized study using a crossover design examined the effects of virtual reality distraction on chemotherapy symptom distress in women age 50 and older ($N = 16$). The results were not statistically significant but trended toward improved symptoms 48 hours after the completion of the chemotherapy. The participants did not experience cybersickness (a complication causing dizziness and nausea) (Schneider et al., 2003).

Possibly Harmful

No applicable published research was found in this category.

OUTCOME MEASUREMENT

NAUSEA CONTROL

Definition: Ability to prevent or alleviate nausea.
Nausea Control as evidenced by the following indicators:
- Reports onset of nausea promptly
- Recognizes stimuli resulting in nausea
- Uses diary to record symptoms over time

Continued

RCT = Randomized Controlled (Clinical) Trial, **NIC** = Nursing Interventions Classification, **NOC** = Nursing Outcomes Classification

OUTCOME MEASUREMENT—*cont'd*

- Uses measures to prevent nausea
- Reduces frequency of nausea
- Reduces intensity of nausea
- Uses antiemetic medications as needed
- Reports continuation of nausea following treatment

(Note: This is not a NOC outcome.)

REFERENCES

Devine EC, Westlake SK. (1995). The effects of psychoeducational care provided to adults with cancer: Meta-analysis of 116 studies. *Oncol Nurs Forum*, 22(9):1369-1381.

Dibble SL, Chapman J, Mack KA, Shih AS. (2000). Acupressure for nausea: Results of a pilot study. *Oncol Nurs Forum*, 27(1):41-47.

Dibble SL, Luce J, Cooper BA, Israel J, Cohen M, Nussey B, et al. (2007). Acupressure for delayed chemotherapy induced nausea & vomiting: A RCT. *Oncol Nurs Forum* (In press).

Ezzo J, Vickers A, Richardson MA, Allen C, Dibble SL, Issell B, et al. (2005). Acupuncture-point stimulation for chemotherapy-induced nausea and vomiting. *J Clin Oncol*, 23(28):7188-7198.

Ezzo JM, Richardson MA, Vickers A, Allen C, Dibble SL, Issell BF, et al. (2006). Acupuncture-point stimulation for chemotherapy-induced nausea or vomiting. *Cochrane Database Syst Rev*, (2)CD002285.

Luebbert K, Dahme B, Hasenbring M. (2001). The effectiveness of relaxation training in reducing treatment-related symptoms and improving emotional adjustment in acute non-surgical cancer treatment: A meta-analytical review. Psychooncology, 10(6):490-502.

Manusirivithaya S, Sripramote M, Tangjitgamol S, Sheanakul C, Leelahakorn S, Thavaramara T, et al. (2004). Antiemetic effect of ginger in gynecologic oncology patients receiving cisplatin. *Int J Gynecol Cancer*, 14(6):1063-1069.

Molassiotis A, Yung HP, Yam BM, Chan FY, Mok TS. (2002). The effectiveness of progressive muscle relaxation training in managing chemotherapy-induced nausea and vomiting in Chinese breast cancer patients: A randomised controlled trial. Support Care Cancer, 10(3):237-246.

National Comprehensive Cancer Network (NCCN). (2006). Antiemesis practice guidelines in oncology, version 2. Available online: http://www.nccn.org. Retrieved on June 6, 2007.

Pace JC. (1987). Oral ingestion of encapsulated ginger and reported self-care actions for the relief of chemotherapy associated nausea and vomiting. *Dissertation Abstracts Int*, 47:3297-B.

Pearl ML, Fischer M, McCauley DL, Valea FA, Chalas E. (1999). Transcutaneous electrical nerve stimulation as an adjunct for controlling chemotherapy-induced nausea and vomiting in gynecologic oncology patients. *Cancer Nurs*, 22(4):307-311.

Roila F, Hesketh PJ, Herrstedt J; Antiemetic Subcommittee of the Multinational Association of Supportive Care in Cancer. (2006). Prevention of chemotherapy- and radiotherapy-induced emesis: Results of the 2004 Perugia International Antiemetic Consensus Conference. Ann Oncol, 17(1):20-28.

Roscoe JA, Jean-Pierre P, Morrow GR, Hickok JT, Issell B, Wade JL, et al. (2006). Exploratory analysis of the usefulness of acupressure bands when severe chemotherapy-related nausea is expected. *J Soc Integr Oncol*, 4(1):16-20.

Roscoe JA, Morrow GR, Bushunow P, Tian L, Matteson S. (2002). Acustimulation wristbands for the relief of chemotherapy-induced nausea. *Altern Ther Health Med*, 8(4):56-57, 59-63.

Roscoe JA, Morrow GR, Hickok JT, Bushunow P, Pierce HI, Flynn PJ, et al. (2003). The efficacy of acupressure and acustimulation wrist bands for the relief of chemotherapy-induced nausea and vomiting. A University of Rochester Cancer Center Community Clinical Oncology Program multicenter study. *J Pain Symptom Manage*, 26(2):731-742.

Schneider SM, Ellis M, Coombs WT, Shonkwiler EL, Folsom LC. (2003). Virtual reality intervention for older women with breast cancer. *Cyberpsychol Behav*, 6(3):301-307.

NR = Nursing Research, **MR** = Multidisciplinary Research, **SP** = Standard of Practice, **EO** = Expert Opinion, **LOE** = Level of Evidence

Schneider SM, Prince-Paul M, Allen MJ, Silverman P, Talaba D. (2004). Virtual reality as a distraction intervention for women receiving chemotherapy. *Oncol Nurs Forum*, 31(1):81-88.

Sharma SS, Gupta YK. (1998). Reversal of cisplatin induced delay in gastric emptying in rats by ginger *(Zingiber officinale)*. *J Ethnopharmacol*, 62(1):49-55.

Sharma SS, Kochupillai V, Gupta SK, Seth SD, Gupta YK. (1997). Antiemetic efficacy of ginger *(Zingiber officinale)* against cisplatin-induced emesis in dogs. *J Ethnopharmacol*, 57(2):93-96.

Shin YH, Kim TI, Shin MS, Juon HS. (2004). Effect of acupressure on nausea and vomiting during chemotherapy cycle for Korean postoperative stomach cancer patients. *Cancer Nurs*, 27(4):267-274.

Treish I, Shord S, Valgus J, Harvey D, Nagy J, Stegal J, et al. (2003). Randomized double-blind study of the ReliefBand as an adjunct to standard antiemetics in patients receiving moderately-high to highly emetogenic chemotherapy. *Support Care Cancer*, 11(8):516-521.

Williams SA, Schreier AM. (2004). The effect of education in managing side effects in women receiving chemotherapy for treatment of breast cancer. Oncol Nurs Forum, *31(1)*:E16-E23.

Yoo HJ, Ahn SH, Kim SB, Kim WK, Han OS. (2005). Efficacy of progressive muscle relaxation training and guided imagery in reducing chemotherapy side effects in patients with breast cancer and in improving their quality of life. *Support Care Cancer*, 13(10):826-833.

NAUSEA MANAGEMENT: POSTOPERATIVE NAUSEA AND VOMITING

Ruth G. McCaffrey, DNP, ARNP-BC; Paulette C. Chiravalle, MSN, APRN-BC, CCRN

Definition: Prevention and alleviation of nausea in the postoperative patient.

NURSING ACTIVITIES

Effective

■ *Use acupressure at pressure points to decrease nausea and vomiting following some surgeries.* **LOE = I**

NR An RCT (*N* = 50) demonstrated that Korean K-9 hand acupressure was effective in reducing postoperative vomiting in children after strabismus repair (Schlager et al., 2000).

NR An RCT (*N* = 150) demonstrated that acupressure was effective in preventing postoperative nausea and vomiting (PONV) in functional endoscopic sinus surgery (Ming et al., 2002).

MR An RCT (*N* = 80) demonstrated acupressure seeds at Korean hand acupoint K-9 was effective in reducing PONV in women after minor gynecological surgery (Boehler et al., 2002).

■ *Use acupressure in combination with antiemetic medication compared with usual treatment of PONV.* **LOE = I**

NR An RCT (*N* = 80) established that use of the ReliefBand, an acustimulation device, in combination with ondansetron significantly reduced nausea, vomiting, and the need for rescue antiemetics (White et al., 2002).

MR An RCT (*N* = 120) demonstrated that stimulation of the P6 acupoint with capsicum plaster was effective for prevention of PONV after middle ear surgery and that its efficacy was comparable to that of ondansetron for the first 6 hours after surgery (Misra et al., 2005).

RCT = Randomized Controlled (Clinical) Trial, **NIC** = Nursing Interventions Classification, **NOC** = Nursing Outcomes Classification

■ *Use acupoint injections to decrease PONV.* **LOE = I**

(MR) An RCT ($N = 187$) showed that using P6 acupoint injections significantly lowered the incidence of PONV in the postanesthesia care unit and 24 hours after surgery in children. In children, P6 acupoint injections were as effective as droperidol in controlling early PONV (Wang & Kain, 2002).

Possibly Effective

■ *Use P6 acupressure for patients having vaginal and breast surgery.* **LOE = II**

(NR) An RCT ($N = 410$) comparing patients who underwent gynecological surgery (vaginal and laparoscopic) found a complete response to P6 acupressure. However, there was a more marked decrease in PONV in the vaginal surgery patients, whereas in the laparoscopic group it was not statistically significant (Alkaissi et al., 2002).

(NR) An RCT ($N = 220$) comparing patients who underwent gynecological surgery or breast surgery demonstrated that the use of P6 acupuncture might be effective for prophylactic treatment of PONV (Streitberger et al., 2004).

■ *Use aromatherapy with inhaled isopropyl alcohol.* **LOE = I**

(NR) An RCT ($N = 100$) demonstrated that inhaled isopropyl alcohol was faster in relieving postoperative nausea than the IV medication ondansetron (Winston et al., 2003).

(NR) A randomized double-blind placebo-controlled study ($N = 33$) compared aromatherapy with peppermint, alcohol, or placebo and found that saline "placebo" was as effective as alcohol or peppermint, suggesting that the beneficial effect may be more related to controlled breathing patterns than to the actual aroma inhaled (Anderson & Gross, 2004).

(NR) A quasi-experimental, blinded ($N = 111$) study to determine the effectiveness of isopropyl alcohol treatment of PONV showed no significant difference between the standard treatment protocol and treatment with isopropyl alcohol (Merritt et al., 2002).

■ *Use ginger preparations to prevent/treat PONV.* **LOE = III**

(MR) A systemic review and meta-analysis of trials comparing ginger with placebo for the prevention of PONV was done. Five randomized trials included 363 patients and found relative risks of 0.69 to 0.61, respectively, to demonstrate that 1 g of ginger was more effective than placebo for the prevention of PONV and that the use of ginger was an effective means for reducing PONV (Chaiyakunapruk et al., 2006).

(MR) An RCT ($N = 80$) demonstrated that ginger was effective in preventing nausea after outpatient gynecological laparoscopy (Pongrojpaw & Chiamchanya, 2003).

(MR) An RCT ($N = 180$) revealed that two different doses of herbal remedy ginger did not reduce the incidence of PONV in patients who underwent gynecological laparoscopic surgery (Eberhart et al., 2003).

(MR) A Cochrane systematic review demonstrated that ginger was not a clinically relevant antiemetic in the PONV setting (Morin et al., 2004).

■ *Combine dexamethasone and ginger for prevention of PONV.* **LOE = III**

(MR) An RCT ($N = 120$) found that combining dexamethasone and ginger was not clinically or statistically superior to dexamethasone alone in preventing PONV in patients undergoing thyroidectomy (Tavlan et al., 2006).

NR = Nursing Research, **MR** = Multidisciplinary Research, **SP** = Standard of Practice, **EO** = Expert Opinion, **LOE** = Level of Evidence

Not Effective

■ *Using acupressure band(s) along with antiemetic medications for treatment of PONV from urological surgeries, laparoscopic cholecystectomy, or cardiac surgery.* **LOE = I**

(MR) An RCT (*N* = 200) using beads at P6 points appropriately or inappropriately did not decrease the incidence of PONV in urological patients (Agarwal et al., 2000).

(MR) An RCT application of P6 was not an effective treatment of PONV in laparoscopic cholecystectomy (*N* = 50) (Samad et al., 2003).

(NR) An RCT (*N* = 157) demonstrated that neither unilateral nor bilateral application of acupressure using a Sea-Band significantly affected the incidence of nausea and vomiting in gynecologic, plastic, and urologic surgery patients (Windle et al., 2001).

(NR) An RCT (*N* = 143) demonstrated that acupressure bands or droperidol was not effective in reducing PONV in gynecologic surgical patients (Schultz et al., 2003).

(MR) An RCT using acupressure treatment or placebo (*N* = 152) demonstrated that acupressure bands (Sea-Bands) did not lead to a reduction in nausea, vomiting, or antiemetic requirements in patients after cardiac surgery (Klein et al., 2004).

Possibly Harmful

No applicable published research was found in this category.

OUTCOME MEASUREMENT

NAUSEA AND VOMITING SEVERITY   (NOC)

Definition: Severity of nausea, retching and vomiting symptoms.
Nausea and Vomiting Severity as evidenced by the following selected NOC indicators:
• Frequency of nausea
• Intensity of nausea
• Distress of nausea
• Frequency of retching
• Intensity of retching
• Distress of retching
(Rate each indicator of **Nausea and Vomiting Severity:** 1 = severe, 2 = substantial, 3 = moderate, 4 = mild, 5 = none) (Moorhead et al., 2004).

REFERENCES

Agarwal A, Pathak A, Gaur A. (2000). Acupressure wristbands do not prevent postoperative nausea and vomiting after urological endoscopic surgery. *Can J Anaesth,* 47(4):319-324.

Alkaissi A, Evertsson K, Johnsson V, Ofenbartl L, Kalman S. (2002). P6 acupressure may relieve nausea and vomiting after gynecological surgery: An effectiveness study in 410 women. *Can J Anaesth,* 49(10): 1034-1039.

Anderson LA, Gross J. (2004). Aromatherapy with peppermint, isopropyl alcohol, or placebo is equally effective in relieving postoperative nausea. *J Perianesth Nurs,* 19(1):29-35.

Boehler M, Mitterschiffthaler G, Schlager A. (2002). Korean hand acupressure reduces postoperative nausea and vomiting after gynecological laparoscopic surgery. *Anesth Analg*, 94(4):872-875.

Chaiyakunapruk N, Kitikannakorn N, Nathisuwan S, Leeprakobboon K, Leelasettagool C. (2006). The efficacy of ginger for the prevention of postoperative nausea and vomiting: A meta-analysis. *Am J Obstet Gynecol*, 194(1):95-99.

Eberhart LH, Mayer R, Betz O, Tsolakidis S, Hilpert W, Morin AM, et al. (2003). Ginger does not prevent postoperative nausea and vomiting after laparoscopic surgery. *Anesth Analg*, 96(4):995-998.

Klein AA, Djaiani G, Karski J, Carroll J, Karkouti K, McCluskey S, et al. (2004). Acupressure wristbands for the prevention of postoperative nausea and vomiting in adults undergoing cardiac surgery. *J Cardiothorac Vasc Anesth*, 18(1):68-71.

Merritt BA, Okyere CP, Jasinski DM. (2002). Isopropyl alcohol inhalation: Alternative treatment of postoperative nausea and vomiting. *Nurs Res*, 51(2):125-128.

Ming JL, Kuo BI, Lin JG, Lin LC. (2002). The efficacy of acupressure to prevent nausea and vomiting in postoperative patients. *J Adv Nurs*, 39(4):343-351.

Misra MN, Pullani AJ, Mohamed ZU. (2005). Prevention of PONV by acustimulation with capsicum plaster is comparable to ondansetron after middle ear surgery. *Can J Anaesth*, 52(5):485-489.

Morin AM, Betz O, Kranke P, Geldner G, Wulf H, Eberhart LH. (2004). Is ginger a relevant antiemetic for postoperative nausea and vomiting? *Anasthesiol Intensivmed Notfallmed Schmerzther*, 39(5): 281-285.

Moorhead, M., Johnson, M., & Maas, M. (Eds.) (2004). *Nursing Outcomes Classification (NOC)* (3rd ed). St. Louis, MO: Mosby.

Pongrojpaw D, Chiamchanya C. (2003). The efficacy of ginger in prevention of post-operative nausea and vomiting after outpatient gynecological laparoscopy. *J Med Assoc Thai*, 86(3):244-250.

Samad K, Afshan G, Kamal R. (2003). Effect of acupressure on postoperative nausea and vomiting in laparoscopic cholecystectomy. *J Pak Med Assoc*, 53(2):68-72.

Schlager A, Boehler M, Puhringer F. (2000). Korean hand acupressure reduces postoperative vomiting in children after strabismus surgery. *Br J Anaesth*, 85(2):267-270.

Schultz AA, Andrews AL, Goran SF, Mathew T, Sturdevant N. (2003). Comparison of acupressure bands and droperidol for reducing PONV in gynecologic surgery patients. *Appl Nurs Res*, 16(4): 256-265.

Streitberger K, Diefenbacher M, Bauer A, Conradi R, Bardenheuer H, Martin E, et al. (2004). Acupuncture compared to placebo-acupuncture for postoperative nausea and vomiting prophylaxis: A randomised placebo-controlled patient and observer blind trial. *Anesthesia*, 59(2):142-149.

Tavlan A, Tuncer S, Erol A, Reisli R, Aysolmaz G, Otelcioglu S. (2006). Prevention of postoperative nausea and vomiting after thyroidectomy: Combined antiemetic treatment with dexamethasone and ginger versus dexamethasone alone. *Clin Drug Invest*, 26(4):209-214.

Wang SM, Kain ZN. (2002). P6 acupoint injections are as effective as droperidol in controlling early postoperative nausea and vomiting in children. *Anesthesiology*, 97(2):359-366.

White PF, Issioui T, Hu J, Jones SB, Coleman JE, Waddle JP, et al. (2002). Comparative efficacy of acustimulation (ReliefBand) versus ondansetron (Zofran) in combination with droperidol for preventing nausea and vomiting. *Anesthesiology*, 97(5):1075-1081.

Windle PE, Borromeo A, Robles H, Ilacio-Uy V. (2001). The effects of acupressure on the incidence of postoperative nausea and vomiting in postsurgical patients. *J Perianesth Nurs*, 16(3):158-162.

Winston AW, Rinehart RS, Riley GP, Vacchiano CA, Pellegrini JE. (2003). Comparison of inhaled isopropyl alcohol and intravenous ondansetron for the treatment of postoperative nausea. *AANA J*, 71(2): 127-132.

NEUROLOGICAL MONITORING

 NIC

Kathleen A. Clark, MSN, RN, APN-BC; Beth Ann Swan, PhD, CRNP, FAAN

NIC   **Definition:** Collection and analysis of patient data to prevent or minimize neurologic complications (Dochterman & Bulechek, 2004).

NR = Nursing Research, **MR** = Multidisciplinary Research, **SP** = Standard of Practice, **EO** = Expert Opinion, **LOE** = Level of Evidence

NURSING ACTIVITIES

Effective

■ ⓢ *Conduct a baseline neurological assessment on admission and when there is a change in patients' status including level of consciousness, orientation, motor skills, pupils, speech/language ability, vital signs, and blood glucose.* **LOE = VII**

ⓔ A focused neurological assessment including pertinent history and physical examination is conducted to determine nervous system dysfunction and an individual's response to actual or potential health problems (Crimlisk & Grande, 2004).

ⓔ The most important evaluation of neurological status is determining level of consciousness (LOC); a change in LOC is the most sensitive indicator and the first indicator of neurological deterioration (Noah, 2004).

ⓔ Nurses should recognize that signs in decline of neurological status may be related to neurological or secondary medical complications (Crimlisk & Grande, 2004).

ⓔ Neurological changes may be subtle, and without a baseline assessment the changes may not be recognized (Lower, 2002).

■ ⓢ *Use the Glasgow Coma Scale (GCS) to screen for level of consciousness.* **LOE = VII**

ⓔ The GCS is the most widely recognized LOC assessment tool. It is a neurological scale that provides a reliable method to assess for LOC and includes three tests: eye opening response, verbal response, and motor response (Teasdale & Jennett, 1974).

ⓔ The GCS is useful in evaluating patients in the acute stages of illness (Noah, 2004).

■ ⓢ *Screen patients for alterations in cognitive, perceptual, and language function using validated tools such as the Mini-Mental State Examination (MMSE).* **LOE = VII**

ⓔ Alteration in mental status, perceptual, or language function may impair patients' safety. The MMSE has been used to detect impairment, follow the course of an illness, and monitor response to treatment (Haymore, 2004).

ⓔ The MMSE is a widely used method for assessing cognitive functioning and is important in clinical settings because of the recognized high prevalence of cognitive impairment in medical patients (Folstein et al., 1975).

ⓔ The MMSE is a brief, standardized method that assesses orientation, attention, immediate and short-term recall, language, and the ability to follow simple verbal and written commands (Folstein et al., 1975).

■ **NIC** ⓢ *Monitor vital signs: temperature, pulse, blood pressure, and respirations.* **LOE = VII**

ⓔ Increased intracranial pressure can be suspected from specific changes in vital signs such as (1) increasing systolic blood pressure with a widening pulse pressure, (2) bradycardia, and (3) irregular breathing pattern (Crimlisk & Grande, 2004).

RCT = Randomized Controlled (Clinical) Trial, **NIC** = Nursing Interventions Classification, **NOC** = Nursing Outcomes Classification

EO Respiratory patterns that may indicate neurological causes include Cheyne-Stokes breathing, central hyperventilation, apneustic, cluster, and ataxic breathing patterns (Crimlisk & Grande, 2004).

EO Other vital changes suggesting a neurological injury can include bradycardia, hypertension then hypotension, and loss of thermal control with hypothermia or hyperthermia (Crimlisk & Grande, 2004).

SP *Check pupillary responses and eye movement.* **LOE = VII**

EO Neurological changes can be reflected in pupil responses; dilated pupils can indicate compressed cranial nerve III, or bilateral pinpoint pupils may indicate pons damage or drugs (Crimlisk & Grande, 2004).

EO Cranial nerves III and IV arise from the midbrain, and cranial nerve VI originates in the pons. Because of their location, the pupils and eyes reflect the function of the upper and middle brainstem (Haymore, 2004).

EO Metabolic disturbances rarely cause papillary changes; abnormal papillary findings are usually due to a nervous system lesion (Haymore, 2004).

SP *Perform an evaluation including dermatomes, reflexes, and cranial nerves.* **LOE = VII**

EO Such an evaluation provides information about sensory functioning and reflexes (Crimlisk & Grande, 2004).

EO Facial asymmetry is indicative of a lesion of cranial nerve VII. Complete hemifacial involvement is usually seen in peripheral dysfunction (Haymore, 2004).

EO Diminished or absent oropharyngeal reflexes, cranial nerves IX and X, is indicative of lower brainstem damage (Haymore, 2004).

SP *Assess motor activity of the body and limbs.* **LOE = VII**

EO Assessment of extremities and body movement provides valuable information about the patient with a decreased LOC (Haymore, 2004).

EO Asymmetrical examination of motor ability/tone may indicate a lesion in the contralateral hemisphere or brainstem (Haymore, 2004).

Document findings of neurological assessment and identify emerging patterns. **LOE = VI**

NR A quantitative study that included an evaluation of nursing assessments of neurological patients through 25 chart reviews revealed that 30% of the records contained incomplete documentation of the neurological assessment (Lehman et al., 2003).

EO Many patients with alterations in neurological status are not assessed consistently and/or not assessed accurately; therefore, patterns and/or subtle changes may not be recognized (Lower, 2002).

Possibly Effective

No applicable published research was found in this category.

NR = Nursing Research, **MR** = Multidisciplinary Research, **SP** = Standard of Practice, **EO** = Expert Opinion, **LOE** = Level of Evidence

Not Effective

No applicable published research was found in this category.

Possibly Harmful

No applicable published research was found in this category.

OUTCOME MEASUREMENT

NEUROLOGICAL STATUS

Definition: Ability of the peripheral and central nervous system to receive, process, and respond to internal and external stimuli.

Neurological Status as evidenced by the following selected NOC indicators:

- Consciousness
- Central motor control
- Cranial sensory/motor function
- Cognitive ability
- Blood pressure
- Respiratory rate
- Hyperthermia
- Breathing pattern
- Pupil reactivity
- Eye movement pattern

(Rate each indicator of **Neurological Status:** 1 = severely compromised, 2 = substantially compromised, 3 = moderately compromised, 4 = mildly compromised, 5 = not compromised) (Moorhead et al., 2004).

REFERENCES

Crimlisk JT, Grande MM. (2004). Neurologic assessment skills for the acute medical surgical nurse. *Orthop Nurs,* 23(1):3-9.

Dochterman JM, Bulechek GM (Eds). (2004). *Nursing Interventions Classification (NIC),* 4th ed. St. Louis: Mosby.

Folstein MF, Folstein SE, McHugh PR. (1975). "Mini-mental state." A practical method for grading the cognitive state of patients for the clinician. *J Psychiatr Res,* 12(3):189-198.

Haymore J. (2004). A neuron in a haystack: Advanced neurologic assessment. *AACN Clin Issues,* 15(4):568-581.

Lehman CA, Hayes JM, LaCroix M, Owen SV, Nauta HJ. (2003). Development and implementation of a problem-focused neurological assessment system. *J Neurosci Nurs,* 35(4):185-192.

Lower J. (2002). Facing neuro assessment fearlessly. *Nursing,* 32(2):58-64.

Moorhead M, Johnson M, Maas M (Eds). (2004). *Nursing Outcomes Classification (NOC),* 3rd ed. St. Louis: Mosby.

Noah P. (2004). Neurological assessment: A refresher. *RN,* Suppl:18-23.

Teasdale G, Jennett B. (1974). Assessment of coma and impaired consciousness. A practical scale. *Lancet,* 2(7872):81-84.

NUTRITION MANAGEMENT

Joseph T. DeRanieri, MSN, RN, CPN, BCECR

> **NIC** **Definition:** Assisting with or providing a balanced dietary intake of foods and fluids (Dochterman & Bulechek, 2004).

NURSING ACTIVITIES

Effective

■ *Address dietary changes and demands during acute illness.* **LOE = V**

> NR A systematic review of the literature stated that during acute illness, catabolic processes elevated metabolic demands, often exceeding nutrient intake (Gary & Fleury, 2002).

■ **NIC** SP *Inquire if patient has any food allergies.* **LOE = VII**

> EO Inquire whether the patient has any food allergies as outlined in institutional policy (Wilkes, 2000).

■ **NIC** *Ascertain the patient's food preferences.* **LOE = V**

> NR A systematic review of the literature stated that including a patient's likes and dislikes in a nutritional screening allowed a focused therapeutic plan and evaluation process (Gary & Fleury, 2002).

■ *Assess nutritional requirements in collaboration with the dietician.* **LOE = V**

> MR A systematic review of the literature stated that nutritional interventions and screenings ensured that patients at nutritional risk achieved optimal health outcomes (McGee & Jensen, 2000).
>
> NR A systematic review of the literature stated that a nutritional assessment integrated medical, social, and nutritional histories as well as anthropometric, biochemical, clinical, and dietary measurements. It also identified the patients who needed nutritional supportive therapy (Gary & Fleury, 2002).

■ **NIC** *Encourage a calorie intake appropriate for body type and lifestyle.* **LOE = V**

> MR A systematic review of the literature stated that derangement in energy balance would result in under- or overnutrition, so it was important to correlate energy expenditure with dietary intake (McGee & Jensen, 2000).
>
> MR Energy intake should be matched with energy needs with appropriate changes, taking into consideration when weight loss or weight gain is a concern (Krauss et al., 2000).

■ **NIC** *Provide the patient with high-protein, high-calorie, nutritious finger foods and drinks that can be readily consumed, as appropriate.* **LOE = VII**

> EO Have patients eat small, frequent, high-calorie, high-protein snacks. Stay away from "empty" food choices (e.g., lettuce, diet soda, and bouillon) (Wilkes, 2000).

NR = Nursing Research, **MR** = Multidisciplinary Research, **SP** = Standard of Practice, **EO** = Expert Opinion, **LOE** = Level of Evidence

■ **NIC** *Teach the patient how to keep a food diary, as needed.* **LOE = V**

(NR) A systematic review of the literature stated that 24-hour dietary recall and food frequency questionnaires were useful when used together because one addressed not only food intake but also dietary patterns. This could be difficult to assess in older patients because of memory recall requirements (Gary & Fleury, 2002).

■ **NIC** *Weigh the patient at appropriate intervals.* **LOE = VII**

(EO) Measure body weight at least once a week in standard clothing (empty bowel and bladder) (Rotilio et al., 2004).

■ **NIC** *Encourage the patient to wear properly fitted dentures and/or obtain dental care.* **LOE = V**

(MR) A systematic review of the literature stated that ill-fitting dentures as well as an edentulous state could make it difficult to obtain adequate nutrition (McGee & Jensen, 2000).

■ **NIC** *Provide appropriate information about nutritional needs and how to meet them.* **LOE = V**

(NR) A systematic review of the literature stated that difficulty with walking, shopping, and buying and cooking food, especially as patients get older, could cause nutritional problems (Gary & Fleury, 2002).

■ **NIC** *Determine the patient's ability to meet nutritional needs.* **LOE = V**

(NR) A systematic review of the literature stated that poverty, lack of help with food shopping and preparation, and isolation at mealtimes could negatively affect nutrition (McGee & Jensen, 2000).

(NR) A systematic review of the literature stated that the Nutrition Screening Initiative's nutrition checklist was available to assess patients' ability to meet their own nutritional needs (Gary & Fleury, 2002).

Possibly Effective

■ **NIC** *Provide a sugar substitute, as appropriate.* **LOE = V**

(MR) A systematic review of the literature stated that there was evidence supporting that nonnutritive sweeteners were safe for people when consumed within the acceptable daily intake levels established by the FDA (Franz et al., 2002).

■ **NIC** *Ensure that diet includes foods high in fiber content to prevent constipation.* **LOE = V**

(NR) A systematic review of the literature stated that poor fiber intake, poor hydration, stress, medication, and inactivity could lead to constipation. Increase in dietary fiber could help to avoid this negative consequence (Gary & Fleury, 2002).

■ **NIC** *Offer herbs and spices as an alternative to salt.* **LOE = VII**

(EO) Season foods with pepper, basil, oregano, or rosemary. Marinate meats with sweet and sour sauce or sweet wine (Wilkes, 2000).

RCT = Randomized Controlled (Clinical) Trial, **NIC** = Nursing Interventions Classification, **NOC** = Nursing Outcomes Classification

Not Effective

No applicable published research was found in this category.

Possibly Harmful

No applicable published research was found in this category.

OUTCOME MEASUREMENT

NUTRITIONAL STATUS

Definition: Extent to which nutrients are available to meet metabolic needs.
Nutritional Status as evidenced by the following selected NOC indicators:
• Nutrient intake
• Food intake
• Fluid intake
(Rate each indicator of **Nutritional Status:** 1 = severe deviation from normal range, 2 = substantial deviation from normal range, 3 = moderate deviation from normal range, 4 = mild deviation from normal range, 5 = no deviation from normal range) (Moorhead et al., 2004).

REFERENCES

Dochterman JM, Bulechek GM (Eds). (2004). *Nursing Interventions Classification (NIC)*, 4th ed. St. Louis: Mosby.

Franz MJ, Bantle JP, Beebe CA, Brunzell JD, Chiasson JL, Garg A, et al. (2002). Evidence-based nutrition principles and recommendations for the treatment and prevention of diabetes and related complications. *Diabetes Care*, 25(1):148-198.

Gary R, Fleury J. (2002). Nutritional status: Key to preventing functional decline in hospitalized older adults. *Top Geriatr Rehabil*, 17(3):40-71.

Krauss RM, Eckel RH, Howard BP, Appel LJ, Daniels S, Deckelbaum RJ, et al. (2000). AHA dietary guidelines: Revision 2000: A statement for healthcare professionals from the Nutrition Committee of the American Heart Association. *Stroke*, 31(11):2751-2766.

McGee M, Jensen GL. (2000). Nutrition in the elderly. *J Clin Gastroenterol*, 30(4):372-380.

Moorhead M, Johnson M, Maas M (Eds). (2004). *Nursing Outcomes Classification (NOC)*, 3rd ed. St. Louis: Mosby.

Rotilio G, Berni Canani R, Branca F, Cairella G, Fieschi C, Garbagnati F, et al. (2004). Nutritional recommendations for the prevention of ischemic stroke. *Nutr Metab Cardiovasc Dis*, 14(2), 115-120.

Wilkes GM. (2000). Nutrition: The forgotten ingredient in cancer care. *Am J Nurs*, 100(4):46-51.

 # NUTRITIONAL COUNSELING

Joseph T. DeRanieri, MSN, RN, CPN, BCECR

NIC Definition: Use of an interactive helping process focusing on the need for diet modification (Dochterman & Bulechek, 2004).

NR = Nursing Research, **MR** = Multidisciplinary Research, **SP** = Standard of Practice, **EO** = Expert Opinion, **LOE** = Level of Evidence

NURSING ACTIVITIES

Effective

- **NIC** *Determine the patient's food intake and eating habits.* **LOE = VII**

  EO Review with the patient the importance of maintaining a balanced diet; preventing malnutrition is easier than reversing it (Wilkes, 2000).

- **NIC** *Facilitate identification of eating behaviors to be changed.* **LOE = VII**

  EO A statement from the U.S. Preventive Services Task Force (USPSTF) stated that effective behavioral interventions result when nutrition education with behaviorally oriented counseling is used (USPSTF, 2003).

- **NIC** *Use accepted nutritional standards to assist the client in evaluating adequacy of dietary intake.* **LOE = VII**

  EO It is important for patients to maintain a balanced diet with all food groups represented. This needs to be established over a period of time and not necessarily based on one meal (Krauss et al., 2000).

- **NIC** *Provide information, as necessary, about the health need for diet modification: weight loss, weight gain, sodium restriction, cholesterol reduction, fluid restriction, and so on.* **LOE = VII**

  EO General principles for maintaining a healthy diet and lifestyle can have a positive effect on health promotion (Krauss et al., 2000).

- **NIC** *Help the patient to consider factors of age, stage of growth and development, past eating experiences, injury, disease, culture, and finances in planning ways to meet nutritional requirements.* **LOE = VII**

  EO Good nutritional guidelines form a framework with specific dietary recommendations that are based on an individual's health status, dietary preferences, and cultural background (Krauss et al., 2000).

- **NIC** *Discuss nutritional requirements and the patient's perceptions of prescribed/recommended diet.* **LOE = VII**

  EO Good nutritional guidelines form a framework with specific dietary recommendations that are based on an individual's health status, dietary preferences, and cultural background (Krauss et al., 2000).

- **NIC** *Discuss the patient's food likes and dislikes.* **LOE = VII**

  EO Good nutritional guidelines form a framework with specific dietary recommendations that are based on an individual's health status, dietary preferences, and cultural background (Krauss et al., 2000).

- **NIC** *Discuss food buying habits and budget constraints.* **LOE = V**

  NR A systematic review of the literature stated that difficulty with walking, shopping, and buying and cooking food, especially as patients get older, could cause nutritional problems (Gary & Fleury, 2002).

RCT = Randomized Controlled (Clinical) Trial, **NIC** = Nursing Interventions Classification, **NOC** = Nursing Outcomes Classification

■ **NIC** *Provide referral/consultation with other members of the health care team, as appropriate.* **LOE = V**

MR A systematic review of the literature stated that a multidisciplinary approach was essential in order to address properly the impact that nutritional status had on patients (McGee & Jensen, 2000).

EO Nutrition assessments should be completed by a registered dietitian with experience with that disease process or one who consults with one who has experience in that area (Nerad et al., 2003).

EO A multidisciplinary consensus paper revealed that family caregivers as well as the patient needed to be trained on the complications of nutritional therapy (Rotilio et al., 2004).

Possibly Effective

■ **NIC** *Discuss the patient's knowledge of the four basic food groups, as well as perceptions of the needed diet modification.* **LOE = VII**

EO It is important that patients maintain a balanced diet with all food groups represented. This needs to be established over a period of time and not necessarily based on one meal (Krauss et al., 2000).

Not Effective

■ **NIC** *Assist the patient to record what is usually eaten in a 24-hour period.* **LOE = V**

NR A systematic review of the literature stated that the 24-hour recall method required remembering food consumption, which could be difficult; it was a less reliable method of data collection (Gary & Fleury, 2002).

Possibly Harmful

No applicable published research was found in this category.

OUTCOME MEASUREMENT

KNOWLEDGE: DIET **NOC**

Definition: Extent of understanding conveyed about recommended diet.
Knowledge: Diet as evidenced by the following selected NOC indicators:
• Description of diet
• Description of dietary goals
• Description of relationships among diet, exercise, and body weight
• Description of foods allowed in diet
• Description of menu planning using dietary guidelines
(Rate each indicator of **Knowledge: Diet:** 1 = none, 2 = limited, 3 = moderate, 4 = substantial, 5 = extensive) (Moorhead et al., 2004).

NR = Nursing Research, **MR** = Multidisciplinary Research, **SP** = Standard of Practice, **EO** = Expert Opinion, **LOE** = Level of Evidence

REFERENCES

Dochterman JM, Bulechek GM (Eds). (2004). *Nursing Interventions Classification (NIC)*, 4th ed. St. Louis: Mosby.

Gary R, Fleury J. (2002). Nutritional status: Key to preventing functional decline in hospitalized older adults. *Top Geriatr Rehabil*, 17(3):40-71.

Krauss RM, Eckel RH, Howard B, Appel LJ, Daniels SR, Deckelbaum RJ, et al. (2000). AHA Dietary Guidelines: Revision 2000: A statement for healthcare professionals from the Nutrition Committee of the American Heart Association. *Stroke*, 31(11):2751-2766.

McGee M, Jensen GL. (2000). Nutrition in the elderly. *J Clin Gastroenterol* 30(4):372-380.

Moorhead M, Johnson M, Maas M (Eds). (2004). *Nursing Outcomes Classification (NOC)*, 3rd ed. St. Louis: Mosby.

Nerad J, Romeyn M, Silverman E, Allen-Reid J, Dieterich D, Merchant J, et al. (2003). General nutrition management in patients infected with human immunodeficiency virus. *Clin Infect Dis*, 36(Suppl 2): S52-S62.

Rotilio G, Berni Canani R, Branca F, Cairella G, Fieschi C, Garbagnati F, et al. (2004). Nutritional recommendations for the management of stroke patients. *Riv Ital Nutr Parent Ent*, 22(4):227-236.

US Preventive Service Task Force. (2003). Behavioral counseling in primary care to promote a healthy diet: Recommendations and rationale. *Am J Nurs*, 103(8):81-92.

Wilkes GM. (2000). Nutrition: The forgotten ingredient in cancer care. *Am J Nurs*, 100(4):46-51.

 # NUTRITIONAL MONITORING

Joseph T. DeRanieri, MSN, RN, CPN, BCECR

NIC **Definition:** Collection and analysis of patient data to prevent or minimize malnourishment (Dochterman & Bulechek, 2004).

NURSING ACTIVITIES

Effective

■ **NIC** *Weigh the patient at specified intervals.* **LOE = VII**

EO A multidisciplinary consensus paper that was compiled measured body weight at least once a week in standard clothing (empty bowel and bladder) (Rotilio et al., 2004).

■ **NIC** *Monitor the type and amount of usual exercise.* **LOE = VII**

EO Energy intake should be matched with energy needs with appropriate changes, taking into consideration when weight loss or weight gain is a concern (Krauss et al., 2000).

■ **NIC** *Monitor the patient's emotional response when placed in situations that involve food and eating.* **LOE = VII**

MR A review of the literature stated that poverty, lack of help with food shopping and preparation, and isolation at mealtimes could negatively affect nutrition (McGee & Jensen, 2000).

RCT = Randomized Controlled (Clinical) Trial, **NIC** = Nursing Interventions Classification, **NOC** = Nursing Outcomes Classification

■ **NIC** *Monitor the environment where eating occurs.* **LOE = VII**

NR A review of the literature stated that being with people daily had a positive effect on morale, well-being, and eating (Gary & Fleury, 2002).

■ **NIC** *Monitor gums for swelling, sponginess, receding, and increased bleeding.* **LOE = VII**

NR A review of the literature stated that physical signs of nutritional deficiency included receding gums, spongy bleeding gums, missing teeth, and loose teeth (Gary & Fleury, 2002).

■ *Monitor prealbumin levels.* **LOE = VII**

MR A systematic review of the literature showed that prealbumin levels seemed to be a better choice to use to measure nutritional progress (Jacobs et al., 2004).

NR A review of the literature stated that prealbumin levels were more sensitive in determining acute changes in nutritional status and were an important measure to ascertain effectiveness of nutritional management (Gary & Fleury, 2002).

NR A case study showed that a prealbumin level was the best for nutritional monitoring; by tracking their levels, nutritional deficiencies could be identified early. Prealbumin levels indicated visceral protein status. These levels are less influenced by liver disease, so they have a broader application to patients (Kuszajewski & Clontz, 2005).

■ **NIC** *Monitor for pale, reddened, and dry conjunctival tissue.* **LOE = VII**

NR A review of the literature stated that physical signs of nutritional deficiency included pale conjunctiva, conjunctival dryness, corneal dullness, redness and fissuring of eyelids, and corneal softening (Gary & Fleury, 2002).

■ **NIC** *Note any sores, edema, and hyperemic and hypertrophic papillae of the tongue and oral cavity.* **LOE = VII**

NR A review of the literature stated that physical signs of nutritional deficiency included angular stomatitis, red tongue, magenta tongue, atrophy, or hypertrophy. They also include receding gums, spongy bleeding gums, missing teeth, and loose teeth (Gary & Fleury, 2002).

■ **NIC** *Initiate a dietary consult as appropriate.* **LOE = V**

MR A systematic review of the literature stated that nutritional interventions and screenings were important to ensure that patients at nutritional risk achieved optimal health outcomes (McGee & Jensen, 2000).

NR A review of the literature stated that a nutritional assessment integrated medical, social, and nutritional histories as well as anthropometric, biochemical, clinical, and dietary measurements. It also identified the patients who needed nutritional supportive therapy (Gary & Fleury, 2002).

■ **NIC** *Provide nutritional food and fluid, as appropriate.* **LOE = VII**

NR A review of the literature stated that in acute illness, without adequate dietary protein, immune responses would be minimized, new tissue could not be formed, and muscle strength

NR = Nursing Research, **MR** = Multidisciplinary Research, **SP** = Standard of Practice, **EO** = Expert Opinion, **LOE** = Level of Evidence

may not be regained; this could all cause a decrease in functioning for the patient (Gary & Fleury, 2002).

Possibly Effective

■ **NIC** *Monitor for dry, flaky skin with depigmentation.* **LOE = VII**

> **NR** A review of the literature stated that flaking dermatitis, bruising, pigmentation changes, psoriasis from rash, and eczematous scaling may result from nutritional deficiency (Gary & Fleury, 2002).

■ **NIC** *Monitor for dry, thin hair that is easy to pluck.* **LOE = VII**

> **NR** A review of the literature stated that easily plucked hair with no pain, dull and dry hair, and thin and sparse hair could also result from nutritional deficiency (Gary & Fleury, 2002).

■ *Assess for ethnic considerations.* **LOE = VII**

> **NR** A review of the literature stated that certain populations may be at risk for specific diet-related diseases; poverty, religious beliefs, lifestyle, and dietary practices may all have an influence (Gary & Fleury, 2002).

■ **NIC** *Monitor caloric and nutrient intake.* **LOE = VII**

> **NR** A review of the literature stated that optimal nutritional status was important to ensure health and well-being, which were directly dependent on nutrient intakes and nutrient requirements. Malnutrition could be a nutritional deficit, excess, or imbalance. Calorie counts during hospitalization and dietary recall after discharge were most effective (Gary & Fleury, 2002).

■ **NIC** *Monitor for spoon-shaped, brittle, ridged nails.* **LOE = VII**

> **NR** A review of the literature stated that spooning of the nails could also result from nutritional deficiency (Gary & Fleury, 2002).

Not Effective

■ *Monitoring albumin levels.* **LOE = V**

> **MR** A systematic review of the literature showed that albumin was unsuitable as a marker of the acute efficacy of nutritional support (Jacobs et al., 2004).

■ *Monitoring protein levels.* **LOE = V**

> **MR** A systematic review of the literature showed that serum protein levels may be related more to restoration of hepatic constitutive protein synthesis than to nutritional progress (Jacobs et al., 2004).

Possibly Harmful

No applicable published research was found in this category.

RCT = Randomized Controlled (Clinical) Trial, **NIC** = Nursing Interventions Classification, **NOC** = Nursing Outcomes Classification

OUTCOME MEASUREMENT

NUTRITIONAL STATUS

Definition: Extent to which nutrients are available to meet metabolic needs.

Nutritional Status as evidenced by the following selected NOC indicators:

- Nutrient intake
- Fluid intake
- Food intake
- Energy
- Weight/height ratio
- Muscle tone
- Hydration

(Rate each indicator of **Nutritional Status:** 1 = severe deviation from normal range, 2 = substantial deviation from normal range, 3 = moderate deviation from normal range, 4 = mild deviation from normal range, 5 = no deviation from normal range) (Moorhead et al., 2004).

REFERENCES

Dochterman JM, Bulechek GM (Eds). (2004). *Nursing Interventions Classification (NIC)*, 4th ed. St. Louis: Mosby.

Gary R, Fleury J. (2002). Nutritional status: Key to preventing functional decline in hospitalized older adults. *Top Geriatr Rehabil*, 17(3):40-71.

Jacobs DG, Jacobs DO, Kudsk KA, Moore FA, Oswanski MF, Poole GV, et al. (2004). Practice management guidelines for nutritional support of the trauma patient. *J Trauma*, 57(3):660-679.

Krauss RM, Eckel RH, Howard BP, Appel LJ, Daniels S, Deckelbaum RJ, et al. (2000). AHA dietary guidelines: Revision 2000: A statement for healthcare professionals from the Nutrition Committee of the American Heart Association. *Stroke*, 31(11):2751-2766.

Kuszajewski M, Clontz A. (2005). Prealbumin is best for nutritional monitoring. *Nursing*, 35(5):70-71.

McGee M, Jensen G. (2000). Nutrition in the elderly. *J Clin Gastroenterol* 30(4):372-380.

Moorhead M, Johnson M, Maas M (Eds). (2004). *Nursing Outcomes Classification (NOC)*, 3rd ed. St. Louis: Mosby.

Rotilio G, Berni Canani R, Branca F, Cairella G, Fieschi C, Garbagnati F, et al. (2004). Nutritional recommendations for the management of stroke patients. *Riv Ital Nutr Parent Ent*, 22(4):227-236.

 # ORAL HEALTH MAINTENANCE

Dianna S. Weikel, RDH, MS

Definition: Maintenance and promotion of oral hygiene and dental health for the patient at risk for developing oral or dental lesions (Dochterman & Bulechek, 2004).

Note: This is usually the patient with chemotherapy, head and neck radiation therapy, or acquired immunodeficiency syndrome (AIDS).

NR = Nursing Research, **MR** = Multidisciplinary Research, **SP** = Standard of Practice, **EO** = Expert Opinion, **LOE** = Level of Evidence

NURSING ACTIVITIES

Effective

■ **SP** *Perform a comprehensive oral examination before initiation of chemotherapy or radiation, with aggressive preventive dental care as needed.* **LOE = V**

MR In a review from the first proceedings regarding oral complications of cancer therapies, a panel of experts convened to review the literature and present their findings, which included recommendations for diagnosis, prevention, and treatment of oral complications in pediatric and adult cancer patients. Recommendations included a comprehensive dental examination with radiographs, dental prophylaxis, and restorative dental care as needed prior to treatment (NIH, Consensus Development Conference, 1990).

MR An international survey (questionnaire) ($N = 74$) regarding practice methods of dental and medical providers working with cancer patients evaluated knowledge and current practice for preventing and managing side effects in the oral cavity associated with chemotherapy, hematopoietic cell transplant, and radiation therapy. Findings included a wide variation in clinical practice and significant variation in preventive/palliative care related to complications associated with cancer therapies. The authors cautioned the interpretation of findings because of a limited response rate (Barker et al., 2005).

■ **NIC** **SP** *Recommend the use of a soft-bristle toothbrush.* **LOE = V**

EO Use of a soft toothbrush replaced at regular intervals is recommended based on a comprehensive review of the literature by experts in the fields of nursing and dentistry (McGuire et al., 2006).

EO Use of a soft toothbrush is accepted as the standard of care from the American Dental Association (ADA) to maintain healthy dentition (ADA, 2006).

■ **SP** *Recommend use of dental floss once a day to assist in plaque control.* **LOE = VII**

EO A self-care intervention model, the PRO-SELF program, which includes didactic information related to daily oral care, development of self-care exercises, and supportive communication with a nurse, was used in both outpatient chemotherapy and radiation therapy settings. The authors found that teaching patients self-care instructions was an important contribution during their cancer therapy (Larson et al., 1998).

EO Use of dental floss is accepted by the ADA as a standard of care to assist in daily oral hygiene (ADA, 2006).

■ **SP** *Reinforce daily self-care to the mouth, including application of topical fluoride for the head/neck radiation patient.* **LOE = V**

EO Use of topical fluoride is accepted as standard practice by the ADA and the National Institute of Dental and Craniofacial Research, National Oral Health Information Clearinghouse (ADA, 2006; NOHIC, 2007).

MR An RCT of patients receiving radiation to the head/neck to one of three arms found that patients receiving oral hygiene and topical fluoride experienced a reduction in dental decay (Dreizen et al., 1977).

RCT = Randomized Controlled (Clinical) Trial, **NIC** = Nursing Interventions Classification, **NOC** = Nursing Outcomes Classification

■ (SP) *Provide instruction regarding cleaning and assist with care of dental appliances as needed.* **LOE = VII**

(EO) A self-care intervention model, the PRO-SELF program, which includes didactic information related to daily oral care, development of self-care exercises, and supportive communication with a nurse, was used in both outpatient chemotherapy and radiation therapy settings. The authors found that teaching patients self-care instructions was an important contribution during their cancer therapy (Larson et al., 1998).

(EO) Daily cleansing of dental appliances is accepted by the ADA as a standard of care to assist in daily oral hygiene (ADA, 2006).

Possibly Effective

■ *Instruct about the need for and method of providing frequent oral care to the patient 1 week before radiotherapy.* **LOE = III**

(MR) An RCT ($N = 30$) demonstrated that instructions on oral care given 1 week prior to radiation resulted in reduced mucositis as opposed to instructions given 1 day before or no instructions (Shieh et al., 1997).

■ *Use salivary substitutes to assist in maintaining mouth moisture.* **LOE = VII**

(MR) A review of the literature regarding oral complications of cancer and its therapies examined strategies related to diagnosis, prevention, and treatment of complications such as xerostomia. Results recommended the use of salivary substitutes for symptomatic relief of xerostomia (NIH, 1990).

(EO) The National Institute of Dental and Craniofacial Research (NIDCR) supports the use of salivary substitutes (NIDCR, 2002).

■ *Instruct patients to use sugarless gum or sugarless sour candy to promote salivary flow.* **LOE = VII**

(EO) The ADA and NIDCR support the use of sugarless gum or candy to promote salivary flow (ADA, 2006; NIDCR, 2002).

■ *Rinse with a bland mouthwash such as normal saline as part of daily oral care.* **LOE = IV**

(NR) An RCT of outpatient cancer patients with mucositis ($N = 142$) evaluated one of three mouthwashes. The study found the effectiveness of the three rinses to be equal and thus recommended the use of the most economical rinse, which was a combination of salt and soda mouthwash (Dodd et al., 2000).

■ *Use chlorhexidine mouthwash to assist in oral microbial control in intubated patients and patients receiving chemotherapy.* **LOE = II**

(NR) Intubated patients ($N = 34$) were randomly assigned to two different forms of chlorhexidine or placebo, and oral cultures were obtained. Data suggested that use of chlorhexidine gluconate in the early postintubation period may delay development of pneumonia (Grap et al., 2004).

(MR) An RCT evaluated the effect of 0.12% chlorhexidine mouth rinse in a prospective, double-blind trial as prophylaxis against cytotoxic therapy–induced damage to oral soft

---

NR = Nursing Research, **MR** = Multidisciplinary Research, **SP** = Standard of Practice, **EO** = Expert Opinion, **LOE** = Level of Evidence

tissues. Of 70 cancer patients, 40 received high-dose chemotherapy and 30 received high-dose radiation to the head and neck. Reductions in oral streptococci and yeast were found in patients receiving chemotherapy. No benefit was found in the patients with head and neck radiation (Ferretti et al., 1990).

(MR) A comprehensive literature review cited the use of chlorhexidine as part of an oral care protocol for the reduction of plaque (Rubenstein et al., 2004).

Note: Use of chlorhexidine mouthwash is intended to reduce the microbial burden in patients whose daily self-care may be compromised and is *not* intended for the prevention of mucositis.

Not Effective

■ *Use of foam swabs for removing dental plaque.* **LOE = III**

(NR) A crossover controlled trial with 34 volunteers demonstrated that use of a toothbrush was more effective than use of foam sticks in removal of plaque (Pearson & Hutton, 2002).

■ *Use of chlorhexidine mouthwash to prevent mucositis in patients diagnosed with head and neck cancer undergoing radiation therapy.* **LOE = II**

(MR) An RCT ($N = 52$) of patients treated with radiation involving at least one third of the oral cavity mucosa found no benefit to the use of this agent in reducing mucositis (Foote et al., 1994).

Possibly Harmful

■ *Use of hydrogen peroxide as a mouthwash or cleansing agent.* **LOE = II**

(NR) An RCT ($N = 35$) of the use of one-quarter-strength hydrogen peroxide versus one-half-strength hydrogen peroxide versus normal saline mouth rinsing agent demonstrated that the use of hydrogen peroxide was associated with development of mucosal abnormalities, and participants found the use of hydrogen peroxide overwhelmingly a negative experience (Tombes & Gallucci, 1993).

(MR) A controlled trial ($N = 150$) of the use of five different mouth care products, including a 1.5% hydrogen peroxide solution, demonstrated that use of the hydrogen peroxide solution did not result in any pathological changes in the oral cavity or cause adverse changes in the microflora in the mouth (Shibly et al., 1997).

■ *Use of lemon and glycerin swabs to give oral care.* **LOE = II**

(NR) A controlled trial involving nursing home patients ($N = 136$) comparing the effects of lemon-glycerin versus normal saline as a mouthwash found that the lemon-glycerin solution resulted in decreased moisture in the mouth (Van Drimmelen & Rollins, 1969).

(NR) An RCT of the use of lemon-glycerin swabs versus Moi-Stir swabs ($N = 20$) found the lemon-glycerin swabs did not relieve mouth dryness and resulted in decreased dentition and gingival scores (Poland et al., 1987).

(MR) An in vitro RCT of the use of three commercially available swab sticks on bovine teeth demonstrated significant erosion of the teeth soaked in the lemon-glycerin solution for 4 hours (Meurman et al., 1996).

RCT = Randomized Controlled (Clinical) Trial, **NIC** = Nursing Interventions Classification, **NOC** = Nursing Outcomes Classification

OUTCOME MEASUREMENT

ORAL MUCOSITIS ASSESSMENT SCALE

This instrument has two components: clinicians' assessment—objective measures of mucositis: erythema and ulceration of multiple anatomic locations; and patients' report of pain, difficulty swallowing, and ability to eat (Sonis et al., 1999). For details regarding measurement of oral mucositis, please refer to Eilers and Epstein (2004).

ORAL HYGIENE   (NOC)

Definition: Condition of the mouth, teeth, gums, and tongue.
Oral Hygiene as evidenced by the following selected NOC indicators:
• Cleanliness of mouth
• Cleanliness of teeth
• Cleanliness of gums
• Moisture of oral mucosa and tongue
• Moistness of lips
• Color of mucosa membranes
• Oral mucosa integrity
(Rate each indicator of **Oral Hygiene:** 1 = severely compromised, 2 = substantially compromised, 3 = moderately compromised, 4 = mildly compromised, 5 = not compromised) (adapted from Moorhead et al., 2004).

REFERENCES

American Dental Association (ADA). (2006). Cleaning your teeth and gums. Available online: www.ada. org. Retrieved on June 5, 2007.

Barker GJ, Epstein JB, Williams KB, Gorsky M, Raber-Durlacher JE. (2005). Current practice and knowledge of oral care for cancer patients: A survey of supportive health care providers. *Support Care Cancer,* 13(1):32-41.

Dochterman JM, Bulechek GM (Eds). (2004). *Nursing Interventions Classification (NIC),* 4th ed. St. Louis: Mosby.

Dodd MJ, Dibble SL, Miaskowski C. (2000). Randomized clinical trial of the effectiveness of 3 commonly used mouthwashes to treat chemotherapy-induced mucositis, *Oral Surg Oral Med Oral Pathol Oral Radiol Endod,* 90(1): 39-47.

Dreizen S, Brown LR, Daly TE, Drane JB. (1977). Prevention of xerostomia-related dental caries in irradiated cancer patients. *J Dent Res,* 56(2):99-104.

Eilers J, Epstein JB. (2004). Assessment and measurement of oral mucositis. *Semin Oncol Nurs,* 20(1): 22-29.

Ferretti GA, Raybould TP, Brown AT, Macdonald JS, Greenwood M, Maruyama Y, et al. (1990). Chlorhexidine prophylaxis for chemotherapy- and radiotherapy-induced stomatitis: A randomized double-blind trial. *Oral Surg Oral Med Oral Pathol,* 69(3):331-338.

Foote RL, Loprinzi CL, Frank AR, O'Fallon JR, Gulavita S, Tewfik HH, et al. (1994). Randomized trial of a chlorhexidine mouthwash for alleviation of radiation-induced mucositis. *J Clin Oncol,* 12(12): 2630-2633.

Grap MJ, Munro CL, Elswick RK Jr, Sessler CN, Ward KR. (2004). Duration of action of a single, early oral application of chlorhexidine on oral microbial flora in mechanically ventilated patients: A pilot study. *Heart Lung,* 33(2):83-91.

Larson PJ, Dodd MJ, Aksamit I. (1998). A symptom-management program for patients undergoing cancer treatment: The Pro-Self Program. *J Cancer Educ,* 13(4):248-252.

NR = Nursing Research, **MR** = Multidisciplinary Research, **SP** = Standard of Practice, **EO** = Expert Opinion, **LOE** = Level of Evidence

McGuire DB, Correa ME, Johnson J, Wienandts P. (2006). The role of basic oral care and good clinical practice principles in the management of oral mucositis. *Support Care Cancer,* 14(6):541-547.

Meurman JH, Sorvari R, Pelttari A, et al. (1996). Hospital mouth-cleaning aids may cause dental erosion, *Spec Care Dentist,* 16(6): 247-250.

Moorhead M, Johnson M, Maas M (Eds). (2004). *Nursing Outcomes Classification (NOC),* 3rd ed. St. Louis: Mosby.

National Institute of Dental and Craniofacial Research (NIDCR). (2002). Cancer treatment and oral health. Available online: http://www.nidcr.nih.gov. Retrieved on June 6, 2007.

National Institutes of Health (NIH). (1990). National Institutes of Health Consensus Development Conference on Oral Complications of Cancer Therapies: Diagnosis, prevention, and treatment. Bethesda, MD, April 17-19, 1989. *NCI Monogr,* 9:1-184.

NOHIC, National Oral Health Information Clearinghouse (2007). Fluoride and Fluoridation Available online: http://www.ada.org/prof/resources/topics/fluoride.asp. Retrieved on June 6, 2007.

Pearson LS, Hutton JL. (2002). A controlled trial to compare the ability of foam swabs and toothbrushes to remove dental plaque. *J Adv Nurs,* 39(5):480-489.

Poland JM, Dugan M, Parashos P, Irick N, Dugan W, Tracey M. (1987). Comparing Moi-Stir to lemon-glycerin swabs. *Am J Nurs,* 87(4):422, 424.

Rubenstein EB, Peterson DE, Schubert M, et al. (2004). Clinical practice guidelines for the prevention and treatment of cancer therapy-induced oral and gastrointestinal mucositis. *Cancer,* 100(9) Suppl: 2026-2046.

Shibly O, Ciancio SG, Kazmierczak M, et al. (1997). Clinical evaluation of the effect of a hydrogen peroxide mouth rinse, sodium bicarbonate dentifrice, and mouth moisturizer on oral health. *J Clin Dent,* 8(5): 145-149.

Shieh SH, Wang ST, Tsai ST, Tseng CC. (1997). Mouth care for nasopharyngeal cancer patients undergoing radiotherapy. *Oral Oncol,* 33(1):36-41.

Sonis ST, Eilers JP, Epstein JB, LeVeque FG, Liggett WH Jr, Mulagha MT, et al. (1999). Validation of a new scoring system for the assessment of clinical trial research of oral mucositis induced by radiation or chemotherapy. Mucositis Study Group. *Cancer,* 85(10):2103-2113.

Tombes MB, Gallucci B. (1993). The effects of hydrogen peroxide rinses on the normal oral mucosa. *Nurs Res,* 42(6):332-337.

Van Drimmelen J, Rollins HF. (1969). Evaluation of a commonly used oral hygiene agent. *Nurs Res,* 18(4): 327-332.

ORAL HEALTH PROMOTION

Betty J. Ackley, MSN, EdS, RN; Dianna S. Weikel, RDH, MS

NIC Definition: Promotion of oral hygiene and dental care for a patient with normal oral and dental health (Dochterman & Bulechek, 2004).

NURSING ACTIVITIES

Effective

■ *Use a soft toothbrush two times per day to remove dental plaque and to decrease formation of caries and gingivitis.* **LOE = I**

 A crossover controlled trial (*N* = 34) demonstrated that use of a toothbrush was more effective than use of foam sticks for removal of plaque (Pearson & Hutton, 2002).

A systematic review demonstrated that regular tooth brushing with a fluoride toothpaste could help decrease or eliminate caries and periodontal disease (Kay, 1998).

(MR) A controlled study on older patients in nursing homes in Japan ($N = 417$ patients) demonstrated that an experimental group of patients who received tooth brushing after each meal plus professional care from a dental hygienist or a dentist once a week, versus a control group who did not receive oral care, had decreased febrile days, decreased incidence of pneumonia, decreased deaths from pneumonia, increased activities of daily living, and increased cognitive function (Yoneyama et al., 2002).

■ *Use a powered toothbrush to remove dental plaque and prevent gingivitis.* LOE = I

(MR) A Cochrane systematic review found that powered toothbrushes with a rotation oscillation action reduced plaque and incidence of gingivitis more than manual toothbrushes (Robinson et al., 2005).

(MR) An RCT comparing the Braun 3D Excel versus the Cybersonic power toothbrush versus a manual toothbrush demonstrated that both power toothbrushes were more effective in removing plaque and reducing papillary bleeding than a manual toothbrush (Zimmer et al., 2005).

(MR) An RCT comparing fluoride toothpaste along with manual brushing only, manual brushing and daily flossing, electric brushing using a rotational oscillation toothbrush, and electric brushing using a sonic toothbrush demonstrated that the amount of interproximal plaque was lowest with the sonic brushing (Sjögren et al., 2004).

■ *Use fluoride-containing toothpaste.* LOE = I

(MR) A Cochrane review demonstrated that the benefits of fluoride toothpaste in preventing caries in children and adolescents had been firmly established by many high-quality RCTs (Marinho et al., 2003).

(MR) A systematic review of the literature demonstrated that brushing teeth twice daily with fluoride toothpaste was helpful in reducing dental caries (CDC, 2001).

■ (NIC) *Teach and encourage flossing.* LOE = I

(MR) A review of the literature of mechanical oral hygiene practices found that there was good evidence to recommend flossing for adults (Brothwell et al., 1998).

(MR) In a controlled trial of participants ($N = 39$) in which the experimental group used manual tooth brushing plus daily flossing versus a control group that used manual tooth brushing alone, the group that combined tooth brushing with flossing had a significant reduction in the amount of plaque present between teeth (Bellamy et al., 2004).

Possibly Effective

■ *Use an essential oil–containing mouthwash after brushing teeth and flossing.* LOE = II

(MR) A controlled trial ($N = 237$) comparing three groups—(1) tooth brushing and control mouth rinse; (2) tooth brushing, flossing, and control mouthwash; and (3) tooth brushing, flossing, and use of an essential oil mouthwash—demonstrated that there was significantly less plaque and gingivitis with use of the essential oil mouthwash plus tooth brushing and flossing (Sharma et al., 2004).

NR = Nursing Research, **MR** = Multidisciplinary Research, **SP** = Standard of Practice, **EO** = Expert Opinion, **LOE** = Level of Evidence

(MR) An RCT ($N = 362$) comparing three groups—(1) tooth brushing with control mouth rinse, (2) tooth brushing with flossing, and (3) tooth brushing with twice-daily rinsing with an essential oil mouth rinse (Cool Mint Listerine Antiseptic)—demonstrated that the group using tooth brushing plus the essential oil mouth rinse had lower plaque and gingivitis scores than the tooth brushing and flossing group (Bauroth et al., 2003).

▪ *Use a tongue scraper to clean the tongue as part of oral hygiene care.* **LOE = II**

(MR) A controlled trial of participants ($N = 10$) using a tongue scraper versus using a soft toothbrush to cleanse the tongue demonstrated that the use of a tongue scraper resulted in a 75% reduction in volatile sulfur compounds versus a 45% reduction with use of the toothbrush (Pedrazzi et al., 2004). (Note: Volatile sulfur compounds are associated with halitosis.)

(MR) An RCT ($N = 60$) of three treatments—(1) tongue scraping following brushing, (2) placement of a Listerine Oral Care Strip on the tongue after brushing, and (3) rinsing with normal saline following brushing—demonstrated that the count of mutans streptococci (a cariogenic pathogen) was reduced most effectively in the tongue scraping group (White & Armaleh, 2004).

Not Effective

▪ *Use of foam swabs for removing dental plaque.* **LOE = I**

(Note: Foam swabs may be used when tooth brushing is not appropriate, such as when a patient has bleeding tendencies.)

(NR) A controlled trial ($N = 34$) demonstrated that use of a toothbrush was more effective than use of foam sticks in removal of plaque (Pearson & Hutton, 2002).

(MR) A systematic review demonstrated that there was moderate evidence *not* to recommend use of foam brushes for caries prevention (Brothwell et al., 1998).

Possibly Harmful

▪ *Use of hydrogen peroxide as a mouthwash or cleansing agent.* **LOE = II**

(NR) An RCT ($N = 35$) of use of $\frac{1}{4}$-strength hydrogen peroxide versus $\frac{1}{2}$-strength hydrogen peroxide versus normal saline mouth rinsing agent demonstrated that the use of hydrogen peroxide was associated with development of mucosal abnormalities, and subjects found the use of hydrogen peroxide overwhelmingly a negative experience (Tombes & Gallucci, 1993).

(NR) A controlled trial ($N = 150$) comparing five different mouth care products, including a 1.5% hydrogen peroxide solution, demonstrated that use of the hydrogen peroxide solution did not result in any pathological changes in the oral cavity or cause adverse changes in the microflora in the mouth (Shibly et al., 1997).

▪ *Use of lemon and glycerin swabs to give oral care.* **LOE = II**

(NR) In a controlled trial of nursing home patients ($N = 136$) comparing the effects of lemon-glycerin versus normal saline as a mouthwash, the lemon-glycerin solution resulted in decreased moisture in the mouth (Van Drimmelen & Rollins, 1969).

(NR) In an RCT of the use of lemon-glycerin swabs versus Moi-Stir swabs ($N = 20$), the lemon-glycerin swabs did not relieve mouth dryness and resulted in decreased dentition and gingival scores (Poland et al., 1987).

RCT = Randomized Controlled (Clinical) Trial, **NIC** = Nursing Interventions Classification, **NOC** = Nursing Outcomes Classification

(MR) An in vitro RCT of the use of three commercially available swab sticks on bovine teeth demonstrated significant erosion of the teeth soaked in the lemon-glycerin solution for 4 hours (Meurman et al., 1996).

OUTCOME MEASUREMENT

ORAL HYGIENE (NOC)

Definition: Condition of the mouth, teeth, gums, and tongue.

Oral Hygiene as evidenced by the following selected NOC indicators:
- Cleanliness of mouth
- Cleanliness of teeth
- Cleanliness of gums
- Moisture of oral mucosa and tongue
- Moistness of lips
- Color of mucosa membranes
- Oral mucosa integrity

(Rate each indicator of **Oral Hygiene**: 1 = severely compromised, 2 = substantially compromised, 3 = moderately compromised, 4 = mildly compromised, 5 = not compromised) (Moorhead et al., 2004).

REFERENCES

Bauroth K, Charles CH, Mankodi SM, Simmons K, Zhao Q, Kumar LD. (2003). The efficacy of an essential oil antiseptic mouthrinse vs. dental floss in controlling interproximal gingivitis: A comparative study. *J Am Dent Assoc,* 134(3):359-365.

Bellamy P, Barlow A, Puri G, Wright KI, Mussett A, Zhou X. (2004). A new in vivo interdental sampling method comparing a daily flossing regime versus a manual brush control. *J Clin Dent,* 15(3):59-65.

Brothwell DJ, Jutai DK, Hawkins RJ. (1998). An update of mechanical oral hygiene practices: Evidence-based recommendations for disease prevention. *J Can Dent Assoc,* 64(4):295-306.

Centers for Disease Control and Prevention (CDC). (2001). Recommendations for using fluoride to prevent and control dental caries in the United States. Centers for Disease Control and Prevention. *MMWR Recomm Rep,* 50(RR-14):1-42.

Dochterman JM, Bulechek GM (Eds). (2004). *Nursing Interventions Classification (NIC),* 4th ed. St. Louis: Mosby.

Kay EJ. (1998). Caries prevention—Based on evidence? Or an act of faith? *Br Dent J,* 185(9):432-433.

Marinho VC, Higgins JP, Sheiham A, Logan S. (2003). Fluoride toothpastes for preventing dental caries in children and adolescents. *Cochrane Database Syst Rev,* (1):CD002278.

Meurman JH, Sorvari R, Pelttari A, Rytomaa I, Franssila S, Kroon L. (1996). Hospital mouth-cleaning aids may cause dental erosion. *Spec Care Dentist,* 16(6):247-250.

Moorhead M, Johnson M, Maas M (Eds). (2004). *Nursing Outcomes Classification (NOC),* 3rd ed. St. Louis: Mosby.

Pearson LS, Hutton JL. (2002). A controlled trial to compare the ability of foam swabs and toothbrushes to remove dental plaque. *J Adv Nurs,* 39(5):480-489.

Pedrazzi V, Sato S, de Mattos Mda G, Lara EH, Panzeri H. (2004). Tongue-cleaning methods: A comparative clinical trial employing a toothbrush and a tongue scraper. *J Periodontol,* 75(7):1009-1012.

Poland JM, Dugan M, Parashos, P, Irick N, Dugan W, Tracey M. (1987). Comparing Moi-Stir to lemon-glycerin swabs. *Am J Nurs,* 87(4):422, 424.

Robinson PG, Deacon SA, Deery C, Heanue M, Walmsley AD, Worthington HV, et al. (2005). Manual versus powered toothbrushing for oral health. *Cochrane Database Syst Rev,* (2):CD002281.

NR = Nursing Research, **MR** = Multidisciplinary Research, **SP** = Standard of Practice, **EO** = Expert Opinion, **LOE** = Level of Evidence

Sharma N, Charles CH, Lynch MC, Qagish J, McGuire JA, Galustians JG, et al. (2004). Adjunctive benefit of an essential oil-containing mouthrinse in reducing plaque and gingivitis in patients who brush and floss regularly: A six-month study. *J Am Dent Assoc,* 135(4):496-504.

Shibly O, Ciancio SG, Kazmierczak M, Cohen RE, Mather ML, Ho A, et al. (1997). Clinical evaluation of the effect of a hydrogen peroxide mouth rinse, sodium bicarbonate dentifrice, and mouth moisturizer on oral health. *J Clin Dent,* 8(5):145-149.

Sjögren K, Lundberg AB, Birkhed D, Dudgeon DJ, Johnson MR. (2004). Interproximal plaque mass and fluoride retention after brushing and flossing—A comparative study of powered toothbrushing, manual toothbrushing and flossing. *Oral Health Prev Dent,* 2(2):119-124.

Tombes MB, Gallucci B. (1993). The effects of hydrogen peroxide rinses on the normal oral mucosa. *Nurs Res,* 42(6):332-337.

Van Drimmelen J, Rollins HF. (1969). Evaluation of a commonly used oral hygiene agent. *Nurs Res,* 18(4):327-332.

White GE, Armaleh MT. (2004). Tongue scraping as a means of reducing oral mutans streptococci. *J Clin Pediatr Dent,* 28(2):163-166.

Yoneyama T, Yoshida M, Ohrui T, Mukaiyama H, Okamoto H, Hoshiba K, et al. (2002). Oral care reduces pneumonia in older patients in nursing homes. *J Am Geriatr Soc,* 50(3):430-433.

Zimmer S, Strauss J, Bizhang M, Krage T, Raab WH, Barthel C. (2005). Efficacy of the Cybersonic in comparison with the Braun 3D Excel and a manual toothbrush. *J Clin Periodontol,* 32(4):360-363.

ORAL HEALTH RESTORATION

Dianna S. Weikel, RDH, MS

NIC   **Definition:** Promotion of healing for a patient who has an oral mucosa or dental lesion (Dochterman & Bulechek, 2004).

NURSING ACTIVITIES

Effective

■ *Use benzydamine hydrochloride (HCl) mouthwash as ordered for the prevention of radiation-induced mucositis in patients with head and neck cancer receiving radiotherapy.* **LOE = I**

MR A multicenter, randomized, placebo-controlled trial evaluated 172 patients with head and neck cancer receiving external beam radiation and prophylactic use of benzydamine mouth rinse during radiation treatment. Results showed that benzydamine was safe and effective for prophylactic treatment of radiation-induced oral mucositis (Epstein et al., 2001).

MR A systematic review of the literature recommended use of benzydamine for prevention of radiation-induced mucositis (Rubenstein et al., 2004).

(Note: Benzydamine HCl has not been approved for use in the United States.)

■ *Use amifostine as ordered to reduce the incidence of acute and late xerostomia in patients treated with standard fractionated radiation to the head and neck.* **LOE = I**

MR A systematic review found that amifostine, a cytoprotectant, has been shown to reduce the incidence of xerostomia, both acute and chronic, in head and neck cancer patients. The

American Society for Clinical Oncology recommended its use for reducing the effects of xerostomia in this population of patients (Schuchter et al., 2002).

(EO) Support for the use of amifostine is expressed by the experts (Brizel & Overgaard, 2003).

■ *Use palifermin in the prevention of mucositis in patients undergoing total body irradiation and chemotherapy prior to autologous transplantation.* **LOE = I**

(MR) A double-blind study (*N* = 212) of patients with hematologic cancers compared the effect of palifermin versus placebo in the development of mucositis. Palifermin reduced the duration and severity of oral mucositis after intensive chemotherapy and radiotherapy for patients with hematologic malignancies (Spielberger et al., 2004).

(EO) The use of palifermin for the prevention of mucositis in patients undergoing peripheral blood stem cell transplantation is supported by experts (von Bultzingslowen et al., 2006).

■ *Use ice chips (cryotherapy) to prevent chemotherapy-induced oral mucositis in patients being treated with 5-fluorouracil (5-FU).* **LOE = II**

(MR) An RCT randomly allocated 84 cancer patients treated with 5-FU to receive oral cryotherapy with 5-FU administration or to a control group that did not receive cryotherapy. A reduction in mucositis of approximately 50% was observed among those who received oral cryotherapy (Cascinu et al., 1994).

(MR) An earlier RCT of cancer patients receiving 5-FU (*N* = 178) using oral cryotherapy for either 30 minutes or 60 minutes reported that extending the duration of the intervention did not yield additional benefit. Therefore, 30 minutes of cryotherapy prior to initiation of 5-FU was recommended (Rocke et al., 1993).

■ *Use ice chips (cryotherapy) to prevent chemotherapy-induced oral mucositis in patients being treated with edatrexate administered in bolus doses.* **LOE = III**

(MR) Nonrandomized controlled trials (*N* = 46 cancer patients) suggested that oral cryotherapy may reduce oral mucositis related to edatrexate administration. Rationale for use in this instance is the short half-life of edatrexate (Edelman et al., 1998).

(MR) A nonrandomized study of 46 solid tumor patients being treated with edatrexate and prophylactic cryotherapy found less grade 3 and 4 mucositis. Thus, the dose-limiting toxicity did not occur, allowing escalation of edatrexate above levels previously reported. The authors attributed this finding to the prophylactic use of ice chips (Edelman et al., 1998).

■ *Use ice chips (cryotherapy) to prevent chemotherapy-induced oral mucositis in hematopoietic stem cell transplant patients receiving melphalan during conditioning treatment.* **LOE = III**

(MR) In a controlled study of 18 allogenic stem cell transplant patients receiving oral cryotherapy, it was shown that 2 of the 18 patients developed mucositis versus six of seven historical controls (Aisa et al., 2005).

(MR) A convenience sample of 22 patients receiving high-dose melphalan and treated with cryotherapy 30 minutes prior to the infusion showed less grade 3 mucositis compared with previous reports in the literature. The authors suggested the benefit of cryotherapy in this population of patients (Tartarone et al., 2005).

(MR) A meta-analysis reviewed the use of oral prophylactic agents to affect the incidence of oral mucositis in cancer patients. The authors examined 11 randomized trials and found ice

---

NR = Nursing Research, **MR** = Multidisciplinary Research, **SP** = Standard of Practice, **EO** = Expert Opinion, **LOE** = Level of Evidence

chips to be the only agent to show efficacy in preventing mucositis (Worthington & Clarkson, 2002).

■ (SP) *Rinse with a bland mouthwash such as normal saline as part of daily oral care.* **LOE = IV**

(NR) A randomized (*N* = 142) outpatient study of cancer patients with mucositis evaluated one of three mouthwashes. The study found the effectiveness of the three rinses to be equal and thus recommended use of the most economical rinse, which was a combination of salt and soda mouthwash (Dodd et al., 2000).

(MR) An RCT (*N* = 30) evaluated head and neck patients receiving radiation therapy. Patients were randomly assigned to a mouthwash containing sucralfate or a salt/soda mouth rinse at the onset of oral mucositis. The authors found no difference in duration of mucositis between the two groups and thus recommended the less costly salt/soda mouth rinse (Dodd et al., 2003).

■ (NIC) (SP) *Remove dentures in case of severe stomatitis.* **LOE = VII**

(EO) In the patient at risk for oral mucositis, the recommendation is to wear dental prostheses only to assist in eating of solid food. If the intraoral tissues are severely ulcerated, preventing the patient from eating solid foods, the dentures should not be worn at all to prevent further trauma to the intraoral tissues (NIDCR, 2005).

Possibly Effective

■ *Use bioadhesive products (Gelclair) for pain control in patients with oral ulcerations/mucositis.* **LOE = VI**

(MR) Preliminary studies of bioadhesive products have shown that they decrease pain and may decrease the severity of the mucositis (Buchsel, 2003; Innocenti et al., 2002). (Note: Studies were open-label trials; RCTs are needed before the product can be deemed effective.)

Not Effective

■ *Using topical preparations such as viscous lidocaine, milk of magnesia, kaolin, pectin, chlorhexidine, and diphenhydramine for the prevention or reduction of cancer treatment–induced mucositis.* **LOE = V**

(MR) A systematic review of the literature stated that there was not enough evidence to support the use of coating agents or chlorhexidine for the prevention of oral mucositis (Rubenstein et al., 2004).

(MR) An RCT (*N* = 30) evaluated head and neck patients receiving radiation therapy. Patients were randomly assigned to a mouthwash containing sucralfate or salt/soda at the onset of oral mucositis. The authors found no difference in duration of mucositis between the two groups and thus recommended the less costly salt/soda mouth rinse (Dodd et al., 2003).

(MR) In an RCT (*N* = 200) where patients received one of three mouthwashes and instructions for oral self-care, no significant differences in cessation of oral symptoms were observed among the three groups. The authors recommended the use of the least costly product, which was a mixture of salt and soda suspended in solution (Dodd et al., 2000).

RCT = Randomized Controlled (Clinical) Trial, **NIC** = Nursing Interventions Classification, **NOC** = Nursing Outcomes Classification

■ *Using foam swabs for removing dental plaque.* **LOE = III**

(NR) A crossover controlled trial with 34 volunteers demonstrated that the use of a toothbrush was more effective than the use of foam sticks in removal of plaque (Pearson & Hutton, 2002).

Possibly Harmful

■ *Using hydrogen peroxide as a daily mouthwash.* **LOE = II**

(NR) An RCT ($N = 35$) using $\frac{1}{4}$-strength hydrogen peroxide versus $\frac{1}{2}$-strength hydrogen peroxide versus a normal saline mouth rinsing agent demonstrated that the use of hydrogen peroxide was associated with development of mucosal abnormalities. Subjects also found the use of hydrogen peroxide overwhelmingly a negative experience (Tombes & Gallucci, 1993).

(NR) A controlled trial ($N = 150$) of the use of five different mouth care products including a 1.5% hydrogen peroxide solution demonstrated that the use of the hydrogen peroxide solution did not result in any pathological changes in the oral cavity or cause adverse changes in the microflora in the mouth (Shibly et al., 1997).

OUTCOME MEASUREMENT

ORAL MUCOSITIS ASSESSMENT SCALE

This instrument has two components: clinician assessment—objective measures of mucositis: erythema and ulceration of multiple anatomic locations, and patients' report of pain, difficulty swallowing, and ability to eat (Sonis et al., 1999). For details regarding measurement of oral mucositis, please refer to Eilers and Epstein (2004).

ORAL HYGIENE (NOC)

Definition: Condition of the mouth, teeth, gums, and tongue.
Oral Hygiene as evidenced by the following indicators:
• Halitosis
• Bleeding
• Pain
• Oral mucosa lesions
• Gingivitis
• Periodontal disease
(Rate each indicator of **Oral Hygiene:** 1 = severe, 2 = substantial, 3 = moderate, 4 = mild, 5 = none) (Moorhead et al., 2004).

REFERENCES

Aisa Y, Mori T, Kudo M, Yashima T, Dondo S, Yokoyama A, et al. (2005). Oral cryotherapy for the prevention of high-dose melphalan-induced stomatitis in allogeneic hematopoietic stem cell transplant recipients. *Support Care Cancer,* 13(4):266-269.

Brizel DM, Overgaard J. (2003). Does amifostine have a role in chemoradiation treatment? *Lancet Oncol,* 4(6):378-381.

Buchsel PC. (2003). Gelclair oral gel. *Clin J Oncol Nurs,* 7(1):109-110.

Cascinu S, Fedeli A, Fedeli SL, Catalano G. (1994). Oral cooling (cryotherapy), an effective treatment for prevention of 5-fluorouracil-induced stomatitis. *Eur J Cancer B Oral Oncol,* 30B(4):234-236.

Clarkson JE, Worthington HV, Eden OB. (2003). Interventions for preventing oral mucositis for patients with cancer receiving treatment. *Cochrane Database Syst Rev,* (3):CD000978.

Dochterman JM, Bulechek GM (Eds). (2004). *Nursing Interventions Classification (NIC),* 4th ed. St. Louis: Mosby.

Dodd MJ, Dibble SL, Miaskowski C, MacPhail L, Greenspan D, Paul SM, et al. (2000). Randomized clinical trial of the effectiveness of 3 commonly used mouthwashes to treat chemotherapy-induced mucositis. *Oral Surg Oral Med Oral Pathol Oral Radiol Endod,* 90(1):39-47.

Dodd MJ, Miaskowski C, Greenspan D, MacPhail L, Shih AS, Shiba G, et al. (2003). Radiation-induced mucositis: A randomized clinical trial of micronized sucralfate versus salt and soda mouthwashes. *Cancer Invest,* 21(1):21-33.

Edelman MJ, Gandara DR, Perez EA, et al. (1998). Phase I trial of edatrexate plus carboplatin in advanced solid tumors: Amelioration of dose-limiting mucositis by ice chip cryotherapy. *Invest New Drugs,* 16(1):69-75.

Eilers J, Epstein JB. (2004). Assessment and measurement of oral mucositis. *Semin Oncol Nurs,* 20(1):22-29.

Epstein JB, Silverman S Jr, Paggiarino DA, Crockett S, Schubert MM, Senzer NN, et al. (2001). Benzydamine HCl for prophylaxis of radiation-induced oral mucositis: Results from a multi-center, randomized, double-blind, placebo-controlled clinical trial. *Cancer,* 92(4):875-885.

Innocenti M, Moscatelli G, Lopez S. (2002). Efficacy of gelclair in reducing pain in palliative care patients with oral lesions: Preliminary findings from an open pilot study. *J Pain Symptom Manage,* 24(5):456-457.

Moorhead M, Johnson M, Maas M (Eds). (2004). *Nursing Outcomes Classification (NOC),* 3rd ed. St. Louis: Mosby.

National Institute of Dental and Craniofacial Research (NIDCR). (2005). Oral complications of cancer treatment: What the oncology team can do. Available online: http://www.nidcr.nih.gov/. Retrieved on June 6, 2007.

Pearson LS, Hutton JL. (2002). A controlled trial to compare the ability of foam swabs and toothbrushes to remove dental plaque. *J Adv Nurs,* 39(5):480-489.

Rocke LK, Loprinzi CL, Lee JK, Kunselman SJ, Iverson RK, Finck G, et al. (1993). A randomized clinical trial of two different durations of oral cryotherapy for prevention of 5-fluorouracil-related stomatitis. *Cancer,* 72(7):2234-2238.

Rubenstein EB, Peterson DE, Schubert M, Keefe D, McGuire D, Epstein J, et al. (2004). Mucositis: Clinical practice guidelines for the prevention and treatment of cancer therapy-induced oral and gastrointestinal mucositis. *Cancer,* 100(9 Suppl):2026-2046.

Schuchter LM, Hensley ML, Meropol NJ, et al. (2002). American Society of Clinical Oncology Chemotherapy and Radiotherapy Expert Panel, 2002 update of recommendations for the use of chemotherapy and radiotherapy protectants: Clinical practice guidelines of the American Society of Clinical Oncology. *J Clin Oncol,* 20(12):2895-2903.

Shibly O, Ciancio SG, Kazmierczak M, Cohen RE, Mather ML, Ho A, et al. (1997). Clinical evaluation of the effect of a hydrogen peroxide mouth rinse, sodium bicarbonate dentifrice, and mouth moisturizer on oral health. *J Clin Dent,* 8(5):145-149.

Sonis ST, Eilers JP, Epstein JB, LeVeque FG, Liggett WH, Mulagha MT, et al. (1999). Validation of a new scoring system for the assessment of clinical trial research of oral mucositis induced by radiation or chemotherapy. Mucositis Study Group. *Cancer,* 85(10):2103-2113.

Spielberger R, Stiff P, Bensinger W, Gentile T, Weisdorf D, Kewalramani T, et al. (2004). Palifermin for oral mucositis after intensive therapy for hematologic cancers. *N Engl J Med,* 351(25):2590-2598.

Tartarone A, Matera R, Romano G, et al. (2005). Prevention of high-dose melphalan-induced mucositis by cryotherapy. *Leuk Lymphoma,* 46(4):633-634.

Tombes MB, Gallucci B. (1993). The effects of hydrogen peroxide rinses on the normal oral mucosa. *Nurs Res,* 42(6):332-337.

RCT = Randomized Controlled (Clinical) Trial, **NIC** = Nursing Interventions Classification, **NOC** = Nursing Outcomes Classification

von Bultzingslowen I, Brennan M, Spijkervet FK, Logan R, Stringer A, Raber-Durlacher JE, et al. (2006). Growth factors and cytokines in the prevention and treatment of oral and gastrointestinal mucositis. *Support Care Cancer*, 14(6):519-527.

Worthington HV, Clarkson JE. (2002). Prevention of oral mucositis and oral candidiasis for patients with cancer treated with chemotherapy: Cochrane systematic review. *J Dent Educ* 66(8):903-911.

PAIN MANAGEMENT: ACUTE PAIN

Yvonne D'Arcy, MS, CRNP, CNS; Claudia E. Campbell, BSN, RN-BC;
Betty J. Ackley, MSN, EdS, RN

NIC **Definition:** Alleviation of pain or a reduction in pain to a level of comfort that is acceptable to the patient (Dochterman & Bulechek, 2004).

Acute pain is the result of tissue damage and alerts the body that injury has occurred. It has a short duration and an identifiable cause such as trauma, surgery, or injury (APS, 2003; ASPMN, 2004).

NURSING ACTIVITIES

Effective

■ **NIC** **SP** *Perform a comprehensive assessment of pain to include location, characteristics, onset/duration, frequency, quality, intensity or severity of pain, and precipitating factors.* **LOE = VII**

EO Systematic ongoing assessment and documentation provide direction for the pain treatment plan; adjustments are based on the patient's response (Berry et al., 2006). The patient's report of pain is the single most reliable indicator of pain (APS, 2003; ASPMN, 2004).

■ *Assess pain using a simple unidimensional, valid, and reliable rating tool such as the numeric rating scale (NRS), the visual analogue scale, or the verbal descriptor scale.* **LOE = I**

MR A systematic review of 164 articles on pain measures found that single-item ratings of pain intensity are valid and reliable as measures of pain intensity (Jensen, 2003).

EO The Joint Commission (TJC) requires regular assessment and reassessment of pain in hospitalized patients as a part of the JCAHO Pain Management Standard (The Joint Commission, 2000).

■ **SP** *Utilize the FACES scale for pediatric and elderly patients including those who are unable to speak.* **LOE = VI**

EO The FACES scale uses six faces that range from smiling to one with tears. It can provide an accurate pain assessment in a population of pediatric patients (APS, 2003; ASPMN, 2004; AGS, 2002; D'Arcy, 2003, 2006).

MR In a Spanish comparison study, elderly patients preferred the FACES scale to the pain thermometer to record level of pain (Miro et al., 2005).

NR In a comparison study, three methods of pain measurement in patients with head and neck pain, including patients who were unable to speak, were evaluated including the FACES scale, the numeric pain rating scale, and the visual analogue scale. All three scales

NR = Nursing Research, **MR** = Multidisciplinary Research, **SP** = Standard of Practice, **EO** = Expert Opinion, **LOE** = Level of Evidence

demonstrated comparable reporting of pain. Patients preferred the numeric pain rating scale (Rodriquez et al., 2004).

(NR) In a comparison study of 130 long-term care patients with cognitive impairment, results of the use of three pain assessment tools were varied in response. The Present Pain Intensity and Numerical Rating Scales were the preferred choices by patients versus the FACES pain scale, which was more challenging for the cognitively impaired elderly patients to use (Kaas-alainen & Crook, 2004).

(NR) A prospective, correlational descriptive study was conducted using children from various cultures, Chinese ($N = 132$), Japanese ($N = 173$), and Thai ($N = 151$), to determine whether the FACES scale was reliable and valid in cultures other than Caucasian. The scale was found to be reliable, valid, and the preferred pain scale for all of the Asian children in the study (Wong & DiVito-Thomas, 2006).

■ (SP) *If the patient is cognitively impaired and unable to report pain or use a pain rating scale, assess and document behaviors that might be indicative of pain (e.g., change in activity, loss of appetite, guarding, grimacing, or moaning).*
LOE = III

(NR) Using a Checklist of Nonverbal Pain Indicators (CNPI) in a controlled study with impaired and nonimpaired older adults, it was found that pain report and intensity did not differ significantly between the two groups. In addition, it was found that impaired older adults received significantly less pain medication than cognitively intact patients in the early postoperative period (Feldt et al., 1998).

(EO) The absence of behaviors thought to be indicative of pain does not necessarily mean that pain is absent (Pasero, 2003; Pasero & McCaffery, 2004; McCaffery & Pasero, 1999).

(EO) Certain behaviors have been shown to be indicative of pain and can be used to assess pain in patients who cannot use a self-report pain rating tool (e.g., the cognitively impaired patient). The clinician should be aware that pain expression is highly individual and what may be a pain behavior in one client may not be in another. Pain assessment must be individualized (Herr, 2002).

■ (SP) *Question the patient regarding pain at frequent intervals, often at the same time as taking vital signs.* **LOE = VII**

(EO) Pain assessment is as important as taking vital signs, and the American Pain Society suggests applying the concept of pain assessment as the "fifth vital sign" (APS, 2004; Berry et al., 2006).

(EO) The Joint Commission requires the assessment and reassessment of pain intensity at regular intervals (The Joint Commission, 2000).

(EO) The American Society of Perianesthesia Nurses recommends the assessment of pain regularly in the postanesthesia care unit (Krenzischek et al., 2003).

■ *Assume that pain is present and treat accordingly in a patient who has a pathological condition or who is undergoing a procedure thought to be painful.*
LOE = I

(EO) Pain is associated with certain pathological conditions (e.g., fractures) and procedures (e.g., surgery). In the absence of the patient's report of pain (e.g., anesthetized, critically ill, or cognitively impaired patients), the clinician should assume pain is present and treat accordingly (Pasero, 2003; Herr et al., 2006; McCaffery & Pasero, 1999).

RCT = Randomized Controlled (Clinical) Trial, **NIC** = Nursing Interventions Classification, **NOC** = Nursing Outcomes Classification

(EO) Prevent pain when possible during procedures such as venipuncture. Use a topical local anesthetic as ordered such as EMLA cream or LMX-4. Venipuncture pain is often not minor pain to the adult experiencing the pain. Nurses are obligated to minimize all kinds of pain (Wong, 2003).

(NR) A crossover placebo-controlled study ($N = 18$) demonstrated that multiple sclerosis patients receiving the application of EMLA cream before intramuscular injection of interferon had reduced fear of injection scores and reduced pain of injection scores (Buhse, 2006).

(NR) A meta-analysis of 20 studies analyzing the effectiveness of a topical anesthetic (2.5% lidocaine and 2.5% prilocaine mixture, EMLA cream) concluded that the use of EMLA significantly decreased venipuncture and IV insertion pain in 85% of the population (Fetzer, 2002).

(Please refer to the guideline on Procedural Pain Alleviation.)

■ (SP) *Question patients about what level of pain they think is appropriate to achieve a state of comfort and appropriate function. Attempt to keep pain level no higher than that level, preferably much lower.* **LOE = VII**

(EO) The pain rating that allows the patient to have comfort and appropriate function should be determined; this allows a tangible way to measure outcomes of pain management (Pasero & McCaffery, 2004; Griffie, 2003).

(EO) Monitoring of postoperative pain should reflect not only pain intensity at rest but also activity-associated, dynamic pain (Dahl & Kehlet, 2006).

■ (SP) *Ensure that the patient receives prompt analgesic care before the pain becomes severe and includes optimal pain relief with medications.* **LOE = VII**

(EO) Patients have a right to pain assessment and adequate treatment (The Joint Commission, 2000).

(EO) When pain is treated aggressively in the acute care setting with adequate analgesia, patients suffer less and experience less stress and less impact overall on their physiologic functioning (Page, 2005).

■ *Explore the need for medications from the three classes of analgesics: opioids (narcotics), nonopioids (acetaminophen, nonselective nonsteroidal anti-inflammatory drugs), and adjuvant medications.* **LOE = I**

(EO) Some types of pain respond to nonopioid drugs alone. If the pain is not responding, however, consider increasing the dosage or adding an opioid. At any level of pain, analgesic adjuvants may be useful (APS, 2003).

(EO) Use the World Health Organization Analgesic Ladder to determine which level of pain medication to use for mild, moderate, or severe pain. Continue to use the adjuvant medications such as antidepressants or antiseizure medications with each step (Dalton & Youngblood, 2000).

(EO) Acute pain, especially postoperative pain, is a result of multiple nociceptive mechanisms and is best treated with a combination of treatment modalities, each working with a different pain mechanism to improve analgesia and reduce analgesic side effects (Curatolo & Sveticic, 2002; Kehlet, 2002).

NR = Nursing Research, **MR** = Multidisciplinary Research, **SP** = Standard of Practice, **EO** = Expert Opinion, **LOE** = Level of Evidence

(EO) The American Society of Anesthesiologists recommends combining various types of pain relief for postoperative pain relief (ASA, 2004).

(EO) Combining analgesics can result in acceptable pain relief with lower dosages of each analgesic than would be possible with one analgesic alone. Lower dosages can result in fewer or less severe side effects (Pasero, 2003).

(MR) A meta-analysis demonstrated that use of acetaminophen plus patient-controlled analgesia (PCA) with opioids in the postoperative period resulted in a 20% reduction in the use of opioids but no documented decrease in pain or decrease in morphine side effects (Remy et al., 2005).

(MR) A meta-analysis of randomized clinical trials determined that peripheral nerve catheters with local anesthetic provided statistically significant improved postoperative pain control compared with opioids with a decrease in opioid-related side effects (Richman et al., 2006).

■ (SP) *When opioids are administered, assess pain intensity, sedation, and respiratory status at regular intervals. Assess sedation and respiratory status every 1 to 2 hours in opioid-naive patients (those who have not been taking regular daily doses of opioids) during the first 24 hours of therapy. Decrease the opioid dose if the patient is excessively sedated.* **LOE = IV**

(MR) A retrospective case-control analysis found that 77.4% of 62 patients' respiratory events occurred in the first 24 hours postoperatively (Taylor et al., 2005).

(EO) Opioids may cause respiratory depression because they reduce the responsiveness of carbon dioxide chemoreceptors located in the respiratory centers of the brain. Because even more opioid is required to produce respiratory depression than is required to produce sedation, patients with clinically significant respiratory depression are usually also sedated. Respiratory depression can be prevented by assessing sedation and decreasing the opioid dose when the patient is arousable but has difficulty staying awake (Pasero & McCaffery, 2002).

(EO) In opioid-naive patients, once the pain is relieved, the patient may fall asleep, which can increase the opioid depressant effect on the respiratory center with an increased risk of airway obstruction by the tongue. Exercise close observation of the patient for at least 3 hours past the time of expected peak analgesic blood concentrations (APS, 2003).

■ (SP) *Ask the patient to describe past experiences with pain and the effectiveness of methods used to manage pain, including experiences with side effects, typical coping responses, and the way the patient expresses pain.* **LOE = VI**

(NR) An observational study involving 270 people with cancer pain revealed that those surveyed had a number of concerns (barriers) that affected their willingness to report pain and use analgesics (Ward et al., 1993). Many harbored fears and misconceptions regarding the use of analgesics, management of side effects, and risk of addiction.

■ (SP) *For chronic neuropathic pain, consider adjuvant medications that are analgesic, such as anticonvulsants and antidepressants. Patients who use descriptors for pain such as burning, painful tingling, numbness, or shooting pain are describing neuropathic pain.* **LOE = VII**

(EO) Neuropathic pain requires a specialized medication regimen; the pain is a result of damage to nerves, not muscles (APS 2003; Marcus, 2000; Staats et al., 2004).

RCT = Randomized Controlled (Clinical) Trial, **NIC** = Nursing Interventions Classification, **NOC** = Nursing Outcomes Classification

■ SP *Administer analgesics using the least invasive route available; avoid the intramuscular route of administration when possible.* **LOE = VI**

EO The least invasive route of administration capable of providing adequate pain control is recommended (APS, 2004; Pasero, 2003).

NR A descriptive study done as an audit ($N = 115$) found that postoperative patients receiving intramuscular injections received much less pain medication than patients who received PCA in the early postoperative period (Everett & Salamonson, 2005).

■ *Provide PCA and intraspinal routes of administration when appropriate and ordered.* **LOE = I**

NR A comparative study demonstrated that PCA was more effective in controlling pain than on-demand IM injections (Chang et al., 2004).

MR A meta-analysis demonstrated that PCA significantly reduced the visual analogue scores of pain when compared with nurse-controlled analgesia (Bainbridge et al., 2006).
(Please refer to the guideline on Patient-Controlled Analgesia.)

■ SP *Question the patient about any disruption in sleep.* **LOE = VII**

EO Patients should be assessed for sleep disruption (AGS, 2002).

EO Regional anesthesia options should be considered to reduce opioid requirements for patients with obstructive sleep apnea in the postoperative setting (Gross et al., 2006).

■ NIC *Explore the patient's knowledge and beliefs about pain. Consider cultural influences on pain response.* **LOE = VII**

EO Each patient has a right to have pain assessed and adequately treated. Language barriers to pain management must be addressed (The Joint Commission, 2000).

Possibly Effective

■ *Monitor for nonverbal signs of discomfort in nonverbal populations such as Alzheimer's and intubated patients using the Checklist of Nonverbal Pain Indicators.* **LOE = VI**

NR A comparison descriptive study of the CNPI with impaired and cognitively intact patients ($N = 88$) demonstrated significant correlation with observed pain behaviors in the instrument and self-report of pain in both cognitively intact and cognitively impaired older adults. Findings demonstrated that the cognitively impaired patients received less pain medication than the intact patients (Feldt et al., 1998), although pain behaviors were similar in both groups. More pain behaviors were noted in the cognitively impaired patients with movement (Feldt et al., 1998; Feldt, 2000).

■ *Monitor for nonverbal signs of discomfort in patients with dementia using the Pain Assessment in Patients with Advanced Dementia (PAINAD) scale.* **LOE = VI**

EO The PAINAD scale includes the elements of breathing, negative vocalizations, facial expressions, body language, and consolability. Scores go from 0 (no pain) to 10 (maximum pain). The scale is a combination of the FLACC (faces, legs, activity, cry, and consolability) scale with the NRS of 0 to 10 (Lane et al., 2003).

NR = Nursing Research, **MR** = Multidisciplinary Research, **SP** = Standard of Practice, **EO** = Expert Opinion, **LOE** = Level of Evidence

(NR) A review of 10 behavior pain scales for use with demented patients demonstrated that there was no standardized behavioral pain scale that is well developed and researched; they are in early stages of development and testing (Herr et al., 2006).

(NR) In a study of 105 critical care patients, 33 were evaluated while intubated and unconscious and 99 were evaluated while intubated and conscious. All 105 were evaluated after extubation. The Critical Care Pain Observation tool was found to be reliable, valid, and supported by patients' reports of pain after extubation when compared with the Pain Observation Tool ratings while intubated (Gelinas et al., 2006).

(MR) The Payen Behavioral Pain Scale was developed using 30 intubated and sedated critical care patients. The groups were divided into mild sedation, moderate sedation, and heavy sedation. The tool measured behaviors with an added dimension of tolerance for ventilation. This 12-point scale was found to be reliable and valid (Payen et al., 2001).

▪ *Discuss the patient's fears of undertreated pain, overdose, and addiction.* **LOE = VII**

(EO) All patients have the right to pain management, including addicts, and they may experience undertreated pain related to their history of substance abuse (The Joint Commission, 2000; APS, 2001; ASPMN, 2004).

(EO) Because of the many misconceptions regarding pain and its treatment, education about the ability to control pain effectively and correction of myths about the use of opioids should be included as part of the treatment plan. Addiction is unlikely when patients use opioids for pain management in the postoperative setting (APS, 2004; McCaffery et al., 2004).

(NR) A survey study of 270 people with cancer pain revealed that many harbored fears and misconceptions regarding the use of analgesics, management of side effects, and risk of addiction (Ward et al., 1993).

▪ *Use a pain equivalency chart when switching from one medication to another.* **LOE = VII**

(EO) When switching from one drug to another or from one route to another (e.g., intravenous to oral), use of an equivalency chart can ensure that the two doses of medication are equivalent for pain relief (Anderson et al., 2001; Golembiewski, 2002; ASPMN, 2004).

▪ (SP) *Recognize that oral opioid medications begin to work in about 1 hour and intravenous medications in 5 to 30 minutes depending on the medication; transdermal medication becomes effective in 12 to 16 hours with steady blood levels within 48 hours (APS, 2003).* **LOE = VII**

(EO) Knowing when the medication becomes effective helps guide nursing practice to checking back on the patient, ensuring that adequate pain relief has been obtained, and also planning nursing activities.

▪ *Utilize music of the patient's choice to help decrease pain.* **LOE = I**

(MR) A Cochrane review demonstrated that listening to music reduced pain intensity and opioid use, "but the magnitude of these benefits is small and the clinical importance is unclear" (Cepeda et al., 2006).

RCT = Randomized Controlled (Clinical) Trial, **NIC** = Nursing Interventions Classification, **NOC** = Nursing Outcomes Classification

■ *Suggest massage therapy for treatment of pain.* **LOE = VII**

> (MR) Both massage therapy and aromatherapy massage have short-term benefits for psychological well-being for the client with cancer (Fellowes et al., 2004).
> (Note: For information on guided imagery, hand massage, healing touch, therapeutic touch, heat/cold application, anxiety reduction, distraction, music therapy, and progressive muscle relaxation/autogenic therapy, refer to the guidelines available in this text.)

Not Effective

■ *Intramuscular injections are no longer recommended for pain relief.* **LOE = VI**

> (EO) Intramuscular injections result in irregular medication absorption (ASPMN, 2004; APS, 2003).
> (EO) Intramuscular injections are painful, provide unreliable absorption, and are inconvenient (Pasero, 2003).
> (NR) A descriptive study done as an audit ($N = 115$) found that postoperative patients receiving intramuscular injections received much less pain medication than patients who received PCA in the early postoperative period (Everett & Salamonson, 2005).
> (NR) A comparative study demonstrated that PCA was more effective in controlling pain than on-demand IM injections (Chang et al., 2004).
> (EO) Repeated IM injections can cause sterile abscesses and fibrosis of muscle and soft tissue. In addition, IM injection may lead to nerve injury with persistent neuropathic pain (APS, 2003).

■ *Use of a placebo as an analgesic.* **LOE = VII**

> (EO) An analgesic effect from a placebo such as an injection of saline solution does not provide any useful information about the genesis or severity of pain (APS, 2003).
> (EO) Placebo use for the assessment and/or treatment of pain, including the evaluation of response to pain treatments, constitutes fraud and deception (Coggins et al., 2004).

Possibly Harmful

■ *Avoid the use of opioids with toxic metabolites, such as meperidine (Demerol) and propoxyphene (Darvon, Darvocet), in older patients.* **LOE = VII**

> (EO) Meperidine's metabolite, normeperidine, can produce central nervous system irritability, seizures, and even death; propoxyphene's metabolite, norpropoxyphene, can produce cardiotoxicity. Both of these metabolites are eliminated by the kidneys, which makes meperidine and propoxyphene particularly poor choices for older patients, many of whom have at least some degree of renal insufficiency (Ardery et al., 2003; Fick et al., 2003).

OUTCOME MEASUREMENT

PAIN LEVEL (NOC)

Definition: Severity of observed or reported pain.
Pain Level as evidenced by the following NOC indicators:

NR = Nursing Research, **MR** = Multidisciplinary Research, **SP** = Standard of Practice, **EO** = Expert Opinion, **LOE** = Level of Evidence

OUTCOME MEASUREMENT—*cont'd*

- Reported pain
- Length of pain episodes
- Moaning and crying
- Facial expressions of pain
- Restlessness
- Pacing
- Narrowed focus
- Muscle tension
- Loss of appetite

(Rate each indicator of **Pain Level:** 1 = severe, 2 = substantial, 3 = moderate, 4 = mild, 5 = none) (Moorhead et al., 2004).

REFERENCES

American Geriatric Society (AGS) Panel on Persistent Pain in Older Persons. (2002). The management of persistent pain in older persons. *J Am Geriatr Soc,* 50(6 Suppl):S205-S224.

American Pain Society (APS). (2003). *Principles of analgesic use in the treatment of acute and cancer pain,* 5th ed. Glenview IL: APS.

American Pain Society (APS). (2004). *Progress and directions for the agenda for pain management.* Available at http://www.ampainsoc.org/pub/bulletin/sep04/pres2.htm. Retrieved on June 6, 2007.

American Pain Society (APS), American Academy of Pain Medicine (AAPM), American Society of Addiction Medicine (ASAM). (2001). Definitions related to the use of opioids for the treatment of pain. *WMJ,* 100(5):28-29.

American Society of Anesthesiologists (ASA) Task Force on Acute Pain Management. (2004). Practice guidelines for acute pain management in the perioperative setting: An updated report by the American Society of Anesthesiologists Task Force on Acute Pain Management. *Anesthesiology,* 100(6):1573-1581.

American Society of Pain Management Nursing (ASPMN). (2004). ASPMN position statement: Pain management in patients with addictive disease. *J Vasc Nurs,* 22(3):99-101.

Anderson R, Saiers JH, Abram S, Schlicht C. (2001). Accuracy in equianalgesic dosing. Conversion dilemmas. *J Pain Symptom Manage,* 21(5):397-406.

Ardery G, Herr KA, Titler MG, Sorofman BA, Schmitt MB. (2003). Assessing and managing acute pain in older adults: A research base to guide practice. *Medsurg Nurs,* 12(1):7-18.

Bainbridge D, Martin JE, Cheng DC. (2006). Patient-controlled versus nurse-controlled analgesia after cardiac surgery—A meta-analysis. *Can J Anaesth,* 53(5):492-499.

Berry PH, Covington ED, Dahl J, et al. (2006). *Pain: Current understanding of assessment, management, and treatment.* Reston, VA: National Pharmaceutical Council, Inc.

Buhse M. (2006). Efficacy of EMLA cream to reduce fear and pain associated with interferon beta-1a injection in patients with multiple sclerosis. *J Neurosci Nurs,* 38(4):222-226.

Cepeda MS, Carr DB, Lau J, Alvarez H. (2006). Music for pain relief. *Cochrane Database Syst Rev,* (2): CD004843.

Chang AM, Ip WY, Cheung TH. (2004). Patient-controlled analgesia versus conventional intramuscular injection: A cost effectiveness analysis. *J Adv Nurs,* 46(5):531-541.

Coggins C, Arnstein P, Leahy S. (2004). Position Statement on Use of Placebos in Pain Management. American Society for Pain Management Nursing (ASPMN). Available online: http://www.aspmn.org. Retrieved on June 6, 2007.

Curatolo M, Sveticic G. (2002). Drug combinations in pain treatment: A review of the published evidence and a method for finding the optimal combination. *Best Pract Res Clin Anaesthiol,* 16(4):507-519.

Dahl JB, Kehlet H. (2006). Postoperative pain and its management. In McMahon SB, Koltzenburg M (Eds). *Wall and Melzack's textbook of pain,* 5th ed. Philadelphia: Churchill Livingstone, p 639.

Dalton JA, Youngblood R. (2000). Clinical application of the World Health Organization analgesic ladder. *J Intraven Nurs,* 23(2):118-124.

D'Arcy Y. (2003). Pain assessment. In Iyer P, Levin B, Shea M (Eds). *Medical legal aspects of pain and suffering.* Tucson, AZ: Lawyers and Judges Publishers, pp 19-35.

D'Arcy Y. (2006). Pain assessment and management. In Iyer P, Levin B, Shea M (Eds). *Medical legal aspects of medical records.* Tucson, AZ: Lawyers and Judges Publishers, pp 605-637.

Dochterman JM, Bulechek GM (Eds). (2004). *Nursing Interventions Classification (NIC),* 4th ed. St. Louis: Mosby.

Everett B, Salamonson Y. (2005). Differences in postoperative opioid consumption in patients prescribed patient-controlled analgesia versus intramuscular injection. *Pain Manag Nurs,* 6(4):137-144.

Feldt KS. (2000). The checklist of nonverbal pain indicators (CNPI). *Pain Manag Nurs,* 1(1):13-21.

Feldt KS, Ryden MB, Miles S. (1998). Treatment of pain in cognitively impaired compared with cognitively intact older patients with hip-fracture. *J Am Geriatr Soc,* 46(9):1079-1085.

Fellowes D, Barnes K, Wilkinson S. (2004). Aromatherapy and massage for symptom relief in patients with cancer. *Cochrane Database Syst Rev,* (2):CD002287.

Fetzer SJ. (2002). Reducing venipuncture and intravenous insertion pain with eutectic mixture of local anesthetic: A meta-analysis. *Nurs Res,* 51(2):119-124.

Fick DM, Cooper JW, Wade WE, Waller JL, Maclean JR, Beers MH. (2003). Updating the Beers criteria for potentially inappropriate medication use in older adults: Results of a US consensus panel of experts. *Arch Intern Med,* 163(22):2716-2724.

Gelinas C, Fillion L, Puntillo KA, Viens C, Fortier M. (2006). Validation of the critical-care pain observation tool in adult patients. *Am J Crit Care,* 15(4):420-427.

Golembiewski J. (2002). Equianalgesic dosing: Implications for the perianesthesia setting. *J Perianesth Nurs,* 17(5):341-343.

Griffie J. (2003). Addressing inadequate pain relief. *Am J Nurs,* 103(8):61-63.

Gross JB, Bachenberg KL, Benumof JL, Caplan RA, Connis RT, Cote CJ, et al. (2006). Practice guidelines for the perioperative management of patients with obstructive sleep apnea: A report by the American Society of Anesthesiologists Task Force on Perioperative Management of Patients with Obstructive Sleep Apnea. *Anesthesiology,* 104(5):1081-1093.

Herr K. (2002). Pain assessment in cognitively impaired older adults. *Am J Nurs,* 102(12):65-67.

Herr K, Bjoro K, Decker S. (2006). Tools for assessment of pain in nonverbal older adults with dementia: A state-of-the-science review. *J Pain Symptom Manage,* 31(2):170-192.

Jensen MP. (2003). The validity and reliability of pain measures in adults with cancer. *J Pain,* 4(1): 2-21.

The Joint Commission. (2000). *Pain assessment and management: An organizational approach.* Oakbrook Terrace, IL: The Joint Commission.

Kaasalainen S, Crook J. (2004). An exploration of seniors' ability to report pain. *Clin Nurs Res,* 13(3): 199-215.

Kehlet H. (2002). Approach to the patient with postoperative pain. In American College of Surgeons (ACS): *Principles and practice 2.* New York: WebMD, pp 1-14.

Krenzischek DA, Wilson L; American Society of Perianesthesia Nurses (ASPAN). (2003). An introduction to the ASPAN pain and comfort clinical guideline. *J Perianesth Nurs,* 18(4):228-236.

Lane P, Kuntupis M, MacDonald S, McCarthy P, Panke JA, Warden V, et al. (2003). A pain assessment tool for people with advanced Alzheimer's and other progressive dementias. *Home Healthc Nurse,* 21(1):32-37.

Marcus D. (2000). Treatment of nonmalignant chronic pain. *Am Fam Physician,* 61(5):1331-1338, 1345-1346.

McCaffery M, Pasero C. (1999). *Pain: Clinical manual.* Philadelphia: Mosby.

McCaffery M, Pasero C, Portenoy RK. (2004). *Understanding your pain: Taking oral opioid analgesics.* Chadds Ford, PA: Endo Pharmaceuticals.

Miro J, Huguet A, Nieto R, Paredes S, Baos J. (2005). Evaluation of reliability, validity, and preference for a pain intensity scale for use with the elderly. *J Pain,* 6(11):727-735.

Moorhead M, Johnson M, Maas M (Eds). (2004). *Nursing Outcomes Classification (NOC),* 3rd ed. St. Louis: Mosby.

Page GG. (2005). Surgery-induced immunosuppression and postoperative pain management. *ACCN Clin Issues,* 16(3):302-309.

Pasero C. (2003). Multimodal balanced analgesia in the PACU. *J Perianesth Nurs,* 18(4):265-268.

Pasero C, McCaffery M. (2002). Monitoring sedation. *Am J Nurs,* 102(2):67-69.

Pasero C, McCaffery M. (2004). Comfort-function goals: A way to establish accountability for pain relief. *Am J Nurs,* 104(9):77-78, 81.

Payen JF, Bru O, Bosson JL, Lagrasta A, Novel E, Deschaux I, et al. (2001). Assessing pain in critically ill sedated patients by using a behavioral pain scale. *Crit Care Med,* 29(12):2258-2263.

Remy C, Marret E, Bonnet F. (2005). Effects of acetaminophen on morphine side-effects and consumption after major surgery: Meta-analysis of randomized controlled trials. *Br J Anaesth,* 94(4):505-513.

Richman J, Liu S, Courpas G, Wong R, Rowlingson A, McGready J, et al. (2006). Does continuous peripheral nerve block provide superior pain control to opioids? A meta-analysis. *Anesth Analg,* 102(1): 248-257.

Rodriguez CS, McMillan S, Yarandi H. (2004). Pain measurement in older adults with head and neck cancer and communication impairments. *Cancer Nurs,* 27(6):425-433.

Staats PS, Argoff CE, Brewer R, D'Arcy Y, Gallagher RM, McCarberg W, et al. (2004). Neuropathic pain: Incorporating new consensus guidelines into the reality of clinical practice. *Adv Stud Med,* 4(7B): S542-S582.

Taylor S, Kirton OC, Staff I, Kozol RA. (2005). Postoperative day one: A high risk period for respiratory events. *Am J Surg,* 190(5):752-756.

Ward SE, Goldberg N, Miller-McCauley V, Mueller C, Nolan A, Pawlik-Plank D, et al. (1993). Patient-related barriers to management of cancer pain. *Pain,* 52(3):319-324.

Wong D. (2003). Topical local anesthetics. *Am J Nurs,* 103(6):42-45.

Wong D, DiVito-Thomas P. (2006). The validity, reliability, and preference of the Wong-Baker FACES Pain Rating Scale among Chinese, Japanese, and Thai children. Abstract available from authors.

 # PAIN MANAGEMENT: CHRONIC PAIN

Yvonne D'Arcy, MS, CRNP, CNS

NIC **Definition:** Alleviation of pain or a reduction in pain to a level of comfort that is acceptable to the patient (Dochterman & Bulechek, 2004).

Chronic or persistent pain is pain that lasts beyond the normal healing period, usually longer than 3 to 6 months (Elliot et al., 2002). There are many different types of chronic pain. The following information provides research-based indications for use with the more common chronic pain conditions. Chronic pain has many sources and may be present without physical evidence of damage (Marcus, 2000).

NURSING ACTIVITIES

Effective

■ **NIC** **SP** *Perform a comprehensive assessment of pain to include location, characteristics, onset/duration, frequency, quality, intensity or severity of pain, and precipitating factors.* **LOE = VII**

EO Systematic ongoing assessment and documentation provide direction for the pain treatment plan; adjustments are based on the patient's response. The patient's report of pain is the single most reliable indicator of pain (APS, 2003; Berry et al., 2006; ASPMN, 2002; D'Arcy, 2003).

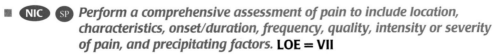
RCT = Randomized Controlled (Clinical) Trial, **NIC** = Nursing Interventions Classification, **NOC** = Nursing Outcomes Classification

■ (SP) *Use the Brief Pain Inventory (BPI) chronic pain assessment tool.* **LOE = V**

(EO) Pain assessment tools have all the elements of the required assessment information and have additional survey questions to assess for distress, impaired functionality, and a physical diagram to draw the pain locations (D'Arcy, 2003).

(EO) The BPI has a scale for indicating pain intensity, present pain, worst pain, best pain in the past 24 hours, and a body diagram to draw the location of the pain. There are questions related to function and pain medication efficacy. The tool can be used as either an interview or a self-report form, and it is used internationally in a variety of countries (Daut et al., 1983).

(MR) A review of two studies of the BPI assessing osteoarthritis pain using controlled-release oxycodone (study 1, $N = 133$; study 2, $N = 107$) found adequate test-retest reliability and excellent correlation with sleep interference subscale, confirming the reliability and validity of the tool in noncancer patients (Williams et al., 2006).

(MR) In a comparison study of two tools, patients with spinal cord injuries ($N = 127$) compared pain ratings with two pain tools: the Graded Chronic Pain Disability scale and the BPI. The daily pain intensity ratings and functional status compared favorably with similar ratings using the BPI. The BPI was found to be a reliable and valid measure of the pain interference subscale (Raichle et al., 2006).

(NR) In a comparison study of medical ($N = 229$) and surgical ($N = 159$) cancer patients, pain ratings using a visual analogue scale (VAS) and the BPI were compared. The reliability scores and validity scores were equally high. The BPI was found to be a reliable and valid tool for rating pain in male Caucasian patients with cancer (Tittle et al., 2003).

(MR) In a comparison study using two pain tools with a group of patients with chronic non-malignant pain ($N = 440$), the BPI was tested for reliability and validity. A factor analysis revealed a good correlation of the two scales—the BPI and the Roland-Morris Disability Questionnaire—finding that both scales assessed related and distinct dimensions of pain. The findings also indicated that the BPI was an effective tool for measuring improvement of pain over time in patients with chronic pain (Tan et al., 2004).

(MR) In a descriptive study, the Norwegian BPI was used with 300 hospitalized Norwegian cancer patients with findings of satisfactory psychometric properties, but it was difficult to complete for some patients (Klepstad et al., 2002).

Additional research: Ger et al.,1999; Radbruch et al., 1999; Mystakidou et al., 2002.

■ (SP) *Use the McGill Pain Questionnaire (MPQ) (both short and long forms) chronic pain assessment tool.* **LOE = V**

(EO) Pain assessment tools have all the elements of the required assessment information and have additional survey questions to assess for distress, impaired functionality, and a physical diagram to draw the pain locations (D'Arcy, 2003).

(EO) The MPQ has a scale for pain intensity and a body diagram to locate the pain. It has three classes of verbal descriptors that are scored and weighted. It has been used to study postprocedural pain, experimentally induced pain, and a large number of medical and surgical areas. It has been translated into many different languages for use internationally (Melzack, 1975, 1987).

(MR) In a descriptive study, the MPQ was used to assess pain in 30 postoperative patients. The descriptors on the MPQ were felt to help patients who had difficulty describing their pain. The MPQ was found to be clinically relevant for assessing postoperative pain and support for the sensory and affective subscales (McDonald & Weiskopf, 2001).

NR = Nursing Research, **MR** = Multidisciplinary Research, **SP** = Standard of Practice, **EO** = Expert Opinion, **LOE** = Level of Evidence

(MR) In a comparison study of the VAS with the MPQ in patients with back pain, the two tools were found to be reliable and sensitive to changes in pain. The MPQ was noted to be able to detect both the emotional and cognitive aspects of the pain experience (Chok, 1998).

(MR) In a comparison study using the Functional Index Questionnaire and the MPQ with a group of patients with patellofemoral pain syndrome, the MPQ was found to be reliable and valid with strong correlations in the sensory and affective classes (McIntyre et al., 1995).

(MR) In a descriptive study of 114 Greek cancer patients, the Greek MPQ was found to be reliable and valid in evaluating the qualities of cancer pain in palliative care patients (Mystakidou et al., 2002).

■ (SP) *If the patient has fibromyalgia, use the Fibromyalgia Impact Questionnaire (FIQ) to assess fibromyalgia pain and functionality.* **LOE = VI**

(EO) Pain assessment tools have all the elements of the required assessment information and have additional survey questions to assess for distress and impaired functionality and a physical diagram to draw the pain locations (D'Arcy, 2003).

(EO) The FIQ is a 20-item self-administered questionnaire that covers the elements of function, fatigue, pain, anxiety, and depression (APS, 2005; Burckhardt et al., 1991; D'Arcy & McCarberg, 2005).

(MR) In a descriptive study with 73 Swedish female fibromyalgia patients, the FIQ was found to be a reliable and valid measure of pain and functionality (Hedin et al., 1995).

■ (SP) *If the patient is cognitively impaired and unable to report pain and use a pain rating scale, assess and document behaviors that might be indicative of pain (e.g., change in activity, loss of appetite, guarding, grimacing, or moaning).* **LOE = III**

(NR) Using a Checklist of Nonverbal Pain Indicators (CNPI) in a controlled study with impaired and nonimpaired older adults, it was found that pain report and intensity did not differ significantly between the two groups. In addition, impaired older adults received significantly less pain medication than cognitively intact patients in the early postoperative period (Feldt et al., 1998; Feldt, 2000).

(EO) Certain behaviors have been shown to be indicative of pain and can be used to assess pain in patients who cannot use a self-report pain rating tool (e.g., in the cognitively impaired patient). The clinician should be aware that pain expression is highly individual and what may be a pain behavior in one patient may not be in another. Pain assessment must be individualized (Herr, 2002).

■ *Assess pain in a patient using a simple, valid, and reliable rating tool such as the numeric rating scale (NRS), the visual analogue scale (VAS), or the verbal descriptor scale.* **LOE = I**

(MR) A systematic review of 164 articles on pain measures found that single-item ratings of pain intensity were valid and reliable as measures of pain intensity (Jensen, 2003).

(EO) The Joint Commission requires regular assessment and reassessment of pain in hospitalized patients as a part of the Joint Commission Pain Management Standards (The Joint Commission, 2000).

(EO) The patient's report of the pain is considered the single most reliable piece of data (APS, 2005; The Joint Commission, 2000).

RCT = Randomized Controlled (Clinical) Trial, **NIC** = Nursing Interventions Classification, **NOC** = Nursing Outcomes Classification

■ ⓢⓟ *Question the patient regarding pain at frequent intervals, often at the same time as checking vital signs or at every office visit.* **LOE = VII**

ⒺⓄ Pain assessment is as important as taking vital signs, and the American Pain Society suggests applying the concept of pain assessment as the "fifth vital sign" (APS, 2003).

■ ⓢⓟ *Question patients regarding the level of pain that they think is appropriate to achieve a state of comfort and appropriate function. Attempt to keep pain level no higher than that level, preferably much lower.* **LOE = VII**

ⒺⓄ The pain rating that allows the patient to have comfort and appropriate function should be determined, and this allows a tangible way to measure outcomes of pain management (Pasero & McCaffery, 2004; Griffie, 2003).

ⒺⓄ Setting pain goals and assessing increases in functionality are key to assessing progress in pain control for patients with persistent pain (AGS, 2002; Marcus, 2000; ASPMN, 2002).

■ ⓃⒾⒸ ⓢⓟ *Ensure that the patient receives attentive analgesic care. Provide the person optimal pain relief with prescribed analgesics. Encourage the patient to use adequate pain medication. Use pain control measures before pain becomes severe.* **LOE = VII**

ⒺⓄ Recommendations from experts in pain management and national guidelines (The Joint Commission) support the need to address pain promptly and provide adequate pain medication to control pain (Berry et al., 2006; Gordon et al., 2002; The Joint Commission, 2000).

■ ⓢⓟ *Ask the patient to maintain a diary of pain ratings, timing, precipitating events, medications, treatments, and steps that work best to relieve pain.* **LOE = VI**

ⓃⓇ In a controlled study of nursing pain assessment using a control group ($N = 23$) for comparison, a population of oncology patients ($N = 20$) was assessed using standardized assessment tools. Eight-five percent of the patients in the study group had significantly lower pain intensity ratings from day 1 of hospitalization (Faries, 1991).

■ ⓢⓟ *Explore the need for medications from the three classes of analgesic: opioids (narcotics), nonopioids (acetaminophen, nonselective nonsteroidal anti-inflammatory drugs), and adjuvant medications.* **LOE = VII**

ⒺⓄ The analgesic regimen for treating chronic pain should include a nonopioid drug around the clock, even if pain is severe enough to require the use of an opioid (APS, 2003). Some types of pain respond to nonopioid drugs alone. If the pain is not responding, however, adding an opioid is an option. At any level of pain, adding analgesic adjuvants may be useful (APS, 2003).

ⒺⓄ The World Health Organization Analgesic Ladder can determine which level of pain medication to use for mild, moderate, or severe pain. Continue to use the adjuvant medications such as antidepressants or antiseizure medications with each step (Dalton & Youngblood, 2000).

ⒺⓄ The American Society of Anesthesiologists recommends a combination of medications to treat chronic pain (Wilson et al, 1997).

NR = Nursing Research, **MR** = Multidisciplinary Research, **SP** = Standard of Practice, **EO** = Expert Opinion, **LOE** = Level of Evidence

EO A review of pharmacotherapy for chronic pain recommends therapy that provides a combination of medications designed to address all types of chronic pain presentations (Lynch & Watson, 2006).

EO A multimodal treatment approach is encouraged combining opioids, nonopioids, and other forms of pain relief to optimize the level of pain control for patients (Berry et al., 2006; Gordon et al., 2002).

■ SP *Recognize that patients who use descriptors for pain such as burning, painful tingling, numbness, or shooting pain are describing neuropathic pain. For chronic neuropathic pain, consider adjuvant medications that are analgesic, such as anticonvulsants and antidepressants.* **LOE = VII**

EO Neuropathic pain requires a specialized medication regimen. The pain is a result of damage to nerves, not muscles (APS, 2003; Marcus, 2002).

■ SP *Question the patient about any disruption in sleep.* **LOE = VI**

EO Patients should be assessed for sleep disruption (AGS, 2002; Marcus, 2000).

MR In a prospective cross-sectional survey, 268 patients with low back pain completed the Short-Form MPQ (SF-MPQ) and the Pittsburgh Sleep Quality Index (PSQI) and rated their pain using a VAS for numeric pain intensity. Fifty-five percent of the patients reported restless/light sleep after pain onset. There was a correlation between SF-MPQ and the PSQI and between PSQI and the VAS. The overall findings indicated that pain significantly affected sleep (Marin et al., 2006).

■ SP *Watch for signs of depression in the patient with chronic pain, including sleeplessness, not eating, flat affect, statements of depression, or suicidal ideation.* **LOE = V**

EO Depression is common in patients with chronic pain and should be assessed regularly (Marcus, 2000; AGS, 2002).

MR A systematic review demonstrated that patients with chronic pain had twice the rate of suicide of the people without pain (Tang & Crane, 2006).

MR A case-control study ($N = 154$) of people aged 60 or older who committed suicide versus a control group who did not, found that physical illness, especially pain, breathlessness, and disability, was most commonly associated with suicide (Harwood et al., 2006).

■ NIC *Explore the patient's knowledge and beliefs about pain. Consider cultural influences on pain response.* **LOE = VII**

EO Each patient has a right to have pain assessed and adequately treated. Language barriers to pain management must be addressed (The Joint Commission, 2000).

Possibly Effective

■ *Use the Checklist of Nonverbal Pain Indicators, a behavior pain scale that is indicated to assess pain in nonverbal populations such as Alzheimer's patients.* **LOE = III**

NR In a controlled study using the CNPI with impaired and nonimpaired older adults, it was found that pain report and intensity did not differ significantly between the two groups.

RCT = Randomized Controlled (Clinical) Trial, **NIC** = Nursing Interventions Classification, **NOC** = Nursing Outcomes Classification

In addition, impaired older adults received significantly less pain medication than cognitively intact patients in the early postoperative period (Feldt et al., 1998; Feldt, 2000).

■ *Use the Pain Assessment in Patients with Advanced Dementia (PAINAD) scale, which is indicated to assess pain in nonverbal populations such as Alzheimer's patients.* **LOE = VI**

(EO) The PAINAD combines the FLACC scale (faces, legs, activity, cry, and consolability scale) with the NRS 0 to 10 and wording from the literature defining pain behaviors. It includes the elements of breathing, negative vocalizations, facial expressions, body language, and consolability. Scores go from 0 (no pain) to 10 (maximum pain) (Lane et al., 2003).

(NR) A review of 10 behavior pain scales for use with demented patients demonstrated that there is no standardized behavioral pain scale that is well developed and researched; they are in early stages of development and testing (Herr et al., 2006).

■ *Discuss fears of addiction and the terms addiction, dependence, tolerance, and pseudoaddiction with the patient.* **LOE = VII**

(EO) Addiction is a primary, chronic, neurobiologic disease with genetic, psychosocial, and environmental factors influencing its development and manifestations. It is characterized by the four Cs: impaired control over drug use, compulsive use, continued use despite harm, and craving (APS, 2003; Staats et al., 2004; APS et al., 2001).

(EO) Dependence is a universal physiological and pharmacologic phenomenon following regular use of opioids for 2 weeks. Withdrawal occurs if the opioids are abruptly stopped. It is not evidence of opioid addiction (APS, 2003; APS et al., 2001). Dependent patients should not be classified as addicted.

(EO) Tolerance is a state of adaptation in which a drug's clinical effect diminishes over time (APS et al., 2001; Staats et al., 2004). It does signal addiction.

(EO) Pseudoaddiction refers to drug-seeking behaviors such as doctor shopping, lost prescriptions, or frequent trips to the emergency room that appear to be addictive behavior but are in reality attempts to achieve adequate pain relief (Weissman & Haddox, 1989; Staats et al., 2004). Behaviors should resolve with adequate treatment. These behaviors do not signal addiction unless behaviors persist after pain is adequately relieved.

■ *Use a pain equivalency chart when switching from one medication to another.* **LOE = VII**

(EO) Using medications and doses that are equivalent in the ability to relieve pain provides that the patient will not suffer increased pain when conversions are made from one opioid to another or one form of medication to another such as from intravenous to oral pain medication (ASPMN, 2002; Anderson et al., 2001).

■ *Use around-the-clock medication administration when pain is present most of the day.* **LOE = VII**

(EO) For patients who have consistent pain levels on a daily basis, using around-the-clock medication provides consistent pain relief (APS, 2003).

NR = Nursing Research, **MR** = Multidisciplinary Research, **SP** = Standard of Practice, **EO** = Expert Opinion, **LOE** = Level of Evidence

■ *Use long-acting medication or extended-release medication when the patient is taking short-acting medication regularly and pain is present consistently.* **LOE = VII**

(EO) When a patient has persistent pain on a daily basis and is using short-acting pain medication to relieve pain, a long-acting medication without acetaminophen should be considered. Many of the short-acting pain medications contain acetaminophen, and the use of these short-acting pain medications is limited by the recommended daily dose of acetaminophen (4000 mg per day and less for patients with impaired organ function) (APS, 2003).

(MR) A randomized, placebo-controlled double-blind study of extended-release morphine with 295 osteoarthritis patients found that pain control and sleep were improved compared with placebo (Caldwell et al., 2002).

(MR) A randomized controlled trial of 159 patients with diabetic neuropathy found that extended-release oxycodone decreased pain intensity compared with placebo (Gimbel et al., 2003).

■ *Use short-acting medications for breakthrough pain when the patient is taking long-acting or extended-release medication.* **LOE = VII**

(EO) When a patient has increased pain with increased activity or during the day, a breakthrough medication is indicated to maintain a consistent level of pain control (APS, 2003).

■ (SP) *Recognize that oral opioid medications begin to work in about 1 hour and intravenous medications in 5 to 30 minutes depending on the medication; transdermal medication becomes effective in 12 to 16 hours with steady blood levels within 48 hours (APS, 2003).* **LOE = VII**

(EO) Knowing when pain medication becomes effective can help the nurse plan nursing care activities and provide breakthrough pain medication as needed (D'Arcy, 2006).

■ *Suggest acupuncture for treatment of pain.* **LOE = II**

(NR) Systematic reviews indicated that acupuncture for fibromyalgia may be effective (APS, 2005; D'Arcy & McCarberg, 2005).

■ *Suggest massage therapy for treatment of pain.* **LOE = VII**

(MR) A Cochrane review found that both massage and aromatherapy massage have short-term benefits for psychological well-being for the patient with cancer (Fellowes et al., 2004).

(EO) In a Cochrane review of randomized and quasi-randomized trials of massage for relief of low back pain, massage was found to be superior to relaxation therapy, acupuncture, and self-care education (Furlan et al., 2002).

(Note: For information on guided imagery, hand massage, healing touch, therapeutic touch, heat/cold application, anxiety reduction, distraction, music therapy, and progressive muscle relaxation/autogenic therapy, refer to guidelines available in this text.)

Not Effective

■ *Intramuscular injections for pain relief.* **LOE = VI**

(EO) Intramuscular injections result in irregular medication absorption (ASPMN, 2002; APS, 2003).

(EO) Repeated IM injections can cause sterile abscesses, tissue fibrosis, and nerve injury with persistent neuropathic pain (APS, 2003).

RCT = Randomized Controlled (Clinical) Trial, **NIC** = Nursing Interventions Classification, **NOC** = Nursing Outcomes Classification

■ *Use of lumbar supports to relieve back pain.* **LOE = I**

(MR) A Cochrane review demonstrated that lumbar supports were not effective in relieving back pain (Van Tulder et al., 2000).

Possibly Harmful

■ *Use of opioids with toxic metabolites such as meperidine (Demerol) and propoxyphene (Darvon, Darvocet) in older patients.* **LOE = VII**

(EO) Meperidine's metabolite, normeperidine, can produce central nervous system irritability and seizures; propoxyphene's metabolite, norpropoxyphene, can produce cardiotoxicity. Both of these metabolites are eliminated by the kidneys, which makes meperidine and propoxyphene particularly poor choices for older patients, many of whom have at least some degree of renal insufficiency (APS, 2003; Ardery et al., 2003; Fick et al., 2003).

■ *Unrelieved pain can result in depression and suicide.* **LOE = V**

(MR) A systematic review demonstrated that patients with chronic pain had twice the rate of suicide of people without pain (Tang & Crane, 2006).

(MR) A case-control study ($N = 154$) of people aged 60 or older who committed suicide versus a control group who did not, found that physical illness, especially pain, breathlessness, and disability, was most commonly associated with suicide (Harwood et al., 2006).

OUTCOME MEASUREMENT

PAIN LEVEL (NOC)

Definition: Severity of observed or reported pain.
Pain Level as evidenced by the following NOC indicators:
• Reported pain
• Length of pain episodes
• Moaning and crying
• Facial expressions of pain
• Restlessness
• Pacing
• Narrowed focus
• Muscle tension
• Loss of appetite
(Rate each indicator of **Pain Level:** 1 = severe, 2 = substantial, 3 = moderate, 4 = mild, 5 = none) (Moorhead et al., 2004).

REFERENCES

American Geriatric Society (AGS) Panel on Persistent Pain in Older Persons.** (2002). The management of persistent pain in older persons. *J Am Geriatr Soc,* 50(6 Suppl):S205-S224.
American Pain Society (APS). (2003). *Principles of analgesic use in the treatment of acute and cancer pain,* 5th ed. Glenview, IL: APS. Available online: http://www.ampainsoc.org/pub/bulletin/jan03/reso3.htm. Retrieved on October 17, 2007.

American Pain Society (APS). (2005). *Fibromyalgia pain guideline.* Glenview, IL: APS. Available online: http://www.ampainsoc.org/enews/feb05/. Retrieved on October 17, 2007.

American Pain Society (APS), American Academy of Pain Medicine (AAPM), American Society of Addiction Medicine (ASAM). (2001). Definitions related to the use of opioids for the treatment of pain. *WMJ,* 100(5):28-29.

American Society of Pain Management Nurses (ASPMN). (2002). *Core curriculum for pain management nursing.* Philadelphia: Saunders.

Anderson R, Saiers JH, Abram S, Schlicht C. (2001). Accuracy in equianalgesic dosing. Conversion dilemmas. *J Pain Symptom Manage,* 21(5):397-406.

Ardery G, Herr KA, Titler MG, Sorofman BA, Schmitt MB. (2003). Assessing and managing acute pain in older adults: A research base to guide practice. *Medsurg Nurs,* 12(1):7-18.

Berry PH, Covington ED, Dahl J, et al. (2006). *Pain: Current understanding of assessment, management, and treatment.* Reston, VA: National Pharmaceutical Council, Inc.

Burckhardt CS, Clark SR, Bennett RM. (1991). The fibromyalgia impact questionnaire: Development and validation. *J Rheumatol,* 18(5):728-733.

Caldwell JR, Rapoport RJ, Davis JC, Offenberg HL, Marker HW, Roth SH, et al. (2002). Efficacy and safety of a once-daily morphine formulation in chronic, moderate-to-severe osteoarthritis pain: Results from a randomized, placebo-controlled, double-blind trial and an open-label extension trial. *J Pain Symptom Manage,* 23(4):278-291.

Chok B. (1998). An overview of the Visual Analogue Scale and the McGill Pain Questionnaire. *Physiother Singapore,* 1(3):88-93.

Dalton JA, Youngblood R. (2000). Clinical application of the World Health Organization analgesic ladder. *J Intraven Nurs,* 23(2):118-124.

D'Arcy Y. (2003). Pain assessment. In Iyer P, Levin B, Shea M (Eds). *Medical legal aspects of pain and suffering.* Tucson, AZ: Lawyers and Judges Publishers, pp 19-35.

D'Arcy Y. (2006). Pain assessment and management. In Iyer P, Levin B, Shea M (Eds). *Medical legal aspects of medical records.* Tucson, AZ: Lawyers and Judges Publishers, pp 605-637.

D'Arcy Y, McCarberg BH. (2005). New fibromyalgia: Pain management recommendations. *J Nurse Pract,* 1(4):218-225.

Daut RL, Cleeland CS, Flanery RC. (1983). Development of the Wisconsin Brief Pain Questionnaire to assess pain in cancer and other diseases. *Pain,* 17(2):197-210.

Dochterman JM, Bulechek GM (Eds). (2004). *Nursing Interventions Classification (NIC),* 4th ed. St. Louis: Mosby.

Elliot et al. (2002). In B. St. Marie (Ed): *Core curriculum for pain management nursing.* Philadelphia: Saunders, p 272.

Faries JE, Mills DS, Goldsmith KW, Phillips KD, Orr J. (1991). Systematic pain records and their impact on pain control. A pilot study. *Cancer Nurs,* 14(6):306-313.

Feldt KS. (2000). The checklist of nonverbal pain indicators (CNPI). *Pain Manag Nurs,* 1(1):13-21.

Feldt KS, Ryden MB, Miles S. (1998). Treatment of pain in cognitively impaired compared with cognitively intact older patients with hip-fracture. *J Am Geriatr Soc,* 46(9):1079-1085.

Fellowes D, Barnes K, Wilkinson S. (2004). Aromatherapy and massage for symptom relief in patients with cancer. *Cochrane Database Syst Rev,* (2):CD002287.

Fick DM, Cooper JW, Wade WE, Waller JL, Maclean JR, Beers MH. (2003). Updating the Beers criteria for potentially inappropriate medication use in older adults: Results of a US consensus panel of experts. *Arch Intern Med,* 163(22):2716-2724.

Furlan AD, Brosseau L, Imamura M, Irvin E. (2002). Massage for low back pain. *Cochrane Database Syst Rev,* (2):CD001929.

Ger LP, Ho ST, Sun WZ, Wang MS, Cleeland CS. (1999). Validation of the Brief Pain Inventory in a Taiwanese population. *J Pain Symptom Manage,* 18(5):316-322.

Gimbel JS, Richards P, Portenoy RK. (2003). Controlled-release oxycodone for pain in diabetic neuropathy: A randomized controlled trial. *Neurology,* 60(6):927-934.

Gordon DB, Pellino TA, Miaskowski C, McNeill JA, Paice JA, Laferriere D, et al. (2002). A 10-year review of quality improvement monitoring in pain management: Recommendations for standardized outcome measures. *Pain Manag Nurs,* 3(4):116-130.

Griffie J. (2003). Addressing inadequate pain relief. *Am J Nurs,* 103(8):61-63.

Harwood DM, Hawton K, Hope T, Harriss L, Jacoby R. (2006). Life problems and physical illness as risk factors for suicide in older people: A descriptive and case-control study. *Psychol Med,* 36(9):1265-1274.

Hedin PJ, Hamne M, Burckhardt CS, Engstrom-Laurent A. (1995). The Fibromyalgia Impact Questionnaire, a Swedish translation of a new tool for evaluation of the fibromyalgia patient. *Scand J Rheumatol,* 24(2):69-75.

Herr K. (2002). Pain assessment in cognitively impaired older adults. *Am J Nurs,* 102(12):65-67.

Herr K, Bjoro K, Decker S. (2006). Tools for assessment of pain in nonverbal older adults with dementia: A state-of-the-science review. *J Pain Symptom Manage,* 31(2):170-192.

Herr K, Coyne PJ, Key T, Manworren R, McCaffery M, Merkel S, et al. (2006). Pain assessment in the nonverbal patient: Position statement with clinical practice recommendations. *Pain Manag Nurs,* 7(2):44-52.

Jensen MP. (2003). The validity and reliability of pain measures in adults with cancer. *J Pain,* 4(1):2-21.

The Joint Commission. (2000). *Pain assessment and management: An organizational approach.* Oakbrook Terrace, IL: The Joint Commission.

Klepstad P, Loge JH, Borchgrevink PC, Mendoza TR, Cleeland C, Kaasa S. (2002). The Norwegian Brief Pain Inventory Questionnaire: Translation and validation in cancer pain patients. *J Pain Symptom Manage,* 24(5):517-525.

Lane P, Kuntupis M, MacDonald S, McCarthy P, Panke JA, Warden V, et al. (2003). A pain assessment tool for people with advanced Alzheimer's and other progressive dementias. *Home Healthc Nurse,* 21(1):32-37.

Lynch ME, Watson CP. (2006). The pharmacotherapy of chronic pain: A review. *Pain Res Manage,* 11(1): 11-38.

MacIntyre DL, Hopkins PM, Harris SR. (1995). Evaluation of pain and functional activity in patellofemoral pain syndrome: Reliability and validity of two assessment tools. *Physiother Can,* 47(3):164-170.

Marcus D. (2000). Treatment of nonmalignant chronic pain. *Am Fam Physician,* 61(5):1331-1338, 1345-1346.

Marin R, Cyhan T, Miklos W. (2006). Sleep disturbance in patients with chronic low back pain. *Am J Phys Med Rehabil,* 85(5):430-435.

McDonald DD, Weiskopf CS. (2001). Adult patients' postoperative pain descriptions and responses to the Short-Form McGill Pain Questionnaire. *Clin Nurs Res,* 10(4):442-452.

Melzack R. (1975). The McGill Pain Questionnaire: Major properties and scoring methods. *Pain,* 1(3):277-299.

Melzack R. (1987). The Short-Form McGill Pain Questionnaire. *Pain,* 30(2):191-197.

Moorhead M, Johnson M, Maas M (Eds). (2004). *Nursing Outcomes Classification (NOC),* 3rd ed. St. Louis: Mosby.

Mystakidou K, Mendoza T, Tsilika E, Befon S, Parpa E, Bellos G, et al. (2001). Greek brief pain inventory: Validation and utility in cancer pain. *Oncology,* 60(1):35-42.

Mystakidou K, Parpa E, Tsilika E, Kalaidopoulou O, Georgaki S, Galanos A, et al. (2002). Greek McGill Pain Questionnaire: Validation and utility in cancer patients. *J Pain Symptom Manage,* 24(4):379-387.

Page GG, Ben-Eliyahu S. (1997). The immune-suppressive nature of pain. *Semin Oncol Nurs,* 13(1):10-15.

Payen JF, Bru O, Bosson JL, Lagrasta A, Novel E, Deschaux I, et al. (2001). Assessing pain in critically ill sedated patients by using a behavioral pain scale. *Crit Care Med,* 29(12):2258-2263.

Pasero C, McCaffery M. (2004). Comfort-function goals: A way to establish accountability for pain relief. *Am J Nurs,* 104(9):77-78, 81.

Radbruch L, Loick G, Kiencke P, Lindena G, Sabatowski R, Grond S, et al. (1999). Validation of the German version of the Brief Pain Inventory. *J Pain Symptom Manage,* 18(3):180-187.

Raichle KA, Osborne TL, Jensen MP, Cardenas D. (2006). The reliability and validity of pain interference measures in persons with spinal cord injury. *J Pain,* 7(3):179-186.

Staats PS, Argoff CE, Brewer R, D'Arcy Y, Gallagher RM, McCarberg W, et al. (2004). Neuropathic pain: Incorporating new consensus guidelines into the reality of clinical practice. *Adv Stud Med,* 4(7B):S550-S566, S580-S582.

Tan G, Jensen MP, Thornby JI, Shanti BF. (2004). Validation of the Brief Pain Inventory for chronic nonmalignant pain. *J Pain,* 5(2):133-137.

Tang NK, Crane C. (2006). Suicidality in chronic pain: A review of the prevalence, risk factors and psychological links. *Psychol Med,* 36(5):575-586.

Tittle MB, McMillan SC, Hagan S. (2003). Validating the Brief Pain Inventory for use with surgical patients with cancer. *Oncol Nurs Forum,* 30(2):325-330.

Van Tulder MW, Jellema P, van Poppel MN, Nachemson AL, Bouter LM. (2000). Lumbar supports for prevention and treatment of low back pain. *Cochrane Database Syst Rev*, (2):CD001823.

Weissman DE, Haddox JD. (1989). Opioid pseudoaddiction—An iatrogenic syndrome. *Pain*, 36(3):363-366.

Williams VS, Smith MY, Fehnel SE. (2006). The validity and utility of the BPI interference measures for evaluating the impact of osteoarthritic pain. *J Pain Symptom Manage*, 31(1):48-57.

Wilson P, Caplan R, Connis R, Gilbert H, Grigsaby E, Haddox D, et al. (1997). Practice Guidelines for Chronic Pain Management: A report by the American Society of Anesthesiologists Task Force on Pain Management, Chronic Pain Section. *Anesthesiology*, 86(4):995-1004.

 # PATIENT CONTRACTING

Celia E. Wills, PhD, RN; Catherine E. Lein, MS, APRN, FNP-BC;
Kathleen Gaskill Bappert, BSN, RN, MS

NIC **Definition:** Negotiating an agreement with an individual that reinforces a specific behavior change (Dochterman & Bulechek, 2004).

NURSING ACTIVITIES

Effective

■ SP *Involve patients (mutuality) in care planning, identify expected outcomes, and evaluate outcomes.* **LOE = VII**

EO Nurses should involve patients in planning their own care (ANA, 2004).

■ *Craft an individualized mutual agreement (health action plan) with active patient's involvement and formulation of short-term goals to improve treatment adherence, health promotion goals, and clinical outcomes.* **LOE = II**

MR A controlled study of exercise contracting ($N = 233$) demonstrated improvements in lowering of cholesterol and decreased exercising heart rate for patients ($N = 96$) who contracted to do aerobic exercise three times per week compared with those who did not (Neale, 1991).

MR A meta-analysis of interventions to improve compliance showed that educational strategies ($N = 7$ studies involving verbal patient's contracting) improved treatment adherence, health outcomes, and utilization of services, especially for diabetes, hypertension, mental health, and cancer populations (Roter et al., 1998).

MR A descriptive study of an action plan intervention with primary care patients with coronary heart disease risk factors ($N = 274$) demonstrated that, of those who made an action plan ($N = 228$), at least 53% made a behavior change that was consistent with their own action plan (Handley et al., 2006).

Possibly Effective

■ *Contract to reduce behaviors known to be harmful to health.* **LOE = III**

MR In an RCT of a multicomponent smoking cessation intervention in lower income African Americans ($N = 650$), submitting a quit-smoking contract was significantly associated with quitting smoking (Resnicow et al., 1997).

RCT = Randomized Controlled (Clinical) Trial, **NIC** = Nursing Interventions Classification, **NOC** = Nursing Outcomes Classification

■ *Use "no suicide" contracts to foster control and commitment of patients to actions other than self-harm, if certain essential elements are included.* **LOE = V**

(MR) A systematic review of interventions for preventing self-harm in adolescents concluded that patient contracting may foster personal control and commitment of adolescents to avoiding self-harm (Brent, 1997).

(NR) In a descriptive survey of inpatient psychiatric hospitals ($N = 84$), it was concluded that no-suicide contracting was used in 79% of the hospitals in the context of patients' suicidal ideation or acts (Drew, 1999).

(MR) In an integrative review, it was concluded that no-suicide contracts could be useful adjuncts to other treatments, provided that the contract was sufficiently specific to the individual, collaboratively developed, positive, and context sensitive and the patient was provided with a copy of the contract (Range et al., 2002).

■ *Use no-suicide contracts to build a trusting therapeutic relationship and to assess the quality of the therapeutic alliance.* **LOE = V**

(EO) The use of contracting may foster the therapist-patient relationship and be associated with positive outcomes (Sills, 1997).

(NR) In an integrative review of assessment strategies for psychiatric inpatient suicide, it was concluded that contracts can provide useful information about the therapeutic alliance status (Billings, 2003).

Not Effective

■ *Contracting with patients with developmental limitations, cognitive impairment, inability or unwillingness to control behaviors, or during severe illnesses or medical emergencies.* **LOE = V**

(NR) An integrative review of patient contracting determined that patients with certain cognitive, behavioral, and medical issues may not be suitable candidates for contracting (Simons, 1999).

(MR) In an integrative review, it was concluded that contracting was not effective unless appropriately developmentally tailored for an individual (Range et al., 2002).

■ *Use of no-suicide contracts as a guarantee of patients' safety.* **LOE = V**

(NR) A brief review of the literature on patient contracting for safety concluded that no-suicide contracts had not been shown to be effective for suicide prevention and should not be used on a solo basis for suicide prevention (Egan et al., 1997).

Possibly Harmful

■ *Use of no-suicide contracts for building therapeutic relationships with selected populations of patients.* **LOE = V**

(NR) A brief review concluded that certain patients may interpret contracting as a lack of caregiver empathy (Egan et al., 1997).

(MR) In an integrative review, it was concluded that the use of no-suicide contacts with patients carried a potential for negative patients' perceptions (anger and feeling coerced) and a "false security" perception in caregivers (Range et al., 2002).

NR = Nursing Research, **MR** = Multidisciplinary Research, **SP** = Standard of Practice, **EO** = Expert Opinion, **LOE** = Level of Evidence

(MR) In an integrative review, it was concluded that no-suicide contracts should not be used as a substitute for clinical judgment and other means of assessing suicide potential (Range et al., 2002).

OUTCOME MEASUREMENT

ADHERENCE BEHAVIOR (NOC)

Definition: Self-initiated actions to promote wellness, recovery, and rehabilitation.
Adherence Behavior as evidenced by the following selected NOC indicators:
• Asks health-related questions when indicated
• Uses strategies to eliminate unhealthy behavior
• Uses strategies to maximize health
• Uses health services congruent with need
• Describes rationale for deviating from a recommended health regimen
(Rate each indicator of **Adherence Behavior:** 1 = never demonstrated, 2 = rarely demonstrated, 3 = sometimes demonstrated, 4 = often demonstrated, 5 = consistently demonstrated) (Moorhead et al., 2004).

SUICIDE SELF-RESTRAINT (NOC)

Definition: Personal actions to refrain from gestures and attempts at killing self.
Suicide Self-Restraint as evidenced by the following selected NOC indicators:
• Seeks help when feeling self-destructive
• Verbalizes suicidal ideas
• Refrains from gathering means for suicide
• Refrains from attempting suicide
• Discloses plan for suicide if present
• Refrains from inflicting serious injury
(Rate each indicator of **Suicide Self-Restraint:** 1 = never demonstrated, 2 = rarely demonstrated, 3 = sometimes demonstrated, 4 = often demonstrated, 5 = consistently demonstrated) (Moorhead et al., 2004).

REFERENCES

American Nurses Association (ANA). (2004). *Nursing: Scope & standards of practice.* Washington, DC: ANA.

Billings CV. (2003). Psychiatric inpatient suicide: Assessment strategies. *J Am Psychiatr Nurs Assoc,* 9(5): 176-178.

Brent DA. (1997). The aftercare of adolescents with deliberate self-harm. *J Child Psychol Psychiatry,* 38(3): 277-286.

Dochterman JM, Bulechek GM (Eds). (2004). *Nursing Interventions Classification (NIC),* 4th ed. St. Louis: Mosby.

Drew BL. (1999). No-suicide contracts to prevent suicidal behavior in inpatient psychiatric settings. *J Am Psychiatr Nurs Assoc,* 5(1):23-28.

Egan MP, Rivera SG, Robillard RR, Hanson A. (1997). The "no suicide" contract: Helpful or harmful? *J Psychosoc Nurs Ment Health Serv,* 35(3):31-33.

RCT = Randomized Controlled (Clinical) Trial, **NIC** = Nursing Interventions Classification, **NOC** = Nursing Outcomes Classification

Handley M, MacGregor K, Schillinger D, Sharifi C, Wong S, Bodenheimer T. (2006). Using action plans to help primary care patients adopt healthy behaviors: A descriptive study. *J Am Board Fam Med,* 19(3):224-231.

Moorhead M, Johnson M, Maas M (Eds). (2004). *Nursing Outcomes Classification (NOC),* 3rd ed. St. Louis: Mosby.

Neale AV. (1991). Behavioural contracting as a tool to help patients achieve better health. *Fam Pract,* 8(4):336-342.

Range LM, Campbell C, Kovac SH, Marion-Jones M, Aldridge H, Kogos S, et al. (2002). No-suicide contracts: An overview and recommendations. *Death Stud,* 26(1):51-74.

Resnicow K, Royce J, Vaughan R, Orlandi MA, Smith M. (1997). Analysis of multicomponent smoking cessation project: What worked and why. *Prev Med,* 26(3):373-381.

Roter DL, Hall JA, Merisca R, Nordstrom B, Cretin D, Svarstad B. (1998). Effectiveness of interventions to improve patient compliance: A meta-analysis. *Med Care,* 36(8):1138-1161.

Sills C. (1997). Contracts and contract making. In Sills C (Ed). *Contracts in counseling.* Thousand Oaks, CA: Sage, pp 11-35.

Simons MR. (1999). Patient contracting. In Bulechek GM, McCloskey JC (Eds). *Nursing interventions: Effective nursing treatments,* 3rd ed. Philadelphia: Saunders, pp 385-397.

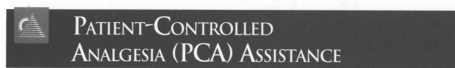

PATIENT-CONTROLLED ANALGESIA (PCA) ASSISTANCE   NIC

Debra B. Gordon, MS, RN-C, APRN-BC, FAAN

NIC **Definition:** Facilitating patient control of analgesic administration and regulation (Dochterman & Bulechek, 2004).

(Note: This guideline includes new devices and strategies including intravenous, oral, intranasal, transdermal, spinal, and regional PCA.)

NURSING ACTIVITIES

Effective

■ *Assess for adequacy of analgesia and patients' satisfaction with PCA.* **LOE = I**

MR A Cochrane review of 55 studies with 2023 patients receiving PCA and 1838 patients assigned to a control group found that PCA provided better pain control and greater patients' satisfaction than conventional "as-needed" analgesia, although patients with PCA consumed more opioids and had a higher incidence of pruritus (Hudcova et al., 2006).

MR A descriptive study (*N* = 36) found that patients using oral PCA attained their pain rating goal within 1 hour after 93% of the doses they took, compared with only 65% for patients who received nurse-administered oral analgesia, even though the PCA patients took less doses of medication (Riordan et al., 2004).

NR A descriptive study (*N* = 30) of children who received IV PCA found bedside documentation of pain intensity, failed attempts, and hourly analgesia intake helpful to assess efficacy of PCA (Ellis et al., 1999).

NR = Nursing Research, **MR** = Multidisciplinary Research, **SP** = Standard of Practice, **EO** = Expert Opinion, **LOE** = Level of Evidence

■ **SP** *When opioid PCA is used, assess risk factors for respiratory depression and monitor sedation level and respiratory rate every 1 to 2 hours for the first 12 to 24 hours of PCA therapy.* **LOE = I**

MR A descriptive study of patients ($N = 32$) following total hip arthroplasty who received IV PCA found that a significant degree of nocturnal hypoxemia occurred in half of the patients while they breathed room air (Stone et al., 1999).

MR A review of the literature from 1990 to 2004 identified risk factors for respiratory depression with IV PCA including age older than 70; basal infusion with IV PCA; renal, hepatic, pulmonary, or cardiac impairment; sleep apnea (suspected or history); concurrent central nervous system depressants; obesity; upper abdominal or thoracic surgery; and IV PCA bolus greater than 1 mg (Hagle et al., 2004).

MR Pooled data from165 original papers representing 20,000 patients found that the incidence of respiratory depression using hypoventilation and oxygen desaturation to monitor IV PCA varied between 1.2 (0.7% to 1.9%) and 11.5 (5.6% to 22%) (Cashman & Dolin, 2004).

■ *Monitor respiratory rate, depth, and rhythm with serial sedation assessments. If available, capnography (E_tCO_2) or oxygen saturation (SpO_2) may be monitored for patients with increased risk of respiratory depression.* **LOE = I**

MR A review of the literature from 1990 to 2004 found no single parameter to be superior to detect respiratory depression, including mechanical monitoring such as pulse oximetry (SpO_2) or end-tidal carbon dioxide (E_tCO_2) (Hagle et al., 2004).

MR A prospective convenience study ($N = 60$) of procedural sedation found abnormal capnography before changes in oxygen saturation or clinically observed hypoventilation in 70% of patients with acute respiratory events (Burton et al., 2006).

■ **SP** *Double check programming of the pump using a second-person separate check process as outlined in institutional policy.* **LOE = IV**

MR An evidence-based estimate using a search of incidents in the Food and Drug Administration Medical Device Reporting (MDR) database and other sources (denominator of 22,000,000) found that the probability of death from user programming errors associated with PCA was 1 in 33,000 to 1 in 338,800 or 65 to 667 deaths (Vicente et al., 2003).

MR A review of the USP Medication Errors Reporting (MER) Program ($N = 5377$ records) found the patients' harm rate for error reports increased more than 3.5 times when PCA pumps were involved, and the most frequent type of error involving PCA pumps was improper dose/quantity (38.9%) (USP, 2004).

■ *Teach patients how to use the designated PCA system. Include information about how and when to administer a dose, potential side effects of the analgesic, safety mechanisms, and low risk of addiction (if opioids are used).* **LOE = II**

MR Seven focus groups ($N = 100$) found that the type of information patients wanted about PCA included whether the drug used was morphine, the range of possible side effects, reassurance that PCA was safe and that they could not overdose or become addicted, and detailed instructions and diagrams about the technique (Chumbley et al., 2002).

MR An RCT ($N = 60$) to investigate the effectiveness of a structured preoperative education program in patients receiving PCA found improved patients' satisfaction in the education group but no differences in severity of postoperative pain, side effects, or morphine consumption (Lam et al., 2001).

■ *Assess for potential technical complications including, if present, the catheter site and delivery system.* **LOE = II**

(MR) A laboratory study found that infusion rate accuracy differed significantly among four electronic pumps and one elastomeric pump (used for PCA perineural local anesthetic infusions), exhibiting flow rates within ±15% of their expected rate for 29% to 100% of their infusion duration (Ilfeld et al., 2003).

(NR) A descriptive study ($N = 40$) of adult sickle cell patients aimed at improving the delivery of IV PCA found a significant number of problems related to the pump or IV cannulae threatening PCA effectiveness, and participants unanimously equated PCA use with poorer personal attention from the nurse (Johnson, 2003).

(MR) An RCT ($N = 60$) compared two forms of local anesthetic PCA regional analgesia and reported a low incidence of technical complications including catheter dislodgement and leakage (Rawal et al., 2002).

Possibly Effective

■ *Assess patients' attitudes about PCA.* **LOE = II**

(MR) A randomized quasi-experimental design ($N = 120$) of three different PCA regimens examined the effect of perceived versus actual control and found that a complex pattern of psychological cognitive factors including patients' perceptions, beliefs, and expectations affected the outcomes of PCA (Shiloh et al., 2003).

(MR) An RCT ($N = 70$) comparing IV versus epidural morphine PCA following thoracic or abdominal surgery demonstrated that preoperative expectations of patients' satisfaction and expectations of medication efficacy postoperatively predicted postoperative satisfaction with pain control (Lebovits et al., 2001).

■ *Instruct family members and caregivers not to administer doses for the patient (i.e., "by proxy") unless otherwise authorized and specifically instructed.* **LOE = IV**

(MR) A prospective, 1-year observational study of parent/nurse IV PCA ($N = 212$) found an 8% incidence of pruritus, 15% incidence of vomiting, and 1.7% incidence of apnea or desaturation, reinforcing the need for close monitoring of patients (Monitto et al., 2000).

(MR) A review of the U.S. Pharmacopeia medication error database contained a total of 6069 PCA errors, including 460 that resulted in fatality or some level of harm to the patient, and 15 of these (including one death) were the direct result of PCA by proxy (JCICPS, 2004).

(MR) A descriptive study ($N = 1011$) of children and young adults with cancer who received PCA between 1999 and 2003 reported several events of respiratory depression from PCA by proxy and recommended careful selection of patients, education of proxy users, documentation, and institutional guidelines (Anghelescu et al., 2005).

(EO) The use of PCA by proxy, in which an unauthorized person activates the dosing mechanism of an analgesic infusion pump, increases the risk for potential harm to patients (ASPMN, 2006).

Not Effective

No applicable published research was found in this category.

NR = Nursing Research, **MR** = Multidisciplinary Research, **SP** = Standard of Practice, **EO** = Expert Opinion, **LOE** = Level of Evidence

Possibly Harmful

- *Family members and caregivers administering doses for the patient by proxy unless otherwise authorized and specifically instructed.* **LOE = IV**

    (MR) A prospective 1-year observational study of parent/nurse IV PCA ($N = 212$) found an 8% incidence of pruritus, 15% incidence of vomiting, and 1.7% incidence of apnea or desaturation, reinforcing the need for close monitoring of patients (Monitto et al., 2000).

    (MR) A review of the U.S. Pharmacopeia medication error database contained a total of 6069 PCA errors, including 460 that resulted in fatality or some level of harm to the patient, and 15 of these (including one death) were the direct result of PCA by proxy (JCICPS, 2004).

    (MR) A descriptive study ($N = 1011$) of children and young adults with cancer who received PCA between 1999 and 2003 reported several events of respiratory depression from PCA by proxy and recommended careful selection of patients, education of proxy users, documentation, and institutional guidelines (Anghelescu et al., 2005).

    (EO) The use of PCA by proxy, in which an unauthorized person activates the dosing mechanism of an analgesic infusion pump, increases the risk for potential patient harm (ASPMN, 2006).

OUTCOME MEASUREMENT

PAIN LEVEL   (NOC)

Definition: Severity of observed or reported pain.

Pain Level as evidenced by the following selected NOC indicators:

- Reported pain
- Length of pain episodes
- Facial expressions
- Restlessness

(Rate each indicator of **Pain Level:** 1 = severe, 2 = substantial, 3 = moderate, 4 = mild, 5 = none) (Moorhead et al., 2004).

REFERENCES

American Society for Pain Management Nursing (ASPMN). (2006). Authorized and Unauthorized ("PCA by Proxy") Dosing of Analgesic Infusion Pumps. Available online: http://www.aspmn.org. Retrieved on June 6, 2007.

Anghelescu DL, Burgoyne LL, Oakes LL, Wallace DA. (2005). The safety of patient-controlled analgesia by proxy in pediatric oncology patients. *Anesth Analg,* 101(6):1623-1627.

Burton JH, Harrah JD, Germann CA, Dillon DC. (2006). Does end-tidal carbon dioxide monitoring detect respiratory events prior to current sedation monitoring practices? *Acad Emerg Med,* 13(5): 500-504.

Cashman JN, Dolin SJ. (2004). Respiratory and haemodynamic effects of acute postoperative pain management: Evidence from published data. *Br J Anaesth,* 93(2):212-223.

Chumbley GM, Hall GM, Salmon P. (2002). Patient-controlled analgesia: What information does the patient want? *J Adv Nurs,* 39(5):459-471.

Dochterman JM, Bulechek GM (Eds). (2004). *Nursing Interventions Classification (NIC),* 4th ed. St. Louis: Mosby.

Ellis JA, Blouin R, Lockett J. (1999). Patient-controlled analgesia: Optimizing the experience. *Clin Nurs Res*, 8(3):283-294.

Hagle ME, Lehr VT, Brubakken K, Shippee A. (2004). Respiratory depression in adult patients with intravenous patient-controlled analgesia. *Orthop Nurs*, 23(1):18-27.

Hudcova J, McNicol E, Quah C, Lau J, Carr DB. (2006). Patient controlled opioid analgesia versus conventional opioid analgesia for postoperative pain. *Cochrane Database Syst Rev*, (4):CD003348.

Ilfeld BM, Morey TE, Enneking FK. (2003). Delivery rate accuracy of portable, bolus-capable infusion pumps used for patient-controlled continuous regional analgesia. *Reg Anesth Pain Med*, 28(1):17-23.

Johnson L. (2003). Sickle cell disease patients and patient-controlled analgesia. *Br J Nurs*, 12(3):144-153.

Joint Commission International Center for Patient Safety (JCICPS). (2004). Patient controlled analgesia by proxy. *Sentinel Event Alert*, (33):1-2. Available online: http://www.jcipatientsafety.org/. Retrieved on June 6, 2007.

Lam KK, Chan MT, Chen PP, Kee WD. (2001). Structured preoperative patient education for patient-controlled analgesia. *J Clin Anesth*, 13(6):465-469.

Lebovits AH, Zenetos P, O'Neill DK, Cox D, Dubois MY, Jansen LA, et al. (2001). Satisfaction with epidural and intravenous patient-controlled analgesia. *Pain Med*, 2(4):280-286.

Monitto CL, Greenberg RS, Kost-Byerly S, Wetzel R, Billett C, Lebet RM, et al. (2000). The safety and efficacy of parent-/nurse-controlled analgesia in patients less than six years of age. *Anesth Analg*, 91(3):573-579.

Moorhead M, Johnson M, Maas M (Eds). (2004). *Nursing Outcomes Classification (NOC)*, 3rd ed. St. Louis: Mosby.

Rawal N, Allvin R, Axelsson K, Hallen J, Ekback G, Ohlsson T, et al. (2002). Patient-controlled regional analgesia (PCRA) at home: Controlled comparison between bupivacaine and ropivacaine brachial plexus analgesia. *Anesthesiology*, 96(6):1290-1296.

Riordan SW, Beam K, Okabe-Yamamura T. (2004). Introducing patient-controlled oral analgesia. *Nursing*, 34(9):20.

Shiloh S, Zukerman G, Butin B, Deutch A, Yardeni I, Benyamini Y, et al. (2003). Postoperative patient-controlled analgesia (PCA): How much control and how much analgesia? *Psychol Health*, 18(6):753-770.

Stone JG, Cozine KA, Wald A. (1999). Nocturnal oxygenation during patient-controlled analgesia. *Anesth Analg*, 89(1):104-110.

United States Pharmacopeia (USP). (2004). Patient-controlled analgesia pumps. *USP Quality Review*, 81:1-3.

Vicente KJ, Kada-Bekhaled K, Hillel G, Cassano A, Orser BA. (2003). Programming errors contribute to death from patient-controlled analgesia: Case report and estimate of probability. *Can J Anesth*, 50(4):328-332.

 ## PELVIC MUSCLE EXERCISE

Angelina A. Arcamone, DNSc, RN, CCE

> **NIC** **Definition:** Strengthening and training the levator ani and urogenital muscles through voluntary, repetitive contraction to decrease stress, urge, or mixed types of urinary incontinence (Dochterman & Bulechek, 2004).

NURSING ACTIVITIES

Effective

■ **NIC** *Determine the ability to recognize the urge to void.* **LOE = VII**

> **EO** A thorough continence assessment can help to diagnose the cause of incontinence and leads to effective management to relieve symptoms (Benson, 2003).

NR = Nursing Research, **MR** = Multidisciplinary Research, **SP** = Standard of Practice, **EO** = Expert Opinion, **LOE** = Level of Evidence

■ **NIC** *Instruct the individual to tighten, then relax, the ring of muscle around the urethra and anus, as if trying to prevent urination or bowel movement.* **LOE = I**

MR A Cochrane systematic review found that the use of pelvic floor muscle training was better than no treatment or placebo treatment for women with stress or mixed incontinence (Hay-Smith et al., 2001).

EO Contracting the pelvic floor muscles several seconds after the onset of urination helps determine whether the patient is able to stop or slow urinary flow (Gray, 2004).

■ *Counsel women to perform pelvic floor muscle exercises while seated upright in a chair with a firm seat.* **LOE = VII**

EO The contraction of the levator ani is perceived as the tightening of the U-shaped muscle in direct contact with the chair and is accompanied by a very slight elevation of the anus from the firm surface of the chair (Gray, 2004).

■ *Counsel men to stand with feet apart and tighten and lift the pelvic floor muscles, as if controlling flatus or preventing urine flow, and practice in front of a mirror.* **LOE = VII**

EO Standing allows men to observe for the base of the penis moving nearer to the abdomen, and testicles should rise (Dorey, 2003).

■ **NIC** *Instruct the individual to avoid contracting the abdomen, thighs, and buttocks; holding the breath, or straining down during the exercise.* **LOE = V**

NR A review of the literature supported that patients must learn to relax abdominal muscles while contracting the pelvic floor muscles because when abdominal muscles are contracted, they press on the bladder and may contribute to loss of urine (Burgio, 2004).

■ **NIC** *Ensure that the individual can differentiate between the desired drawing up-and-in muscle contraction and the nondesired bearing-down effort.* **LOE = V**

EO The most critical variables in the success of pelvic floor muscle exercises are the correct identification of the pelvic floor muscles and adherence to the exercise regimen (Wyman, 2003).

NR A systematic review found that although numerous variations in the protocol for pelvic floor muscle exist, all concurred on three basic components: (1) setting aside a devoted time to exercise, (2) graduating the amount or intensity of exercise, and (3) striving to induce structural change in the muscles (Miller, 2002).

EO In women during an examination by gently inserting one or two gloved fingers into the vagina, a proper contraction can be assessed by asking the woman to contract the pelvic floor muscles around the examiner's finger (Gray, 2005).

EO In men during an examination, a proper contraction creates a circumferential tightening of the anal sphincter, drawing the finger in and toward the rectal vault (Gray, 2005).

■ **NIC** *Instruct the individual to perform muscle tightening exercises, working up to 300 contractions each day, holding the contractions for 10 seconds each, and resting at least 10 seconds each between each contraction, per agency protocol.* **LOE = II**

MR An RCT ($N = 747$) to assess urinary incontinence in women who had assessment by nurses and conservative advice on pelvic floor muscles exercises at 5, 7, and 9 months after

RCT = Randomized Controlled (Clinical) Trial, **NIC** = Nursing Interventions Classification, **NOC** = Nursing Outcomes Classification

delivery compared with a control group found that women in the intervention group had significantly less urinary incontinence (Glazener et al., 2006).

(NR) A systematic review demonstrated that a typical schedule for pelvic floor muscle exercises was 36 to 50 pelvic floor muscle contractions divided into two to three exercise sets and performed either daily or three times per week (Wyman, 2003).

(NR) A review of the literature supported instructing patients to start by holding a contraction for 2 to 3 seconds and gradually progressing to a goal of 10 seconds (Burgio, 2004).

■ **(NIC)** *Inform the individual that it takes 6 to 12 weeks for exercises to be effective.* **LOE = I**

(MR) A Cochrane systematic review found that women who did pelvic floor muscle exercises for 12 weeks were more likely to report their incontinence was cured or improved than women who did not do the pelvic floor muscle exercises (Hay-Smith & Dumoulin, 2006).

(NR) A systematic review found that a typical regimen for pelvic floor muscle exercises should be performed for 12 to 16 weeks (Wyman, 2003).

Possibly Effective

■ **(NIC)** *Provide positive feedback for doing exercises as prescribed.* **LOE = V**

(NR) A systematic review of the effectiveness of pelvic floor muscle exercises found that the evidence on giving the patient feedback about exercise effectiveness was not conclusive (Haddow et al., 2005).

(NR) A qualitative study identified factors that facilitated pelvic floor muscle exercises as (1) realistic goals, (2) positive affirmation, (3) follow-up, and (4) maintaining an exercise routine (Milne & Moore, 2006).

■ **(NIC)** *Incorporate biofeedback or electrical stimulation for selected individuals when assistance is indicated to identify correct muscles to contract and/or to elicit desired strength of muscle contraction.* **LOE = I**

(MR) A Cochrane systematic review found that the effectiveness of biofeedback-assisted pelvic floor muscle training was not clear, but based on the evidence available, there did not appear to be any benefit over pelvic floor muscle training alone at post-treatment assessment. In addition, the effect of adding pelvic floor muscle training to other treatments such as electrical stimulation was not clear because of the limited amount of evidence that existed (Hay-Smith et al., 2001).

(MR) A systematic review demonstrated that strengthening the pelvic floor muscles significantly improved postprostatectomy urinary incontinence, postmicturition dribble, and erectile function. There was no evidence that biofeedback enhanced the treatment effect (Dorey et al., 2005).

(MR) A systematic review found that the value of the various approaches to the conservative management of postprostatectomy incontinence remained unclear. There may be some benefit of offering pelvic floor muscle training with biofeedback early in the postoperative period (Hunter et al., 2004).

(MR) An RCT ($N = 55$) to compare the efficacy of pelvic floor muscle exercises and manometric biofeedback with lifestyle changes for men with erectile dysfunction found that at 3 months, compared with controls, men in the intervention group showed significant mean increases in erectile functioning and significant progress in reducing or eliminating postmicturition dribble (Dorey et al., 2004).

(MR) A clinical trial ($N = 20$) to evaluate the strength of pelvic floor muscles in women with urinary incontinence and to evaluate relief of symptoms using biofeedback therapy found that biofeedback training objectively improved pelvic floor exercises in the cohort who performed them incorrectly and improved urinary continence in the majority of subjects (Russell et al., 2005).

■ **(NIC)** *Provide written instructions describing the intervention and the recommended number of repetitions.* **LOE = V**

(NR) A systematic review found that the effectiveness of providing the patient with take-home materials and reminder phone calls was unclear (Haddow et al., 2005).

(NR) A quasi-experimental study ($N = 100$) that compared the effectiveness of a new education tool for pelvic floor muscle exercises in the form of a refrigerator magnet compared with written instructions found that the women in the magnet group had a higher rate of compliance with the pelvic floor muscle exercises (Ip, 2004).

■ *Discuss with the patient the importance of keeping a daily record of continence to provide reinforcement.* **LOE = VI**

(MR) A descriptive study found that significant predictors of adherence to pelvic floor muscle exercise therapy were the amount of urine loss per incontinent episode and women's perception of their ability to do the exercises as recommended under various circumstances (Alewijnse et al., 2001).

Not Effective

No applicable published research was found in this category.

Possibly Harmful

■ **(NIC)** *Teach the individual to monitor the response to exercise by attempting to stop urine flow no more often than once a week.* **LOE = V**

(MR) A review of the literature recommended that patients should not practice pelvic floor muscle exercises by routinely starting and stopping the flow of urine, as this may disrupt the micturition reflex (National Guidelines Clearinghouse, 2005).

(NR) A review of the literature revealed that some patients may benefit from interruption or slowing of the urinary stream during voiding once per day; however, some clinicians hesitated to recommend this exercise because it may lead to incomplete emptying of the bladder (Burgio, 2004).

OUTCOME MEASUREMENT

KNOWLEDGE: TREATMENT REGIMEN   (NOC)

Definition: Extent of understanding conveyed about a specific treatment regimen.
Knowledge: Treatment Regimen as evidenced by the following selected NOC indicators:

Continued

OUTCOME MEASUREMENT—*cont'd*

- Description of rationale for treatment regimen
- Description of self-care responsibilities for ongoing treatment
- Description of self-monitoring techniques
- Description of prescribed procedure(s)

(Rate each indicator of **Knowledge: Treatment Regimen:** 1 = none, 2 = limited, 3 = moderate, 4 = substantial, 5 = extensive) (Moorhead et al., 2004).

REFERENCES

Alewijnse D, Mesters I, Metsemakers J, Adriaans J, van den Borne B. (2001). Predictors of intention to adhere to physiotherapy among women with urinary incontinence. *Health Educ Res*, 16(2):173-186.

Benson D. (2003). The importance of a thorough continence assessment. *Nurs Times*, 99(29):53-54.

Burgio KL. (2004). Current perspectives on management of urgency using bladder and behavioral training. *J Am Acad Nurse Pract*, 16(10 Suppl):4-7.

Dochterman JM, Bulechek GM (Eds). (2004). *Nursing Interventions Classification (NIC)*, 4th ed. St. Louis: Mosby.

Dorey G. (2003). Pelvic floor muscle exercises for men. *Nurs Times*, 99(19):46-48.

Dorey G, Speakman M, Feneley R, Swinkels A, Dunn C. (2005). Pelvic floor exercises for erectile dysfunction. *BJU Int*, 96(4):595-597.

Dorey G, Speakman M, Feneley R, Swinkels A, Dunn C, Ewings P. (2004). Randomised controlled trial of pelvic floor muscle exercises and manometric biofeedback for erectile dysfunction. *Br J Gen Pract*, 54(508):819-825.

Glazener CM, Herbison GP, MacArthur C, Lancashire R, McGee MA, Grant AM, Wilson PD. (2006). New postnatal urinary incontinence: Obstetric and other risk factors in primiparae. *BJOG*, 113(2):208-217.

Gray M. (2004). Stress urinary incontinence in women. *J Am Acad Nurse Pract*, 16(5):188-190, 192-197.

Gray M. (2005). Assessment and management of urinary incontinence. *Nurs Pract*, 30(7):32-33, 36-43.

Haddow G, Watts R, Robertson J. (2005). Effectiveness of a pelvic floor muscle exercise program on urinary incontinence following childbirth. *Int J Evid Based Healthc*, 3(5):103-146.

Hay-Smith EJ, Bo K, Berghmans LC, Hendriks HJ, de Bie RA, van Waalwijk van Doorn ES. (2001). Pelvic floor muscle training for urinary incontinence in women. *Cochrane Database Syst Rev*, (1):CD001407.

Hay-Smith EJ, Dumoulin C. (2006). Pelvic floor muscle training versus no treatment, or inactive control treatments, for urinary incontinence in women. *Cochrane Database Syst Rev*, (1):CD005654.

Hunter KF, Moore KN, Cody DJ, Glazener CM. (2004). Conservative management for postprostatectomy urinary incontinence. *Cochrane Database Syst Rev*, (2), CD001843.

Ip V. (2004). Evaluation of a patient education tool to reduce the incidence of incontinence post-prostrate surgery. *Urol Nurs*, 24(5):401-407.

Miller JM. (2002). Criteria for the therapeutic use of pelvic floor muscle training in women. *J Wound Ostomy Continence Nurs*, 29(6):301-311.

Milne JL, Moore KN. (2006). Factors impacting self-care for urinary incontinence. *Urol Nurs*, 26(1):41-51.

Moorhead M, Johnson M, Maas M (Eds). (2004). *Nursing Outcomes Classification (NOC)*, 3rd ed. St. Louis: Mosby.

National Guidelines Clearinghouse. (2005). Urinary incontinence: Guide to diagnosis and management. Available online: http://www.guideline.gov. Retrieved on May 6, 2007.

Russell AL, Grigo HM, Joseph NS, Niu J, Bachmann G. (2005). Evaluating the performance of pelvic floor exercises in women with urinary incontinence. *J Reprod Med*, 50(7):529-532.

Wyman JF. (2003). Treatment of urinary incontinence in men and older women: The evidence shows the efficacy of a variety of techniques. *Am J Nurs*, 103(Suppl):26-35.

PERINEAL CARE   NIC

Angelina A. Arcamone, DNSc, RN, CCE

NIC **Definition:** Maintenance of perineal skin integrity and relief of perineal discomfort (Dochterman & Bulechek, 2004).

NURSING ACTIVITIES

Effective

■ **NIC** *Clean the perineum thoroughly at regular intervals.* **LOE = III**

MR A controlled study determined the effectiveness of a new cleanser protectant lotion (Baza Cleanse and Protect) in reducing perineal erythema and pain in patients (N = 19) with incontinence. Patients demonstrated significant improvement in erythema and reported significant improvement in pain (Warshaw et al., 2002).

NR A review of the literature recommended instructing patients to clean and direct the flow of water from front to back to minimize the risk of washing fecal material from the anus onto the perineum (Steen, 2001).

MR A review of the literature on incontinent patients recommended cleansing the entire perineum daily with a skin cleanser and after each major incontinent episode (Gray, 2004; National Guideline Clearinghouse, 2003).

NR A review of the literature on incontinent patients recommended using a soft moist cloth and avoiding brisk scrubbing of the perineum. In addition, no-rinse cleansers were particularly useful because they simplified the care regimen and eliminated the risk of irritation associated with incomplete removal of traditional cleansers from the skin (Gray, 2004).

■ **NIC** *Keep the perineum dry.* **LOE = V**

NR A review of the literature on incontinent patients recommended assisting patients in choosing a containment device (pad, incontinence brief, condom catheter) that absorbed urine or contained stool and minimized skin exposure to irritants (Gray et al., 2002).

NR A review of the literature on incontinent patients recommended using moisture barriers after cleansing to shield the perineal area from exposure to irritants or moisture (Gray et al., 2002; Gray & Jones, 2004).

NR A review of the literature on incontinent patients recommended using a barrier paste that absorbed drainage and protected skin from irritants for incontinent patients with extensive skin erosion with exudates (Gray et al., 2002; Gray & Jones, 2004).

■ *Inspect the condition of the perineum.* **LOE = VII**

EO Inspect the genital-perineal area daily and note skin integrity, any signs of contact dermatitis, skin excoriation, and drainage (National Guideline Clearinghouse, 2003).

■ **NIC** *Apply a cold pack as appropriate.* **LOE = II**

NR A systematic review demonstrated that cooling treatments (ice packs) applied locally to the perineum were effective at reducing perineal pain, swelling, and bruising without any adverse effects on wound healing (Steen & Cooper, 1998).

RCT = Randomized Controlled (Clinical) Trial, **NIC** = Nursing Interventions Classification, **NOC** = Nursing Outcomes Classification

(NR) An RCT ($N = 316$) involving postpartum women in which an experimental group used a cooling gel pad on the perineum, versus an ice pack, versus no treatment (control group) found that the gel pad could alleviate symptoms of perineal trauma and associated pain during the first and second postpartum weeks without adverse effects on healing (Steen, 2002).

■ *Use topical wound treatment products.* **LOE = II**

(NR) An RCT ($N = 30$) compared the safety and efficacy of Xenaderm ointment versus Granulex spray and saline for the treatment of perineal dermatitis secondary to urinary and fecal incontinence. Wounds managed with the ointment-based product had significantly lower edema, scabbing, and erythema and higher epithelialization than the spray- or saline-managed wounds (Gray & Jones, 2004).

(MR) A prospective randomized controlled study was conducted to investigate the efficacy and safety of a new mode of local antibiotic administration in patients after abdominoperineal excision of rectal cancer ($N = 49$) compared with patients ($N = 43$) who received standard treatment. Patients in the experimental group had significantly lower perineal infection rates (Gruessner et al., 2001).

■ *Assess the patient's level of perineal pain.* **LOE = VII**

(EO) Pain cannot be properly controlled and treated if it is not assessed. The severity and quality of perineal pain must be routinely assessed (Steen, 2003).

Possibly Effective

■ *Use sitz baths in managing anorectal disorders.* **LOE = I**

(MR) A systematic review of the literature demonstrated that there was a lack of scientific data to support the use of sitz baths in the treatment of anorectal disorders (Tejirian & Abbas, 2005).

(MR) A Cochrane review found that there was insufficient evidence either to support or undermine the routine use of tap water for wound cleansing (Fernandez et al., 2002).

■ *Use therapeutic ultrasound for perineal pain.* **LOE = I**

(MR) A Cochrane systematic review found that there was not enough evidence to evaluate the use of ultrasound in treating perineal pain following childbirth (Hay-Smith, 2000).

■ (NIC) *Apply a heat cradle/heat lamp as appropriate.* **LOE = VII**

(EO) After the use of a sitz bath, the patient should allow the perineum to dry thoroughly either by air or the aid of a small light bulb (Leeds, 2003).

■ (NIC) *Provide scrotal support, as appropriate.* **LOE = VII**

(EO) Pelvic and acetabular fractures are associated with severe perineal soft tissue injury, and there is risk of significant insult to the perineal soft tissue during operative stabilization of these fractures. A canvas sail lined with soft cotton under the scrotum and then elevated by using a traction cord over a pulley can be used to reduce the swelling (Raman et al., 2004).

Not Effective

No applicable published research was found in this category.

NR = Nursing Research, **MR** = Multidisciplinary Research, **SP** = Standard of Practice, **EO** = Expert Opinion, **LOE** = Level of Evidence

Possibly Harmful

■ *Using bar soaps, antibacterial agents, and scented skin cleansers for perineal cleansing.* **LOE = V**

(NR) A review of the literature recommended not using soap or detergent bars when caring for incontinent patients because they required application with a washcloth, they were frequently alkaline, and they removed needed oils from the skin, further diminishing its barrier function (Gray, 2004).

(NR) A review of the literature suggested that the use of skin cleansers that contained antibacterial agents was controversial because of concerns related to bacterial resistance (Gray, 2004).

(NR) A review of the literature suggested that scented skin cleansers must be used with caution in incontinent patients because they could act as irritants and sensitizers, particularly when perineal skin integrity was compromised (Gray, 2004).

OUTCOME MEASUREMENT

TISSUE INTEGRITY: SKIN AND MUCOUS MEMBRANES   (NOC)

Definition: Structural intactness and normal physiological function of skin and mucous membranes.

Tissue Integrity: Skin and Mucous Membranes as evidenced by the following selected NOC indicators:

• Sensation
• Skin temperature
• Tissue perfusion
• Skin intactness

(Rate each indicator of **Tissue Integrity: Skin and Mucous Membranes:** 1 = severely compromised, 2 = substantially compromised, 3 = moderately compromised, 4 = mildly compromised, 5 = not compromised) (Moorhead et al., 2004).

REFERENCES

Dochterman JM, Bulechek GM (Eds). (2004). *Nursing Interventions Classification (NIC)*, 4th ed. St. Louis: Mosby.

Fernandez R, Griffiths R, Ussia C. (2002). Water for wound cleansing. *Cochrane Database Syst Rev*, (4): CD003861.

Gray M. (2004). Preventing and managing perineal dermatitis: A shared goal for wound and continence care. *J Wound Ostomy Continence Nurs*, 31(1 Suppl):S2-S9.

Gray M, Jones DP. (2004). The effect of different formulations of equivalent active ingredients on the performance of two topical wound treatment products. *Ostomy Wound Manage*, 50(3):34-38, 40, 42-44.

Gray M, Ratliff C, Donovan A. (2002). Tender mercies: Providing skin care for an incontinent patient. *Nursing*, 32(7):51-54.

Gruessner U, Clemens M, Pahlplatz PV, Sperling P, Witte J, Rosen HR, et al. (2001). Improvement of perineal wound healing by local administration of gentamicin-impregnated collagen fleeces after abdominoperineal excision of rectal cancer. *Am J Surg*, 182(5):502-509.

RCT = Randomized Controlled (Clinical) Trial, **NIC** = Nursing Interventions Classification, **NOC** = Nursing Outcomes Classification

Hay-Smith EJ. (2000). Therapeutic ultrasound for postpartum perineal pain and dyspareunia. *Cochrane Database Syst Rev,* (2):CD000495.

Hedayati H, Parsons J, Crowther CA. (2005). Topically applied anaesthetics for treating perineal pain after childbirth. *Cochrane Database Syst Rev,* (2):CD004223.

Leeds A. (2003). The art of the sitz bath. *Midwifery Today Int Midwife,* (65):25-26.

Moorhead M, Johnson M, Maas M (Eds). (2004). *Nursing Outcomes Classification (NOC),* 3rd ed. St. Louis: Mosby.

National Guideline Clearinghouse. (2003). *Nursing management of patients with urinary incontinence. Complete summary.* King of Prussia, PA: National Guideline Clearinghouse.

Raman R, Senior C, Segura P, Giannoudis PV. (2004). Management of scrotal swelling after pelvic and acetabular fractures. *Br J Nurs,* 13(8):458-461.

Steen M. (2001). Product focus. Do we care enough about perineal wounds? *Br J Midwifery,* 9(5):316.

Steen M. (2002). A randomised controlled trial to evaluate the effectiveness of localised cooling treatments in alleviating perineal trauma: The APT study. *MIDIRS Midwifery Digest,* 12(3):373-376.

Steen M. (2003). Postnatal breast and perineal pain. *Br J Midwifery,* 11(5):318.

Steen M, Cooper K. (1998). Clinical cold therapy and perineal wounds: Too cool or not too cool? *Br J Midwifery,* 6(9):572-579.

Tejirian T, Abbas MA. (2005). Sitz bath: Where is the evidence? Scientific basis of a common practice. *Dis Colon Rectum,* 48(12):2336-2340.

Warshaw E, Nix D, Kula J, Markon CE. (2002). Clinical and cost effectiveness of a cleanser protectant lotion for treatment of perineal skin breakdown in low-risk patients with incontinence. *Ostomy Wound Manage,* 48(6):44-51.

 # PERIPHERAL SENSATION MANAGEMENT NIC

Teresa J. Kelechi, PhD, RN

NIC Definition: Prevention or minimization of injury or discomfort in the patient with altered sensation (Dochterman & Bulechek, 2004).

NURSING ACTIVITIES

Effective

■ *Use skin protection measures such as moisturizers, bathing products, and garments specifically designed to reduce the incidence of skin tears.* **LOE = I**

MR A systematic review of the literature demonstrated that to help prevent skin tears, all patients should be assessed on admission to medical facilities using a skin tear risk assessment tool and placed on a risk reduction program if indicated (O'Regan, 2002).

NR In a descriptive study of patients (N = 30) on a residential Alzheimer's disease unit, the majority of patients (N = 26) remained with tear-free skin through a 10-month preventive skin care regimen (Brillhart, 2005).

MR A descriptive study of 29 bed-bound residents at a long-term care facility demonstrated that changing from soap and water to a no-rinse formula for bathing significantly reduced the occurrence of skin tears (Birch & Coggins, 2003).

EO Bag baths versus traditional bed baths reduce dryness and potential for skin injury of impaired skin (Sheppard & Brenner, 2000).

EO Padded arm sleeves and/or armrests, bedrails, and lifts prevent skin tears associated with contact with friable skin (Baranoski, 2001).

NR = Nursing Research, **MR** = Multidisciplinary Research, **SP** = Standard of Practice, **EO** = Expert Opinion, **LOE** = Level of Evidence

■ (SP) *Use burn prevention strategies to reduce the incidence of burn injuries.*
   LOE = III

(MR) A quasi-experimental trial ($N = 209$) of older adults residing in a multicultural metropolitan city demonstrated that a community-based burn prevention campaign was effective in improving burn prevention knowledge (Tan et al., 2004).

(EO) Thermometers are an effective way to test water temperature (Redlick et al., 2002).

(EO) Water temperature for bathing older adults should be no warmer than 105°F (Rader et al., 2006). Water heater temperature should be set no higher than 120°F (Huyer & Corkum, 1997).

(EO) Thermal insulated mitts should be used when handling cooking utensils (Lieberman, 2004).

(EO) The use of heat or cold, such as heating pads, hot water bottles, and ice packs, should be avoided or carefully monitored (Grant, 2004).

Possibly Effective

■ *Use higher sun protection factor (SPF) sunscreens to reduce the incidence of thermal injuries.* **LOE = II**

(MR) An RCT ($N = 367$) of sunscreens demonstrated that the use of higher SPF sunscreens resulted in fewer sunburns (Dupuy et al., 2005).

(EO) Body parts should be protected from extreme temperature changes by the use of gloves and other protective clothing (Blach & Ignatavicius, 2006).

■ *Use quantitative sensory testing for monitoring vibration and warm and cold discrimination.* **LOE = I**

(MR) A Cochrane systematic review found that the use of quantitative sensory testing (QST) of vibration and thermal perception threshold was probably an effective tool in the documentation of diabetic sensory neuropathy (Shy et al., 2003).

(MR) A Cochrane review demonstrated that the QST was possibly useful in detecting thermal threshold abnormalities in patients with small fiber neuropathy (Shy et al., 2003).

(MR) An RCT ($N = 82$) of individuals with diabetic peripheral neuropathy indicated that the use of the Semmes-Weinstein monofilament (5.07/10 g) was useful in detecting sensory loss of the plantar surface of the feet (Kamei et al., 2005).

(EO) Test temperature sensation only when pain sensation is abnormal (Bickley & Szilagyi, 2005).

Not Effective

No applicable published research was found in this category.

Possibly Harmful

No applicable published research was found in this category.

(Note: For care of the feet, please refer to the guideline on Foot Care.)

RCT = Randomized Controlled (Clinical) Trial, **NIC** = Nursing Interventions Classification, **NOC** = Nursing Outcomes Classification

OUTCOME MEASUREMENT

PHYSICAL INJURY SEVERITY   NOC

(Please refer to *Nursing Outcomes Classification* [Moorhead et al., 2004] for the **Physical Injury Severity** outcome.)

REFERENCES

Baranoski S. (2001). Skin tears. *Nurs Manage,* 32(8):25-31.

Bickley LS, Szilagyi PG. (2005). *Bates' guide to physical examination and history taking,* 9th ed. Philadelphia: Lippincott Williams & Wilkins.

Birch S, Coggins T. (2003). No-rinse, one-step bed bath: The effects on the occurrence of skin tears in a long-term care setting. *Ostomy Wound Manage,* 49(1):64-67.

Blach DA, Ignatavicius DD. (2006). Interventions for clients with vascular problems. In Ignatavicius DD, Workman ML (Eds). *Medical-surgical nursing: Critical thinking for collaborative care,* 5th ed. St. Louis: Saunders.

Brillhart B. (2005). Pressure sore and skin tear prevention and treatment during a 10-month program. *Rehabil Nurs,* 30(3):85-91.

Dochterman JM, Bulechek GM (Eds). (2004). *Nursing Interventions Classification (NIC),* 4th ed. St. Louis: Mosby.

Dupuy A, Dunant A, Grob JJ; Reseau d'Epidemiologie en Dermatologie. (2005). Randomized controlled trial testing the impact of high-protection sunscreens on sun-exposure behavior. *Arch Dermatol,* 141(8):950-956.

Grant EJ. (2004). Burn prevention. *Crit Care Nurs Clin North Am,* 16(1):127-138.

Huyer DW, Corkum SH. (1997). Reducing the incidence of tap-water scalds: Strategies for physicians. *CMAJ,* 156(6):841-844.

Kamei N, Yamane K, Nakanishi S, Yamashita Y, Tamura T, Ohshita K, et al. (2005). Effectiveness of Semmes-Weinstein monofilament examination for diabetic peripheral neuropathy screening. *J Diabetes Complications,* 19(1):47-53.

Lieberman S. (2004). Too hot to handle: Burn prevention for home care & hospice clients. *Caring,* 23(4):28-30.

Moorhead M, Johnson M, Maas M (Eds). (2004). *Nursing Outcomes Classification (NOC),* 3rd ed. St. Louis: Mosby.

O'Regan A. (2002). Skin tears: A review of the literature. *World Counc Enterostom Therapists J,* 22(2): 26-31.

Rader J, Barrick AL, Hoeffer B, Sloane PD, McKenzie D, Talerico KA, et al. (2006). The bathing of older adults with dementia. *Am J Nurs,* 106(4):40-48.

Redlick F, Cooke A, Gomez M, Banfield J, Cartotto RC, Fish JS. (2002). A survey of risk factors for burns in the elderly and prevention strategies. *J Burn Care Rehabil,* 23(5):351-356.

Sheppard CM, Brenner PS. (2000). The effects of bathing and skin care practices on skin quality and satisfaction with an innovative product. *J Gerontol Nurs,* 26(10):36-45.

Shy ME, Frohman EM, So YT, Arezzo JC, Cornblath DR, Giuliani MJ, et al. (2003). Quantitative sensory testing: Report of the Therapeutics and Technology Assessment Subcommittee of the American Academy of Neurology. *Neurology,* 60(6):898-904.

Tan J, Banez C, Cheung Y, Gomez M, Nguyen H, Banfield J, et al. (2004). Effectiveness of a burn prevention campaign for older adults. *J Burn Care Rehabil,* 25(5):445-451.

PERIPHERALLY INSERTED CENTRAL CATHETER CARE

Lisa Gorski, MS, APRN-BC, CRNI, FAAN

NIC **Definition:** Insertion and maintenance of a peripherally inserted central catheter, either midline or centrally located (Dochterman & Bulechek, 2004).

NURSING ACTIVITIES

Effective

■ (SP) *Place and monitor peripherally inserted central catheter (PICC) or midline catheters by a registered nurse who is educated and has demonstrated competency in performing the procedure.* **LOE = VI**

(EO) Strict entry criteria related to nursing experience, education, and competency along with adoption of technology and continuous data collection have resulted in increased PICC placement success rates over a 5-year period. Data were collected and retrospectively analyzed on more than 12,500 PICCs in the specialty nursing program (Burns, 2005).

(MR) A prospective quality assurance study conducted to evaluate the impact of a PICC team found an increase in success of bedside PICC placement with the use of ultrasound, decreased patients' waiting time, and decreased PICC placement costs including less use of expensive interventional radiology facilities (Robinson et al., 2005).

(NR) In a descriptive study, the presence of a dedicated PICC insertion team and education of nurses in PICC maintenance resulted in a decrease in PICC-related complication rates over a 2-year period (Funk et al., 2001).

(EO) Placement of central vascular access devices should meet the criteria established by the state's nurse practice act, rules and regulations promulgated by the state board of nursing, organizational policies and procedures, and practice guidelines (INS, 2006).

■ (SP) *Use ultrasonography to visualize the blood vessel and surrounding structures prior to vein cannulation to improve success of PICC placement.* **LOE = V**

(NR) A descriptive study compared usual PICC placement by palpation of the intended vein to implementation of ultrasound-guided PICC placement by nursing IV teams in two acute care settings ($N = 1338$ PICCs) and found an increase in the success rate of PICC placement, referrals to the PICC team, and cost savings related to a reduced need for interventional radiologists to place PICCs (Anstett & Royer, 2003).

(NR) A descriptive retrospective study ($N = 757$) comparing usual selection of the vein for PICC placement (vision/palpation of the potential vein) with ultrasound-guided placement by a registered nurse demonstrated a 25% decrease in the number of attempts required to access the vein using ultrasound-guided placement (LaRue, 2000).

(NR) A descriptive study that was part of a quality improvement project at an acute care hospital reported an improvement in the success rate of PICC placement and a decrease in the need to refer patients to interventional radiology for PICC placement when ultrasound guidance techniques were implemented by the nursing PICC team (McMahon, 2002).

RCT = Randomized Controlled (Clinical) Trial, **NIC** = Nursing Interventions Classification, **NOC** = Nursing Outcomes Classification

(MR) A systematic review of prospective, randomized studies found decreased complications during attempted central venous catheter placements and a reduction in the number of venipuncture attempts. Although the major focus of this review was related to subclavian catheter placement, ultrasound guidance was also demonstrated to improve insertion of PICCs (Rothschild, 2001).

(MR) A systematic review of safety practices found that use of real-time ultrasound guidance during central line insertion to prevent complications was listed as one of the 11 practices rated most highly in terms of strength of the evidence supporting more widespread implementation (Shojania et al., 2001).

■ *Use a local intradermal or topical anesthetic cream to decrease pain associated with PICC insertion.* **LOE = II**

(NR) An RCT involving adult patients who required PICC placement ($N = 42$) comparing use of intradermal injection of buffered lidocaine, a topical anesthetic (EMLA cream), and no anesthetic found that the buffered lidocaine was significantly more effective than EMLA cream or no anesthetic in relieving pain associated with PICC insertion (Fry & Aholt, 2001).

■ *Implement the "central line bundle," which includes all of the following: hand hygiene, maximal barrier precautions (use of sterile gown, sterile powder-free gloves, cap, mask, protective eyewear, and large sterile drapes) during placement, use of chlorhexidine for skin antisepsis, and daily review of the necessity of the catheter with prompt removal when no longer needed to reduce the risk of catheter-related bloodstream infection.* **LOE = I**

(MR) A descriptive study of the implementation of the central line bundle in critical care units in a level one trauma full-service hospital demonstrated a reduction in catheter-related bloodstream infections (IHI, 2006a).

(MR) The use of maximum sterile barriers while placing central venous catheters to prevent infection was listed as one of the 11 practices rated most highly in terms of strength of the evidence supporting more widespread implementation (Shojania et al., 2001).

(MR) A systematic, evidence-based review of the literature to determine the value of maximal sterile barriers was undertaken and yielded three studies for inclusion. The evidence supported the use of maximal sterile barriers in ambulatory oncology patients but was incomplete for other settings. More prospective studies are needed (Hu et al., 2004).

(MR) A meta-analysis of studies ($N = 8$ studies involving 4143 catheters) comparing chlorhexidine gluconate with povidone iodine solutions for catheter site care found that the incidence of bloodstream infections was significantly reduced when chlorhexidine gluconate was used (Chaiyakunapruk et al., 2002).

Additional references: O'Grady et al., 2002; IHI, 2006b.

■ *Verify PICC placement ensuring that the distal tip is located in the lower one third of the superior vena cava (SVC) to the junction of the SVC and the right atrium as determined radiographically prior to administering any IV medications or solutions to reduce the risk of complications.* **LOE = II**

(MR) A randomized study ($N = 39$) compared placement of the PICC catheter tip in the SVC with placement in the axillosubclavian-innominate vein. Significant findings included

NR = Nursing Research, **MR** = Multidisciplinary Research, **SP** = Standard of Practice, **EO** = Expert Opinion, **LOE** = Level of Evidence

a reduction in the incidence of catheter-related thrombosis, improved catheter survival, and reduced risk for infection when the catheter tip was placed in the SVC (Kearns et al., 1996).

(EO) Central catheter tip location should be determined radiographically and documented prior to initiation of the prescribed therapy (INS, 2006).

(EO) The most appropriate location for the tip of PICCs is the lower one third of the SVC, close to the junction of the SVC and the right atrium (NAVAN, 1998).

■ *Use a manufactured catheter securement device instead of tape or sutures to reduce risk of complications.* **LOE = II**

(MR) A systematic review of prospective or prospective randomized studies that compared tape and suture versus other methods of securing peripheral IV catheters or PICCs was performed. Five studies involving PICCs, midlines, or other central venous catheters comparing tape or sutures with a manufactured catheter securement device demonstrated a reduction in overall complications (Frey & Schears, 2006).

(MR) A prospective randomized study ($N = 170$) comparing suturing of PICCs with a manufactured securement device demonstrated a significant decrease in the rate of catheter-related bloodstream infections (Yamamoto et al., 2002).

■ *Wash hands using conventional antiseptic soap and water or with waterless alcohol-based gels or foams before and after inserting and when caring for the PICC or midline catheter to reduce the risk of intravenous device–related infections.* **LOE = I**

(Please refer to the guideline on Infection Control: Hand Hygiene.)

■ (SP) *Maintain aseptic technique including sterile gloves and masks while providing site care for the PICC or midline catheter to reduce the risk of intravenous device–related infections.* **LOE = VII**

(MR) A retrospective descriptive study of PICC ($N = 322$) outcomes in a group of patients who received a variety of types of infusions, but primarily parenteral nutrition, found a low rate of complications including infection. Site care was provided using aseptic technique including the use of sterile gloves and masks (Loughran & Borzatta, 1995).

(EO) Catheter site care consists of sterile cleansing of the catheter-skin junction, application of a new stabilization device, and application of a sterile dressing (INS, 2006).

(EO) Sterile gloves and a mask should be worn to provide site care when the catheter tip is centrally located (INS, 2006).

■ *Disinfect the skin utilizing a 2% chlorhexidine-based preparation as part of catheter site care prior to dressing changes to reduce the risk of infection.* **LOE = I**

(MR) A meta-analysis of studies ($N = 8$ studies involving 4143 catheters) comparing chlorhexidine gluconate with povidone iodine solutions for catheter site care found that the incidence of bloodstream infections is significantly reduced when chlorhexidine gluconate is used (Chaiyakunapruk et al., 2002).

RCT = Randomized Controlled (Clinical) Trial, **NIC** = Nursing Interventions Classification, **NOC** = Nursing Outcomes Classification

■ *Use either a transparent or gauze dressing to protect the catheter insertion site; change the dressing as part of routine site care; change the transparent dressing at least every 7 days; change the gauze dressing at least every 2 days.* **LOE = II**

(NR) A systematic review of controlled trials ($N = 6$ studies) comparing the effects of gauze and tape versus transparent dressings found no evidence of difference in the incidence of infectious complications between dressing types. However, the studies were from small samples and there was a high level of uncertainty regarding risk for infection related to type of dressing. Patients' preference can be used to base decisions; more studies are needed (Gillies et al., 2003).

(MR) In an RCT, 339 bone marrow transplant patients with a tunneled (group A, 230 patients) or a nontunneled central venous catheter (group B, 169 patients) received a dressing change using a transparent dressing every 5 or 10 days (group A) or every 2 or 5 days (group B). Patients in both groups who received central venous catheter dressing changes at the longer interval did not show a significant increase in the rate of local infections, whereas those who received a dressing change every 2 days had a significant increase in local skin toxicity (Rasero et al., 2000).

Additional research: O'Grady et al., 2002; INS, 2006.

■ (SP) *Replace the catheter site dressing if it becomes damp, loosened, or soiled or when inspection of the site is necessary.* **LOE = VII**

(EO) The risk for infection or catheter dislodgement is increased when the catheter site dressing is not intact or is compromised (Gorski & Czaplewski, 2004).

■ (SP) *Routinely flush intermittently used PICCs and midline catheters to maintain patency; flush a PICC with an open-ended distal tip with a low concentration of heparin to maintain patency; flush a PICC with a built-in antireflux valve with saline.* **LOE = VI**

(NR) A process improvement study was undertaken to improve the occlusion rate with central venous catheters. Creative nursing education, user-friendly order sets, and eventually changing technology to a positive-pressure valve including daily heparin flush orders for PICCs resulted in a reduction of declotting interventions from about 8% to 3% over a 2-year period (Feehery et al., 2003).

(NR) A retrospective descriptive study of PICC placements ($N > 12,500$ PICCs) found a significant reduction in the incidence of PICC occlusions and infections when a PICC with proximal valve technology (PASV) with saline-only flushing was implemented (Burns, 2005).

(EO) The minimum volume of the flush solution should be equal to at least twice the volume capacity of the catheter and any add-on devices (e.g., extension tubing) (INS, 2006).

(EO) The concentration of heparin should not be in amounts that cause systemic anticoagulation; heparin should be in the lowest possible concentration to maintain patency (INS, 2006).

(MR) In three cases described in a report, heparin-induced thrombocytopenia, although rare, could result from heparin flushes of central venous access devices (Kadidal et al., 1999).

(EO) Flush an intermittently used PICC that has an integral three-position valve with saline at intervals according to the manufacturer's directions (INS, 2006; Bard Access Systems, 2006; Boston Scientific, 2005).

NR = Nursing Research, **MR** = Multidisciplinary Research, **SP** = Standard of Practice, **EO** = Expert Opinion, **LOE** = Level of Evidence

■ (SP) *Use a 10-mL or larger size syringe to reduce excessive force with flushing.* **LOE = VII**

(EO) To prevent catheter damage, the size of the syringe used for flushing should be in accordance with the catheter manufacturer's directions (INS, 2006).

(EO) Excessive force when flushing the catheter can result in catheter damage including catheter fracture (Bowe-Geddes & Nichols, 2005; Gorski & Czaplewski, 2004).

■ *Use a catheter cap/valve with positive-pressure technology.* **LOE = II**

■ (EO) *Use a positive-pressure flushing technique to reduce the risk of blood reflux into the catheter and the risk of catheter occlusion.* **LOE = VII**

(NR) A randomized study ($N = 302$) comparing two positive-pressure cap/valves (CLC2000, PASV) with a standard cap/valve (CLAVE) found a significant reduction in PICC occlusions with use of the positive-pressure valves. Although both positive-pressure caps were approved for saline-only flushing, heparin was used to flush the PICCs to eliminate saline-only flushing as a variable (Buehrle, 2004).

(EO) Flushing using a positive-pressure technique such as clamping the catheter while maintaining pressure on the syringe plunger minimizes reflux of blood into the distal tip of the catheter and reduces risk of catheter occlusion (INS, 2006; Gorski & Czaplewski, 2004).

Possibly Effective

■ *Flush the PICC with saline only when a positive-pressure cap/valve is used because this type of valve reduces blood reflux into the distal catheter tip.* **LOE = VI**

(MR) A two-phase sequential study including use of a standard catheter cap with a heparin flush in phase one and a positive-pressure cap (CLC2000) with a saline flush in phase two ($N = 312$ catheter lumens) found a significant reduction in the rate of complete central venous catheter occlusion in the positive-pressure cap/saline flush group. There were no significant differences between the two groups in partial occlusions or catheter-related bloodstream infections (Jacobs et al., 2004).

(NR) A quality improvement study undertaken at an acute care hospital found a decrease in the incidence of occlusion using a saline-only flush when a positive-pressure valve (CLC 2000) was implemented (Lenhart, 2001).

Not Effective

No applicable published research was found in this category.

Possibly Harmful

■ *Placing a PICC or midline catheter in a patient with chronic or impending renal failure; this may prevent the ability to construct an arteriovenous fistula, which is the preferred access for hemodialysis.* **LOE = V**

(MR) A retrospective analysis of PICCs ($N = 354$) found an overall thrombosis rate of 38% with no significant differences noted in the rates of thrombosis by age, sex, or catheter size.

RCT = Randomized Controlled (Clinical) Trial, **NIC** = Nursing Interventions Classification, **NOC** = Nursing Outcomes Classification

Because of the relatively high rate of venous thrombosis associated with PICCs, an alternative mode of access should be considered in current or potential hemodialysis patients (Allen et al., 2000).

(MR) A prospective study to investigate the incidence of venous thrombosis ($N = 26$) in the upper limbs of patients who had PICCs inserted found venous thrombosis in 38.5% of the patients and concluded that PICCs were associated with a significant risk of upper extremity deep vein thrombosis (Abdullah et al., 2005).

(EO) There is increased risk of venous thrombosis with peripherally placed catheters that may cause vessel damage; preservation of these veins by avoiding peripheral catheter placement increases the ability to create an arteriovenous fistula, the preferred vascular access for hemodialysis (Saad & Vesely, 2003; INS, 2006).

(EO) Instruct hospital staff, patients with progressive kidney disease (serum creatinine >3 mg/dL), and all patients with conditions that are likely to lead to end-stage renal disease to protect the arms from venipuncture and intravenous catheters (NKF/KDOQI, 2000).

■ **(SP)** *Placing a PICC or midline catheter in the arm of a patient who has undergone breast surgery requiring axillary node dissection or who has an existing fistula or graft.* **LOE = VII**

(EO) Altered venous and lymphatic circulation can cause or exacerbate edema or increase risk for infection (INS, 2006; Lubelchek & Weinstein, 2006).

■ **(SP)** *Advancing a PICC or midline catheter.* **LOE = VII**

(EO) The risk for infection or phlebitis is increased if the catheter is advanced back into the insertion site. Any changes in the length of catheter extruding from the site require radiographic confirmation for distal tip location (INS, 2006; Gorski & Czaplewski, 2004).

OUTCOME MEASUREMENT

PICC CATHETER FREE OF COMPLICATIONS

Definition: PICC catheter free of complications of clotting, infection, leakage, and swelling of involved extremity.

PICC Catheter Free of Complications as evidenced by the following indicators:
- Catheter site condition
- Skin around catheter insertion
- Swelling around catheter site
- Swelling in involved extremity
- Drainage around catheter site
- WBC count
- Temperature

(Rate each indicator of **PICC Catheter Free of Complications:** 1 = severely compromised, 2 = substantially compromised, 3 = moderately compromised, 4 = mildly compromised, 5 = not compromised.) (Note: This is not a NOC outcome.)

NR = Nursing Research, **MR** = Multidisciplinary Research, **SP** = Standard of Practice, **EO** = Expert Opinion, **LOE** = Level of Evidence

REFERENCES

Abdullah BJ, Mohammad N, Sangkar JV, Abd Aziz YF, Gan GG, Goh KY, et al. (2005). Incidence of upper limb venous thrombosis associated with peripherally inserted central catheters (PICC). *Br J Radiol,* 78(931):596-600.

Allen AW, Megargell JL, Brown DB, Lynch FC, Singh H, Singh Y, et al. (2000). Venous thrombosis associated with the placement of peripherally inserted central catheters. *J Vasc Interv Radiol,* 11(10): 1309-1314.

Anstett M, Royer TI. (2003). The impact of ultrasound on PICC placement. *J Assoc Vasc Access,* 8(3): 24-28.

Bard Access Systems. (2006). *Frequently asked questions regarding Bard catheters & ports.* Available online: http://www.bardaccess.com. Retrieved on June 4, 2007.

Boston Scientific. (2005). *Vaxcel® PICC with PASV® Valve Technology.* Available online: http://www. bostonscientific.com. Retrieved on June 4, 2007.

Bowe-Geddes LA, Nichols HA. (2005). An overview of peripherally inserted central catheters. *Top Adv Pract Nurs,* 5(3). Available online: http://www.medscape.com/nursingejournal. Retrieved on June 4, 2007.

Buehrle DC. (2004). A prospective, randomized comparison of three needleless IV systems used in conjunction with peripherally inserted central catheters. *J Assoc Vasc Access,* 9(1):35-38.

Burns D. (2005). The Vanderbilt PICC Service: Program, procedural, and patient outcomes successes. *J Assoc Vasc Access,* 10(4):183-192.

Chaiyakunapruk N, Veenstra DL, Lipsky BA, Saint S. (2002). Chlorhexidine compared with povidone-iodine solution for vascular catheter-site care: A meta-analysis. *Ann Intern Med,* 136(11):792-801.

Dochterman JM, Bulechek GM (Eds). (2004). *Nursing Interventions Classification (NIC),* 4th ed. St. Louis: Mosby.

Feehery PA, Allen S, Bey J. (2003). Flushing 101: Using a FOCUS-PDCA quality improvement model to reduce catheter occlusions with standardized protocols. *J Assoc Vasc Access,* 8(2):38-45.

Frey AM, Schears GJ. (2006). Why are we stuck on tape and suture? A review of catheter securement devices. *J Infus Nurs,* 29(1):34-38.

Fry C, Aholt D. (2001). Local anesthesia prior to the insertion of peripherally inserted central catheters. *J Infus Nurs,* 24(6):404-408.

Funk D, Gray J, Plourde PJ. (2001). Two-year trends of peripherally inserted central catheter-line complications at a tertiary-care hospital: Role of nursing expertise. *Infec Control Hosp Epidemiol,* 22(6): 377-379.

Gillies D, O'Riordan L, Carr D, Frost J, Gunning R, O'Brien I. (2003). Gauze and tape and transparent polyurethane dressings for central venous catheters. *Cochrane Database Syst Rev,* (4):CD003827.

Gorski LA, Czaplewski L. (2004). Peripherally inserted central & midline catheters for the home care nurse. *Home Healthc Nurse,* 22(11):758-771.

Hu KK, Lipsky BA, Veenstra DL, Saint S. (2004). Using maximal sterile barriers to prevent central venous catheter-related infection: A systematic evidence-based review. *Am J Infect Control,* 32(3):142-146.

Infusion Nurses Society (INS). (2006). Infusion Nursing Standards of Practice. *J Infus Nurs,* 29(1 Suppl): S1-S92.

Institute for Healthcare Improvement (IHI). (2006a). *Implement the central line bundle.* Available online: http://www.ihi.org/ihi. Retrieved on June 4, 2007.

Institute for Healthcare Improvement (IHI). (2006b). Pursuing perfection: Report from HealthPartners' regions hospital on reducing hospital-acquired infection: Ventilator-associated pneumonia and catheter-related bloodstream infection. Available online: http://www.ihi.org/ihi. Retrieved on June 4, 2007.

Jacobs BR, Schilling S, Doellman D, et al. (2004). Central venous catheter occlusion: A prospective, controlled trial examining the impact of a positive-pressure valve device. *JPEN J Parenter Enteral Nutr,* 28(2):113-118.

Kadidal VV, Mayo DJ, Horne MK. (1999). Heparin-induced thrombocytopenia (HIT) due to heparin flushes: A report of three cases. *J Intern Med,* 246(3):325-329.

Kearns PJ, Coleman S, Wehner JH. (1996). Complications of long arm-catheters: A randomized trial of central vs peripheral tip location. *JPEN J Parenter Enteral Nutr,* 20(1):20-24.

LaRue GD. (2000). Efficacy of ultrasonography in peripheral venous cannulation. *J Infus Nurs,* 23(1): 29-34.

Lenhart C. (2001). Preventing central venous access device occlusions with saline only flush by use of an adapter. *J Vasc Access Devices,* 6(2):29-31.

Loughran SC, Borzatta M. (1995). Peripherally inserted central catheters: A report of 2506 catheter days. *J Parenter Enteral Nutr,* 19(2):133-136.

Lubelchek RJ, Weinstein RA. (2006). Strategies for preventing catheter-related bloodstream infections: the role of new technologies. *Crit Care Med,* 34(3):905-907.

McMahon DD. (2002). Evaluating new technology to improve patient outcomes: A quality improvement approach. *J Infus Nurs,* 25(4):250-255.

National Association of Vascular Access Networks (NAVAN). (1998). Tip location of peripherally inserted central catheters. *J Vasc Access Devices,* 3(2):8-10.

National Kidney Foundation/Kidney Disease Outcomes Quality Initiative (NKF/KDOQI). (2000). *Guidelines for vascular access.* Available online: http://www.kidney.org/professionals/KDOQI/. Retrieved on June 4, 2007.

O'Grady NP, Alexander M, Dellinger EP, Gerberding JL, Heard SO, Maki DG, et al. (2002). Guidelines for the prevention of intravascular catheter-related infections. Centers for Disease Control and Prevention. *MMWR Recomm Rep,* 51(RR-10):1-29.

Rasero L, Degl'Innocenti M, Mocali M, Alberani F, Boschi S, Giraudi A, et al. (2000). Comparison of two different protocols on change of medication in central venous catheterization in patients with bone marrow transplantation: Results of a randomized multicenter study. *Assist Inferm Ric,* 19(2):112-119.

Robinson MK, Mogensen KM, Grudinskas GF, Kohler S, Jacobs DO. (2005). Improved care and reduced costs for patients requiring peripherally inserted central catheters: The role of bedside ultrasound and a dedicated team. *J Parenter Enteral Nutr,* 29(5):374-379.

Rothschild JM. (2001). Ultrasound guidance of central vein catheterization. In *Making Health Care Safer: A Critical Analysis of Patient Safety Practices.* Evidence Report/Technology Assessment: Number 43. AHRQ Publication No. 01-E058, July 2001. Agency for Healthcare Research and Quality, Rockville, MD. Available online: http://www.ahrq.gov. Retrieved on June 4, 2007.

Saad TF, Vesely TM. (2003). Venous access for patients with chronic renal failure or end-stage renal disease: What is the role for peripherally inserted central catheters? *J Assoc Vasc Access,* 8(4):27-32.

Shojania KG, Duncan BW, McDonald KM, Wachter RM, Markowitz AJ. (2001). Making health care safer: A critical analysis of patient safety practices. *Evid Rep Techno Assess,* 43:i-x, 1-668.

Yamamoto AJ, Solomon JA, Soulen MC, Tang J, Parkinson K, Lin R, et al. (2002). Sutureless securement device reduces complications of peripherally inserted central venous catheters. *J Vasc Interv Radiol,* 13(1):77-81.

POSITIONING

NIC

Deborah Gavin-Dreschnack, PhD; Lee Barks, PhD, ARNP, CDDN

NIC **Definition:** Deliberative placement of the patient or a body part to promote physiological and/or psychological well-being (Dochterman & Bulechek, 2004).

NURSING ACTIVITIES

Effective

■ SP *Use continuous lateral rotation therapy (continuous rotation around long axis with the patient in a horizontal supine, prone, or side-lying position) to improve oxygenation and resolve pneumonia and acute respiratory distress syndrome.* **LOE = III**

NR = Nursing Research, **MR** = Multidisciplinary Research, **SP** = Standard of Practice, **EO** = Expert Opinion, **LOE** = Level of Evidence

(MR) A controlled trial ($N = 70$) demonstrated increased oxygenation and decreased incidence of ventilator-associated pneumonia in ICU patients who received continuous lateral rotation therapy (Wang et al., 2003).

(MR) A controlled trial ($N = 37$) found that use of continuous lateral rotation therapy resulted in decreased incidence of pneumonia in critically ill patients (Kirschenbaum et al., 2002).

■ (SP) *Use upright positioning with coughing and huffing to improve maximal expiratory pressure and peak expiratory flow rate (preferable to head-down positioning).* **LOE = III**

(MR) A controlled study ($N = 36$) measuring the maximal expiratory pressure and flow in both normal patients and patients with chronic obstructive pulmonary disease demonstrated that sitting upright increased peak expiratory flow rate (Badr et al., 2002).

■ (SP) *For patients with raised intracranial pressure, cautiously use 30-degree head-up position, avoid extreme hip flexion for prolonged periods, and avoid undue neck flexion, rotation, and/or extension.* **LOE = V**

(NR) A systematic review of research concerning positioning of patients with raised intracranial pressure recommended use of the head-up position, based on intracranial pressure readings, and avoidance of hip flexion, neck flexion, and rotation/extension (Fan, 2004; Grap & Munro, 2004; McLean, 2001).

■ (SP) *For children with neurogenic disorders and swallowing problems, position the head in a chin tuck where the head is in midline with the trunk in upright alignment and the neck flexed, so that the chin is directed slightly downward and inward.* **LOE = V**

(NR) A review of the literature on postural control for feeding recommended the chin tuck position to facilitate swallowing (Redstone & West, 2004).

■ (SP) *Use a consistent practice method of logrolling in the different patients' care settings.* **LOE = VII**

(EO) A multidisciplinary group of health care providers who developed regional policies and procedures for logrolling methods and staff unanimously chose the lifting sheet method of turning, stating that it was easier and more comfortable (Groeneveld et al., 2001).

■ *Proactively manage pain by encouraging regular analgesics, promotion of hot packs, and regular position changes in the immediate postoperative period to decrease low back pain following transurethral resection of the prostate (TURP) in the lithotomy position. This approach is preferable to using a sacral wedge intraoperatively.* **LOE = II**

(NR) An RCT of males ($N = 236$) undergoing TURP using a sacral wedge found that the incidence and severity of back pain increased after surgery in 28% of patients. There was no evidence to support positioning with a sacral wedge intraoperatively to reduce incidence of postoperative back pain (Pietrocola et al., 2004).

RCT = Randomized Controlled (Clinical) Trial, **NIC** = Nursing Interventions Classification, **NOC** = Nursing Outcomes Classification

Possibly Effective

■ *Position patients with acute unilateral lung pathology in the lateral position with the sick lung uppermost.* **LOE = V**

(NR) Review and analysis of the literature demonstrated the beneficial effect (i.e., improving suboptimal ventilation/perfusion V/Q relationships) of lateral positioning on oxygenation in acute unilateral lung disease (Moore, 2002).

■ *Position seated patients with back support but no neck support.* **LOE = IV**

(NR) A controlled crossover design study ($N = 7$) demonstrated that sitting in a position with back support but no neck support increased the function of the autonomic nervous system more than sitting in a position with both back and neck support. This increase in sympathetic nerve function enhanced blood flow to heart, skeletal muscles, and brain and promoted increased supply of oxygen to cells (Okubo & Hishinuma, 2005).

■ *Use continuous lateral rotation therapy (continuous rotation around long axis with the patient in a horizontal supine, prone, or side-lying position) as an adjunct to good wound care practices in managing partial-thickness (superficial, stage I or II) and full-thickness (stage III or IV) wounds.* **LOE = VI**

(MR) A descriptive study of the rate of wound healing ($N = 30$) demonstrated that continuous lateral rotation therapy delivered in a 40-degree arc to the selected undiluted population of home care and long-term care patients appeared to assist in closing of pressure ulcers with results comparable to those with low-air-loss mattresses and outcomes of larger studies (Anderson & Rappl, 2004).

■ *Use prone positioning as a trial for patients with acute respiratory distress syndrome (ARDS) in the early course of the disease.* **LOE = I**

(NR) A systematic review of the literature on prone positioning showed that 70% of all patients studied who had ARDS responded to prone positioning, with a 20% increase in Pao_2 or an increase in Pao_2/FiO_2 (P/F) ratio greater than 20 within 2 hours of the turn (Essat, 2005; Voggenreiter et al., 2005; Vollman, 2004; Relvas et al., 2003; Beuret et al., 2002).

Not Effective

■ *Use of thoracopelvic supports during prone positioning in patients with acute lung injury/ARDS.* **LOE = II**

(NR) An RCT ($N = 11$) showed that application of thoracopelvic supports decreased chest wall compliance, increased pleural pressure, and caused a slight deterioration in hemodynamics without any advantage in gas exchange (Chiumello et al., 2006).

■ *Having the patient recline to relieve pressure on ischial tuberosities.* **LOE = III**

(MR) A controlled trial without randomization ($N = 10$ with spinal cord injury) found no effective reduction in pressure on ischial tuberosities (Henderson et al., 1994).

NR = Nursing Research, **MR** = Multidisciplinary Research, **SP** = Standard of Practice, **EO** = Expert Opinion, **LOE** = Level of Evidence

■ *Positioning the patient in an upright posture (defined in study as 30 degrees from supine/horizontal posture) after a coronary artery bypass graft (CABG) procedure.* **LOE = II**

> **MR** In an RCT ($N = 16$) measuring the effect of positioning on selected hemodynamic parameters following a CABG procedure, there was no effect of the study position (30 degrees from supine/horizontal) at 1 hour after the procedure (Belcher, 1991).

Possibly Harmful

No applicable published research was found in this category.

OUTCOME MEASUREMENT

MOBILITY   **NOC**

> (Please refer to *Nursing Outcomes Classification* [Moorhead et al., 2004] for the **Mobility** outcome.)

REFERENCES

Anderson C, Rappl L. (2004). Lateral rotation mattresses for wound healing. *Ostomy Wound Manage*, 50(4):50-54, 56, 58.

Badr C, Elkins MR, Ellis ER. (2002). The effect of body position on maximal expiratory pressure and flow. *Aust J Physiother*, 48(2):95-102.

Belcher R. (1991). *Effects of upright posturing on selected physiologic parameters at twenty-four hours post coronary artery bypass surgery*. A dissertation submitted to the Graduate School of the University of Southern Mississippi in partial fulfillment of the requirements for the degree of Doctor of Philosophy. University of Southern Mississippi, Hattiesburg, Mississippi, 1991.

Beuret P, Carton M, Nourdine K, Kaaki M, Tramoni G, Ducreux J. (2002). Prone position as prevention of lung injury in comatose patients: A prospective, randomized, controlled study. *Intensive Care Med*, 28(5):564-569.

Chiumello D, Cressoni M, Racagni M, Landi L, Li Bassi G, Polli F, et al. (2006). Effects of thoraco-pelvic supports during prone position in patients with acute lung injury/acute respiratory distress syndrome: A physiological study. *Crit Care*, 10(3):R87.

Dochterman JM, Bulechek GM (Eds). (2004). *Nursing Interventions Classification (NIC)*, 4th ed. St. Louis: Mosby.

Essat Z. (2005). Prone positioning in patients with acute respiratory distress syndrome. *Nurs Stand*, 20(9):52-55.

Fan JY. (2004). Effect of backrest position on intracranial pressure and cerebral perfusion pressure in individuals with brain injury: A systematic review. *J Neurosci Nurs*, 36(5):278-288.

Grap MJ, Munro CL, Elswick RK Jr, et al. (2004). Duration of action of a single, early oral application of chlorhexidine on oral microbial flora in mechanically ventilated patients: A point study. *Heart Lung*, 33(2):83-91.

Groeneveld A, McKenzie ML, Williams D. (2001). Logrolling: Establishing consistent practice. *Orthop Nurs*, 20(2):45-49.

Henderson JL, Price SH, Brandstater ME, Mandac BR. (1994). Efficacy of three measures to relieve pressure in seated persons with spinal cord injury. *Arch Phys Med Rehabil*, 75(5):535-539.

Kirschenbaum L, Azzi E, Sfeir T, Tietjen P, Astiz M. (2002). Effect of continuous lateral rotational therapy on the prevalence of ventilator-associated pneumonia in patients requiring long-term ventilatory care. *Crit Care Med*, 30(9):1983-1986.

McLean C. (2001). Moving and positioning patients with altered intracranial haemodynamics. *Nurs Crit Care*, 6(5):239-244.

Moore T. (2002). The effect of lateral positioning on oxygenation in acute unilateral lung disease. *Nurs Crit Care,* 7(6):278-282.

Moorhead M, Johnson M, Maas M (Eds). (2004). *Nursing Outcomes Classification (NOC),* 3rd ed. St. Louis: Mosby.

Okubo N, Hishinuma M. (2005). Effects of aided and unaided support of the neck while sitting (with back support), on autonomic nervous system activities. *Japan J Nurs Sci,* 2(1):33-39.

Pietrocola P, Riley RG, Beanland CJ, Kelly C, Radnell J. (2004). A randomized controlled trial to measure the effectiveness of a sacral wedge in preventing postoperative back pain following trans-urethral resection of the prostate (TURP) in lithotomy position. *J Clin Nurs,* 13(8):977-985.

Redstone F, West JF. (2004). The importance of postural control for feeding. *Pediatr Nurs,* 30(2):97-100.

Relvas MS, Silver PC, Sagy M. (2003). Prone positioning of pediatric patients with ARDS results in improvement in oxygenation if maintained >12 h daily. *Chest,* 124(1):269-274.

Voggenreiter G, Aufmkolk M, Stiletto R, Baacke M, Waydhas C, Ose C, et al. (2005). Prone positioning improves oxygenation in post-traumatic lung injury—A prospective randomized trial. *J Trauma,* 59(2):333-341.

Vollman KM. (2004). Prone positioning in the patient who has acute respiratory distress syndrome: The art and science. *Crit Care Nurs Clin North Am,* 16(3):319-336, viii.

Wang JY, Chuang PY, Lin CJ, Yu CJ, Yang PC. (2003). Continuous lateral rotational therapy in the medical intensive care unit. *J Formos Med Assoc,* 102(11):788-792.

POSITIONING: WHEELCHAIR   NIC

Deborah Gavin-Dreschnack, PhD; Lee Barks, PhD, ARNP, CDDN

NIC **Definition:** Placement of a patient in a properly selected wheelchair to enhance comfort, promote skin integrity, and foster independence (Dochterman & Bulechek, 2004).

NURSING ACTIVITIES

Effective

■ *Refer to therapy or a seating specialist for an individualized fitting of an appropriate wheelchair and seating components (including pressure-relieving cushions) for individuals who use a wheelchair as their primary means of mobility.* **LOE = I**

 An RCT evaluating the use of individually prescribed wheelchairs versus standard regularly assigned wheelchairs in elderly nursing home residents (*N* = 24) demonstrated that all subjects benefited from receiving an individually prescribed wheelchair in one or more ways (i.e., able to propel their wheelchairs better and faster, increased forward reach, increased quality of life, and increased satisfaction with assistive technology) (Trefler et al., 2004).

 An analysis of the effects of an individualized wheelchair seating intervention on wheelchair users (*N* = 38) confirmed the possibility of reducing or eliminating common problems such as back pain and discomfort (Samuelsson et al., 2001).

 An intervention study demonstrated the benefits of individualized wheelchair seating for improved posture and function in frail older adults residing in a long-term care setting (Rader et al., 2000).

 An analysis of data from an RCT indicated that higher interface pressure was associated with a higher incidence of sitting-acquired pressure ulcers for high-risk elderly persons (Brienza et al., 2001).

(MR) An RCT ($N = 32$) showed that segmented foam cushions were more likely to produce pressure ulcers than pressure-reducing cushions (Geyer et al., 2001).

■ *Follow a safe sequence of repositioning a patient in a wheelchair or dependency chair at defined intervals for comfort and prevention of skin breakdown.* **LOE = II**

(NR) A systematic review of the existing evidence for positioning with an algorithm for safe nursing practice showed effective repositioning techniques (Nelson et al., 2003).

■ (SP) *Assess posture in the patient's designated wheelchair.* **LOE = III**

(MR) A controlled trial without randomization showed that any level of nursing staff could perform a simple but reliable assessment of patients' posture when seated in a wheelchair using the Resident Ergonomic Assessment Profile for Seating (Gavin-Dreschnack et al., 2005).

■ (SP) *Monitor the skin of seated patients to prevent breakdown by checking pressure points on the elbow, sacrum, coccyx, ischial tuberosities, and heels and by ensuring full contact of thighs with the seat, with lack of pressure on the fibular head.* **LOE = VII**

(EO) Monitoring the skin of wheelchair-seated patients is a safe nursing care practice (Jacobs, 1994).

Possibly Effective

■ *Use the wheelbarrow technique (in which the push handles are used to lift the locked rear wheels off the floor) versus conventional technique (bending to release and apply wheel locks) to move empty wheelchairs short distances.* **LOE = III**

(MR) A within-subject controlled study demonstrated that the wheelbarrow technique was a superior method of moving an empty wheelchair short distances (Woolfrey & Kirby, 1998).

■ *Reposition a slumped person upward in a wheelchair by using a two-person horizontally assisted lift (HAL) technique (where one person lifts upward from behind the patient holding the patient under the armpits and the second person pushes the patient's legs toward the back of wheelchair) or a one-person transfer technique.* **LOE = II**

(MR) A controlled study ($N = 16$) with randomized order of three lifting interventions (unassisted lift, two-person vertically assisted lift [VAL], and HAL), showed that use of HAL was better than the two-person technique, providing the least amount of force on caregivers' spines, and the unassisted lift was safer than VAL. A fourth technique, the mechanical lift, was not tested (Varcin-Coad & Barrett, 1998).

■ *Observe while positioning the patient in a wheelchair to provide deformity prevention, independence, alignment, symmetry around the midline, and base of support.* **LOE = VII**

(EO) Interdisciplinary training materials recommend these clinical guidelines (Gerber et al., 1991).

RCT = Randomized Controlled (Clinical) Trial, **NIC** = Nursing Interventions Classification, **NOC** = Nursing Outcomes Classification

■ *Position hips and trunk first (proximally) and then position extremities (distally).*
LOE = VII

(EO) It is an interdisciplinary clinical practice axiom of physical therapists to stabilize posture proximally, then distally (Knott & Voss, 1968).

■ *Position the patient in a wheelchair with (sagittal view) the center of head, arm, and trunk over ischial tuberosities and buttocks touching the chair back.*
LOE = VII

(EO) This is proper positioning for good alignment (Zacharkow, 1988).

■ *Position the patient in a wheelchair with a comfortable, symmetrical midline posture: the head in midline, trunk erect, hips flexed to 90 to 105 degrees, knees flexed at 90 to 100 degrees, feet neutral, spine stable, and pelvis level.*
LOE = VII

(EO) Clinical guidelines recommend this as proper positioning for good alignment (Braddon, 2000).

■ *Relieve pressure in long-sitters by eliciting patients to lean forward, chest to thighs, with pressure off ischial tuberosities.* **LOE = IV**

(MR) A controlled trial without randomization ($N = 10$) compared three methods of pressure relief in patients with spinal cord injury. The greatest pressure relief over the ischial tuberosities was found in the forward-leaning position. There was significant pressure relief with the 65-degree backward tip, but only a small drop in ischial pressure was observed with a backward tip of 35 degrees (Henderson et al., 1994).

(MR) A case-control study ($N = 30$) showed the effect of leaning forward on interface pressure in children with myelomeningocele, which was less than the neutral position (Vaisbuch et al., 2000).

■ *Position the patient for activity and interaction with the environment with the neck at 11 to 27 degrees of flexion with eyes looking straight ahead.*
LOE = III

(MR) A controlled trial of wheelchair users ($N = 20$) demonstrated that the most comfortable position was with the neck slightly flexed, about 11 degrees and 27 degrees more flexed, respectively, than when looking at an average-height sitting or standing person (Kirby et al., 2004).

(EO) Adequate seating with appropriate neck flexion affects visual orientation and tracking (Padula, 1989).

Not Effective

■ *Reclining the patient to relieve pressure on ischial tuberosities.* **LOE = III**

(MR) A controlled trial without randomization ($N = 10$ with spinal cord injury) found no effective reduction in pressure on ischial tuberosities with patients in a reclined position of 35 degrees (Henderson et al., 1994).

NR = Nursing Research, **MR** = Multidisciplinary Research, **SP** = Standard of Practice, **EO** = Expert Opinion, **LOE** = Level of Evidence

Possibly Harmful

■ *Positioning using towels, linens, or bandages to "tie the person into the chair" and support posture in the wheelchair.* **LOE = V**

(NR) A systematic review told of the dangers of these measures, including entrapment, as risks in positioning using restraints (Nelson et al., 2004).

■ *Use of the vertically assisted lift to lift the patient up in the wheelchair.* **LOE = III**

(MR) A controlled study (*N* = 16) with randomized order of three lifting interventions (unassisted lift, two-person VAL, and HAL) showed that use of HAL was better than the two-person technique, providing the least amount of force on caregivers' spines, and the unassisted lift was safer than VAL. A fourth technique, the mechanical lift, was not tested (Varcin-Coad & Barrett, 1998).

MEASUREMENT OUTCOME

WHEELCHAIR POSITIONING

Definition: Correct positioning and care in a wheelchair to increase comfort, protect from harm, and promote ease of use.

Wheelchair Positioning as evidenced by the following indicators:
• Sits upright in midline position
• Free of pressure ulcers
• Wheelchair fitted well to body
• Appropriate cushioning used to protect skin
(Note: This is not a NOC outcome.)

REFERENCES

Braddon R. (2000). *Physical medicine and rehabilitation,* 2nd ed. Philadelphia: Saunders, p 387.

Brienza DM, Karg PE, Geyer MJ, Kelsey S, Trefler E. (2001). The relationship between pressure ulcer incidence and buttock-seat cushion interface pressure in at-risk elderly wheelchair users. *Arch Phys Med Rehabil,* 82(4):529-533.

Dochterman JM, Bulechek GM (Eds). (2004). *Nursing Interventions Classification (NIC),* 4th ed. St. Louis: Mosby.

Gavin-Dreschnack D, Schonfeld L, Nelson A, Luther S. (2005). Development of a screening tool for safe wheelchair seating. Agency for Healthcare Research and Quality. *Adv Patient Safety,* 4:127-137.

Gerber D, McAllister S, Tencza K. (1991). *Challenges in physical management.* Training program produced for the Oklahoma Department of Human Services by Therapeutic Concepts, Inc., Winter Park, FL (out of print).

Geyer MJ, Brienza DM, Karg P, Trefler E, Kelsey S. (2001). A randomized control trial to evaluate pressure-reducing seat cushions for elderly wheelchair users. *Adv Skin Wound Care,* 14(3):120-129.

Henderson JL, Price SH, Brandstater ME, Mandac BR. (1994). Efficacy of three measures to relieve pressure in seated persons with spinal cord injury. *Arch Phys Med Rehabil,* 75(5):535-539.

Jacobs BW. (1994). Working on the right moves. *Nursing,* 24(11):52-54.

Kirby RL, Fahie CL, Smith C, et al. (2004). Neck discomfort of wheelchair users: Effect of neck position. *Disabil Rehabil,* 26(1):9-15.

Knott M, Voss D. (1968). *Proprioceptive neuromuscular facilitation,* 2nd ed. Philadelphia: Harper & Row, pp 111-116.

Nelson A, Lloyd JD, Menzel N, Gross C. (2003). Preventing nursing back injuries: Redesigning patient handling tasks. *AAOHN J,* 51(3):126-134.

Nelson A, Powell-Cope G, Gavin-Dreschnack D, Quigley P, Bulat T, Baptiste AS, et al. (2004). Technology to promote safe mobility in the elderly. *Nurs Clin North Am,* 39(3):649-671.

Padula W. (1989). *Post trauma vision syndrome affecting seating posture.* Proceedings of the 5th International Seating Symposium. Memphis, TN, February 1989.

Rader J, Jones D, Miller L. (2000). The importance of individualized wheelchair seating for frail older adults. *J Gerontol Nurs,* 26(11):24-32.

Samuelsson K, Larsson H, Thyberg M, Girdle B. (2001). Wheelchair seating intervention. Results from a client-centred approach. *Disabil Rehabil,* 23(15):677-682.

Trefler E, Fitzgerald SG, Hobson DA, Bursick T, Joseph R. (2004). Outcomes of wheelchair systems intervention with residents of long-term care facilities. *Assist Technol,* 16(1):18-27.

Vaisbuch N, Meyer S, Weiss PL. (2000). Effect of seated posture on interface pressure in children who are able-bodied and who have myelomeningocele. *Disabil Rehabil,* 22(17):749-755.

Varcin-Coad L, Barrett R. (1998). Repositioning a slumped person in a wheelchair. A biomechanical analysis of three transfer techniques. *AAOHN J,* 46(11):530-536.

Woolfrey PG, Kirby RL. (1998). Ergonomics in rehabilitation: a comparison of two methods of moving an empty manual wheelchair short distances. *Arch Phys Med Rehabil,* 79(8):955-958.

Zacharkow D. (1988). *Posture: Sitting, standing, chair design and exercise.* Springfield, IL: Charles C Thomas.

 # POSTMORTEM CARE

Tracy A. Szirony, PhD, RN-C, CHPN

NIC **Definition:** Providing physical care of the body of an expired patient and support for the family viewing the body (Dochterman & Bulechek, 2004).

NURSING ACTIVITIES

Effective

■ **SP** *Follow agency policy for postmortem care.* **LOE = VII**

EO Professional nursing staff provide assistance in postmortem care when nursing assistants or other unlicensed personnel have been delegated to perform this task. The majority of unlicensed personnel have minimal training or experience performing postmortem care. This lack of knowledge and experience can lead to unnecessary stress on the unlicensed caregiver as well as the deceased's family (Confidentially, *Nursing,* 2000).

■ **SP** *Prepare the body with respect and dignity to the deceased.* **LOE = VII**

EO Family members can begin the grieving process in an appropriate manner when their loved one is treated with respect, as this communicates continued care and concern on the part of the nurse (Sewell, 2002).

■ **SP** *Consider religious and cultural practices of the deceased and the family.* **LOE = VII**

EO These practices can assist in the initial process of grief and bereavement (Kuebler et al., 2002).

NR = Nursing Research, **MR** = Multidisciplinary Research, **SP** = Standard of Practice, **EO** = Expert Opinion, **LOE** = Level of Evidence

■ (SP) *Remove all tubes unless an autopsy will be performed.* **LOE = VII**

(EO) All tubes must be left in place, as the goal of the autopsy is to determine the cause of death (Berry & Griffie, 2006).

■ (SP) *Cleanse the body if the body is soiled and comb the hair.* **LOE = VII**

(EO) These interventions may enhance the family viewing process and initial grief reactions (Potter & Perry, 2005).

■ (SP) *Replace any soiled or odorous wound dressings with clean ones.* **LOE = VII**

(EO) The presence of clean dressings enhances the family viewing process (Matzo & Sherman, 2001).

■ (NIC) (SP) *Place incontinent pad securely under buttocks and between legs.* **LOE = VII**

(EO) Incontinent pads prevent potential stool or urine from soiling the sheets (Matzo & Sherman, 2001).

■ (NIC) (SP) *Raise the head of the bed slightly to prevent pooling of fluids in head or face.* **LOE = VII**

(EO) As normal blood circulation stops after death, the skin begins to turn a reddish-purple color. This is called livor mortis and begins within 20 minutes of death. Heme molecules then begin to break down, causing further discoloration of the skin, called postmortem stain. Placing the patient in a semi-Fowler's position reduces this type of discoloration. This is important if viewing of the deceased is a request of the family, as cosmetics only cover the stain. Families often want to view the deceased in as natural a state as possible, and elevating the head of the bed or the stretcher for transfer assists in decreasing the potential for livor mortis or postmortem stain (Mayer, 2006).

■ (SP) *Be familiar with agency policy on what types of death require notification of the coroner.* **LOE = VII**

(EO) Examples of deaths that may involve a coroner's investigation include deaths that occur within 24 hours of admission to an acute care setting, a violent death, or an unnatural death (Potter & Perry, 2005).

■ (SP) *Follow agency policy if an autopsy will be performed.* **LOE = VII**

(EO) Obtain consent, prepare the body, and transport to the morgue (Sewell, 2002).

■ (SP) *Place dentures or a partial plate in a denture cup labeled with the patient's name.* **LOE = VII**

(EO) Do not put dentures back in the mouth of the deceased, as jaw muscles normally relax after death and dentures may be broken or lost in the process of the transfer to the funeral home (Kuebler et al., 2002).

■ (NIC) (SP) *Close the eyes.* **LOE = VII**

(EO) Closing the eyes makes the appearance of the body more natural to those who will be viewing the body (Kuebler et al., 2002).

RCT = Randomized Controlled (Clinical) Trial, **NIC** = Nursing Interventions Classification, **NOC** = Nursing Outcomes Classification

■ **NIC** ⓢ *Maintain proper body alignment.* **LOE = VII**

ⓔ Proper body alignment is more aesthetically pleasing and allows the mortician to complete his or her tasks in a most efficient manner (Berry & Griffie, 2006).

■ **NIC** ⓢ *Label personal belongings and place in the appropriate place.* **LOE = VII**

ⓔ Family may want to retain personal items of the deceased, depending on their value and sentiment (Potter & Perry, 2005).

■ **NIC** ⓢ *Notify clergy as requested by family.* **LOE = VII**

ⓔ Identification and implementation of families' needs related to spirituality and religion at the time of death is often a necessary component of the bereavement process (Lomas et al., 2004).

■ **NIC** ⓢ *Facilitate and support the family's viewing of the body.* **LOE = VII**

Consider the circumstance of the death as it relates to the viewing by grieving family members:
• Was the death related to an acute or traumatic event or a chronic condition?
• Was the death sudden and unexpected or expected?
• What was the age of the deceased?
• What is the relationship of the bereaved?
Be available to listen and support the family as they begin to experience the grief process.
ⓔ Effective communication at this time requires attentive listening skills. Professional nursing staff has the obligation to prepare and educate the family prior to viewing the body of the deceased (Vacarolis et al., 2006).

■ ⓢ *Prepare the room and the environment for the viewing of the deceased. Remove all equipment, unnecessary medical items, turn off monitors, and have Kleenex available.* **LOE = VII**

Creating a comfortable environment for family viewing of the deceased may assist in the facilitation of the grieving process (Marthaler, 2005).

■ ⓢ *Ensure a member of the professional nursing staff is with the family when they first view the body of their loved one.* **LOE = VII**

ⓔ Nurses have the ability to support the care of the family, ensuring that the early process of grieving can be facilitated (Kuebler et al., 2002).

■ ⓢ *Provide education to families, as a prerequisite to viewing the deceased, about what they can expect when they first view their loved one after death has occurred.* **LOE = VII**

ⓔ Efforts toward educating the family are necessary as each person present will have a different experience in the initial phase of the grieving process (Davies, 2006).

NR = Nursing Research, **MR** = Multidisciplinary Research, **SP** = Standard of Practice, **EO** = Expert Opinion, **LOE** = Level of Evidence

■ ⒮ᴾ *Consider the family's wishes related to the provision of postmortem care.*
LOE = VII

Ⓔᴼ A thorough assessment of the family's level of involvement may assist them in accepting the reality of the death. The easiest way to determine family wishes is to simply ask them how they would like to be involved. One way that families can become involved is to ask if they would like to help bathe their loved one (Pessagno, 1997).

■ ⒮ᴾ *Assess individual family members' needs to be with the deceased and be available for support while also allowing the family time alone with their loved one if they are comfortable.* **LOE = VII**

Ⓔᴼ Some people find comfort in being alone with the deceased. Assessing comfort levels of the families may allow the initial grieving process to progress in a manner that is acceptable to the family (Berry & Griffie, 2006).

■ Ⓝᴵᶜ ⒮ᴾ *Answer questions concerning organ donation.* **LOE = VII**

Ⓔᴼ Nurses can be helpful to the family by providing education and support for those who have make the decision to donate organs (Potter & Perry, 2005).

■ Ⓝᴵᶜ ⒮ᴾ *Label the body, according to policy, after the family has left.* **LOE = VII**

Note: It is not necessary to use all of the ties that you may find in a "shroud kit." The ties often do not stay in place and may actually damage the skin of the decreased.
Ⓔᴼ Proper identification is essential (Potter & Perry, 2005).

■ ⒮ᴾ *Provide support to other patients and families in the surrounding area who may be aware that a death has occurred.* **LOE = VII**

Ⓔᴼ Families of other patients may be experiencing grief reactions themselves (Vacarolis et al., 2006).

■ ⒮ᴾ *Transfer the body to the morgue after explaining the process to the family while assessing their needs for continued care of their loved one.* **LOE = VII**

Ⓔᴼ Family knowledge of the procedures after death will assist in the grieving process (Ufema, 2000).

■ Ⓝᴵᶜ ⒮ᴾ *Notify the mortician as appropriate.* **LOE = VII**

Ⓔᴼ Deaths that occur in the home, as with a hospice team, will negate the need to transport the body to a morgue. It is then up to the nurse to evaluate when the family has spent their private time with the patient and when the funeral home should be notified (Matzo & Sherman, 2001).

■ ⒮ᴾ *Document the care provided.* **LOE = VII**

Ⓔᴼ Documentation of the death is important and must be clear. Include the patient's name, date, and time of death; who was present at the time of death; any unusual circumstances or unusual findings on physical exam; all persons who were notified; and plans for disposition of the body (Berry & Griffie, 2006).
   Note: There is no current research related to postmortem care, which includes care of the body as well as care of the deceased's family members or significant others. There is a

RCT = Randomized Controlled (Clinical) Trial, **NIC** = Nursing Interventions Classification, **NOC** = Nursing Outcomes Classification

tremendous need for nurses to expand their knowledge base of needs of the family related to their involvement and understanding of postmortem care. Nursing must go beyond current published anecdotal reports of effective family involvement in postmortem care and begin focused research in the area of family needs during this most difficult time. Interventions could then be developed and further researched as their applicability to evidence-based practice. The overarching goal is to assist families and enhance the initial grieving process.

Postmortem care of the body is clearly described in textbooks of fundamental nursing. Interventions rarely deviate from one text to the next. In addition, institutional-based policies and procedures are utilized to guide nursing practice.

There is a need for nurses who provide postmortem care to gain a greater understanding of the rationale for the specific interventions that they provide during care of the patient after death. Funeral home directors are in a perfect position to share their knowledge and needs for what is essential to their role after death. If nurses have the knowledge and a greater understanding of the needs of morticians related to quality embalming, the desire of the family for the "natural look" may be better achieved.

OUTCOME MEASUREMENT

POSTMORTEM CARE

Definition: The family of the deceased feels support from the nursing staff, the body is presented in the best manner possible, and all necessary procedures are followed.
Postmortem Care as evidenced by the following indicators:
- The family is comfortable viewing the body
- The family is able to talk about the death with nursing staff
- The body is clean
- The body is positioned properly
- Valuables are taken care of appropriately
- Postmortem care is documented appropriately
(**Note:** This is not a NOC outcome.)

REFERENCES

Berry P, Griffie J. (2006). Planning for actual death. In Ferrell BR, Coyle N (Eds). *Textbook of palliative nursing*, 2nd ed. New York: Oxford University Press, pp 561-577.
Confidentially. Postmortem care: Delegation complication. (2000). *Nursing*, 30(3):80.
Davies DE. (2006). Parental suicide after the expected death of a child at home. *Brit Med J*, 332:647-648.
Dochterman JM, Bulechek GM (Eds). (2004). *Nursing Interventions Classification (NIC)*, 4th ed. St. Louis: Mosby.
Kuebler KK, Berry PH, Heidrich DE. (2002). *End of life care: Clinical practice guidelines*. Philadelphia: Saunders.
Lomas D, Timmins J, Harley B, Mates A. (2004). The use of pastoral and spiritual support in bereavement care. *Nurs Times*, 100(31):34-35.
Marthaler MT. (2005). End-of-life care: Practical tips. *Dimens Crit Care Nurs*, 24(5):215-218.
Matzo ML, Sherman DW (Eds). (2001). *Palliative care nursing: Quality care to the end of life*. New York: Springer.
Mayer R. (2006). *Embalming: History, theory and practice*, 4th ed. New York: McGraw-Hill.
Pessagno RA. (1997). Postmortem care: Healing's first step. *Nursing*, 27(4):32a-32b.

NR = Nursing Research, **MR** = Multidisciplinary Research, **SP** = Standard of Practice, **EO** = Expert Opinion, **LOE** = Level of Evidence

Potter PA, Perry AG. (2005). *Fundamentals of nursing*, 6th ed. St. Louis: Mosby.

Sewell P. (2002). Respecting a patient's care needs after death. *Nurs Times*, 98(39):36-37.

Ufema J. (1999). Reflections on death and dying. *Nurs*, 29(6):56-59.

Vacarolis EM, Carson VB, Shoemaker NC. (2006). *Foundations of psychiatric mental health nursing: A clinical approach*, 5th ed. St. Louis: Saunders.

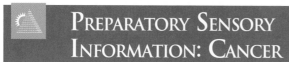

PREPARATORY SENSORY INFORMATION: CANCER

Jean E. Johnson, PhD, FAAN; Miriam O. Ezenwa, MS, RN

Definition: Describing the typical sensory experiences and events associated with chemotherapy and radiation during the treatment of cancer.

The descriptions include the sequence of events; the causes of the sensory experiences; how long the sensations, symptoms, and procedural events are expected to last (or when they may be expected to change); and the environment associated with the procedure/treatment. The comprehensive description is labeled *concrete objective information*.

NURSING ACTIVITIES

Effective

■ *Use concrete objective information to prepare patients for chemotherapy experiences.* **LOE = II**

(NR) An RCT ($N = 109$ cancer chemotherapy patients) of computer-based intervention that included concrete objective information delivered in nine visits over 18 weeks versus usual care demonstrated that the experimental intervention group had less depression than the control group (Rawl et al., 2002).

(MR) An RCT ($N = 60$ cancer chemotherapy patients) compared a standard control group with a group that received concrete objective information conveyed by way of a tour of the clinic, a videotape about receiving a treatment, a discussion with a question-and-answer session, and a booklet before the first treatment. It was demonstrated that the concrete objective information reduced anticipatory side effects, negative affect, vomiting, and negative impact on daily activities as compared with the results seen in the control group (Burish et al., 1991).

■ *Use concrete objective information to prepare patients for radiation therapy experiences.* **LOE = I**

(NR) An RCT ($N = 50$ patients receiving radiation therapy) of concrete objective information delivered by a researcher about the planning procedures, treatment phase, side effects, and self-care versus standard care demonstrated that the members of the concrete objective information group reported less anxiety during treatments and were more satisfied with the information received and their nursing care than members of the control group (Poroch, 1995).

(NR) An RCT ($N = 84$ radiation therapy patients) of an intervention consisting of four audiotapes of concrete objective information about treatment planning procedures, receiving treatments, experiences during the weeks of treatment, and experiences after therapy as compared with usual care demonstrated that the concrete objective information group reported less disruption in usual activities during and after therapy than the control group did (Johnson et al., 1988).

(NR) An RCT (N = 62 radiation therapy patients) of three audiotapes of concrete objective information about the treatment planning procedure, the side effects during the weeks of treatment, and changes in side effects after therapy as compared with three audiotapes of messages about the cancer center and staff demonstrated that the concrete objective information group of patients had less disruption in usual life activities during the last week of treatment (when side effects were most severe) and that patients who received the intervention and who tended to be pessimistic had less mood disturbance during therapy than the control group (Johnson, 1996).

(NR) A controlled trial (N = 226 radiation therapy patients) of the preparation of patients by staff nurses instructed in the theoretic basis of concrete objective information interventions as compared with care given by the nurses before their instruction showed that patients whose nurses were prepared with concrete objective information showed less disruption in their usual activities during and after radiation therapy. When patients who tended to be pessimistic were prepared with concrete objective information, they had a more positive mood than the control group patients (Johnson et al., 1997).

(NR) An RCT (N = 76 radiation therapy patients) of combinations of audiotapes of concrete objective information, relaxation instruction, and control information as preparation for radiation therapy showed that patients who received concrete objective information engaged in more social activities during the weeks that they received therapy than the control group did (Christman & Cain, 2004).

Possibly Effective

No applicable research was found in this category.

Not Effective

No applicable research was found in this category.

Possibly Harmful

No applicable research was found in this category.

OUTCOME MEASUREMENT

COPING   (NOC)

Definition: Personal actions to manage stressors that tax an individual's resources.
Coping as evidenced by the following selected NOC indicators:
• Identifies effective coping patterns
• Verbalizes sense of control
• Reports decrease in stress
• Uses available social support
(Rate each indicator of **Coping:** 1 = never demonstrated, 2 = rarely demonstrated, 3 = sometimes demonstrated, 4 = often demonstrated, 5 = consistently demonsrated) (Moorhead et al., 2004).

NR = Nursing Research, **MR** = Multidisciplinary Research, **SP** = Standard of Practice, **EO** = Expert Opinion, **LOE** = Level of Evidence

REFERENCES

Burish TG, Snyder SL, Jenkins RA. (1991). Preparing patients for cancer chemotherapy: Effect of coping preparation and relaxation interventions. *J Consult Clin Psychol,* 59(4):518-525.

Christman NJ, Cain LB. (2004). The effects of concrete objective information and relaxation on maintaining usual activity during radiation therapy. *Oncol Nurs Forum,* 31(2):E39-E45.

Johnson JE. (1996). Coping with radiation therapy: Optimism and the effect of preparatory interventions. *Res Nurs Health,* 19(1):3-12.

Johnson JE, Fieler VK, Wlasowicz GS, Mitchell ML, Jones LS. (1997). The effects of nursing care guided by self-regulation theory on coping with radiation therapy. *Oncol Nurs Forum,* 24(6):1041-1050.

Johnson JE, Nail LM, Lauver D, King KB, Keys H. (1988). Reducing the negative impact of radiation therapy on functional status. *Cancer,* 61(1):46-51.

Moorhead S, Johnson M, Maas M (Eds). (2004). *Nursing Outcomes Classification (NOC),* 3rd ed. St Louis: Mosby.

Poroch D. (1995). The effect of preparatory patient education on the anxiety and satisfaction of cancer patients receiving radiation therapy. *Cancer Nurs,* 18(3):206-214.

Rawl SM, Given BA, Given CW, Champion VL, Kozachik SL, Barton D, et al. (2002). Intervention to improve psychological functioning for newly diagnosed patients with cancer. *Oncol Nurs Forum,* 29(6):967-975.

PREPARATORY SENSORY INFORMATION: PROCEDURES

Jean E. Johnson, PhD, FAAN; Miriam O. Ezenwa, MS, RN

NIC **Definition:** Describing in concrete and objective terms the typical sensory experiences and events associated with an upcoming stressful health care procedure/treatment (Dochterman & Bulechek, 2004).

The descriptions can include the sequence of events; the causes of the sensory experiences; how long the sensations and procedural events are expected to last (or when they may be expected to change); and the environment associated with the procedure. The comprehensive description is labeled *concrete objective information.* Interventions limited to descriptions of sensory experience are labeled *sensory information.*

NURSING ACTIVITIES

Effective

■ *Use concrete objective information to prepare patients for experience with cardiac catheterization.* **LOE = I**

NR An RCT (*N* = 40 cardiac catheterization patients) demonstrated that, as compared with patients receiving usual care, patients who were prepared with an audiotape of concrete objective information reported less negative moods 1 to 2 hours before and the morning after the procedure and that they displayed fewer distress behaviors during the examination (Rice et al., 1988).

RCT = Randomized Controlled (Clinical) Trial, **NIC** = Nursing Interventions Classification, **NOC** = Nursing Outcomes Classification

(MR) An RCT (N = 44 cardiac catheterization patients) showed that patients who were prepared with concrete objective information received better behavioral ratings of adjustment during the procedure, reported lower anxiety during the procedure, and used more positive coping self-statements than did patients in the standard care control group (Kendall et al., 1979).

(MR) An RCT (N = 72 cardiac catheterization patients) of an audiotape of concrete objective information demonstrated that, as compared with control information, concrete objective information increased the number of positive coping self-statements and reduced the time it took to complete the cardiac catheterization (Ludwick-Rosenthal & Neufeld, 1993).

■ *Use concrete objective information to prepare patients for experience with endoscopy.* **LOE = I**

(MR) An RCT (N = 45 endoscopy patients) of concrete objective information interventions delivered verbally in an interactive manner as compared with a control intervention demonstrated that patients in the experimental groups showed a reduction in distress during the procedure and in the amount of time required for scope induction (Maguire et al., 2004).

(MR) An RCT (N = 42 endoscopy patients) of preparation with an audiotape of concrete objective information, instruction in relaxation, and a control group showed that patients who received concrete objective information exhibited less distress during the insertion of the endoscope, that they had smaller increases in heart rate during tube insertion, that they experienced insertion failures less frequently, that they found the procedure to be less uncomfortable than they expected, that they thought they would be less frightened during future hospital experiences, and that they were more positive about being informed about future hospital experiences (Wilson et al., 1982).

(NR) An RCT (N = 48 endoscopy patients) of audiotapes of concrete objective information, instruction in breathing techniques, and a control group showed that patients in the concrete objective information group required fewer milligrams of diazepam, had more stable heart rates, and had fewer episodes of gagging (Johnson & Leventhal, 1974).

(NR) A controlled trial (N = 99 endoscopy patients) of preparation with audiotapes of sensory information, procedure information, or a control message showed that patients who received sensory information required less diazepam and had less tension in their hands and arms during the examination (Johnson et al., 1973).

■ *Use concrete objective information to prepare patients for experience with other procedures.* **LOE = I**

(NR) An RCT (N = 60 pyelography patients) demonstrated that, as compared with a usual care control group, patients who received an audiotape of concrete objective information about the experience plus slides reported that they felt more calm, safer, more relaxed, and more in control of the situation. They also experienced less pain and discomfort from the contrast dye, compression, and the entire examination (Hjelm-Karlsson, 1989).

(MR) An RCT (N = 50 nasogastric intubation patients) of filmstrips of four different types of information showed that sensory information alone led to greater willingness to repeat the procedure and that sensory information plus procedure information in combination with coping behavior information decreased discomfort, pain, and anxiety during and after the procedure (Padilla et al., 1981).

NR An RCT (N = 24 pelvic examination patients) of four types of information interventions (sensory only, sensory plus relaxation instruction, health only, or health plus relaxation) demonstrated that patients who received the interventions that contained sensory information displayed fewer distress behaviors and had lower pulse increases during the examination, as compared with the patients who received health information (Fuller et al., 1978).

Possibly Effective

■ *Use concrete objective information to prepare patients for experience with a barium enema.* **LOE = III**

NR A controlled trial (N = 24 barium enema patients) of preparation with audiotapes of sensory information, procedural information, and a control group showed that, when patients who tended to be anxious received sensory information, they had reduced anxiety during the barium enema (Hartfield et al., 1982).

NR An RCT (N = 20 barium enema patients) of preparatory audiotapes of sensory information as compared with control information showed reduced anxiety during the procedure for the group who received the sensory information (Hartfield & Cason, 1981).

Not Effective

■ *Using procedural sensory information to prepare patients for experience with cardiac catheterization.* **LOE = II**

NR An RCT (N = 145 cardiac catheterization patients) of three preparatory interventions—(1) a videotape of procedural modeling information; (2) a videotape of procedure-sensory modeling information; and (3) procedural-sensory information booklet—produced no clear support for the procedural-sensory information (Davis et al., 1994).

MR An RCT (N = 60 cardiac catheterization patients) of five types of psychological preparatory interventions, including concrete objective information, showed that patients who received any one of the preparatory interventions had lower autonomic arousal during and after the catheterization than control patients (Anderson & Masur, 1989).

Possibly Harmful

No applicable research was found in this category.

OUTCOME MEASUREMENT

COPING

Definition: Personal actions to manage stressors that tax an individual's resources.
Coping as evidenced by the following selected NOC indicators:
• Identifies multiple coping strategies
• Uses behaviors to reduce stress

Continued

RCT = Randomized Controlled (Clinical) Trial, **NIC** = Nursing Interventions Classification, **NOC** = Nursing Outcomes Classification

OUTCOME MEASUREMENT—*cont'd*

- Verbalizes need for assistance
- Seeks help from a health care professional as appropriate

(Rate each indicator of **Coping:** 1 = never demonstrated, 2 = rarely demonstrated, 3 = sometimes demonstrated, 4 = often demonstrated, 5 = consistently demonstrated) (Moorhead et al., 2004).

REFERENCES

Anderson KO, Masur FT III. (1989). Psychologic preparation for cardiac catheterization. *Heart Lung*, 18(2):154-163.

Davis TM, Maguire TO, Haraphongse M, Schaumberger MR. (1994). Undergoing cardiac catheterization: The effects of informational preparation and coping style on patient anxiety during the procedure. *Heart Lung*, 23(2):140-150.

Dochterman JM, Bulechek GM (Eds). (2004). *Nursing Interventions Classification (NIC)*, 4th ed. St Louis: Mosby.

Fuller SS, Endress MP, Johnson JE. (1978). The effects of cognitive and behavioral control on coping with an aversive health examination. *J Human Stress*, 4(4):18-25.

Hartfield MJ, Cason CL. (1981). Effect of information on emotional responses during barium enema. *Nurs Res*, 30(3):151-155.

Hartfield MT, Cason CL, Cason GJ. (1982). Effects of information about a threatening procedure on patients' expectations and emotional distress. *Nurs Res*, 31(4):202-206.

Hjelm-Karlsson K. (1989). Effects of information to patients undergoing intravenous pyelography: An intervention study. *J Adv Nurs*, 14(10):853-862.

Johnson JE, Leventhal H. (1974). Effects of accurate expectations and behavioral instructions during a noxious medical examination. *J Pers Soc Psychol*, 29(5):710-718.

Johnson JE, Morrissey JF, Leventhal H. (1973). Psychological preparation for an endoscopic examination. *Gastrointest Endosc*, 19(4):180-182.

Kendall PC, Williams L, Pechacek TF, Graham LE, Shisslak C, Herzoff N. (1979). Cognitive-behavioral and patient education interventions in cardiac catheterization procedures: The Palo Alto Medical Psychology Project. *J Consult Clin Psychol*, 47(1):49-58.

Ludwick-Rosenthal R, Neufeld RW. (1993). Preparation for undergoing an invasive medical procedure: Interacting effects of information and coping style. *J Consult Clin Psychol*, 61(1):156-164.

Maguire D, Walsh JC, Little CL. (2004). The effect of information and behavioural training on endoscopy patients' clinical outcomes. *Patient Educ Counsel*, 54(1):61-65.

Moorhead S, Johnson M, Maas M (Eds). (2004). *Nursing Outcomes Classification (NOC)*, 3rd ed. St Louis: Mosby.

Padilla GV, Grant MM, Rains BL, Hansen BC, Bergstrom N, Wong HL, et al. (1981). Distress reduction and the effects of preparatory teaching films and patient control. *Res Nurs Health*, 4(4):375-387.

Rice VH, Sieggreen M, Mullin M, Williams J. (1988). Development and testing of an arteriography information intervention for stress reduction. *Heart Lung*, 17(1):23-28.

Wilson JF, Moore RW, Randolph S, Hanson BJ. (1982). Behavioral preparation of patients for gastrointestinal endoscopy: Information, relaxation, and coping style. *J Human Stress*, 8(4):13-23.

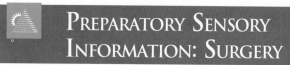

PREPARATORY SENSORY INFORMATION: SURGERY

Jean E. Johnson, PhD, FAAN; Miriam O. Ezenwa, MS, RN

Definition: Describing the typical sensory experiences and events associated with an upcoming surgery.

The descriptions include the sequence of events; the causes of the sensory experiences; how long the sensations, symptoms, and procedural events are expected to last (or when they may be expected to change); and the environment associated with the surgical experience. The comprehensive description is labeled *concrete objective information*. Interventions limited to descriptions of the sensory experience are labeled *sensory information*.

NURSING ACTIVITIES

Effective

■ *Use concrete objective information to prepare total joint replacement surgical patients for their experiences.* **LOE = II**

MR An RCT ($N = 100$ total hip replacement patients) of a videotape of concrete objective information before surgery versus usual care control demonstrated that concrete objective information reduced anxiety and the secretion of cortisol the day of surgery and 2 days after surgery. Also, the percentage of patients who had an increase of 15% in systolic blood pressure intraoperatively was lower (Doering et al., 2000).

MR An RCT ($N = 222$ total hip and knee replacement patients) of preoperative audiotape and slides of concrete objective information versus usual care demonstrated that concrete objective information reduced the uses of pain medication and the length of hospital stay for patients who used denial as a coping strategy and reduced mental confusion postoperatively among patients who were not highly anxious before surgery as compared with the control group (Daltroy et al., 1998).

NR A controlled trial ($N = 82$ total hip replacement patients) of concrete objective information pre- and postoperatively versus control information demonstrated that the patients who received concrete objective information received less pain medication after surgery, mobilized sooner, and had, on average, 2 fewer days of hospitalization (Gammon & Mulholland, 1996a).

NR A controlled trial ($N = 82$ total hip replacement patients) of concrete objective information provided by a nurse pre- and postoperatively versus control demonstrated that, at the time of hospital discharge, the patients who received concrete objective information reported lower anxiety, less depression, higher self-esteem, a higher sense of control, and a higher ability to cope (Gammon & Mulholland, 1996b).

RCT = Randomized Controlled (Clinical) Trial, **NIC** = Nursing Interventions Classification, **NOC** = Nursing Outcomes Classification

■ *Use concrete objective information to prepare cardiac surgery patients for their experiences.* **LOE = II**

(NR) An RCT ($N = 60$ cardiac surgery patients) comparing a concrete objective information videotape plus audiotape, concrete objective information plus instruction in postoperative exercises, and control information demonstrated that both experimental groups had less anxiety and fears after receiving the intervention and before surgery. These patients were rated by nurses as having made a better psychological and physical recovery after surgery, and they had a lower incidence of acute postoperative hypertension as compared with the control group (Anderson, 1987).

(NR) A controlled trial ($N = 43$ cardiac surgery patients) of concrete objective information related to mechanical ventilation delivered preoperatively by a nurse and a booklet versus a control group showed that the concrete objective information group reported less anxiety, a less negative mood, and less difficulty communicating during mechanical ventilation (Kim et al., 1999).

(NR) A controlled trial ($N = 82$ cardiac surgery patients) of an audiotape of concrete objective information given to patients on the fifth or sixth postoperative day (patients also took the tape home) versus a control group showed that the concrete objective information group had better physical functioning 1 month after discharge (Moore, 1996).

(NR) A controlled trial ($N = 83$ cardiac surgery patients) of preparation for the intensive care unit experience with an audiotape of concrete objective information about the experience versus a control group demonstrated that patients who received concrete objective information perceived the intensive care unit environment to be less stressful and had reduced cognitive confusion (Shi et al., 2003).

(NR) A controlled trial ($N = 101$ cardiac surgery patients) of a video of a model patient presenting behavioral instructions and concrete objective information about what patients experienced pre- and postoperatively versus a control video demonstrated that the video containing concrete objective information about the experience helped patients to better prepare for the operation, and that patients would like to be prepared again by such a video in other similar situations (Roth-Isigkeit et al., 2002).

■ *Use concrete objective information to prepare patients for other surgical experiences.* **LOE = I**

(NR) An RCT ($N = 42$ cesarean delivery patients) of preparatory concrete objective information delivered by slides and audiotape as compared with control information about parent-infant interaction delivered by slides and audiotape demonstrated that patients who received concrete objective information had lower systolic blood pressure intraoperatively and recovered from surgery more rapidly (Greene et al., 1989).

(MR) An RCT ($N = 141$ day-stay cataract surgery patients) of a videotape of concrete objective information about what to expect versus a videotape of an explanation of the anatomy of cataracts as the control group demonstrated that, after surgery, the concrete objective information group was less anxious, understood better what was happening, and was more satisfied than the control group (Pager, 2005).

(NR) An RCT ($N = 81$ cholecystectomy patients) of preparation with audiotaped combinations of sensory information, descriptions of events during the surgical experience, and instructions for coping activities showed that, as compared with a control group, sensory information reduced the length of postoperative hospitalization and time after discharge before patients ventured from their homes (Johnson et al., 1978a).

(NR) A controlled trial (*N* = 83 cholecystectomy patients) compared combinations of preadmission booklets about admission procedures and postoperative exercises; audiotapes of concrete objective information about pre- and postoperative experiences that were provided to patients preoperatively; and a restatement of concrete objective information about postoperative experiences that was provided on the first postoperative day. It was demonstrated that, as compared with the control groups, concrete objective information groups reported less helplessness, had shorter hospital stays, and ventured from home sooner after discharge (Johnson et al., 1978b).

(NR) An RCT (*N* = 40 cataract surgery patients) of combinations of audiotapes of sensory information and behavioral instructions showed that, as compared with the control information group, the group that received the combination of sensory information and behavioral instructions ventured from their homes sooner after discharge (Hill, 1982).

Possibly Effective

No applicable published research was found in this category.

Not Effective

- *Using an audiotape for preoperative preparation for a hysterectomy.* **LOE = II**

  (NR) An RCT (*N* = 168 hysterectomy patients) of preoperative preparation with audiotapes of combinations of concrete objective information, instructions for distraction from negative aspects and attending to positive aspects of the experience, behavioral-coping techniques, and concrete objective information about typical experiences after discharge from the hospital showed that there were no consistent differences between the experimental and control groups (Johnson et al., 1985).

Possibly Harmful

No applicable published research was found in this category.

OUTCOME MEASUREMENT

COPING (NOC)

Definition: Personal actions to manage stressors that tax an individual's resources.
Coping as evidenced by the following selected NOC indicators:
- Reports decrease in physical symptoms of stress
- Seeks information concerning illness and treatment
- Uses effective coping patterns
- Uses behaviors to reduce stress

(Rate each indicator of **Coping:** 1 = never demonstrated, 2 = rarely demonstrated, 3 = sometimes demonstrated, 4 = often demonstrated, 5 = consistently demonstrated) (Moorhead et al., 2004).

RCT = Randomized Controlled (Clinical) Trial, **NIC** = Nursing Interventions Classification, **NOC** = Nursing Outcomes Classification

REFERENCES

Anderson EA. (1987). Preoperative preparation for cardiac surgery facilitates recovery, reduces psychological distress, and reduces the incidence of acute postoperative hypertension. *J Consult Clin Psychol,* 55(4):513-520.

Daltroy LH, Morlino CI, Eaton HM, Poss R, Liang MH. (1998). Preoperative education for total hip and knee replacement patients. *Arthritis Care Res,* 11(6):469-478.

Doering S, Katzlberger F, Rumpold G, Roessler S, Hofstoetter B, Schatz DS, et al. (2000). Videotape preparation of patients before hip replacement surgery reduces stress. *Psychosom Med,* 62(3):365-373.

Gammon J, Mulholland CW. (1996a). Effect of preparatory information prior to elective total hip replacement on post-operative physical coping outcomes. *Int J Nurs Stud,* 33(6):589-604.

Gammon J, Mulholland CW. (1996b). Effect of preparatory information prior to elective total hip replacement on psychological coping outcomes. *J Adv Nurs,* 24(2):303-308.

Greene PG, Zeichner A, Roberts NL, Callahan EJ, Granados JL. (1989). Preparation for cesarean delivery: A multicomponent analysis of treatment outcome. *J Consult Clin Psychol,* 57(4):484-487.

Hill BJ. (1982). Sensory information, behavioral instructions and coping with sensory alteration surgery. *Nurs Res,* 31(1):17-21.

Johnson JE, Christman NJ, Stitt C. (1985). Personal control interventions: Short- and long-term effects on surgical patients. *Res Nurs Health,* 8(2):131-145.

Johnson JE, Fuller SS, Endress MP, Rice VH. (1978a). Altering patients' responses to surgery: An extension and replication. *Res Nurs Health,* 1(3):111-121.

Johnson JE, Rice VH, Fuller SS, Endress MP. (1978b). Sensory information, instruction in a coping strategy and recovery from surgery. *Res Nurs Health,* 1(1):4-17.

Kim H, Garvin BJ, Moser DK. (1999). Stress during mechanical ventilation: Benefit of having concrete objective information before cardiac surgery. *Am J Crit Care,* 8(2):118-126.

Moore SM. (1996). The effects of a discharge information intervention on recovery outcomes following coronary artery bypass surgery. *Int J Nurs Stud,* 33(2):181-189.

Moorhead S, Johnson M, Maas M. (Eds). (2004). *Nursing Outcomes Classification (NOC),* 3rd ed. St Louis: Mosby.

Pager CK. (2005). Randomised controlled trial of preoperative information to improve satisfaction with cataract surgery. *Br J Ophthalmol,* 89(1):10-13.

Roth-Isigkeit A, Ocklitz E, Bruckner S, Ros A, Dibbelt L, Friedrich HJ, et al. (2002). Development and evaluation of a video program for presentation prior to elective cardiac surgery. *Acta Anaesthesiol Scand,* 46(4):415-423.

Shi SF, Munjas BA, Wan TT, Cowling WR III, Grap MJ, Wang BB. (2003). The effects of preparatory sensory information on ICU patients. *J Med Syst,* 27(2):191-204.

 ## PRESENCE

Barbara A. Caldwell, PhD, APRN-BC

NIC **Definition:** Being with another, both physically and psychologically, during times of need (Dochterman & Bulechek, 2004).

NURSING ACTIVITIES

Effective

No applicable published research was found in this category.

NR = Nursing Research, **MR** = Multidisciplinary Research, **SP** = Standard of Practice, **EO** = Expert Opinion, **LOE** = Level of Evidence

Possibly Effective

■ *Use a healing and dignified conscious awareness and connection in the interpersonal experience.* **LOE = V**

(NR) A systematic review demonstrated that a caring conversation was defined by connection (listening, connective and caring touch, being with) and contact (hearing, task-oriented touch, and being with) (Fredriksson, 1999).

(NR) A systematic review demonstrated that the use of a midwife/nurse to act as a guide and a companion in a willing and desired relationship with a woman in labor supported the woman's psychological, physical, spiritual, and emotional needs (Hunter, 2002).

(NR) A systematic review found that the essence of nurse/midwife care was to protect the woman's dignity, mutual process, trust, ongoing dialogue, shared responsibility, and enduring presence (Berg, 2005).

(NR) A systemic review demonstrated five outcomes of nursing presence: (1) the achievement of client goals; (2) nursing care satisfaction; (3) growth; (4) comfort; and (5) enhanced healing (Godkin, 2001).

(NR) A systematic review demonstrated that a caring presence was defined as the interpersonal, intersubjective experience during which conscious awareness (intentionality) and connection allowed for a mutual transformation of the nurse and patient to unfold (Covington, 2003).

(MR) A systematic review demonstrated that components of healing presence were love, spiritual grace, focused awareness, openness to healing, creativity, imagination, connectedness, good intention, belief, and listening (Jonas & Crawford, 2004).

(NR) A systematic review demonstrated that proper study design (the appropriate assignment of variables, quantitative and qualitative design structure) was an essential element of research fostering healing at bio-psycho-social-spiritual levels of the individual (McDonough-Means et al., 2004).

■ *Convey understanding, personal connection, and a sense of being valued through human touch and spiritual comfort to patients in the here and now.* **LOE = IV**

(NR) A cohort study ($N = 21$) of therapeutic presence within a population of low-income pregnant women demonstrated an interpersonal reciprocity to work together, attention to the here and now, and expert care delivery via telephone social support. This qualitative, randomized, controlled investigation revealed expert nursing practice outcomes, including the maintenance of psychological presence and diminished maternal stress (Finfgeld-Connett, 2005).

(NR) A cohort study ($N = 7$) demonstrated that presence during tele- or video-consultation was effective when nurses working within a nursing home paid particular attention to sensory variability and facilitated a safe, secure, and familiar environment. Participants included 18 residents within the nursing home. Teleconsultations provided a snapshot of the residents' living experiences (Savenstedt et al., 2004).

(MR) A qualitative cohort study ($N = 15$) with participants from a community-based breast cancer support group found that active listening, honesty, partnership, interest, and use of touch were effective for enhancing perceptions of being cared for by health practitioners (Harris & Templeton, 2001).

RCT = Randomized Controlled (Clinical) Trial, **NIC** = Nursing Interventions Classification, **NOC** = Nursing Outcomes Classification

(NR) A cohort study ($N = 23$) consisting of a population of nursing staff within a state psychiatric hospital demonstrated that presence involved knowing the uniqueness of the person, listening intently, involving the person, mobilizing resources, and mutually defining changes in the provision of confident caring (Caldwell et al., 2005).

(MR) A qualitative case study ($N = 1$) involving the process of child psychotherapy demonstrated that presence involved a holding environment in which the patient and the caregiver formed a mutual regulation and synchrony with each other in which the world was experienced as both safe and immediately meaningful (Binder, 2005).

▪ *Convey trust, support, and awareness of personal suffering through the use of touch and spiritual bonding during periods of living and dying.* **LOE = IV**

(NR) A cohort study ($N = 6$) composed of six female volunteers from an urban center verbally demonstrated that nursing presence within the childbirth process was contextualized in the place of care and subject to mutual knowing (attentive gaze and heartfelt listening), trusting, supporting, and advocacy (MacKinnon et al., 2005).

(NR) A cohort study ($N = 10$) composed of chronically ill volunteers who were treated by a nurse practitioner at least once that year indicated that caring presence was found between two individuals with mutual trust, sharing, spiritual bonding, and accessibility to a higher and deeper energy source as a place to share the illness (Covington, 2005).

(NR) A qualitative cohort study ($N = 3$) composed of nurses' clinical accounts defined presence as a moment of understanding (intuitive experience) during which the nurse was open and willingly responded by listening attentively, instilling trust, and providing encouragement. The nurse was vigilant with respect to patient needs and used touch that was intended to support and comfort (Hawley, 2000).

(NR) A cohort study ($N = 9$) found that meditation in action supported intention and being aware, presence in the in-between spaces of living and dying, seeing differently, cultivating the unknown, and continuous change to hospice caregivers (Bruce & Davies, 2005).

(MR) A cohort study ($N = 2$) composed of two accounts of patient-therapist interaction within a clinical environment found that presence involved meaningful interpretations or communicated understanding using personal languages that guided the person to feeling valued by the other (Viederman, 1999).

(NR) A cohort study ($N = 10$) found that critical-care patients reflected five themes that substantiated the presence of the nurse: (1) perceptual presence (availability and vigilance); (2) knowing the patient; (3) intimacy in suffering; (4) appreciation for details; and (5) honoring the body (Gramling, 2004).

(NR) A cohort study ($N = 12$) composed of volunteer health care providers working at an acute psychiatric facility found that presence in the face of violence or fear was composed of an inner dialogue (reflection of the here and now) and of a tension of distance and earlier experiences that may color one's capacity to take responsibility for care (Carlsson et al., 2004).

(NR) A cohort study ($N = 11$) composed of recently discharged patients demonstrated four themes as being central to presence: (1) being with the nurse in a calm, gentle, courteous, kind, attentive, and available manner; (2) competence in care; (3) supporting and facilitating meaningful (spiritual) interactions; and (4) appreciation of the time allotted to care (Davis, 2005).

NR = Nursing Research, **MR** = Multidisciplinary Research, **SP** = Standard of Practice, **EO** = Expert Opinion, **LOE** = Level of Evidence

Not Effective

No applicable published research was found in this category.

Possibly Harmful

No applicable published research was found in this category.

OUTCOME MEASUREMENT

CAREGIVER-PATIENT RELATIONSHIP 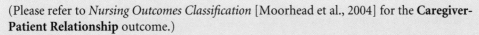 NOC

(Please refer to *Nursing Outcomes Classification* [Moorhead et al., 2004] for the **Caregiver-Patient Relationship** outcome.)

REFERENCES

Berg M. (2005). A midwifery model of care for childbearing women at high risk: Genuine caring in caring for the genuine. *J Perinat Educ,* 14(1):9-21.

Binder PE. (2005). The meaning bearing other—A relational view of the child psychotherapeutic process. *J Am Acad Psychoanal Dyn Psychiatry,* 33(4):657-670.

Bruce A, Davies B. (2005). Mindfulness in hospice care: Practicing meditation-in-action. *Qual Health Res,* 15(10):1329-1344.

Caldwell B, Doyle M, Morris M, McQuaide T. (2005). Presencing: Channeling therapeutic effectiveness with the mentally ill in a state psychiatric hospital. *Issues Ment Health Nurs,* 26(8):853-871.

Carlsson G, Dahlberg K, Lutzen K, Nystrom M. (2004). Violent encounters in psychiatric care: A phenomenological study of embodied caring knowledge. *Issues Ment Health Nurs,* 25(2):191-217.

Covington H. (2003). Caring presence. Delineation of a concept for holistic nursing. *J Holist Nurs,* 21(3):301-317.

Covington H. (2005). Caring presence: Providing a safe space for patients. *Holist Nurs Pract,* 19(4): 169-172.

Davis LA. (2005). A phenomenological study of patient expectations concerning nursing care. *Holist Nurs Pract,* 19(3):126-133.

Dochterman JM, Bulechek GM (Eds). (2004). *Nursing Interventions Classification (NIC),* 4th ed. St. Louis: Mosby.

Finfgeld-Connett D. (2005). Telephone social support or nursing presence? Analysis of a nursing intervention. *Qual Health Res,* 15(1):19-29.

Fredriksson L. (1999). Modes of relating in a caring conversation: A research synthesis on presence, touch and listening. *J Adv Nurs,* 30(5):1167-1176.

Godkin J. (2001). Healing presence. *J Holist Nurs,* 19(1):5-21.

Gramling KL. (2004). A narrative study of nursing art in critical care. *J Holist Nurs,* 22(4):379-398.

Harris SR, Templeton E. (2001). Who's listening? Experiences of women with breast cancer in communicating with physicians. *Breast J,* 7(6):444-449.

Hawley PM. (2000). Moments in nursing practice: An interpretive analysis. *Int J Human Caring,* 4(3):18-22.

Hunter LP. (2002). Being with woman: A guiding concept for the care of laboring women. *J Obstet Gynecol Neonatal Nurs,* 31(6):650-657.

Jonas WB, Crawford CC. (2004). The healing presence: Can it be reliably measured? *J Altern Complement Med,* 10(5):751-756.

MacKinnon K, McIntyre M, Quance M. (2005). The meaning of the nurse's presence during childbirth. *J Obstet Gynecol Neonatal Nurs,* 34(1):28-36.

McDonough-Means SI, Kreitzer MJ, Bell IR. (2004). Fostering a healing presence and investigating its mediators. *J Altern Complement Med,* 10(Suppl 1):S25-S41.

Moorhead S, Johnson M, Mass M (Eds). (2004). *Nursing Outcomes Classification (NOC).* 3rd ed. St. Louis: Mosby.

Savenstedt S, Zingmark K, Sandman PO. (2004). Being present in a distant room: Aspects of teleconsultations with older people in a nursing home. *Qual Health Res,* 14(8):1046-1057.

Viederman M. (1999). Presence and enactment as a vehicle of psychotherapeutic change. *J Psychother Pract Res,* 8(4):274-283.

PRESSURE ULCER CARE STAGE I

Diane K. Langemo, PhD, RN, FAAN; Julie Anderson, PhD, RN, CCRC

Definition: The facilitation of healing of a stage I pressure ulcer.

A pressure ulcer is an area of localized tissue destruction that occurs as the result of the compression of soft tissue, usually between a bony prominence and an external surface, for a prolonged period of time. A stage I pressure ulcer is a localized, reddened area with nonblanchable skin. The skin's epidermal layer is still intact.

NURSING ACTIVITIES

Effective

■ *Reduce the risk of developing additional pressure ulcers.*

(Refer to the guideline on Pressure Ulcer Prevention.)

■ *Reposition individuals who are in bed and who are at risk for the development of pressure ulcers at least every 2 hours (if this is consistent with the overall goals of care). Maintain a written schedule.* **LOE = II**

(NR) In a clinical trial, patients who were at risk for the development of pressure ulcers who were turned every 2 to 3 hours developed fewer pressure ulcers than those who were not turned as frequently (Norton et al., 1975).

(NR) In an RCT, with the experimental group receiving small body shifts and the control group not receiving them, there was no significant effect on pressure ulcer incidence among 19 long-term care residents. However, residents in both groups were turned every 2 hours (Smith & Malone, 1990).

(NR) In a quasi-experimental study of 838 nursing home residents, four different turning schedules were tested: every 2 hours and every 3 hours on a standard institutional mattress and every 4 hours and every 6 hours on a viscoelastic foam (VEF) mattress. There was a significant reduction in pressure ulcer incidence among residents who were turned every 4 hours on the VEF mattress (Defloor et al., 2005).

(EO) Data support a negative relationship between the number of spontaneous movements made by elderly individuals who are confined to bed and pressure ulcer incidence (Exton-Smith & Sherwin, 1961).

(EO) Clinicians are generally taught to change the patient's position every 2 hours. This in fact may not be frequent enough, depending on an individual's tissue tolerance (e.g., an elderly patient with frail skin; Maklebust, 2005).

(Also refer to the guideline on Pressure Ulcer Prevention.)

NR = Nursing Research, **MR** = Multidisciplinary Research, **SP** = Standard of Practice, **EO** = Expert Opinion, **LOE** = Level of Evidence

■ *Redistribute pressure surfaces for a stage I pressure ulcer. This may include therapeutic mattress replacements, static and dynamic surfaces, and, for critically ill patients, low air loss (LAL) beds and mattresses. The appropriate support surface may change as the patient's condition and setting change. Although cost and product availability are considerations, monitoring current product evaluations is helpful for determining the appropriate device.* **LOE = I**

(EO) An LAL support surface provides pressure redistribution via cyclic changes in loading and unloading as characterized by frequency, duration, amplitude, and rate of change parameters over the "active area" of the surface (NPUAP, 2006).

(NR) In an RCT, 447 patients were treated on either a VEF plus turning every 4 hours or on an alternating pressure air mattress (APAM) with identical sitting protocols. Although there was no significant difference between the two groups with regard to developing stage II, III, or IV pressure ulcers, fewer patients developed heel ulcers if they were treated on APAMs (Vanderwee et al., 2005).

(NR) An RCT of 40 at-risk nursing home residents who were randomly assigned to a foam mattress overlay or a foam mattress replacement found the foam mattress replacement to be more effective in preventing a pressure ulcer. This was also more cost-effective (Vyhlidal et al., 1997).

(NR) A prospective RCT divided 95 intensive care unit patients into three groups: standard mattress, foam mattress, and LAL mattress. There was a significant difference between the LAL mattress and both the foam and standard mattresses (Sterzi et al., 2003).

(MR) A Cochrane review supported the use of higher-specification foam mattresses for individuals who were at risk for skin breakdown (Cullum et al., 2004).

(NR) In a controlled study ($N = 70$), a comparison between APAMs and standard hospital beds in the United Kingdom was inconclusive (Keogh & Dealey, 2001).

(NR) LAL beds and fluid-filled nonpowered mattresses were compared in a laboratory and in a retrospective clinical study. The laboratory study showed significantly lower interface pressures only at the sacral site in those patients treated on the LAL mattress. The clinical study ($N = 73$) showed no significant differences in breakdown between the mattresses (Hardin et al., 2000).

■ *Check support surfaces daily for inadequate support or "bottoming out." Adequate support can be monitored by placing a hand palm up under the mattress or cushion below the area that is at risk for the development of a pressure ulcer. Bottoming out has occurred when less than an inch of support material is felt; in those cases, the support surface is inadequate.* **LOE = III**

(NR) A multisite study ($N = 200$) determined that, for a support surface to remain effective, a patient should not bottom out on it (Bergstrom et al., 1996).

(EO) A support surface loses its effectiveness if a patient bottoms out on it (Bergstrom et al., 1994; WOCN, 2003).

■ *Use redistribution devices and repositioning in conjunction with one another to provide optimal patient care. Pressure redistribution devices should not replace repositioning protocols.* **LOE = II**

(NR) An RCT ($N = 838$) compared four different preventative regimens for 28 days each: a 2-hour turning schedule on a standard institutional mattress (SI), a 3-hour turning schedule on a standard institutional mattress, and 4- and 6-hour turning schedules on a pressure-reducing mattress (VEF). The authors concluded that turning every 4 hours on a VEF mattress resulted in a significant reduction in the development of pressure ulcers (Defloor et al., 2005; WOCN, 2003).

■ *Cleanse stage I pressure ulcers with water, saline, or a noncytotoxic wound cleanser during each dressing change.* **LOE = V**

(EO) Saline is noncytotoxic to tissue, and it can be used to cleanse the site along with tap water or other noncytotoxic cleansers (Bergstrom et al., 1994; WOCN, 2003; Baranoski & Ayello, 2003; Maklebust & Sieggreen, 2001).

■ *Use topical treatments, including barrier creams and skin protectants.* **LOE = III**

(NR) In a controlled study ($N = 19$), researchers demonstrated that using a protectant lotion significantly reduced average scores for perineal erythema and pain (Warshaw et al., 2002).

(NR) A controlled trial ($N = 18$) documented that a petrolatum-containing product demonstrated protection against irritants and maceration and provided some skin hydration, whereas protectants that contained zinc oxide provided protection only against irritation (Hoggarth et al., 2005).

(NR) A prospective clinical trial ($N = 136$) documented that a product containing petrolatum was effective in reducing the incidence of perineal dermatitis in incontinent patients (Thompson et al., 2004).

(NR) A prospective clinical trial ($N = 136$) found that the prophylactic use of a skin cleanser and a skin protectant resulted in a significant decrease in skin breakdown and in stage I and II pressure ulcers from before to after the intervention (Hunter et al., 2003).

■ *Provide a protective dressing (e.g., semipermeable film, thin hydrocolloid sheets, foam) to protect the stage I pressure ulcer.* **LOE = I**

(NR) A random convenience sample ($N = 44$) of stage II pressure ulcers showed that polymeric membrane dressings were more effective than antibiotic ointment and dry sterile gauze dressings (Yastrub, 2004).

(MR) An RCT ($N = 83$) of patients with spinal cord injuries with stage I or II pressure ulcers that compared hydrocolloid, phenytoin cream, and gauze dressings found that hydrocolloid was more effective for treatment (Hollisaz et al., 2004).

(MR) A meta-analysis of 21 peer-reviewed, published, randomized quasi-experimental and controlled clinical trials showed moderate superiority of hydrocolloid dressings as compared with conventional dressings with regard to size efficacy for pressure ulcer treatment (Bouza et al., 2005).

(MR) Studies have demonstrated no significant difference in overall pressure ulcer healing rates or outcomes among a variety of moist wound dressings (e.g., hydrocolloids, hydrogels, foams, normal saline, dextranomer paste, combinations of dressings; Bale et al., 1997; Banks et al., 1997; Belmin et al., 2002; Hondé et al., 1994; Motta et al., 1999; Muller et al., 2001; Ovington, 1999; Seeley et al., 1999; Thomas, 1997; Thomas et al., 1998).

NR = Nursing Research, **MR** = Multidisciplinary Research, **SP** = Standard of Practice, **EO** = Expert Opinion, **LOE** = Level of Evidence

Possibly Effective

■ *Provide education to the patient and/or the caregiver regarding causative/risk factors for the development of pressure ulcers.* **LOE = IV**

(EO) Educational programs should include information that address the following: skin monitoring, devices to assist with the prevention of pressure ulcers, risk assessment, factors that place an individual at risk, and the prevention of pressure ulcers (Bergstrom et al., 1992, 1994; WOCN, 2003).

(EO) The patient and his or her family are integral to the prevention and management of pressure ulcers (Andberg et al., 1983; Barnes, 1987; Sebern, 1987).

■ *Provide education to the patient, including information about minimizing friction and shear forces; not using donut-type devices or rings; ensuring the maintenance of adequate nutrition; turning and repositioning on a regular basis; using pressure-reducing devices if he or she has limited mobility and/or is confined to a bed or a chair; avoiding vigorous massage over bony prominences; regularly inspecting the skin over bony prominences; reporting changes in health status or nutrition; and following prescribed skin care protocols.* **LOE = III**

(EO) It is important that the patient know and understand the measures that need to be taken to protect the skin (Bergstrom et al., 1992, 1994; WOCN, 2003).

Not Effective

■ *Using sheepskin for pressure reduction.* **LOE = VII**

(EO) There is no evidence that sheepskin has pressure-reducing properties (Pieper, 2007; WOCN, 2003).

Possibly Harmful

■ *Massaging the skin over bony prominences.* **LOE = IV**

(NR) A study using a convenience sample ($N = 13$) found that extended massage resulted in a significantly lower skin temperature than standard massage (Olson, 1989).

(NR) A cohort study ($N = 54$) demonstrated that massage over bony prominences with skin discoloration resulted in a lower skin blood flow than was present before massage (Ek et al., 1985).

(NR) In a descriptive study, postmortem biopsies documented macerated, degenerated tissue in areas that were exposed to massage that were not documented on individuals who were not massaged (Dyson, 1978).

■ *Using donut-type devices or rings (such devices concentrate pressure to the surrounding tissue).* **LOE = VI**

(NR) A survey study documented that ring cushions had a greater tendency to cause pressure ulcers than to prevent them (Crewe, 1987).

RCT = Randomized Controlled (Clinical) Trial, **NIC** = Nursing Interventions Classification, **NOC** = Nursing Outcomes Classification

OUTCOME MEASUREMENT

SKIN INTEGRITY

Definition: Maintenance of intact skin, especially in areas that are prone to pressure ulcers (e.g., heels, buttocks).

Skin Integrity as evidenced by the following indicators:

- Skin is intact and of appropriate texture/turgor for the age and health of the patient.
- There are no areas of deep purple/black discoloration of the skin.
- There are no areas of nonblanchable erythema.

(Note: This is not a NOC outcome.)

REFERENCES

Allman RM. (1998). The impact of pressure ulcers on health care costs and mortality. *Adv Wound Care,* 11(3 Suppl):2.

Allman RM, Goode PS, Patrick MM, et al. (1995). Pressure ulcer risk factors among hospitalized patients with activity limitation. *JAMA,* 273(11):865-870.

American Medical Directors Association (AMDA). (1996). *Pressure ulcers.* Columbia, MD: AMDA. Available online: www.guideline.gov. Retrieved on July 9, 2007.

Andberg MM, Rudolph A, Anderson TP. (1983). Improving skin care through patient and family training. *Top Clin Nurs,* 5(2):45-54.

Aronovitch SA, Wilber M, Slezak S, Martin T, Utter D. (1999). A comparative study of an alternating air mattress for the prevention of pressure ulcers in surgical patients. *Ostomy Wound Manage,* 45(3):34-40, 42-44.

Ayello EA, Braden B. (2002). How and why to do pressure ulcer risk assessment. *Adv Skin Wound Care,* 15(3):125-131.

Bale S, Squires D, Varnon T, Walker A, Benbow M, Harding KG. (1997). A comparison of two dressings in pressure sore management. *J Wound Care,* 6(10):463-466.

Banks V, Bale S, Harding K, Harding EF. (1997). Evaluation of a new polyurethane foam dressing. *J Wound Care,* 6(6):266-269.

Baranoski S, Ayello EA. (2003). *Wound care essentials: Practice principles.* Philadelphia: Lippincott Williams & Wilkins.

Barnes SH. (1987). Patient/family education for the patient with a pressure necrosis. *Nurs Clin North Am,* 22(2):463-474.

Barr JE, Day AL, Weaver VA, Taler GM. (1995). Assessing clinical efficacy of a hydrocolloid/alginate dressing on full-thickness pressure ulcers. *Ostomy Wound Manage* 41(3):28-30, 32, 34-36 passim.

Belmin J, Meaume S, Rabus M, Bohbot S; Investigators of the Sequential Treatment of the Elderly with Pressure Sores (STEPS) Trial. (2002). Sequential treatment with calcium alginate dressings and hydrocolloid dressings accelerates pressure ulcer healing in older subjects: A multicenter randomized trial of sequential versus nonsequential treatment with hydrocolloid dressings alone. *J Am Geriatr Soc,* 50(2):269-274.

Bergstrom N, Allman R, Alvarez O, et al. (1994). *Treatment of pressure ulcers.* Clinical practice guideline No. 15. Rockville, MD: Agency for Health Care Policy and Research, AHCPR Publication No. 95-0652.

Bergstrom N, Allman R, Carlson C, et al. (1992). *Pressure ulcers in adults: Prediction and prevention.* Clinical practice guideline No. 3. Rockville, MD: Agency for Health Care Policy and Research, AHCPR Publication No. 92-0047.

Bergstrom N, Braden B. (1992). A prospective study of pressure sore risk among institutionalized elderly. *J Am Geriatr Soc,* 40(8):747-758.

Bergstrom N, Braden B, Kemp M, Champagnes M, Ruby E. (1996). Multi-site study of incidence of pressure ulcers and the relationship between risk level, demographic characteristics, diagnoses, and prescription of preventive interventions. *J Am Geriatric Soc,* 44(1):22-30.

Berlowitz DR, Brandeis GH, Anderson J, et al. (1997). Effect of pressure ulcers on the survival of long-term care residents. *J Gerontol A Biol Sci Med Sci,* 52(2):M106-M110.

Berlowitz DR, Wilking SV. (1989). Risk factors for pressure sores. A comparison of cross-sectional and cohort-derived data. *J Am Geriatr Soc,* 37(11):1043-1050.

Bourdel-Marchasson I, Barateau M, Rondeau V, et al. (2000). A multi-center trial of the effects of oral nutritional supplementation in critically ill older inpatients. GAGE Group. Groupe Aquitain Geriatrique d'Evaluation. *Nutrition,* 16(1):1-5.

Bouza C, Saz Z, Munoz A, Amate JM. (2005). Efficacy of advanced dressings in the treatment of pressure ulcers: A systematic review. *J Wound Care,* 14(5):193-199.

Brandeis GH, Berlowitz DR, Hossain M, Morris JN. (1995). Pressure ulcers: The minimum data set and the resident assessment protocol. *Adv Wound Care,* 8(6):18-25.

Breslow RA, Hallfrisch J, Guy DG, Crawley B, Goldberg AP. (1993). The importance of dietary protein in healing pressure ulcers. *J Am Geriatr Soc,* 41(4):357-362.

Brienza DM, Karg PE, Geyer MJ, Kelsey S, Trefler E. (2001). The relationship between pressure ulcer incidence and buttock-seat cushion interface pressure in at-risk elderly wheelchair users. *Arch Phys Med Rehabil,* 82(4):529-533.

Brown J, McElvenny D, Nixon J, Bainbridge J, Mason S. (2000). Some practical issues in the design, monitoring and analysis of a sequential randomized trial in pressure sore prevention. *Stat Med,* 19(24):3389-3400.

Collins N. (2002). Glutamine and wound healing. *Adv Skin Wound Care,* 15(5):233-234.

Colwell JC, Foreman MD, Trotter JP. (1993). A comparison of the efficacy and cost-effectiveness of two methods of managing pressure ulcers. *Decubitus,* 6(4):28-36.

Cooper P, Gray D. (2001). Comparison of two skin care regimes for incontinence. *Br J Nurs,* 10(6 Suppl): S6, S8, S10 passim.

Crewe RA. (1987). Problems of rubber ring nursing cushions and a clinical survey of alternative cushions for ill patients. *Care Sci Pract* 5(2):9-11.

Cullum N, Deeks J, Sheldon TA, Song F, Fletcher AW. (2000). Beds, mattresses and cushions for pressure sore prevention and treatment. *Cochrane Database Syst Rev,* (2):CD001735.

Cullum N, McInnes E, Bell-Syer SE, Legood R. (2004). Support surfaces for pressure ulcer prevention. *Cochrane Database Syst Rev,* (3):CD001735.

Darkovich SL, Brown-Etris M, Spencer M. (1990). Biofilm hydrogel dressing: A clinical evaluation in the treatment of pressure sores. *Ostomy Wound Manage,* 29:47-60.

Day A, Dombranski S, Farkas C, Foster C, Godin J, Moody M. (1995). Managing sacral pressure ulcers with hydrocolloid dressings: Results of a controlled, clinical study. *Ostomy Wound Manage,* 41(2):52-54, 56, 58 passim.

Defloor T, De Bacquer D, Grypdonck MH. (2005). The effect of various combinations of turning and pressure reducing devices on the incidence of pressure ulcers. *Int J Nurs Stud,* 42(1):37-46.

De Keyser G, Dejaeger E, De Meyst H, Eders GC. (1994). Pressure-reducing effects of heel protectors. *Adv Wound Care,* 7(4):30-32, 34.

Delmi M, Rapin CH, Bengoa JM, Delmas PD, Vasey H, Bonjour JP. (1990). Dietary supplementation in elderly patients with fractured neck of the femur. *Lancet,* 335(8696):1013-1016.

Dinsdale SM. (1973). Decubitus ulcers in swine: Light and electron microscopy study of pathogenesis. *Arch Phys Med Rehabil,* 54(2):51-56 passim.

Dinsdale SM. (1974). Decubitus ulcers: Role of pressure and friction in causation. *Arch Phys Med Rehabil,* 55(4):147-152.

Dyson R. (1978). Bed sores—the injuries hospital staff inflict on patients. *Nurs Mirror,* 146(24):30-32.

Eckman KL. (1989). The prevalence of dermal ulcers among persons in the U.S. who have died. *Decubitus,* 2(2):36-40.

Ek AC, Gustavsson G, Lewis DH. (1985). The local skin blood flow in areas at risk for pressure sores treated with massage. *Scand J Rehabil Med,* 17(2):81-86.

Exton-Smith AN, Sherwin RW. (1961). The prevention of pressure sores. Significance of spontaneous bodily movements. *Lancet,* 2(7212):1124-1126.

Flemister BG. (1991). A pilot study of interface pressure with heel protectors used for pressure reduction. *J ET Nurs,* 18(5):158-161.

Gebhardt K. (1994). Preventing pressure sores. *Elder Care,* 6(2):23-28.

Geyer M, Brienza D, Karg P, Kelsey S, Trefler E. (2001). A randomized control trial to evaluate pressure-reducing seat cushions for elderly wheelchair users. *Adv Skin Wound Care,* 14(3):120-129.

Guin P, Hudson A, Gallo J. (1991). The efficacy of six heel pressure reducing devices. *Decubitus,* 4(3):15-16, 18, 20 passim.

Gunningberg L, Lindholm C, Carlsson M, Sjödén PO. (2000). Effect of visco-elastic foam mattresses on the development of pressure ulcers in patients with hip fractures. *J Wound Care,* 9(10):455-460.

Gunningberg L, Lindholm C, Carlsson M, Sjödén PO. (2001). Reduced incidence of pressure ulcers in patients with hip fractures: A 2-year follow-up of quality indicators. *Int J Qual Health Care,* 13(5):399-407.

Harada C, Shigematsu T, Hagisawa S. (2002). The effect of 10-degree leg elevation and 30-degree head elevation on body displacement and sacral interface pressures over a 2-hour period. *J Wound Ostomy Continence Nurs,* 29(3):143-148.

Hardin JB, Cronin SN, Cahill K. (2000). Comparison of the effectiveness of two pressure-relieving surfaces: Low-air-loss versus static fluid. *Ostomy Wound Manage,* 46(9):50-56.

Hartgrink HH, Wille J, Konig P, Hermans J, Breslau PJ. (1998). Pressure sores and tube feeding in patients with a fracture of the hip: A randomized clinical trial. *Clin Nutr,* 17(6):287-292.

Hoggarth A, Waring M, Alexander J, Greenwood A, Callaghan T. (2005). A controlled, three-part trial to investigate the barrier function and skin hydration properties of six skin protectants. *Ostomy Wound Manage,* 51(12):30-42.

Hollisaz MT, Khedmat H, Yari F. (2004). A randomized clinical trial comparing hydrocolloid, phenytoin and simple dressings for the treatment of pressure ulcers [ISRCTN33429693]. *BMC Dermatol,* 4(1):18.

Hondé C, Derks C, Tudor D. (1994). Local treatment of pressure sores in the elderly: Amino acid copolymer membrane versus hydrocolloid dressings. *J Am Geriatr Soc,* 42(11):1180-1183.

Horn SD, Bender SA, Ferguson ML, Smout RJ, Bergstrom N, Taler G, et al. (2004). The National Pressure Ulcer Long-Term Care Study: Pressure ulcer development in long-term care residents. *J Am Geriatr Soc,* 52(3):359-367.

Houwing R, Rozendaal M, Wouters-Wesseling W, Beulens JW, Buskens E, Haalboom J. (2003). A randomised, double-blind assessment of the effect of nutritional supplementation on the prevention of pressure ulcers in hip-fracture patients. *Clin Nutr,* 22(4):401-405.

Hunter S, Anderson J, Hanson D, Thompson P, Langemo D, Klug MG. (2003). Clinical trial of a prevention and treatment protocol for skin breakdown in two nursing homes. *J Wound Ostomy Continence Nurs,* 30(5):250-258.

Iglesias C, Nixon J, Cranny G, Nelson EA, Hawkins K, Phillips A, et al. (2006). Pressure relieving support surfaces (PRESSURE) trial: Cost effectiveness and analysis. *BMJ,* 332(7555):1416.

Jeter KF, Lutz JB. (1996). Skin care in the frail, elderly, dependent, incontinent patient. *Adv Wound Care,* 9(1):29-34.

Jolley DJ, Wright R, McGowan S, Hickey MB, Campbell DA, Sinclair RD, et al. (2004). Preventing pressure ulcers with the Australian Medical Sheepskin: An open-label randomised controlled trial. *Med J Aust,* 180(7):324-327.

Keogh A, Dealey C. (2001). Profiling beds versus standard hospital beds: Effects on pressure ulcer incidence outcomes. *J Wound Care,* 10(2):15-19.

Knox DM, Anderson TM, Anderson PS. (1994). Effects of different turning intervals on skin of healthy older adults. *Adv Wound Care,* 7(1):48-52, 54-56.

Kuflik A, Stillo J, Sanders D, Roland K, Sweeney T, Lemke P. (2001). Petrolatum versus Resurfix ointment in the treatment of pressure ulcers. *Ostomy Wound Manage,* 47(2):52-56.

Leyden JJ, Katz S, Stewart R, Kligman AM. (1977). Urinary ammonia and ammonia-producing microorganisms in infants with and without diaper dermatitis. *Arch Dermatol,* 113(12):1678-1680.

Ljungberg S. (1998). Comparison of dextranomer paste and saline dressings for management of decubitus ulcers. *Clin Ther,* 20(4):737-743.

Maklebust J. (2005). Choosing the right support surface. *Adv Skin Wound Care,* 18(3):158-161.

Maklebust J, Sieggreen M. (2001). *Pressure ulcers: Guidelines for prevention and nursing management,* 3rd ed. Springhouse, PA: Springhouse.

Matzen S, Peschardt A, Alsbjorn B. (1999). A new amorphous hydrocolloid for the treatment of pressure sores: A randomised controlled study. *Scand J Plast Reconstr Surg Hand Surg,* 33(1):13-15.

Motta G, Dunham L, Dye T, Mentz J. (1999). Clinical efficacy and cost-effectiveness of a new synthetic polymer sheet wound dressing. *Ostomy Wound Manage,* 45(10):41, 44-46, 48-49.

Mulder GD, Altman M, Seeley JE, Tintle T. (1993). Prospective randomized study of the efficacy of hydrogel, hydrocolloid, and saline-solution moistened dressings on the management of pressure ulcers. *Wound Repair Regen,* 1(4):213-218.

Muller E, van Leen MW, Bergemann R. (2001). Economic evaluation of collagenase-containing ointment and hydrocolloid dressing in the treatment of pressure ulcers. *Pharmacoeconomics*, 19(12):1209-1216.

National Pressure Ulcer Advisory Panel. (2006). Support surface standards initiative: Terms and definitions. Wahsington D.C. Available online: http://www.npuap.org/PDF/NPUAP%20S31%20Terms%20and%20Definitions%5B1%5D.pdf. Retrieved on July 7, 2007.

Newman DK, Wallace DW, Wallace J. (2001). Moisture control and incontinence management. In Krasner D, Rodeheaver G, Sibbald G (Eds). *Chronic wound care: A clinical source book for health care professionals*, 3rd ed. Wayne, PA: HMP Communications.

Nixon J, Cranny G, Iglesias C, Nelson EA, Hawkins K, Phillips A, et al. (2006). Randomised, controlled trial of alternating pressure mattresses compared with alternating pressure overlays for the prevention of pressure ulcers: PRESSURE (pressure relieving support surfaces) trial. *BMJ*, 332(7555):1413.

Norris JR, Reynolds RE. (1971). The effect of oral zinc sulfate therapy on decubitus ulcers. *J Am Geriatr Soc*, 19:793-797.

Norton D, McLaren R, Exton-Smith AN. (1975). *An investigation of geriatric nursing problems in hospital*. London: Churchill Livingstone.

Olson B. (1989). Effects of massage for prevention of pressure ulcers. *Decubitus*, 2(4):32-37.

Ovington LG. (1999). Dressings and adjunctive therapies: AHCPR guidelines revisited. *Ostomy Wound Manage*, 45(1A Suppl):94S-106S.

Pieper B. (2007). Mechanical forces: Pressure, shear, and friction. In Bryant RA, Nix DP (Eds). *Acute and chronic wounds: Current management concepts*, 3rd ed. St. Louis: Mosby.

Pinchcofsky-Devin GD, Kaminski MV Jr. (1986). Correlation of pressure sores and nutritional status. *J Am Geriatr Soc*, 34(6):435-440.

Pinzur MS, Schumacher D, Reddy N, Osterman H, Havey R, Patwardin A. (1991). Preventing heel ulcers: A comparison of prophylactic body-support systems. *Arch Phys Med Rehabil*, 72(7):508-510.

Ratliff CR, Rodeheaver GT. (1999). Pressure ulcer assessment and management. *Lippincotts Prim Care Pract*, 3(2):242-258.

Reichel SM. (1958). Shearing force as a factor in decubitus ulcers in paraplegics. *JAMA*, 166(7):762-763.

Russell JA, Lichtenstein SL. (2000). Randomized controlled trial to determine the safety and efficacy of a multi-cell pulsating dynamic mattress system in the prevention of pressure ulcers in patients undergoing cardiovascular surgery. *Ostomy Wound Manage*, 46(2):46-51, 54-55.

Sayag J, Meaume S, Bohbot S. (1996). Healing properties of calcium alginate dressings. *J Wound Care*, 5(8):357-362.

Sebern M. (1987). Home-team strategies for treating pressure sores. *Nursing*, 17(4):50-53.

Seeley J, Jensen JL, Hutcherson J. (1999). A randomized clinical study comparing a hydrocellular dressing to a hydrocolloid dressing in the management of pressure ulcers. *Ostomy Wound Manage*, 45(6):39-44, 46-47.

Smith AM, Malone JA. (1990). Preventing pressure ulcers in institutionalized elders: Assessing the effects of small, unscheduled shifts in body position. *Decubitus*, 3(4):20-24.

Stratton RJ, Ek AC, Engfer M, Moore Z, Rigby P, et al. (2005). Enteral nutritional support in prevention and treatment of pressure ulcers: A systematic review and meta-analysis. *Ageing Res Rev*, 4(3):422-450.

Sterzi S, Selvaggi G, Romanelli A, Valente P, Bertolini C. (2003). Evaluation of prevalence and incidence of pressure ulcers and their relationship with mattresses used in a general hospital intensive care unit. *Eur J Plast Surg*, 25(7-8):401-404.

Taylor TV, Rimmer S, Day B, Butcher J, Dymock IW. (1974). Ascorbic acid supplementation in the treatment of pressure sores. *Lancet*, 2(7880):544-546.

Ter Riet G, Kessels AG, Knipschild PG. (1995). Randomized clinical trial of ascorbic acid in the treatment of pressure ulcers. *J Clin Epidemiol*, 48(12):1453-1460.

Thomas DR. (1997). Existing tools: Are they meeting the challenges of pressure ulcer healing? *Adv Wound Care*, 10(5):86-90.

Thomas DR, Goode PS, LaMaster K, Tennyson T. (1998). Acemannan hydrogel dressing versus saline dressing for pressure ulcers. A randomized, controlled trial. *Adv Wound Care*, 11(6):273-276.

Thompson P, Anderson J, Langemo D, Hanson D, Hunter S. (2005). Skin care protocol for pressure ulcers and incontinence in long-term care: a quasi-experimental study. *Adv Skin Wound Care*, 18(8):422-429.

Tymec AC, Pieper B, Vollman K. (1997). A comparison of two pressure-relieving devices on the prevention of heel pressure ulcers. *Adv Wound Care*, 10(1):39-44.

RCT = Randomized Controlled (Clinical) Trial, **NIC** = Nursing Interventions Classification, **NOC** = Nursing Outcomes Classification

Vanderwee K, Grypdonck MH, Defloor T. (2005). Effectiveness of an alternating pressure air mattress for the prevention of pressure ulcer. *Age Ageing,* 34(3):261-267.

Vyhlidal SK, Moxness D, Bosak KS, Van Meter FG, Bergstrom N. (1997). Mattress replacement or foam overlay? A prospective study on the incidence of pressure ulcers. *Appl Nurs Res,* 10(3):111-120.

Warshaw E, Nix D, Kula J, Markon CE. (2002). Clinical and cost effectiveness of a cleanser protectant lotion for treatment of perineal skin breakdown in low-risk patients with incontinence. *Ostomy Wound Manage,* 48(6):44-51.

Whittemore R. (1998). Pressure reduction support surfaces: A review of the literature. *J Wound Ostomy Continence Nurs,* 25(1):6-25.

Wound Ostomy Continence Nursing (WOCN). (2003). *Guideline for prevention and management of pressure ulcers.* Glenview, IL: WOCN.

Xakellis GC, Chrischilles EA. (1992). Hydrocolloid versus saline-gauze dressings in treating pressure ulcers: A cost-effectiveness analysis. *Arch Phys Med Rehabil,* 73(5):463-469.

Yastrub DJ. (2004). Relationship between type of treatment and degree of wound healing among institutionalized geriatric patients with stage II pressure ulcers. *Care Manag J,* 5(4):213-218.

Zimmerer RE, Lawson KD, Calvert CJ. (1986). The effects of wearing diapers on skin. *Pediatr Dermatol,* 3(2):95-101.

PRESSURE ULCER CARE STAGE II

Karen Zulkowski, DNS, RN, CWS; Elizabeth A. Ayello, PhD, RN, APRN-BC, FAPWCA, FAAN

Definition: The facilitation of healing of a stage II pressure ulcer.

A pressure ulcer is a localized wound that develops over bony prominences as a result of excessive pressure and that leads to ischemia, necrosis, and, eventually, skin ulceration (NPUAP, 2003).

A stage II pressure ulcer is a partial-thickness skin loss that involves the epidermis, the dermis, or both. The ulcer is superficial, and it presents clinically as an abrasion, a blister, or a shallow crater. Pressure ulcer treatment must be individualized for each person. It includes the proper cleansing of the wound, the application of dressings, and pressure redistribution and positioning, and it may involve other therapeutic modalities.

NURSING ACTIVITIES

Effective

■ *Reduce the risk of developing additional pressure ulcers and use pressure-relieving activities to help the existing pressure ulcer heal.* **LOE = I**

(Refer to the guideline on Pressure Ulcer Prevention.)

Wound Cleansing

■ *Cleanse the wound to remove debris and contaminants from the wound without damaging healthy tissue using water, saline, or a noncytotoxic wound cleanser at each dressing change.* **LOE = I**

 A Cochrane review identified three studies that addressed the cleansing of pressure ulcers. One noted a statistically significant improvement in pressure ulcer healing for wounds that were cleansed with saline spray that contained aloe vera, silver chloride, and decyl glucoside (Vulnopur) as compared with isotonic saline solution. Overall, there was not good evidence

NR = Nursing Research, **MR** = Multidisciplinary Research, **SP** = Standard of Practice, **EO** = Expert Opinion, **LOE** = Level of Evidence

to support the use of any particular wound cleansing solution or technique for pressure ulcers (Moore & Cowman, 2005).

(MR) An in vitro controlled study of the toxicity of skin and wound cleansers demonstrated that Shur-Clens, Saf-Clens, and saline were the least toxic to fibroblasts and that Biolex, Shur-Clens, and Techni-Care were the least toxic to keratinocytes. Both fibroblasts and keratinocytes are needed for tissue repair to occur in wounds (Wilson et al., 2005).

Wound Dressing

Dressings that are appropriate for stage II wounds include transparent films, hydrocolloid dressings, hydrogels, and foams. The dressing should be chosen on the basis of wound characteristics rather than just the stage of the wound. Modern wound dressings are more effective than gauze dressings. If the wound is infected, only silver-impregnated dressings should be used (Baranoski & Ayello, 2007).

■ *Use transparent films (e.g., Tegaderm, Op-site, Bioclusive) to dress wounds.*
LOE = II

(EO) Transparent dressings create a moist healing environment for granulating wounds as a result of trapped moisture (Baranoski & Ayello, 2007).

(NR) A random convenience sample ($N = 44$) of stage II pressure ulcers showed that polymeric membrane dressings were more effective than antibiotic ointment and dry sterile gauze dressings (Yastrub, 2004).

■ *Use hydrocolloid dressings (Duoderm) to dress wounds.* **LOE = I**

(EO) Hydrocolloid dressings consist of absorptive ingredients (typically carboxymethylcellulose, pectin, or gelatin) that are used as a primary dressing for partial-thickness pressure ulcers, and they are also used as a preventive dressing (Baranoski & Ayello, 2007).

(MR) An RCT ($N = 65$) of stage II and III pressure ulcers showed similar ulcer healing for both hydrocolloid and topical collagen treatments, with an 8-week complete healing rate for the hydrocolloid dressings of 50% (Graumlich et al., 2003).

(MR) An RCT ($N = 83$) of patients with spinal cord injuries with stage I or II pressure ulcers that compared hydrocolloid, phenytoin cream, and gauze dressings found that hydrocolloid was a more effective treatment (Hollisaz et al., 2004).

(MR) A meta-analysis of 21 peer-reviewed, published, randomized quasi-experimental and controlled clinical trials showed moderate superiority of hydrocolloid dressings as compared with conventional dressings with regard to size efficacy for pressure ulcer treatment (Bouza et al., 2005).

(MR) A randomized convenience sample ($N = 40$) showed no difference in healing, odor, or pain between hydrocolloid and foam dressings (Seeley et al., 1999).

■ *Use hydrogel (e.g., Carrington) to dress wounds.* **LOE = II**

(EO) A water- or glycerin-based product that is usually clear or translucent in color and that varies in viscosity or thickness is used for stage II, III, and IV pressure ulcers and necrotic wounds. These hydrogels are nonadherent to the wound base, and they maintain a moist wound environment on a clean, healthy, granulating wound (Baranoski & Ayello, 2007).

(NR) A randomized pilot study ($N = 10$) of stage II and III pressure ulcers showed that polymer hydrogel dressings may be a favorable alternative to hydrocolloid dressings (Motta et al., 1999).

RCT = Randomized Controlled (Clinical) Trial, **NIC** = Nursing Interventions Classification, **NOC** = Nursing Outcomes Classification

(MR) An RCT (*N* = 26) of noninfected stage II, III, and IV pressure ulcers found that hydrogel reduced the healing time of pressure ulcers as compared with wet saline compresses (Matzen et al., 1999).

■ *Use a hydrogel dressing with aloe vera to dress wounds.* **LOE = II**

(EO) A review indicated that hydrogel dressings were as effective as saline gauze dressings for stage II, III, and IV pressure ulcers (Baranoski & Ayello, 2007).

(MR) An RCT (*N* = 41) demonstrated that a hydrogel dressing with aloe vera was equal to but not superior to a saline moist gauze dressing (Thomas et al., 1998).

■ *Use foam dressings (e.g., Lyofoam) to dress wounds.* **LOE = II**

(EO) Foam dressings rely on exudate to achieve an optimum healing environment. They are used for partial-thickness wounds with heavy drainage and for surgical wounds, and they are used under compression wraps (Baranoski & Ayello, 2007).

(MR) A retrospective descriptive study of 5 years (*N* = 1891 people with 4200 wounds) of patients with stage II and III pressure ulcers in 30 nursing homes showed that most chronic wounds that were treated with either adhesive hydrocellular foam or soft silicone foam dressing healed in approximately 70 days (Viamontes et al., 2003).

(MR) A prospective, multicenter trial (*N* = 32) of stage II and III pressure ulcers compared a foam dressing with a contact layer and a foam dressing without a contact layer. It was found that the dressing with the contact layer was less likely to delaminate, that it handled exudate better, and that it was more comfortable (Amione et al., 2005).

(MR) A case study (*N* = 6) of venous leg or pressure ulcers showed that foam was both effective and comfortable (Charles et al., 2004).

(MR) A prospective, randomized, stratified, parallel group study (*N* = 39) of stage II and III pressure ulcers showed that adhesive foam was easier to remove but that otherwise outcomes were similar to those of hydrocolloid (Seeley et al., 1999).

(MR) An RCT of elderly patients with skin tears demonstrated better healing with a foam dressing as compared with a transparent film dressing (Thomas et al., 1999).

Possibly Effective

No applicable published research was found in this category.

Not Effective

■ *Using dry gauze directly on wounds.* **LOE = I**

(MR) A meta-analysis of 21 peer-reviewed, published, randomized quasi-experimental and controlled clinical trials showed moderate superiority of hydrocolloid dressings as compared with conventional dressings with regard to size efficacy for pressure ulcer treatment (Bouza et al., 2005).

(NR) A random convenience sample (*N* = 44) of stage II pressure ulcers showed that polymeric membrane dressings were more effective than antibiotic ointment and dry sterile gauze dressings (Yastrub, 2004).

Possibly Harmful

■ *Using the cleansing agent betadine (povidone-iodine) or betadine ointment.* **LOE = III**

NR = Nursing Research, **MR** = Multidisciplinary Research, **SP** = Standard of Practice, **EO** = Expert Opinion, **LOE** = Level of Evidence

(MR) In a controlled laboratory study of the use of betadine and Elase on wounds, the use of betadine resulted in reduced functional capillary density and decreased arteriolar diameters; the use of Elase resulted in capillary flow, and arteriolar diameters were significantly increased (Peter et al., 2002).

Using concentrated hydrogen peroxide to cleanse wounds. LOE = VII

(EO) A review of hydrogen peroxide use stated that hydrogen peroxide can cause a cytotoxic effect to the wound and that this may include inflammation and blistering after contact with skin. When it is used to irrigate wounds in a closed body cavity, hydrogen peroxide can result in gas embolism from the release of oxygen (Watt et al., 2004).

Massaging skin over bony prominences. LOE = IV

(NR) A study using a convenience sample ($N = 20$) found that extended massage over bony prominences resulted in a significantly lower skin temperature than standard massage (Olson, 1989).

(MR) A cohort study demonstrated that massage over bony prominences with skin discoloration resulted in a lower skin blood flow than was present before massage (Ek et al., 1985).

(MR) Postmortem biopsies documented macerated, degenerated tissue in areas that had been exposed to massage that were not documented on individuals that were not massaged individuals (Dyson, 1978).

OUTCOME MEASUREMENT

SKIN INTEGRITY

Definition: Re-establishment of intact skin.

Skin Integrity as evidenced by the following indicators:

- Intact skin
- Skin that is without redness or nonblanchable erythema
- Skin that is free of purulent drainage, odor, or other signs of infection
- Involved area kept free of pressure and moisture

(Rate each indicator of **Skin Integrity:** 1 = severely compromised, 2 = substantially compromised, 3 = moderately compromised, 4 = mildly compromised, 5 = not compromised.) (Note: This is not a NOC outcome.)

REFERENCES

Amione P, Ricci E, Topo F, Izzo L, Pirovano R, Rega V, et al. (2005). Comparison of Allevyn Adhesive and Biatain Adhesive in the management of pressure ulcers. *J Wound Care,* 14(8):365-370.

Baranoski S, Ayello E. (2007). *Wound care essentials: Practice principles.* Philadelphia: Lippincott Williams & Wilkins.

Bouza C, Saz Z, Munoz A, Amate JM. (2005). Efficacy of advanced dressings in the treatment of pressure ulcers: A systematic review. *J Wound Care,* 14(5):193-199.

Charles H, Corser R, Varrow S, Hart J. (2004). A non-adhesive foam dressing for exuding venous leg ulcers and pressure ulcers: Six case studies. *J Wound Care,* 13(2):58-62.

Dyson R. (1978). Bed sores—the injuries hospital staff inflict on patients. *Nurs Mirror,* 146(24):30-32.

Ek AC, Gustavsson G, Lewis DH. (1985). The local skin blood flow in areas at risk for pressure sores treated with massage. *Scand J Rehabil Med,* 17(2):81-86.

RCT = Randomized Controlled (Clinical) Trial, **NIC** = Nursing Interventions Classification, **NOC** = Nursing Outcomes Classification

Graumlich JF, Blough LS, McLaughlin RG, Milbrandt JC, Calderon CL, Agha SA, et al. (2003). Healing pressure ulcers with collagen or hydrocolloid: A randomized, controlled trial. *J Am Geriatr Soc,* 51(2): 147-154.

Hollisaz MT, Khedmat H, Yari F. (2004). A randomized clinical trial comparing hydrocolloid, phenytoin and simple dressings for the treatment of pressure ulcers [ISRCTN33429693]. *BMC Dermatol,* 4(1): 18.

Matzen S, Peschardt A, Alsbjorn B. (1999). A new amorphous hydrocolloid for the treatment of pressure sores: A randomised controlled study. *Scand J Plast Reconstr Surg Hand Surg,* 33(1):13-15.

Moore ZE, Cowman S. (2005). Wound cleansing for pressure ulcers. *Cochrane Database Syst Rev,* (4): CD004983.

Motta G, Dunham L, Dye T, Mentz J, O'Connell-Gifford E, Smith E. (1999). Clinical efficacy and cost-effectiveness of a new synthetic polymer sheet wound dressing. *Ostomy Wound Manage,* 45(10):41, 44-46, 48-49.

National Pressure Ulcer Advisory Panel (NPUAP). (2003). NPUAP staging report. Available online: http://www.npuap.org. Retrieved on July 13, 2007.

Olson B. (1989). Effects of massage for prevention of pressure ulcers. *Decubitus,* 2(4):32-37.

Peter FW, Li-Peuser H, Vogt PM, Muehlberger T, Homann HH, Steinau HU. (2002). The effect of wound ointments on tissue microcirculation and leucocyte behaviour. *Clin Exp Dermatol,* 27(1):51-55.

Seeley J, Jensen JL, Hutcherson J. (1999). A randomized clinical study comparing a hydrocellular dressing to a hydrocolloid dressing in the management of pressure ulcers. *Ostomy Wound Manage,* 45(6):39-44, 46-47.

Thomas DR, Goode PS, LaMaster K, Tennyson T. (1998). Acemannan hydrogel dressing versus saline dressing for pressure ulcers. A randomized, controlled trial. *Adv Wound Care,* 11(6):273-276.

Thomas DR, Goode PS, LaMaster K, Tennyson T, Parnell LK. (1999). A comparison of an opaque foam dressing versus a transparent film dressing in the management of skin tears in institutionalized subjects. *Ostomy Wound Manage,* 45(6):22-24, 27-28.

Viamontes L, Temple D, Wytall D, Walker A. (2003). An evaluation of an adhesive hydrocellular foam dressing and a self-adherent soft silicone foam dressing in a nursing home setting. *Ostomy Wound Manage,* 49(8):48-52, 54-56, 58.

Watt BE, Proudfoot AT, Vale JA. (2004). Hydrogen peroxide poisoning. *Toxicol Rev,* 23(1):51-57.

Wilson JR, Mills JG, Prather ID, Dimitrijevich SD. (2005). A toxicity index of skin and wound cleansers used on in vitro fibroblasts and keratinocytes. *Adv Skin Wound Care,* 18(7):373-378.

Yastrub DJ. (2004). Relationship between type of treatment and degree of wound healing among institutionalized geriatric patients with stage II pressure ulcers. *Care Manag J,* 5(4):213-218.

 # PRESSURE ULCER CARE STAGE III

Karen Zulkowski, DNS, RN, CWS; Elizabeth A. Ayello, PhD, RN, APRN-BC, FAPWCA, FAAN

Definition: The facilitation of healing of a stage III pressure ulcer.

A pressure ulcer is a localized wound that develops over bony prominences as a result of excessive pressure and that leads to ischemia, necrosis, and, eventually, skin ulceration (NPUAP, 2003). A stage III pressure ulcer is a full-thickness skin loss that involves damage to or necrosis of subcutaneous tissue that may extend down to (but not through) underlying fascia. The ulcer presents clinically as a deep crater with or without the undermining of adjacent tissue. Pressure ulcer treatment must be individualized for each person. It includes the proper cleansing of the wound, the application of dressings, and pressure redistribution and positioning, and it may involve other therapeutic modalities.

NR = Nursing Research, **MR** = Multidisciplinary Research, **SP** = Standard of Practice, **EO** = Expert Opinion, **LOE** = Level of Evidence

NURSING ACTIVITIES

Effective

■ *Reduce the risk of the development of additional pressure ulcers.*

(Refer to the guideline on Pressure Ulcer Prevention.)

■ *If the wound is painful, use eutectic mixture of local anesthetics (EMLA) cream for at least 20 minutes before cleansing, debriding, or dressing the wound.* **LOE = I**

(NR) A systematic review found that research findings supported the use of topical analgesic EMLA cream applied to the wound bed for the chronic pain associated with the treatment of the wound (Evans & Gray, 2005).

(MR) A Cochrane review found that EMLA cream was effective in decreasing pain with the debridement of venous leg ulcers (Briggs & Nelson, 2003).

Wound Cleansing

■ *Cleanse the wound to remove debris and contaminants from the wound without damaging healthy tissue using water, saline, or a noncytotoxic wound cleanser at each dressing change.* **LOE = II**

(MR) A Cochrane review identified three studies that addressed the cleansing of pressure ulcers. One noted a statistically significant improvement in pressure ulcer healing for wounds that were cleansed with saline spray that contained aloe vera, silver chloride, and decyl glucoside (Vulnopur) as compared with isotonic saline solution. Overall, the research evidence did not support the use of any particular wound cleansing solution or technique for pressure ulcers (Moore & Cowman, 2005).

(MR) An in vitro controlled study of the toxicity of skin and wound cleansers demonstrated that Shur-Clens, Saf-Clens, and saline were the least toxic to fibroblasts and that Biolex, Shur-Clens, and Techni-Care were the least toxic to keratinocytes. Both fibroblasts and keratinocytes are needed for tissue repair to occur in wounds (Wilson et al., 2005).

■ *Use pressure irrigation to remove microbes and debris at pressures between 8 and 15 psi (13 psi is recommended) to cleanse wounds.* **LOE = II**

(NR) A systematic review from the Joanna Briggs Institute recommended 13 psi for irrigation pressure for adults and children with traumatic wounds on the basis of one RCT with a sample size of 335 and significant reductions in inflammation and infection. Another RCT with 208 patients found similar infection rates (1% and 4%, not significant) with two irrigation devices that delivered the solution in less than 4 minutes and with 1.5 and 2 psi. The amount and rate of irrigation still need to be studied (Fernandez et al., 2002).

(EO) An international expert panel summarized the best practices for wound care and recommended irrigation pressures of 8 to 15 psi (Schultz et al., 2003).

(EO) Wound care experts recommend a 30-mL syringe and a 19-gauge needle to achieve sufficient pressure (8 psi) for effective irrigation; 60 mL per cm of wound length is one suggestion for the amount of irrigating fluid, although this requires further study (Howell & Chisholm, 1997).

RCT = Randomized Controlled (Clinical) Trial, **NIC** = Nursing Interventions Classification, **NOC** = Nursing Outcomes Classification

■ *Use Vulnopur (a saline spray that contains aloe vera, silver chloride, and decyl glucoside) for effective pressure ulcer wound cleansing.* **LOE = II**

(NR) A systematic review cautiously recommended Vulnopur on the basis of an RCT with 133 patients and improved wound healing using a valid and reliable tool (Moore & Cowman, 2005).

Wound Dressing

Dressings appropriate for stage III wounds include transparent films, hydrocolloid dressings, hydrogels, and foams. Modern wound dressings are more appropriate than gauze dressings. If the wound is infected, only silver-impregnated dressings should be used.

■ *Use transparent films (e.g., Tegaderm, Op-site, Bioclusive) to dress wounds.* **LOE = II**

(EO) Transparent dressings allow for the autolytic debridement of necrotic wounds and for the creation of a moist healing environment for granulating wounds as a result of trapped moisture (Baranoski & Ayello, 2007).

(NR) A random convenience sample ($N = 44$) of stage II pressure ulcers showed that polymeric membrane dressing was more effective than antibiotic ointment and dry sterile gauze dressings (Yastrub, 2004).

■ *Use hydrocolloid dressings (Duoderm) to dress wounds.* **LOE = II**

(EO) Hydrocolloid dressings consist of absorptive ingredients (typically carboxymethylcellulose, pectin, or gelatin) that are used as secondary dressings for full-thickness pressure ulcers as well as for granulating or necrotic wounds (Baranoski & Ayello, 2007).

(MR) An RCT ($N = 65$) of stage II and III pressure ulcers showed similar ulcer healing for both hydrocolloid and topical collagen treatments, with an 8-week complete healing rate for the hydrocolloid dressings of 50% (Graumlich et al., 2003).

(MR) A meta-analysis of 21 peer-reviewed, published, randomized quasi-experimental and controlled clinical trials showed moderate superiority of hydrocolloid dressings as compared with conventional dressings with regard to size efficacy for pressure ulcer treatment (Bouza et al., 2005).

(MR) A randomized convenience sample ($N = 40$) showed no difference in healing, odor, or pain between hydrocolloid and foam dressings (Seeley et al., 1999).

■ *Use hydrogel (e.g., Carrington) to dress wounds.* **LOE = II**

(EO) A water- or glycerin-based product that is usually clear or translucent in color and that varies in viscosity or thickness is used for stage II, III, and IV pressure ulcers and necrotic wounds. These hydrogels are nonadherent to the wound base, and they maintain a moist wound environment on a clean, healthy, granulating wound (Baranoski & Ayello, 2007).

(NR) An RCT using a convenience sample ($N = 50$) of people with necrotic pressure ulcers found that hydrogels were effective for debridement, regardless of the manufacturer (Bale et al., 1998).

(NR) A randomized pilot study ($N = 10$) of stage II and III pressure ulcers showed that polymer hydrogel dressings may be a favorable alternative to hydrocolloid dressings (Motta et al., 1999).

NR = Nursing Research, **MR** = Multidisciplinary Research, **SP** = Standard of Practice, **EO** = Expert Opinion, **LOE** = Level of Evidence

(MR) An RCT ($N = 26$) of noninfected stage II, III, and IV pressure ulcers found that hydrogel reduced the healing time of pressure ulcers as compared with wet saline compresses (Matzen et al., 1999).

▪ *Use hydrogel dressing with aloe vera to dress wounds.* **LOE = II**

(MR) An RCT ($N = 41$) demonstrated that a hydrogel dressing with aloe vera was equal to but not superior to saline-moistened gauze (Thomas et al., 1998).

▪ *Use foam dressings (e.g., Lyofoam) to dress wounds.* **LOE = II**

(EO) Foam dressings rely on exudate to achieve an optimum healing environment. They are used for full-thickness wounds with heavy drainage, stage IV pressure ulcers, and surgical wounds, and they are used under compression wraps (Baranoski & Ayello, 2007).

(MR) A retrospective descriptive study of 5 years ($N = 1891$ people with 4200 wounds) of patients with stage II and III pressure ulcers in 30 nursing homes showed that most chronic wounds that were treated with either adhesive hydrocellular foam or soft silicone foam dressing healed in approximately 70 days (Viamontes et al., 2003).

(MR) A prospective, multicenter trial ($N = 32$) of stage II and III pressure ulcers compared a foam dressing with a contact layer and a foam dressing without a contact layer. It was found that the dressing with the contact layer was less likely to delaminate, that it handled exudate better, and that it was more comfortable (Amione et al., 2005).

(MR) A case study ($N = 6$) of venous leg or pressure ulcers showed that foam was both effective and comfortable (Charles et al., 2004).

(MR) A prospective, randomized, stratified, parallel group study ($N = 39$) of stage II and III pressure ulcers showed that adhesive foam was easier to remove but that otherwise outcomes were similar to those of hydrocolloid (Seeley et al., 1999).

▪ *Use calcium alginate dressings (e.g., Sorbsan, Kaltostat) to dress wounds.* **LOE = III**

(EO) Calcium alginate dressing is a highly absorptive dressing that is made from brown seaweed and that acts via an ion exchange mechanism, absorbing the serous fluid or exudate that forms a hydrophilic gel and conforms to the shape of the wound. It is used for full-thickness wounds, stage III and IV pressure ulcers that have moderate to heavy drainage, and dermal and surgical wounds. It is indicated for moderate to heavily exuding wounds and moist wounds with slough, and it is capable of absorbing up to 20 times its own weight in fluid (Baranoski & Ayello, 2007).

(MR) A randomized, multicenter, parallel group trial ($N = 110$) of older adults with stage III and IV pressure ulcers showed faster healing with calcium alginate dressings among frail older adults (Belmin et al., 2002).

▪ *Use silver dressings to dress wounds that have signs of infection.* **LOE = III**

(EO) Silver dressings are used for any type of infected wound. They are also used when there is a need to reduce the risk of infection or to decrease the bacterial burden of a wound (Baranoski & Ayello, 2007).

(MR) A study of a randomized, multicenter stratified parallel group ($N = 99$) with pressure ulcers ($N = 28$) and venous leg ulcers ($N = 71$) suggested that silver-releasing hydroalginate dressings may be effective for wounds with a high risk of infection (Meaume et al., 2005).

RCT = Randomized Controlled (Clinical) Trial, **NIC** = Nursing Interventions Classification, **NOC** = Nursing Outcomes Classification

(EO) Topical silver dressings provide an excellent reduction of bacteria in wounds, and they may also decrease wound pain (Tomaselli, 2006).

■ *Use combination dressings to dress wounds.* LOE = II

(EO) Sequential treatment with calcium alginate and hydrocolloid dressings is more effective for debridement and healing than hydrocolloid alone for older people (Baranoski & Ayello, 2007).

(MR) A randomized, multicenter, parallel group trial ($N = 110$) of older adults with stage III and IV pressure ulcers showed faster healing with combination dressings among frail older adults (Belmin et al., 2002).

■ *Use collagen/collagenase dressings to dress wounds.* LOE = II

(EO) Collagen dressings, which are available as sheets, pads, particles, and gels, consist of predominately type I collagen with small amounts of type II and type IV fibers. These dressings enhance granulation, reduce pain, and promote healing (Baranoski & Ayello, 2007).

(MR) An RCT ($N = 65$) of patients with stage II or III pressure ulcers showed similar ulcer healing for both hydrocolloid and topical collagen treatment, with an 8-week complete healing rate for the collagen paste of 51% (Graumlich et al., 2003).

(MR) A prospective randomized trial using a convenience sample ($N = 24$) of hospital patients with stage IV pressure ulcers on the heel found that collagenase ointment cost 5% less than hydrocolloid treatment and that it healed wounds in 10 weeks (as compared with 14 weeks for hydrocolloid treatment; Muller et al., 2001).

■ *Use growth factors for wound healing.* LOE = II

(EO) Nerve growth factors stimulate the growth and differentiation of epithelialization for wound healing (Baranoski & Ayello, 2007).

(MR) A 12-month follow-up for a 35-day placebo-controlled trial ($N = 61$) showed that long-term outcomes were better for those patients who received growth factors (Payne et al., 2001).

(MR) In a randomized, double-blind, placebo-controlled trial of a convenience sample ($N = 36$) of nursing home patients with foot ulcers, half received nerve growth factors, and half received "conventional therapy." The study found that, at 6 weeks, the nerve growth factor group had a significantly greater reduction in ulcer size (Landi et al., 2003).

■ *Use vacuum (VAC) therapy for wound healing.* LOE = II

(EO) VAC therapy is the application of a controlled level of subatmospheric pressure to a wound at 50 mm Hg to 175 mm Hg that is generated by a portable programmable pump. The suction effect is applied to the entire interior surface of a clean wound through open-cell polyurethane or polyvinyl alcohol foam. VAC therapy is effective for healing full-thickness stage III and IV pressure ulcers (Baranoski & Ayello, 2007).

(MR) A randomized convenience sample ($N = 22$ patients) with 35 stage II, III, and IV pressure ulcers showed that VAC was more effective for healing than wound gel products were (Ford et al., 2002).

(MR) A randomized convenience sample ($N = 22$) of patients showed similar results between a VAC therapy group and a group using wet-to-dry/wet-to-wet gauze soaked in Ringer's solution (Wanner et al., 2003).

NR = Nursing Research, **MR** = Multidisciplinary Research, **SP** = Standard of Practice, **EO** = Expert Opinion, **LOE** = Level of Evidence

(MR) An RCT of patients ($N = 65$) with acute or chronic wounds received either VAC-assisted closure or modern wound dressings. Results indicated no significant difference in time to wound closure, except among patients with cardiovascular disease and diabetes, in whom wounds did heal faster with VAC therapy. Patients who underwent VAC therapy experienced less pain, and the time of nursing care was reduced (Braakenburg et al., 2006).

■ *Use radiant heat with the application of moist, warm topical dressings for wound healing.* **LOE = II**

(EO) Radiant heat will improve rates of wound healing in stage III and IV pressure ulcers (Baranoski & Ayello, 2007).

(MR) In an RCT ($N = 40$ patients with 43 stage II, III, and IV pressure ulcers), noncontact normothermic wound therapy provided significantly faster healing than moist retentive dressings (Kloth et al., 2000).

(MR) In a convenience sample ($N = 14$ patients with 15 stage III and IV pressure ulcers), results showed that wounds treated with radiant heat healed significantly faster than those treated with standard care (Kloth et al., 2002).

(NR) In a prospective single-site randomized trial ($N = 50$), patients treated with radiant heat demonstrated an accelerated rate of healing (Price et al., 2000).

(MR) A randomized convenience sample ($N = 41$) of stage II, III, and IV pressure ulcers did not show significantly different healing rates between the radiant-heat method and hydrocolloid dressings (Thomas et al., 2005).

Possibly Effective

■ *Use honey dressings for wound healing.* **LOE = IV**

(EO) Honey is an ancient remedy that is effective for treating wounds that are infected and for reducing odor, debriding, and healing wounds (Baranoski & Ayello, 2007).

(NR) A case study ($N = 2$) using honey-impregnated alginate gauze demonstrated the effective treatment of full-thickness or necrotic wounds (Van der Weyden, 2003).

Not Effective

■ *Using dry gauze directly on wounds.* **LOE = I**

(MR) A meta-analysis of 21 peer-reviewed, published, randomized quasi-experimental and controlled clinical trials showed moderate superiority of hydrocolloid dressings as compared with conventional dressings with regard to size efficacy for pressure ulcer treatment (Bouza et al., 2005).

(NR) A random convenience sample ($N = 44$) of stage II pressure ulcers showed that polymeric membrane dressings were more effective than antibiotic ointment and dry sterile gauze dressings (Yastrub, 2004).

Possibly Harmful

■ *Using concentrated hydrogen peroxide to cleanse wounds.* **LOE = VII**

(MR) A review of hydrogen peroxide use stated that hydrogen peroxide can cause a cytotoxic effect to the wound and that this may include inflammation and blistering after contact with skin. When it is used to irrigate wounds in a closed body cavity, hydrogen peroxide can result in gas embolism from the release of oxygen (Watt et al., 2004).

■ *Using high pressure for wound irrigation (≥20 psi), with or without pulsatile lavage.* **LOE = IV**

(MR) A case-control study in a 1000-bed hospital concluded that an infectious outbreak among 11 patients within 2 months was associated with pulsatile lavage therapy. Infection control precautions are needed with lavage therapy (Maragakis et al., 2004).

(MR) A narrative review cautioned about the use of high-pressure pulsatile lavage for all types of wounds and recommended the Agency for Health Care Policy and Research guideline pressures of 4 to 15 psi for wound irrigation. Early studies support pulsatile lavage for wound cleansing, but more RCTs are needed (Luedtke-Hoffmann & Schafer, 2000).

■ *Using the cleansing agent betadine (povidone-iodine) or betadine ointment.* **LOE = III**

(MR) In a controlled animal study of the use of betadine and Elase on wounds, the use of betadine resulted in reduced functional capillary density and decreased arteriolar diameters; the use of Elase resulted in capillary flow, and arteriolar diameters were significantly increased (Peter et al., 2002).

■ *Massaging skin over bony prominences.* **LOE = IV**

(NR) A study using a convenience sample ($N = 20$) found that extended massage over bony prominences resulted in a significantly lower skin temperature than standard massage (Olson, 1989).

(MR) A cohort study demonstrated that massage over bony prominences with skin discoloration resulted in a lower skin blood flow than was present before massage (Ek et al., 1985).

(MR) Postmortem biopsies documented macerated, degenerated tissue in areas that had been exposed to massage that were not documented on individuals that were not massaged individuals (Dyson, 1978).

OUTCOME MEASUREMENT

SKIN AND TISSUE INTEGRITY

Definition: Re-establishment of intact skin and tissues in the area in which the epidermis and dermis are no longer intact.
Skin and Tissue Integrity as evidenced by the following indicators:
- Intact skin
- Wound is decreasing in size
- Formation of granulation tissue
- Skin is without redness or nonblanchable erythema
- Wound is free of purulent drainage, odor, or other signs of infection
- Involved area is kept free of pressure and moisture

(Rate each indicator of **Skin and Tissue Integrity:** 1 = severely compromised, 2 = substantially compromised, 3 = moderately compromised, 4 = mildly compromised, 5 = not compromised.) (Note: This is not a NOC outcome.)

NR = Nursing Research, **MR** = Multidisciplinary Research, **SP** = Standard of Practice, **EO** = Expert Opinion, **LOE** = Level of Evidence

REFERENCES

Amione P, Ricci E, Topo F, Izzo L, Pirovano R, Rega V, et al. (2005). Comparison of Allevyn Adhesive and Biatain Adhesive in the management of pressure ulcers. *J Wound Care,* 14(8):365-370.

Bale S, Banks V, Haglestein S, Harding KG. (1998). A comparison of two amorphous hydrogels in the debridement of pressure sores. *J Wound Care,* 7(2):65-68.

Baranoski S, Ayello E. (2007). *Wound care essentials: Practice principles.* Philadelphia: Lippincott Williams & Wilkins.

Belmin J, Meaume S, Rabus MT, Bohbot S; Investigators of the Sequential Treatment of the Elderly with Pressure Sores (STEPS) Trial. (2002). Sequential treatment with calcium alginate dressings and hydrocolloid dressings accelerates pressure ulcer healing in older subjects: A multicenter randomized trial of sequential versus nonsequential treatment with hydrocolloid dressings alone. *J Am Geriatr Soc,* 50(2):269-274.

Bouza C, Saz Z, Munoz A, Amate JM. (2005). Efficacy of advanced dressings in the treatment of pressure ulcers: A systematic review. *J Wound Care,* 14(5):193-199.

Braakenburg A, Obdeijn MC, Feitz R, van Rooij IA, van Griethuysen AJ, Klinkenbijl JH. (2006). The clinical efficacy and cost effectiveness of the vacuum-assisted closure technique in the management of acute and chronic wounds: A randomized controlled trial. *Plast Reconstr Surg,* 118(2): 390-397.

Briggs M, Nelson EA. (2003). Topical agents or dressings for pain in venous leg ulcers. *Cochrane Database Syst Rev,* (1):CD001177.

Charles H, Corser R, Varrow S, Hart J. (2004). A non-adhesive foam dressing for exuding venous leg ulcers and pressure ulcers: Six case studies. *J Wound Care,* 13(2):58-62.

Dyson R. (1978). Bed sores—the injuries hospital staff inflict on patients. *Nurs Mirror,* 146(24):30-32.

Ek AC, Gustavsson G, Lewis DH. (1985). The local skin blood flow in areas at risk for pressure sores treated with massage. *Scand J Rehabil Med,* 17(2):81-86.

Evans E, Gray M. (2005). Do topical analgesics reduce pain associated with wound dressing change or debridement of chronic wounds? *J Wound Ostomy Continence Nurs,* 32(5):287-290.

Fernandez R, Griffiths R, Ussia C. (2002). Water for wound cleansing. *Cochrane Database Syst Rev,* (4): CD003861.

Ford CN, Reinhard ER, Yeh D, Syrek D, De Las Morenas A, Bergman SB, et al. (2002). Interim analysis of a prospective, randomized trial of vacuum-assisted closure versus the healthpoint system in the management of pressure ulcers. *Ann Plast Surg,* 49(1):55-61.

Graumlich JF, Blough LS, McLaughlin RG, Milbrandt JC, Calderon CL, Agha SA, et al. (2003). Healing pressure ulcers with collagen or hydrocolloid: A randomized, controlled trial. *J Am Geriatr Soc,* 51(2): 147-154.

Hollisaz MT, Khedmat H, Yari F. (2004). A randomized clinical trial comparing hydrocolloid, phenytoin and simple dressings for the treatment of pressure ulcers [ISRCTN33429693]. *BMC Dermatol,* 4(1): 18.

Howell JM, Chisholm CD. (1997). Wound care. *Emerg Med Clin North Am,* 15(2):417-425.

Kloth LC, Berman JE, Dumit-Minkel S, Sutton CH, Papanek PE, Wurzel J. (2000). Effects of a normothermic dressing on pressure ulcer healing. *Adv Skin Wound Care,* 13(2):69-74.

Kloth LC, Berman JE, Nett M, Papanek PE, Dumit-Minkel S. (2002). A randomized controlled clinical trial to evaluate the effects of noncontact normothermic wound therapy on chronic full-thickness pressure ulcers. *Adv Skin Wound Care,* 15(6):270-276.

Landi F, Aloe L, Russo A, Cesari M, Onder G, Bonini S, et al. (2003). Topical treatment of pressure ulcers with nerve growth factor: A randomized clinical trial. *Ann Intern Med,* 139(8):635-641.

Luedtke-Hoffmann KA, Schafer DS. (2000). Pulsed lavage in wound cleansing. *Phys Ther,* 80(3):292-300.

Maragakis LL, Cosgrove S, Song X, Kim D, Rosenbaum P, Ciesla N, et al. (2004). An outbreak of multi-drug-resistant *Acinetobacter baumannii* associated with pulsatile lavage wound treatment. *JAMA,* 292(24):3006-3011.

Matzen S, Peschardt A, Alsbjorn B. (1999). A new amorphous hydrocolloid for the treatment of pressure sores: A randomised controlled study. *Scand J Plast Reconstr Surg Hand Surg,* 33(1):13-15.

Meaume S, Vallet D, Morere MN, Teot L. (2005). Evaluation of a silver-releasing hydroalginate dressing in chronic wounds with signs of local infection. *J Wound Care,* 14(9):411-419.

RCT = Randomized Controlled (Clinical) Trial, **NIC** = Nursing Interventions Classification, **NOC** = Nursing Outcomes Classification

Moore ZE, Cowman S. (2005). Wound cleansing for pressure ulcers. *Cochrane Database Syst Rev*, (4): CD004983.

Motta G, Dunham L, Dye T, Mentz J, O'Connell-Gifford E, Smith E. (1999). Clinical efficacy and cost-effectiveness of a new synthetic polymer sheet wound dressing. *Ostomy Wound Manage*, 45(10):41, 44-46, 48-49.

Muller E, van Leen MW, Bergemann R. (2001). Economic evaluation of collagenase-containing ointment and hydrocolloid dressing in the treatment of pressure ulcers. *Pharmacoeconomics*, 19(12): 1209-1216.

National Pressure Ulcer Advisory Panel (NPUAP). (2003). NPUAP staging report. Available online: http://www.npuap.org. Retrieved on July 13, 2007.

Olson B. (1989). Effects of massage for prevention of pressure ulcers. *Decubitus*, 2(4):32-37.

Payne WG, Ochs DE, Meltzer DD, Hill DP, Mannari RJ, Robson LE, et al. (2001). Long-term outcome study of growth factor-treated pressure ulcers. *Am J Surg*, 181(1):81-86.

Peter FW, Li-Peuser H, Vogt PM, Muehlberger T, Homann HH, Steinau HU. (2002). The effect of wound ointments on tissue microcirculation and leucocyte behaviour. *Clin Exp Dermatol*, 27(1): 51-55.

Price P, Bale S, Crook H, Harding KG. (2000). The effect of a radiant heat dressing on pressure ulcers. *J Wound Care*, 9(4):201-205.

Schultz GS, Sibbald RG, Falanga V, Ayello E, Dowsett C, Harding K, et al. (2003). Wound bed preparation: A systematic approach to wound management. *Wound Repair Regen*, 11(Suppl 1):S1-S28.

Seeley J, Jensen JL, Hutcherson J. (1999). A randomized clinical study comparing a hydrocellular dressing to a hydrocolloid dressing in the management of pressure ulcers. *Ostomy Wound Manage*, 45(6):39-44, 46-47.

Thomas DR, Diebold MR, Eggemeyer LM. (2005). A controlled, randomized, comparative study of a radiant heat bandage on the healing of stage 3-4 pressure ulcers: A pilot study. *J Am Med Dir Assoc*, 6(1):46-49.

Thomas DR, Goode PS, LaMaster K, Tennyson T. (1998). Acemannan hydrogel dressing versus saline dressing for pressure ulcers. A randomized, controlled trial. *Adv Wound Care*, 11(6):273-276.

Tomaselli N. (2006). The role of topical silver preparations in wound healing. *J Wound Ostomy Continence Nurs*, 33(4):367-378.

Van der Weyden EA. (2003). The use of honey for the treatment of two patients with pressure ulcers. *Br J Community Nurs*, 8(12):S14-S20.

Viamontes L, Temple D, Wytall D, Walker A. (2003). An evaluation of an adhesive hydrocellular foam dressing and a self-adherent soft silicone foam dressing in a nursing home setting. *Ostomy Wound Manage*, 49(8):48-52, 54-56, 58.

Wanner MB, Schwarzl F, Strub B, Zaech GA, Pierer G. (2003). Vacuum-assisted wound closure for cheaper and more comfortable healing of pressure sores: A prospective study. *Scand J Plast Reconstr Surg Hand Surg*, 37(1):28-33.

Watt BE, Proudfoot AT, Vale JA. (2004). Hydrogen peroxide poisoning. *Toxicol Rev*, 23(1):51-57.

Wilson JR, Mills JG, Prather ID, Dimitrijevich SD. (2005). A toxicity index of skin and wound cleansers used on in vitro fibroblasts and keratinocytes. *Adv Skin Wound Care*, 18(7):373-378.

Yastrub DJ. (2004). Relationship between type of treatment and degree of wound healing among institutionalized geriatric patients with stage II pressure ulcers. *Care Manag J*, 5(4):213-218.

 # PRESSURE ULCER CARE STAGE IV

Karen Zulkowski, DNS, RN, CWS; Elizabeth A. Ayello, PhD, RN, APRN-BC, FAPWCA, FAAN

Definition: The facilitation of healing of a stage IV pressure ulcer.

A pressure ulcer is a localized wound that develops over bony prominences as a result of excessive pressure and that leads to ischemia, necrosis, and, eventually, skin ulceration (NPUAP, 2003).

NR = Nursing Research, **MR** = Multidisciplinary Research, **SP** = Standard of Practice, **EO** = Expert Opinion, **LOE** = Level of Evidence

A stage IV pressure ulcer is a full-thickness skin loss that involves damage to or necrosis of subcutaneous tissue that may extend down to (but not through) underlying fascia. The ulcer presents clinically as a deep crater with or without the undermining of adjacent tissue. Pressure ulcer treatment must be individualized for each person. It includes the proper cleansing of the wound, the application of dressings, and pressure redistribution and positioning, and it may involve other therapeutic modalities.

NURSING ACTIVITIES

Effective

▧ *Reduce the risk of the development of additional pressure ulcers.*

(Refer to the guideline on Pressure Ulcer Prevention.)

▧ *If the wound is painful, use eutectic mixture of local anesthetics (EMLA) cream for at least 20 minutes before cleansing, debriding, or dressing the wound.* **LOE = I**

(NR) A systematic review found that research findings supported the use of topical analgesic EMLA applied to the wound bed for the chronic pain associated with the treatment of the wound (Evans & Gray, 2005).

(MR) A Cochrane review found that EMLA cream was effective in decreasing pain with the debridement of venous leg ulcers (Briggs & Nelson, 2003).

Wound Cleansing

▧ *Cleanse the wound to remove debris and contaminants from the wound without damaging healthy tissue using water, saline, or a noncytotoxic wound cleanser at each dressing change.* **LOE = II**

(MR) A Cochrane review identified three studies that addressed the cleansing of pressure ulcers. One noted a statistically significant improvement in pressure ulcer healing for wounds that were cleansed with saline spray that contained aloe vera, silver chloride, and decyl glucoside (Vulnopur) as compared with isotonic saline solution. Overall, the research evidence did not support the use of any particular wound cleansing solution or technique for pressure ulcers (Moore & Cowman, 2005).

(MR) An in vitro controlled study of the toxicity of skin and wound cleansers demonstrated that Shur-Clens, Saf-Clens, and saline were the least toxic to fibroblasts and that Biolex, Shur-Clens, and Techni-Care were the least toxic to keratinocytes. Both fibroblasts and keratinocytes are needed for tissue repair to occur in wounds (Wilson et al., 2005).

▧ *Use pressure irrigation to remove microbes and debris at pressures between 8 and 15 psi (13 psi is recommended) to cleanse wounds.* **LOE = II**

(NR) A systematic review from the Joanna Briggs Institute recommended 13 psi for irrigation pressure for adults and children with traumatic wounds on the basis of one RCT with a sample size of 335 and significant reductions in inflammation and infection. Another RCT with 208 patients found similar infection rates (1% and 4%, not significant) with two irrigation devices that delivered the solution in less than 4 minutes and with 1.5 and 2 psi. The amount and rate of irrigation still need to be studied (Fernandez et al., 2002).

RCT = Randomized Controlled (Clinical) Trial, **NIC** = Nursing Interventions Classification, **NOC** = Nursing Outcomes Classification

(EO) An international expert panel summarized best practices for wound care and recommended irrigation pressures of 8 to 15 psi (Schultz et al., 2003).

(EO) Wound care experts recommend a 30-mL syringe and a 19-gauge needle to achieve sufficient pressure (8 psi) for effective irrigation; 60 mL per cm of wound length is one suggestion for the amount of irrigating fluid, although this requires further study (Howell & Chisholm, 1997).

■ *Use Vulnopur (a saline spray that contains aloe vera, silver chloride, and decyl glucoside) for effective pressure ulcer wound cleansing.* **LOE = II**

(NR) A systematic review cautiously recommended Vulnopur on the basis of an RCT with 133 patients and improved wound healing using a valid and reliable tool (Moore & Cowman, 2005).

Wound Dressing

Dressings appropriate for stage IV wounds include hydrogels, foams, calcium alginate, transparent films, and hydrocolloid dressings. Modern wound dressings are more appropriate than gauze dressings. If the wound is infected, silver dressings are appropriate for use (Baranoski & Ayello, 2007).

■ *Use hydrogel (e.g., Carrington) to dress wounds.* **LOE = II**

(EO) A water- or glycerin-based product that is usually clear or translucent in color and that varies in viscosity or thickness is used for stage II, III, and IV pressure ulcers and necrotic wounds. These hydrogels are nonadherent to the wound base, and they maintain a moist wound environment on a clean, healthy, granulating wound (Baranoski & Ayello, 2007).

(NR) An RCT using a convenience sample ($N = 50$) of people with necrotic pressure ulcers found that hydrogels were effective for debridement, regardless of the manufacturer (Bale et al., 1998).

(NR) A randomized pilot study ($N = 10$) of stage II and III pressure ulcers showed that polymer hydrogel dressings may be a favorable alternative to hydrocolloid dressings (Motta et al., 1999).

■ *Use hydrogel dressing with aloe vera to dress wounds.* **LOE = II**

(MR) An RCT ($N = 41$) demonstrated that a hydrogel dressing with aloe vera was equal to but not superior to saline-moistened gauze (Thomas et al., 1998).

■ *Use foam dressings (e.g., Lyofoam) to dress wounds.* **LOE = II**

(EO) Foam dressings rely on exudate to achieve an optimum healing environment. They are used for full-thickness wounds with heavy drainage, stage IV pressure ulcers, and surgical wounds, and they are used under compression wraps (Baranoski & Ayello, 2007).

(MR) A retrospective descriptive study of 5 years ($N = 1891$ people with 4200 wounds) of patients with stage II and III pressure ulcers in 30 nursing homes showed that most chronic wounds that were treated with either adhesive hydrocellular foam or soft silicone foam dressing healed in approximately 70 days (Viamontes et al., 2003).

(MR) A prospective, multicenter trial ($N = 32$) of stage II and III pressure ulcers compared a foam dressing with a contact layer and a foam dressing without a contact layer. It was found that the dressing with the contact layer was less likely to delaminate, that it handled exudate better, and that it was more comfortable (Amione et al., 2005).

(MR) A case study ($N = 6$) of venous leg or pressure ulcers showed that foam was both effective and comfortable (Charles et al., 2004).

(MR) A prospective, randomized, stratified, parallel group study ($N = 39$) of stage II and III pressure ulcers showed that adhesive foam was easier to remove but that outcomes were similar to those of hydrocolloid (Seeley et al., 1999).

■ *Use calcium alginate dressings (e.g., Sorbsan, Kaltostat) to dress wounds.*
LOE = III

(EO) Calcium alginate dressing is a highly absorptive dressing that is made from brown seaweed and that acts via an ion exchange mechanism, absorbing the serous fluid or exudate that forms a hydrophilic gel and conforms to the shape of the wound. It is used for full-thickness wounds, stage III and IV pressure ulcers that have moderate to heavy drainage, and dermal and surgical wounds. It is indicated for moderate to heavily exuding wounds and moist wounds with slough, and it is capable of absorbing up to 20 times its own weight in fluid (Baranoski & Ayello, 2007).

(MR) A randomized, multicenter, parallel group trial ($N = 110$) of older adults with stage III and IV pressure ulcers showed faster healing with calcium alginate dressings among frail older adults (Belmin et al., 2002).

■ *Use silver dressings to dress wounds that have signs of infection.* **LOE = III**

(EO) Silver dressings are used for any type of infected wound. They are also used when there is a need to reduce the risk of infection or to decrease the bacterial burden of a wound (Baranoski & Ayello, 2007).

(MR) A study of a randomized, multicenter stratified parallel group ($N = 99$) with pressure ulcers ($N = 28$) and venous leg ulcers ($N = 71$) suggested that silver-releasing hydroalginate dressings may be effective for wounds with a high risk of infection (Meaume et al., 2005).

(EO) Topical silver dressings provide an excellent reduction of bacteria in wounds, and they may also decrease wound pain (Tomaselli, 2006).

■ *Use combination dressings to dress wounds.* **LOE = II**

(EO) Sequential treatment with calcium alginate and hydrocolloid dressings is more effective for debridement and healing than hydrocolloid alone for older people (Baranoski & Ayello, 2007).

(MR) A randomized, multicenter parallel group trial ($N = 110$) of older adults with stage III and IV pressure ulcers showed faster healing with combination dressings among frail older adults (Belmin et al., 2002).

■ *Use collagen/collagenase dressings to dress wounds.* **LOE = II**

(EO) Collagen dressings, which are available as sheets, pads, particles, and gels, consist of predominately type I collagen with small amounts of type II and type IV fibers. These dressings enhance granulation, reduce pain, and promote healing (Baranoski & Ayello, 2007).

(MR) An RCT ($N = 65$) of patients with stage II or III pressure ulcers showed similar ulcer healing for both hydrocolloid and topical collagen treatment, with an 8-week complete healing rate for the collagen paste of 51% (Graumlich et al., 2003).

RCT = Randomized Controlled (Clinical) Trial, **NIC** = Nursing Interventions Classification, **NOC** = Nursing Outcomes Classification

(MR) A prospective randomized trial using a convenience sample ($N = 24$) of hospital patients with stage IV pressure ulcers on the heel found that collagenase ointment cost 5% less than hydrocolloid treatment and that it healed wounds in 10 weeks (as compared with 14 weeks for hydrocolloid treatment; Muller et al., 2001).

▪ *Use growth factors for wound healing.* **LOE = II**

(EO) Nerve growth factors stimulate the growth and differentiation of epithelialization for wound healing (Baranoski & Ayello, 2007).

(MR) A 12-month follow-up for a 35-day placebo-controlled trial ($N = 61$) showed that long-term outcomes were better for those patients who received growth factors (Payne et al., 2001).

(MR) In a randomized, double-blind, placebo-controlled trial of a convenience sample ($N = 36$) of nursing home patients with foot ulcers, half received nerve growth factors, and half received "conventional therapy." The study found that, at 6 weeks, the nerve growth factor group had a significantly greater reduction in ulcer size (Landi et al., 2003).

▪ *Use vacuum therapy (VAC) therapy for wound healing.* **LOE = II**

(EO) VAC therapy is the application of a controlled level of subatmospheric pressure to a wound at 50 mm Hg to 175 mm Hg that is generated by a portable programmable pump. The suction effect is applied to the entire interior surface of a clean wound through open-cell polyurethane or polyvinyl alcohol foam. VAC therapy is effective for healing full-thickness stage III and IV pressure ulcers (Baranoski & Ayello, 2007).

(MR) A randomized convenience sample ($N = 22$ patients) with 35 stage II, III, and IV pressure ulcers showed that VAC was more effective for healing than wound gel products were (Ford et al., 2002).

(MR) A randomized convenience sample ($N = 22$) of patients showed similar results between a VAC therapy group and a group using wet-to-dry/wet-to-wet gauze soaked in Ringer's solution (Wanner et al., 2003).

(MR) An RCT of patients ($N = 65$) with acute or chronic wounds received either VAC-assisted closure or modern wound dressings. Results indicated no significant difference in time to wound closure, except among patients with cardiovascular disease and diabetes, in whom wounds did heal faster with VAC therapy. Patients who underwent VAC therapy experienced less pain, and the time of nursing care was reduced (Braakenburg et al., 2006).

▪ *Use radiant heat with the application of moist, warm topical dressings for wound healing.* **LOE = II**

(EO) Radiant heat will improve rates of wound healing in stage III and IV pressure ulcers (Baranoski & Ayello, 2007).

(MR) In an RCT ($N = 40$ patients with 43 stage II, III, and IV pressure ulcers), noncontact normothermic wound therapy provided significantly faster healing than moist retentive dressings (Kloth et al., 2000).

(MR) In a convenience sample ($N = 14$ patients with 15 stage III and IV pressure ulcers), results showed that wounds treated with radiant heat healed significantly faster than those treated with standard care (Kloth et al., 2002).

(NR) In a prospective single-site randomized trial ($N = 50$), patients treated with radiant heat demonstrated an accelerated rate of healing (Price et al., 2000).

NR = Nursing Research, **MR** = Multidisciplinary Research, **SP** = Standard of Practice, **EO** = Expert Opinion, **LOE** = Level of Evidence

(MR) A randomized convenience sample ($N = 41$) of stage II, III, and IV pressure ulcers did not show significantly different healing rates between the radiant-heat method and hydrocolloid dressings (Thomas et al., 2005).

■ Use transparent films (e.g., Tegaderm, Op-site, Bioclusive) to dress wounds. LOE = II

(EO) Transparent dressings allow for the autolytic debridement of necrotic wounds and for the creation of a moist healing environment for granulating wounds as a result of trapped moisture (Baranoski & Ayello, 2007).

(NR) A random convenience sample ($N = 44$) of stage II pressure ulcers showed that polymeric membrane dressing was more effective than antibiotic ointment and dry sterile gauze dressings (Yastrub, 2004).

■ Use hydrocolloid dressings (e.g., Duoderm) to dress wounds. LOE = II

(EO) Hydrocolloid dressings consist of absorptive ingredients (typically carboxymethylcellulose, pectin, or gelatin) that are used as secondary dressings for full-thickness pressure ulcers as well as for granulating or necrotic wounds (Baranoski & Ayello, 2007).

(MR) An RCT ($N = 65$) of stage II and III pressure ulcers showed similar ulcer healing for both hydrocolloid and topical collagen treatments, with an 8-week complete healing rate for the hydrocolloid dressings of 50% (Graumlich et al., 2003).

(MR) An RCT ($N = 26$) of noninfected stage II, III, and IV pressure ulcers found that hydrogel reduced the healing time of pressure ulcers as compared with wet saline compresses (Matzen et al., 1999).

(MR) A meta-analysis of 21 peer-reviewed, published, randomized quasi-experimental and controlled clinical trials showed moderate superiority of hydrocolloid dressings as compared with conventional dressings with regard to size efficacy for pressure ulcer treatment (Bouza et al., 2005).

(MR) A randomized convenience sample ($N = 40$) showed no difference in healing, odor, or pain between hydrocolloid and foam dressings (Seeley et al., 1999).

Possibly Effective

■ Use honey dressings for wound healing. LOE = IV

(EO) Honey is an ancient remedy that is effective for treating wounds that are infected and for reducing odor, debriding, and healing wounds (Baranoski & Ayello, 2007).

(NR) A case study ($N = 2$) using honey-impregnated alginate gauze demonstrated the effective treatment of full-thickness or necrotic wounds (Van der Weyden, 2003).

Not Effective

■ Using dry gauze directly on wounds. LOE = I

(MR) A meta-analysis of 21 peer-reviewed, published, randomized quasi-experimental and controlled clinical trials showed moderate superiority of hydrocolloid dressings as compared with conventional dressings with regard to size efficacy for pressure ulcer treatment (Bouza et al., 2005).

RCT = Randomized Controlled (Clinical) Trial, **NIC** = Nursing Interventions Classification, **NOC** = Nursing Outcomes Classification

NR A random convenience sample ($N = 44$) of stage II pressure ulcers showed that polymeric membrane dressings were more effective than antibiotic ointment and dry sterile gauze dressings (Yastrub, 2004).

Possibly Harmful

■ *Using concentrated hydrogen peroxide to cleanse wounds.* **LOE = VII**

MR A review of hydrogen peroxide use stated that hydrogen peroxide can cause a cytotoxic effect to the wound and that this may include inflammation and blistering after contact with skin. When it is used to irrigate wounds in a closed body cavity, hydrogen peroxide can result in gas embolism from the release of oxygen (Watt et al., 2004).

■ *Using high pressure for wound irrigation (≥20 psi), with or without pulsatile lavage.* **LOE = IV**

MR A case-control study in a 1000-bed hospital concluded that an infectious outbreak among 11 patients within 2 months was associated with pulsatile lavage therapy. Infection control precautions are needed with lavage therapy (Maragakis et al., 2004).

MR A narrative review cautioned about the use of high-pressure pulsatile lavage for all types of wounds and recommended the Agency for Health Care Policy and Research guideline pressures of 4 to 15 psi for wound irrigation. Early studies support pulsatile lavage for wound cleansing, but more RCTs are needed (Luedtke-Hoffmann & Schafer, 2000).

■ *Using the cleansing agent betadine (povidone-iodine) or betadine ointment.* **LOE = III**

MR In an in vitro animal controlled study of the use of betadine and Elase on wounds, the use of betadine resulted in reduced functional capillary density and decreased arteriolar diameters; the use of Elase resulted in capillary flow, and arteriolar diameters were significantly increased (Peter et al., 2002).

■ *Massaging skin over bony prominences.* **LOE = IV**

NR A study using a convenience sample ($N = 20$) found that extended massage over bony prominences resulted in a significantly lower skin temperature than standard massage (Olson, 1989).

MR A cohort study demonstrated that massage over bony prominences with skin discoloration resulted in a lower skin blood flow than was present before massage (Ek et al., 1985).

MR Postmortem biopsies documented macerated, degenerated tissue in areas that had been exposed to massage that were not documented on individuals that were not massaged individuals (Dyson, 1978).

OUTCOME MEASUREMENT

SKIN AND TISSUE INTEGRITY

Definition: Re-establishment of intact skin and tissues in the area in which the epidermis and dermis are no longer intact.

Skin and Tissue Integrity as evidenced by the following indicators:

NR = Nursing Research, **MR** = Multidisciplinary Research, **SP** = Standard of Practice, **EO** = Expert Opinion, **LOE** = Level of Evidence

OUTCOME MEASUREMENT—*cont'd*

- Intact skin
- Wound is decreasing in size
- Formation of granulation tissue
- Skin around the wound is without redness or nonblanchable erythema
- Wound is free of purulent drainage, odor, or other signs of infection
- Involved area is kept free of pressure and moisture

(Note: This is not a NOC outcome.)

REFERENCES

Amione P, Ricci E, Topo F, Izzo L, Pirovano R, Rega V, et al. (2005). Comparison of Allevyn Adhesive and Biatain Adhesive in the management of pressure ulcers. *J Wound Care,* 14(8):365-370.

Bale S, Banks V, Haglestein S, Harding KG. (1998). A comparison of two amorphous hydrogels in the debridement of pressure sores. *J Wound Care,* 7(2):65-68.

Baranoski S, Ayello E. (2007). *Wound care essentials: Practice principles.* Philadelphia: Lippincott Williams & Wilkins.

Belmin J, Meaume S, Rabus MT, Bohbot S; Investigators of the Sequential Treatment of the Elderly with Pressure Sores (STEPS) Trial. (2002). Sequential treatment with calcium alginate dressings and hydrocolloid dressings accelerates pressure ulcer healing in older subjects: A multicenter randomized trial of sequential versus nonsequential treatment with hydrocolloid dressings alone. *J Am Geriatr Soc,* 50(2):269-274.

Bouza C, Saz Z, Munoz A, Amate JM. (2005). Efficacy of advanced dressings in the treatment of pressure ulcers: A systematic review. *J Wound Care,* 14(5):193-199.

Braakenburg A, Obdeijn MC, Feitz R, van Rooij IA, van Griethuysen AJ, Klinkenbijl JH. (2006). The clinical efficacy and cost effectiveness of the vacuum-assisted closure technique in the management of acute and chronic wounds: A randomized controlled trial. *Plast Reconstr Surg,* 118(2):390-397.

Briggs M, Nelson EA. (2003). Topical agents or dressings for pain in venous leg ulcers. *Cochrane Database Syst Rev,* (1):CD001177.

Charles H, Corser R, Varrow S, Hart J. (2004). A non-adhesive foam dressing for exuding venous leg ulcers and pressure ulcers: Six case studies. *J Wound Care,* 13(2):58-62.

Dyson R. (1978). Bed sores—the injuries hospital staff inflict on patients. *Nurs Mirror,* 146(24):30-32.

Ek AC, Gustavsson G, Lewis DH. (1985). The local skin blood flow in areas at risk for pressure sores treated with massage. *Scand J Rehabil Med,* 17(2):81-86.

Evans E, Gray M. (2005). Do topical analgesics reduce pain associated with wound dressings changes or debridement of chronic wounds? *J Wound Ostomy Continence Nurs,* 32(5):287-290.

Fernandez R, Griffiths R, Ussia C. (2002). Water for wound cleansing. *Cochrane Database Syst Rev,* (4): CD003861.

Ford CN, Reinhard ER, Yeh D, Syrek D, De Las Morenas A, Bergman SB, et al. (2002). Interim analysis of a prospective, randomized trial of vacuum-assisted closure versus the healthpoint system in the management of pressure ulcers. *Ann Plast Surg,* 49(1):55-61.

Graumlich JF, Blough LS, McLaughlin RG, et al. (2003). Healing pressure ulcers with collagen or hydrocolloid: A randomized, controlled trial. *J Am Geriatr Soc,* 51(2):147-154.

Hollisaz MT, Khedmat H, Yari F. (2004). A randomized clinical trial comparing hydrocolloid, phenytoin and simple dressings for the treatment of pressure ulcers [ISRCTN33429693]. *BMC Dermatol,* 4(1): 18.

Howell JM, Chisholm CD. (1997). Wound care. *Emerg Med Clin North Am,* 15(2):417-425.

Kloth LC, Berman JE, Dumit-Minkel S, Sutton CH, Papanek PE, Wurzel J. (2000). Effects of a normothermic dressing on pressure ulcer healing. *Adv Skin Wound Care,* 13(2):69-74.

Kloth LC, Berman JE, Nett M, Papanek PE, Dumit-Minkel S. (2002). A randomized controlled clinical trial to evaluate the effects of noncontact normothermic wound therapy on chronic full-thickness pressure ulcers. *Adv Skin Wound Care*, 15(6):270-276.

Landi F, Aloe L, Russo A, Cesari M, Onder G, Bonini S, et al. (2003). Topical treatment of pressure ulcers with nerve growth factor: A randomized clinical trial. *Ann Intern Med*, 139(8):635-641.

Luedtke-Hoffmann KA, Schafer DS. (2000). Pulsed lavage in wound cleansing. *Phys Ther*, 80(3):292-300.

Maragakis LL, Cosgrove S, Song X, Kim D, Rosenbaum P, Ciesla N, et al. (2004). An outbreak of multidrug-resistant *Acinetobacter baumannii* associated with pulsatile lavage wound treatment. *JAMA*, 292(24):3006-3011.

Matzen S, Peschardt A, Alsbjorn B. (1999). A new amorphous hydrocolloid for the treatment of pressure sores: A randomised controlled study. *Scand J Plast Reconstr Surg Hand Surg*, 33(1):13-15.

Meaume S, Vallet D, Morere MN, Teot L. (2005). Evaluation of a silver-releasing hydroalginate dressing in chronic wounds with signs of local infection. *J Wound Care*, 14(9):411-419.

Moore ZE, Cowman S. (2005). Wound cleansing for pressure ulcers. *Cochrane Database Syst Rev*, (4): CD004983.

Motta G, Dunham L, Dye T, Mentz J, O'Connell-Gifford E, Smith E. (1999). Clinical efficacy and cost-effectiveness of a new synthetic polymer sheet wound dressing. *Ostomy Wound Manage*, 45(10):41, 44-46, 48-49.

Muller E, van Leen MW, Bergemann R. (2001). Economic evaluation of collagenase-containing ointment and hydrocolloid dressing in the treatment of pressure ulcers. *Pharmacoeconomics*, 19(12): 1209-1216.

National Pressure Ulcer Advisory Panel (NPUAP). (2003). NPUAP staging report. Available online: http://www.npuap.org. Retrieved on July 7, 2007.

Olson B. (1989). Effects of massage for prevention of pressure ulcers. *Decubitus*, 2(4):32-37.

Payne WG, Ochs DE, Meltzer DD, Hill DP, Mannari RJ, Robson LE, et al. (2001). Long-term outcome study of growth factor-treated pressure ulcers. *Am J Surg*, 181(1):81-86.

Peter FW, Li-Peuser H, Vogt PM, Muehlberger T, Homann HH, Steinau HU. (2002). The effect of wound ointments on tissue microcirculation and leucocyte behaviour. *Clin Exp Dermatol*, 27(1):51-55.

Price P, Bale S, Crook H, Harding KG. (2000). The effect of a radiant heat dressing on pressure ulcers. *J Wound Care*, 9(4):201-205.

Schultz GS, Sibbald RG, Falanga V, Ayello E, Dowsett C, Harding K, et al. (2003). Wound bed preparation: A systematic approach to wound management. *Wound Repair Regen*, 11(Suppl 1):S1-S28.

Seeley J, Jensen JL, Hutcherson J. (1999). A randomized clinical study comparing a hydrocellular dressing to a hydrocolloid dressing in the management of pressure ulcers. *Ostomy Wound Manage*, 45(6):39-44, 46-47.

Thomas DR, Diebold MR, Eggemeyer LM. (2005). A controlled, randomized, comparative study of a radiant heat bandage on the healing of stage 3-4 pressure ulcers: A pilot study. *J Am Med Dir Assoc*, 6(1):46-49.

Thomas DR, Goode PS, LaMaster K, Tennyson T. (1998). Acemannan hydrogel dressing versus saline dressing for pressure ulcers. A randomized, controlled trial. *Adv Wound Care*, 11(6):273-276.

Tomaselli N. (2006). The role of topical silver preparations in wound healing. *J Wound Ostomy Continence Nurs*, 33(4):367-378.

Van der Weyden EA. (2003). The use of honey for the treatment of two patients with pressure ulcers. *Br J Community Nurs*, 8(12):S14-S20.

Viamontes L, Temple D, Wytall D, Walker A. (2003). An evaluation of an adhesive hydrocellular foam dressing and a self-adherent soft silicone foam dressing in a nursing home setting. *Ostomy Wound Manage*, 49(8):48-52, 54-56, 58.

Wanner MB, Schwarzl F, Strub B, Zaech GA, Pierer G. (2003). Vacuum-assisted wound closure for cheaper and more comfortable healing of pressure sores: A prospective study. *Scand J Plast Reconstr Surg Hand Surg*, 37(1):28-33.

Watt BE, Proudfoot AT, Vale JA. (2004). Hydrogen peroxide poisoning. *Toxicol Rev*, 23(1):51-57.

Wilson JR, Mills JG, Prather ID, Dimitrijevich SD. (2005). A toxicity index of skin and wound cleansers used on in vitro fibroblasts and keratinocytes. *Adv Skin Wound Care*, 18(7):373-378.

Yastrub DJ. (2004). Relationship between type of treatment and degree of wound healing among institutionalized geriatric patients with stage II pressure ulcers. *Care Manag J*, 5(4):213-218.

NR = Nursing Research, **MR** = Multidisciplinary Research, **SP** = Standard of Practice, **EO** = Expert Opinion, **LOE** = Level of Evidence

PRESSURE ULCER PREVENTION

NIC **Definition:** Prevention of pressure ulcers for an individual at high risk for developing them (Dochterman & Bulechek, 2004).

Julie Anderson, PhD, RN, CCRC; Diane K. Langemo, PhD, RN, FAAN; Karen Zulkowski, DNS, RN, CWS; Elizabeth A. Ayello, PhD, RN, APRN-BC, FAPWCA, FAAN

NURSING ACTIVITIES

Effective

Positioning

■ *Reposition individuals who are in bed and who are at risk for the development of pressure ulcers at least every 2 hours (if this is consistent with the overall goals of care). Maintain a written schedule.* **LOE = II**

(NR) In a controlled clinical trial, patients who were at risk for the development of pressure ulcers who were turned every 2 to 3 hours developed fewer pressure ulcers than those who were not turned as frequently (Norton et al., 1975).

(NR) In an RCT with an experimental group receiving small body position shifts versus a control group that did not, there was no significant effect on pressure ulcer incidence among 19 long-term care residents. However, residents in both groups were turned every 2 hours (Smith & Malone, 1990).

(MR) Data support a negative relationship between the number of spontaneous movements made by elderly individuals who are confined to bed and pressure ulcer incidence (Exton-Smith & Sherwin, 1961).

(EO) Clinicians are generally taught to change the patient's position every 2 hours. This in fact may not be frequent enough, depending on an individual's tissue tolerance (e.g., an elderly patient with frail skin; Maklebust, 2005).

(NR) In a quasi-experimental study of 838 nursing home residents, four different turning schedules were tested: every 2 hours and every 3 hours on a standard institutional mattress and every 4 hours and every 6 hours on a viscoelastic foam (VEF) mattress. There was a significant reduction in pressure ulcer incidence among residents who were turned every 4 hours on the VEF mattress (Defloor et al., 2005).

■ (SP) *Minimize friction and shearing forces by using lift sheets and lifting devices to turn or transfer patients.* **LOE = III**

(MR) In a controlled study, it was determined in animal models that continuous shear on a site of constant axial pressure lowered the threshold for ulceration sixfold (Dinsdale, 1973).

(EO) Minimizing friction will decrease or prevent injuries that are caused by pulling or dragging (Bergstrom et al., 1994; Dinsdale, 1974; Maklebust & Sieggreen, 1996; WOCN, 2003).

RCT = Randomized Controlled (Clinical) Trial, **NIC** = Nursing Interventions Classification, **NOC** = Nursing Outcomes Classification

■ *Limit the elevation of the head of the bed to 30 degrees or to the lowest elevation that is consistent with the patient's condition.* **LOE = VII**

(EO) The elevation of the head of the bed beyond 30 degrees increases the amount of friction and shear to which the sacrum, coccyx, and buttocks are exposed. Elevating the head of the bed as little as necessary and for as short a time as possible is recommended (Bergstrom et al., 1994; Maklebust & Sieggreen, 1996; Reichel, 1958; WOCN, 2003).

■ *Use overhead trapeze bars as much as possible to facilitate patient mobility.* **LOE = VII**

(EO) A lifting device promotes independence in the patient and assists the patient with not dragging the body across the bed (Bergstrom et al., 1994; WOCN, 2003).

■ *Reposition chair- and bed-bound individuals frequently and regularly. Small and frequent position changes using pillows or wedges reduce pressure on bony prominences.* **LOE = IV**

(NR) A quasi-experimental study (*N* = 16) comparing 1-, 1.5-, and 2-hour turning schedules for healthy adults found that the greatest increase in skin surface temperature occurred at the end of the 2-hour turning schedule and when the patient was in the trochanteric position. However, no significant tissue interface pressure differences were found with regard to the length of the turning interval or the body position (Knox et al., 1994).

(NR) In a controlled study, turning patients (*N* = 62) every 4 hours in combination with the use of a pressure-reducing mattress was shown to decrease the occurrence of pressure ulcers as compared with turning patients every 6 hours with the use of a pressure-reducing mattress or with turning patients every 2 to 4 hours without a pressure-reducing mattress (Defloor, 2001).

Positioning Seated Patients

■ *Position individuals who are seated with attention to anatomy, postural alignment, weight distribution, and support of the feet.* **LOE = II**

(NR) In a controlled study, it was found that posture influenced ischial pressures and that the final sitting surface pressure was dependent on lateral pelvic tilt (Hobson, 1992).

(EO) Briefly stand and reseat seated patients to relieve pressure. Small weight shifts may include leg elevation (Bergstrom et al., 1994; WOCN, 2003).

(NR) A quasi-experimental pilot study (*N* = 10) examining the effects of leg elevation demonstrated that leg elevation at 10 degrees in the 30-degree head-up position effectively reduced body displacement at the acromium but not at the sacrum (Harada et al., 2002).

■ *Reposition individuals who are unable to change their chair positions every hour.* **LOE = VII**

(EO) Small and frequent position changes using pillows or wedges reduce pressure on bony prominences (Bergstrom et al., 1994; Brand, 1976; Kosiak, 1959; Krouskop et al., 1983; Reddy & Cochran, 1979; WOCN, 2003).

(EO) Encourage seated individuals who are able to reposition themselves to provide pressure relief every 15 minutes with chair push-ups (Bergstrom et al., 1994; WOCN, 2003).

NR = Nursing Research, **MR** = Multidisciplinary Research, **SP** = Standard of Practice, **EO** = Expert Opinion, **LOE** = Level of Evidence

Managing Incontinence

■ **NIC** **SP** *Remove excessive moisture on the skin resulting from perspiration, wound drainage, and fecal or urinary incontinence.* **LOE = VII**

EO Moisture from incontinence can macerate the skin and contribute to the development of pressure ulcers. Stool is an even greater risk factor for pressure ulcer development, because it contains bacteria and enzymes that are chemical irritants to the skin. When both urinary and fecal incontinence are present, fecal enzymes convert urea to ammonia, which raises the skin pH. As the skin pH becomes more alkaline, the permeability of the skin to irritants increases. Keep the skin as clean and dry as possible after each episode of incontinence, because the presence of moisture enhances the effect of friction and shearing (Leyden et al., 1977; Ratliff & Rodeheaver, 1999; Zimmerer et al., 1986).

■ **SP** *Develop bowel and/or bladder training programs for individuals with urinary and/or fecal incontinence to control sources of moisture and skin irritation.* **LOE = IV**

EO Bowel and bladder training programs are needed to decrease moisture and to protect the skin from stool (WOCN, 2003).

NR A prospective clinical trial found that 33% of participants in both unstructured and structured care groups had perineal dermatitis. When fecal and urinary continence were both present, a pressure ulcer developed within 2 days (Lyder et al., 1992).

■ **SP** *Use absorbent briefs and underpads when urine and fecal sources of skin moisture and irritation cannot be controlled to provide a quick-drying surface to the skin.* **LOE = VII**

EO "Cloth or disposable adult-size diapers are the current standard of practice for care of frail, elderly patients with intractable incontinence who have not responded to bowel and bladder programs" (Jeter & Lutz, 1996, p 29; Bergstrom et al., 1994; WOCN, 2003).

■ *Promptly cleanse the skin after each soiling episode with warm water and pH-balanced cleansers while minimizing trauma to the skin.* **LOE = II**

NR A prospective RCT ($N = 93$) of two cleansing protocols used after episodes of incontinence was conducted in nursing home residents. Thirty-three patients in each group had healthy skin at the outset. More participants retained healthy skin in the Clinisan group (27 of 44) than in the group who received soap-and-water cleansing (17 of 49; Cooper & Gray, 2001).

NR An evaluative study ($N = 9$) documented that using a cleanser protectant lotion significantly reduced the average scores of perineal erythema and pain (Warshaw, 2002).

EO Nonionic cleansers with surfactants are gentler to the skin than the anionic surfactants that are found in the soaps that are typically used for bathing. The pH of normal skin is slightly acidic; most bar soaps have an alkaline pH, thereby disturbing the normal acid mantle of the skin and leaving it more permeable to water-soluble irritants (Jeter & Lutz, 1996).

RCT = Randomized Controlled (Clinical) Trial, **NIC** = Nursing Interventions Classification, **NOC** = Nursing Outcomes Classification

(EO) Warm water rather than hot is recommended to minimize drying and irritation (Bergstrom et al., 1994; CSCM, 2001).

(EO) Perineal cleansers that contain topical antimicrobials such as benzalkonium chloride have been shown to be effective for decreasing microbial counts on perineal skin (Newman et al., 2001).

■ (SP) *Use topical agents that act as skin barriers, including creams, ointments, pastes, and film-forming protectants as well as products that contain petrolatum, to curb moisture and prevent skin irritation.* **LOE = III**

(NR) An evaluative study ($N = 19$) documented that using a protectant lotion significantly reduced average scores for perineal erythema and pain (Warshaw, 2002).

(NR) A controlled trial ($N = 18$) documented that a petrolatum-containing product demonstrated protection against irritants and maceration and that it provided some skin hydration, whereas zinc-oxide-containing protectants provided protection only against irritation (Hoggarth et al., 2005).

(NR) A prospective clinical trial ($N = 136$) documented that a product containing petrolatum was effective for reducing the incidence of perineal dermatitis in incontinent patients (Thompson et al., 2004).

(NR) A prospective clinical trial ($N = 136$) found that the prophylactic use of a skin cleanser and a skin protectant resulted in a significant decrease in skin breakdown and stage I and II pressure ulcers from before to after the intervention (Hunter et al., 2003).

■ *Change bed linens promptly when they are wet or soiled.* **LOE = VII**

(EO) The skin barrier function will become impaired by moisture and irritants from soiled bed linens as a result of skin maceration (Hoggarth et al., 2005; Bergstrom et al., 1994; WOCN, 2003).

■ (SP) *Apply a pouch system or a collection device for urine or stool to contain the waste matter and to protect the skin when other interventions fail.* **LOE = VII**

(EO) Pouch systems or collection devices for urine and stool can be effective for containing waste matter from incontinent patients (Bergstrom et al., 1994; Jeter & Lutz, 1996; WOCN, 2003).

■ *Consider an indwelling catheter as a short-term, last-resort measure when the severity of the incontinence has contributed to or may contaminate a pressure ulcer.* **LOE = VII**

(EO) Typically, urinary catheters are used to manage incontinence only if patients have ulcerated areas that must be kept free from urine contamination or saturation or if repositioning is painful (Bergstrom et al., 1994; Jeter & Lutz, 1996).

(Refer to the guidelines on Bowel Training, Bowel Incontinence Care, Urinary Habit Training, and Prompted Voiding.)

Minimizing Pressure Using a Pressure Relieving System

(Refer to the guidelines on Pressure Ulcer Care.)

NR = Nursing Research, **MR** = Multidisciplinary Research, **SP** = Standard of Practice, **EO** = Expert Opinion, **LOE** = Level of Evidence

Nutrition

■ (SP) *Conduct a nursing nutritional assessment for individuals who are at risk for malnutrition.* **LOE = IV**

(NR) In a retrospective cohort study, 1524 residents of 95 long-term care facilities were followed for 12 weeks. Twenty-nine residents developed pressure ulcers, and characteristics that were associated with a greater likelihood of developing a pressure ulcer included significant weight loss and oral eating problems (Horn et al., 2004).

(NR) A prospective study ($N = 200$) of pressure ulcer risk among elderly nursing home residents found that malnutrition was correlated with pressure ulcer development (Bergstrom & Braden, 1992).

(EO) Nutritional support is believed to be an important component of pressure ulcer prevention and healing (AMDA, 1996; Bergstrom et al., 1992, 1994; Blackburn et al., 1992; CSCM, 2001).

■ (SP) *Ensure the maintenance of adequate nutrition that is appropriate to the patient's condition and personal wishes.* **LOE = VII**

(EO) Although adequate nutrition is known to be important (particularly in situations in which the skin is at risk of breakdown), insufficient evidence exists to prove the value of specific nutritional support for individuals who are at risk for the development of pressure ulcers (EPUAP, 1998; WOCN, 2003).

■ *Provide dietary supplementation to prevent pressure ulcers among elderly patients who are acutely ill.* **LOE = I**

(MR) In a multicenter RCT ($N = 672$), individuals 65 years old and older who were in the acute phase of an illness and who were immobile and unable to eat independently had nutritional interventions for up to 15 days. It was found that nutritional supplementation reduced the number of new pressure ulcers (Bourdel-Marchasson et al., 2000).

(MR) A meta-analysis of 15 studies, including 10 RCTs, found that high-protein enteral support could significantly reduce the risk of pressure ulcer development by 25% (Stratton et al., 2005).

(MR) A controlled study found that a high-protein diet with a higher calorie content may enhance pressure ulcer healing in nursing home patients who were malnourished ($N = 28$; Breslow et al., 1993).

(NR) Observational studies reported that vitamin and mineral deficiencies were demonstrated in the majority of nursing home residents (Bergstrom & Braden, 1992 [$N = 200$]; Pinchcofsky-Devin & Kaminski, 1986 [$N = 232$]).

■ (SP) *Provide nutrition and dietary supplements, including zinc and vitamin C, to prevent and/or treat pressure ulcers.* **LOE = IV**

(MR) An open enrollment study ($N = 39$) of patients with stage III and IV pressure ulcers who were given supplements with protein, arginine, vitamin C, and zinc for 3 weeks showed a reduction in wound area and an improvement in wound condition (Frias Soriano et al., 2004).

(NR) An observational study found that vitamin and mineral deficiencies were demonstrated in the majority of nursing home residents (Bergstrom & Braden, 1992; Pinchcofsky-Devin & Kaminski, 1986).

RCT = Randomized Controlled (Clinical) Trial, **NIC** = Nursing Interventions Classification, **NOC** = Nursing Outcomes Classification

(EO) Supplementation with a daily high-potency vitamin and mineral supplement is recommended for patients who are suspected of having a vitamin deficiency (Bergstrom et al., 1994).

(MR) A systematic review of actions that proved to be helpful for the prevention of pressure ulcers found that four actions were appropriate: (1) using support surfaces to decrease pressure; (2) turning and repositioning the patient; (3) optimizing nutritional status; and (4) keeping the skin on the sacral area moisturized (Reddy et al., 2006).

(EO) A patient with a pressure ulcer who is underweight or losing weight should receive calorie and protein supplementation (NPUAP, 2003).

(MR) An RCT of inpatients ($N = 16$) with stage II, III, and IV pressure ulcers were randomized to receive either the standard hospital diet, the standard diet plus two high-protein supplements, or the standard diet plus two high-protein supplements plus additional arginine, vitamin C, and zinc. There were no significant reported changes in weight, biochemical markers, or oral dietary intake among the groups. However, those patients who received protein supplementation and additional supplements demonstrated improved wound healing (Desneves et al., 2005).

Additional research: Delmi et al., 1990; Hartgrink et al., 1998; Bourdel-Marchasson et al., 2000; Houwing et al., 2003.

■ (SP) *Request a nutritional consultation when nutritional deficiencies are suspected or identified or when nutritional supplementation is needed to prevent or treat malnutrition.* **LOE = VII**

(EO) Nutritional consultation is recommended for patients with suspected or identified nutritional deficiencies or to prevent malnutrition (Bergstrom et al., 1994; WOCN, 2003).

Possibly Effective

■ *Provide education to the patient and/or caregiver regarding causative/risk factors for the development of pressure ulcers.* **LOE = VII**

(EO) Educational programs should include information about the following: skin monitoring; minimizing friction and shear forces; not using donut-type devices or rings; ensuring the maintenance of adequate nutrition; turning and repositioning patients on a regular basis; using pressure-reducing devices if the patient has limited mobility and/or is confined to a bed or chair; avoiding vigorous massage over bony prominences; regularly inspecting the skin over bony prominences; reporting any changes in health status or nutrition; following prescribed skin care protocols; and preventing pressure ulcers (Bergstrom et al., 1994; WOCN, 2003).

(EO) The patient and his or her family are integral to the prevention and management of pressure ulcers (Andberg et al., 1983; Barnes, 1987; Sebern, 1987).

Not Effective

■ *Reclining the patient to relieve pressure on ischial tuberosities.* **LOE = III**

(MR) A controlled trial without randomization ($N = 10$ patients with spinal cord injury) found no effective reduction in pressure on ischial tuberosities with patients in a reclined position at 35 degrees (Henderson et al., 1994).

NR = Nursing Research, **MR** = Multidisciplinary Research, **SP** = Standard of Practice, **EO** = Expert Opinion, **LOE** = Level of Evidence

■ *Using sheepskin for pressure reduction.* **LOE = VII**

(EO) There is inadequate evidence that sheepskin has pressure-reducing properties (Pieper, 2007; WOCN, 2003).

(MR) In a controlled study ($N = 44$) that compared genuine sheepskin with synthetic sheepskin, results found that genuine sheepskin was more effective for improving outcomes (Marchand, 1993).

(MR) An open label RCT ($N = 441$) evaluating low to moderate risks of pressure ulcer development found a lower incidence of pressure ulcers among the group using high-performance sheepskin as compared with the group that received usual care (Jolley, 2004).

Possibly Harmful

■ *Massaging skin over bony prominences.* **LOE = IV**

(NR) A controlled study using a convenience sample ($N = 13$) found that extended massage resulted in a significantly lower skin temperature than standard massage (Olson, 1989).

(MR) A cohort study ($N = 54$) demonstrated that massage over immobile patients' bony prominences with skin discoloration resulted in a lower skin blood flow than was present before massage (Ek et al., 1985).

(MR) In a descriptive study, postmortem biopsies documented macerated, degenerated tissue in areas that were exposed to massage that were not documented on individuals that were not massaged (Dyson, 1978).

(MR) A review of the literature found no evidence that massage was appropriate for pressure ulcers in at-risk individuals (Buss, 1997).

(MR) A review of the literature found that effleurage applied with moderate pressure is the most preferred massage for the treatment of pressure ulcers, but more research is needed (Duimel-Peeters, 2005).

■ *Using donut-type devices or rings (such devices concentrate pressure to the surrounding tissue).* **LOE = VI**

(NR) A survey study documented that ring cushions had a greater tendency to cause pressure ulcers than to prevent them (Crewe, 1987).

OUTCOME MEASUREMENT

SKIN INTEGRITY

Definition: Maintenance of intact skin, especially in areas that are prone to pressure ulcers, particularly over bony prominences.
Skin Integrity as evidenced by the following indicators:
• Intact skin
• Skin is without redness or nonblanchable erythema
(Rate each indicator of **Skin Integrity**: 1 = severely compromised, 2 = substantially compromised, 3 = moderately compromised, 4 = mildly compromised, 5 = not compromised.) (Note: This is not a NOC outcome.)

RCT = Randomized Controlled (Clinical) Trial, **NIC** = Nursing Interventions Classification, **NOC** = Nursing Outcomes Classification

REFERENCES

American Medical Directors Association (AMDA). (1996). *Pressure ulcers.* Columbia, MD: AMDA. Available online: www.guideline.gov. Retrieved on July 7, 2007.

Andberg MM, Rudolph A, Anderson TP. (1983). Improving skin care through patient and family training. *Top Clin Nurs,* 5(2):45-54.

Barnes SH. (1987). Patient/family education for the patient with a pressure necrosis. *Nurs Clin North Am,* 22(2):463-474.

Bergstrom N, Allman R, Alvarez O, et al. (1994). *Treatment of pressure ulcers.* Clinical practice guideline No. 15. Rockville, MD: Agency for Health Care Policy and Research, AHCPR Publication No. 95-0652.

Bergstrom N, Allman R, Carlson C, et al. (1992). *Pressure ulcers in adults: Prediction and prevention.* Clinical practice guideline No. 3. Rockville, MD: Agency for Health Care Policy and Research, AHCPR Publication No. 92-0047.

Bergstrom N, Braden B. (1992). A prospective study of pressure sore risk among institutionalized elderly. *J Am Geriatr Soc,* 40(8):747-758.

Berlowitz DR, Brandeis GH, Anderson J, et al. (1997). Effect of pressure ulcers on the survival of long-term care residents. *J Gerontol A Biol Sci Med Sci,* 52(2):M106-M110.

Blackburn GL, Dwyer JT, Wellman NS (Eds). (1992). *Nutrition interventions manual for professionals caring for older Americans.* Washington DC: The Nutrition Screening Initiative.

Brand PW. (1976). Pressure sores—the problem. In Kenedi RM, Cowden JM, Scales JT (Eds). *Bed sore biomechanics.* London: MacMillan Press, pp. 19-23.

Breslow RA, Hallfrisch J, Guy DG, et al. (1993). The importance of dietary protein in healing pressure ulcers. *J Am Geriatr Soc,* 41(4):357-362.

Buss IC, Halfens RJ, Abu-Saad HH. (1997). The effectiveness of massage in preventing pressure sores: A literature review. *Rehabil Nurs,* 22(5):229-234, 242.

Consortium for Spinal Cord Medicine (CSCM) Clinical Practice Guidelines. (2001). Pressure ulcer prevention and treatment following spinal cord injury: A clinical practice guideline for health-care professionals. *J Spinal Cord Med,* 24(Suppl 1):S40-S101.

Cooper P, Gray D. (2001). Comparison of two skin care regimes for incontinence. *Br J Nurs,* 10(6) Suppl: S6, S8, S10.

Crewe RA. (1987). Problems of rubber ring nursing cushions and a clinical survey of alternative cushions for ill patients. *Care Sci Pract,* 5(2):9-11.

Defloor T. (2001). Less frequent turning intervals and yet less pressure ulcers. *Tijdschr Gerontol Geriatr,* 32(4):174-177.

Defloor T, De Bacquer D, Grypdonck MH. (2005). The effect of various combinations of turning and pressure reducing devices on the incidence of pressure ulcers. *Int J Nurs Stud,* 42(1):37-46.

Delmi M, Rapin CH, Bengoa JM, et al. (1990). Dietary supplementation in elderly patients with fractured neck of the femur. *Lancet,* 335(8696):1013-1016.

Desneves KJ, Todorovic BE, Cassar A, Crowe TC. (2005). Treatment with supplementary arginine, vitamin C and zinc in patients with pressure ulcers: A randomised controlled trial. *Clin Nutr,* 24(6):979-987.

Dinsdale SM. (1973). Decubitus ulcers in swine: Light and electron microscopy study of pathogenesis. *Arch Phys Med Rehabil,* 54(2):51-56 passim.

Dinsdale SM. (1974). Decubitus ulcers: Role of pressure and friction in causation. *Arch Phys Med Rehabil,* 55(4):147-152.

Dochterman JM, Bulechek GM (Eds). (2004). *Nursing interventions classification (NIC),* 4th ed. St Louis: Mosby.

Duimel-Peeters IG, Halfens RJ, Berger MP, et al. (2005) The effects of massage as a method to prevent pressure ulcers. A review of the literature. *Ostomy Wound Manage,* 51(4):70-80.

Dyson R. (1978). Bed sores—the injuries hospital staff inflict on patients. *Nurs Mirror,* 146(24):30-32.

Ek AC, Gustavsson G, Lewis DH. (1985). The local skin blood flow in areas at risk for pressure sores treated with massage. *Scand J Rehabil Med,* 17(2):81-86.

European Pressure Ulcer Advisory Panel (EPUAP). (1998). *Pressure ulcer prevention guidelines.* Available online: www.epuap.org. Retrieved on July 7, 2007.

Exton-Smith AN, Sherwin RW. (1961). The prevention of pressure sores: Significance of spontaneous bodily movements. *Lancet* 2(7212):1124-1126.

Frias Soriano L, Lage Vazquez MA, Maristany CP, Xandri Graupera JM, Wouters-Wesseling W, Wagenaar L. (2004). The effectiveness of oral nutritional supplementation in the healing of pressure ulcers. *J Wound Care*, 13(8):319-322.

Harada C, Shigematsu T, Hagisawa S. (2002). The effect of 10-degree leg elevation and 30-degree head elevation on body displacement and sacral interface pressures over a 2-hour period. *J Wound Ostomy Continence Nurs* 29(3):143-148.

Hartgrink HH, Wille J, Konig P, et al. (1998). Pressure sores and tube feeding in patients with a fracture of the hip: A randomized clinical trial. *Clin Nutr*, 17(6):287-292.

Henderson JL, Price SH, Brandstater ME, et al. (1994). Efficacy of three measures to relieve pressure in seated persons with spinal cord injury. *Arch Phys Med Rehabil*, 75:535-539.

Hobson DA. (1992). Comparative effects of posture on pressure and shear at the body-seat interface. *J Rehabil Res Devel*, 29(4):21-31.

Hoggarth A, Waring M, Alexander J, Greenwood A, Callaghan T. (2005). A controlled, three-part trial to investigate the barrier function and skin hydration properties of six skin protectants. *Ostomy Wound Manage*, 51(12):30-42.

Horn SD, Bender SA, Ferguson ML, et al. (2004). The National Pressure Ulcer Long-Term Care Study: Pressure ulcer development in long-term care residents. *J Am Geriatr Soc*, 52(3):359-367.

Houwing R, Rozendaal M, Wouters-Wesseling W, et al. (2003). A randomized, double-blind assessment of the effect of nutritional supplementation on the prevention of pressure ulcers in hip-fracture patients. *Clin Nutr*, 22(4):401-405.

Hunter S, Anderson J, Hanson D, et al. (2003). Clinical trial of a prevention and treatment protocol for skin breakdown in two nursing homes. *J Wound Ostomy Continence Nurs*, 30(5):250-258.

Jeter KF, Lutz JB. (1996). Skin care in the frail, elderly, dependent, incontinent patient. *Adv Wound Care*, 9(1):29-34.

Jolley DJ, Wright R, McGowan S, et al. (2004). Preventing pressure ulcers with the Australian Medical Sheepskin: An open-label randomised controlled trial. *Med J Aust* 180(7):324-327.

Kosiak M. (1959). Etiology and pathology of ischemic ulcers. *Arch Phys Med Rehabil*, 40(2):62-69.

Knox DM, Anderson TM, Anderson PS. (1994). Effects of different turn intervals on skin of healthy older adults. *Adv Wound Care*, 7(1):48-52, 54-56.

Krouskop TA, Noble PC, Garber SL, Spencer WA. (1983). The effectiveness of preventive management in reducing the occurrence of pressure sores. *J Rehabil R D*, 20(1):74-83.

Leyden JJ, Katz S, Stewart R, Kligman AM. (1977). Urinary ammonia and ammonia-producing microorganisms in infants with and without diaper dermatitis. *Arch Dermatol*, 113(12):1678-1680.

Lyder CH, Clemes-Lowrance C, Davis A, Sullivan L, Zucker A. (1992). Structured skin care regimen to prevent perineal dermatitis. *J ET Nurs*, 19(1):12-16.

Maklebust J, Sieggreen MY. (1996). Attacking on all fronts. How to conquer pressure ulcers. *Nursing*, 26(12):34-39.

Maklebust, J. (2005). Choosing the right support surface. *Adv Skin Wound Care*, 18(3):158-161.

Maklebust J, Sieggreen M. (2001). *Pressure ulcers: Guidelines for prevention and management* (3rd ed). Springhouse, PA: Springhouse.

Marchand AC, Lidowski H. (1993). Reassessment of the use of genuine sheepskin for pressure ulcer prevention and treatment. *Decubitus*, 6(1):44-47.

Moorhead M, Johnson M, Maas M (Eds). (2004). *Nursing outcomes classification (NOC)*, 3rd ed. St Louis: Mosby.

National Pressure Ulcer Advisory Panel. (2003). *Frequently asked questions.* Available online: www.npuap.org/npuap-faq.htm. Retrieved on September 24, 2006.

Newman DK, Wallace DW, Wallace J. (2001). Moisture control and incontinence management. In Krasner D, Rodeheaver G, Sibbald G (Eds). *Chronic wound care: A clinical source book for health care professionals,* 3rd ed. Wayne, PA: HMP Communications.

Norton D, McLaren R, Exton-Smith AN. (1975). *An investigation of geriatric nursing problems in hospital.* London: Churchill Livingstone.

Olson B. (1989). Effects of massage for prevention of pressure ulcers. *Decubitus*, 2(4):32-37.

Pieper B. (2007). Mechanical forces: Pressure, shear, and friction. In Bryant RA, Nix DP (Eds). *Acute and chronic wounds: Current management concepts,* 3rd ed. St Louis: Mosby.

Pinchofsky-Devin GD, Kaminski MV Jr. (1996). Correlation of pressure sores and nutritional status. *J Am Geriatr Soc*, 34(6):435-440.

RCT = Randomized Controlled (Clinical) Trial, **NIC** = Nursing Interventions Classification, **NOC** = Nursing Outcomes Classification

Ratliff CR, Rodeheaver GT. (1999). Pressure ulcer assessment and management. *Lippincotts Prim Care Pract*, 3(2):242-258.

Reddy N, Cochran G. (1979). Phenomenological theory underlying pressure-time relationship in decubitus ulcer formation. *Fed Proc*, 38:1153.

Reddy M, Gill SS, Rochon PA. (2006). Preventing pressure ulcers: A systematic review. *JAMA*, 296(8):974-984.

Reichel SM. (1958). Shearing force as a factor in decubitus ulcers in paraplegics. *JAMA*, 166(7):762-763.

Sebern M. (1987). Home-team strategies for treating pressure sores. *Nursing*, 17(4):50-53.

Smith AM, Malone JA. (1990). Preventing pressure ulcers in institutionalized elders: Assessing the effects of small, unscheduled shifts in body position. *Decubitus* 3(4):20-24.

Stratton RJ, Ek AC, Engfer M, et al. (2005). Enteral nutritional support in prevention and treatment of pressure ulcers: A systematic review and meta-analysis. *Ageing Res Rev*, 4(3):422-450.

Thompson P, Langemo DK, Hunter S, Olson B, Hanson D. (2004). Prevalence of diabetes and related complications in migrant farm workers. *Tex J Community Health*, 22(1):20-27.

Warshaw E, Nix D, Kula J, Markon CE. (2002). Clinical and cost effectiveness of a cleanser protectant lotion for treatment of perineal skin breakdown in low-risk patients with incontinence. *Ostomy Wound Manage*, 48(6):44-51.

Wound Ostomy Continence Nursing (WOCN). (2003). *Guideline for prevention and management of pressure ulcers.* Glenview, IL: WOCN.

Zimmerer RE, Lawson KD, Calvert CJ. (1986). The effects of wearing diapers on skin. *Pediatr Dermatol*, 3(2):95-101.

 # PROCEDURAL PAIN ALLEVIATION

Yvonne D'Arcy, MS, CRNP, CNS; Betty J. Ackley, MSN, EdS, RN

Definition: Prevention or reduction of pain experienced with an invasive or noxious diagnostic or therapeutic procedure.

The Joint Commission requires that all patients be assessed for pain and that they receive adequate treatment for pain (Joint Commission, 2001). This includes all patients who are undergoing procedures as a part of their treatment plan.

NURSING ACTIVITIES

Effective

■ (SP) *Assess pain and medicate the patient for pain just before a procedure and as needed during the procedure.* **LOE = IV**

(EO) Sedation is not analgesia. Medicate patients just before the procedure, and use opioids such as fentanyl to control pain during the procedure. Establish signals that the patient can use to indicate increasing pain and the need for pain medication (D'Arcy, 2004).

(EO) Assess and document the pain intensity rating before, during, and after the procedure using a simple pain rating tool such as the 0-to-10 pain intensity scale (D'Arcy, 2004).

(NR) A comparative descriptive study of 6201 patients in the intensive care unit, including children and adults, found that pain intensity scores for children 12 years old or younger were 28 to 60 during turning and 52 to 56 during tracheal suctioning on a 0-to-100 pain intensity scale. Adolescents reported pain scores for wound dressing changes, turning, tracheal suctioning, and wound drain removal from 5 to 7 on a 0-to-10 pain intensity scale. Adults reported scores of 2.65 and 4.93 during procedures on a 0-to-10 scale, with turning in bed being the most painful experience. Of note is that less than 20% of the patients received opiates before their procedures (Puntillo et al., 2001).

(NR) A descriptive study of 31 surgical patients who had drains removed indicated that pain was the most common sensation during drain removal, with a visual analog scale score of 40 (this was equivalent to a score of 4 on a 0-to-10 pain intensity rating scale; Mimnaugh et al., 1999).

(NR) In a prospective, descriptive study, 45 adult patients rated their pain during endotracheal suctioning. More than one third of the patients reported a pain level of more than 7 on a 0-to-10 pain intensity rating scale (Puntillo, 1994).

■ (SP) *Assess patients for pain using a recognized behavioral pain rating tool as an adjunct or as a replacement for a numeric pain rating if a self-report is not possible.* **LOE = IV**

(NR) In a group of 5957 adult patients who were undergoing procedures, a 30-item behavioral observation tool was used to assess patients' behaviors before and during the procedure. Pain behaviors that were noted were moaning, grimacing, rigidity, wincing, closed eyes, and clenched fists. Patients with procedural pain were at least three times more likely to have increased behavioral responses. A regression model found that 33% of the variance in pain behaviors was explained by three factors: (1) the degree of procedural pain intensity; (2) the degree of procedural distress; and (3) undergoing a procedure in which turning was involved (Puntillo et al., 2004).

(MR) A prospective study evaluated 30 mechanically ventilated intensive care patients either undergoing non-nociceptive procedures (e.g., compression stocking application) or experiencing a nociceptive stimulus (e.g., nasotracheal suctioning). Using the Payen Behavioral Pain Scale with the elements of facial expression, the movements of the upper limbs, and compliance with ventilation, scores on all three correlated well with ratings on the 0-to-10 pain intensity scale, and increased pain was noted during the procedures. The tool was found to be a valid measure of pain for this patient population, and it could be used to help with the titration of analgesia (Payen et al., 2001).

■ *Use a topical anesthetic cream or a local intradermal anesthetic to decrease the pain associated with the insertion of an intravenous (IV) tube.* **LOE = I**

(NR) A meta-analysis of 20 studies analyzing the effectiveness of a topical anesthetic (2.5% lidocaine and 2.5% prilocaine mixture; eutectic mixture of local anesthetics [EMLA] cream) concluded that the use of EMLA cream significantly decreased venipuncture and IV insertion pain in 85% of the population (Fetzer, 2002).

(NR) A randomized double-blinded study involving surgical adult patients ($N = 47$) that compared the use of intradermal injections of either lidocaine hydrochloride 1% with sodium bicarbonate or sodium chloride 0.9% with benzyl alcohol demonstrated that there was no significant difference between the anesthetic effects. Both were safe and effective for reducing pain (Brown, 2004).

(NR) A quasi-experimental study involving surgical adult patients ($N = 30$) that compared the intradermal injection of lidocaine, the use of EMLA cream, and the Numby Stuff system (local anesthetic iontocaine with the use of mild electrical current to deliver the medication through the skin) found the Numby Stuff system to be superior to the other methods of decreasing IV insertion pain (Miller et al., 2001).

RCT = Randomized Controlled (Clinical) Trial, **NIC** = Nursing Interventions Classification, **NOC** = Nursing Outcomes Classification

(NR) A descriptive study involving adult medical-surgical patients ($N = 180$) was designed to determine patient preferences regarding the use of intradermal lidocaine before peripheral IV insertions. Significant findings were that patients who had any type of experience with lidocaine preferred to have it used for future IV insertions and that the pain associated with lidocaine injection was less than the pain associated with IV insertion (Brown, 2003).

(NR) A randomized, double-blind study involving adult inpatients on medical units ($N = 33$) compared the subcutaneous injection of buffered lidocaine hydrochloride 1%, sodium chloride 0.9% with benzyl alcohol, and no treatment and found a significantly improved pain rating associated with use of lidocaine hydrochloride 1%. There was no significant difference between no treatment and the use of sodium chloride with benzyl alcohol (Hattula et al., 2002).

■ *When inserting a nasogastric tube, use lidocaine spray alone or in combination with lidocaine gel as ordered.* **LOE = II**

(MR) A double-blind, placebo-controlled, randomized trial of adult patients ($N = 70$) was conducted to determine whether nebulized lidocaine reduced patient discomfort during nasogastric tube insertion. Twenty-nine patients received the nebulized lidocaine, and 21 received nebulized normal saline. Patients rated their discomfort on a 100-mm visual analog scale (0 = no discomfort, 100 = severe discomfort), and the difficulty of insertion was rated on a 5-point Likert scale. The results indicated a significant decrease in pain for those who received lidocaine. There was no difference in the difficulty in tube passage as identified by the nurses. Patients who received the lidocaine had more complications, including epistaxis, dyspnea, and chest tightness in one patient (Cullen et al., 2004).

(MR) A double-blind, double-dummy, randomized, triple-crossover design was performed with healthy volunteers ($N = 30$). Each subject had three nasogastric tubes placed and acted as their own control for the three study medications: lidocaine gel, lidocaine spray, and atomized cocaine. A visual analog scale (0 to 100) was used for pain and for global discomfort. Participants were asked to identify which study medication they preferred. The volunteers rated all the medications as equally effective for pain control, but the lidocaine gel was identified as being preferred and being significantly better for overall discomfort (Ducharme & Matheson, 2003).

(MR) In an RCT conducted on adult patients ($N = 40$) in the emergency department, patients were randomized to receive either atomized lidocaine ($N = 20$) or normal saline ($N = 20$) into their oropharynx. All patients received lidocaine gel intranasally during the insertion. A visual analog scale (0 = least possible pain, 100 = worst possible pain) was used immediately after securing the tube. Mean pain scores for the lidocaine group were statistically and clinically significantly lower than the scores of the placebo group (Wolfe et al., 2000).

■ *Medicate the patient for pain or ensure that the patient receives an anesthetic agent as ordered before a bone marrow aspiration.* **LOE = II**

(NR) In a two-part study, first a descriptive study ($N = 132$) was done that found that patients having a bone marrow aspiration experienced moderate to severe pain. In the second part of the study, a controlled study was done that compared the pain associated with a bone marrow aspiration when tramadol was given before the procedure ($N = 100$) with the pain of a control group that did not receive preprocedure medication. Results indicated that patients who were pretreated with tramadol had significantly less pain and that the medication was well tolerated (Vanhelleputte et al., 2003).

NR = Nursing Research, **MR** = Multidisciplinary Research, **SP** = Standard of Practice, **EO** = Expert Opinion, **LOE** = Level of Evidence

(MR) In a controlled study of patients who received a bone marrow aspiration ($N = 136$), one group of patients received inhaled nitrous oxide (Entonox) during the procedure, whereas the other group received local anesthesia only. Patients who received nitrous oxide had significantly less pain with the procedure and preferred to receive nitrous oxide again for future bone marrow aspirations (Steedman et al., 2006).

(MR) In an RCT, patients ($N = 50$) undergoing a bone marrow biopsy were divided into two groups. The group that received lorazepam before the procedure remembered significantly less pain, and one third of the patients did not remember the procedure at all. The control group that did not receive lorazepam reported remembering significant pain (Milligan et al., 1987).

(MR) In a controlled study of patients undergoing a bone marrow aspiration/trephine biopsy ($N = 102$), one group of patients received IV midazolam, whereas the control group received local anesthesia only. The group receiving midazolam experienced amnesia for the procedure and mild pain only. The control group experienced intense pain during the biopsy, and more than half of the patients had lingering discomfort in the area (Mainwaring et al., 1996).

■ *Medicate the patient for pain or ensure that the patient receives an analgesic agent as ordered before the removal of a chest tube.* **LOE = II**

(NR) In a controlled study, patients who had undergone coronary artery bypass graft surgery ($N = 40$) received either opioids plus slow breathing relaxation exercise or opioids alone. The group that received the breathing relaxation exercise plus opioids had a significant reduction in pain rating after the procedure (Friesner et al., 2006). (Note: At the time of the actual chest tube removal, the patient is generally advised to take a deep breath and to hold it while the tube is removed.)

(NR) In an RCT of patients experiencing chest tube removal, four groups received differing treatments: (1) IV morphine and procedural information; (2) IV ketorolac and procedural information; (3) IV morphine plus procedural and sensory information; or (4) IV ketorolac plus procedural and sensory information. Results were low pain intensity and pain distress for all four groups (Puntillo & Ley, 2004).

(MR) In an RCT of patients experiencing chest tube removal ($N = 53$), patients receiving topical valdecoxib experienced significantly less pain than patients receiving liquid paraffin at the chest tube site (Singh & Gopinath, 2005).

■ *When performing wound care, use EMLA cream as ordered for at least 20 minutes before cleansing, debriding, or dressing the wound.* **LOE = I**

(NR) A systematic review found that research supported the use of topical analgesic EMLA cream applied to the wound bed for the chronic wound pain associated with the treatment of the wound (Evans & Gray, 2005).

(MR) A Cochrane review found that EMLA cream was effective for decreasing the pain associated with the debridement of venous leg ulcers (Briggs & Nelson, 2003).

Possibly Effective

■ *Use a topical anesthetic cream or a local anesthetic to decrease the pain associated with intramuscular injection or the pain from femoral catheter removal or suctioning.* **LOE = IV**

(NR) A crossover, placebo-controlled study ($N = 18$) demonstrated that multiple sclerosis patients who received an application of EMLA cream before the intramuscular injection of interferon had reduced fear-of-injection scores and reduced pain-from-injection scores (Buhse, 2006).

(NR) In an observational study, 105 of 111 patients undergoing femoral sheath removal reported that they had an acceptable level of pain without the local anesthetic infiltration before sheath removal. Patients rated their pain from 0 to 3 on the 0-to-10 pain intensity scale (Bowden & Worrey, 1995).

(MR) In an RCT, 20 patients were randomized to two groups, with one group receiving a new angioplasty catheter and the other receiving a standard catheter. Lidocaine was injected through the port of the new sheath. These 10 patients reported less pain during catheter insertion and removal. Patients in the standard catheter group reported their pain at 5.2 overall on the 0-to-10 pain intensity scale. Patients who received the new sheath with lidocaine infiltration reported a pain intensity of 1.2 at insertion and of 2.6 at removal on a scale of 0 to 10 (Lambert et al., 1996).

■ *Offer adjuvant methods of pain control if the patient is able to use them.*
LOE = VI

(EO) In addition to pain medication, offer distraction techniques such as music, relaxation tapes, and guided imagery (D'Arcy, 2004).

(NR) In a group of 26 postoperative patients with abdominal wound packing postoperatively, a comparison study found that pain ratings were significantly lower when music was used during the procedure. All patients had all received preprocedure pain medication (Angus & Faux, 1989).

Not Effective

■ *Using ice therapy before the removal of a chest tube.* **LOE = II**

(NR) In an RCT of patients experiencing chest tube removal ($N = 50$), patients in the experimental group received ice therapy, whereas the control group received a placebo. Differences in pain reports between the groups were not significant (Sauls, 2002).

Possibly Harmful

■ *Using Demerol, which is no longer recommended as a first-line pain medication.*
LOE = VII

(EO) Demerol is no longer recommended for use for pain relief because of the risk of seizures from the accumulation of the neurotoxic metabolite normeperidine (APS, 2003).

OUTCOME MEASUREMENT

PAIN LEVEL (NOC)

Definition: Severity of observed or reported pain.
Pain Level as evidenced by the following NOC indicators:
• Reported pain
• Length of pain episodes

NR = Nursing Research, **MR** = Multidisciplinary Research, **SP** = Standard of Practice, **EO** = Expert Opinion, **LOE** = Level of Evidence

OUTCOME MEASUREMENT—*cont'd*

- Moaning and crying
- Facial expressions of pain
- Restlessness
- Pacing
- Narrowed focus
- Muscle tension
- Loss of appetite

(Rate each indicator of **Pain Level:** 1 = severe, 2 = substantial, 3 = moderate, 4 = mild, 5 = none) (Moorhead et al., 2004).

REFERENCES

American Pain Society (APS). (2003). *Principles of analgesic use in the treatment of acute and cancer pain,* 5th ed. Glenview, IL: APS.

Angus JE, Faux S. (1989). The effect of music on postoperative patients' pain during a nursing procedure. In Funk SG, Tournquist EM, Champagne MT, et al (Eds). *Key aspects of comfort: Management of pain fatigue and nausea.* New York: Springer, pp. 166-172.

Bowden SM, Worrey JA. (1995). Assessing patient comfort: Local infiltration of lidocaine during femoral sheath removal. *Am J Crit Care,* 4(5):368-369.

Briggs M, Nelson EA. (2003). Topical agents or dressings for pain in venous leg ulcers. *Cochrane Database Syst Rev,* (1):CD001177.

Brown J. (2003). Using lidocaine for peripheral I.V. insertions: Patients' preferences and pain experiences. *Med Surg Nurs,* 12(2):95-100.

Brown D. (2004). Local anesthesia for vein cannulation: A comparison of two solutions. *J Infus Nurs,* 27(2):85-88.

Buhse M. (2006). Efficacy of EMLA cream to reduce fear and pain associated with interferon beta-1a injection in patients with multiple sclerosis. *J Neurosci Nurs,* 38(4):222-226.

Cullen L, Taylor D, Taylor S, Chu K. (2004). Nebulized lidocaine decreases the discomfort of nasogastric tube insertion: A randomized, double-blind trial. *Ann Emerg Med,* 44(2):131-137.

D'Arcy Y. (2004). Managing procedural pain. *Nursing,* 34(12):76.

Ducharme J, Matheson K. (2003). What is the best topical anesthetic for nasogastric insertion? A comparison of lidocaine gel, lidocaine spray, and atomized cocaine. *J Emerg Nurs,* 29(5):427-430.

Evans E, Gray M. (2005). Do topical analgesics reduce pain associated with wound dressing changes or debridement of chronic wounds? *J Wound Ostomy Continence Nurs,* 32(5):287-290.

Fetzer SJ. (2002). Reducing venipuncture and intravenous insertion pain with eutectic mixture of local anesthetic: A meta-analysis. *Nurs Res,* 51(2):119-124.

Friesner SA, Curry DM, Moddeman GR. (2006). Comparison of two pain-management strategies during chest tube removal: Relaxation exercise with opioids and opioids alone. *Heart Lung,* 35(4):269-276.

Hattula JL, McGovern EK, Neumann TL. (2002). Comparison of intravenous cannulation injectable preanesthetics in an adult medical inpatient population. *App Nurs Res,* 15(3):189-193.

The Joint Commission. (2001). Pain management standards. Available online: www.jointcommission.org. Retrieved on July 7, 2007.

Lambert CR, Bikkina M, Shakoor A, Korzun WJ. (1996). New vascular sheath for subcutaneous drug administration: Design, animal testing, and clinical application for pain prevention after angioplasty. *Cathet Cardiovasc Diagn,* 37(1):68-72.

Mainwaring CJ, Wong C, Lush RJ, et al. (1996). The role of midazolam-induced sedation in bone marrow aspiration/trephine biopsies. *Clin Lab Haematol,* 18(4):285-288.

RCT = Randomized Controlled (Clinical) Trial, **NIC** = Nursing Interventions Classification, **NOC** = Nursing Outcomes Classification

Miller KA, Balakrishnan G, Eichbauer G, Betley K. (2001). 1% lidocaine injection, EMLA cream, or "numby stuff" for topical analgesia associated with peripheral intravenous cannulation. *AANA J*, 69(3):185-187.

Milligan DW, Howard MR, Judd A. (1987). Premedication with lorazepam before bone marrow biopsy. *J Clin Pathol*, 40(6):696-698.

Mimnaugh L, Winegar M, Mabrey Y, Davis JE. (1999). Sensations experienced during removal of tubes in acute postoperative patients. *Appl Nurs Res*, 12(2):78-85.

Moorhead M, Johnson M, Maas M (Eds). (2004). *Nursing Outcomes Classification (NOC)*, 3rd ed. St Louis: Mosby.

Payen JF, Bru O, Bosson JL, et al. (2001). Assessing pain in critically ill sedated patients by using a behavioral pain scale. *Crit Care Med*, 29(12):2258-2263.

Puntillo KA. (1994). Dimensions of procedural pain and its analgesic management in critically ill surgical patients. *Am J Crit Care*, 3(2):116-122.

Puntillo K, Ley SJ. (2004). Appropriately timed analgesics control pain due to chest tube removal. *Am J Crit Care*, 13(4):292-301.

Puntillo KA, Morris A, Thompson C, et al. (2004). Pain behaviors observed during six common procedures: Results from Thunder Project II. *Crit Care Med*, 32(2):421-427.

Puntillo KA, White C, Morris A, et al. (2001). Patients' perceptions and responses to procedural pain: Results from the Thunder Project II. *Am J Crit Care*, 10(4):238-251.

Sauls J. (2002). The use of ice for pain associated with chest tube removal. *Pain Manag Nurs*, 3(2):44-52.

Singh M, Gopinath R. (2005). Topical analgesia for chest tube removal in cardiac patients. *J Cardiothorac Vasc Anesth*, 19(6):719-722.

Steedman B, Watson J, Ali S, et al. (2006). Inhaled nitrous oxide (Entonox) as a short acting sedative during bone marrow examination. *Clin Lab Haematol*, 28(5):321-324.

Vanhelleputte P, Nijs K, Delforge M, et al. (2003). Pain during bone marrow aspiration: Prevalence and prevention. *J Pain Symptom Manage*, 26(3):860-866.

Wolfe TR, Fosnocht DE, Linscott MS. (2000). Atomized lidocaine as topical anesthesia for nasogastric tube placement: A randomized, double-blind, placebo-controlled trial. *Ann Emerg Med*, 35(5):421-425.

 # PROGRESSIVE MUSCLE RELAXATION

Carolyn B. Yucha, PhD, RN, FAAN, CNE, BCIA

NIC **Definition:** Facilitating the tensing and releasing of successive muscle groups while attending to the resulting differences in sensation (Dochterman & Bulechek, 2004).

NURSING ACTIVITIES

Effective

■ *Use progressive muscle relaxation (PMR) to reduce chronic pain.* **LOE = II**

NR An RCT evaluating guided imagery coupled with PMR in women with osteoarthritis (*N* = 28) showed that the treatment group reported a significant reduction in pain and mobility difficulty at week 12 as compared with the control group (Baird & Sands, 2004).

MR An RCT comparing Internet-delivered combination therapy (PMR, biofeedback, autogenic training, and stress management) to waitlist control in those with chronic headache (*N* = 86) showed a significant reduction in headache symptoms and associated medication usage (Devineni & Blanchard, 2005).

MR A controlled study of women with menstruation-related tension-type headache (*N* = 6) showed that nine sessions of PMR had no effect on headache activity or medication taken for headaches (Blanchard & Kim, 2005).

NR = Nursing Research, **MR** = Multidisciplinary Research, **SP** = Standard of Practice, **EO** = Expert Opinion, **LOE** = Level of Evidence

- *Use PMR for people with cancer.* **LOE = II**

  (NR) An RCT designed to assess the effects of PMR on chemotherapy-related nausea and vomiting in breast cancer patients ($N = 71$) showed that, as compared with the control group, those patients trained in PMR had a decreased duration of nausea and vomiting but no change in nausea and vomiting frequency or intensity (Molassiotis et al., 2002).

  (NR) A four-group RCT that compared PMR, guided imagery, both, and neither in community patients with advanced cancer ($N = 56$) showed positive changes in depression and quality of life but no changes in anxiety (Sloman, 2002).

  (NR) An RCT that compared three groups (concrete objective information, PMR, control) of patients undergoing radiation therapy ($N = 76$) showed that those receiving either intervention reported more social activity and that those who received PMR reported more household activity during treatment (Christman & Cain, 2004).

  (MR) An RCT studying PMR coupled with guided imagery for patients with breast cancer undergoing chemotherapy ($N = 60$) reported that, as comparison with the control group, the members of the intervention group were less anxious, depressive, and hostile, and they reported less anticipatory and postchemotherapy nausea and vomiting and improved quality of life (Yoo et al., 2005).

  (MR) An RCT evaluating the effects of PMR in colorectal cancer patients after stoma surgery ($N = 59$) reported that PMR significantly decreased anxiety and improved quality of life (Cheung et al., 2003).

  (MR) A controlled study comparing PMR, massage therapy, and standard care over 5 weeks in women with breast cancer ($N = 58$) found that those in the treatment groups reported less depression, anxiety, and pain. However, the massage group also had higher dopamine levels, natural killer cells, and lymphocytes at the end of the study (Hernandez-Reif et al., 2005).

  (MR) In an RCT involving patients with localized cancer ($N = 116$), those who were treated with PMR coupled with guided imagery showed a modest improvement with regard to psychological distress as compared with the control group and as measured using the Global Severity Index (Baider et al., 2001).

- *Use PMR to reduce blood pressure.* **LOE = II**

  (NR) A controlled study of biofeedback including PMR and autogenic training in hypertensive patients ($N = 54$) showed that this combination resulted in a small reduction in both systolic and diastolic blood pressures. The effect of PMR could not be distinguished from other program components (Yucha et al., 2005).

  (NR) A controlled study of people with hypertension ($N = 40$) showed that PMR practiced at home daily reduced systolic and diastolic blood pressures as compared with those of a control group (Sheu et al., 2003).

  (NR) An RCT comparing PMR, stretch release relaxation, and cognitive imagery relaxation in patients with hypertension ($N = 9$) showed that all three led to blood pressure reduction, with the first two being more effective than the third technique (Yung et al., 2001).

Possibly Effective

- *Use PMR to promote sleep.* **LOE = II**

  (MR) An RCT of adult cancer patients that compared PMR ($N = 80$) with autogenic training ($N = 71$) and a control group ($N = 78$) showed that both treatment groups had moderate- to

---

RCT = Randomized Controlled (Clinical) Trial, **NIC** = Nursing Interventions Classification, **NOC** = Nursing Outcomes Classification

large-scale improvements in sleep latency, duration, efficiency, and quality (Simeit et al., 2004).

(MR) A four-group RCT that compared PMR plus cognitive distraction, sleep restriction/stimulus control, sleep hygiene education, and flurazepam reported that the drug was better than other treatments and that PMR had a greater effect on sleep onset, whereas sleep restriction had a greater effect on sleep maintenance (Waters et al., 2003).

■ Use PMR to reduce anxiety. **LOE = II**

(NR) A controlled study examining the effect of PMR on participants in cardiac rehabilitation ($N = 14$) revealed positive effects of PMR on heart rate and anxiety as compared with results seen in the control group (Wilk & Turkoski, 2001).

(MR) A systematic review of the literature showed that relaxation training may be effective for generalized anxiety, panic disorder, dental phobia, and test anxiety (Jorm et al., 2004).

(MR) An RCT of patients who had undergone stoma surgery ($N = 18$) compared PMR at home using an audiotape with a control group. The results showed that those in the experimental group reported less anxiety and an enhanced quality of life (Cheung et al., 2001).

(MR) An RCT of abused women residing in domestic violence shelters ($N = 28$) addressed the results of PMR paired with music as compared with no treatment. The women in the treatment group experienced reduced anxiety levels and improved sleep quality (Hernandez-Ruiz, 2005).

■ Use PMR for people with asthma. **LOE = III**

(MR) An RCT comparing medication plus cognitive behavior therapy (including PMR) with medication alone in patients with asthma ($N = 10$) showed that those in the experimental group reported a decrease in asthma symptoms, anxiety, and depression and an increase in quality of life (Grover et al., 2002).

(MR) An RCT comparing PMR training with placebo in female adolescents with asthma ($N = 31$) demonstrated a reduction in systolic blood pressure and a rise in forced expiratory volume and peak expiratory flow in the experimental group (Nickel et al., 2005).

(MR) A systematic review of studies exploring the emotional stress of asthma patients ($N = 15$ total, $N = 5$ PMR) concluded that there was a lack of evidence for the efficacy of relaxation therapies for the management of asthma (Huntley et al., 2002).

Not Effective

■ Using PMR to reduce acute pain. **LOE = II**

(MR) An RCT comparing guided imagery, PMR, and control groups of patients undergoing colorectal resections ($N = 60$) showed no significant differences in pain or analgesic consumption, although patients responded favorably to both interventions (Haase et al., 2005).

(MR) A controlled study of patients with post-traumatic headache ($N = 14$) evaluated combined biofeedback, PMR, education, and cognitive therapy and found no significant differences as compared with a wait list control group (Tatrow et al., 2003).

(MR) A descriptive study of patients undergoing abdominal surgery ($N = 61$) showed that PMR training decreased the self-reported pain levels of these patients (de Paula et al., 2002).

NR = Nursing Research, **MR** = Multidisciplinary Research, **SP** = Standard of Practice, **EO** = Expert Opinion, **LOE** = Level of Evidence

■ *Using PMR to reduce depression.* **LOE = II**

(MR) An RCT that compared massage, PMR, and standard prenatal care alone in depressed pregnant women ($N = 84$) showed no effect of PMR on anxiety, depressed mood, or pain (Field et al., 2004).

Possibly Harmful

No applicable published research was found in this category.

OUTCOME MEASUREMENT

PERSONAL WELL-BEING (NOC)

Definition: Extent of positive perception of one's health status and life circumstances.
Personal Well-Being as evidenced by the following selected NOC indicators:
• Psychological health
• Physical health
• Ability to cope
• Ability to relax
(Rate each indicator of **Personal Well-Being:** 1 = not at all satisfied, 2 = somewhat satisfied, 3 = moderately satisfied, 4 = very satisfied, 5 = completely satisfied) (Moorhead et al., 2004).

REFERENCES

Baider L, Peretz T, Hadani PE, Koch U. (2001). Psychological intervention in cancer patients: A randomized study. *Gen Hosp Psychiatry,* 23(5):272-277.

Baird CL, Sands L. (2004). A pilot study of the effectiveness of guided imagery with progressive muscle relaxation to reduce chronic pain and mobility difficulties of osteoarthritis. *Pain Manag Nurs,* 5(3):97-104.

Blanchard EB, Kim M. (2005). The effect of the definition of menstrually-related headache on the response to biofeedback treatment. *Appl Psychophysiol Biofeedback,* 30(1):53-63.

Cheung YL, Molassiotis A, Chang AM. (2001). A pilot study on the effect of progressive muscle relaxation training of patients after stoma surgery. *Eur J Cancer Care,* 10(2):107-114.

Cheung YL, Molassiotis A, Chang AM. (2003). The effect of progressive muscle relaxation training on anxiety and quality of life after stoma surgery in colorectal cancer patients. *Psychooncology,* 12(3):254-266.

Christman NJ, Cain LB. (2004). The effects of concrete objective information and relaxation on maintaining usual activity during radiation therapy. *Oncol Nurs Forum,* 31(2):E39-E45.

de Paula AA, de Carvalho EC, dos Santos CB. (2002). The use of the "progressive muscle relaxation" technique for pain relief in gynecology and obstetrics. *Rev Lat Am Enferm,* 10(5):654-659.

Deviveni T, Blanchard EB. (2005). A randomized controlled trial of an Internet-based treatment for chronic headache. *Behav Res Ther,* 43(3):277-292.

Dochterman JM, Bulechek GM (Eds). (2004). *Nursing Interventions Classification (NIC),* 4th ed. St Louis: Mosby.

Field T, Diego MA, Hernandez-Reif M, et al. (2004). Massage therapy effects on depressed pregnant women. *J Psychosom Obstet Gynaecol,* 25(2):115-122.

Grover N, Kumaraiah V, Prasadrao PS, D'souza G. (2002). Cognitive behavioural intervention in bronchial asthma. *J Assoc Physicians India,* 50:896-900.

Haase O, Schwenk W, Hermann C, Muller JM. (2005). Guided imagery and relaxation in conventional colorectal resections: A randomized, controlled, partially blinded trial. *Dis Colon Rectum,* 48(10):1955-1963.

Hernandez-Reif M, Field T, Ironson G, et al. (2005). Natural killer cells and lymphocytes increase in women with breast cancer following massage therapy. *Int J Neurosci,* 115(4):495-510.

RCT = Randomized Controlled (Clinical) Trial, **NIC** = Nursing Interventions Classification, **NOC** = Nursing Outcomes Classification

Hernandez-Ruiz E. (2005). Effect of music therapy on the anxiety levels and sleep patterns of abused women in shelters. *J Music Ther,* 42(2):140-158.

Huntley A, White AR, Ernst E. (2002). Relaxation therapies for asthma: A systematic review. *Thorax,* 57(2):127-131.

Jorm AF, Christensen H, Griffiths KM, et al. (2004). Effectiveness of complementary and self-help treatments for anxiety disorders. *Med J Aust,* 181(7 Suppl):S29-S46.

Molassiotis A, Yung HP, Yam BM, et al. (2002). The effectiveness of progressive muscle relaxation training in managing chemotherapy-induced nausea and vomiting in Chinese breast cancer patients: A randomised controlled trial. *Support Care Cancer,* 10(3):237-246.

Moorhead M, Johnson M, Maas M (Eds). (2004). *Nursing Outcomes Classification (NOC),* 3rd ed. St Louis: Mosby.

Nickel C, Kettler C, Muehlbacher M, et al. (2005). Effect of progressive muscle relaxation in adolescent female bronchial asthma patients: A randomized, double-blind, controlled study. *J Psychosom Res,* 59(6):393-398.

Sheu S, Irvin BL, Lin HS, Mar CL. (2003). Effects of progressive muscle relaxation on blood pressure and psychosocial status for clients with essential hypertension in Taiwan. *Holist Nurs Pract,* 17(1):41-47.

Simeit R, Deck R, Conta-Marx B. (2004). Sleep management training for cancer patients with insomnia. *Support Care Cancer,* 12(3):176-183.

Sloman R. (2002). Relaxation and imagery for anxiety and depression control in community patients with advanced cancer. *Cancer Nurs,* 25(6):432-435.

Tatrow K, Blanchard EB, Silverman DJ. (2003). Posttraumatic headache: An exploratory treatment study. *Appl Psychophysiol Biofeedback,* 28(4):267-278.

Waters WF, Hurry MJ, Binks PG, et al. (2003). Behavioral and hypnotic treatments for insomnia subtypes. *Behav Sleep Med,* 1(2):81-101.

Wilk C, Turkoski B. (2001). Progressive muscle relaxation in cardiac rehabilitation: A pilot study. *Rehabil Nurs,* 26(6):238-243.

Yoo HJ, Ahn SH, Kim SB, et al. (2005). Efficacy of progressive muscle relaxation training and guided imagery in reducing chemotherapy side effects in patients with breast cancer and in improving their quality of life. *Support Care Cancer,* 13(10):826-833.

Yucha CB, Tsai P, Calderon KS, Tian L. (2005). Biofeedback assisted relaxation training for essential hypertension: Who is most likely to benefit? *J Cardiovasc Nurs,* 20(3):198-205.

Yung P, French P, Leung B. (2001). Relaxation training as complementary therapy for mild hypertension control and the implications of evidence-based medicine. *Complement Ther Nurs Midwifery,* 7(2):59-65.

PROMPTED VOIDING   NIC

Jean F. Wyman, PhD, APRN-BC, GNP, FAAN

NIC   **Definition:** Promotion of urinary continence through the use of timed verbal toileting reminders and positive social feedback for successful toileting (Dochterman & Bulechek, 2004).

NURSING ACTIVITIES

Effective

■ *Use prompted voiding to reduce urinary incontinence.* **LOE = I**

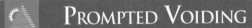 A Cochrane systematic review found that there was suggestive evidence of short-term benefit from prompted voiding with respect to increasing self-initiated voiding and decreasing incontinent episodes. However, longer-term effects and whether effects persisted after stopping prompted voiding were not known (Eustice et al., 2000).

NR = Nursing Research, **MR** = Multidisciplinary Research, **SP** = Standard of Practice, **EO** = Expert Opinion, **LOE** = Level of Evidence

(MR) An International Consultation on Incontinence systematic review found that prompted voiding was effective for the short-term treatment of daytime urinary incontinence among nursing home residents and home-care clients if caregivers complied with the protocol. Findings varied with regard to the characteristics of patients who responded to prompted voiding (e.g., cognitive status, mobility, bladder capacity, appropriate toileting rates, and baseline urinary incontinence severity; Fonda et al., 2005).

(NR) An RCT of an 8-week prompted voiding program in cognitively impaired homebound older adults ($N = 15$) found a greater reduction in incontinent episodes (day and night) for those in the experimental group than for those in the control group. There were no differences between groups with regard to any changes in self-initiated toileting or reduction in daytime incontinence (Engberg et al., 2002).

(MR) An RCT of a 6-week prompted voiding program with female nursing home residents ($N = 133$) found a significant reduction of wet episodes (26%) among those who were on a 1-hour prompting schedule versus the control group, which remained essentially the same. Although self-initiated toileting requests increased in both groups, this was greater in the experimental group, the members of which continued to have higher toileting requests than their own baseline period and than the control group, even after the program was terminated (Hu et al., 1989).

(Note: Using a voiding diary that includes space to record the time of voluntary voiding and incontinent episodes is very helpful when initiating prompted voiding. Other information that can be collected would be the fluid intake, the precipitating circumstances of incontinence, the amount of leakage, whether an urge was present at the time of voiding, whether a request to toilet was made, and/or pad changes.)

Possibly Effective

No applicable published research was found in this category.

Not Effective

■ *Using prompted voiding to reduce nighttime urinary incontinence.* **LOE = VI**

(MR) A prospective case series with nursing home residents ($N = 61$) did not find a reduction in nighttime incontinence or an increase in nighttime appropriate toileting rates with prompted voiding in the overall group or in those who responded well to daytime voiding (Ouslander et al., 2001).

Possibly Harmful

No applicable published research was found in this category.

OUTCOME MEASUREMENT

URINARY CONTINENCE (NOC)

Definition: Control of elimination of urine from the bladder.
Urinary Continence as evidenced by the following selected NOC indicators:
• Maintains predictable pattern of voiding
• Responds to urge in a timely manner

Continued

RCT = Randomized Controlled (Clinical) Trial, **NIC** = Nursing Interventions Classification, **NOC** = Nursing Outcomes Classification

OUTCOME MEASUREMENT—*cont'd*

- Gets to toilet between urge and passage of urine
- Voids >150 cc each time
- Recognizes urge to void
- Urine leakage between voidings
- Wets underclothing or bedding during night

(Rate each indicator of **Urinary Continence:** 1 = never demonstrated, 2 = rarely demonstrated, 3 = sometimes demonstrated, 4 = often demonstrated, 5 = consistently demonstrated) (Moorhead et al., 2004).

REFERENCES

Dochterman JM, Bulechek GM (Eds). (2004). *Nursing Interventions Classification (NIC)*, 4th ed. St Louis: Mosby.

Engberg S, Sereika SM, McDowell BJ, Weber E, Brodak I. (2002). Effectiveness of prompted voiding in treating urinary incontinence in cognitively impaired homebound older adults. *J Wound Ostomy Continence Nurs,* 29(5):252-265.

Eustice S, Roe B, Paterson J. (2000). Prompted voiding for the management of urinary incontinence in adults. *Cochrane Database Syst Rev,* (2):CD002113.

Fonda D, DuBeau CE, Harari D, Ouslander JG, Palmer M, Roe B. (2005). Incontinence in the frail elderly. In Abrams P, Cardozo L, Khoury S, Wein A (Eds): *Incontinence: Management,* Volume 2. Paris: Health Publication Ltd, pp 1163-1240.

Hu TW, Igou JF, Kaltreider DL, Yu LC, Rohner TJ, Dennis PJ, et al. (1989). A clinical trial of a behavioral therapy to reduce urinary incontinence in nursing homes. Outcome and implications. *JAMA,* 261(18):2656-2662.

Moorhead M, Johnson M, Maas M (Eds). (2004). *Nursing Outcomes Classification (NOC)*, 3rd ed. St Louis: Mosby.

Ouslander JG, Ai-Samarrai N, Schnelle JF. (2001). Prompted voiding for nighttime incontinence in nursing homes: Is it effective? *J Am Geriatr Soc,* 49(6):706-709.

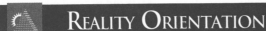

REALITY ORIENTATION   **NIC**

Dorothy A. Forbes, PhD, RN

NIC   **Definition:** Promotion of the patient's awareness of personal identity, time, and environment (Dochterman & Bulechek, 2004).

NURSING ACTIVITIES

Effective

■ *Use reality orientation to promote cognition.* **LOE = I**

 A Cochrane review (six studies, $N = 125$) and a systematic review found that reality orientation (RO) resulted in a significant change in cognition among patients with mild to severe dementia. Activities during the RO sessions included an RO board that displayed the day, weather, photographs, newspapers, and so on; orientation discussions; food preparations; exercises; and clocks, calendars, maps, posters, and the like (Spector et al., 2000a, b).

(MR) An RCT ($N = 201$) examined the effectiveness of cognitive stimulation therapy based on the concepts of RO for improving cognition among individuals with mild to moderate dementia. Topics included using money, word games, the present day, and famous faces. An RO board displayed both personal and orientation information. The treatment group significantly improved relative to the control group on the Mini-Mental State Examination and the Alzheimer's Disease Assessment Scale—Cognition. This degree of benefit for cognitive function appeared to be similar to that that can be attributed to acetylcholinesterase inhibitors (Spector et al., 2003). The effectiveness of 16 weekly maintenance sessions after the original cognitive stimulation therapy program was shown to result in continuous significant improvement in cognition (Orrell et al., 2005).

(MR) A retrospective study ($N = 74$) examined the impact of continued RO for delaying the symptoms of dementia progression. Data from 46 patients who completed from two to ten RO cycles were compared with 28 patients who completed only one RO cycle. The treatment group showed higher estimated survival rates than the control group with regard to cognitive decline and rates of institutionalization. Thus, continued RO classes during the early to middle stages of dementia may delay institutionalization and slow down the progression of cognitive decline (Metitieri et al., 2001).

(MR) An RCT ($N = 156$) evaluated the effect of combining RO with cholinesterase inhibitors with informal caregivers trained to offer RO at home. The treatment group showed improvement in Mini-Mental State Examination scores as compared with a decline in the control group and in the Alzheimer's Disease Assessment Scale—Cognition. RO was shown to enhance the effects of donepezil on cognition (Onder et al., 2005).

(MR) A retrospective study ($N = 38$) examined predictors of cognitive improvement after RO in outpatients with Alzheimer's disease and found that a lower Mini-Mental State Examination score and the absence of euphoric behavior in patients with mild to moderate dementia may predict a good cognitive outcome of RO therapy (Zanetti et al., 2002).

■ *Use RO to promote increased quality of life.* **LOE = II**

(MR) An RCT ($N = 201$) examined the effectiveness of RO for improving quality of life in individuals with mild to moderate dementia. The treatment group significantly improved relative to the control group on the Quality of Life—Alzheimer's Disease scales. The quality of life for women in the treatment group improved to a greater extent than was found for men. This result may be related to men being in the minority in most groups, which could have created discomfort and a reluctance to participate (Spector et al., 2003).

Possibly Effective

No applicable published research was found in this category.

Not Effective

■ *Using RO to promote improved mood.* **LOE = II**

(MR) A clinical controlled trial ($N = 34$) compared three groups of residents with dementia who received either RO, validation therapy, or no formal therapy and found no significant differences in rates of depression, functional status, and cognition between the groups (Scanland & Emershaw, 1993).

RCT = Randomized Controlled (Clinical) Trial, **NIC** = Nursing Interventions Classification, **NOC** = Nursing Outcomes Classification

(MR) Studies in a Cochrane review (Spector et al., 2000a) found similar nonsignificant results when changes in depression scores were compared between the experimental groups and the control groups (Baldelli et al., 1993; Ferrario et al., 1991).

■ *Using RO to promote appropriate behaviors.* **LOE = II**

(MR) A Cochrane review and a systematic review (three studies, $N = 45$) demonstrated that RO significantly improved behavior (Spector et al., 2000a, b). However, more recent RCTs found no significant changes in behavior and function (Spector et al., 2003; Onder et al., 2005).

Possibly Harmful

■ *Using RO that is provided in a mechanical, insensitive, or confrontational manner.* **LOE = VII**

(EO) If RO is applied in a mechanical, inflexible, insensitive, and/or confrontational manner, then the positive small cognitive improvements would be outweighed by the negative impact on the individual's well-being (APA, 1997; Woods et al., 2005).

(MR) A pilot study that developed a cognitive-based therapies program attempted to address the insensitivity and rigidity that was associated with some applications of RO. Recognizing the "personhood" of individuals with dementia, harnessing implicit memory, emphasizing active engagement with materials, and providing positive retrieval cues were emphasized (Spector et al., 2001).

OUTCOME MEASUREMENT

COGNITIVE ORIENTATION (NOC)

Definition: Ability to identify person, place, and time accurately.
Cognitive Orientation as evidenced by the following selected NOC indicators:
- Identifies self
- Identifies significant other
- Identifies current place
- Identifies correct season

(Rate each indicator of **Cognitive Orientation:** 1 = severely compromised, 2 = substantially compromised, 3 = moderately compromised, 4 = mildly compromised, 5 = not compromised) (Moorhead et al., 2004).

REFERENCES

American Psychiatric Association (APA). (1997). Practice guideline for the treatment of patients with Alzheimer's disease and other dementias of late life. *Am J Psychiatry,* 154(5 Suppl):1-39.

Baldelli MV, Pirani A, Motta M, Abati E, Mariani E, Manzi V. (1993). Effects of reality orientation therapy on elderly patients in the community. *Arch Gerontol Geriatr,* 17(3):211-218.

Dochterman JM, Bulechek GM (Eds). (2004). *Nursing Interventions Classification (NIC),* 4th ed. St Louis: Mosby.

Ferrario E, Cappa G, Molaschi M, Rocco M, Fabris F. (1991). Reality orientation therapy in institutionalized elderly patients: Preliminary results. *Arch Gerontol Geriatr,* 12(Suppl 2):139-142.

Metitieri T, Zanetti O, Geroldi C, Frisoni GB, De Leo D, Dello Buono M, et al. (2001). Reality orientation therapy to delay outcomes of progression in patients with dementia: A retrospective study. *Clin Rehabil,* 15(5):471-478.

Moorhead M, Johnson M, Maas M (Eds). (2004). *Nursing Outcomes Classification (NOC),* 3rd ed. St Louis: Mosby.

Onder G, Zanetti O, Giacobini E, Frisoni GB, Bartorelli L, Carbone G, et al. (2005). Reality orientation therapy combined with cholinesterase inhibitors in Alzheimer's disease: Randomised controlled trial. *Br J Psychiatry,* 187:450-455.

Orrell M, Spector A, Thorgrimsen L, Woods B. (2005). A pilot study examining the effectiveness of maintenance cognitive stimulation therapy (MCST) for people with dementia. *Int J Geriatr Psychiatry,* 20(5):446-451.

Scanland SG, Emershaw LE. (1993). Reality orientation and validation therapy. Dementia, depression, and functional status. *J Gerontol Nurs,* 19(6):7-11.

Spector A, Davies S, Woods B, Orrell M. (2000a). Reality orientation for dementia: A systematic review of the evidence of effectiveness from randomized controlled trials. *Gerontologist,* 40(2):206-212.

Spector A, Orrell M, Davies S, Woods B. (2000b). Reality orientation for dementia. *Cochrane Database Syst Rev,* (4):CD001119.

Spector A, Orrell M, Davies S, Woods B. (2001). Can reality orientation be rehabilitated? Development and piloting of an evidence-based programme of cognition-based therapies for people with dementia. *Neuropsychol Rehabil,* 11(3-4):377-397.

Spector A, Thorgrimsen L, Woods B, Royan L, Davies S, Butterworth M, et al. (2003). Efficacy of an evidence-based cognitive stimulation therapy programme for people with dementia: Randomised controlled trial. *Br J Psychiatry,* 183:248-254.

Woods B, Spector A, Jones C, Orrell M, Davies S. (2005). Reminiscence therapy for dementia. *Cochrane Database Syst Rev,* (2):CD001120.

Zanetti O, Oriani M, Geroldi C, Binetti G, Frisoni GB, Di Giovanni G, et al. (2002). Predictors of cognitive improvement after reality orientation in Alzheimer's disease. *Age Ageing,* 31(3):193-196.

RELIGIOUS RITUAL ENHANCEMENT   NIC

Lisa Burkhart, PhD, RN

> **NIC** **Definition:** Facilitating participation in religious practices (Dochterman & Bulechek, 2004).

NURSING ACTIVITIES

Effective

■ *Encourage the use of prayer/religious meditation as appropriate.* **LOE = II**

 In a descriptive correlation study of 111 individuals with fibromyalgia, 23% used spirituality and prayer as a coping strategy for pain (Nicassio et al., 1997).

 A descriptive random sample household survey of 679 African American women living in an urban area found that respondents who prayed less often reported a greater number of depressive symptoms, with social support mediating the positive relationship (van Olphen et al., 2003).

 A qualitative study of 32 participants in a weight-loss program in five focus groups identified spiritual interventions (including prayer and scripture reading) that helped with weight loss (Reicks et al., 2004).

(MR) In a controlled study with one control and two experimental groups of 84 college students, both experimental groups participated in a spiritual meditation exercise (one had a religious focus and the other had a nonreligious focus). Both experimental groups experienced significantly less anxiety and increases in positive mood, spiritual health, spiritual experiences, and pain tolerance. The religious experimental group had variables that were affected significantly higher than those seen in the other two groups (Wachholtz & Pargament, 2005).

(EO) Forgiveness therapy, adapted cognitive-behavioral therapy with a religious focus, prayer, meditation, and 12-step fellowship are recommended as spiritual interventions (Harris et al., 1999).

Additional research: Benson et al., 1990; Mullen et al., 1993.

Possibly Effective

■ *Determine and encourage the patient's religious practices (if used) to promote health and to cope with disease.* **LOE = V**

(NR) A qualitative phenomenological study of inner strength with a sample of five Hispanic women found that Hispanic women drew strength from spiritual and religious resources (Dingley & Roux, 2003).

(NR) A qualitative study of 55 adult female survivors of child abuse identified spiritual connection as a positive value for coping with negative experiences, church as a location for accessing God and communing with others, and a growing relationship with the natural world and the body (Hall, 2003).

(NR) A qualitative study of 13 African American women living with breast cancer and undergoing initial treatment identified spirituality (relationships with and reliance on God) as one of the three major themes, which were experience trajectory, femininity, and spirituality (Lackey et al., 2001).

(NR) A qualitative study of 15 chronically ill patients identified spiritual coping mechanisms as reaching out to God in the belief and faith that help would be forthcoming; feeling connected to God through prayer; finding meaning and purpose; following a strategy of privacy; and developing connectedness with others (Narayanasamy, 2002).

(NR) A qualitative survey of 115 nurses regarding when and how spiritual needs were identified and the impact of spiritual care indicated that nurses commonly supported religious beliefs and practices and a cultural approach that integrated nonmainstream religious practices into care. Spiritual care was also associated with positive feelings of patients and relatives (Narayanasamy & Owens, 2001).

(MR) A descriptive cross-sectional survey of 838 patients of a general medical service and who were 50 years old and older correlated religiousness and spirituality with greater social support, fewer depressive symptoms, better cognitive function, and greater cooperativeness. Internal religiosity was associated with better physical functioning (Koenig et al., 2004).

(MR) A qualitative study of 14 hospice patients, cancer survivors, caregivers, and health care professionals indicated that religious beliefs were strengthened during crises only if the participants had a history of religious beliefs. However, all participants expressed strong spiritual beliefs as defined in terms of meaning and purpose in life (McGrath, 2003).

(MR) A qualitative study of 26 older women who had not experienced a recent loss or terminal illness identified a need to feel connected, spiritual questioning, existential angst, thoughts about death and dying, and reliance on organized religion as important. Those who relied on religion did not experience the other themes (Moremen, 2005).

NR = Nursing Research, **MR** = Multidisciplinary Research, **SP** = Standard of Practice, **EO** = Expert Opinion, **LOE** = Level of Evidence

A qualitative study of 70 African American women with type 2 diabetes identified spirituality and religiousness as important factors in general health, disease adjustment, and coping (Samuel-Hodge et al., 2000).

A qualitative study of 19 former runaway and homeless youth identified spiritual practices as important in coping, including having a personal relationship with a nonjudgmental higher power, using prayer, participating in traditional and nontraditional religious practices, and finding meaning and purpose in life, including a desire to "give back" to the community. Spirituality played an important role in their resilience, nourished them, and gave them a feeling of being rescued (Williams & Lindsey, 2005).

Additional research: Yates et al., 1981; Larson et al., 1989; Oxman et al., 1995; Bush et al., 1999; Harris et al., 1999; Strawbridge et al., 1997.

■ *Determine and encourage the family's religious practices (if used) to help cope with loss.* LOE = VI

A descriptive, cross-sectional survey of 84 caregivers of dementia patients and 81 non-caregivers (matched sample by age) determined that unmet spiritual needs predicted more stress and less well-being. Caregivers had greater unmet needs for religious contact, and both groups had unmet spiritual needs (Burgener, 1994).

A qualitative study of 30 survivors regarding final conversations that they had with loved ones identified religious faith and spirituality as being helpful for coping with life's challenges after the loved one is gone (Keeley, 2004).

Not Effective

No applicable published research was found in this category.

Possibly Harmful

■ *Encouraging religious expression if the patient has no religious preference.* LOE = VI

A qualitative study of 10 people with advanced HIV disease identified three themes related to spirituality: purpose and life emerged from stigmatization, opportunities for meaning arose from a disease without a cure, and, after suffering, spirituality framed the life. In this study, subjects clearly differentiated spirituality from religiosity; many rejected faith belief systems, but spirituality became an organizing framework for life (Denzin, 1989).

A qualitative study of 14 hospice patients, cancer survivors, caregivers, and health care professionals indicated that religious beliefs were strengthened during crises only if participants had a history of religious beliefs. However, all participants expressed strong spiritual beliefs as defined in terms of meaning and purpose in life (McGrath, 2003).

A qualitative study of eight self-identified lesbians diagnosed with cancer identified spirituality as important in their lives and their illness journeys. However, religion could be a barrier. All of these patients sought and valued spirituality during treatment (Varner, 2004).

RCT = Randomized Controlled (Clinical) Trial, **NIC** = Nursing Interventions Classification, **NOC** = Nursing Outcomes Classification

OUTCOME MEASUREMENT

PERSONAL HEALTH STATUS   NOC

Definition: Overall physical, psychological, social, and spiritual functioning of an adult 18 years or older.

Personal Health Status as evidenced by the following selected NOC indicators:

- Spiritual life
- Ability to cope
- Adjustment to chronic conditions

(Rate each indicator of **Personal Health Status:** 1 = severely compromised, 2 = substantially compromised, 3 = moderately compromised, 4 = mildly compromised, 5 = not compromised) (Moorhead et al., 2004).

CLIENT SATISFACTION: CULTURAL NEEDS FULFILLMENT   NOC

Definition: Extent of positive perception of integration of cultural beliefs, values, and social structures into nursing care.

Client Satisfaction: Cultural Needs Fulfillment as evidenced by the following selected NOC indicators:

- Respect for religious beliefs
- Respect for spiritual beliefs
- Respect for personal values

(Rate each indicator of **Client Satisfaction: Cultural Needs Fulfillment:** 1 = not at all satisfied, 2 = somewhat satisfied, 3 = moderately satisfied, 4 = very satisfied, 5 = completely satisfied) (Moorhead et al., 2004).

REFERENCES

Burgener SC. (1994). Caregiver religiosity and well-being in dealing with Alzheimer's dementia. *J Relig Health*, 33(2):175-189.

Bush EG, Rye MS, Brant CR, Emery E, Pargament KI, Riessinger CA. (1999). Religious coping with chronic pain. *Appl Psychophysiol Biofeedback*, 24(4):249-260.

Denzin N. (1989). *Interpretive interactionism*. Newbury Park, CA: Sage.

Dingley C, Roux G. (2003). Inner strength in older Hispanic women with chronic illness. *J Cult Divers*, 10(1):11-22.

Dochterman JM, Bulechek GM (Eds). (2004). *Nursing Interventions Classification (NIC)*, 4th ed. St Louis: Mosby.

Hall JM. (2003). Positive self-transitions in women child abuse survivors. *Issues Ment Health Nurs*, 24(6-7): 647-666.

Harris AH, Thoresen CE, McCullough ME, Larson DB. (1999). Spiritually and religiously oriented health interventions. *J Health Psychol*, 4(3):413-433.

Keeley MP. (2004). Final conversations: Survivors' memorable messages concerning religious faith and spirituality. *Health Commun*, 16(1):87-104.

Koenig HG, George LK, Titus P. (2004). Religion, spirituality, and health in medically ill hospitalized older patients. *J Am Geriatr Soc*, 52(4):554-562.

Lackey NR, Gates MF, Brown G. (2001). African American women's experiences with the initial discovery, diagnosis, and treatment of breast cancer. *Oncol Nurs Forum*, 28(3):519-527.

Larson DB, Koenig HG, Kaplan BH, Greenberg RS, Logue E, Tyroler HA. (1989). The impact of religion on men's blood pressure. *J Religious Health*, 28(4):265-278.

McGrath P. (2003). Religiosity and the challenge of terminal illness. *Death Stud*, 27(10):881-899.

Moorhead M, Johnson M, Maas M (Eds). (2004). *Nursing Outcomes Classification (NOC)*, 3rd ed. St Louis: Mosby.

Moremen RD. (2005). What is the meaning of life? Women's spirituality at the end of life span. *Omega*, 50(4):309-330.

Narayanasamy A. (2002). Spiritual coping mechanisms in chronically ill patients. *Br J Nurs*, 11(22):1461-1470.

Narayanasamy A, Owens J. (2001). A critical incident study of nurses' responses to the spiritual needs of their patients. *J Adv Nurs*, 33(4):446-455.

Nicassio PM, Schuman C, Kim J, Cordova A, Weisman MH. (1997). Psychosocial factors associated with complementary treatment use in fibromyalgia. *J Rheumatol*, 24(10):2008-2013.

Oxman TE, Freeman DH Jr, Manheimer ED. (1995). Lack of social participation or religious strength and comfort as risk factors for death after cardiac surgery in the elderly. *Psychosom Med*, 57(1):5-15.

Reicks M, Mills J, Henry H. (2004). Qualitative study of spirituality in a weight loss program: Contribution to self-efficacy and locus of control. *J Nutr Educ Behav*, 36(1):13-15.

Samuel-Hodge CD, Headen SW, Skelly AH, Ingram AF, Keyserling TC, Jackson EJ, et al. (2000). Influences on day-to-day self-management of type 2 diabetes among African-American women: Spirituality, the multi-caregiver role, and other social context factors. *Diabetes Care*, 23(7):928-933.

Strawbridge WJ, Cohen RD, Shema SJ, Kaplan GA. (1997). Frequent attendance at religious services and mortality over 28 years. *Am J Public Health*, 87(6):957-961.

van Olphen J, Schulz A, Israel B, Chatters L, Klem L, Parker E, et al. (2003). Religious involvement, social support, and health among African-American women on the east side of Detroit. *J Gen Intern Med*, 18(7):549-557.

Varner A. (2004). Spirituality and religion among lesbian women diagnosed with cancer: A qualitative study. *J Psychosoc Oncol*, 22(1):75-89.

Wachholtz AB, Pargament KI. (2005). Is spirituality a critical ingredient of meditation? Comparing the effects of spiritual meditation, secular meditation, and relaxation on spiritual, psychological, cardiac, and pain outcomes. *J Behav Med*, 28(4):369-384.

Williams NR, Lindsey E. (2005). Spirituality and religion in the lives of runaway and homeless youth: Coping with adversity. *J Religion Spirituality Soc Work*, 24(4):19-38.

Yates JW, Chalmer BJ, St. James P, Follansbee M, McKegney FP. (1981). Religion in patients with advanced cancer. *Med Pediatr Oncol*, 9(2):121-128.

 # RELOCATION STRESS REDUCTION

Rebecca A. Johnson, PhD, RN, FAAN

NIC **Definition:** Assisting the individual to prepare for and cope with movement from one environment to another (Dochterman & Bulechek, 2004).

NURSING ACTIVITIES

Effective

Note: Do not expect that all older adults will experience relocation stress syndrome.

■ *Prepare for relocation with early and careful discharge planning.* **LOE = II**

MR Case studies revealed the importance of using an integrated approach to planning, with clear communication among practitioners (LeClerc & Wells, 2001).

NR An RCT ($N = 100$) showed that early discharge planning enhanced elders' information levels and decreased their concerns (Kleinpell, 2004).

NR A one-group experiment ($N = 11$) showed that even demented elders benefited from relocation preparation (Dickinson, 1996).

EO Using a standardized model of relocation preparation is beneficial (Cortes et al., 2004).

RCT = Randomized Controlled (Clinical) Trial, **NIC** = Nursing Interventions Classification, **NOC** = Nursing Outcomes Classification

(NR) A descriptive study ($N = 106$) of older adults moved from one nursing home to another showed no symptoms of the syndrome (Mallick & Whipple, 2000).

(NR) A large cohort study ($N = 7512$) showed only short-term limitations in functional ability (Chen & Wilmoth, 2004).

Additional research: Castle, 2001; Popejoy, 2005; Jordan-Marsh & Harden, 2005.

■ *Assess for and address depression in response to this major life transition, both before and after the relocation.* **LOE = III**

(MR) A longitudinal study ($N = 5082$) found that changes in social milieu were more likely to affect mood than somatic symptoms (Fonda & Herzog, 2001).

(MR) A cohort controlled study ($N = 186$) compared the level of depression in three groups after their relocation to either living alone, living with others, or living in a nursing home. The group relocated to a nursing home had increased depressive symptoms (Loeher et al., 2004).

(NR) A controlled clinical trial ($N = 77$) showed that elders who were anticipating relocation had more depression and anxiety than those who had moved (Hodgson et al., 2004).

■ *After relocation, provide adequate rest, minimize exposure to infection, and watch for signs of infection.* **LOE = III**

(MR) A two-group, nonrandomized study ($N = 58$) showed that, 2 weeks after relocation, elders had decreased natural killer cell cytotoxicity, decreased vigor, and more intrusive thoughts, thus identifying the importance of postrelocation care lasting a minimum of 2 weeks (Lutgendorf et al., 2001).

(MR) A controlled study ($N = 58$) of healthy older adults versus a control group found that older adults who sustained a move had decreased natural killer cell activity, especially if they also had a low sense of coherence with a lower mood (Lutgendorf et al., 1999).

■ *Carefully monitor the neuroleptic prescriptions of relocated patients.* **LOE = IV**

(MR) A cohort study ($N = 3299$) showed that 60% of nursing home admissions were prescribed neuroleptic drugs (most commonly haloperidol) and that 10% received doses that were over the recommended levels within 100 days of admission (Bronskill et al., 2004).

Possibly Effective

■ *Assess elders' ability to self-manage their medications.* **LOE = VI**

(MR) A descriptive study ($N = 78$) showed that the ability to self-manage medications was highly predictive of further relocation to more supportive housing levels in the same retirement facility (Lieto & Schmidt, 2005).

■ *Implement grief-management strategies.* **LOE = V**

(NR) A qualitative study ($N = 10$) defined grief as "aching solitude amid enduring cherished affiliations" (Pilkington, 2005).

■ *Assess for relocation transition style.* **LOE = V**

(MR) A qualitative study ($N = 31$) showed that more than half of elders who relocated to a retirement facility had only partial or minimal transition styles, thereby increasing their vulnerability and likelihood of unhealthy adjustment (Rossen & Knafl, 2003).

NR = Nursing Research, **MR** = Multidisciplinary Research, **SP** = Standard of Practice, **EO** = Expert Opinion, **LOE** = Level of Evidence

(MR) A case study ($N = 5$) showed that elders and their families benefited from use of information and technology (Magnusson & Hanson, 2005).

■ *Identify and respect ethnic differences with regard to social support and views about care.* **LOE = VII**

(EO) Facilitating elders' self-control and maintaining their identity is beneficial (Johnson & Tripp-Reimer, 2001).

Not Effective

No applicable published research was found in this category.

Possibly Harmful

■ *Overlooking elders' personality and motivation in making housing recommendations.* **LOE = VI**

(MR) External validation of a mathematical model of housing decision making ($N = 68$) showed that such models may overlook personality factors and relocation motivation (Unsworth & Thomas, 2003).

(Note: For further interventions to help the relocated elderly patient, refer to the guidelines on Reminiscence Therapy, Reality Orientation, Music Therapy, Self-Esteem Enhancement, Animal-Assisted Therapy, and Exercise Therapy: Balance Training, as appropriate.)

OUTCOME MEASUREMENT

PSYCHOSOCIAL ADJUSTMENT: LIFE CHANGE   (NOC)

(Please refer to *Nursing Outcomes Classification* [Moorhead et al., 2004] for the **Psychosocial Adjustment: Life Change** outcome.)

REFERENCES

Bronskill SE, Anderson GM, Sykora K, Wodchis WP, Gill S, Shulman KI, et al. (2004). Neuroleptic drug therapy in older adults newly admitted to nursing homes: Incidence, dose, and specialist contact. *J Am Geriatr Soc,* 52(5):749-755.

Castle NG. (2001). Relocation of the elderly. *Med Care Res Rev,* 58(3):291-333.

Chen PC, Wilmoth JM. (2004). The effects of residential mobility on ADL and IADL limitations among the very old living in the community. *J Gerontol B Psychol Sci Soc Sci,* 59(3):S164-S172.

Cortes TA, Wexler S, Fitzpatrick JJ. (2004). The transition of elderly patients between hospitals and nursing homes. Improving nurse-to-nurse communication. *J Gerontol Nurs,* 30(6):10-15.

Dickinson D. (1996). Can elderly residents with memory problems be prepared for relocation? *J Clin Nurs,* 5(2):99-104.

Dochterman JM, Bulechek GM (Eds). (2004). *Nursing Interventions Classification (NIC),* 4th ed. St Louis: Mosby.

Fonda SJ, Herzog AR. (2001). Patterns and risk factors of change in somatic and mood symptoms among older adults. *Ann Epidemiol,* 11(6):361-368.

Hodgson N, Freedman VA, Granger DA, Erno A. (2004). Biobehavioral correlates of relocation in the frail elderly: Salivary cortisol, affect, and cognitive function. *J Am Geriatr Soc,* 52(11):1856-1862.

RCT = Randomized Controlled (Clinical) Trial, **NIC** = Nursing Interventions Classification, **NOC** = Nursing Outcomes Classification

Johnson RA, Tripp-Reimer T. (2001). Relocation among ethnic elders: A review—part 2. *J Gerontol Nurs*, 27(6):22-27.

Jordan-Marsh M, Harden JT. (2005). Fictive kin: Friends as family supporting older adults as they age. *J Gerontol Nurs*, 31(2):24-31.

Kleinpell R. (2004). Randomized trial of an intensive care unit-based early discharge planning intervention for critically ill elderly patients. *Am J Crit Care*, 13(4):335-345.

LeClerc M, Wells DL. (2001). Process evaluation of an integrated model of discharge planning. *Can J Nurs Leadersh*, 14(2):19-26.

Lieto JM, Schmidt KS. (2005). Reduced ability to self-administer medication is associated with assisted living placement in a continuing care retirement community. *J Am Med Dir Assoc*, 6(4):246-249.

Loeher KE, Bank AL, MacNeill SE, Lichtenberg PA. (2004). Nursing home transition and depressive symptoms in older medical rehabilitation patients. *Clin Gerontol*, 27(1/2):59-70.

Lutgendorf SK, Reimer TT, Harvey JH, Marks G, Hong SY, Hillis SL, et al. (2001). Effects of housing relocation on immunocompetence and psychosocial functioning in older adults. *J Gerontol A Biol Sci Med Sci*, 56(2):M97-M105.

Lutgendorf SK, Vitaliano PP, Tripp-Reimer T, Harvey JH, Lubaroff DM. (1999). Sense of coherence moderates the relationship between life stress and natural killer cell activity in healthy older adults. *Psychol Aging*, 14(4):552-563.

Magnusson L, Hanson E. (2005). Supporting frail older people and their family carers at home using information and communication technology: Cost analysis. *J Adv Nurs*, 51(6):645-657.

Mallick MJ, Whipple TW. (2000). Validity of the nursing diagnosis of relocation stress syndrome. *Nurs Res*, 49(2):97-100.

Moorhead M, Johnson M, Maas M (Eds). (2004). *Nursing Outcomes Classification (NOC)*, 3rd ed. St Louis: Mosby.

Pilkington FB. (2005). Grieving a loss: The lived experience for elders residing in an institution. *Nurs Sci Q*, 18(3):233-242.

Popejoy, L. (2005). Health-related decision-making by older adults and their families: How clinicians can help. *J Gerontol Nurs*, 31(9):12-18.

Rossen EK, Knafl KA. (2003). Older women's response to residential relocation: Description of transition styles. *Qual Health Res*, 13(1):20-36.

Unsworth C, Thomas S. (2003). External validation of a housing recommendation model for clients following stroke rehabilitation. *Disabil Rehabil*, 25(21):1208-1218.

REMINISCENCE THERAPY   NIC

William J. Puentes, DNSc, RN, CNS-BC

NIC **Definition:** Using the recall of past events, feelings, and thoughts to facilitate pleasure, quality of life, or adaptation to present circumstances (Dochterman & Bulechek, 2004).

NURSING ACTIVITIES

Effective

■ **NIC** *Inform family members about the benefits of reminiscence.* **LOE = II**

 A one-group pre-/posttest study ($N = 36$) showed that participation in six reminiscence therapy sessions positively affected family coping (Comana et al., 1998).

 A systematic review found that caregivers who participated in reminiscence groups with their relatives with dementia exhibited a significant decrease in caregiving strain (Woods et al., 2005).

NR = Nursing Research, **MR** = Multidisciplinary Research, **SP** = Standard of Practice, **EO** = Expert Opinion, **LOE** = Level of Evidence

Possibly Effective

▪ (NIC) *Select an appropriate small number of participants for group reminiscence therapy.* **LOE = I**

(NR) Nine RCTs examined in a systematic review varied with regard to person, outcome measurement, control, and exposure/intervention. The results were also diverse, with only about half showing that reminiscence therapy decreased depression (Hsieh & Wang, 2003).

(NR) A systematic review identified a lack of consistent research findings resulting from differences in therapeutic goals, types of reminiscence, dependent measures, data collection tools, and populations, thus indicating that concept refinement and measurement standardization were essential (Lin et al., 2003).

▪ *Determine the number of weekly (or more) sessions by the patient's response and willingness to continue.* **LOE = III**

(NR) A controlled study with a twice-weekly group reminiscence intervention over 6 weeks demonstrated that reminiscence did not significantly affect self-transcendence or depression in a group of older women ($N = 24$) living in an assisted-living facility (Stinson & Kirk, 2006).

(NR) A controlled study with weekly individual reminiscence therapy sessions with institutionalized and noninstitutionalized older adults ($N = 58$) showed no significant impact between groups in terms of self-esteem, self-health perception, and depressive symptoms. However, these sessions did significantly affect mood status in the institutionalized group (Wang, 2004).

▪ (NIC) *Determine which method of reminiscence (e.g., taped autobiography, journal, structured life review, scrapbook, open discussion, and storytelling) is most effective.* **LOE = VII**

(NR) In a theoretically based discussion, a model of reminiscence as a coping mechanism within a stress adaptation framework was developed (Puentes, 2002).

(MR) In a qualitative study, narrative discourse by individuals with Alzheimer's disease in loosely structured reminiscence group environments was qualitatively better than discourse elicited during a formal language function evaluation (Moss et al., 2002).

(EO) A seminal analysis of life review and reminiscence developed by two nurse experts in the field discussed their use as therapeutic modalities and elucidated their application in nursing practice (Burnside & Haight, 1992).

(MR) Broad functions of autobiographic memory (self, social, and directive) were identified, described, and correlated with functions identified in the reminiscence literature (Bluck & Alea, 2002).

(EO) A discussion by an expert in the field described a model that proposed that reminiscence was a source of self-referent knowledge, which influenced a person's self-worth involving a process of acquiring personal existential meaning and as a mechanism for adapting to stress (Kovach, 1991).

Additional research: Haight & Gibson, 2005; Peplau, 1991; Watt & Wong, 1991.

▪ (NIC) *Introduce props that address all five senses (e.g., music for auditory, photo albums for visual, perfume for olfactory) to stimulate recall.* **LOE = V**

(EO) Olfactory stimulation is often used as an impetus for reminiscence therapy. However, numerous neurologic studies show that adults with Alzheimer's disease and related dementia

RCT = Randomized Controlled (Clinical) Trial, **NIC** = Nursing Interventions Classification, **NOC** = Nursing Outcomes Classification

perform poorly on tests of smell detection and identification as a result of cell death in the olfactory bulb (Vance, 2002).

(MR) In a descriptive study, the impact of group reminiscence therapy using familiar objects and photographs on the well-being of individuals with mild to moderate dementia using day hospital services ($N = 25$) was significantly greater than participation in general group activities or unstructured time (Brooker & Duce, 2000).

■ (NIC) *Use culturally sensitive props, themes, and techniques.* **LOE = VII**

(EO) Clinician-directed language activities that make use of autobiographic reminiscence are well suited for adults from culturally and linguistically diverse backgrounds (Harris, 1997).

■ (NIC) *Encourage writing about past events.* **LOE = VI**

(MR) An exploratory case study found that writing within a reminiscence framework may positively affect the psychological well-being of older adults (Elford et al., 2005).

■ (NIC) *Identify with the patient a theme for each session (e.g., work life).* **LOE = VI**

(NR) A case study illustrated the integration of reminiscence and cognitive therapy techniques within a life-span perspective to effectively treat affective symptoms in community-residing older adults (Puentes, 2004).

■ (NIC) *Encourage the verbal expression of both positive and negative feelings about past events.* **LOE = VI**

(MR) In a descriptive study ($N = 420$), reminiscence to revive old problems, provide stimulation, or maintain connection with a departed person was predictive of distress, whereas reminiscence for death preparation or to foster conversation was related to higher life satisfaction (Cappeliez et al., 2005).

(MR) In two descriptive studies ($N = 710$, $N = 399$), the development and validation of the Reminiscence Functions Scale identified eight different functions of reminiscence: boredom reduction, death preparation, identity/problem solving, conversation, intimacy maintenance, bitterness revival, and teaching/informing (Webster, 1993, 1997).

Not Effective

No applicable published research was found in this category.

Possibly Harmful

No applicable published research was found in this category.

OUTCOME MEASUREMENT

COPING (NOC)

Definition: Personal actions to manage stressors that tax an individual's resources.
Coping as evidenced by the following selected NOC indicators:
• Verbalizes sense of control
• Reports decrease in stress
• Verbalizes acceptance of situation

NR = Nursing Research, **MR** = Multidisciplinary Research, **SP** = Standard of Practice, **EO** = Expert Opinion, **LOE** = Level of Evidence

OUTCOME MEASUREMENT—*cont'd*

- Adapts to life changes
- Uses available social support
- Uses effective coping strategies
- Reports decrease in negative feelings
- Reports increase in psychological comfort

(Rate each indicator of **Coping:** 1 = never demonstrated, 2 = rarely demonstrated, 3 = sometimes demonstrated, 4 = often demonstrated, 5 = consistently demonstrated) (Moorhead et al., 2004).

REFERENCES

Bluck S, Alea N. (2002). Exploring the functions of autobiographical memory: Why do I remember the autumn? In Webster JD, Haight BK (Eds). *Critical advances in reminiscence work: From theory to application.* New York: Springer.

Brooker D, Duce L. (2000). Wellbeing and activity in dementia: A comparison of group reminiscence therapy, structured goal-directed group activity and unstructured time. *Aging Ment Health,* 4(4): 354-358.

Burnside I, Haight BK. (1992). Reminiscence and life review: Analysing each concept. *J Adv Nurs,* 17(7):855-862.

Cappeliez P, O'Rourke N, Chaudhury H. (2005). Functions of reminiscence and mental health in later life. *Aging Ment Health,* 9(4):295-301.

Comana MT, Brown VM, Thomas JD. (1998). The effect of reminiscence therapy on family coping. *J Fam Nurs,* 4(2):182-197.

Dochterman JM, Bulechek GM (Eds). (2004). *Nursing Interventions Classification (NIC),* 4th ed. St Louis: Mosby.

Elford H, Wilson F, McKee KJ, Chung MC, Bolton G, Goudie F. (2005). Psychosocial benefits of solitary reminiscence writing: An exploratory study. *Aging Ment Health,* 9(4):305-314.

Haight B, Gibson F (Eds). (2005). *Burnside's working with older adults: Group process and techniques,* 4th ed. Sudbury, MA: Jones & Bartlett.

Harris JL. (1997). Reminiscence: A culturally and developmentally appropriate language intervention for older adults. *Am J Speech Lang Pathol,* 6(3):19-26.

Hsieh H, Wang J. (2003). Effect of reminiscence therapy on depression in older adults: A systematic review. *Int J Nurs Stud,* 40(4):335-345.

Kovach C. (1991). Reminiscence: Exploring the origins, processes, and consequences. *Nurs Forum,* 26(3):14-20.

Lin YC, Dai YT, Hwang SL. (2003). The effect of reminiscence on the elderly population: A systematic review. *Public Health Nurs,* 20(4):297-306.

Moorhead M, Johnson M, Maas M (Eds). (2004). *Nursing Outcomes Classification (NOC),* 3rd ed. St Louis: Mosby.

Moss SE, Polignano E, White CL, Minichiello MD, Sunderland T. (2002). Reminiscence group activities and discourse interaction in Alzheimer's disease. *J Gerontol Nurs,* 28(8):36-44.

Peplau HE. (1991). *Interpersonal relations in nursing: A conceptual frame of reference for psychodynamic nursing.* New York: Springer.

Puentes WJ. (2002). Simple reminiscence: A stress-adaptation model of the phenomenon. *Issues Ment Health Nurs,* 23(5):497-511.

Puentes WJ. (2004). Cognitive therapy integrated with life review techniques: An eclectic treatment approach for affective symptoms in older adults. *J Clin Nurs,* 13(1):84-89.

Stinson CK, Kirk E. (2006). Structured reminiscence: An intervention to decrease depression and increase self-transcendence in older women. *J Clin Nurs,* 15(2):208-218.

RCT = Randomized Controlled (Clinical) Trial, **NIC** = Nursing Interventions Classification, **NOC** = Nursing Outcomes Classification

Vance DE. (2002). Implications of olfactory stimulation in activities for adults with age-related dementia. *Act Adapt Aging*, 27(2):17-25.

Wang JJ. (2004). The comparative effectiveness among institutionalized and non-institutionalized elderly people in Taiwan of reminiscence therapy as a psychological measure. *J Nurs Res*, 12(3):237-245.

Watt L, Wong PT. (1991). A taxonomy of reminiscence and therapeutic implications. *J Ment Health Counsel*, 12:270-278.

Webster JD. (1993). Construction and validation of the Reminiscence Functions Scale. *J Gerontol*, 48(5): P256-P262.

Webster JD. (1997). The Reminiscence Functions Scale: A replication. *Int J Aging Hum Dev*, 44(2):137-148.

Woods B, Spector A, Jones C, Orrell M, Davies S. (2005). Reminiscence therapy for dementia. *Cochrane Database Syst Rev*, (2):CD001120.

 # RESILIENCY PROMOTION

Della J. Derscheid, MSN, RN, CNS

> **NIC** **Definition:** Assisting individuals, families, and communities in the development, use, and strengthening of protective factors to be used in coping with environmental and societal stressors (Dochterman & Bulechek, 2000).

NURSING ACTIVITIES

Effective

■ **NIC** *Assist youth/families/communities in developing optimism for the future.* **LOE = III**

MR A quasi-experimental study of students and families (*N* = 75) who received the Safe Schools/Healthy Students treatment initiative, which makes use of multisystemic therapy, resulted in significant improvements in behavior at school, home, and the community; behavior toward others; moods; self-harm; and substance use (Timmons-Mitchell et al., 2006).

MR A quasi-experimental study of a 10-session cognitive behavior therapy program (FRIENDS) with primary school-aged children (*N* = 213) promoted emotional resilience, reduced anxiety, and increased self-esteem (Stallard et al., 2005).

■ **NIC** *Motivate youth to pursue academic achievement and goals.* **LOE = III**

MR A quasi-experimental study of children (*N* = 569) who were referred for emotional and behavioral problems tested a school-based prevention intervention using social-skill development, problem-solving skills training, behavior management, and parent skills training. The study found reductions in child impairment in the categories of school problems, pervasive problems with mood, and school and home problems clusters (Rosas, 2006).

MR A quasi-experimental study of seventh-grade Hispanic students (*N* = 525) tested an educational school-based intervention, Going for the Goal, during 10 weekly workshops that focused on goal setting. As compared with a wait-listed control group, the intervention group had significantly increased knowledge of goal-setting skills and means-ends problem-solving skills (O'Hearn, 2002).

MR A quasi-experimental study of preschool children compared the Chicago Child-Parent Center Program (*N* = 989) delivered for 1 to 2 years with a control group (*N* = 550) on a number of academic and social outcomes. The intervention group was significantly more likely to complete high school, to complete more years of education, and to have lower rates of juvenile and violent arrests, special education, grade retention, and school dropout (Reynolds et al., 2001).

(MR) A quasi-experimental study of three school-based depression-prevention programs for ninth-grade students ($N = 260$) found that participation in the Resourceful Adolescent Program—Adolescents and the Resourceful Adolescent Program—Family resulted in decreased depressive symptomatology and hopelessness after the intervention and at 10-month follow-up among adolescents who participated in the program (Shochet et al., 2001).

(MR) A quasi-experimental study of 13- to 18-year-old adolescents ($N = 19$) with anxiety and depression who participated in the Resourceful Adolescent Program (a school-based early intervention program) found significantly reduced anxiety and depression in addition to increasing self-efficacy (Muris et al., 2001).

■ (NIC) *Assist youth in viewing family as a resource for advice and support.*
   LOE = I

(MR) An RCT of three intervention programs ($N = 218$ families)—a mother program, a mother-plus-child program, and a control group for children and mothers—found that significantly fewer children in the mother-plus-child program had a 1-year prevalence of mental health diagnosis and that they also had fewer sexual partners. As compared with controls, children with more initial mental health problems had significantly lower externalizing problems and fewer symptoms of mental health disorders, whereas children with more initial mental health problems with mothers in the mother program had significantly fewer externalizing problems and symptoms of mental disorders as well as less alcohol, marijuana, and other drug use (e.g, heroin) (Wolchik et al., 2002).

(MR) An RCT used a family-based prevention counseling intervention for inner-city, at-risk, African American youth ($N = 124$) and demonstrated significant improvements in self-confidence and attitudes about drug use along with a decrease in both externalizing and internalizing symptoms with less school behavior problems (Hogue et al., 2002).

(MR) A quasi-experimental study tested the impact of the Adolescent and Family Rites of Passage Program (which emphasizes the African and African American cultures and makes use of an after-school component, family enhancement and empowerment activities, and individual and family counseling) with at-risk African American boys ($N = 57$) between the ages of 11.5 and 14.5 years. Three-year program results showed these adolescents to have increased self-esteem and accurate knowledge regarding the dangers of drug use (Harvey & Hill, 2004).

■ (NIC) *Promote quality, caring schools in the community.* **LOE = II**

(MR) An RCT studied three family- and school-based competency training programs with students between the ages of 10 and 14 years at rural schools ($N = 36$). Findings showed that the Life Skills Training program in combination with the Strengthening Families Program as well as the Life Skills Training program alone both resulted in significant reduction rates for marijuana initiation 1 year after the program intervention (Spoth et al., 2002).

(MR) An RCT of two interventions—the Preparing for the Drug Free Years Program and the Iowa Strengthening Families Program—with sixth graders and their families ($N = 667$) at 33 public schools found significant differences between brief family skills training intervention and control groups for decreased rates of the initiation and use of substances (Spoth et al., 2001).

RCT = Randomized Controlled (Clinical) Trial, **NIC** = Nursing Interventions Classification, **NOC** = Nursing Outcomes Classification

■ *Counsel family members about additional effective coping skills for their own use.* **LOE = II**

⬤ An RCT of the Family Bereavement Program ($N = 90$ families, $N = 135$ children and adolescents) and a self-study control group ($N = 66$ families, $N = 109$ children and adolescents) resulted in a decrease of child-related symptoms of anxiety, depression, and externalizing behaviors. Improved skills of the surviving parent were positive parenting, coping, reduced stressful events, improved expression of feelings, and improved mental health (Sandler et al., 2002).

⬤ A quasi-experimental study tested the effects of the Title I Child-Parent Centers, which provided child education and family support services to preschool children ($N = 913$) and found significantly reduced rates of child maltreatment as compared with children who did not receive the intervention (Reynolds & Robertson, 2003).

⬤ In an RCT of Hispanic immigrant families of sixth and seventh graders ($N = 167$), the Familias Unidas intervention program, which uses a multifamily group format, resulted in greater parental investment and a greater decline of child behavior problems than in the control group (Coatsworth et al., 2002).

⬤ A quasi-experimental study of a support program, Strength to Strength, with referred families of children between the ages of 7 and 14 years with a depressed parent ($N = 10$) found significant child improvements with increased out-of-home networks and general social functioning and significant family improvements with improved balance in family interactions (Place et al., 2002).

■ *Use a relationship-training program to create a positive workplace.* **LOE = II**

⬤ An RCT of the Personal Resilience and Resilient Relationships training program with allied health personnel ($N = 123$) resulted in improved self-esteem, locus of control, purpose in life, and interpersonal relations as compared with the control group, which showed no positive effects ($N = 109$) (Waite & Richardson, 2004).

Possibly Effective

■ ⬤ⁿᵢᶜ *Link youth to interested adults in the community.* **LOE = VI**

⬤ A qualitative grounded theory study concluded that individuals ($N = 28$ adolescents; $N = 4$ adults) who used the technique of "envisioning the future" via adults who modeled reaching goals, coached commitment follow through, and countered negative stereotypes promoted resilience such that the adolescents were the participants with increased competence and elevated expectations (Aronowitz, 2005).

Not Effective

■ *Appraising the patient's needs/desires for social support.* **LOE = VI**

⬤ A descriptive and exploratory correlation design of homeless adolescents ($N = 59$) found that connectedness was significantly negatively associated with resilience (Rew et al., 2001).

■ *Assisting patients with identifying appropriate short- and long-term goals.* **LOE = III**

NR = Nursing Research, **MR** = Multidisciplinary Research, **SP** = Standard of Practice, **EO** = Expert Opinion, **LOE** = Level of Evidence

(MR) A quasi-experimental study of seventh-grade Hispanic students ($N = 525$) received an educational school-based intervention, Going for the Goal, during 10 weekly workshops that focused on goal setting. The intervention group demonstrated a greater improvement in locus of control when not receiving the intervention. However, the control group did as well (O'Hearn, 2002).

- **(NIC)** *Encourage family involvement with the child's schoolwork and activities.*
  LOE = II

(MR) In an RCT of Hispanic immigrant families of sixth and seventh graders ($N = 167$), the Familias Unidas intervention program, which uses a multifamily group format, did not affect the child's school bonding experience or academic achievement (Pantin et al., 2003).

Possibly Harmful

No applicable published research was found in this category.

OUTCOME MEASUREMENT

COPING   (NOC)

Definition: Personal actions to manage stressors that tax an individual's resources.
Coping as evidenced by the following selected NOC indicators:
- Uses effective coping strategies
- Modifies lifestyle as needed
- Uses available social support
- Seeks help from a health care professional as appropriate

(Rate each indicator of **Coping:** 1 = never demonstrated, 2 = rarely demonstrated, 3 = sometimes demonstrated, 4 = often demonstrated, 5 = consistently demonstrated) (Moorhead et al., 2004).

REFERENCES

Aronowitz T. (2005). The role of "envisioning the future" in the development of resilience among at-risk youth. *Public Health Nurs,* 22(3):200-208.

Coatsworth JD, Pantin H, Szapocznik J. (2002). Familias Unidas: A family-centered ecodevelopmental intervention to reduce risk for problem behavior among Hispanic adolescents. *Clin Child Fam Psychol Rev,* 5(2):113-132.

Dochterman JM, Bulechek GM (Eds). (2000). *Nursing Interventions Classification (NIC),* 4th ed. St Louis: Mosby.

Harvey AR, Hill RB. (2004). Africentric youth and family rites of passage program: Promoting resilience among at-risk African American youths. *Soc Work,* 49(1):65-74.

Hogue A, Liddle HA, Becker D, Johnson-Leckrone J. (2002). Family-based prevention counseling for high-risk young adolescents: Immediate outcomes. *J Community Psychol,* 30(1):1-22.

Luthar SS (Ed). (2003). *Resilience and vulnerability.* Cambridge, UK: University Press.

Moorhead S, Johnson M, Maas M (Eds). (2004). *Nursing Outcomes Classification (NOC),* 3rd ed. St Louis: Mosby.

Muris P, Bogie N, Hoogsteder A. (2001). Effects of an early intervention group program for anxious and depressed adolescents: A pilot study. *Psychol Rep,* 88(2):481-482.

O'Hearn TC. (2002). Going for the goal: Improving youths' problem-solving skills through a school-based intervention. *J Community Psychol,* 30(3):281-303.

RCT = Randomized Controlled (Clinical) Trial, **NIC** = Nursing Interventions Classification, **NOC** = Nursing Outcomes Classification

Pantin H, Coatsworth JD, Feaster DJ, Newman FL, Briones E, Prado G, et al. (2003). Familias Unidas: The efficacy of an intervention to promote parental investment in Hispanic immigrant families. *Prev Sci*, 4(3):189-201.

Place M, Reynolds J, Cousins A, O'Neill S. (2002). Developing a resilience package for vulnerable children. *Child Adolesc Ment Health*, 7(4):162-167.

Rew L, Taylor-Seehafer M, Thomas NY, Yockey RD. (2001). Correlates of resilience in homeless adolescents. *J Nurs Scholarsh*, 33(1):33-40.

Reynolds AJ, Robertson DL. (2003). School-based early intervention and later child maltreatment in the Chicago Longitudinal Study. *Child Dev*, 74(1):3-26.

Reynolds AJ, Temple JA, Robertson DL, Mann EA. (2001). Long-term effects of an early childhood intervention on educational achievement and juvenile arrest: A 15-year follow-up of low-income children in public schools. *JAMA*, 285(18):2339-2346.

Rosas S. (2006). *Functional impairment outcomes for children served by a school-based preventive intervention.* Paper presented at the A System of Care for Children's Mental Health: Expanding the Research Base, Tampa, Florida.

Sandler IN, Ayers TS, Romer AL. (2002). Fostering resilience in families in which a parent has died. *J Palliat Med*, 5(6):945-956.

Shochet IM, Dadds MR, Holland D, Whitefield K, Harnett PH, Osgarby SM. (2001). The efficacy of a universal school-based program to prevent adolescent depression. *J Clin Child Psychol*, 30(3):303-315.

Spoth RL, Redmond C, Shin C. (2001). Randomized trial of brief family interventions for general populations: Adolescent substance use outcomes 4 years following baseline. *J Consult Clin Psychol*, 69(4):627-642.

Spoth RL, Redmond C, Trudeau L, Shin C. (2002). Longitudinal substance initiation outcomes for a universal preventive intervention combining family and school programs. *Psychol Addict Behav*, 16(2):129-134.

Stallard P, Simpson N, Anderson S, Carter T, Osborn C, Bush S. (2005). An evaluation of the FRIENDS programme: A cognitive behaviour therapy intervention to promote emotional resilience. *Arch Dis Child*, 90(10):1016-1019.

Timmons-Mitchell J, Husset D, Buckeye L, Usaj K, Mitchell C. (2006). *The Child and Adolescent Functional Assessment Scale (CAFAS), multi-systemic therapy (MST), and Safe Schools Healthy Students: Resilience in action.* Paper presented at the A System of Care for Children's Mental Health: Expanding the Research Base, Tampa, Florida.

Waite PJ, Richardson GE. (2004). Determining the efficacy of resiliency training in the work site. *J Allied Health*, 33(3):178-183.

Wolchik SA, Sandler IN, Millsap RE, Plummer BA, Greene SM, Anderson ER, et al. (2002). Six-year follow-up of preventive interventions for children of divorce: A randomized controlled trial. *JAMA*, 288(15):1874-1881.

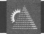 # SECURITY ENHANCEMENT   NIC

Kathleen L. Patusky PhD, APRN-BC

NIC **Definition:** Intensifying a patient's sense of physical and psychological safety (Dochterman & Bulechek, 2004).

NURSING ACTIVITIES

Effective

■ **SP** *Use physical restraint for patient safety judiciously, with consideration of other alternatives as appropriate.* **LOE = VII**

NR = Nursing Research, **MR** = Multidisciplinary Research, **SP** = Standard of Practice, **EO** = Expert Opinion, **LOE** = Level of Evidence

(NR) A review of current research on the use of bed rails as a means of restraint that would promote patient safety noted that U.S. Food and Drug Administration reports of related deaths and injuries prompted new guidelines for the use of bed rails, including the nurse's individual and comprehensive assessment of patient risk and a weighing of the risks and benefits of other interventions, with bed rails to be used as a last resort (Marcy-Edwards, 2005).

(NR) A systematic review of studies relating to the use of restraints described potential injuries, patient experiences, and best practice guidelines for the appropriate use or minimization of restraints on the basis of level II, III, and IV studies (Evans et al., 2002a).

(NR) A systematic review of studies relating to the minimization of restraint use described restraint alternatives, the management of specific populations, and organizational activities to minimize the use of restraints on the basis of one level II RCT (Evans et al., 2002b).

(NR) A systematic review of physical restraint from the patient's and family's perspectives reported a principally negative impact of the procedure, with the authors concluding that restraint should be used minimally (Evans & Fitzgerald, 2002).

(MR) A controlled study ($N = 571$) of an interdisciplinary intervention (Fall Clinic) with patients who had a history of falls, gait or balance problems, or multiple medical issues demonstrated a significant threefold decrease in falls at 3-month follow-up, with treatment plans (in descending order of referral numbers) that included medication modification, prosthetics, home exercise, rehabilitative services referral, specialty clinics referral, home evaluation, primary care clinic referral, hip protectors, and exercise/education classes (Hart-Hughes et al., 2004).

■ (SP) *Evaluate the use of physical interventions relative to their safety and efficacy.*
   LOE = V

(NR) A systematic review of the use of resistance training with patients with congestive heart failure concluded that, although clinicians still avoided this type of exercise with patients who experienced congestive heart failure, controlled studies showed that resistance training increased strength and functional ability while improving hemodynamic function. Resistance training was deemed safe, with no negative cardiovascular consequences found (Benton, 2005).

(NR) A review of the literature regarding safe patient handling and maintaining patient dignity discussed the limitations of existing research and identified the following competencies for skillful patient handling: safe use of equipment; appropriate leadership of staff; negotiation skills that include patients; awareness of organizational policies; and accurate record keeping to manage risk assessment and patient care plans (Pellatt, 2005).

■ (NIC) (SP) *Provide a nonthreatening environment.* **LOE = V**

(NR) A systematic review of the risks and opportunities for patient safety that are inherent in managed care identified the fact that, although little of the managed care literature had addressed patient safety, managed care organizations were in the position to influence patient safety through selective contracting, financial incentives for performance, quality improvement programs, consumer education, and the integration of care delivery. Providers could reduce patient safety risks through the adoption of relevant patient education materials, the development of a culture of patient safety, and the promotion of patient safety through consumer safety education programs, continuous program improvements, and the routine disclosure of quality and safety data (Unruh et al., 2005).

RCT = Randomized Controlled (Clinical) Trial, **NIC** = Nursing Interventions Classification, **NOC** = Nursing Outcomes Classification

(NR) In a qualitative study ($N = 45$) of critically ill patients, patients reported that they needed to feel safe, with safety determined by family, friends, intensive care unit staff, religious beliefs, feeling in control, hoping, and trusting (Hupcey, 2000).

(NR) A qualitative study of 40 patients and 12 nurses exploring patient perceptions of care in an effort to develop a theory of nurses' interpersonal competence found that four themes predominated: (1) "translation," with nurses thoroughly explaining medical procedures and instructions regarding treatment; (2) "getting to know you," with nurses' personal sharing and connecting; (3) "establishing trust," with nurses demonstrating their abilities to take charge and enjoy their work; and (4) "going the extra mile," with nurses providing care that went beyond the norm (Fosbinder, 1994).

(MR) A systematic review of the elements in organizational culture that are necessary to maintain patient safety identified five dimensions: (1) leadership; (2) policies and procedures; (3) staffing; (4) communication; and (5) reporting. Research was recommended on the basis of relationships between patient safety measures and patient outcomes (Colla et al., 2005).

(MR) A systematic review of patient safety practices prepared for the Agency for Healthcare Research and Quality described the 11 most highly rated patient safety practices of 79 that were reviewed (Shojania et al., 2001):

- Appropriate prophylaxis to prevent venous thromboembolism
- Use of perioperative beta-blockers as appropriate
- Use of optimal sterile barriers when placing central intravenous catheters
- Appropriate prophylactic antibiotics use for surgical patients
- Requesting that patients restate their understanding of what they are told during the informed consent process
- Continuous aspiration of subglottic secretions in ventilator patients
- Use of pressure-relieving bedding
- Use of ultrasound verification during central line insertion
- Patient self-management for warfarin therapy
- Provision of nutrition, especially early enteral nutrition, with critically ill and surgical patients
- Use of antibiotic-saturated central venous catheters

■ (SP) *Anticipate patient/family needs.* **LOE = V**

(NR) A qualitative study ($N = 8$) conducted after hospitalization asked medical-surgical patients to identify methods that can be used to seek nursing care while in the hospital. Patients reported three strategies that were used with nurses: (1) "make them your friend"; (2) "be an easy patient"; and (3) "try to get them to listen," although patients recognized that trying to get nurses to listen may conflict with the intention of being a good patient (Shattell, 2005).

(NR) A case study of a man with cancer illustrated that denial was not entirely maladaptive and that it may assist patients with dealing with threats to their physical health, relationships, or sense of control. The authors concluded that nurses could promote the safety and trust of the patient environment by exercising patience and understanding in the face of denial, by becoming knowledgeable about denial, and by approaching maladaptive denial gently and appropriately (Stephenson, 2004).

(NR) A qualitative study of 15 parents of hospitalized children identified that the key variable of trust in health care providers was meeting parents' expectations for care, which included preexisting trust, an evaluation of technical skills and care provision, and caring behaviors (Thompson et al., 2003).

NR = Nursing Research, **MR** = Multidisciplinary Research, **SP** = Standard of Practice, **EO** = Expert Opinion, **LOE** = Level of Evidence

NR A qualitative study of 50 adult inpatients identified that the key variable of trust in health care providers was meeting patients' expectations for care (Hupcey et al., 2000).

NR A qualitative study found that anticipating family needs contributed to a sense of trust. A lack of trust in nurse-patient interactions could lead to the refusal of treatment or withdrawing from the nurse-patient relationship. The presence of trust occurred with secure relationships, in which patients and relatives were more relaxed and more willing to accept care without vigilance (Morse, 1991).

■ SP ***Assist the patient and family with developing a sense of trust in the nurse, the health care system, and the care to be provided.*** **LOE = V**

NR A descriptive study of pediatric intensive care unit parents (N = 96) and their stressors during children's hospitalization concluded that parental trust was enhanced when nurses shared their credentials and expertise with parents, including their number of years of experience and their relevant certifications (Huckabay & Tilem-Kessler, 1999).

NR A qualitative study using unstructured interviews of intensive care unit nurses and family members of intensive care unit patients found that families who trusted the nurse were truthful, asked for advice or guidance, refrained from questioning the nurse's actions, and willingly accepted that the patient would be cared for in the family's absence. Families who did not trust the nurse were rude and demanding while questioning the care that was being given (Hupcey, 1998).

■ NIC SP ***Help the patient/family identify what factors increase their sense of security.*** **LOE = V**

NR A case study of a man with cancer illustrated that denial was not entirely maladaptive and that it may assist patients with dealing with threats to their physical health, relationships, or sense of control. The authors concluded that nurses could promote the safety and trust of the patient environment by exercising patience and understanding in the face of denial, by becoming knowledgeable about denial, and by approaching maladaptive denial gently and appropriately (Stephenson, 2004).

NR A qualitative study (N = 34 acute medical patients, N = 7 family members) found that "good quality care" was described as individualized, patient-focused, need-focused, humanistic, and demonstrative of involvement, commitment, and concern. "Not so good" care was described as unrelated to need, impersonal, distant, and unable to involve patients. The authors concluded that patients placed greater emphasis on relational rather than technical aspects of care, which was contrary to the previously perceived view (Attree, 2001).

MR A qualitative study (N = 51 Danish participants, N = 35 American participants) encouraged patients with multiple sclerosis to identify ways in which they managed their symptoms during periods of remission. Self-care strategies included using individualized methods of following their medical regimen, alternative treatments, lay referral networks, and accessing information about their illness, with these coping strategies aimed at achieving a sense of control over their illness, their increasing dependence, and their declining medical status (McLaughlin & Zeeberg, 1993).

■ NIC SP ***Listen to the patient's/family's fears.*** **LOE = V**

NR A qualitative study (N=8) conducted after hospitalization asked medical-surgical patients to identify methods that can be used to seek nursing care while in the hospital. Patients

RCT = Randomized Controlled (Clinical) Trial, **NIC** = Nursing Interventions Classification, **NOC** = Nursing Outcomes Classification

reported three strategies that were used with nurses: (1) "make them your friend"; (2) "be an easy patient"; and (3) "try to get them to listen," although patients recognized that trying to get nurses to listen may conflict with the intention of being a good patient (Shattell, 2005).

NR A qualitative study ($N = 8$) of patient's experiences of nurses' communication found that "lack of communication" (failure to provide information, task orientation) was frequently reported, along with "attending" (accessibility and readiness to listen), "empathy" (emotional engagement), and "friendliness/humor." The authors noted that patients felt reassured and safe when they experienced attending (McCabe, 2004).

NR A case study of a man with cancer illustrated that denial was not entirely maladaptive and that it may assist patients with dealing with threats to their physical health, relationships, or sense of control. The authors concluded that nurses could promote the safety and trust of the patient environment by exercising patience and understanding in the face of denial, by becoming knowledgeable about denial, and by approaching maladaptive denial gently and appropriately (Stephenson, 2004).

NR A descriptive study of parents' ($N = 32$ [10 males, 22 females]) stressors during their children's hospitalization in the pediatric intensive care unit of a children's hospital identified multiple stressors, including the child's appearance, the unfamiliar and frightening environment, the unfamiliar procedures, and the displacement from their parental role (Heuer, 1993).

■ NIC SP *Assist the patient to identify usual coping responses.* LOE = III

NR A controlled study ($N = 175$) of older adults who were at risk for repeated hospitalizations demonstrated that coping assistance was a function of nursing case management that could improve the functional status of frail elderly patients, despite declining health (Schein et al., 2005).

NR A systematic review of the patient's/family's and the nurse's identifications of interventions for supporting hope identified the following strategies or themes that were common to both groups: the support of family and friends; cognitive strategies; spiritual/religious activities; relationship with caregivers; finding meaning; inner resources; setting goals; self-worth; living in the present; humor; role models; sense of normalcy; symptom relief (comfort); and giving the patient control (Holt, 2001).

MR A qualitative study ($N = 51$ Danish participants, $N = 35$ American participants) encouraged patients with multiple sclerosis to identify ways in which they managed their symptoms during periods of remission. Self-care strategies included using individualized methods of following their medical regimen, alternative treatments, lay referral networks, and accessing information about their illness, with these coping strategies aimed at achieving a sense of control over their illness, their increasing dependence, and their declining medical status (McLaughlin & Zeeberg, 1993).

Possibly Effective

■ NIC *Facilitate a parent's staying overnight with a hospitalized child.* LOE = VI

NR A qualitative study of 15 parents of hospitalized children identified that keeping parents separate from children, not allowing shared meals, and not permitting nearby sleeping arrangements were nurse behaviors that inhibited trust (Thompson et al., 2003).

NR = Nursing Research, **MR** = Multidisciplinary Research, **SP** = Standard of Practice, **EO** = Expert Opinion, **LOE** = Level of Evidence

Not Effective

No applicable published research was found in this category.

Possibly Harmful

■ *Using bed rails as physical restraint for patient safety.* **LOE = VII**

(NR) A review of current research on the use of bed rails as a means of restraint that would promote patient safety noted that US Food and Drug Administration reports of related deaths and injuries prompted new guidelines for the use of bed rails, including the nurse's individual and comprehensive assessment of patient risk and a weighing of the risks and benefits of other interventions, with bed rails to be used as a last resort (Marcy-Edwards, 2005).

(MR) A systematic review of research related to the use of bed rails conducted by a US Food and Drug Administration work group determined specific clinical guidelines that should be applied if all other alternatives had been exhausted and bed rails were required (HBSW, 2003).

OUTCOME MEASUREMENT

CLIENT SATISFACTION: SAFETY   (NOC)

(Please refer to *Nursing Outcomes Classification* [Moorhead et al., 2004] for the **Client Satisfaction: Safety** outcome.)

REFERENCES

Attree M. (2001). Patients' and relatives' experiences and perspectives of "Good" and "Not so Good" quality care. *J Adv Nurs,* 33(4):456-466.

Benton MJ. (2005). Safety and efficacy of resistance training in patients with chronic heart failure: Research-based evidence. *Prog Cardiovasc Nurs,* 20(1):17-23.

Colla JB, Bracken AC, Kinney LM, Weeks WB. (2005). Measuring patient safety climate: A review of surveys. *Qual Saf Health Care,* 14(5):364-366.

Dochterman JM, Bulechek GM (Eds). (2004). *Nursing Interventions Classification (NIC),* 4th ed. St Louis: Mosby.

Evans D, Fitzgerald M. (2002). The experience of physical restraint: A systematic review of qualitative research. *Contemp Nurse,* 13(2-3):126-135.

Evans D, Wood J, Lambert L. (2002a). Physical restraint—Part 1: Use in acute and residential care facilities. *Best Pract,* 6(3):1-6. Available online: http://www.joannabriggs.edu.au/best_practice/bp11.php. Retrieved on 7/19/07.

Evans D, Wood J, Lambert L. (2002b). Physical restraint—Part 2: Minimisation in acute and residential care facilities. *Best Pract,* 6(4):1-6. Available online: http://www.joannabriggs.edu.au/best_practice/bp12.php. Retrieved on 7/19/07.

Fosbinder D. (1994). Patient perceptions of nursing care: An emerging theory of interpersonal competence. *J Adv Nurs,* 20(6):1085-1093.

Hart-Hughes S, Quigley P, Bulat T, Palacios P, Scott S. (2004). An interdisciplinary approach to reducing fall risks and falls. *J Rehabil,* 70(4):46-51.

Heuer L. (1993). Parental stressors in a pediatric intensive care unit. *Pediatr Nurs,* 19(2):128-131.

Holt J. (2001). A systematic review of the congruence between *people's* needs and nurses' interventions for supporting hope. *Online J Knowl Synth Nurs,* 8:1.

Hospital Bed Safety Workgroup (HBSW). (2003). Clinical guidance for the assessment and implementa-tion of bed rails in hospitals, long term care facilities, and home care settings. *Crit Care Nurs Q,* 26(3):244-262.

Huckabay LM, Tilem-Kessler D. (1999). Patterns of parental stress in PICU emergency admission. *Dimens Crit Care Nurs,* 18(2):36-42.

Hupcey JE. (1998). Establishing the nurse-family relationship in the intensive care unit. *West J Nurs Res,* 20(2):180-194.

Hupcey JE. (2000). Feeling safe: The psychosocial needs of ICU patients. *J Nurs Scholarsh,* 32(4):361-367.

Hupcey JE, Penrod J, Morse JM. (2000). Establishing and maintaining trust during acute care hospitaliza-tions. *Sch Inq Nurs Pract,* 14(3):227-242.

Marcy-Edwards D. (2005). Bed rails. Is there an up side? *Can Nurse,* 101(1):30-34.

McCabe C. (2004). Nurse-patient communication: An exploration of patients' experiences. *J Clin Nurs,* 13(1):41-49.

McLaughlin J, Zeeberg I. (1993). Self-care and multiple sclerosis: A view from two cultures. *Soc Sci Med,* 37(3):315-329.

Moorhead M, Johnson M, Maas M (Eds). (2004). *Nursing Outcomes Classification (NOC),* 3rd ed. St Louis: Mosby.

Morse JM. (1991). Negotiating commitment and involvement in the nurse-patient relationship. *J Adv Nurs,* 16(4):455-468.

Pellatt GC. (2005). The safety and dignity of patients and nurses during patient handling. *Br J Nurs,* 14(21):1150-1156.

Schein C, Gagnon AJ, Chan L, Morin I, Grondines J. (2005). The association between specific nurse case management interventions and elder health. *J Am Geriatr Soc,* 53(4):597-602.

Shattell M. (2005). Nurse bait: Strategies hospitalized patients use to entice nurses within the context of the interpersonal relationship. *Issues Ment Health Nurs,* 26(2):205-223.

Shojania KG, Duncan BW, McDonald KM, Wachter RM, Markowitz AJ. (2001). Making health care safer: A critical analysis of patient safety practices. *Evid Rep Technol Assess (Summ),* (43):i-x, 1-668.

Stephenson PS. (2004). Understanding denial. *Oncol Nurs Forum,* 31(5):985-988.

Thompson VL, Hupcey JE, Clark MB. (2003). The development of trust in parents of hospitalized children. *J Spec Pediatr Nurs,* 8(4):137-147.

Unruh L, Lugo NR, White SV, Byers JF. (2005). Managed care and patient safety. Risks and opportunities. *Health Care Manag,* 24(3):245-256.

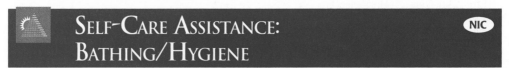

Self-Care Assistance: Bathing/Hygiene

NIC

Linda Williams, MSN, RN-BC; Scott Chisholm Lamont, BSN, RN, CCRN, CFRN; Betty J. Ackley, MSN, EdS, RN

NIC **Definition:** Assisting the patient to perform personal hygiene (Dochterman & Bulechek, 2004).

NURSING ACTIVITIES

Effective

■ *Use a person-centered care technique when bathing a cognitively impaired patient. Foster the development of an understanding relationship with the patient, plan for the patient's comfort and preferences, personalize care, show respect in communications, critically think to solve issues that arise, and use a gentle approach.* **LOE = II**

(NR) A crossover controlled study that included 15 nursing homes tested two interventions and compared their results with those of a control group. Certified nursing assistants (CNAs) who received specialized training in a person-centered approach when bathing patients (*N* = 69 nursing home residents) demonstrated the increased use of gentleness and verbal support and showed ease when accomplishing the bathing as compared with a control group (Hoeffer et al., 2006).

(NR) An RCT that included 15 nursing homes (*N* = 69 nursing home residents) tested two interventions and compared the results with those of a control group. The first intervention was the use of CNAs who received specialized training in a person-centered approach when bathing patients, which demonstrated a 53% decrease in aggressive incidents as compared with the control group. A second intervention, which was the use of a towel bath, demonstrated a 60% decrease in aggressive incidents as compared with the control group (Sloane et al., 2004).

(MR) In a controlled pilot study using specially trained CNAs, it was demonstrated that creating opportunities for guiding personal care honored long-standing routines, increased control, and made bath time more pleasant for caregivers. In the study, warm, soapy towels were used for bathing as the patient preferred, and privacy was maintained. It was found that patient aggression (a defensive patient response) was increased with shower and tub bathing (Perlmutter & Camberg, 2004).

■ *Use a towel bath to bathe the patient, if desired.* **LOE = II**

(MR) In a controlled pilot study using specially-trained CNAs, it was demonstrated that creating opportunities for guiding personal care honored long-standing routines, increased control, and made bath time more pleasant for caregivers. In the study, warm, soapy towels were used for bathing as the patient preferred, and privacy was maintained. It was found that patient aggression (a defensive patient response) was increased with shower and tub bathing (Perlmutter & Camberg, 2004).

(NR) An RCT that included 15 nursing homes (*N* = 69 nursing home residents) tested two interventions and compared the results with those of a control group. The first intervention was the use of CNAs who received specialized training in a person-centered approach when bathing patients, which demonstrated a 53% decrease in aggressive incidents as compared with the control group. A second intervention, which was the use of a towel bath, demonstrated a 60% decrease in aggressive incidents as compared with the control group (Sloane et al., 2004).

Possibly Effective

■ *Use comforting words to describe the bathing experience, such as "warm," "relaxing," or "massage." For example, "I'm going to give you a massage and get you clean at the same time."* **LOE = VII**

(EO) For cognitively impaired patients, avoid using upsetting words that are associated with bathing. Instead of using terms like "bath," "shower," or "wash," use comforting words like "warm," "relaxing," or "massage." Some words are associated with unpleasant bathing experiences, whereas others convey a pleasant bathing experience (Rader et al., 2006).

RCT = Randomized Controlled (Clinical) Trial, **NIC** = Nursing Interventions Classification, **NOC** = Nursing Outcomes Classification

■ *Avoid using triggers for assaultive behavior (a defensive response) by the patient with dementia while assisting the patient with bathing. These triggers may include the following:*

- *Spraying water without a verbal warning*
- *Touching the patient's axilla or perineum (instead, place the washcloth in the patient's hand and place your hand over the washcloth to wash the area, if needed)*
- *Touching the patient's feet without warning*
- *Confrontational communication*
- *Invalidation*
- *Failure to alert the resident of an impending action*
- *Disrespectful speech*
- *Washing the face first*
- *Hair washing that results in water dripping in the face* **LOE = VI**

(NR) A descriptive study performed by videotaping the bathing of patients with dementia with incidences of assault of caregivers found that, within 5 seconds of the behaviors listed above, defensive behaviors often occurred, such as hitting, kicking, spitting, throwing objects, or biting (Somboontanont et al., 2004).

(EO) Beginning bathing with the face or hair first is distressing to the patient as a result of water in the face and having a cold, wet head (Rader et al., 2006).

■ *Ensure that bathing assistance preserves patient dignity through the conveyance of honor and the recognition of the deservedness of respect and the maintenance of esteem of all people, regardless of their dependency and infirmity.* **LOE = VI**

(NR) In a cross-sectional observational study of terminal cancer patients ($N = 213$), needing assistance with bathing, being hospitalized, and having pain were among the most significant issues that fractured the terminally ill patient's sense of dignity, which resulted in a higher desire for death and a loss of the will to live (Chochinov et al., 2002).

■ *Use nondetergent, no-rinse, prepackaged bathing products as a cost-effective means of providing skin care that is equivalent or superior to a traditional soap-and-water bed bath.* **LOE = IV**

(NR) A nonrandomized controlled comparison trial of a traditional basin bath with a prepackaged disposable bed bath for critically ill patients ($N = 40$) in three intensive care units found no difference in quality scores or microbial counts. Nurses rated the prepackaged product more highly, and it significantly reduced both time and cost (Larson et al., 2004).

(NR) A retrospective pretest/post-test study of bed-bound long-term care residents ($N = 29$) found fewer skin tears after switching from traditional soap-and-water bathing to a no-rinse formula, which was suggested to result in significant cost savings associated with care of skin tears (Birch & Coggins, 2003). However, the study was noted to be quite small and underpowered by the authors of a systematic review article on skin care (Hodgkinson & Nay, 2005).

NR = Nursing Research, **MR** = Multidisciplinary Research, **SP** = Standard of Practice, **EO** = Expert Opinion, **LOE** = Level of Evidence

(NR) A nonrandomized controlled study of skin dryness associated with bathing among elderly long-term care residents ($N = 32$) found that mean skin condition was better for the group bathed with the prepackaged product and that skin flaking and scaling were significantly reduced for that group (Sheppard & Brenner, 2000).

(NR) A review article regarding the use of a specific prepackaged bathing product for the home care setting noted that this form of bathing product was demonstrated to be inexpensive, convenient, quick drying, and time effective (Collins & Hampton, 2003).

■ *Apply moisturizing ointments or creams to the skin within 3 minutes of exiting the shower or bath.* **LOE = VII**

(EO) Applying moisturizers before the skin dries completely helps trap moisture in the upper layers of the skin, thereby reducing skin dryness and irritation (AAD, 2002).

■ *Assess bathing ability and use environmental adaptations for community-living people who may require assistance with activities of daily living.* **LOE = VI**

(MR) A descriptive study of the prevalence of environmental adaptations used for bathing among elderly people living in a community setting ($N = 566$) demonstrated that adaptations were present in less than 50% of homes (Anaissie et al., 2002).

(EO) The assessment of a person's ability to bathe themselves should occur in a typical setting for that person, and the teaching of adaptive equipment should include follow-up in the home setting (Williams, 2008).

■ *Support bathing practices that may have culturally specific significance for social well-being for members of that culture.* **LOE = V**

(MR) A qualitative review article regarding the provision of bathing assistance as a social service for long-term care in Japan noted the importance of cultural considerations in both individual- and policy-level decision making for long-term care (Traphagan, 2004).

■ *Add lavender oil to the bathwater to improve psychological well-being.* **LOE = III**

(MR) A two-part, single-blind RCT involving female volunteers ($N = 80$) compared the effects of placebo oil versus lavender oil added to bathwater with regard to two aspects of psychological well-being. Psychologically positive mood changes were demonstrated in the first study group ($N = 40$), and reduced negative responses regarding the future were demonstrated in the second study group ($N = 40$; Morris, 2002).

■ *If tub baths are tolerated by an elderly person, use warm (40°C) bath water to assist with passive body heating to improve sleep onset, duration, and quality in the elderly.* **LOE = V**

(MR) A systematic review of three controlled studies of the effects on sleep of passive heating by bathing among participants 60 years old and older ($N = 53$), all using a randomized cross-over design, found that participants had improved subjective quality of sleep and quantitative measures of sleep. However, male and female genders were not reported separately in the one mixed-gender study, so results could only be considered definitively positive for females (Liao, 2002).

■ *Briefly immerse patients in a 40°C hot tub as tolerated, which is as safe for stable, treated hypertensive people as for normotensive people.* **LOE = VI**

RCT = Randomized Controlled (Clinical) Trial, **NIC** = Nursing Interventions Classification, **NOC** = Nursing Outcomes Classification

(MR) A case-controlled descriptive study of participants ($N = 44$) comparing blood pressure and heart rate changes during and after a 10-minute immersion in a public hot tub found that, although diastolic blood pressure fell and heart rate increased in both the hypertensive and normotensive groups, no adverse symptoms were reported. The study concluded that brief bathing in hot tubs should be safe for most treated hypertensive people (Shin et al., 2003).

- ■ *Clean shower facilities immediately before use by immunocompromised patients.* **LOE = III**

   (MR) A pretest/post-test descriptive study of randomly selected patient shower facilities ($N = 11$) on a bone marrow transplantation unit found a significant reduction in the concentration of airborne filamentous fungi, including pathogenic species, even if only the floor of the shower was cleaned (Anaissie et al., 2002).

Not Effective

No applicable published research was found in this category.

Possibly Harmful

- ■ *Using forced bathing with showers and tub baths for patients with dementia if patient aggression occurs. Forced bathing should be considered a form of abuse.* **LOE = VII**

   (MR) In a pilot controlled study ($N = 8$), patient aggression and agitation were increased among dementia patients during showers and tub baths. It may be preferable to use a towel bath for these patients; this is a comforting, warm, private, more gentle, and more dignified approach (Perlmutter & Camberg, 2004).

   (EO) Forced bathing that results in patient aggression, which is a defensive patient response, should be eliminated in extended-care facilities, as restraints have been. Instead, person-centered care should be instituted; this better meets the needs of the patients and is safer for caregivers (Rader et al., 2006).

- ■ *Exposing central venous catheters to hospital tap water during the course of bathing or showering.* **LOE = IV**

   (NR) A case-control study of bone marrow transplant and oncology patients ($N = 18$) after an outbreak of *Mycobacterium mucogenicum* bacteremias found a DNA match between isolates from one patient's blood and the shower in that patient's room, and *Mycobacterium* isolates were found from numerous water sources in the facility. The poststudy follow-up of recommendations to protect central venous catheters from water during bathing resulted in a reduction of *Mycobacterium* bacteremia cases from six in a 4-month period to one in a 30-month period (Kline et al., 2004).

- ■ *Using shower gel, antiseptic agents, or shampoo in the bath for women who are being treated for bacterial vaginosis.* **LOE = VII**

   (EO) A clinical practice guideline promulgated by the British Association for Sexual Health and HIV recommends that this population avoid these products (Hay, 2006).

NR = Nursing Research, **MR** = Multidisciplinary Research, **SP** = Standard of Practice, **EO** = Expert Opinion, **LOE** = Level of Evidence

■ *Exposing patients who are at risk for infection to tap water, including those who are immunocompromised or who have open wounds.* **LOE = V**

(NR) A systematic review of select literature on bathwater as a source of infection concluded that following recommendations such as using sterile water for drinking, using sterile sponges for bathing, educating staff and families about infection control practices related to waterborne infections, implementing targeted surveillance, and following Centers for Disease Control and Prevention guidelines to suppress organisms present in water systems may improve patient outcomes. However, significantly more study is needed to determine best practices (John, 2006).

■ *Bathing or showering people with dry skin with hot water as opposed to warm water.* **LOE = VII**

(EO) Hot water strips the skin of oils that help maintain skin moisture, thereby resulting in increased dryness and irritation (AAD, 2002).

■ *Bathing a patient in hot water (40°C or greater) for a prolonged period of time, thus increasing risk of syncope.* **LOE = V**

(MR) A descriptive study that compared young men ($N = 9$; mean age 27 years) with older men ($N = 9$; mean age 75 years) found that heart rate variability changed after 4 minutes of immersion in 40°C water, possibly reflecting decreased sympathetic tone and risk for syncope (Nagasawa et al., 2001).

(MR) A second descriptive study of heart rate variability experienced by young men bathing in 38°C and 41°C water ($N = 14$) led the authors to conclude that immersion time should be limited to 10 minutes at 38°C or 5 minutes at 41°C (Kataoka & Yoshida, 2005).

OUTCOME MEASUREMENT

SELF-CARE: ACTIVITIES OF DAILY LIVING   (NOC)

Definition: Ability to perform the most basic physical tasks and personal care activities independently with or without assistive device.

Self-Care: Activities of Daily Living as evidenced by the following selected NOC indicators:
- Bathing
- Grooming
- Hygiene

(Rate each indicator of **Self-Care: Activities of Daily Living:** 1 = severely compromised, 2 = substantially compromised, 3 = moderately compromised, 4 = mildly compromised, 5 = not compromised) (Moorhead et al., 2004).

REFERENCES

American Academy of Dermatology (AAD). (2002). Protecting your skin as the snow flies: Separating the myth from the fact about dry winter skin. Available online: http://www.aad.org. Retrieved on July 7, 2007.

Anaissie EJ, Stratton SL, Dignani MC, Lee CK, Mahfouz TH, Rex JH, et al. (2002). Cleaning patient shower facilities: A novel approach to reducing patient exposure to aerosolized Aspergillus species and other opportunistic molds. *Clin Infect Dis,* 35(8):E86-E88.

Birch S, Coggins T. (2003). No-rinse, one-step bed bath: The effects on the occurrence of skin tears in a long-term care setting. *Ostomy Wound Manage,* 49(1):64-67.

Chochinov HM, Hack T, Hassard T, Kristjanson LJ, McClement S, Harlos M. (2002). Dignity in the terminally ill: A cross-sectional, cohort study, *Lancet,* 360(9350):2026-2030.

Collins F, Hampton S. (2003). BagBath: The value of simplistic care in the community. *Br J Community Nurs,* 8(10):470-475.

Dochterman JM, Bulechek GM (Eds). (2004). *Nursing Interventions Classification (NIC),* 4th ed. St Louis: Mosby.

Hay P. (2006). National guideline for the management of bacterial vaginosis. Clinical Effectiveness Group, British Association for Sexual Health and HIV. Available online: http://www.bashh.org. Retrieved on July 7, 2007.

Hodgkinson B, Nay R. (2005). Effectiveness of topical skin care provided in aged care facilities. *Int J Evid Based Healthc,* 3(4):65-101.

Hoeffer B, Talerico KA, Rasin J, Mitchell CM, Stewart BJ, McKenzie D, et al. (2006). Assisting cognitively impaired nursing home residents with bathing: Effects of two bathing interventions on caregiving. *Gerontologist,* 46(4):524-532.

John LD. (2006). Nosocomial infections and bath water: Any cause for concern? *Clin Nurse Spec,* 20(3): 119-123.

Kataoka Y, Yoshida F. (2005). The change of hemodynamics and heart rate variability on bathing by the gap of water temperature. *Biomed Pharmacother,* 59(Suppl 1):S92-S99.

Kline S, Cameron S, Streifel A, Yakrus MA, Kairis F, Peacock K, et al. (2004). An outbreak of bacteremias associated with Mycobacterium mucogenicum in a hospital water supply. *Infect Control Hosp Epidemiol,* 25(12):1042-1049.

Larson EL, Ciliberti T, Chantler C, Abraham J, Lazaro EM, Venturanza M, et al. (2004). Comparison of traditional and disposable bed baths in critically ill patients. *Am J Crit Care,* 13(3):235-241.

Liao WC. (2002). Effects of passive body heating on body temperature and sleep regulation in the elderly: A systematic review. *Int J Nurs Stud,* 39(8):803-810.

Moorhead M, Johnson M, Maas M (Eds). (2004). *Nursing Outcomes Classification (NOC),* 3rd ed. St Louis: Mosby.

Morris N. (2002). The effects of lavender (Lavendula angusifolium) baths on psychological well-being: Two exploratory randomized control trials. *Complement Ther Med,* 10(4):223-228.

Nagasawa Y, Komori S, Sato M, Tsuboi Y, Umetani K, Watanabe Y, et al. (2001). Effects of hot bath immersion on autonomic activity and hemodynamics: Comparison of the elderly patient and the healthy young. *Jpn Circ J,* 65(7):587-592.

Perlmutter JS, Camberg L. (2004). Better bathing for residents with Alzheimer's. *Nurs Homes Long Term Care Manage,* 53(4):40, 42-43.

Rader J, Barrick AL, Hoeffer B, Sloane PD, McKenzie D, Talerico KA, et al. (2006). The bathing of older adults with dementia. *Am J Nurs,* 106(4):40-48.

Sheppard CM, Brenner PS. (2000). The effects of bathing and skin care practices on skin quality and satisfaction with an innovative product. *J Gerontol Nurs,* 26(10):36-45.

Shin TW, Wilson M, Wilson TW. (2003). Are hot tubs safe for people with treated hypertension? *CMAJ,* 169(12):1265-1268.

Sloane PD, Hoeffer B, Mitchell CM, McKenzie DA, Barrick AL, Rader J, et al. (2004). Effect of person-centered showering and the towel bath on bathing-associated aggression, agitation, and discomfort in nursing home residents with dementia: A randomized, controlled trial. *J Am Geriatr Soc,* 52(11): 1795-1804.

Somboontanont W, Sloane PD, Floyd FJ, Holditch-Davis D, Hogue CC, Mitchell CM. (2004). Assaultive behavior in Alzheimer's disease: Identifying immediate antecedents during bathing. *J Gerontol Nurs,* 30(9):22-29.

Traphagan JW. (2004). Culture and long-term care: The bath as social service in Japan. *Care Manag J,* 5(1):53-60.

Williams LS. (2008). Bathing/hygiene self-care deficit. In Ackley BJ, Ladwig GB (Eds). *Nursing diagnosis handbook: A guide to planning care,* 8th ed. St Louis: Mosby.

NR = Nursing Research, **MR** = Multidisciplinary Research, **SP** = Standard of Practice, **EO** = Expert Opinion, **LOE** = Level of Evidence

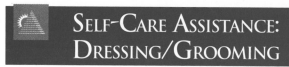

SELF-CARE ASSISTANCE: DRESSING/GROOMING

Cornelia Beck, PhD, RN, FAAN; Valorie M. Shue, BA

NIC **Definition:** Assisting the patient with clothes and makeup (Dochterman & Bulechek, 2004).

NURSING ACTIVITIES

Effective

■ *Provide graded assistance for patients with dementia as needed. For example, ask the patient to "pick up your sock, put the sock on your foot, pick up the other sock, put that sock on the other foot. . . ."* **LOE = III**

(MR) An evidence-based review of controlled studies classified graded assistance (from verbal prompts to physical demonstration, physical guidance, practical physical assistance, and complete physical assistance) as a guideline (a recommendation that reflects moderate clinical certainty) for activities of daily living (ADLs) in people with dementia (Doody et al., 2001).

(MR) A controlled study comparing usual care and functional rehabilitation in 17 nursing home residents with dementia found that functional rehabilitation, which included substituting nondirective and directive verbal assists for physical assists, could reduce functional decline during dressing and grooming (Rogers et al., 2000).

(NR) In a case study, a decrease in assistance occurred for washing the face, brushing the teeth, and combing the hair in eight nursing home residents with mild cognitive impairment after systematic prompting and social reinforcement through one-step commands (Lim, 2003).

(MR) A case study showed that certified nursing assistants learned and used a system of least prompts at each step of a task beginning with less intrusive prompts and gradually proceeding to more intrusive prompts with three nursing home residents with dementia. The residents' independence in dressing increased (Engelman et al., 2002).

■ (SP) *Obtain clothing that is larger-sized and easier to put on, including clothing with elastic waistbands, wide sleeves and pant legs, dresses that open down the back for women in wheelchairs, and Velcro fasteners or larger buttons.* **LOE = VII**

(EO) Simplifying the clothing that is put on facilitates dressing for those with an impaired ability to perform ADLs (Williams, 2008).

■ *Refer the patient to occupational therapy for learning to dress and groom him- or herself.* **LOE = II**

(MR) An RCT of 100 people recovering from hip fractures in Stockholm, Sweden, found that early individualized postoperative occupational training that began during the person's

RCT = Randomized Controlled (Clinical) Trial, **NIC** = Nursing Interventions Classification, **NOC** = Nursing Outcomes Classification

hospital stay and included a home visit before discharge sped up the patient's ability to perform ADLs. As compared with the control group, members of the intervention group significantly improved in their ability to dress and take care of personal hygiene (Hagsten et al., 2004).

(MR) An RCT of 319 older community dwellers who reported difficulty with one or more ADLs involved home modifications and training in their use; instructions in problem solving, energy conservation, safe performance, and fall-recovery techniques; and balance and muscle strength training. After 6 months, the treatment group had significantly less difficulty with dressing and grooming (Gitlin et al., 2006).

(MR) A controlled study involved 50 people who had ischemic stroke and who were consecutively admitted to two postacute units in Rome, Italy. One randomly chosen unit added two occupational therapists to the rehabilitation team, whereas the other unit received only physiotherapy. The team constructed individualized plans of treatment that could include strengthening and range-of-motion exercises, musculoskeletal control, trunk and upper extremity positioning, transfer training, postural and gait training, functional and self-care retraining, and adaptive equipment training. The intervention group demonstrated significantly better performance with regard to dressing and personal hygiene than the control group (Landi et al., 2006).

Possibly Effective

■ *Provide nurse education and training in how to help patients learn to dress and groom themselves.* **LOE = III**

(NR) In a controlled study, nurse educators supported three nursing homes over a 2-year period by helping the staff match the correct care practice with the residents' capacity for self-care. The rate of resident dressing decline decreased four times more than it did in 10 control facilities that provided usual care (Goldman et al., 2004).

(NR) In a controlled study with repeated measures of 40 nursing home residents with dementia, one unit was randomly selected to receive a comprehensive education program on abilities-focused morning care; three units served as controls. Results revealed that residents whose caregivers received the intervention improved in their levels of functioning with regard to morning care (i.e., bathing, grooming, dressing, and toileting) (Wells et al., 2000).

■ *Provide goal-focused therapy.* **LOE = IV**

(MR) In a controlled study with a pretest/post-test design, 31 patients who were receiving treatment for neurologic, cardiopulmonary, and orthopedic deficits, back injury, and debilitation at a rehabilitation hospital received physical therapy and occupational therapy. However, participants in the experimental group also received a goal notebook and discussed goals with their therapists daily. The experimental group made significantly greater gains in upper-body dressing than the control group (Gagné & Hoppes, 2003).

Not Effective

No applicable published research was found in this category.

NR = Nursing Research, **MR** = Multidisciplinary Research, **SP** = Standard of Practice, **EO** = Expert Opinion, **LOE** = Level of Evidence

Possibly Harmful

No applicable published research was found in this category.

OUTCOME MEASUREMENT

SELF-CARE: ACTIVITIES OF DAILY LIVING NOC

Definition: Ability to perform the most basic physical tasks and personal care activities independently with or without assistive device.

Self-Care: Activities of Daily Living as evidenced by the following selected NOC indicators:

• Dressing

• Grooming

(Rate each indicator of **Self-Care: Activities of Daily Living:** 1 = severely compromised, 2 = substantially compromised, 3 = moderately compromised, 4 = mildly compromised, 5 = not compromised) (Moorhead et al., 2004).

REFERENCES

Dochterman JM, Bulechek GM (Eds). (2004). *Nursing Interventions Classification (NIC),* 4th ed. St Louis: Mosby.

Doody RS, Stevens JC, Beck C, Dubinsky RM, Kaye JA, Gwyther L, et al. (2001). Practice parameter: Management of dementia (an evidence-based review). Report of the Quality Standards Subcommittee of the American Academy of Neurology. *Neurology,* 56(9):1154-1166.

Engelman KK, Mathews RM, Altus DE. (2002). Restoring dressing independence in persons with Alzheimer's disease: A pilot study. *Am J Alzheimers Dis Other Demen,* 17(1):37-43.

Gagné DE, Hoppes S. (2003). The effects of collaborative goal-focused occupational therapy on self-care skills: A pilot study. *Am J Occup Ther,* 57(2):215-219.

Gitlin LN, Winter L, Dennis MP, Corcoran M, Schinfeld S, Hauck WW. (2006). A randomized trial of a multicomponent home intervention to reduce functional difficulties in older adults. *J Am Geriatr Soc,* 54(5):809-816.

Goldman B, Balgobin S, Bish R, Lee RH, McCue S, Morrison MH, et al. (2004). Nurse educators are key to a best practices implementation program. *Geriatr Nurs,* 25(3):171-174.

Hagsten B, Svensson O, Gardulf A. (2004). Early individualized postoperative occupational therapy training in 100 patients improves ADL after hip fracture: A randomized trial. *Acta Orthop Scand,* 75(2): 177-183.

Landi F, Cesari M, Onder G, Tafani A, Zamboni V, Cocchi A. (2006). Effects of an occupational therapy program on functional outcomes in older stroke patients. *Gerontology,* 52(2):85-91.

Lim YM. (2003). Nursing intervention for grooming of elders with mild cognitive impairments in Korea. *Geriatr Nurs,* 24(1):11-15.

Moorhead M, Johnson M, Maas M (Eds). (2004). *Nursing Outcomes Classification (NOC),* 3rd ed. St Louis: Mosby.

Rogers JC, Holm MB, Burgio LD, Hsu C, Hardin JM, McDowell BJ. (2000). Excess disability during morning care in nursing home residents with dementia. *Int Psychogeriatr,* 12(2):267-282.

Wells DL, Dawson P, Sidani S, Craig D, Pringle D. (2000). Effects of an abilities-focused program on morning care on residents who have dementia and on caregivers. *J Am Geriatr Soc,* 48(4):442-449.

Williams L. (2008). Self-care deficit, dressing/grooming. In Ackley B, Ladwig G (Eds): *Nursing diagnosis handbook: A guide to planning care,* 7th ed. St Louis: Mosby.

RCT = Randomized Controlled (Clinical) Trial, **NIC** = Nursing Interventions Classification, **NOC** = Nursing Outcomes Classification

Self-Esteem Enhancement

Judith R. Gentz, RN, CS, NP

> **NIC** **Definition:** Assisting a patient to increase his/her personal judgment of self-worth (Dochterman & Bulecheck, 2004).

NURSING ACTIVITIES

Effective

■ *Encourage the identification of thoughts and feelings via talking, journaling, or other modes of expression.* **LOE = I**

NR In a controlled study ($N = 51$), the participants in a cognitive behavioral treatment group raised self-esteem significantly by verbalizing and gaining understanding of their feelings (Chen et al., 2006).

EO Journal writing prompts mood-elevating activities and reduces reactive depression (Smith et al., 2003).

NR A small ($N = 3$) descriptive study found that patients being understood and understanding the care provider fostered a sense of caring (Sundin et al., 2002).

EO A theoretical analysis of self-concept has cognitive and affective (feeling) components and is a determinant of both behavior and feelings (LeMone, 1991).

■ *Identify and encourage the use of social supports.* **LOE = I**

NR A descriptive study ($N = 10$) found that health care providers' ability to confirm and care for patients increased patients' positive emotions and ultimately their self-esteem (Raty & Gustafsson, 2006).

MR In an RCT, young mothers ($N = 116$) receiving group social support and education had significantly higher self-esteem than those mothers who did not receive social support (Lipman & Boyle, 2005).

NR In a descriptive study ($N = 27$) using telephone nursing interventions with people with schizophrenia, social support was identified as increasing the patient's ability to deal with problems (Beebe, 2002).

NR In a descriptive study designed to predict well-being among breast cancer survivors ($N = 84$), social support was a strong predictor of resourcefulness, self-esteem, and well-being among postmastectomy patients (Dirsken, 2000).

NR A descriptive study ($N = 94$) found that social involvement and work were predictors of higher self-esteem among people with mental illness (Van Dongen, 1998).

■ *Encourage physical activity and well-being.* **LOE = I**

MR A Cochrane systematic review found some evidence that exercise had positive short-term effects on the self-esteem of children and youth (Ekeland et al., 2004).

MR A descriptive study of 174 older adults over a 4-year period found that higher levels of self-efficacy and physical activity were significantly related to self-esteem (McAuley et al., 2005).

NR = Nursing Research, **MR** = Multidisciplinary Research, **SP** = Standard of Practice, **EO** = Expert Opinion, **LOE** = Level of Evidence

(MR) A controlled study of 143 veterans compared fallers and nonfallers and found that the exercise intervention positively affected the psychosocial status—including self-esteem—of the fallers (Means et al., 2003).

(MR) In a descriptive study of adolescents receiving mental health treatment ($N = 39$), short-term goal setting and achievement increased a sense of competence and self-esteem (Willoughby et al., 2000).

▨ *Actively listen to the patient and provide validation.* LOE = I

(NR) A descriptive study supported the importance of presence and caring during communication with patients, although the sample size was small ($N = 3$; Sundin et al., 2002).

(MR) A descriptive study of 80 women living with breast cancer found that validation and feelings of reassurance were identified as important psychosocial needs by the women (Marlow et al., 2003).

Possibly Effective

▨ *Teach mindfulness techniques.* LOE = II

(NR) A descriptive study ($N = 15$) involving the use of grounded theory found that patients' development of mindfulness strategies increased the resolution of internal conflicts and that conflict resolution may, in turn, increase self-esteem (Horton-Deutsch & Horton, 2003).

(MR) The results of a longitudinal study ($N = 930$) of adolescents determined that clinicians assisted the patients with being mindful of current behaviors, because low self-esteem increased the risk for unhealthy behaviors (McGee & Williams, 2000).

Not Effective

▨ *Allowing patients to work on their self-esteem after the depression subsides.* LOE = I

(MR) A systematic review of the literature found that low self-esteem contributed to the incidence of depression, so raising self-esteem may reduce depressive symptoms (Mann et al., 2004).

▨ *Identifying and improving coping with acute stressors rather than chronic stressors.* LOE = II

(MR) In a descriptive study of college students ($N = 88$), chronic life experiences contributed more to negative self-esteem that acute stress (Wilburn & Smith, 2005).

Possibly Harmful

▨ *Providing "time alone" to work out problems.* LOE = III

(MR) In a descriptive study of 88 college students, acute stress was more detrimental to self-esteem in those individuals with suicidal ideation. Isolation increased the risk of suicide (Wilburn & Smith, 2005).

(EO) Withdrawal and isolation are detrimental to feelings of self-worth (Stuart-Shor et al., 2003).

RCT = Randomized Controlled (Clinical) Trial, **NIC** = Nursing Interventions Classification, **NOC** = Nursing Outcomes Classification

■ *Addressing grief and loss during the acute phase of treatment.* **LOE = V**

(EO) Maladjustment to loss or change can have detrimental effects on the entire concept of self (Drench, 1994).

OUTCOME MEASUREMENT

SELF-ESTEEM   (NOC)

(Please refer to *Nursing Outcomes Classification* [Moorhead et al., 2004] for the **Self-Esteem** outcome.)

REFERENCES

Beebe LH. (2002). Problems in community living identified by people with schizophrenia. *J Psychosoc Nurs Ment Health Serv,* 40(2):38-45.

Chen TH, Lu RB, Chang AJ, Chu DM, Chou KR. (2006). The evaluation of cognitive-behavioral group therapy on patient depression and self-esteem. *Arch Psychiatr Nurs,* 20(1):3-11.

Dirksen SR. (2000). Predicting well-being among breast cancer survivors. *J Adv Nurs,* 32(4):937-943.

Dochterman JM, Bulechek GM (Eds). (2004). *Nursing Interventions Classification (NIC),* 4th ed. St Louis: Mosby.

Drench ME. (1994). Changes in body image secondary to disease and injury. *Rehabil Nurs,* 19(1):31-36.

Ekeland E, Heian F, Hagen KB, Abbott J, Nordheim L. (2004). Exercise to improve self-esteem in children and young people. *Cochrane Database Syst Rev,* (1):CD003683.

Horton-Deutsch SL, Horton JM. (2003). Mindfulness: Overcoming intractable conflict. *Arch Psychiatr Nurs,* 17(4):186-193.

LeMone P. (1991). Analysis of a human phenomenon: Self-concept. *Nurs Diagn,* 2(3):126-130.

Lipman EL, Boyle MH. (2005). Social support and education groups for single mothers: A randomized controlled trial of a community-based program. *CMAJ,* 173(12):1451-1456.

Mann M, Hosman CM, Schaalma HP, de Vries NK. (2004). Self-esteem in a broad-spectrum approach for mental health promotion. *Health Educ Res,* 19(4):357-372.

Marlow B, Cartmill T, Cieplucha H, Lowrie S. (2003). An interactive process model of psychosocial support needs for women living with breast cancer. *Psychooncology,* 12(4):319-330.

McAuley E, Elavsky S, Motl RW, Konopack JF, Hu L, Marquez DX. (2005). Physical activity, self-efficacy, and self-esteem: Longitudinal relationships in older adults. *J Gerontol B Psychol Sci Soc Sci,* 60(5): P268-P275.

McGee R, Williams S. (2000). Does low self-esteem predict health compromising behaviours among adolescents? *J Adolesc,* 23(5):569-582.

Means KM, O'Sullivan PS, Rodell DE. (2003). Psychosocial effects of an exercise program in older persons who fall. *J Rehabil Res Dev,* 40(1):49-58.

Moorhead M, Johnson M, Maas M (Eds). (2004). *Nursing Outcomes Classification (NOC),* 3rd ed. St Louis: Mosby.

Raty L, Gustafsson B. (2006). Emotions in relation to healthcare encounters affecting self-esteem. *J Neurosci Nurs,* 38(1):42-50.

Smith CE, Leenerts MH, Gajewski BJ. (2003). A systematically tested intervention for managing reactive depression. *Nurs Res,* 52(6):401-409.

Stuart-Shor EM, Buselli EF, Carroll DL, Forman DE. (2003). Are psychosocial factors associated with the pathogenesis and consequences of cardiovascular disease in the elderly? *J Cardiovasc Nurs* 18(3):169-183.

Sundin K, Jansson L, Norberg A. (2002). Understanding between care providers and patients with stroke and aphasia: A phenomenological hermeneutic inquiry. *Nurs Inq,* 9(2):93-103.

Van Dongen CJ. (1998). Self-esteem among persons with severe mental illness. *Issues Ment Health Nurs,* 19(1):29-40.

NR = Nursing Research, **MR** = Multidisciplinary Research, **SP** = Standard of Practice, **EO** = Expert Opinion, **LOE** = Level of Evidence

Wilburn VR, Smith DE. (2005). Stress, self-esteem, and suicidal ideation in late adolescents. *Adolescence,* 40(157):33-45.

Willoughby C, Polatajko H, Currado C, Harris K, King G. (2000). Measuring the self-esteem of adolescents with mental health problems: Theory meets practice. *Can J Occup Ther,* 67(4):230-238.

 # SELF-RESPONSIBILITY FACILITATION

Deborah R. Gillum, MSN, RN, ANP-C, FNP-C

> **NIC** **Definition:** Encouraging a patient to assume more responsibility for his or her own behavior (Dochterman & Bulechek, 2004).

NURSING ACTIVITIES

Effective

■ *Recognize differing perceptions regarding health issues between health care workers and patients.* **LOE = V**

> **MR** In a descriptive study of 70 injured-worker rehabilitation patients and 70 health care workers, each selected the most influential psychosocial variables that affected recovery. The health care staff rated self-responsibility as the most important variable, whereas the patients ranked it eleventh out of a total of 17 variables (Antoniazzi et al., 2002).

> **MR** A qualitative study (*N* = 9) described the thoughts and rationalizations of smoking mothers of children who had respiratory illnesses when the risk factors of smoking were previously known. Their attempts to minimize the risks to a more acceptable level and their perceived responsibility regarding these risks were captured in the authors' notes (Coxhead & Rhodes, 2006).

■ *Recognize the effect of culture on health care practices and adherence to medical regimens.* **LOE = II**

> **NR** A cross-sectional convenience sample of 200 Chinese subjects examined the cultural factors affecting adherence to antihypertensive medications. Low perceived susceptibility, high perceived benefits of herbal treatments, lower perceived benefits of Western medications, and length of stay in the emigrated country were significant predictors of medication nonadherence (Li et al., 2006).

> **MR** An RCT of 1227 lower-income African American women from 10 urban public health centers received a series of women's magazines that were specifically tailored to meet the educational needs of the participants regarding mammography screening and fruit and vegetable intake. Researchers found that information designed to meet the unique characteristics of the individual through behavioral construct tailoring and culturally relevant tailoring increased the adherence rate of the interventions significantly (Kreuter et al., 2005).

> **MR** A two-stage qualitative (*N* = 28) and quantitative (*N* = 46) study of a convenience sample described the cultural interpretation of the causes of type II diabetes mellitus and analyzed the relationship between cultural knowledge and diabetes control in a Mexican community. Results demonstrated that emotional distress and the deteriorating quality of modern foods were seen as primary causes of the disease. The individuals who were in better control of their

diabetes had a stronger cultural knowledge of the disease rather than a medical knowledge (Daniulaityte, 2004).

Possibly Effective

■ *Discuss personal and social health responsibilities with the patient.* **LOE = VI**

(MR) A controlled study over a 4-month period of time determined that patients ($N = 528$) were more motivated by social responsibility than personal responsibility messages regarding the increase of their daily fruit and vegetable intake to five servings per day (Williams-Piehota et al., 2004).

(EO) Competent patients have the obligation of and should take responsibility for looking after their health for their own benefit as well as for the benefit of society (Draper & Sorell, 2002).

■ *Help the patient to explore the benefits of assuming more responsibility.* **LOE = VI**

(NR) A small qualitative study ($N = 4$) explored adolescents' experiences of gaining more independence in the management of their diabetes. These teens gained freedom by becoming more involved in the management of their disease and accepting self-responsibility (Christian et al., 1999).

Not Effective

■ *Associating unhealthy behaviors with irresponsibility, "badness," or immorality.* **LOE = VII**

(MR) A descriptive study of four focus groups explored attitudes toward health and unhealthy behaviors. The unhealthy behaviors, which could be associated with irresponsibility, could lead to resistance in health promotion, because the participants asserted their own independence over the socially acceptable value of good health (Crossley, 2003).

(EO) When exploring the personal and moral responsibility associated with an individual's state of health and the lack of evidence that supports causality, it was found that deciding who was responsible for their negative health consequences was subjective and a value judgment (Yoder, 2002).

Possibly Harmful

No applicable published research was found in this category.

Note: There is a tremendous lack of research regarding self-responsibility facilitation. The knowledge base regarding this subject would benefit greatly from nursing research focused on this area, and this would also help to determine further relationships between the culture and the role of self-responsibility in health care practices.

OUTCOME MEASUREMENT

HEALTH BELIEFS: PERCEIVED CONTROL   (NOC)

(Please refer to *Nursing Outcomes Classification* [Moorhead et al., 2004] for the **Health Beliefs: Perceived Control** outcome.)

NR = Nursing Research, **MR** = Multidisciplinary Research, **SP** = Standard of Practice, **EO** = Expert Opinion, **LOE** = Level of Evidence

REFERENCES

Antoniazzi M, Celinski M, Alcock J. (2002). Self-responsibility and coping with pain: Disparate attitudes toward psychosocial issues in recovery from work place injury. *Disabil Rehabil,* 24(18):948-953.

Christian BJ, D'Auria JP, Fox LC. (1999). Gaining freedom: Self-responsibility in adolescents with diabetes. *Pediatr Nurs,* 25(3):255-260, 266.

Coxhead L, Rhodes T. (2006). Accounting for risk and responsibility associated with smoking among mothers of children with respiratory illness. *Sociol Health Illn,* 28(1):98-121.

Crossley ML. (2003). Would you consider yourself a healthy person? Using focus groups to explore health as a moral phenomenon. *J Health Psychol,* 8(5):501-514.

Daniulaityte R. (2004). Making sense of diabetes: Cultural models, gender and individual adjustment to Type 2 diabetes in a Mexican community. *Soc Sci Med,* 59(9):1899-1912.

Dochterman JM, Bulechek GM (Eds). (2004). *Nursing Interventions Classification (NIC),* 4th ed. St Louis: Mosby.

Draper H, Sorell T. (2002). Patients' responsibilities in medical ethics. *Bioethics,* 16(4):335-352.

Kreuter MW, Sugg-Skinner C, Holt CL, Clark EM, Haire-Joshu D, Fu Q, et al. (2005). Cultural tailoring for mammography and fruit and vegetable intake among low-income African-American women in urban public health centers. *Prev Med,* 41(1):53-62.

Li WW, Stewart AL, Stotts N, Froelicher ES. (2006). Cultural factors associated with antihypertensive medication adherence in Chinese immigrants. *J Cardiovasc Nurs,* 21(5):354-362.

Moorhead S, Johnson M, Maas M (Eds). (2004). *Nursing Outcomes Classification (NOC),* 3rd ed. St Louis: Mosby.

Williams-Piehota P, Cox A, Silvera SN, Mowad L, Garcia S, Katulak N, et al. (2004). Casting health messages in terms of responsibility for dietary change: Increasing fruit and vegetable consumption. *J Nutr Educ Behav,* 36(3):114-120.

Yoder SD. (2002). Individual responsibility for health: Decision, not discovery. *Hastings Cent Rep,* 32(2):22-31.

SEPSIS PREVENTION

Deborah Pool, MS, RN, CCRN

Definition: Early detection and treatment of infection with sepsis in patients who are at risk.

NURSING ACTIVITIES

Effective

■ **SP** *Monitor for systemic and localized signs and symptoms of infection.* **LOE = VII**

EO Any infection may result in the development of sepsis, but the most likely causes in hospitalized patients include community-acquired pneumonia, intra-abdominal infections, central nervous system infections, urinary tract infections, wound infections, and intravenous catheter-related infections (Robson & Newell, 2005; Vincent & Abraham, 2006).

EO The assessment of the patient's clinical picture, in conjunction with laboratory studies, is used to determine the diagnosis of sepsis (Dettenmeier et al., 2003; MacIntyre, 2001).

■ **SP** *Facilitate the early diagnosis of sepsis through the use of cultures, white blood cell counts, the clinical picture, and the hemodynamic status.* **LOE = I**

EO Early diagnosis to facilitate the rapid administration of appropriate antibiotics is crucial to improving outcomes. Collect two to three peripheral blood samples from peripheral sites

RCT = Randomized Controlled (Clinical) Trial, **NIC** = Nursing Interventions Classification, **NOC** = Nursing Outcomes Classification

simultaneously (to avoid delaying the administration of initial broad-spectrum antibiotics) and then change antibiotics appropriately when culture and sensitivity results are available (Cohen et al., 2004; Vincent & Abraham, 2006; Robson & Newell, 2005).

■ **(SP)** *Suspect the presence of sepsis with a new-onset change in the level of consciousness in a patient who is immunodepressed, elderly, or malnourished or who has a number of comorbidities, even if there is not a significant rise in temperature.* **LOE = VII**

(EO) Some patients with septic shock have normal or subnormal temperatures, especially elderly patients, neonates, and patients with renal failure or alcoholism (Kasper et al., 2005).

■ **(SP)** *Administer ordered antibiotics as quickly as possible, preferably within 2 hours or less, when the presence of sepsis is suspected.* **LOE = I**

(MR) A systematic review of the literature by critical care experts from 11 international organizations determined that the prompt administration of the appropriate antimicrobial agent was the best predictor of outcome. Practitioners must be cognizant of the most likely infective organisms and the antimicrobials that are most likely to be appropriate for the organism in an effort to administer the medications as quickly as possible (within 2 hours) after suspicion and/or after the diagnosis of sepsis is made (Bochud et al., 2004; Dellinger et al., 2004).

(EO) The initial approach to the treatment of sepsis is empiric antibiotics based on the location of the patient, the site of infection, the geographic area, and local resistance patterns (MacIntyre, 2001).

■ **(SP)** *Monitor the following aspects of circulatory status: blood pressure, heart rate, skin color, skin temperature, cardiac rhythm, capillary refill, and presence and quality of peripheral pulses.* **LOE = VII**

(EO) Monitoring vital signs and cardiac output will facilitate the early recognition of changes in tissue perfusion and blood flow. Increased body temperature in conjunction with tachycardia and/or tachypnea may be the first clinical indications of sepsis (Kleinpell, 2003, 2004; Rivers et al., 2005; Robson & Newell, 2005).

■ **(SP)** *Monitor for signs of inadequate tissue and organ perfusion, such as decreased urine output or an altered level of consciousness.* **LOE = III**

(MR) A prospective observational study (342 videos from a total of 26 patients obtained via orthogonal polarization spectral imaging) demonstrated that, even when mean arterial pressure was maintained at ≥65 mm Hg, regional hypoperfusion occurred (Abate et al., 2006).

(EO) The development of organ dysfunction as a result of inadequate perfusion and oxygenation is associated with increased morbidity and mortality in the patient with sepsis. Early recognition is crucial to determine the development of inadequate organ function and to facilitate early treatment (Aird, 2003; Rivers et al., 2005; Robson & Newell 2005; Bridges & Dukes, 2005).

(EO) The outcomes of sepsis are directly related to the degree of organ dysfunction (Vincent & Abraham, 2006; MacIntyre, 2001).

NR = Nursing Research, **MR** = Multidisciplinary Research, **SP** = Standard of Practice, **EO** = Expert Opinion, **LOE** = Level of Evidence

■ (SP) *Monitor coagulation studies, including prothrombin time, partial thromboplastin time, fibrinogen levels, fibrin degradation/split products, and platelet counts, as appropriate.* **LOE = VII**

(EO) Septic patients are in a procoagulant state that is related to alterations in coagulation and fibrinolytic pathways and decreased protein C. Alterations in measures of coagulation and fibrinolysis and platelet levels may be correlated with outcomes (Ely et al., 2003; Kleinpell, 2003; Robson & Newell, 2005; Bridges & Dukes, 2005).

(EO) Disseminated intravascular coagulation is a condition that is frequently found in the patient with sepsis; fibrin deposits in the microvasculature result in occlusion and hypoperfusion, which contribute to organ failure and death. Monitoring coagulation and fibrinolysis levels can facilitate the diagnosis and treatment of the patient with sepsis (Zeeleder et al., 2005).

■ (SP) *Monitor serum lactate levels and report elevated levels as appropriate.* **LOE = III**

(MR) A prospective observational study ($N = 111$) of patients presenting to the emergency department with a diagnosis of severe or septic shock suggested that patients who were resuscitated successfully with fluids and vasopressors and whose serum lactate levels returned to normal within 6 hours of presentation were more likely to survive (Nguyen et al., 2004).

(MR) In a prospective, nonrandomized convenience sample ($N = 20$), it was learned that resuscitating patients to a standard end point of mean arterial pressure >65 mm Hg with the use of fluid challenges and vasopressors did not ensure adequate tissue perfusion. The serum lactate level was likely to be a more accurate method of assessing tissue perfusion (Ledoux et al., 2000).

(EO) An elevated serum lactate level during the initial resuscitation of patients presenting in early sepsis is an indicator of tissue hypoperfusion (Dellinger et al., 2004; Rivers et al., 2005; Robson & Newell, 2005).

■ *With an early diagnosis of sepsis, consider the administration of fluids as ordered to achieve a central venous pressure of 8 to 12 mm Hg and/or a mean arterial pressure of ≥65 mm Hg.* **LOE = II**

(MR) A randomized trial ($N = 263$) comparing traditional resuscitation in the emergency department to resuscitation with a goal of central venous pressure of 8 to 12 mm Hg and mean arterial pressure of ≥65 mm Hg through the use of intravenous fluids and vasopressors within the first 6 hours demonstrated improved outcomes for patients receiving what is known as *early goal-directed therapy* (Rivers et al., 2001).

(EO) The use of a modified Delphi method by experts from 11 international organizations determined that fluid challenges of either crystalloids or colloids should be administered and titrated to patient response (Vincent & Gerlach, 2004).

(EO) Fluid administration is the initial treatment of choice for patients who are septic and hypotensive (Bridges & Dukes, 2005; Dellinger et al., 2004).

■ *Administer vasopressors as ordered, if appropriate, to maintain a mean arterial pressure of ≥65 mm Hg if fluid resuscitation is not successful.* **LOE = I**

(MR) A systematic review of the literature by critical care experts from 11 international organizations determined that the use of vasopressors, after the placement of an arterial line for

RCT = Randomized Controlled (Clinical) Trial, **NIC** = Nursing Interventions Classification, **NOC** = Nursing Outcomes Classification

patients with a mean arterial pressure of ≤65 mm Hg, was appropriate both during and after fluid resuscitation. Norepinephrine and dopamine were determined to be the agents of choice (Beale et al., 2004).

(MR) An observational study that included patients from 198 European intensive care units (N = 3497) who were admitted with sepsis found that dopamine may be associated with increased mortality overall (Sakr et al., 2006).

(EO) If fluid resuscitation does not improve hemodynamic or lactate levels, consider adding norepinephrine, epinephrine, phenylephrine, or vasopressin (Bridges & Dukes, 2005; Dellinger et al., 2004).

■ *Maintain the blood sugar level at ≤150 mg/dL as ordered and appropriate.* **LOE = I**

(MR) A systematic review of the literature by critical care experts from 11 international organizations determined that the maintenance of the glucose level at ≤150 mg/dL was associated with improved outcomes (Cariou et al., 2004).

(MR) An RCT comparing patients whose blood sugars were kept between 80 and 110 mg/dL (N = 1548 mechanically ventilated patients) with patients who did not receive antihyperglycemic therapy until glucose levels were >250 mg/dL suggested that tight glycemic control in critically ill patients who were being treated with mechanical ventilators resulted in improved outcomes as compared with patients whose blood sugar levels were maintained at the standard level of <250 mg/dL (Van den Berghe et al., 2006).

(MR) In a prospective, randomized, controlled study (N = 1548 patients), participants were randomized either to receive insulin to maintain glucose levels of ≤110 mg/dL or to receive insulin only for glucose levels of ≥215 mg/dL to maintain glucose levels overall between 180 and 200 mg/dL. Patients with glucose levels that were maintained below 110 mg/dL had decreased morbidity and mortality as compared with patients in the group whose blood sugars remained between 180 and 210 mg/dL (Van den Berghe et al., 2001).

(MR) A meta-analysis of research pertaining to blood glucose levels in critically ill patients suggested that tight glycemic control through the use of insulin reduced inflammation and improved outcomes in critically ill medical and surgical patients (Nasraway, 2006).

■ (SP) *Anticipate the need for mechanical ventilation.* **LOE = VII**

(EO) Respiratory failure requiring mechanical ventilation in the patient with sepsis is a frequent complication and should be anticipated in these patients (Rivers et al., 2005; Dellinger et al., 2004; Ely et al., 2003; MacIntyre, 2001).

Possibly Effective

■ *Anticipate the invasive monitoring of venous oxygen saturation in patients who have been diagnosed with sepsis.* **LOE = II**

(MR) In an RCT, patients who were admitted to the intensive care unit with sepsis or septic shock (N = 236) were randomly assigned to goal-directed therapy or standard therapy. The goal was attaining a central venous oxygen saturation of ≥70% within 6 hours of presentation in critical care through the use of fluid resuscitation, vasopressors, red blood cell administration, and supplemental oxygen. Goal-directed therapy was associated with decreased morbidity and mortality (Rivers et al., 2001).

NR = Nursing Research, **MR** = Multidisciplinary Research, **SP** = Standard of Practice, **EO** = Expert Opinion, **LOE** = Level of Evidence

(EO) Mean arterial pressure is a poor indicator of global oxygenation; it is possible for a patient to have a mean arterial pressure above 65 mm Hg and to still have elevated serum lactate levels. Incorporating a device to measure venous oxygen saturation is a more accurate measurement of tissue oxygenation than blood pressure (Shorr, 2005; Rivers et al., 2005; Martin, 2005; Bridges & Dukes, 2005).

(EO) Cellular metabolism requiring oxygen may be altered in the septic patient; this may be assessed by comparing venous oxygen saturation with arterial oxygen saturation (Vincent & Abraham, 2006).

■ *Administer corticosteroids as indicated.* **LOE = II**

(MR) An RCT ($N = 299$) compared the outcomes of patients in septic shock with adrenal insufficiency and demonstrated that, in those patients with known adrenal insufficiency, the administration of corticosteroids improved 28-day outcomes (Beigel & Eichacker, 2003).

(MR) A double-blind, randomized, placebo-controlled crossover study ($N = 40$) determined that hydrocortisone administration during septic shock promoted hemodynamic stability and enhanced immune function by decreasing inflammation (Keh et al., 2003).

(MR) A retrospective review of a previous RCT ($N = 299$) suggested that low-dose corticosteroids in septic patients with early acute respiratory distress syndrome were linked with lower mortality rates than when they were given to patients without early acute respiratory distress syndrome (Annane et al., 2006).

(MR) A meta-analysis of available clinical trials suggested that the use of low-dose corticosteroids for patients with known adrenal insufficiency or for patients with septic shock may improve outcomes (Luce, 2004).

(MR) A meta-analysis of RCTs of sepsis between 1988 and 2003 that examined the effect of corticosteroids in patients with sepsis suggested that a short course of hydrocortisone with subsequent tapering may result in improved outcomes (Minneci et al., 2004).

(MR) A Cochrane systematic review found that corticosteroids did not change the 28-day mortality and hospital mortality rates of patients with severe sepsis and septic shock (Annane et al., 2004).

■ *For patients with severe sepsis with signs of organ dysfunction, consider administering recombinant activated protein C (drotrecogin alpha, activated) as ordered.* **LOE = II**

(MR) In a randomized, double blind, placebo-controlled, multicenter, international study ($N = 1690$ subjects in 11 countries), it was determined that the use of activated protein C for patients with infection and evidence of organ dysfunction in at least one organ significantly reduced 28-day mortality. This study was originally intended to include 2280 subjects, but it was halted prematurely when interim analysis demonstrated reduced mortality rates as compared with the placebo group (Bernard et al., 2001).

(MR) In a double-blind, placebo-controlled trial of patients diagnosed with severe sepsis ($N = 2613$), it was suggested that recombinant activated protein C was not appropriate for patients with severe sepsis and evidence of dysfunction of only one organ or for those who were at low risk of death (Abraham et al., 2005).

(EO) Experts from 11 countries reviewed all available data to create recommendations for the management of sepsis according to the International Sepsis Forum. They concluded that patients who were at high risk of death related to sepsis and organ dysfunction and who had no absolute risk of bleeding could benefit from the administration of activated protein C (Fourrier, 2004).

■ *Promote adequate nutritional intake as ordered and appropriate.* **LOE = I**

(MR) A meta-analysis of studies addressing enteral feedings ($N = 1557$ subjects totally) suggested that enteral feedings incorporating immunomodulating nutrients such as arginine, nucleotides, and omega-3 fatty acids reduced hospital lengths of stay but did not affect the overall mortality rates of study participants (Beale et al., 1999).

(EO) Enteral nutrition, which includes nutrients such as arginine that are designed to enhance the patient's immune system, do result in a reduction in the overall incidence of infection and multiple organ failure (O'Callaghan & Beale, 2003).

(EO) The appropriate use of enteral nutrition, which may include arginine, glutamine, omega-3 fatty acids, and nucleotides, may be of benefit for reducing the risk of infection and for improving outcomes (Martindale & Cresci, 2005).

Not Effective

No applicable published research was found in this category.

Possibly Harmful

No applicable published research was found in this category.

OUTCOME MEASUREMENT

INFECTION SEVERITY (NOC)

Definition: Severity of infection and associated symptoms.
Infection Severity as evidenced by the following selected NOC indicators:
- Purulent drainage
- Purulent sputum
- Pyuria
- Fever
- Hypothermia
- Chilling
- Unexplained cognitive impairment
- Blood culture colonization
- White blood count elevation
- White blood count depression
- Chest x-ray infiltration

(Rate each indicator of **Infection Severity:** 1 = severe, 2 = substantial, 3 = moderate, 4 = mild, 5 = none) (Moorhead et al., 2004).

REFERENCES

Abate NL, Trzeciak SW, Parrillo JE, Dellinger RP, et al. (2006). Heterogeneity of tissue perfusion in septic shock is a function of microcirculatory flow velocity. *Acad Emerg Med*, 13(5):S151-S153.

NR = Nursing Research, **MR** = Multidisciplinary Research, **SP** = Standard of Practice, **EO** = Expert Opinion, **LOE** = Level of Evidence

Abraham E, Laterre PF, Garg R, Levy H, Talwar D, Trzaskoma BL, et al. (2005). Drotrecogin alfa (activated) for adults with severe sepsis and a low risk of death. *N Engl J Med,* 353(13):1332-1344.

Aird WC. (2003). The hematologic system as a marker of organ dysfunction in sepsis. *Mayo Clin Proc,* 78(7):869-881.

Annane D, Bellissant E, Bollaert PE, Briegel J, Keh D, Kupfer Y. (2004). Corticosteroids for treating severe sepsis and septic shock. *Cochrane Database Syst Rev,* (1):CD002243.

Annane D, Sebille V, Bellissant E; Ger-Inf-05 Study Group. (2006). Effect of low doses of corticosteroids in septic shock patients with or without early acute respiratory distress syndrome. *Crit Care Med,* 34(1):22-30.

Beale RJ, Bryg DJ, Bihari DJ. (1999). Immunonutrition in the critically ill: a systematic review of clinical outcomes. *Crit Care Med,* 27(12):2799-2805.

Beale RJ, Hollenberg SM, Vincent JL, Parrillo JE. (2004). Vasopressor and inotropic support in septic shock: An evidence-based review. *Crit Care Med,* 32(11 Suppl):S455-S465.

Beigel J, Eichacker P. (2003). Hydrocortisone and fludrocortisone improved 28-day survival in septic shock and adrenal insufficiency. *ACP J Club,* 138(2):44.

Bernard GR, Vincent JL, Laterre PF, LaRosa SP, Dhainaut JF, Lopez-Rodriguez A, et al. (2001). Efficacy and safety of recombinant human activated protein C for severe sepsis. *N Engl J Med,* 344(10):699-709.

Bochud PY, Bonten M, Marchetti O, Calandra T. (2004). Antimicrobial therapy for patients with severe sepsis and septic shock: An evidence-based review. *Crit Care Med,* 32(11 Suppl):S495-S512.

Bridges EJ, Dukes S. (2005). Cardiovascular aspects of septic shock: Pathophysiology, monitoring, and treatment. *Crit Care Nurse,* 25(2):14-16, 18-20, 22-24 passim.

Cariou A, Vinsonneau C, Dhainaut JF. (2004). Adjunctive therapies in sepsis: An evidence-based review. *Crit Care Med,* 32(11 Suppl):S562-S570.

Cohen J, Brun-Buisson C, Torres A, Jorgensen J. (2004). Diagnosis of infection in sepsis: An evidenced-based review. *Crit Care Med,* 32(11 Suppl):S466-S494.

Dellinger RP, Carlet JM, Masur H, Gerlach H, Calandra T, Cohen J, et al. (2004). Surviving sepsis campaign guidelines for management of severe sepsis and septic shock. *Crit Care Med,* 32(3):858-873.

Dettenmeier P, Swindell B, Stroud M, Arkins N, Howard A. (2003). Role of activated protein C in the pathophysiology of severe sepsis. *Am J Crit Care,* 121(6):518-524.

Ely EW, Kleinpell RM, Goyette RE. (2003). Advances in the understanding of clinical manifestations and therapy of severe sepsis: An update for critical care nurses. *Am J Crit Care,* 12(2):120-133.

Fourrier F. (2004). Recombinant human activated protein C in the treatment of sepsis: An evidence-based review. *Crit Care Med,* 32(11 Suppl):S534-S541.

Kasper DL, Braunwald E, Fauci AS, Hauser SL, Longo DL, Jameson JL, et al. (2005). *Harrison's principles of internal medicine,* 16th ed. New York: McGraw Hill.

Keh D, Boehnke T, Weber-Cartens S, Schulz C, Ahlers O, Bercker S, et al. (2003). Immunologic and hemodynamic effects of "low-dose" hydrocortisone in septic shock: a double-blind, randomized, placebo-controlled, crossover study. *Am J Respir Crit Care Med,* 167(4):512-520.

Kleinpell RM. (2003). Advances in treating patients with severe sepsis: Role of drotrecogin alfa (activated). *Crit Care Nurse,* 23(3):16-24, 26-29, 67-68.

Kleinpell RM. (2004). Working out the complexities of sepsis. *Nurs Manage,* 35(5):48A-53A.

LeDoux D, Astiz ME, Carpati CM, Rackow EC. (2000). Effects of perfusion pressure on tissue perfusion in septic shock. *Crit Care Med,* 28(8):2729-2732.

Luce JM. (2004). Physicians should administer low-dose corticosteroids selective to septic patients until an ongoing trial is completed. *Ann Intern Med,* 141(1):70-74.

MacIntyre NR. (2001). Diagnosis and management of sepsis. In Balk RA (Ed). *Advances in the diagnosis and management of the patient with severe sepsis.* London: The Royal Society of Medicine Press, pp 17-38.

Martin GS. (2005). An update on septic shock. Highlights of the 35th Critical Care Congress. Available online: www.medscape.com. Retrieved on July 7, 2007.

Martindale RG, Cresci G. (2005). Preventing infectious complications with nutrition intervention. *J Parenter Enteral Nutr,* 29(1 Suppl):S53-S56.

Minneci PC, Deans KJ, Banks SM, Eichacker PQ, Natanson C. (2004). Meta-analysis: The effect of steroids on survival and shock during sepsis depends on the dose. *Ann Intern Med,* 141(1):47-57.

RCT = Randomized Controlled (Clinical) Trial, **NIC** = Nursing Interventions Classification, **NOC** = Nursing Outcomes Classification

Moorhead M, Johnson M, Maas M (Eds). (2004). *Nursing Outcomes Classification (NOC)*, 3rd ed. St Louis: Mosby.

Nasraway SA Jr. (2006). Hyperglycemia during critical illness. *J Parenter Enteral Nutr*, 30(3):254-258.

Nguyen HB, Rivers EP, Knoblich BP, Jacobsen G, Muzzin A, Ressler JA, et al. (2004). Early lactate clearance is associated with improved outcome in severe sepsis and septic shock. *Crit Care Med*, 32(8):1637-1642.

O'Callaghan G, Beale RJ. (2003). The role of immune-enhancing diets in the management of perioperative patients. *Crit Care Resusc*, 5(4):277-283.

Rivers EP, McIntyre L, Morro DC, Rivers KK. (2005). Early and innovative interventions for severe sepsis and septic shock: Taking advantage of a window of opportunity. *CMAJ*, 173(9):1054-1065.

Rivers E, Nguyen B, Haystad S, Ressler J, Muzzin A, Knoblich B, et al. (2001). Early goal-directed therapy in the treatment of severe sepsis and septic shock. *N Engl J Med*, 345(19):1368-1377.

Robson W, Newell J. (2005). Assessing, treating and managing patients with sepsis. *Nurs Stand*, 19(50): 56-64.

Sakr Y, Reinhart K, Vincent JL, Sprung CL, Moreno R, Ranieri VM, et al. (2006). Does dopamine administration in shock influence outcome? Results of the Sepsis Occurrence in Acutely Ill Patients (SOAP) Study. *Crit Care Med*, 34(3):589-597.

Shorr AF. (2005). Current controversies in sepsis. Proceedings from the Society of Critical Care Medicine 35th Critical Care Congress. Available online: www.medscape.com. Retrieved on July 7, 2007.

Van den Berghe G, Wouters PJ, Kesteloot K, Hilleman DE. (2006). Analysis of healthcare resource utilization with intensive insulin therapy in critically ill patients. *Crit Care Med*, 34(3):612-616.

Van den Berghe G, Wouters P, Weekers F, Verwaest C, Bruyninckx F, Schetz M, et al. (2001). Intensive insulin therapy in the critically ill patients. *N Engl J Med*, 345(19):1359-1367.

Vincent JL, Abraham E. (2006). The last 100 years of sepsis. *Am J Respir Crit Care Med*, 173(3):256-264.

Vincent JL, Gerlach H. (2004). Fluid resuscitation in severe sepsis and septic shock: An evidence-based review. *Crit Care Med*, 32(11 Suppl):S451-S454.

Zeeleder S, Hack CE, Wuillemin WA. (2005). Disseminated intravascular coagulation in sepsis. *Chest*, 128(4):2864-2876.

 # SEXUAL COUNSELING

Elaine E. Steinke, PhD, ARNP

NIC **Definition:** Use of an interactive helping process focusing on the need to make adjustments in sexual practice or to enhance coping with a sexual event/disorder (Dochterman & Bulechek, 2004).

NURSING ACTIVITIES

Effective

■ **NIC** *Discuss the patient's knowledge about sexuality in general.* **LOE = V**

MR A descriptive survey of women (*N* = 48) and men (*N* = 188) with known coronary disease revealed that most patients believed that the cardiologist should discuss sexual functioning and that few patients felt adequately informed (Bedell et al., 2002).

MR A descriptive study of 657 community-residing women 50 years old and older demonstrated that sexual participation was positively correlated with life satisfaction, health, self-esteem, liberal sexual attitudes, intimacy, and sexual knowledge but negatively correlated with age (Johnson, 1998).

(MR) A descriptive study of older men ($N = 1202$) showed that age was consistently related to erectile dysfunction (ED) and decreased sexual activity, although a number of older men continued to be sexually active, and health status and perceived partner responsiveness to sexual activity moderated the effect of age (Bortz et al., 1999).

(MR) A systematic review of the effect of age and gender on sexual function in the general population revealed that, for men, a decline in sexual activity with age was related to health and medications, whereas for women it was related to partner limitations. Decreased sexual interest was more related to age for men than for women (Avis, 2000).

■ (NIC) *Encourage the patient to verbalize fears and to ask questions.* **LOE = III**

(MR) A descriptive study of sexual adjustment with regard to myocardial infarction (MI) patients and their partners ($N = 63$) revealed that patients' psychological distress uniquely explained 24% of the variance in decreased sexual activity (Rosal et al., 1994).

(MR) A controlled study ($N = 41$) testing a 12-week exercise program on the quality of life of people with MI, coronary artery bypass surgery, or coronary angioplasty revealed satisfaction with sexual relationships and significant reductions in anxiety and depression (Trzcieniecka-Green & Steptoe, 1994).

(MR) A descriptive study of cardiac patients ($N = 858$) revealed that few reported sexual activity during the 24 hours before MI and that risk with sexual activity was not greater among those with prior angina or MI (Muller et al., 1996).

(MR) A systematic review of sexual activity and cardiac risk showed that, although myocardial oxygen demand and sympathetic nervous system activation with sexual intercourse could result in myocardial ischemia in the presence of coronary artery disease, total body oxygen consumption increased modestly and briefly, thus making MI with sexual activity less likely and rare during the 2 hours before MI (<1%; Cheitlin, 2005).

(NR) A descriptive study of the informational needs of those with coronary artery bypass grafts ($N = 432$) or coronary angioplasty ($N = 183$) found that psychosocial function was the most powerful predictor of information needs at 6 months and 1 year, including the need for sexual information (Kattainen et al., 2004).

■ (NIC) *Provide information about sexual functioning as appropriate.* **LOE = II**

(NR) An RCT of MI patients ($N = 115$) who were evaluated for 5 months tested the effects of an educational videotape on the return to sexual activity and revealed improved knowledge at 1 month after the MI for participants in the experimental group (Steinke & Swan, 2004).

(NR) An RCT of female MI patients ($N = 122$) tested a discharge instructional program, and the results demonstrated that the intervention group had fewer symptoms and concerns with sexual activity (Varvaro, 2000).

(MR) An RCT of MI patients ($N = 50$) matched with controls tested a sexual counseling intervention, and the results demonstrated that the intervention group had improved sexual function and less fear about resuming sexual activity (Dhabuwala et al., 1986).

(NR) A descriptive study of heart failure patients ($N = 62$) revealed a significant positive correlation between the 6-minute walk test and patient levels of sexual function (Jaarsma et al., 1996).

(NR) A descriptive survey of 82 patients with an implantable cardioverter defibrillator and 47 partners showed that less than one third of patients received information about resuming

RCT = Randomized Controlled (Clinical) Trial, **NIC** = Nursing Interventions Classification, **NOC** = Nursing Outcomes Classification

sexual activity, safe levels of activity, problems to report, and what to do if a device shock occurred. In addition, few reported a discussion of fears related to the implantable cardioverter defibrillator and sex (Steinke, 2003).

Additional research: Jaarsma, 2002; Foley et al., 2001

◼ NIC *Discuss necessary modifications in sexual activity, as appropriate.* LOE = I

MR A systematic review reported that in a case-crossover analysis of cardiac risk and sexual activity among MI patients ($N = 1663$), regular physical activity may have a protective effect and that it may eliminate any increased risk of coronary events with sexual activity (Muller, 2000).

EO Joint guidelines from the American College of Cardiology and the American Heart Association state that sexual activity can be resumed a week to 10 days after an uncomplicated MI (i.e., the patient did not experience hypotension, serious dysrhythmia, heart failure, or cardiopulmonary resuscitation; Antman et al., 2004).

NR A descriptive study of MI patients who were sexually active within the last year ($N = 462$ men, $N = 51$ women) demonstrated that sexual activity was resumed within 3 to 6 months after a first MI by 72% of women and 89% of men (Drory et al., 2000).

MR In a systematic review, recent research suggested that ED may be an early marker of atherosclerosis and a precursor of systemic vascular disease, thus making assessment for ED an important component of practice (Billups, 2005).

NR A descriptive study of 258 HIV-seropositive women and 228 HIV-seronegative women revealed condom use by 68% of sexually active women; 65% of these users reported consistent use, with those women with HIV being more likely to report condom use (Wilson et al., 2003).

◼ NIC *Discuss the effect of the illness/health situation on sexuality.* LOE = I

MR A descriptive study of first-time MI patients ($N = 143$) revealed that those who associated a large number of symptoms with their illness were more likely to have later sexual dysfunction (Petrie et al., 1996).

NR A descriptive study of patients with advanced heart failure ($N = 62$) revealed that most had a marked loss of interest in sexual activity, a decreased level of sexual activity, and an inability to perform sexually (Jaarsma et al., 1996).

MR A descriptive study of patients with chronic obstructive pulmonary disease ($N = 53$) found that, although almost half of these patients had no comorbid disease for ED, three fourths of them had ED of varying degrees, and severity was correlated with the physical restrictions and severity of the chronic obstructive pulmonary disease (Koseoglu et al., 2005).

MR A meta-analysis of 36 studies conducted between 1975 and 2000 and that included 2786 cases of testicular cancer revealed that ejaculatory dysfunction occurred most frequently and was related to retroperitoneal surgery and that ED was less frequent and related to irradiation (Jonker-Pool et al., 2001).

MR A meta-analysis of six controlled studies ($N = 709$) and seven uncontrolled studies ($N = 337$) demonstrated significantly reduced or absent orgasm, ED, and ejaculatory dysfunction in patients for up to 2 years after treatment for testicular cancer (Nazareth et al., 2001).

NR = Nursing Research, **MR** = Multidisciplinary Research, **SP** = Standard of Practice, **EO** = Expert Opinion, **LOE** = Level of Evidence

Additional research: Greendale et al., 2001; Lallemand et al., 2002; Kimmo et al., 1998; Borello-France et al., 2004; Koch et al., 2002.

■ **NIC** *Discuss the effect of medication on sexuality as appropriate.* **LOE = I**

MR A descriptive study of MI patients and partners ($N = 63$), sexual adjustment, and the use of beta blockers revealed that beta blockers used alone or in combination with other medication classes was not a significant predictor of changes in sexual behavior patterns after MI (Rosal et al., 1994).

MR An RCT of sexual function in hypertensive patients ($N = 902$) between the ages of 45 and 69 years demonstrated an incidence of ED of 9.5% at 24 months and of 14.7% at 48 months that was related to the type of therapy, with greater erectile problems through 24 months for those taking chlorthalidone (Grimm et al., 1997).

MR A controlled study of 96 males with newly diagnosed cardiovascular disease and no prior ED showed that knowledge of the side effects of beta blockers increased the incidence of ED (Silvestri et al., 2003).

MR A systematic review of the safety of phosphodiesterase 5 inhibitors showed that, although their use was contraindicated for those patients taking nitrates, improved exercise tolerance and coronary dilatation in patients taking phosphodiesterase 5 inhibitors were positive outcomes. The safety profile of the drugs was excellent (Carson, 2005).

MR An RCT of postmenopausal women ($N = 120$) taking valsartan revealed positive improvements in sexual desire, changes in sexual behavior, and sexual fantasies (Fogari et al., 2004).

Possibly Effective

■ **NIC** *Include the spouse/sexual partner in the counseling as much as possible as appropriate.* **LOE = III**

NR A descriptive study of cardiac patients and their partners ($N = 55$) demonstrated that the need to receive specific information about sexual activity was not met for 46% of patients and 49% of partners (Moser et al., 1993).

NR A descriptive study of patients with heart failure and their partners ($N = 63$) showed significant concerns regarding sexual frequency and decline in sexual interest (Westlake et al., 1999).

NR A qualitative study of patients with MI and their partners ($N = 14$) revealed fear of death, inability to function during sexual activity, and inadequate and conflicting information about resuming sexual relations and medications (Stewart et al., 2000).

NR A descriptive study of 26 partners of coronary artery bypass graft patients revealed a low level of satisfaction with the sexual relationship (58%; although only 8% stated that this was a change since before the surgery) and a low level of satisfaction (54%) with the frequency of sexual activity after surgery (Stanley & Frantz, 1988).

MR A controlled study of couples ($N = 84$) after treatment for prostate carcinoma and randomized to counseling sessions showed improved overall male distress, male and female global sexual function at 3 months, and sexual function similar to pretreatment levels at 6 months, although increased use of ED treatments was noted (Canada et al., 2005).

RCT = Randomized Controlled (Clinical) Trial, **NIC** = Nursing Interventions Classification, **NOC** = Nursing Outcomes Classification

■ **NIC** *Provide referral/consultation with other members of the health care team as appropriate.* **LOE = V**

NR A descriptive pilot study of nurses' (*N* = 35) beliefs about sexual counseling revealed that barriers to including sexual assessment and counseling in practice included patient expectations of nurses, time availability, and confidence in one's ability to address sexual issues (Reynolds & Magnan, 2005).

NR A descriptive study of nurses (*N* = 155) demonstrated that, although sexuality was viewed as an important part of practice, few nurses addressed sexual concerns with patients (Matocha & Waterhouse, 1993).

NR A descriptive study of oncology nurses (*N* = 937) revealed that the majority believed that sexual counseling was an important part of routine practice and that most nurses were more comfortable discussing sexual issues if the patient initiated the discussion (Wilson & Williams, 1988).

NR A descriptive study of cardiac nurses (*N* = 171) demonstrated that nurses were somewhat comfortable with and responsible for addressing sexual concerns with MI patients; however, few addressed sexual concerns in practice (Steinke & Patterson-Midgley, 1996).

NR A descriptive study of MI patients (*N* = 91) who were evaluated for 6 months using 14 rated items addressing sexual concerns and areas of sexual counseling demonstrated the importance of sexual counseling and addressing patient concerns (Steinke & Patterson-Midgley, 1998).

Not Effective

No applicable published research was found in this category.

Possibly Harmful

No applicable published research was found in this category.

OUTCOME MEASUREMENT

SEXUAL FUNCTIONING NOC

(Please refer to *Nursing Outcomes Classification* [Moorhead et al., 2004] for the **Sexual Functioning** outcome.)

REFERENCES

Antman EM, Anbe DT, Armstrong PW, Bates ER, Green LA, Hand M, et al. (2004). ACC/AHA guidelines for the management of patients with ST-elevation myocardial infarction: A report of the American College of Cardiology/American Heart Association Task Force on Practice Guidelines (Committee to Revise the 1999 Guidelines for the Management of Patients with Acute Myocardial Infarction). *J Am Coll Cardiol*, 44(3):E1-E211.

Avis NE. (2000). Sexual function and aging in men and women: Community and population-based studies. *J Gend Specif Med*, 3(2):37-41.

Bedell SE, Duperval M, Goldberg R. (2002). Cardiologists' discussions about sexuality with patients with chronic coronary heart disease. *Am Heart J*, 144(2):239-242.

Billups KL. (2005). Sexual dysfunction and cardiovascular disease: Integrative concepts and strategies. *Am J Cardiol*, 96(12B):57M-61M.

Borello-France D, Leng W, O'Leary M, Xavier M, Erickson J, Chancellor MB, et al. (2004). Bladder and sexual function among women with multiple sclerosis. *Mult Scler,* 10(4):455-461.

Bortz WM, II, Wallace DH, Wiley D. (1999). Sexual function in 1,202 aging males: Differentiating aspects. *J Gerontol A Biol Sci Med Sci,* 54(5):M237-M241.

Canada AL, Neese LE, Sui D, Schover LR. (2005). Pilot intervention to enhance sexual rehabilitation for couples after treatment for localized prostate carcinoma. *Cancer,* 104(12):2689-2700.

Carson CC, III. (2005). Cardiac safety in clinical trials of phosphodiesterase 5 inhibitors. *Am J Cardiol,* 96(12B):37M-41M.

Cheitlin MD. (2005). Sexual activity and cardiac risk. *Am J Cardiol,* 96(12B):24M-28M.

Dhabuwala CB, Kumar A, Pierce JM. (1986). Myocardial infarction and its influence on male sexual function. *Arch Sex Behav,* 15(6):499-504.

Dochterman JM, Bulechek GM (Eds). (2004). *Nursing Interventions Classification (NIC),* 4th ed. St Louis: Mosby.

Drory Y, Kravetz S, Weingarten M. (2000). Comparison of sexual activity of women and men after a first acute myocardial infarction. *Am J Cardiol,* 85(11):1283-1287.

Fogari R, Preti P, Zoppi A, Corradi L, Pasotti C, Rinaldi A, et al. (2004). Effect of valsartan and atenolol on sexual behavior in hypertensive postmenopausal women. *Am J Hypertens,* 17(1):77-81.

Foley FW, LaRocca NG, Sanders AS, Zemon V. (2001). Rehabilitation of intimacy and sexual dysfunction in couples with multiple sclerosis. *Mult Scler,* 7(6):417-421.

Greendale GA, Petersen L, Zibecchi L, Ganz PA. (2001). Factors related to sexual function in postmenopausal women with a history of breast cancer. *Menopause,* 8(2):111-119.

Grimm RH Jr, Grandits GA, Prineas RJ, McDonald RH, Lewis CE, Flack JM, et al. (1997). Long-term effects on sexual function of five antihypertensive drugs and nutritional hygienic treatment in hypertensive men and women. Treatment of Mild Hypertension Study (TOMHS). *Hypertension,* 29(1 Pt 1): 8-14.

Jaarsma T. (2002). Sexual problems in heart failure patients. *Eur J Cardiovasc Nurs,* 1(1):61-67.

Jaarsma T, Dracup K, Walden J, Stevenson LW. (1996). Sexual function in patients with advanced heart failure. *Heart Lung,* 25(4):262-270.

Johnson BK. (1998). A correlational framework for understanding sexuality in women age 50 and older. *Health Care Women Int,* 19(6):553-564.

Jonker-Pool G, Van de Wiel HB, Hoekstra HJ, Sleijfer DT, Van Driel MF, Van Basten J, et al. (2001). Sexual functioning after treatment for testicular cancer—review and meta-analysis of 36 empirical studies between 1975-2000. *Arch Sex Behav,* 30(1):55-74.

Kattainen E, Merilainen P, Jokela V. (2004). CABG and PTCA patients' expectations of informational support in health-related quality of life themes and adequacy of information in 1-year follow-up. *Eur J Cardiovasc Nurs,* 3(2):149-163.

Kimmo T, Jyrki V, Sirpa AS. (1998). Health status after recovery from burn injury. *Burns,* 24(4):293-298.

Koch T, Kralik D, Eastwood S. (2002). Constructions of sexuality for women living with multiple sclerosis. *J Adv Nurs,* 39(2):137-145.

Koseoglu N, Koseoglu H, Ceylan E, Cimrin HA, Ozalevli S, Esen A. (2005). Erectile dysfunction prevalence and sexual function status in patients with chronic obstructive pulmonary disease. *J Urol,* 174(1):249-252.

Lallemand F, Salhi Y, Linard F, Giami A, Rozenbaum W. (2002). Sexual dysfunction in 156 ambulatory HIV-infected men receiving highly active retroviral therapy combinations with and without protease inhibitors. *J Acquir Immune Defic Syndr,* 30(2):187-190.

Matocha LK, Waterhouse JK. (1993). Current nursing practice related to sexuality. *Res Nurs Health,* 16(5):371-378.

Moorhead M, Johnson M, Maas M (Eds). (2004). *Nursing Outcomes Classification (NOC),* 3rd ed. St Louis: Mosby.

Moser DK, Dracup KA, Marsden C. (1993). Needs of recovering cardiac patients and their spouses: Compared views. *Int J Nurs Stud,* 30(2):105-114.

Muller JE. (2000). Triggering of cardiac events by sexual activity: Findings from a case-crossover analysis. *Am J Cardiol,* 86(2A):14F-18F.

Muller JE, Mittleman MA, Maclure M, Sherwood JB, Tofler GH. (1996). Triggering myocardial infarction by sexual activity. Low absolute risk and prevention by regular physical exertion. Determinants of Myocardial Infarction Onset Study Investigators. *JAMA,* 275(18):1405-1409.

RCT = Randomized Controlled (Clinical) Trial, **NIC** = Nursing Interventions Classification, **NOC** = Nursing Outcomes Classification

Nazareth I, Lewin J, King M. (2001). Sexual dysfunction after treatment for testicular cancer: A systematic review. *J Psychosom Res,* 51(6):735-743.

Petrie KJ, Weinman J, Sharpe N, Buckley J. (1996). Role of patients' view of their illness in predicting return to work and functioning after myocardial infarction: Longitudinal study. *BMJ,* 312(7040):1191-1194.

Reynolds KE, Magnan MA. (2005). Nursing attitudes and beliefs toward human sexuality: Collaborative research promoting evidence-based practice. *Clin Nurse Spec,* 19(5):255-259.

Rosal MC, Downing J, Littman AB, Ahern DK. (1994). Sexual functioning post-myocardial infarction: Effects of beta-blockers, psychological status and safety information. *J Psychosom Res,* 38(7):655-667.

Silvestri A, Galetta P, Cerquetani E, Marazzi G, Patrizi R, Fini M, et al. (2003). Report of erectile dysfunction after therapy with beta-blockers is related to patient knowledge of side effects and is reversed by placebo. *Eur Heart J,* 24(21):1928-1932.

Stanley MJ, Frantz RA. (1988). Adjustment problems of spouses of patients undergoing coronary artery bypass graft surgery during early convalescence. *Heart Lung,* 17(6 Pt 1):677-682.

Steinke EE. (2003). Sexual concerns of patients and partners after an implantable cardioverter defibrillator. *Dimens Crit Care Nurs,* 22(2):89-96.

Steinke EE, Patterson-Midgley P. (1996). Sexual counseling of MI patients: Nurses' comfort, responsibility, and practice. *Dimens Crit Care Nurs,* 15(4):216-223.

Steinke EE, Patterson-Midgley P. (1998). Importance and timing of sexual counseling after myocardial infarction. *J Cardiopulm Rehabil,* 18(6):401-407.

Steinke EE, Swan JH. (2004). Effectiveness of a videotape for sexual counseling after myocardial infarction. *Res Nurs Health,* 27(4):269-280.

Stewart M, Davidson K, Meade D, Hirth A, Makrides L. (2000). Myocardial infarction: Survivors' and spouses' stress, coping, and support. *J Adv Nurs,* 31(6):1351-1360.

Trzcieniecka-Green A, Steptoe A. (1994). Stress management in cardiac patients: A preliminary study of the predictors of improvement in quality of life. *J Psychosom Res,* 38(4):267-280.

Varvaro FF. (2000). Family role and work adaptation in MI women. *Clin Nurs Res,* 9(3):339-351.

Westlake C, Dracup K, Walden JA, Fonarow G. (1999). Sexuality of patients with advanced heart failure and their spouses or partners. *J Heart Lung Transplant,* 18(11):1133-1138.

Wilson ME, Williams HA. (1988). Oncology nurses' attitude and behaviors related to sexuality of patients with cancer. *Oncol Nurs Forum,* 15(1):49-53.

Wilson TE, Koenig L, Ickovics J, Walter E, Suss A, Fernandez MI, et al. (2003). Contraception use, family planning, and unprotected sex: Few differences among HIV-infected and uninfected postpartum women in four US states. *J Acquir Immune Defic Syndr,* 33(5):608-613.

 # SHOCK MANAGEMENT

Ruth M. Kleinpell, PhD, RN, FAAN, FAANP, FCCM; Thomas Ahrens, DNSc, RN, FAAN

> **NIC** **Definition:** Facilitation of the delivery of oxygen and nutrients to systemic tissue with removal of cellular waste products in a patient with severely altered tissue perfusion (Dochterman & Bulechek, 2004).

NURSING ACTIVITIES

Effective

■ *Perform initial resuscitation for hypotension (systolic blood pressure <90 mm Hg for >30 minutes) despite fluid administration (e.g., crystalloid intravenous fluids*

NR = Nursing Research, **MR** = Multidisciplinary Research, **SP** = Standard of Practice, **EO** = Expert Opinion, **LOE** = Level of Evidence

[0.9% normal saline or lactated Ringer's solution]). During the first 6 hours of resuscitation, the goals of resuscitation should include all of the following as one part of a treatment protocol:

- *Central venous pressure: 8 to 12 mm Hg*
- *Mean arterial pressure: ≥65 mm Hg*
- *Urine output: ≥0.5 mL/kg/hour*
- *Central venous or mixed venous oxygen saturation: ≥70%* **LOE = II**

(MR) A randomized, controlled, single-center study of patients in shock (*N* = 236) demonstrated that early goal-directed therapy with resuscitation of patients with shock directed toward increasing perfusion during the initial 6 hours of resuscitation significantly reduced 28-day mortality (Rivers et al., 2001).

■ *Provide adequate oxygenation and ventilation; anticipate the need for intubation and for the use of a ventilator.* **LOE = I**

(MR) One of the primary management goals for the patient in shock is to ensure adequate oxygenation and ventilation. Several multiple-center RCTs and evidence-based recommendations from a systematic literature review identified that low tidal volume ventilation (6 mL per kg of predicted body weight) in conjunction with maintaining end inspiratory plateau pressures of <30 cm water should be used for the mechanical ventilation of patients with sepsis-induced acute lung injury (Dellinger et al., 2004).

■ *Use rapidly initiated antibiotic therapy for the treatment of sepsis and septic shock.* **LOE = I**

(MR) Recommendations from a systematic literature review identified that intravenous antibiotic therapy should be started within the first hour after the recognition of severe sepsis and septic shock, after appropriate cultures have been obtained (Dellinger et al., 2004).

■ *Find the source of infection that has resulted in sepsis and septic shock.* **LOE = I**

(MR) Recommendations from a systematic literature review identified that every patient with severe sepsis should be evaluated for the presence of a focus of infection that may be amenable to source control measures such as the drainage of an abscess, the debridement of infected necrotic tissue, or the removal of a potentially infected device (Dellinger et al., 2004).

■ *If the hemoglobin level is less than 7 g/dL, administer blood products as ordered.* **LOE = I**

(MR) Recommendations from a systematic literature review outlined that red blood cell transfusion should occur in patients with sepsis and septic shock when the hemoglobin level decreased to <7.0 g/dL to reach a target hemoglobin level of 7.0 to 9.0 g/dL (Dellinger et al., 2004).

■ *Use recombinant human activated protein C for patients with severe sepsis and septic shock as ordered.* **LOE = II**

(MR) An RCT of 1690 patients with severe sepsis demonstrated significant decreases in mortality with the use of recombinant activated protein C, which is an endogenous anticoagulant with antiinflammatory properties (Bernard et al., 2001).

RCT = Randomized Controlled (Clinical) Trial, **NIC** = Nursing Interventions Classification, **NOC** = Nursing Outcomes Classification

■ *Prevent complications of critical illness, including renal failure and stress ulcers.*
LOE = I

(MR) Recommendations from a systematic literature review identified that several measures were effective for reducing the complications associated with shock and critical illness. These included glucose control to maintain a blood glucose level of <150 mg/dL, renal replacement therapy for acute renal failure, deep vein thrombosis prophylaxis, and stress ulcer prophylaxis (Dellinger et al., 2004).

Use measures to prevent the formation of deep vein thrombosis. (Refer to the guideline Deep Vein Thrombosis: Prevention.)

■ *Maintain the blood sugar level at ≤150 mg/dL as ordered and appropriate.*
LOE = I

(MR) A systematic review of the literature by critical care experts from 11 international organizations determined that the maintenance of the glucose level at ≤150 was associated with improved outcomes (Cariou et al., 2004).

(MR) An RCT comparing patients whose blood sugars were kept between 80 and 110 mg/dL (*N* = 1548 mechanically ventilated patients) with patients who did not receive antihyperglycemic therapy until their glucose levels were >250 mg/dL suggested that tight glycemic control in critically ill patients who were being treated with mechanical ventilators resulted in improved outcomes as compared with patients whose blood sugars were maintained at the standard level of <250 mg/dL (van den Berghe et al., 2006).

(MR) In a prospective RCT (*N* = 1548 patients), participants were randomized either to receive insulin to maintain glucose levels of ≤110 mg/dL or to receive insulin only for glucose levels of ≥215 mg/dL to maintain glucose levels overall between 180 and 200 mg/dL. Patients with glucose levels that were maintained below 110 mg/dL had decreased morbidity and mortality as compared with patients in the group whose blood sugars remained between 180 and 210 mg/dL (van den Berghe et al., 2001).

(MR) A meta-analysis of research pertaining to blood glucose levels in critically ill patients suggested that tight glycemic control through the use of insulin reduced inflammation and improved outcomes in critically ill medical and surgical patients (Nasraway, 2006).

■ (SP) *Recognize that the early detection and identification of sepsis can promote the best outcomes.* **LOE = VII**

(EO) Important aspects of early identification include the following:
- Recognition (monitoring for vital sign changes; observing for signs of infection and the presence of systemic inflammatory response syndrome criteria)
- Monitoring for signs of organ system dysfunction (e.g., cardiovascular compromise with tachycardia and hypotension; respiratory compromise requiring mechanical ventilation; onset of acute lung injury and/or acute respiratory distress syndrome; acute renal failure with oliguria; hematologic abnormalities; skin color changes; altered neurological status)
- Providing comprehensive sepsis treatment (circulatory support with fluids, inotropes, and vasopressors; supportive treatment with oxygenation and ventilation; antibiotic administration; recombinant human activated protein C therapy; monitoring and reporting the patient's response to treatment)

NR = Nursing Research, **MR** = Multidisciplinary Research, **SP** = Standard of Practice, **EO** = Expert Opinion, **LOE** = Level of Evidence

- Promoting patient and family comfort care (promoting patient comfort by providing pain relief, sedation, turning, and skin care; providing patient and family teaching; addressing the needs of the families of critically ill patients)
- Enforcing sepsis prevention measures (i.e., handwashing, measures to prevent nosocomial infections, oral care, proper positioning, turning, skin care, invasive catheter care, wound care)

NR Several reviews have highlighted the importance of nursing assessment and monitoring for the promotion of the early identification and treatment of sepsis (Kleinpell, 2003; Ahrens & Vollman, 2003).

Possibly Effective

■ *Use vasopressors to restore blood pressure and organ perfusion when fluid resuscitation fails. The first-line treatment for the symptoms of shock is usually the administration of intravenous fluids. If this method is not successful, vasopressors such as dopamine, dobutamine, adrenaline, noradrenaline, and vasopressin are recommended. However, it is controversial which vasopressor is most effective for increasing perfusion in patients with shock.* **LOE = II**

MR A Cochrane systematic review found that there were very few RCTs of vasopressors for the treatment of shock that assessed patient-related outcomes. The available trials were not designed to investigate such outcomes; rather, they looked at surrogate measures such as blood pressure and cardiac index. The methodological quality of the trials was identified as poor. The existing trials were small, and they did not provide conclusive evidence regarding the best choice of vasopressor for the treatment of shock (Mullner et al., 2004).

MR Recommendations from systematic literature reviews identified that vasopressor agents (e.g., norepinephrine, dopamine) should be started when appropriate fluid resuscitation fails to restore adequate blood pressure and organ perfusion (Dellinger et al., 2004).

■ *Use inotropic therapy for patients with sepsis and septic shock.* **LOE = II**

MR Recommendations from a systematic literature review identified that inotropic therapy with dobutamine was indicated for patients with measured or suspected low cardiac output in the presence of adequate left ventricular filling pressure (or clinical assessment of adequate fluid resuscitation) and adequate mean arterial pressure (Dellinger et al., 2004).

Not Effective

■ *Using colloids rather than crystalloids for resuscitation.* **LOE = I**

MR Three systematic reviews demonstrated no differences between fluid resuscitation with colloid solutions and those with crystalloid solutions for critically ill patients (Schierhout & Roberts, 1998; Choi et al., 1999; Finfer et al., 2004).

■ *Using naloxone for shock.* **LOE = I**

MR A Cochrane systematic review found that naloxone improved blood pressure, especially mean arterial blood pressure. However, the clinical usefulness of naloxone to treat shock remains to be determined, and additional RCTs are needed to assess its usefulness (Boeuf et al., 2003).

RCT = Randomized Controlled (Clinical) Trial, **NIC** = Nursing Interventions Classification, **NOC** = Nursing Outcomes Classification

■ *Using steroids for shock.* **LOE = I**

(MR) A Cochrane systematic review found that corticosteroids did not change 28-day mortality and hospital mortality rates among patients with severe sepsis and septic shock (Annane et al., 2004).

Possibly Harmful

■ *Increasing oxygen delivery to supranormal levels.* **LOE = I**

(MR) A systematic review highlighted the fact that, although increasing oxygen delivery to supranormal levels with packed red blood cell transfusions or inotropic therapy would exceed the critical oxygen delivery threshold and ensure that oxygen consumption is not dependent on delivery, a number of well-controlled RCTs have failed to substantiate a mortality benefit. In addition, one study demonstrated increased mortality with this therapeutic strategy (Balk, 2004; Hayes et al., 1994).

OUTCOME MEASUREMENT

TISSUE PERFUSION: CEREBRAL   (NOC)

Definition: Adequacy of blood flow through the cerebral vasculature to maintain blood function.

Tissue Perfusion: Cerebral as evidenced by the following selected NOC indicators:

- Diastolic blood pressure
- Systolic blood pressure
- Neurological function

(Rate each indicator of **Tissue Perfusion: Cerebral:** 1 = severely compromised, 2 = substantially compromised, 3 = moderately compromised, 4 = mildly compromised, 5 = not compromised) (Moorhead et al., 2004).

(Please refer to *Nursing Outcomes Classification* [Moorhead et al., 2004] for the **Tissue Perfusion: Abdominal Organs; Tissue Perfusion: Cardiac;** and **Tissue Perfusion: Peripheral** outcomes.)

REFERENCES

Ahrens T, Vollman K. (2003). Severe sepsis management: Are we doing enough? *Crit Care Nurse,* 23(5 Suppl):2-15.

Annane D, Bellissant E, Bollaert PE, Briegel J, Keh D, Kupfer Y. (2004). Corticosteroids for treating severe sepsis and septic shock. *Cochrane Database Syst Rev,* (1):CD002243.

Balk RA. (2004). Optimum treatment of severe sepsis and septic shock: Evidence in support of the recommendations. *Dis Mon,* 50(4):168-213.

Bernard GR, Vincent JL, Laterre PF, LaRosa SP, Dhainaut JF, Lopez-Rodriguez A, et al. (2001). Efficacy and safety of recombinant human activated protein C for severe sepsis, *N Engl J Med,* 344(10): 699-709.

Boeuf B, Poirier V, Gauvin F, Guerguerian AM, Roy C, Farrell CA, et al. (2003). Naloxone for shock. *Cochrane Database Syst Rev,* (4):CD004443.

NR = Nursing Research, **MR** = Multidisciplinary Research, **SP** = Standard of Practice, **EO** = Expert Opinion, **LOE** = Level of Evidence

Cariou A, Vinsonneau C, Dhainaut JF. (2004). Adjunctive therapies in sepsis: An evidence-based review. *Crit Care Med*, 32(11 Suppl):S562-S570.

Choi PT, Yip G, Quinonez LG, Cook DJ. (1999). Crystalloids vs. colloids in fluid resuscitation: A systematic review. *Crit Care Med*, **27(1)**:200-210.

Dellinger RP, Carlet JM, Masur H, Gerlach H, Calandra T, Cohen J, et al. (2004). Surviving Sepsis Campaign guidelines for management of severe sepsis and septic shock. *Crit Care Med*, 32(3):858-873.

Dochterman JM, Bulechek GM (Eds). (2004). *Nursing Interventions Classification (NIC)*, 4th ed. St Louis: Mosby.

Finfer S, Bellomo R, Boyce N, French J, Myburgh J, Norton R, et al. (2004). A comparison of albumin and saline for fluid resuscitation in the intensive care unit. *N Engl J Med*, **350(22)**:2247-2256.

Hayes MA, Timmins AC, Yau EH, Palazzo M, Hinds CJ, Watson D. (1994). Elevation of systemic oxygen delivery in the treatment of critically ill patients. *N Eng J Med*, 330(24):1717-1722.

Kleinpell RM. (2003). The role of the critical care nurse in the assessment and management of the patient with severe sepsis. *Crit Care Nurs Clin North Am*, 15(1):27-34.

Moorhead M, Johnson M, Maas M (Eds). (2004). *Nursing Outcomes Classification (NOC)*, 3rd ed. St. Louis: Mosby.

Mullner M, Urbanek B, Havel C, Losert H, Waechter F, Gamper G. (2004). Vasopressors for shock. *Cochrane Database Syst Rev*, (3):CD003709.

Nasraway SA, Jr. (2006). Hyperglycemia during critical illness. *JPEN*, 30(3):254-258.

Rivers E, Nguyen B, Havstad S, Ressler J, Muzzin A, Knoblich B, et al. (2001). Early goal-directed therapy in the treatment of severe sepsis and septic shock. *N Engl J Med*, 345(19):1368-1377.

Schierhout G, Roberts I. (1998). Fluid resuscitation with colloid or crystalloid solutions in critically ill patients: A systematic review of randomised trials. *BMJ*, 316(7136):961-964.

van den Berghe G, Wouters PJ, Kesteloot K, Hilleman DE. (2006). Analysis of healthcare resource utilization with intensive insulin therapy in critically ill patients. *Crit Care Med*, 34(3):612-616.

van den Berghe G, Wouters P, Weekers F, Verwaest C, Bruyninckx F, Schetz M, et al. (2001). Intensive insulin therapy in the critically ill patients. *N Engl J Med*, 345(19):1359-1367.

SHOCK PREVENTION

Ruth M. Kleinpell, PhD, RN, FAAN, FAANP, FCCM; Thomas Ahrens, DNSc, RN, FAAN

NIC   **Definition:** Detecting and treating a patient at risk for impending shock (Dochterman & Bulechek, 2004).

NURSING ACTIVITIES

Effective

- **Use a rapid response team for the early detection of shock. LOE = I**

   In several prospective clinical trials, the use of rapid response teams demonstrated decreases in the incidence of in-hospital cardiac arrest, the bed occupancy of cardiac arrest survivors, and overall in-hospital mortality (Bellomo et al., 2003, 2004; Buist et al., 2002).

  Consensus guidelines regarding the use of rapid response teams recommend that hospitals implement a system that detects urgent unmet medical needs and responds to them rapidly and reliably (DeVita et al., 2006).

RCT = Randomized Controlled (Clinical) Trial, **NIC** = Nursing Interventions Classification, **NOC** = Nursing Outcomes Classification

■ **SP** *Use shock protocols to target the early identification and treatment of shock.* **LOE = IV**

MR In a historical, controlled, single-site study, the use of a hospital-wide comprehensive shock program was associated with decreased mortality rates and better outcomes (i.e., discharge to home or a rehabilitation center). The shock protocols were implemented by nurses to provide the early recognition of shock and the initiation of indicated therapies, including goal-directed resuscitation protocols (Sebat et al., 2005).

■ *Use early goal-directed therapy.* **LOE = I**

MR An RCT of emergency-department-focused resuscitation using goal-directed therapy that targeted the optimization of perfusion with the use of fluid resuscitation, the transfusion of packed red blood cells to achieve a hematocrit level of ≥30%, and/or the administration of a dobutamine infusion (up to a maximum of 20 μg/kg/min) was used to achieve perfusion goals that demonstrated significant improvements in survival (Rivers et al., 2001).

■ *Obtain appropriate cultures.* **LOE = I**

MR Recommendations from a systematic literature review identified that appropriate cultures should be obtained before the administration of antibiotics for evolving septic shock. To optimize the identification of the causative organism, at least two blood cultures are recommended, with at least one drawn percutaneously and one drawn through each vascular access line. Cultures of other sites, such as urine, wounds, and respiratory or other body fluids (as indicated) are also recommended (Dellinger et al., 2004).

■ **SP** *Control bleeding loss during hemorrhage.* **LOE = III**

EO Emergency and critical care treatment guidelines indicate that initial resuscitation requires the rapid restoration of the circulating blood volume along with interventions to control ongoing losses. The initial management of the patient with impending shock requires attention to the "ABCs" of resuscitation: maintaining an airway (A), adequate ventilation (breathing, B), and establishing an adequate blood volume to support the circulation (C). The control of hemorrhage requires immediate attention (Maier, 2005).

■ **SP** *Assess for signs of shock.* **LOE = VII**

EO Emergency and critical care treatment guidelines suggest that mild hypovolemia (≤20% of the blood volume) can result in mild tachycardia, but there are relatively few other signs. With moderate hypovolemia (20% to 40% of the blood volume), increasing tachycardia, postural hypotension, and anxiety may be seen. If hypovolemia is severe (≥40% of the blood volume), the classic signs of shock appear, with hypotension, marked tachycardia, oliguria, and agitation or confusion. The transition from mild to severe hypovolemic shock can be insidious or extremely rapid (Maier, 2005; Kolecki & Menckhoff, 2006).

EO Consensus definitions outlining sepsis and septic shock identify that the clinical signs of sepsis and septic shock include the systemic inflammatory response syndrome. Two or more of the following conditions can indicate sepsis: a temperature of >38°C or <36°C; a heart rate of >90 beats/min; a respiratory rate of >20 breaths/min or a $PaCO_2$ (partial pressure of carbon dioxide in arterial blood) of <32 mm Hg (<4.3 kPa); and a white blood cell count of >12,000 cells/mm^3, <4000 cells/mm^3, or >10% immature (band) forms. Additional signs and symp-

---

NR = Nursing Research, **MR** = Multidisciplinary Research, **SP** = Standard of Practice, **EO** = Expert Opinion, **LOE** = Level of Evidence

toms include chills, hypotension, decreased skin perfusion, decreased urine output, significant edema or positive fluid balance (>20 mL/kg over 24 hours), decreased capillary refill or mottling, hyperglycemia (plasma glucose >120 mg/dL) in the absence of diabetes, and an unexplained change in mental status (Levy et al., 2003).

Possibly Effective

- ### *Use blood substitutes.* **LOE = V**

  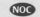 A synthesis review of hemoglobin-based oxygen carriers revealed that, despite numerous clinical trials (predominantly in animal models), there was no consensus with regard to the clinical application of blood substitutes. The critical properties of hemoglobin solutions with regard to oxygen affinity, viscosity, and oncotic pressure require further study (Winslow, 2003).

Not Effective

No applicable published research was found in this category.

Possibly Harmful

No applicable published research was found in this category.

OUTCOME MEASUREMENT

CARDIAC PUMP EFFECTIVENESS   NOC

Definition: Adequacy of blood volume ejected from the left ventricle to support systemic perfusion pressure.

Cardiac Pump Effectiveness as evidenced by the following selected NOC indicators:

- Systolic blood pressure
- Diastolic blood pressure
- Apical heart rate
- Cardiac index
- Ejection fraction
- Activity tolerance
- Peripheral pulses
- Skin color
- Urinary output
- Cognitive status
- 24-hour intake and output balance

(Rate each indicator of **Cardiac Pump Effectiveness:** 1 = severely compromised, 2 = substantially compromised, 3 = moderately compromised, 4 = mildly compromised, 5 = not compromised) (Moorhead et al., 2004).

CIRCULATION STATUS   NOC

Definition: Unobstructed, unidirectional blood flow at an appropriate pressure through large vessels of the systemic and pulmonary circuits.

Continued

RCT = Randomized Controlled (Clinical) Trial, **NIC** = Nursing Interventions Classification, **NOC** = Nursing Outcomes Classification

OUTCOME MEASUREMENT—*cont'd*

Circulation Status as evidenced by the following selected NOC indicators:
- Systolic blood pressure
- Diastolic blood pressure
- Pulse pressure
- Mean blood pressure
- Central venous pressure
- Pulmonary wedge pressure
- PaO_2 (partial pressure of oxygen in arterial blood)
- $PaCO_2$
- Oxygen saturation
- Arterial-venous oxygen difference
- Cognitive status
- Skin temperature
- Skin color
- Urinary output

(Rate each indicator of **Circulation Status:** 1 = severely compromised, 2 = substantially compromised, 3 = moderately compromised, 4 = mildly compromised, 5 = not compromised) (Moorhead et al., 2004).

TISSUE PERFUSION: CEREBRAL   NOC

Definition: Adequacy of blood flow through the cerebral vasculature to maintain brain function.

Tissue Perfusion: Cerebral as evidenced by the following selected NOC indicators:
- Diastolic blood pressure
- Systolic blood pressure
- Neurological function

(Rate each indicator of **Tissue Perfusion: Cerebral:** 1 = severely compromised, 2 = substantially compromised, 3 = moderately compromised, 4 = mildly compromised, 5 = not compromised) (Moorhead et al., 2004).

REFERENCES

Bellomo R, Goldsmith D, Uchino S, Buckmaster J, Hart GK, Opdam H, et al. (2003). A prospective before-and-after trial of a medical emergency team. *Med J Aust,* 179(6):283-287.

Bellomo R, Goldsmith D, Uchino S, Buckmaster J, Hart G, Opdam H, et al. (2004). Prospective controlled trial of effect of medical emergency team on postoperative morbidity and mortality rates. *Crit Care Med,* 32(4):916-921.

Buist MD, Moore GE, Bernard SA, Waxman BP, Anderson JN, Nguyen TV. (2002). Effects of a medical emergency team on reduction of incidence of and mortality from unexpected cardiac arrests in hospital: Preliminary study. *BMJ,* 324(7334):387-390.

Dellinger RP, Carlet JM, Masur H, Gerlach H, Calandra T, Cohen J, et al. (2004). Surviving Sepsis Campaign guidelines for management of severe sepsis and septic shock. *Crit Care Med*, 32(3):858-873.

DeVita MA, Bellomo R, Hillman K, Kellum J, Rotondi A, Teres D, et al. (2006). Findings of the first consensus conference on medical emergency teams. *Crit Care Med*, 34(9):2463-2478.

Dochterman JM, Bulechek GM (Eds). (2004). *Nursing Interventions Classification (NIC)*, 4th ed. St Louis: Mosby.

Kolecki P, Menckhoff CR. (2006). Shock, hypovolemic. eMedicine. Available online: http://www.emedicine.com. Retrieved on July 7, 7007.

Levy MM, Fink MP, Marshall JC, Abraham E, Angus D, Cook D, et al. (2003). 2001 SCCM/ESICM/ACCP/ATS/SIS International Sepsis Definitions Conference. *Crit Care Med*, 31(4):1250-1256.

Maier RV. (2005). Approach to the patient with shock. In Kasper DL, Braunwald E, Fauci AS, Hauser SL, Longo DL, Jameson JL, et al (Eds). *Harrison's principles of internal medicine*, 16th ed. New York: McGraw Hill.

Moorhead M, Johnson M, Maas M (Eds). (2004). *Nursing Outcomes Classification (NOC)*, 3rd ed. St Louis: Mosby.

Rivers E, Nguyen B, Havstad S, Ressler J, Muzzin A, Knoblich B, et al. (2001). Early goal-directed therapy in the treatment of severe sepsis and septic shock. *N Engl J Med*, 345(19):1368-1377.

Sebat F, Johnson D, Musthafa AA, Watnik M, Moore S, Henry K, et al. (2005). A multidisciplinary community hospital program for early and rapid resuscitation of shock in nontrauma patients. *Chest*, 127(5):1729-1743.

Winslow RM. (2003). Current status of blood substitute research: Towards a new paradigm. *J Intern Med*, 253(5):508-517.

SKIN SURVEILLANCE   NIC

Julie Anderson, PhD, RN, CCRC; Diane K. Langemo, PhD, RN, FAAN

NIC Definition: Collection and analysis of patient data to maintain skin and mucous membrane integrity (Dochterman & Bulecheck, 2004).

NURSING ACTIVITIES

Effective

■ ⓢ *Inspect skin and bony prominences on a daily basis for areas of redness and/or breakdown.* LOE = VI

ⓕ Inspecting the skin and bony prominences daily is paramount for the prevention of pressure ulcers (Bergstrom et al., 1992; WOCN, 2003).

ⓡ A cohort study (*N* = 843) recommended the inspection of skin and bony prominences for areas of redness and/or breakdown (Bergstrom et al., 1996).

■ NIC ⓢ *Monitor skin color. Monitor skin temperature.* LOE = VII

ⓕ Skin color normally varies from one body part to another, with normal pigmentation ranging from ivory or light or ruddy pink among light-skinned individuals to light to deep brown or olive among darker-skinned individuals. The skin should also be assessed for cyanosis, jaundice, or erythema. Skin temperature is normally warm, although an increase in

---

RCT = Randomized Controlled (Clinical) Trial, **NIC** = Nursing Interventions Classification, **NOC** = Nursing Outcomes Classification

temperature indicates increased blood flow, and a decrease indicates decreased blood flow (Potter & Perry, 2005).

Possibly Effective

■ *Conduct a pressure ulcer risk assessment using a validated risk assessment scale such as the Braden Scale when the patient is admitted to the health care setting. Repeat the evaluation on a regular basis and when a significant change occurs in the patient's condition.* **LOE = IV**

(NR) A cohort study ($N = 200$) found that the Braden Risk Assessment Scale could predict pressure ulcer development in patients in a skilled nursing facility (Bergstrom & Braden, 1992).

(NR) A cohort study ($N = 301$) determined that there was a need for a formal system of risk assessment (Berlowitz & Wilking, 1989).

(NR) A prospective clinical trial ($N = 74$) determined that the Braden Scale was a valid assessment tool for predicting pressure ulcer risk in black elders who were 75 years old and older (Lyder et al., 1999).

(NR) Three studies of reliability and two prospective studies of predictive validity documented good interrater reliability as well as predictive validity (sensitivity and specificity) for assessing risk for pressure ulcer development among individuals in diverse settings (Bergstrom & Braden, 1992; Bergstrom et al., 1987a, b; Braden & Bergstrom, 1987, 1989).

(NR) In a controlled study ($N = 60$), patients admitted to the intensive care unit were assessed with the Braden Scale within 72 hours of admission. Twenty-four patients subsequently developed pressure ulcers. The scale was predictive at a level of 83% among patients who would develop pressure ulcers (Bergstrom et al, 1987b).

Additional research: Bergstrom et al., 1992; Ayello & Braden, 2002; Berlowitz et al., 1997; Brandeis et al., 1995; WOCN, 2003.

■ (NIC) *Monitor for sources of pressure and friction.* **LOE = VII**

(MR) A descriptive study determined in animal models that continuous shear on a site of constant axial pressure lowered the threshold for ulceration sixfold (Dinsdale, 1974).

(MR) In a descriptive study, it was reported that shear in the sacral area causes blood vessels to become twisted and distorted, thereby leading to ischemia and necrosis (Reichel, 1958).

(EO) Friction is defined as the "mechanical force exerted when skin is dragged across a coarse surface such as bed linens" (AHCPR, 1994). Shear is defined as "the force per unit magnitude of the area acting parallel to the surface of the body" (Bergstrom et al., 1992; WOCN, 2003).

■ *Recognize that the most significant risk factor for pressure ulcer development is immobility.* **LOE = IV**

(MR) A prospective cohort study ($N = 286$) found immobility to be a significant predictor of pressure ulcer development among hospitalized patients (Allman et al., 1995).

(MR) A cohort study ($N = 301$) among nursing home residents identified immobility as a significant predictor of pressure ulcer development (Berlowitz & Wilking, 1989).

NR = Nursing Research, **MR** = Multidisciplinary Research, **SP** = Standard of Practice, **EO** = Expert Opinion, **LOE** = Level of Evidence

■ *Assess the surgical incision, including approximation and the condition of the wound edges; the amount, color, odor, and consistency of drainage present; and the presence of redness, warmth, or swelling of the periwound tissue.* **LOE = VII**

(EO) Wound assessment is necessary to ensure healing of the surgical incision without signs of infection or inflammation, which could hinder healing (Potter & Perry, 2005).

■ **(NIC)** *Monitor for infection, especially of edematous areas.* **LOE = VII**

(EO) Note the presence of warmth, redness, tender skin around the incision, fever and/or chills, and purulent drainage (Potter & Perry, 2005).

■ **(NIC)** *Monitor the skin for rashes and abrasions.* **LOE = VII**

(EO) If rashes or abrasions are detected, note their color, location, size, shape, type, whether they are cluster versus linear, and whether they have localized versus generalized distribution (Potter & Perry, 2005).

■ **(NIC)** *Monitor the skin for excessive dryness and moistness.* **LOE = VII**

(EO) Note any flaking, scaling, or moisture (wetness and oiliness). Skin is normally smooth and dry (Bergstrom et al., 1992; Guralnik et al., 1988; Hardy, 1996; WOCN, 2003).

■ *Document any skin changes.* **LOE = VII**

(EO) Skin changes must be documented (Bergstrom et al., 1992; WOCN, 2003).

■ **(NIC)** *Instruct the family member/caregiver about signs of skin breakdown, as appropriate.* **LOE = V**

(EO) It is important that the family be able to detect signs of skin breakdown early (Bergstrom et al., 1992; Morison, 1989; WOCN, 2003).

Not Effective

No applicable published research was found in this category.

Possibly Harmful

■ *Massaging skin over bony prominences.* **LOE = IV**

(NR) A controlled study ($N = 13$) using a convenience sample found that extended massage resulted in a significantly lower skin temperature than what resulted from standard massage (Olson, 1989).

(MR) A cohort study ($N = 15$) demonstrated that massage over bony prominences with skin discoloration resulted in a lower skin blood flow than was present before massage (Ek et al., 1985).

(MR) In a descriptive study, postmortem biopsies documented macerated, degenerated tissue in areas that had been exposed to massage that was not documented on individuals who had not been massaged (Dyson, 1978).

RCT = Randomized Controlled (Clinical) Trial, **NIC** = Nursing Interventions Classification, **NOC** = Nursing Outcomes Classification

OUTCOME MEASUREMENT

TISSUE INTEGRITY: SKIN & MUCOUS MEMBRANES   NOC

(Please refer to *Nursing Outcomes Classification* [Moorhead et al., 2004] for the **Tissue Integrity: Skin & Mucous Membranes** outcome.)

REFERENCES

Allman RM, Goode PS, Patrick MM, Burst N, Bartolucci AA. (1995). Pressure ulcer risk factors among hospitalized patients with activity limitation. *JAMA,* 273(11):865-870.

Ayello EA, Braden B. (2002). How and why to do pressure ulcer risk assessment. *Adv Skin Wound Care,* 15(3):125-131.

Bergstrom N, Allman R, Carlson C, et al. (1992). *Pressure ulcers in adults: Prediction and prevention.* Clinical practice guideline No. 3. Rockville, MD: Agency for Health Care Policy and Research, AHCPR Publication No. 92-0047.

Bergstrom N, Braden B. (1992). A prospective study of pressure sore risk among institutionalized elderly. *J Am Geriatr Soc,* 40(8):747-758.

Bergstrom N, Braden B, Kemp M, Champagne M, Ruby E. (1996). Multi-site study of incidence of pressure ulcers and the relationship between risk level, demographic characteristics, diagnoses, and prescription of preventive interventions. *J Am Geriatr Soc,* 44(1):22-30.

Bergstrom N, Braden BJ, Laguzza A, Holman V. (1987a). The Braden Scale for predicting pressure sore risk. *Nurs Res,* 36(4):205-210.

Bergstrom N, Demuth PJ, Braden BJ. (1987b). A clinical trial of the Braden Scale for predicting pressure sore risk. *Nurs Clin North Am,* 22(2):417-428.

Berlowitz DR, Brandeis GH, Anderson J, Du W, Brand H. (1997). Effect of pressure ulcers on the survival of long-term care residents. *J Gerontol A Biol Sci Med Sci,* 52(2):M106-M110.

Berlowitz DR, Wilking SV. (1989). Risk factors for pressure sores. A comparison of cross-sectional and cohort-derived data. *J Am Geriatr Soc,* 37(11):1043-1050.

Braden B, Bergstrom N. (1987). A conceptual schema for the study of the etiology of pressure sores. *Rehabil Nurs,* 12(1):8-12.

Braden BJ, Bergstrom N. (1989). Clinical utility of the Braden Scale for predicting pressure sore risk. *Decubitus,* 2(3):44-46, 50-51.

Brandeis GH, Berlowitz DR, Hossain M, Morris JN. (1995). Pressure ulcers: The minimum data set and the resident assessment protocol. *Adv Wound Care,* 8(6):18-25.

Dinsdale SM. (1974). Decubitus ulcers: Role of pressure and friction in causation. *Arch Phys Med Rehabil,* 55(4):147-152.

Dochterman JM, Bulecheck GM (Eds). (2004). *Nursing Outcomes Classification (NOC),* 3rd ed. St Louis: Mosby.

Dyson R. (1978). Bed sores—the injuries hospital staff inflict on patients. *Nurs Mirror,* 146(24):30-32.

Ek AC, Gustavsson G, Lewis DH. (1985). The local skin blood flow in areas at risk for pressure sores treated with massage. *Scand J Rehabil Med,* 17(2):81-86.

Guralnik JM, Harris TB, White LR, Cornoni-Huntley JC. (1988). Occurrence and predictors of pressure sores in the National Health and Nutrition Examination survey follow-up. *J Am Geriatr Soc,* 36(9):807-812.

Hardy MA. (1996). What can you do about your patient's dry skin? *J Gerontol Nurs,* 22(5):10-18.

Lyder CH, Yu C, Emerling J, Mangat R, Stevenson D, Empleo-Frazier O, et al. (1999). The Braden Scale for pressure ulcer risk: Evaluating the predictive validity in Black and Latino/Hispanic elders. *Appl Nurs Res,* 12(2):60-68.

Moorhead M, Johnson M, Maas M (Eds). (2004). *Nursing Outcomes Classification (NOC),* 3rd ed. St Louis: Mosby.

Morison MJ. (1989). Early assessment of pressure sore risk. *Prof Nurse,* 4(9):428-431.

NR = Nursing Research, **MR** = Multidisciplinary Research, **SP** = Standard of Practice, **EO** = Expert Opinion, **LOE** = Level of Evidence

Olson B. (1989). Effects of massage for prevention of pressure ulcers. *Decubitus*, 2(4):32-37.

Potter PA, Perry AG. (2005). *Fundamentals of nursing*, 6th ed. St Louis: Mosby, pp. 1593-1644.

Reichel SM. (1958). Shearing force as a factor in decubitus ulcers in paraplegics. *JAMA*, 166(7):762-763.

Wound Ostomy Continence Nursing (WOCN). (2003). *Guideline for prevention and management of pressure ulcers*. Glenview, IL: WOCN.

 ## SLEEP ENHANCEMENT

Judith A. Floyd, PhD, RN, FAAN; Jean D. Humphries, MSN, RN

NIC **Definition:** Facilitation of regular sleep/wake cycles (Dochterman & Bulechek, 2004).

NURSING ACTIVITIES

Effective

■ *Reduce or eliminate acute or chronic pain.* **LOE = II**

In a descriptive study of cardiac surgery patients ($N = 102$), pain was identified as the factor that most often disturbed their sleep (Simpson et al., 1996).

An RCT of 417 subjects demonstrated that a patient education intervention and nighttime pain assessments significantly reduced overnight pain and improved sleep among adult surgical patients (Closs et al., 1998, 1999).

■ SP *Lower the lights at night.* **LOE = IV**

A controlled study ($N = 843$) demonstrated that decreased sound and light levels increased sleep duration among hospitalized adults (Olson et al., 2001).

■ *Lower the level of noise in patients' sleep areas.* **LOE = II**

An RCT ($N = 105$) demonstrated that audiotaped intensive care unit noise increased the time needed to fall asleep, the waking frequency, and the nighttime waking duration among female volunteers in a sleep laboratory (Topf, 1992).

A controlled study ($N = 60$) demonstrated that audiotaped critical care noise increased the time needed to fall asleep and the frequency of awakening among female volunteers (Topf et al., 1996).

A controlled study ($N = 843$) demonstrated that scheduled quiet time increased sleep duration among hospitalized patients (Olson et al., 2001).

■ *Have patients listen to soothing music.* **LOE = II**

An RCT ($N = 96$) demonstrated that the use of music therapy enhanced sleep among postoperative coronary artery bypass graft patients (Zimmerman et al., 1996).

An RCT ($N = 60$) demonstrated that listening to music resulted in shorter times needed to fall asleep, longer sleep duration, and better sleep quality among older adults (Lai & Good, 2005).

RCT = Randomized Controlled (Clinical) Trial, **NIC** = Nursing Interventions Classification, **NOC** = Nursing Outcomes Classification

■ **_Teach methods for relaxing the body, including progressive muscle relaxation._**
  LOE = I

(MR) An RCT ($N = 30$) demonstrated that physical muscle relaxation shortened time needed to fall asleep but that it did not affect waking after sleep onset among oncology patients (Cannici et al., 1983).

(MR) An RCT ($N = 10$) demonstrated that progressive muscle relaxation shortened the time needed to fall asleep and waking after sleep onset among anxious older women (De Berry, 1982).

(NR) A controlled study ($N = 55$) demonstrated that progressive muscle relaxation shortened the time needed to fall asleep and waking after sleep onset among older women (Johnson, 1991b).

(NR) A controlled study ($N = 176$) demonstrated that progressive muscle relaxation shortened the time needed to fall asleep and waking after sleep onset among older adults (Johnson, 1993).

(MR) A systematic review of 59 studies demonstrated that progressive muscle relaxation shortened the time needed to fall asleep and the frequency and duration of waking after sleep onset among patients with chronic insomnia (Morin et al., 1994).

■ **_Teach methods for calming the mind._** **LOE = I**

(MR) A systematic review of 59 studies demonstrated that techniques such as guided imagery and other forms of meditation shortened the time needed to fall asleep and the frequency and duration of waking after sleep onset among patients with chronic insomnia (Morin et al., 1994).

(NR) An RCT ($N = 36$) demonstrated that guided imagery and relaxation improved the sleep quality of critically ill adults (Richardson, 2003).

(MR) A controlled study ($N = 63$) demonstrated that a type of meditation called *mindfulness meditation* decreased sleep disturbance and increased sleep quality among adult cancer patients (Carlson & Garland, 2005).

Possibly Effective

■ **_Use recordings of soothing sounds (e.g., ocean waves, rainfall, waterfalls) to induce sleep, or use other sources of white noise (e.g., a fan) to block out environmental noises._** **LOE = II**

(NR) An RCT ($N = 60$) demonstrated that white noise in the form of ocean sounds decreased waking frequency and durations among postoperative open-heart surgery patients (Williamson, 1992).

■ **_Consider the use of earplugs to block the level of noise experienced by the wearer._**
  LOE = III

(NR) A descriptive study of female surgical and gynecologic patients who chose to use earplugs ($N = 18$) demonstrated that the use of earplugs was associated with good sleep quality (Haddock, 1994).

(NR) An RCT ($N = 6$) demonstrated that the use of earplugs decreased the effects of simulated intensive care unit noise on sleep, although many patients in the earplug group would not wear them (Wallace et al., 1999).

NR = Nursing Research, **MR** = Multidisciplinary Research, **SP** = Standard of Practice, **EO** = Expert Opinion, **LOE** = Level of Evidence

■ *Use aromatherapy.* **LOE = II**

(NR) A controlled study ($N = 10$) demonstrated that the scent of lavender, juniper, basil, and sweet marjoram improved sleep in elderly persons (Cannard, 1995).

(MR) An RCT ($N = 31$) demonstrated that the scent of lavender increased deep sleep and improved morning energy among young adults (Goel et al., 2005).

(MR) An RCT ($N = 10$) demonstrated that the scent of lavender improved sleep quality among adults with mild insomnia (Lewith et al., 2005).

■ *Encourage bedtime rituals and routines.* **LOE = IV**

(NR) A descriptive study ($N = 42$) suggested that bedtime routines were associated with less time needed to fall asleep and fewer awakenings after sleep onset among older women (Johnson, 1986).

(NR) A descriptive study ($N = 87$) suggested that bedtime routines were associated with less time needed to fall asleep and fewer awakenings after sleep onset among older women in nursing homes (Johnson, 1988).

(NR) A descriptive study ($N = 87$) suggested that bedtime routines were associated with less time needed to fall asleep and fewer awakenings after sleep onset in community-dwelling older men as well as older women (Johnson, 1991a).

Not Effective

■ *Teaching personal control over noise.* **LOE = II**

(NR) An RCT ($N = 105$) demonstrated that instructing adults about how to use and adjust recorded sounds to block out noise was not effective for improving sleep, perhaps because participants had to be responsible for selecting the sounds and turning on/adjusting the volume of the sounds (Topf, 1992).

Possibly Harmful

No applicable published research was found in this category.

OUTCOME MEASUREMENT

SLEEP (NOC)

Definition: Natural periodic suspension of consciousness during which the body is restored.

Sleep as evidenced by the following selected NOC indicators:
- Hours of sleep (at least 5 hr/24 hr)
- Sleep pattern
- Sleep quality
- Sleep efficiency (ratio of sleep time/total time trying)
- Sleeps through the night consistently
- Feels rejuvenated after sleep

(Rate each indicator of **Sleep:** 1 = severely compromised, 2 = substantially compromised, 3 = moderately compromised, 4 = mildly compromised, 5 = not compromised) (Moorhead et al., 2004).

RCT = Randomized Controlled (Clinical) Trial, **NIC** = Nursing Interventions Classification, **NOC** = Nursing Outcomes Classification

REFERENCES

Cannard G. (1995). Complementary therapies: On the scent of a good night's sleep. *Nurs Stand*, 9(34): 17-23.

Cannici J, Malcolm R, Peek LA. (1983). Treatment of insomnia in cancer patients using muscle relaxation training. *J Behav Ther Exp Psychiatry*, 14(3):251-256.

Carlson LE, Garland SN. (2005). Impact of mindfulness-based stress reduction (MBSR) on sleep, mood, stress and fatigue symptoms in cancer outpatients. *Int J Behav Med*, 12(4):278-285.

Closs SJ, Briggs M, Everitt VE. (1999). Implementation of research findings to reduce postoperative pain at night. *Int J Nurs Stud*, 36(1):21-31.

Closs SJ, Gardiner E, Briggs M. (1998). Does improved postoperative pain control improve sleep? *Clin Effect Nurs*, 2:94-97.

De Berry S. (1982). An evaluation of progressive muscle relaxant on stress-related symptoms in a geriatric population. *Int J Aging Hum Dev*, 14(4):255-269.

Dochterman JM, Bulechek GM (Eds). (2004). *Nursing Interventions Classification (NIC)*, 4th ed. St Louis: Mosby.

Goel N, Kim H, Lao RP. (2005). An olfactory stimulus modifies nighttime sleep in young men and women. *Chronobiol Int*, 22(5):889-904.

Haddock J. (1994). Reducing the effects of noise in hospital. *Nurs Stand*, 8:(43):25-28.

Johnson JE. (1986). Sleep and bedtime routines of non-institutionalized aged women. *J Community Health Nurs*, 3(3):117-125.

Johnson JE. (1988). Bedtime routines: Do they influence the sleep of elderly women? *J Appl Gerontol*, 7(1):97-110.

Johnson JE. (1991a). A comparative study of bedtime routines and sleep of older adults. *J Community Health Nurs*, 8(3):129-136.

Johnson JE. (1991b). Progressive relaxation and the sleep of older noninstitutionalized women. *Appl Nurs Res*, 4(4):165-170.

Johnson JE. (1993). Progressive relaxation and the sleep of older men and women. *J Community Health Nurs*, 10(1):31-38.

Lai H, Good M. (2005). Music improves sleep quality in older adults. *J Adv Nurs*, 49(3):234-244.

Lewith GT, Godfrey AD, Prescott P. (2005). A single-blinded, randomized pilot study evaluating the aroma of Lavandula augustifolia as a treatment for mild insomnia. *J Altern Complement Med*, 11(4):631-637.

Moorhead M, Johnson M, Maas M (Eds). (2004). *Nursing Outcomes Classification (NOC)*, 3rd ed. St Louis: Mosby.

Morin CM, Culbert JP, Schwartz SM. (1994). Nonpharmacological interventions for insomnia: A meta-analysis of treatment efficacy. *Am J Psychiatry*, 151(8):1172-1180.

Olson DM, Borel CO, Laskowitz DT, Moore DT, McConnell ES. (2001). Quiet time: A nursing intervention to promote sleep in neurocritical care units. *Am J Crit Care*, 10(2):74-78.

Richardson S. (2003). Effects of relaxation and imagery on the sleep of critically ill adults. *Dimens Crit Care Nurs*, 22(4):182-190.

Simpson T, Lee ER, Cameron C. (1996). Patients' perceptions of environmental factors that disturb sleep after cardiac surgery. *Am J Crit Care*, 5(3):173-181.

Topf M. (1992). Effects of personal control over hospital noise on sleep. *Res Nurs Health*, 15(1):19-28.

Topf M, Bookman M, Arand D. (1996). Effects of critical care noise on the subjective quality of sleep. *J Adv Nurs*, 24(3):545-551.

Wallace CJ, Robins J, Alvord LS, Walker JM. (1999). The effect of earplugs on sleep measures during exposure to simulated intensive care noise. *Am J Crit Care*, 8(4):210-219.

Williamson J. (1992). The effects of ocean sounds on sleep after coronary artery bypass graft surgery. *Am J Crit Care*, 1(1):91-97.

Zimmerman L, Nieveen J, Barnason S, Schmaderer M. (1996). The effects of music interventions on postoperative pain and sleep in coronary artery bypass graft (CABG) patients. *Sch Inq Nurs Pract*, 10(2): 153-174.

SOCIALIZATION ENHANCEMENT

Debra A. Jansen, PhD, RN

NIC **Definition:** Facilitation of another person's ability to interact with others (Dochterman & Bulechek, 2004).

NURSING ACTIVITIES

Effective

■ **NIC** *Refer the patient to an interpersonal skills group or program in which the understanding of transactions can be increased, as appropriate.*
  LOE = I

MR An RCT ($N = 76$) comparing cognitive behavioral social skills training plus usual treatment for outpatients with schizophrenia versus usual treatment alone demonstrated significantly more frequent engagement in social activities and greater cognitive insight for the skills training group (Granholm et al., 2005).

MR An RCT ($N = 51$) of parents with children with Asperger syndrome demonstrated significant parent-rated improvements in the children's social skills after behavior and social communication parent workshops as compared with no improvements for wait-listed control subjects (Sofronoff et al., 2004).

MR An RCT ($N = 67$) of children with social phobia demonstrated significantly more improved social interaction and social skills and decreased social fear and anxiety after social skills training in comparison with a study/test-taking skills training condition (Beidel et al., 2000).

MR An RCT ($N = 28$) of social communication education and training for parents with children with autism versus routine care alone demonstrated significantly greater increases in reciprocal social interaction and communication initiation by the children in the intervention group (Aldred et al., 2004).

MR A controlled study ($N = 24$) of older adults with severe mental illness taking part in a 1-year interpersonal and independent living skills training plus health management intervention versus a health management intervention alone demonstrated significant improvement in social functioning and decreased inappropriate behaviors for the skills training/health management group and no improvements for the health management alone group (Bartels et al., 2004).

Additional research: Erwin et al., 2005; Gresham et al., 2004; Houck & Stember, 2002; Kapp-Simon et al., 2005; LeGoff, 2004; Margolin, 2001; McConnell, 2002; Salt et al, 2002.

■ **NIC** *Use role playing to practice improved communication skills and techniques.*
  LOE = II

NR An RCT of patients with schizophrenia ($N = 78$) demonstrated significantly improved and better conversation and assertiveness skills for those participating in social skills training sessions involving role playing, feedback, and instruction in comparison with those receiving only routine nursing care (Chien et al., 2003).

RCT = Randomized Controlled (Clinical) Trial, **NIC** = Nursing Interventions Classification, **NOC** = Nursing Outcomes Classification

(MR) An RCT ($N = 64$) of adolescents with burns participating in a skills training program involving role playing, education, and feedback versus a usual treatment control condition demonstrated significantly reduced withdrawal and total behavior problems and significantly improved behaviors with others for the intervention group as compared with no significant changes in these areas for the control group (Blakeney et al., 2005).

(MR) A controlled study ($N = 13$ children treated for brain tumors and their parents and teachers) of a social skills training intervention involving role playing resulted in significant improvements in social functioning and significant decreases in behavior problems by the children (Barakat et al., 2003).

(MR) In a case study ($N = 6$), preschoolers at risk for language delays and behavior problems who were taught to plan their play (including using role playing), to use conversational interactions, and to review their play interactions demonstrated increased verbalization and language complexity, usage of descriptive talk, and the making of specific requests (Craig-Unkefer, 2002).

(MR) A case study ($N = 10$) of adolescent boys with autism who participated in social skills training involving role playing, instruction, and games resulted in improvements in social skills (Webb et al., 2004).

Additional research: Hess, 2006; Holsbrink-Engels, 2001; Shearer & Davidhizar, 2003; Timler et al., 2005.

■ (NIC) *Encourage social and community activities.* **LOE = II**

(MR) An RCT ($N = 38$) comparing three groups of patients with AIDS who engaged in tai chi or aerobic exercise versus normal care control only demonstrated significantly improved function and quality of life for both exercise groups, with qualitative reports of improved social interaction (Galantino et al., 2005).

(MR) An RCT ($N = 52$) comparing four groups: (1) exercising patients with multiple sclerosis; (2) nonexercising patients with multiple sclerosis; (3) healthy exercising controls; and (4) healthy nonexercising controls. The results demonstrated significant increases in social functioning as compared with baseline for both exercise groups (Mostert & Kesselring, 2002).

(MR) A controlled study ($N = 15$) of nursing home residents with dementia demonstrated that daily animal-assisted therapy improved social interaction and decreased agitated behaviors (Richeson, 2003).

(MR) A cohort study ($N = 2676$) of residents of Alameda County, California, compared those who in 1965 had weekly religious attendance versus those with less frequent attendance and found significant increases in the number of personal relationships and physical activity in 1994 for those who had been in the weekly religious attendance group (Strawbridge et al., 2001).

(MR) In a controlled study of people with progressive multiple sclerosis ($N = 19$), participants in a 12-week aquatic exercise program showed significant improvements in the quality-of-life domain of social functioning after the intervention (Roehrs & Karst, 2004).

Additional research: Carless & Douglas, 2004; Gentleman & Malozemoff, 2001; Gosline, 2003; Hopman-Rock & Westhoff, 2002; Kunstler, 2002; Miller et al., 2002.

■ *Refer for correction of vision and hearing deficits and assist with the use of compensatory strategies and adaptive devices as needed.* **LOE = III**

(MR) A controlled study ($N = 41$) comparing cochlear implants and hearing aids found improvements in communication and socialization ratings with both devices (no differences between groups) for children with moderately severe to profound hearing loss (Bat-Chava et al., 2005).

(MR) A controlled study ($N = 115$) comparing clinic patients with hearing loss before and after the fitting of hearing aids found improved communication when listening in quiet, noisy, and reverberating environments but no relationship between improved audibility and patient ratings of communication abilities (Souza et al., 2000).

(MR) A controlled study ($N = 58$) comparing children with cochlear implants and children with hearing aids demonstrated significantly better language achievement for those with the implants (Tomblin et al., 1999).

(MR) A cohort study of community-dwelling elders ($N = 1192$) found that, as compared with those using sensory aids, those with uncorrected visual or hearing impairments had significantly poorer social relationships (Appollonio et al., 1996).

(MR) A controlled study ($N = 39$) of an audiologic rehabilitation program for adults involving the fitting and use of hearing aids and amplification devices, role playing, and training resulted in significant improvements in communication techniques (including less use of maladaptive ones) after the intervention but no significant improvements 3 years later (Ringdahl et al., 2001).

Additional research: Binzer, 2000; Crews & Campbell, 2004; Erber & Scherer, 1999; Heine & Browning, 2002; Tolson, 1997.

■ (NIC) (SP) *Encourage respect for the rights of others.* **LOE = VI**

(NR) A controlled study ($N = 20$) demonstrated that training certified nursing assistants to reduce the use of elderspeak (i.e., patronizing talk) decreased the usage of inappropriate terms of endearment and pronouns as well as of controlling speech and increased the usage of more respectful speech by certified nursing assistants, with anecdotal reports of increased dialogue by nursing home residents (Williams et al., 2003).

Possibly Effective

■ *Encourage activity-based therapies, including art, music, and horticultural therapy.* **LOE = III**

(MR) A Cochrane systematic review of the use of music therapy in addition to standard care for people with schizophrenia versus standard care alone found positive effects on global state and social functioning when music therapy was used frequently (Gold et al., 2005).

(MR) In a controlled study ($N = 24$), participants with dementia responded to music significantly longer and engaged in more meaningful activity when listening to live music versus no music or taped music (Sherratt et al., 2004).

(MR) In a qualitative study ($N = 166$), independently living elders who participated in aesthetic activities such as music and art were able to interact with others (family, friends, neighbors) and to be part of a social network (Wikstrom, 2004).

(MR) An RCT ($N = 40$) of a visual art discussion group for elders versus a matched social discussion control group demonstrated significantly increased social interaction for the art group as compared with no increase for the control group (Wikstrom, 2002).

(MR) In a controlled study ($N = 66$), a 5-week indoor gardening intervention was significantly more effective than a 2-week gardening program for increasing socialization (Brown et al., 2004).

RCT = Randomized Controlled (Clinical) Trial, **NIC** = Nursing Interventions Classification, **NOC** = Nursing Outcomes Classification

Additional research: Bober et al., 2002; Pachana et al., 2003; Ruddy & Milnes, 2005; Soderback et al., 2004.

- *Encourage emotion-oriented therapies, including multisensory stimulation/integration (Snoezelen therapy) and reminiscence.* **LOE = III**

(MR) A systematic review found that emotion-oriented approaches including sensory stimulation/integration and reminiscence increased social interaction and decreased behavior problems for people with dementia, although methodologic limitations existed in the reviewed studies (Finnema et al., 2000).

(MR) A Cochrane systematic review of reminiscence therapy found some significant improvements in communication for elders with dementia as compared with no treatment and no significant differences as compared with a social contact intervention, although the limited number of quality studies interfered with the drawing of conclusions (Woods et al., 2005).

(MR) A controlled study ($N = 15$) of a reminiscence group session versus a diagnostic language session demonstrated that narrative and verbal skills were significantly better in the reminiscence setting for people who were being evaluated for probable dementia (Moss et al., 2002).

(MR) A controlled study ($N = 25$) in which elders with dementia participated in three conditions—(1) reminiscence group; (2) activity group; and (3) unstructured time—resulted in significantly higher well-being (sensitivity to others, helpfulness, social contact initiation, and expressions of affection and emotion) in both the reminiscence and activity group conditions, with the reminiscence scores being highest (Brooker & Duce, 2000).

(MR) An RCT ($N = 50$) of the use of 4 weeks of multisensory stimulation versus activity sessions for elders with dementia at a day center resulted in significant improvements in the use of spontaneous speech, better relating to others, greater attention to the environment, and more initiative, activity, alertness, and happiness immediately after each session for both groups. Those in the activity sessions also showed significant improvements in the initiation and amount of speech during the course of the day while at the center, and those in the multisensory stimulation group also showed significant improvements in mood and behavior when at home (Baker et al., 2001).

Additional research: Chitsey et al., 2002; Colling & Buettner, 2002; Lin et al., 2003; Thorgrimsen et al., 2002.

- *Modify the physical and psychosocial environments to promote socialization and choices in activity involvement.* **LOE = VII**

(EO) Alter the physical and psychosocial environments for those with dementia by providing wayfinding and orienting cues, private and social spaces, personalized living areas, appropriate levels of sensory stimulation, and flexible scheduling (e.g., in visiting hours and mealtimes) to promote a therapeutic, socially interactive environment that allows for choices and some degree of control (Werezak & Morgan, 2003).

(EO) Provide environmental options and choices through, for example, making available a variety of subspaces that are conducive to social participation and interaction as well as to independent activity (Moore, 2002).

(EO) Create "home-like" environments in dementia care settings through the use of residential-type furnishings, appliances, and spaces, including kitchens that open into dining and living areas, to promote small-group interaction and the sense of an "extended family" (Nagy, 2002).

NR = Nursing Research, **MR** = Multidisciplinary Research, **SP** = Standard of Practice, **EO** = Expert Opinion, **LOE** = Level of Evidence

E.O. Facilitate social interaction and a sense of community through the arrangement and use of space, including providing pedestrian-friendly sidewalks and trails with adequate way-finding cues, areas where neighbors can meet and become acquainted (e.g., front porches or common areas in apartments where residents get their mail), and natural or green spaces (Kaplan & Kaplan, 2003).

Not Effective

No applicable published research was found in this category.

Possibly Harmful

No applicable published research was found in this category.

OUTCOME MEASUREMENT

LEISURE PARTICIPATION   **NOC**

(Please refer to *Nursing Outcomes Classification* [Moorhead et al., 2004] for the **Leisure Participation** outcome.)

REFERENCES

Aldred C, Green J, Adams C. (2004). A new social communication intervention for children with autism: Pilot randomized controlled treatment study suggesting effectiveness. *J Child Psychol Psychiatry*, 45(8): 1420-1430.

Appollonio I, Carabellese C, Frattola L, Trabucchi M. (1996). Effects of sensory aids on the quality of life and mortality of elderly people: A multivariate analysis. *Age Ageing*, 25(2):89-96.

Baker R, Bell S, Baker E, Gibson S, Holloway J, Pearce R, et al. (2001). A randomized controlled trial of the effects of multi-sensory stimulation (MSS) for people with dementia. *Br J Clin Psychol*, 40(Pt 1): 81-96.

Barakat LP, Hetzke JD, Foley B, Carey ME, Gyato K, Phillips PC. (2003). Evaluation of a social-skills training group intervention with children treated for brain tumors: A pilot study. *J Pediatr Psychol*, 28(5):299-307.

Bartels SJ, Forester B, Mueser KT, Miles KM, Dums AR, Pratt SI, et al. (2004). Enhanced skills training and health care management for older persons with severe mental illness. *Community Ment Health J*, 40(1):75-90.

Bat-Chava Y, Martin D, Kosciw JG. (2005). Longitudinal improvements in communication and socialization of deaf children with cochlear implants and hearing aids: Evidence from parental reports. *J Child Psychol Psychiatry*, 46(12):1287-1296.

Beidel DC, Turner SM, Morris TL. (2000). Behavioral treatment of childhood social phobia. *J Consult Clin Psychol*, 68(6):1072-1080.

Binzer SM. (2000). Self-assessment with the communication profile for the hearing impaired: Pre- and post-cochlear implantation. *J Acad Rehabil Audiol*, 33(1):91-114.

Blakeney P, Thomas C, Holzer C, Rose M, Berniger F, Meyer WJ III. (2005). Efficacy of a short-term, intensive social skills training program for burned adolescents. *J Burn Care Rehabil*, 26(6):546-555.

Bober SJ, McLellan E, McBee L, Westreich L. (2002). The Feelings Art Group: A vehicle for personal expression in skilled nursing home residents with dementia. *J Social Work Long Term Care*, 1(4):73-86.

Brooker D, Duce L. (2000). Well-being and activity in dementia: A comparison of group reminiscence therapy, structured goal-directed group activity and unstructured time. *Aging Ment Health*, 4(4):354-358.

Brown VM, Allen AC, Dwozan M, Mercer I, Warren K. (2004). Indoor gardening and older adults: Effects on socialization, activities of daily living, and loneliness. *J Gerontol Nurs*, 30(10):34-42.

RCT = Randomized Controlled (Clinical) Trial, **NIC** = Nursing Interventions Classification, **NOC** = Nursing Outcomes Classification

Carless D, Douglas K. (2004). A golf programme for people with severe and enduring mental health problems. *J Ment Health Promotion*, 3(4):26-39.

Chien H, Ku C, Lu R, Chu H, Tao Y, Chou K. (2003). Effects of social skills training on improving social skills of patients with schizophrenia. *Arch Psychiatr Nurs*, 17(5):228-236.

Chitsey AM, Haight BK, Jones MM. (2002). Snoezelen: A multisensory environmental intervention. *J Gerontol Nurs*, 28(3):41-49.

Colling KB, Buettner LL. (2002). Simple pleasures: Interventions from the Need-Driven Dementia-Compromised Behavior model. *J Gerontol Nurs*, 28(10):16-20.

Craig-Unkefer LA. (2002). Improving the social communication skills of at-risk social preschool children in a play context. *Top Early Childhood Spec Educ*, 22(1):3-13.

Crews JE, Campbell VA. (2004). Vision impairment and hearing loss among community-dwelling older Americans: Implications for health and functioning. *Am J Public Health*, 94(5):823-829.

Dochterman JM, Bulechek GM (Eds). (2004). *Nursing Interventions Classification (NIC)*, 4th ed. St Louis: Mosby.

Erber N, Scherer S. (1999). Sensory loss and communication difficulties in the elderly. *Aust J Ageing*, 18(1):4-9.

Erwin PG, Purves DG, Johannes CK. (2005). Involvement and outcomes in short-term interpersonal cognitive problem solving groups. *Couns Psychol Q*, 18(1):41-46.

Finnema E, Droes RM, Ribbe M, Van Tilburg W. (2000). The effects of emotion-oriented approaches in the care for persons suffering from dementia: A review of the literature. *Int J Geriatr Psychiatry*, 15(2):141-161.

Galantino ML, Shepard K, Krafft L, LaPerriere A, Ducette J, Sorbello A, et al. (2005). The effect of group aerobic exercise and t'ai chi on functional outcomes and quality of life for persons living with acquired immunodeficiency syndrome. *J Altern Complement Med*, 11(6):1085-1092.

Gentleman B, Malozemoff W. (2001). Falls and feelings: Description of a psychosocial group nursing intervention. *J Gerontol Nurs*, 27(10):35-39.

Gold C, Heldal TO, Dahle T, Wigram T. (2005). Music therapy for schizophrenia or schizophrenia-like illnesses. *Cochrane Database Syst Rev*, (2):CD004025.

Gosline MB. (2003). Client participation to enhance socialization for frail elders. *Geriatr Nurs*, 24(5):286-289.

Granholm E, McQuaid JR, McClure FS, Auslander LA, Perivoliotis D, Pedrelli P, et al. (2005). A randomized, controlled trial of cognitive behavioral social skills training for middle-aged and older outpatients with schizophrenia. *Am J Psychiatry*, 162(3):520-529.

Gresham FM, Cook CR, Crews D. (2004). Social skills training for children and youth with emotional and behavioral disorders: Validity considerations and future directions. *Behav Disord*, 30(1):32-46.

Heine C, Browning CJ. (2002). Communication and psychosocial consequences of sensory loss in older adults: Overview and rehabilitation directions. *Disabil Rehabil*, 24(15):763-773.

Hess L. (2006). I would like to play but I don't know how: A case study of pretend play in autism. *Child Lang Teach Ther*, 22(1):97-116.

Holsbrink-Engels GA. (2001). Using a computer learning environment for initial training in dealing with social-communicative problems. *Br J Educ Technol*, 32(1):53-67.

Hopman-Rock M, Westhoff MH. (2002). Development and evaluation of "Aging Well and Healthily": A health-education and exercise program for community-living older adults. *J Aging Phys Act*, 10(4):364-381.

Houck GM, Stember L. (2002). Small group experience for socially withdrawn girls. *J Sch Nurs*, 18(4):206-211.

Kaplan S, Kaplan R. (2003). Health, supportive environments, and the Reasonable Person Model. *Am J Public Health*, 93(9):1484-1489.

Kapp-Simon KA, McGuire DE, Long BC, Simon DJ. (2005). Addressing quality of life issues in adolescents: Social skills interventions. *Cleft Palate Craniofac J*, 42(1):45-50.

Kunstler R. (2002). Therapeutic recreation in the Naturally Occurring Retirement Community (NORC): Benefiting "Aging in Place". *Ther Recreation J*, 36(2):186-202.

LeGoff DB. (2004). Use of LEGO as a therapeutic medium for improving social competence. *J Autism Dev Disord*, 34(5):557-571.

Lin Y, Dai Y, Hwang S. (2003). The effect of reminiscence on the elderly population: A systematic review. *Public Health Nurs*, 20(4):297-306.

Margolin S. (2001). Interventions for nonaggressive peer-rejected children and adolescents: A review of the literature. *Child Sch,* 23(3):143-159.

McConnell SR. (2002). Interventions to facilitate social interaction for young children with autism: Review of available research and recommendations for educational intervention and future research. *J Autism Dev Disord,* 32(5):351-372.

Miller KD, Schleien SJ, Rider C, Hall C, Roche M, Worsley J. (2002). Inclusive volunteering: Benefits to participants and community. *Ther Recreation J,* 36:247-259.

Moore KD. (2002). Observed affect in a dementia day center: Does the physical setting matter? *Alzheimers Care Q,* 3(1):67-73.

Moorhead M, Johnson M, Maas M (Eds). (2004). *Nursing Outcomes Classification (NOC),* 3rd ed. St Louis: Mosby.

Moss SE, Polignano E, White CL, Minichiello MD, Sunderland T. (2002). Reminiscence group activities and discourse interaction in Alzheimer's disease. *J Gerontol Nurs,* 28(8):36-44.

Mostert S, Kesselring J. (2002). Effects of a short-term exercise training program on aerobic fitness, fatigue, health perception and activity level of subjects with multiple sclerosis. *Mult Scler,* 8(2):161-168.

Nagy JW. (2002). Kitchens that help residents reestablish home. *Alzheimers Care Q,* 3(1):74-77.

Pachana NA, McWha JL, Arathoon M. (2003). Passive therapeutic gardens: A study on an inpatient geriatric ward. *J Gerontol Nurs,* 29(5):4-10.

Richeson NE. (2003). Effects of animal-assisted therapy on agitated behaviors and social interactions of older adults with dementia. *Am J Alzheimers Dis Other Demen,* 18(6):353-358.

Ringdahl A, Brenstaaf E, Simonsson S, Wilroth M, Caprin L, Lyche S, et al. (2001). A three-year follow-up of a four-week multidisciplinary audiological rehabilitation programme. *J Audiol Med,* 10(2):142-157.

Roehrs TG, Karst GM. (2004). Effects of an aquatics exercise program on quality of life measures for individuals with progressive multiple sclerosis. *J Neurol Phys Ther,* 28(2):63-71.

Ruddy R, Milnes D. (2005). Art therapy for schizophrenia or schizophrenia-like illnesses. *Cochrane Database Syst Rev,* (4):CD003728.

Salt J, Shemilt J, Sellars V, Boyd S, Coulson T, McCool S. (2002). The Scottish Centre for Autism preschool treatment programme. II: The results of a controlled treatment outcome study. *Autism,* 6(1):33-46.

Shearer R, Davidhizar R. (2003). Using role play to develop cultural competence. *J Nurs Educ,* 42(6):273-276.

Sherratt K, Thornton A, Hatton C. (2004). Emotional and behavioural responses to music in people with dementia: An observational study. *Aging Ment Health,* 8(3):233-241.

Soderback I, Soderstrom M, Schalander E. (2004). Horticultural therapy: The "healing garden" and gardening in rehabilitation measures at Danderyd Hospital Rehabilitation Clinic, Sweden. *Pediatr Rehabil,* 7(4):245-260.

Sofronoff K, Leslie A, Brown W. (2004). Parent management training and Asperger syndrome: A randomized controlled trial to evaluate a parent based intervention. *Autism,* 8(3):301-317.

Souza PE, Yueh B, Sarubbi M, Loovis CF. (2000). Fitting hearing aids with the Articulation Index: Impact on hearing aid effectiveness. *J Rehabil Res Dev,* 37(4):473-481.

Strawbridge WJ, Shema SJ, Cohen RD, Kaplan GA. (2001). Religious attendance increases survival by improving and maintaining good health behaviors, mental health, and social relationships. *Ann Behav Med,* 23(1):68-74.

Thorgrimsen L, Schweitzer P, Orrell M. (2002). Evaluating reminiscence for people with dementia: A pilot study. *Arts Psychother,* 29(2):93-97.

Timler GR, Olswang LB, Coggins TE. (2005). "Do I know what I need to do?": A social communication intervention for children with complex clinical profiles. *Lang Speech Hear Serv Sch,* 36(1):73-85.

Tolson D. (1997). Age-related hearing loss: A case for nursing intervention. *J Adv Nurs,* 26(6):1150-1157.

Tomblin JB, Spencer L, Flock S, Tyler R, Gantz B. (1999). A comparison of language achievement in children with cochlear implants and children using hearing aids. *J Speech Lang Hear Res,* 42(2):497-511.

Webb BJ, Miller SP, Pierce TB, Strawser S, Jones WP. (2004). Effects of social skill instruction for high-functioning adolescents with autism spectrum disorders. *Focus Autism Other Dev Disabil,* 19(1):53-62.

Werezak LJ, Morgan DG. (2003). Creating a therapeutic psychosocial environment in dementia care: A preliminary framework. *J Gerontol Nurs,* 29(12):18-25.

Wikstrom B. (2002). Social interaction associated with visual art discussions: A controlled intervention study. *Aging Ment Health*, 6(1):82-87.

Wikstrom B. (2004). Older adults and the arts: The importance of aesthetic forms of expression in later life. *J Gerontol Nurs*, 30(9):30-36.

Williams K, Kemper S, Hummert ML. (2003). Improving nursing home communication: An intervention to reduce elderspeak. *Gerontologist*, 43(2):242-247.

Woods B, Spector A, Jones C, Orrell M, Davies S. (2005). Reminiscence therapy for dementia. *Cochrane Database Syst Rev*, (2):CD001120.

 # SPIRITUAL GROWTH FACILITATION

Lisa Burkhart, PhD, RN

> **NIC** **Definition:** Facilitation of growth in the patient's capacity to identify, connect with, and call upon the source of meaning, purpose, comfort, strength, and hope in his/her life (Dochterman & Bulechek, 2004).

NURSING ACTIVITIES

Effective

■ *Use spiritual meditation exercises.* **LOE = II**

MR In a controlled study of two experimental groups and one control group of 84 college students, both experimental groups participated in a spiritual meditation exercise (one had religious focus and the other nonreligious focus). Both experimental groups experienced significantly less anxiety and more positive mood, spiritual health, spiritual experiences, and higher pain tolerance. The religious experimental group affected variables significantly higher than the other two (Wachholtz & Pargament, 2005).

■ **NIC** *Encourage participation in devotional services, retreats, and special prayer/ study programs.* **LOE = II**

MR A controlled study with pre-test/post-test design of 46 students who attended a spirituality course reported significant increases in their spiritual well-being (Bethel, 2004).

MR A controlled study with a pre-test/post-test and 6-month follow-up design of 72 individuals who participated in a cardiac rehabilitation program that included a 2.5-day spiritual retreat revealed a significant increase in well-being, meaning in life, and decreased anger (Kennedy et al., 2002).

MR A controlled study of 48 patients with coronary artery disease ($N = 28$ experimental group members, $N = 20$ control group members) measured spiritual well-being at baseline and 4 years later to measure the relationship between spirituality and the percentage of stenosis from baseline between the experimental and control groups. The program consisted of a vegetarian diet, regular aerobic exercise, and 1 hour of meditation each day. The study found a significant decrease in coronary stenosis in the experimental group (Morris, 2001).

MR In a controlled study with two experimental groups and one control group of 84 college students, both experimental groups participated in a spiritual meditation exercise (one had religious focus and the other a nonreligious focus). Both experimental groups experienced

NR = Nursing Research, **MR** = Multidisciplinary Research, **SP** = Standard of Practice, **EO** = Expert Opinion, **LOE** = Level of Evidence

significantly less anxiety and more positive mood, spiritual health, spiritual experiences, and higher pain tolerance. The religious experimental group affected variables significantly higher than the other two (Wachholtz & Pargament, 2005).

Possibly Effective

■ *Individualize, integrate, and promote the use of spiritual expression in care as a method to promote physical, psychologic, and social health.* LOE = V

(NR) A qualitative study of 25 African American women in five focus groups identified spirituality as an important resource for dealing with health crises. Functions included assisting women to negotiate health crises, undergirding strong families, promoting healing from abusive family situations, and maintaining relationships with ancestors (Banks-Wallace & Parks, 2004).

(NR) A qualitative study of nine stroke survivors participating in a stroke support group identified connectedness as an important theme in hope and determined that spiritual connectedness was a factor in hope-related patterns (Bays, 2001).

(NR) A descriptive study of 256 high school students correlated spiritual health with better self-care initiative and responsibility (Callaghan, 2005).

(NR) A descriptive study of 130 older adults in a suburban senior center correlated spiritual health with more well-being and hope (Davis, 2005).

(NR) A descriptive study of 337 college students correlated higher spiritual health with less marijuana and alcohol use (Ellermann & Reed, 2001).

(NR) A qualitative ethnographic study consisting of 21,806 letters from ovarian cancer survivors from 1994 to 2000 identified that spirituality was used to derive meaning from the life experience. Spiritual themes that emerged were purpose in survivorship, hopefulness, and awareness of mortality (Ferrell et al., 2003).

(NR) A qualitative study of 10 Caucasian women diagnosed with cancer within 5 years of their initial treatment identified a developmental process of spirituality and responses to the diagnosis, treatment, and survival of cancer as a paradox of finding meaning in a belief system but having that belief system challenged as they coped with cure and recurrence. The developmental phases included deciphering the meaning of cancer, realizing human limitations, and learning to live with uncertainty (Halstead & Hull, 2001).

(NR) A qualitative study of 10 older women living in a rural senior high-rise apartment building identified three themes concerning spirituality and health: (1) health was functional and provided a sense of wholeness; (2) the relationship with God or a higher power was a personal one; and (3) death was a part of life (Knestrick & Lohri-Posey, 2005).

(NR) A qualitative study of 15 chronically ill patients identified spiritual coping mechanisms as reaching out to God in the belief and faith that help would be forthcoming, feeling connected to God through prayer, meaning and purpose, strategy of privacy, and connectedness with others (Narayanasamy, 2002).

(NR) A descriptive study of 34 obese individuals correlated spiritual health with a higher quality of life (35% of variance) and self-esteem (47% variance) (Popkess-Vawter et al., 2005).

(NR) A qualitative study of 12 hospice residents identified four themes of spiritual expression: (1) relationships; (2) that which uplifts; (3) spiritual practice; and (4) having hope. Spiritual expression was facilitated by individualized spiritual care. Nurses played an important role in the provision of spiritual care within a hospice setting (Tan et al., 2005).

RCT = Randomized Controlled (Clinical) Trial, **NIC** = Nursing Interventions Classification, **NOC** = Nursing Outcomes Classification

(MR) A descriptive study of 277 geriatric outpatients who rated themselves in good health correlated spiritual health with self-report of health (Daaleman et al., 2004).

(MR) A qualitative study of 30 individuals with musculoskeletal disorders identified spirituality as a component of perceived health. Themes in the health model included reflection, interaction and connection, strength of identity, and bearable pain (Faull et al., 2004).

(MR) A qualitative study of 11 adult patients with pulmonary artery hypertension identified spirituality and making memories as themes (Flattery et al., 2005).

(MR) A descriptive study of 101 recent widows and 87 widowers correlated spiritual health with more psychological well-being, accounting for 28% of the variance (Fry, 2001).

(MR) A descriptive study of 131 rural low-income mothers correlated spiritual health with less depressive symptoms (Garrison et al., 2004).

(MR) A descriptive study of 233 adults living in retirement housing estates in Britain correlated spiritual health with better psychological well-being, personal growth, positive relations with others, and less effects of frailty (Kirby et al., 2004).

(MR) A qualitative research study of 32 participants in a spiritually rooted weight-loss program identified patterns post-program: changes in eating behaviors, self-reported changes in food purchasing and preparation, self-reported changes made when eating out, self-efficacy, and central locus of control (Reicks et al., 2004).

(MR) A descriptive study of 196 undergraduate students correlated spiritual health with less psychological and physical distress (Younger et al., 2004).

(MR) A descriptive 15-year longitudinal population study of 3308 young adults correlated anger and time urgency/impatience with higher blood pressure. Psychosocial interventions were suggested as methods to reduce the risk of hypertension (Yan et al., 2003; Williams et al., 2003).

Additional research: Denzin, 1989.

- ■ **NIC** *Provide an environment that fosters a meditative/contemplative attitude for self-reflection.* **LOE = VI**

(NR) A qualitative study of 25 African American women in five focus groups identified clinicians as assisting in the co-creation of sacred spaces where women could connect with themselves and each other (Banks-Wallace & Parks, 2004).

- ■ *Offer opportunities for prayer, scripture reading, and/or other methods to connect with God if the patient indicates a desire to do so.* **LOE = VI**

(NR) A qualitative study of 13 African American women living with breast cancer and undergoing initial treatment identified spirituality (relationships with and reliance on God) as one of three major themes, which were experience trajectory, femininity, and spirituality (Lackey et al., 2001).

(MR) A qualitative study of 32 participants in a weight-loss program in five focus groups identified that spiritual interventions (including prayer and scripture reading) helped with weight loss (Reicks et al., 2004).

- ■ *Demonstrate caring qualities, provide comfort measures, provide reassurance, and incorporate diversity in care.* **LOE = VI**

(NR) A descriptive study of 44 adults from African American churches identified desired nursing interventions as participating in spiritual activities, demonstrating caring qualities, providing comforting measures, providing reassurance, recognizing the spiritual caregiver role, and incorporating diversity in care (Conner & Eller, 2004).

■ *Integrate family into spiritual practices as appropriate.* **LOE = VI**

(NR) A qualitative study of 425 older adults in three ethnographic studies of rural geriatric communities identified that the emerging themes of transitions were the integration of spirituality, faith, family, and health (Congdon & Magilvy, 2001).

(MR) A qualitative study of 30 survivors that looked at final conversations with loved ones identified religious faith and spirituality as assisting in coping with life's challenges after the loved one is gone (Keeley, 2004).

■ *Encourage the use of and connection with organized religion as appropriate.*
LOE = VI

(NR) A qualitative phenomenologic study of inner strength with a sample of five Hispanic women found that Hispanic women drew strength from spiritual and religious resources (Dingley & Roux, 2003).

(NR) A qualitative study of 55 adult women survivors of child abuse identified spiritual connection as a positive value for coping with negative experiences, church as a location for accessing God and communing with others, and a growing relationship with the natural world and the body (Hall, 2003).

(MR) A qualitative study of 26 older women who had not experienced a recent loss or terminal illness identified a need to feel connected, spiritual questioning, existential angst, thoughts about death and dying, and reliance on organized religion as important. Those who relied on religion did not experience the other themes (Moremen, 2005).

(MR) A qualitative study of 70 African American women with type 2 diabetes identified spirituality and religiousness as important factors in general health, disease adjustment, and coping (Samuel-Hodge et al., 2000).

■ *Integrate the use of humor in care as appropriate.* **LOE = VI**

(NR) A qualitative study of nine breast cancer survivors believed humor was part of their spirituality and that it helped them to find meaning and purpose in life (Johnson, 2002).

■ *Encourage volunteerism as appropriate.* **LOE = VI**

(NR) A qualitative study of 11 individuals receiving hemodialysis identified spirituality as including faith; the presence of God, others, community, and nature; receiving help; and giving back/helping others (Walton, 2002).

Not Effective

No applicable published research was found in this category.

Possibly Harmful

■ *Using religious expression when the patient has no religious preference.* **LOE = VI**

(MR) A qualitative study of 14 hospice patients, cancer survivors, caregivers, and health care professionals indicated that religious beliefs were strengthened during crises only if the patient had a history of religious beliefs. However, all patients expressed strong spiritual beliefs as defined in terms of meaning and purpose in life (McGrath, 2003).

RCT = Randomized Controlled (Clinical) Trial, **NIC** = Nursing Interventions Classification, **NOC** = Nursing Outcomes Classification

OUTCOME MEASUREMENT

SPIRITUAL HEALTH NOC

Definition: Connectedness with self, others, higher power, all life, nature, and the universe that transcends and empowers the self.

Spiritual Health as evidenced by the following selected NOC indicators:

- Meaning and purpose in life
- Ability to pray
- Ability to worship
- Spiritual experiences
- Participation in spiritual rites and passages
- Participation in meditation
- Participation in spiritual reading
- Connectedness with inner self
- Connectedness with others

(Rate each indicator of **Spiritual Health:** 1 = severely compromised, 2 = substantially compromised, 3 = moderately compromised, 4 = mildly compromised, 5 = not compromised) (Moorhead et al., 2004).

REFERENCES

Banks-Wallace J, Parks L. (2004). It's all sacred: African American women's perspectives on spirituality. *Issues Ment Health Nurs,* 25(1):25-45.

Bays CL. (2001). Older adults' description of hope after a stroke. *Rehabil Nurs,* 26(1):18-27.

Bethel JC. (2004). Impact of social work spirituality course on student attitudes, values, and spiritual wellness. *J Religion Spirituality Soc Work,* 23(4):27-45.

Callaghan DM. (2005). The influence of spiritual growth on adolescents' initiative and responsibility for self-care. *Pediatr Nurs,* 31(2):91-95, 115.

Congdon JG, Magilvy JK. (2001). Themes of rural health and aging from a program of research. *Geriatr Nurs,* 22(5):234-238.

Conner NE, Eller LS. (2004). Spiritual perspectives, needs and nursing interventions of Christian African-Americans. *J Adv Nurs,* 46(6):624-632.

Daaleman TP, Perera S, Studenski SA. (2004). Religion, spirituality, and health status in geriatric outpatients. *Ann Fam Med,* 2(1):49-53.

Davis B. (2005). Mediators of the relationship between hope and well-being in older adults. *Clin Nurs Res,* 14(3):253-272.

Denzin N. (1989). *Interpretive interactionism.* Newbury Park, CA: Sage.

Dingley C, Roux G. (2003). Inner strength in older Hispanic women with chronic illness. *J Cult Divers,* 10(1):11-22.

Dochterman JM, Bulechek GM (Eds). (2004). *Nursing Interventions Classification (NIC),* 4th ed. St Louis: Mosby.

Ellermann CR, Reed PG. (2001). Self-transcendence and depression in middle-age adults. *West J Nurs Res,* 23(7):698-713.

Faull K, Hills MD, Cochrane G, Gray J, Hunt M, McKenzie C, et al. (2004). Investigation of health perspectives of those with physical disabilities: The role of spirituality as a determinant of health. *Disabil Rehabil,* 26(3):129-144.

Ferrell BR, Smith SL, Juarez G, Melancon C. (2003). Meaning of illness and spirituality in ovarian cancer survivors. *Oncol Nurs Forum,* 30(2):249-257.

NR = Nursing Research, MR = Multidisciplinary Research, SP = Standard of Practice, EO = Expert Opinion, LOE = Level of Evidence

Flattery MP, Pinson JM, Savage L, Salyer J. (2005). Living with pulmonary artery hypertension: Patients' experiences. *Heart Lung,* 34(2):99-107.

Fry PS. (2001). The unique contribution of key existential factors to the prediction of psychological well-being of older adults following spousal loss. *Gerontologist,* 41(1):69-81.

Garrison ME, Marks LD, Lawrence FC, Braun B. (2004). Religious beliefs, faith community involvement and depression: A study of rural, low-income mothers. *Women Health,* 40(3):51-62.

Hall JM. (2003). Positive self-transitions in women child abuse survivors. *Issues Ment Health Nurs,* 24(6-7):647-666.

Halstead MR, Hull M. (2001). Struggling with paradoxes: The process of spiritual development in women with cancer. *Oncol Nurs Forum,* 28(10):1534-1544.

Johnson P. (2002). The use of humor and its influences on spirituality and coping in breast cancer survivors. *Oncol Nurs Forum,* 29(4):691-695.

Keeley MP. (2004). Final conversations: Survivors' memorable messages concerning religious faith and spirituality. *Health Commun,* 16(1):87-104.

Kennedy JE, Abbott RA, Rosenberg BS. (2002). Changes in spirituality and well-being in a retreat program for cardiac patients. *Altern Ther Health Med,* 8(4):64-73.

Kirby SE, Coleman PG, Daley D. (2004). Spirituality and well-being in frail and nonfrail older adults. *J Gerontol B Psychol Sci Soc Sci,* 59(3):P123-P129.

Knestrick J, Lohri-Posey B. (2005). Spirituality and health: Perceptions of older women in a rural senior high rise. *J Gerontol Nurs,* 31(10):44-50.

Lackey NR, Gates MF, Brown G. (2001). African American women's experiences with the initial discovery, diagnosis, and treatment of breast cancer. *Oncol Nurs Forum,* 28(3):519-527.

McGrath P. (2003). Religiosity and the challenge of terminal illness. *Death Stud,* 27(10):881-899.

Moorhead M, Johnson M, Maas M (Eds). (2004). *Nursing Outcomes Classification (NOC),* 3rd ed. St Louis: Mosby.

Moremen RD. (2005). What is the meaning of life? Women's spirituality at the end of life span. *Omega,* 50(4):309-330.

Morris EL. (2001). The relationship of spirituality to coronary heart disease. *Altern Ther Health Med,* 7(5):96-98.

Narayanasamy A. (2002). Spiritual coping mechanisms in chronic illness. *Br J Nurs,* 11(22):1461-1470.

Popkess-Vawter S, Yoder E, Gajewski B. (2005). The role of spirituality in holistic weight management. *Clin Nurs Res,* 14(2):158-174.

Reicks M, Mills J, Henry H. (2004). Qualitative study of spirituality in a weight loss program: contribution to self-efficacy and locus of control. *J Nutr Educ Behav,* 36(1):13-19.

Samuel-Hodge CD, Headen SW, Skelly AH, Ingram AF, Keyserling TC, Jackson EJ, et al. (2000). Influences on day-to-day self-management of type 2 diabetes among African-American women: Spirituality, the multi-caregiver role, and other social context factors. *Diabetes Care,* 23(7):928-933.

Tan HM, Braunack-Mayer A, Beilby J. (2005). The impact of the hospice environment on patient spiritual expression. *Oncol Nurs Forum,* 32(5):1049-1055.

Wachholtz AB, Pargament KI. (2005). Is spirituality a critical ingredient of meditation? Comparing the effects of spiritual meditation, secular meditation, and relaxation on spiritual, psychological, cardiac, and pain outcomes. *J Behav Med,* 28(4):367-384.

Walton J. (2002). Finding a balance: A grounded theory study of spirituality in hemodialysis patients. *Nephrol Nurs J,* 29(5):447-457.

Williams RB, Barefoot JC, Schneiderman N. (2003). Psychosocial risk factors for cardiovascular disease: more than one culprit at work. *JAMA,* 290(16):2190-2192.

Yan LL, Liu K, Matthews KA, Daviglus ML, Ferguson TF, Kiefe CI. (2003). Psychosocial factors and risk of hypertension: The coronary artery risk development in young adults (CARDIA) study. *JAMA,* 290(16):2138-2148.

Younger JW, Piferi RL, Jobe RL, Lawler KA. (2004). Dimensions of forgiveness: The views of laypersons. *J Soc Pers Relat,* 21(6):837-855.

Spiritual Support

Lisa Burkhart, PhD, RN

NIC **Definition:** Assisting the patient to feel balance and connection with a greater power (Dochterman & Bulechek, 2004).

NURSING ACTIVITIES

Effective

■ *Coordinate or encourage the attending of spiritual retreats, courses, or programming.* **LOE = II**

MR A controlled study of 48 patients with coronary artery disease ($N = 28$ experimental group members, $N = 20$ control group members) measured spiritual well-being at baseline and 4 years later to measure the relationship between spirituality and percentage of stenosis from baseline between the experimental and control groups. The program consisted of a vegetarian diet, regular aerobic exercise, and 1 hour of meditation each day. Results revealed a significant decrease in coronary stenosis in the experimental group (Morris, 2001).

MR A descriptive longitudinal study of 71 patients with advanced cancer who participated in a cancer care and rehabilitation project that included home visits and interventions from nurse practitioners correlated religious belief and measures of religious activity and connections positively with satisfaction with life and negatively with pain (Yates et al., 1981).

EO Forgiveness therapy, adapted cognitive-behavioral therapy with a religious focus, prayer, meditation, and 12-step fellowship are recommended as spiritual interventions (Harris et al., 1999).

Possibly Effective

■ *Encourage spiritual counseling as appropriate.* **LOE = III**

MR A controlled study of 80 cancer patients found that counseling resulted in significantly lowered morality rates (Fawzy et al., 1993; Richardson et al., 1990).

EO Forgiveness therapy, adapted cognitive-behavioral therapy with a religious focus, prayer, meditation, and 12-step fellowship are recommended as spiritual interventions (Harris et al., 1999).

■ *Individualize, integrate, and promote the use of spiritual expression to cope with distress or disease.* **LOE = V**

NR A qualitative study of nine stroke survivors participating in a stroke support group identified connectedness as an important theme in hope and determined that spiritual connectedness was a factor in hope-related patterns (Bays, 2001).

NR A descriptive study of 117 African American men and women living with HIV/AIDS correlated spiritual health with more mental well-being, social functioning, and cognitive functioning and with less severe HIV symptoms (Coleman, 2003).

NR = Nursing Research, **MR** = Multidisciplinary Research, **SP** = Standard of Practice, **EO** = Expert Opinion, **LOE** = Level of Evidence

(NR) A qualitative ethnographic study consisting of 21,806 letters from ovarian cancer survivors from 1994 to 2000 identified that spirituality helped these women to derive meaning from the life experience. Spiritual themes that emerged were purpose in survivorship, hopefulness, and awareness of mortality (Ferrell et al., 2003).

(NR) A qualitative study of 55 adult women survivors of child abuse identified spiritual connection as a positive value for coping with negative experiences, church as a location for accessing God and communing with others, and a growing relationship with the natural world and the body (Hall, 2003).

(NR) A qualitative study of 10 Caucasian women diagnosed with cancer within 5 years of their initial treatments identified a developmental process of spirituality and responses to the diagnosis, treatment, and survival of cancer as a paradox of finding meaning in a belief system but having that belief system challenged as they coped with cure and recurrence. The developmental phases included deciphering the meaning of cancer, realizing human limitations, and learning to live with uncertainty (Halstead & Hull, 2001).

(NR) A qualitative study of 13 African American women living with breast cancer and undergoing initial treatment identified spirituality (relationships with and reliance on God) as one of three major themes, which were experience trajectory, femininity, and spirituality (Lackey et al., 2001).

(NR) A descriptive study of 100 women with breast cancer correlated spiritual health with less symptom distress (Manning-Walsh, 2005).

(NR) A descriptive study of 60 adults with lung cancer correlated spiritual health with more well-being and less cancer symptom distress (Meraviglia, 2004).

(NR) A descriptive study of 184 HIV-positive African American women correlated spiritual health with more quality of life and less emotional distress (Sowell et al., 2000).

(NR) A qualitative study of 12 hospice residents identified four themes of spiritual expression: (1) relationships; (2) that which uplifts; (3) spiritual practice; and (4) having hope. Spiritual expression was facilitated by individualized spiritual care. Nurses played an important role in the provision of spiritual care within the hospice setting (Tan et al., 2005).

(NR) A descriptive study of 52 people living with HIV correlated spiritual health with more emotional well-being, quality of life, social well-being, physical well-being, and functional well-being and with less perceived stress and psychological distress (Tuck et al., 2001).

(MR) A descriptive study of 38 men with prostate cancer ($N = 14$ African American men, $N = 24$ Caucasian men) correlated spiritual health with better coping (Bowie et al., 2004).

(MR) A descriptive study of 1824 individuals with mental illness correlated spiritual health with more psychological well-being, recovery, hope, empowerment, social inclusion, and less depression and symptoms of disabilities (Corrigan et al., 2003).

(MR) A qualitative study 30 individuals with musculoskeletal disorders identified spirituality as a component of perceived health. Themes in the health model included reflection, interaction and connection, strength of identity, and bearable pain (Faull et al., 2004).

(MR) A qualitative study of 11 adult patients with pulmonary artery hypertension identified spirituality and making memories as themes (Flattery et al., 2005).

(MR) A descriptive study of 116 African American breast cancer survivors correlated spiritual health with more hope and a sense of coherence (Gibson & Parker, 2003).

(MR) A systematic review of 29 outcome studies of cancer patients correlated spiritual health with less pain, tumor size, and mortality (Kaplar et al., 2004).

(MR) A descriptive study of 165 patients with end-stage renal disease correlated spiritual health with better quality of life and satisfaction with life (Kimmel et al., 2003).

RCT = Randomized Controlled (Clinical) Trial, **NIC** = Nursing Interventions Classification, **NOC** = Nursing Outcomes Classification

⬤ A descriptive study of 95 cancer patients correlated spiritual health with more quality of life and with less anxiety, depression, and perceived threats (Laubmeier et al., 2004).

⬤ A descriptive study of 160 patients in a palliative care hospital with less than 3 months to live correlated spiritual health with less hopelessness, suicidal ideation, and hastened death (McClain et al., 2003).

⬤ A descriptive study of 162 terminally ill patients with cancer and AIDS correlated spiritual health with more meaning and purpose and with less depression (Nelson et al., 2002).

⬤ A qualitative study of 32 participants in a weight-loss program in five focus groups identified spiritual interventions (including prayer and scripture reading) as helping with weight loss (Reicks et al., 2004).

⬤ A qualitative study of 70 African American women with type 2 diabetes identified spirituality and religiousness as important factors in general health, disease adjustment, and coping (Samuel-Hodge et al., 2000).

Additional research: Pratt et al., 1996.

■ *Integrate the family into spiritual practices as appropriate.* LOE = V

⬤ A qualitative study of 25 African American women in five focus groups identified spirituality as an important resource for dealing with health crises. Functions included assisting women with negotiating health crises, undergirding strong families, promoting healing from abusive family situations, and maintaining relationships with ancestors (Banks-Wallace & Parks, 2004).

⬤ A qualitative study of 20 Caucasian women who had just completed the diagnostic process of breast cancer found that their personal strength and connection to God or their spiritual beliefs were important. When overwhelmed, participants sought out loved ones for support and diversion. The center's staff was found to be supportive, but participants did not wish to see a chaplain (Logan et al., 2006).

⬤ A descriptive, matched sample by age, cross-sectional survey of 84 caregivers of patients with dementia and 81 noncaregivers found that unmet spiritual needs predicted more stress and less well-being. Caregivers had greater unmet needs for religious contact, and both groups had unmet spiritual needs (Burgener, 1994).

⬤ A qualitative study of 30 survivors concerning their final conversations with loved ones identified that religious faith and spirituality were helpful for coping with life's challenges after the loved one is gone (Keeley, 2004).

■ *Use prayer as a method of coping with adverse symptoms as appropriate.* LOE = V

⬤ A descriptive study of 84 women with breast cancer found that these women used prayer more often and that spiritual health and prayer correlated with more meaning in life and psychological well-being and with less physical symptom distress (Meraviglia, 2006).

⬤ A qualitative study of 15 chronically ill patients identified spiritual coping mechanisms as reaching out to God in the belief and faith that help would be forthcoming, feeling connected to God through prayer, meaning and purpose, strategy of privacy, and connectedness with others (Narayanasamy, 2002).

⬤ A qualitative study of 19 former runaway and homeless youth identified spiritual practices as being important in coping, including having a personal relationship with a nonjudgmental higher power, use of prayer, participation in traditional and nontraditional religious practices, and finding meaning and purpose in life, including a desire to "give back" to the community. Spirituality played an important role in resilience for these subjects, nourished them, and provided them with a feeling of being rescued (Williams & Lindsey, 2005).

(MR) A descriptive 15-year longitudinal population study of 3308 young adults correlated anger and time urgency/impatience with higher blood pressure. Psychosocial interventions were suggested as methods to reduce the risk of hypertension (Yan et al., 2003; Williams et al., 2003).

(EO) Forgiveness therapy, adapted cognitive-behavioral therapy with a religious focus, prayer, meditation, and 12-step fellowship are recommended as spiritual interventions (Harris et al., 1999).

Additional research: Mullen et al., 1993, Nicassio et al., 1997.

■ *Determine what provides meaning and purpose in life as a focal point for spiritual care.* **LOE = VI**

(NR) A qualitative survey of 115 nurses concerning when and how spiritual needs were identified and the impact of spiritual care indicated that nurses commonly supported spiritual needs by assisting patients with searching for meaning and purpose in life situations (Narayanasamy & Owens, 2001).

■ *Promote forgiveness as indicated.* **LOE = VI**

(MR) A descriptive study surveying 186 undergraduate college students identified forgiveness as being associated with less physical and psychological distress (Younger et al., 2004).

(EO) Forgiveness therapy, adapted cognitive-behavioral therapy with a religious focus, prayer, meditation, and 12-step fellowship are recommended as spiritual interventions (Harris et al., 1999).

■ *Demonstrate caring qualities, provide comfort measure, provide reassurance, and incorporate diversity in care.* **LOE = VI**

(NR) A descriptive study of 44 adults from African American churches identified desired nursing interventions as participating in spiritual activities, demonstrating caring qualities, providing comforting measures, providing reassurance, recognizing the spiritual caregiver role, and incorporating diversity in care (Conner & Eller, 2004).

■ *Encourage volunteerism.* **LOE = VI**

(NR) A qualitative study of 11 individuals receiving hemodialysis identified spirituality as including faith; the presence of God, others, community, and nature; receiving help; and giving back/helping others (Walton, 2002).

(MR) A qualitative study of 19 former runaway and homeless youth identified spiritual practices as being important in coping, including having a personal relationship with a non-judgmental higher power, use of prayer, participation in traditional and nontraditional religious practices, and finding meaning and purpose in life, including a desire to "give back" to the community. Spirituality played an important role in resilience for these subjects, nourished them, and provided them with a feeling of being rescued (Williams & Lindsey, 2005).

Not Effective

No applicable published research was found in this category.

RCT = Randomized Controlled (Clinical) Trial, **NIC** = Nursing Interventions Classification, **NOC** = Nursing Outcomes Classification

Possibly Harmful

■ *Encouraging religious expression if the patient has no religious preference.*
LOE = VI

(MR) A qualitative study of 10 people with advanced HIV disease identified three themes related to spirituality: (1) purpose and life emerged from stigmatization; (2) opportunities for meaning arose from a disease without a cure; and (3) after suffering, spirituality framed the life. In this study, subjects clearly differentiated spirituality from religiosity; many rejected faith belief systems, but spirituality became an organizing framework for life (Denzin, 1989).

(MR) A qualitative study of 14 hospice patients, cancer survivors, caregivers, and health care professionals indicated that religious beliefs were strengthened during crises only if the subject had a history of religious beliefs. However, all subjects expressed strong spiritual beliefs as defined in terms of meaning and purpose in life (McGrath, 2003).

(MR) A qualitative study of eight self-identified lesbians who had been diagnosed with cancer identified spirituality as being important to life and the illness journey but that religion could be a barrier. All of the subjects studied sought and valued spirituality during treatment (Varner, 2004).

OUTCOME MEASUREMENT

SPIRITUAL HEALTH (NOC)

Definition: Connectedness with self, others, higher power, all life, nature, and the universe that transcends and empowers the self.

Spiritual Health as evidenced by the following selected NOC indicators:
• Meaning and purpose in life
• Ability to pray
• Ability to worship
• Spiritual experiences
• Participation in spiritual rites and passages
• Participation in meditation
• Participation in spiritual reading
• Connectedness with inner self
• Connectedness with others

(Rate each indicator of **Spiritual Health:** 1 = severely compromised, 2 = substantially compromised, 3 = moderately compromised, 4 = mildly compromised, 5 = not compromised) (Moorhead et al., 2004).

REFERENCES

Banks-Wallace J, Parks L. (2004). It's all sacred: African American women's perspectives on spirituality. *Issues Ment Health Nurs,* 25(1):25-45.

Bays CL. (2001). Older adults' descriptions of hope after a stroke. *Rehabil Nurs,* 26(1):18-27.

NR = Nursing Research, **MR** = Multidisciplinary Research, **SP** = Standard of Practice, **EO** = Expert Opinion, **LOE** = Level of Evidence

Bowie JV, Sydnor KD, Granot M, Pargament KI. (2004). Spirituality and coping among survivors of prostate cancer. *J Psychosoc Oncol*, 22(2):41-56.

Burgener SC. (1994). Caregiver religiosity and well-being in dealing with Alzheimer's dementia. *J Religious Health*, 33(2):175-189.

Coleman CL. (2003). Spirituality and sexual orientation: Relationship to mental well-being and functional health status. *J Adv Nurs*, 43(5):457-464.

Conner NE, Eller LS. (2004). Spiritual perspectives, needs and nursing interventions of Christian African-Americans. *J Adv Nurs*, 46(6):624-632.

Corrigan P, McCorkle B, Schell B, Kidder K. (2003). Religion and spirituality in the lives of people with serious mental illness. *Community Ment Heath J*, 39(6):487-499.

Denzin N. (1989). *Interpretive interactionism*. Newbury Park, CA: Sage.

Dochterman JM, Bulechek GM (Eds). (2004). *Nursing Interventions Classification (NIC)*, 4th ed. St Louis: Mosby.

Faull K, Hills MD, Cochrane G, Gray J, Hunt M, McKenzie C, et al. (2004). Investigation of health perspectives of those with physical disabilities: The role of spirituality as a determinant of health. *Disabil Rehabil*, 26(3):129-144.

Fawzy FI, Fawzy NW, Hyun CS, Elashoff R, Guthrie D, Fahey JL, et al. (1993). Malignant melanoma. Effects of an early structured psychiatric intervention, coping, and affective state on recurrence and survival 6 years later. *Arch Gen Psychiatry*, 50(9):681-689.

Ferrell BR, Smith SL, Juarez G, Melancon C. (2003). Meaning of illness and spirituality in ovarian cancer survivors. *Oncol Nurs Forum*, 30(2):249-257.

Flattery MP, Pinson JM, Savage L, Salyer J. (2005). Living with pulmonary artery hypertension: Patients' experiences. *Heart Lung*, 34(2):99-107.

Gibson LM, Parker V. (2003). Inner resources as predictors of psychological well-being in middle-income African American breast cancer survivors. *Cancer Control*, 10(5 Suppl):52-59.

Hall JM. (2003). Positive self-transitions in women child abuse survivors. *Issues Ment Health Nurs*, 24(6-7):647-666.

Halstead MT, Hull M. (2001). Struggling with paradoxes: The process of spiritual development in women with cancer. *Oncol Nurs Forum*, 28(10):1534-1544.

Harris AH, Thoresen CE, McCullough ME, Larson DB. (1999). Spiritually and religiously oriented health interventions. *J Health Psychol*, 4(3):413-433.

Kaplar ME, Wachholtz AB, O'Brien WH. (2004). The effects of religious and spiritual interventions on the biological, psychological, and spiritual outcomes of oncology patients: A meta-analytic review. *J Psychosoc Oncol*, 22(1):39-49.

Keeley MP. (2004). Final conversations: Survivors' memorable messages concerning religious faith and spirituality. *Health Commun*, 16(1):87-104.

Kimmel PL, Emont SL, Newmann JM, Danko H, Moss AH. (2003). ESRD patient quality of life: Symptoms, spiritual beliefs, psychosocial factors, and ethnicity. *Am J Kidney Dis*, 42(4):713-721.

Lackey NR, Gates MF, Brown G. (2001). African American women's experiences with the initial discovery, diagnosis, and treatment of breast cancer. *Oncol Nurs Forum*, 28(3):519-527.

Laubmeier KK, Zakowski SG, Bair JP. (2004). The role of spirituality in the psychological adjustment to cancer: A test of the transactional model of stress and coping. *Int J Behav Med*, 11(1):48-55.

Logan J, Hackbusch-Pinto R, De Grasse CE. (2006). Women undergoing breast diagnostics: The lived experience of spirituality. *Oncol Nurs Forum*, 33(1):121-126.

Manning-Walsh JK. (2005). Psychospiritual well-being and symptom distress in women with breast cancer. *Oncol Nurs Forum*, 32(3):543.

McClain CS, Rosenfeld B, Breitbart W. (2003). Effect of spiritual well-being on end-of-life despair in terminally-ill cancer patients. *Lancet*, 361(9369):1603-1607.

McGrath P. (2003). Religiosity and the challenge of terminal illness. *Death Stud*, 27(10):881-899.

Meraviglia MG. (2004). The effects of spirituality on well-being of people with lung cancer. *Oncol Nurs Forum*, 31(1):89-94.

Meraviglia M. (2006). Effects of spirituality in breast cancer survivors. *Oncol Nurs Forum*, 33(1):E1-E7.

Moorhead M, Johnson M, Maas M (Eds). (2004). *Nursing Outcomes Classification (NOC)*, 3rd ed. St Louis: Mosby.

Morris EL. (2001). The relationship of spirituality to coronary heart disease. *Altern Ther Health Med,* 7(5):96-98.

Mullen PM, Smith RM, Hill EW. (1993). Sense of coherence as a mediator of stress for cancer patients and spouses. *J Psychosoc Oncol,* 11(3):23-46.

Narayanasamy A. (2002). Spiritual coping mechanisms in chronically ill patients. *Br J Nurs,* 11(22): 1461-1470.

Narayanasamy A, Owens J. (2001). A critical incident study of nurses' responses to the spiritual needs of their patients. *J Adv Nurs,* 33(4):446-455.

Nelson CJ, Rosenfeld B, Breitbart W, Galietta M. (2002). Spirituality, religion, and depression in the terminally ill. *Psychosomatics,* 43(3):213-220.

Nicassio PM, Schuman C, Kim J, Cordova A, Weisman MH. (1997). Psychosocial factors associated with complementary treatment use in fibromyalgia. *J Rheumatol,* 24(10):2008-2013.

Pratt LA, Ford DE, Crum RM, Armenian HK, Gallo JJ, Eaton WW. (1996). Depression, psychotropic medication, and risk of myocardial infarction: Prospective data from the Baltimore ECA follow-up. *Circulation,* 94(12):3123-3129.

Reicks M, Mills J, Henry H. (2004). Qualitative study of spirituality in a weight loss program: Contribution to self-efficacy and locus of control. *J Nutr Educ Behav,* 36(1):13-15.

Richardson JL, Shelton DR, Krailo M, Levine AM. (1990). The effect of compliance with treatment on survival among patient with hematologic malignancies, *J Clin Oncol,* 8(2):356-364.

Samuel-Hodge CD, Headen SW, Skelly AH, Ingram AF, Keyserling TC, Jackson EJ, et al. (2000). Influences on day-to-day self-management of type 2 diabetes among African-American women: Spirituality, the multi-caregiver role, and other social context factors. *Diabetes Care,* 23(7):928-933.

Sowell R, Moneyham L, Hennessy M, Guillory J, Demi A, Seals B. (2000). Spiritual activities as a resistance resource for women with human immunodeficiency virus. *Nurs Res,* 49(2):73-82.

Tan HM, Braunack-Mayer A, Beilby J. (2005). The impact of the hospice environment on patient spiritual expression. *Oncol Nurs Forum,* 32(5):1049-1055.

Tuck I, McCain NL, Elswick RK. (2001). Spirituality and psychosocial factors in persons living with HIV. *J Adv Nurs,* 33(6):776-783.

Varner A. (2004). Spirituality and religion among lesbian women diagnosed with cancer: A qualitative study. *J Psychosoc Oncol,* 22(1):75-89.

Walton J. (2002). Finding a balance: A grounded theory study of spirituality in hemodialysis patients. *Nephrol Nurs J,* 29(5):447-457.

Williams RB, Barefoot JC, Schneiderman N. (2003). Psychosocial risk factors for cardiovascular disease: More than one culprit at work. *JAMA,* 290(16):2190-2192.

Williams NR, Lindsey E. (2005). Spirituality and religion in the lives of runaway and homeless youth: Coping with adversity. *J Religion Spirituality Soc Work,* 24(4):19-38.

Yan LL, Liu K, Matthews KA, Daviglus ML, Ferguson TF, Kiefe CI. (2003). Psychosocial factors and risk of hypertension: The Coronary Artery Risk Development in Young Adults (CARDIA) Study. *JAMA,* 290(16):2138-2148.

Yates JW, Chalmer BJ, St. James P, Follansbee M, McKegney FP. (1981). Religion in patients with advanced cancer. *Med Pediatr Oncol,* 9(2):121-128.

Younger JW, Piferi RL, Jobe RL, Lawler KA. (2004). Dimensions of forgiveness: The views of laypersons. *J Soc Personal Relationships,* 21(6):837-855.

 # SUBSTANCE USE PREVENTION

Vicki L. Hicks, MSN, ARNP-CNS

NIC **Definition:** Prevention of an alcoholic or drug use lifestyle (Dochterman & Bulechek, 2004).

NR = Nursing Research, **MR** = Multidisciplinary Research, **SP** = Standard of Practice, **EO** = Expert Opinion, **LOE** = Level of Evidence

NURSING ACTIVITIES

Effective

■ *Use comprehensive, multilevel programs designed to meet the specific needs of a community, address more than one level of influence, and represent varied interests and levels in the community.* **LOE = I**

(MR) A systematic review reported that two large-scale community multilevel trials included prevention strategies such as school programs, parent programs, mass media advertising, community organization, and policy change and found that the Midwestern Prevention Program resulted in significantly lower rates of tobacco, alcohol, and marijuana use at 1- and 3-year follow-up as compared with the control group. Project Northland resulted in lower rates of alcohol use and of the tendency to use alcohol as compared with the control group (Paglia & Room, 1999).

(MR) A cross-sectional national survey of children between the ages of 9 and 18 years old in 48 high-risk communities indicated that multidimensional prevention programming stressing the fostering of multilevel programming (i.e., protective factors, conventional antisubstance use attitudes among parents and peers, the importance of parental supervision, and the development of strong connections between youth and their family, peers, and school) may be the most effective for preventing and reducing substance use patterns among high-risk youth (Sale et al., 2003).

(MR) A systematic review of the literature demonstrated that there were nine characteristics that were consistently associated with effective prevention programs: (1) the programs were comprehensive; (2) they included varied teaching methods; (3) they provided a sufficient dosage of program intensity; (4) they were theory driven; (5) they provided opportunities for positive relationships; (6) they were appropriately timed; (7) they were socioculturally relevant; (8) they included outcome evaluation; and (9) they involved well-trained staff (Nation et al., 2003).

(EO) Although there has been significant development of school-based prevention programs during the last decade (including increases in the number and breadth of evidence-based programs), it remains a challenge to develop models that integrate prevention programming across the institutional structures of schools, community agencies, hospitals, and youth development organizations. This suggests the need for more coordination and dialogue and less duplication of services among these entities (Greenberg, 2004).

■ *Use programs that are focused on the school environment (i.e., the enforcement of school antidrug policies and related activities and curriculums).* **LOE = I**

(MR) An RCT ($N = 4276$) in 55 South Dakota middle schools found that the revised Project Alert curriculum curbed the initiation of cigarette and marijuana use, current and regular cigarette use, and alcohol misuse, thus indicating that school-based drug prevention programs could prevent occasional and more serious drug use, help low- to high-risk adolescents, and be effective in diverse school environments (Ellickson et al., 2003).

(MR) An evidence-based review of 25 long-term adolescent tobacco and other drug-use prevention program evaluations (11 experimental and 14 quasi-experimental) provided empirical evidence of the effectiveness of school- and community-based programs to prevent or reduce adolescent cigarette, alcohol, and marijuana use across follow-up periods ranging from 2 to 15 years. It showed that program effects were less likely to decay among studies that

RCT = Randomized Controlled (Clinical) Trial, **NIC** = Nursing Interventions Classification, **NOC** = Nursing Outcomes Classification

delivered booster programming sessions as a supplement to the program curricula (Skara & Sussman, 2003).

(MR) A meta-analysis of 94 studies of school-based prevention activities suggested that targeting middle-school children was more effective than targeting elementary- or senior-high-school-aged youth, that programs of brief duration (<4.5 months) were as effective as those of longer duration (>4.5 months), and that programs that involved peers alone in program delivery were most effective. However, the analysis suggested that the benefits that accrued for the peer delivery of a program may disappear when the teacher shared the delivery role with the peer (Gottfredson & Wilson, 2003).

(MR) A systematic review reported that effective school-based universal prevention programs included ongoing programs from kindergarten through the first year of high school (including booster sessions if short in duration), different approaches used for various subgroups, the involvement of students in curriculum planning and implementation, more than knowledge-only approaches, the presentation of alternative behaviors, emphasis on active learning (e.g., experiments, role play), leading by peers or teachers that the students trusted, and reinforcement in the community by parents, the media, and health policies (Paglia & Room, 1999).

(MR) A cross-sectional study surveyed 104 school districts to determine if the US Department of Education's Safe and Drug-Free School policy requiring school districts to use research-based substance use prevention programs was being implemented. The study found that the Life Skills Training was the most commonly selected of the research-based programs and the most effectively implemented, along with Project Alert, Project Star, Reconnecting Youth, Project Northland, and Alcohol Misuse Prevention (Hallfors & Godette, 2002).

■ *Use programs that are focused on the family to improve parenting skills and to enhance family communication.* **LOE = I**

(MR) A meta-analysis of family-based preventive interventions found that parent training programs by themselves were useful for creating important changes in children's behavior but that including parent-child sessions and child training broadened the effects and affected more of the associated risk factors. This resulted in increases in prosocial behaviors, decreases in problem behaviors, higher school attachment, greater peer acceptance, and increased positive interaction with parents as well as improved family cohesion, child management, and problem-solving, thereby leading to a positive effect on the onset and prevalence of alcohol use that was evident through 3-year follow-up periods (Lochman & Steenhoven, 2002).

(NR) A controlled study of parents and youth ($N = 42$) from a Native American community found that, after seven intervention sessions and seven booster sessions, the Strengthening Families Program increased skills among Native American youth and their parents and that drug use by youth was neither initiated nor increased during program participation (Erickson & Wagner, 2006).

(MR) An RCT ($N = 672$) of sixth-grade students and their families over a 4-year follow-up period found that embedding family-centered services within a public school context with a focus on family management and school partnerships had a preventive effect on substance use by the first year of high school in both at-risk and typically developing students (Dishion et al., 2002).

(MR) An RCT ($N = 429$) examined the interrelations between substance use and delinquency among sixth-grade students and their families from 33 rural schools using the Preparing for the Drug Free Years Program, a universal family-focused prevention intervention to improve family management skills and parenting behaviors. Boys and girls assigned to the Preparing for the Drug Free Years Program increased polysubstance use and general delinquency at a slower rate than their control group counterparts (Mason et al., 2003).

(MR) A longitudinal school-based trial of middle-school students ($N = 1807$) over 18 months found that nonusing parents had a buffering effect on influence of friends. Substances used by friends did not affect adolescents' use when parents were nonusers, which suggests that parent substance use should be addressed in substance abuse prevention programs and that continued nonuse by parents should be reinforced (Li et al., 2002).

Possibly Effective

■ *Use programs that are focused on community strategies in nonschool settings (e.g., putting out "no use" messages, trying to change community norms, putting up barriers to use).* **LOE = I**

(MR) A Cochrane review demonstrated that the effectiveness of interventions delivered in nonschool settings that were intended to prevent or reduce drug use by young people under the age of 25 years may have some benefit with motivational interviewing and some family intervention, but further research is needed (Gates et al., 2006).

(MR) A controlled trial ($N = 6500$) in which the experimental group completed the PeerCare worksite substance use prevention program resulted in 14% reduced injury rates per month as compared with counts at four other companies (Spicer & Miller, 2005).

(EO) A secondary analysis of National Household Surveys on Drug Abuse revealed that students who were employed full-time demonstrated increased prevalence rates of heavy cigarette smoking, heavy alcohol use, heavy illicit drug use, and any illicit drug use, which suggests that the workplace may be an appropriate venue for establishing substance use prevention and early intervention programs focused on younger workers, including adolescents who work part time (Wu et al., 2003).

(MR) A meta-analysis of 94 studies of prevention activities suggested that "no use" messages that were typically conveyed in universal programs that are effective with general populations may actually increase use among those who are most at risk for using, because these youths were more knowledgeable about drugs and their effects than the curriculum assumed and thus they may reject the messages conveyed (Gottfredson and Wilson, 2003).

■ *Use a harm-reduction approach of controlled drinking or moderation-based treatments may be preferred over abstinence. (However, the public and institutional views of alcohol treatments still support zero tolerance, and US policies support abstinence-only strategies.)* **LOE = I**

(MR) A systematic review of empirical studies of universal prevention programs for young adolescents and college students demonstrated that harm reduction approaches were at least as effective as abstinence-oriented approaches for reducing alcohol consumption and alcohol-related consequences, which suggests that individuals who may benefit the most from a harm-reduction approach to alcohol use are late adolescents and young adults (Marlatt & Witkiewitz, 2002).

(MR) A cross-sectional survey of adolescents in Australia, where harm-reduction policies had been adopted, as compared with adolescents in the United States, with abstinence-focused policies, found that the abstinence policy context was associated with higher levels of illicit drug use whereas the harm-reduction policy context was related to more cigarette and alcohol use (Beyers et al., 2004).

RCT = Randomized Controlled (Clinical) Trial, **NIC** = Nursing Interventions Classification, **NOC** = Nursing Outcomes Classification

(MR) A controlled trial ($N = 2743$) of 13- to 15-year-old adolescents from 14 schools in Australia found that the adolescents who participated in the School Health and Alcohol Harm Reduction Project were more likely to be nondrinkers or supervised drinkers, to consume less alcohol, and to be less likely to drink to risky levels than comparison students and that a harm-reduction program that did not solely advocate nonuse or delayed use could produce larger reductions in alcohol consumption than either classroom-based or comprehensive programs that promoted abstinence and delayed use (McBride et al., 2004).

Not Effective

■ *Using knowledge-only information approaches that include prevention programs that are focused on the individual and that are designed only to increase knowledge or change beliefs (e.g., teaching that alcohol and other drug use is wrong, that it is not the norm).* **LOE = I**

(MR) A systematic review found that "interactive" programs were more effective than "noninteractive" didactic presentations and that individual counseling that was not based on a behavioral or cognitive behavior model, mentoring, tutoring, work-study programs, and recreational programs were found to be ineffective (Gottfredson & Wilson, 2003).

(MR) A cross-sectional national study of substance use prevention programs of private and public middle-school grades ($N = 1795$) in the United States found that content focused on knowledge, affective content (self-esteem, values), drug-refusal skills (communication, coping), and interactive teaching strategies were more effective than programs focused on noninteractive didactic instruction (Ennett et al., 2003).

Possibly Harmful

■ *Grouping high-risk youths for prevention programs, which may actually result in more problem behaviors than are seen among those who had not been grouped with peers, because peers can negatively influence one another through "deviancy training."* **LOE = II**

(MR) An RCT ($N = 158$) of at-risk boys and girls aged between the ages of 11 and 14 years in grades 6 through 8 found that the youth assigned to the peer-only and the parent- and peer-intervention groups of the Adolescent Transitions Program had increased rates of smoking and teacher-reported problem behavior at 1-year follow-up, twice as much tobacco use, and 75% higher teacher-reported delinquency than for the parent-only or control group, thereby suggesting that negative peer influences were most dangerous at the outset of drug use, particularly during the middle-school years (Dishion et al., 1999).

OUTCOME MEASUREMENT

KNOWLEDGE: SUBSTANCE USE CONTROL (NOC)

Definition: Extent of understanding conveyed about controlling the use of drugs, tobacco, or alcohol.

Knowledge: Substance Use Control as evidenced by the following selected NOC indicators:

OUTCOME MEASUREMENT—*cont'd*

- Description of adverse health effects of substance use
- Description of benefits of eliminating substance use
- Description of social consequences of substance use
- Description of personal responsibility in managing substance use
- Description of actions to prevent substance use

(Rate each indicator of **Knowledge: Substance Use Control:** 1 = none, 2 = limited, 3 = moderate, 4 = substantial, 5 = extensive) (Moorhead et al., 2004).

REFERENCES

Beyers JM, Toumbourou JW, Catalano RF, Arthur MW, Hawkins JD. (2004). A cross-national comparison of risk and protective factors for adolescent substance use: The United States and Australia. *J Adolesc Health*, 35(1):3-16.

Dishion TJ, Kavanagh K, Schneiger A, Nelson S, Kaufman NK. (2002). Preventing early adolescent substance use: A family-centered strategy for the public middle school. *Prev Sci*, 3(3):191-201.

Dishion TJ, McCord J, Poulin F. (1999). When interventions harm. Peer groups and problem behavior. *Am Psychol*, 54(9):755-764.

Dochterman JM, Bulechek GM (Eds). (2004). *Nursing Interventions Classification (NIC)*, 4th ed. St Louis: Mosby.

Ellickson PL, McCaffrey DF, Ghosh-Dastidar B, Longshore DL. (2003). New inroads in preventing adolescent drug use: Results from a large-scale trial of project ALERT in middle schools. *Am J Public Health*, 93(11):1830-1836.

Ennett ST, Ringwalt CL, Thorne J, Rohrbach LA, Vincus A, Simons-Rudolph, A et al. (2003). A comparison of current practice in school-based substance use prevention programs with meta-analysis findings. *Prev Sci*, 4(1):1-14.

Erickson JR, Wagner L. (2006). Effects of the strengthening families program with Native American families. Nursing Knowledge International: Virginia Henderson International Nursing Library. Available online: http://www.nursinglibrary.org/Portal/main.aspx?pageid=4024&pid=2670. Retrieved on October 15, 2007.

Gates S, McCambridge J, Smith LA, Foxcroft DR. (2006). Interventions for prevention of drug use by young people delivered in non-school settings. *Cochrane Database Syst Rev*, (1):CD005030.

Gottfredson DC, Wilson DB. (2003). Characteristics of effective school-based substance abuse prevention. *Prev Sci*, 4(1):27-38.

Greenberg MT. (2004). Current and future challenges in school-based prevention: The researcher perspective. *Prev Sci*, 5(1):5-13.

Hallfors D, Godette D. (2002). Will the "principles of effectiveness" improve prevention practice? Early findings from a diffusion study. *Health Educ Res*, 17(4):461-470.

Li C, Pentz MA, Chou CP. (2002). Parental substance use as a modifier of adolescent substance use risk. *Addiction*, 97(12):1537-1550.

Lochman J, Steenhoven A. (2002). Family-based approaches to substance abuse prevention. *J Prim Prev*, 23(1):49-108.

Marlatt GA, Witkiewitz K. (2002). Harm reduction approaches to alcohol use: Health promotion, prevention, and treatment. *Addict Behav*, 27(6):867-886.

Mason WA, Kosterman R, Hawkins JD, Haggerty KP, Spoth RL. (2003). Reducing adolescents' growth in substance use and delinquency: Randomized trial effects of a parent-training prevention intervention. *Prev Sci*, 4(3):203-212.

McBride N, Farringdon F, Midford R, Meuleners L, Phillips M. (2004). Harm minimization in school drug education: Final results of the School Health and Alcohol Harm Reduction Project (SHAHRP). *Addiction*, 99(3):278-291.

Moorhead S, Johnson M, Mass M (Eds). (2004). *Nursing Outcomes Classification (NOC)*, 3rd ed. St Louis: Mosby.

RCT = Randomized Controlled (Clinical) Trial, **NIC** = Nursing Interventions Classification, **NOC** = Nursing Outcomes Classification

Nation M, Crusto C, Wandersman A, Kumpfer KL, Seybolt D, Morrissey-Kane E, et al. (2003). What works in prevention. Principles of effective prevention programs. *Am Psychol,* 58(6-7):449-456.

Paglia A, Room R. (1999). Preventing substance use problems among youth: A literature review and recommendations. *J Prim Prev,* 20(1):3-50.

Sale E, Sambrano S, Springer JF, Turner CW. (2003). Risk, protection, and substance use in adolescents: A multi-site model. *J Drug Educ,* 33(1):91-105.

Skara S, Sussman S. (2003). A review of 25 long-term adolescent tobacco and other drug use prevention program evaluations. *Prev Med,* 37(5):451-474.

Spicer RS, Miller TR. (2005). Impact of a workplace peer-focused substance abuse prevention and early intervention program. *Alcohol Clin Exp Res,* 29(4):609-611.

Wu LT, Schlenger WE, Galvin DM. (2003). The relationship between employment and substance use among students aged 12 to 17. *J Adolesc Health,* 32(1):5-15.

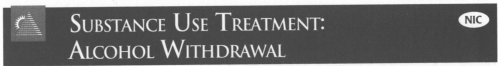

SUBSTANCE USE TREATMENT: ALCOHOL WITHDRAWAL

NIC

Ann McKay, MS, BSN

NIC **Definition:** Care of the patient experiencing sudden cessation of alcohol consumption (Dochterman & Bulechek, 2004).

NURSING ACTIVITIES

Effective

■ **NIC** *Administer anticonvulsants or sedatives, as appropriate.* **LOE = I**

MR A Cochrane systematic review (57 RCTs, $N = 4051$) focusing on evidence of benzodiazepine use for the treatment of alcohol withdrawal syndrome concluded that benzodiazepines were effective against alcohol withdrawal symptoms (particularly seizures) as compared with placebo. No definite conclusions were drawn comparing benzodiazepines with other drugs for alcohol withdrawal (Ntais et al., 2005).

MR Research regarding an evidenced-based guideline for the management of alcohol withdrawal delirium summarized 43 articles involving human subjects, including single case reports and prospective randomized trials. Sedative-hypnotic drugs were recommended as the primary agents for managing alcohol withdrawal syndrome. Sedative-hypnotics decreased mortality, the duration of symptoms, and the complications of withdrawal (Mayo-Smith et al., 2004).

MR A meta-analysis of nine prospective controlled trials found that sedative-hypnotic agents were more effective than neuroleptic agents for reducing the duration of delirium and mortality. Parenteral rapid-acting sedative-hypnotic agents coupled with comprehensive supportive medical care decreased morbidity and mortality (Mayo-Smith et al., 2004).

■ *Use individualized symptom-triggered therapy.* **LOE = I**

MR A controlled study compared a prospective interventional pilot group receiving a standardized alcohol withdrawal program with a retrospective control group managed with a nonstandard approach. The standardized approach was effective for controlling symptoms

NR = Nursing Research, **MR** = Multidisciplinary Research, **SP** = Standard of Practice, **EO** = Expert Opinion, **LOE** = Level of Evidence

with internal medicine patients and used decreased amounts of benzodiazepines (Stanley et al., 2005).

(MR) A prospective randomized treatment trial comparing symptom-triggered therapy ($N =$ 56) and fixed-dose treatment ($N = 61$) concluded that symptom-triggered therapy for alcohol withdrawal was associated with a decrease in the quantity of medication and the duration of treatment (Daeppen et al., 2002).

(MR) A case-controlled study compared patient outcomes before the implementation of symptom-triggered therapy and after the implementation of a program with a protocol. The study found that symptom-triggered therapy was an effective treatment for alcohol withdrawal syndrome and that it was associated with a decreased occurrence of delirium tremens (Jaeger et al., 2001).

(NR) A controlled study comparing a multidisciplinary implementation of a withdrawal protocol using symptom-triggered therapy with retrospective data found a decrease in against-medical-advice dismissals, staff assaults, and length of stay (Patch et al., 1997).

(MR) A double-blind controlled trial of 101 patients who were randomized to receive either a fixed-dose schedule or symptom-triggered therapy determined that symptom-triggered therapy decreased treatment duration and the amount of benzodiazepine used and that it was as effective as standard fixed-schedule therapy for alcohol withdrawal (Saitz et al., 1994).

■ **NIC** *Create a low-stimulation environment for detoxification.* **LOE = VII**

(MR) A meta-analysis of nine prospective controlled trials found support for a quiet room with good lighting to observe environmental cues such as calendars and clocks (Mayo-Smith et al., 2004).

(NR) A controlled descriptive study was the single source cited by multiple authors as the only research involving the variable of supportive nursing care. The study found that 75% of patients without serious medical complications from alcohol withdrawal responded to supportive care that included reducing environmental stimuli by using a private room, a hospital bed, controlled lighting, and controlled contact with the patient (Shaw et al., 1981).

(EO) The key component of supportive withdrawal is a quiet, calm environment with subdued lighting and minimal interpersonal contact (Chang & Steinberg, 2001).

■ **NIC** (SP) *Monitor vital signs during withdrawal.* **LOE = VII**

(EO) Vital signs should be monitored regularly in all patients. The appropriate frequency depends on the frequency of medication administration, the concurrent medical condition, and the degree of abnormality of the vital sign during withdrawal (Mayo-Smith et al., 2004).

(EO) Supportive nursing care including vital sign monitoring should be completed. Increases in heart rate, blood pressure, and respiratory rate can indicate worsening withdrawal symptoms, and heart rhythm should also be noted as an indicator of a possible electrolyte imbalance or a concurrent heart condition (McKay et al., 2004).

■ **NIC** (SP) *Maintain adequate nutrition and fluid intake.* **LOE = VII**

(EO) Fluid and electrolyte balance should be maintained, and the monitoring of input and output may be required. If a patient cannot take oral fluids, intravenous fluids may be necessary (Mayo-Smith et al., 2004).

(EO) It is common for patients in alcohol withdrawal to be dehydrated; intravenous fluids may be necessary if the patient is experiencing vomiting or diarrhea (Chang & Steinberg, 2001).

RCT = Randomized Controlled (Clinical) Trial, **NIC** = Nursing Interventions Classification, **NOC** = Nursing Outcomes Classification

(EO) Patients in alcohol withdrawal are often dehydrated and poorly nourished. Nausea during withdrawal may also contribute to poor oral intake. Intake and output should be monitored, and intravenous fluids should be provided as needed (McKay et al., 2004).

■ (NIC) (SP) *Administer vitamin therapy as appropriate.* **LOE = V**

(EO) Thiamine deficiency is frequently seen in alcoholic patients, and it can lead to Wernicke's encephalopathy. Thus, thiamine should be given until the patient is eating adequately. Many habitual drinkers are also deficient in magnesium, and hypomagnesemia lowers the seizure threshold. Thus, it is important to check the magnesium level and to replace the magnesium if levels are low (Lohr, 2005).

(EO) The parenteral or intravenous administration of thiamine is recommended to prevent or treat Wernicke-Korsakoff syndrome. Also, according to expert opinion and a review of the literature, magnesium therapy has not been shown to specifically benefit the delirium that occurs during alcohol withdrawal. However, magnesium deficiency is common, and magnesium therapy should be provided for hypomagnesemia (Mayo-Smith et al., 2004).

■ (NIC) (SP) *Monitor for delirium tremens (DTs).* **LOE = VII**

(EO) Symptoms of alcohol withdrawal include a clouding of the consciousness and delirium. Episodes of delirium tremens have a mortality rate of between 1% and 5%, and risk factors include concurrent medical illness, daily heavy alcohol use, a history of delirium tremens, older age, abnormal liver function, and more severe withdrawal symptoms on presentation (Bayard et al., 2004).

(EO) Delirium tremens typically begins 48 to 72 hours after the last drink, and it is preceded by the typical signs and symptoms of early withdrawal, although these may be masked or delayed by other illnesses or medications. Signs of sympathetic hyperactivity (e.g., tachycardia, hypertension, fever, diaphoresis) are often profound, and they are hallmarks of alcohol withdrawal delirium (Bayard et al., 2004).

■ (NIC) *Reassure the patient that depression and fatigue commonly occur during withdrawal.* **LOE = VII**

(EO) Depressive symptoms are often observed in alcoholics and those who are withdrawing from alcohol, and up to 15% are at risk for death by suicide. Additionally, sleep is often disturbed with alcohol withdrawal, which can cause daytime drowsiness (Trevisan et al., 1998).

(EO) Dysphoria, insomnia, anxiety, irritability, nausea, agitation, tachycardia, and hypertension are initial symptoms of withdrawal (Kosten & O'Connor, 2003).

Possibly Effective

■ (NIC) *Administer anticonvulsants or sedatives as appropriate.* **LOE = I**

(MR) A Cochrane systematic review (48 RCTs, N = 3610) evaluated the effectiveness and safety of anticonvulsants for the treatment of alcohol withdrawal. Because of the heterogeneity of the trials with regard to both interventions and the assessment of outcomes, it was not possible to draw definite conclusions about the safety and effectiveness of anticonvulsants during alcohol withdrawal (Polycarpou et al., 2005).

NR = Nursing Research, **MR** = Multidisciplinary Research, **SP** = Standard of Practice, **EO** = Expert Opinion, **LOE** = Level of Evidence

Not Effective

No applicable published research was found in this category.

Possibly Harmful

- **NIC** *Administer anticonvulsants or sedatives as appropriate.* **LOE = I**

  MR A guideline on the management of alcohol withdrawal delirium that was based on research summarized from 43 articles involving human subjects and that included single case reports and prospective randomized trials indicated that elderly patients and those with concurrent medical conditions (both acute and chronic) were at higher risk for complications from medication therapy, including excess sedation and seizures (Mayo-Smith et al., 2004).

OUTCOME MEASUREMENT

FLUID BALANCE **NOC**

Definition: Water balance in the intracellular and extracellular compartments of the body.

Fluid Balance as evidenced by the following selected NOC indicators:
- Blood pressure
- Radial pulse rate
- Skin turgor
- Moist mucous membranes
- Serum electrolytes

(Rate each indicator of **Fluid Balance:** 1 = severely compromised, 2 = substantially compromised, 3 = moderately compromised, 4 = mildly compromised, 5 = not compromised) (Moorhead et al., 2004).

CIWA-AR

A clinician instrument to rate acute alcohol withdrawal is the Revised Clinical Institute Withdrawal Assessment for Alcohol Scale (CIWA-AR) (Lohr, 2005).

REFERENCES

Bayard M, McIntyre J, Hill KR, Woodside J Jr. (2004). Alcohol withdrawal syndrome. *Am Fam Physician,* 69(6):1443-1450.

Chang PH, Steinberg MB. (2001). Alcohol withdrawal. *Med Clin North Am,* 85(5):1191-1212.

Daeppen JB, Gache P, Landry U, Sekera E, Schweizer V, Gloor S, et al. (2002). Symptom-triggered vs. fixed-schedule doses of benzodiazepine for alcohol withdrawal: A randomized treatment trial. *Arch Intern Med,* 162(10):1117-1121.

Dochterman JM & Bulechek GM (Eds). (2004). *Nursing Interventions Classification (NIC),* 4th ed. St Louis: Mosby.

Jaeger TM, Lohr RH, Pankratz VS. (2001). Symptom-triggered therapy for alcohol withdrawal syndrome in medical inpatients. *Mayo Clin Proc,* 76(7):695-701.

Kosten TR, O'Connor PG. (2003). Management of drug and alcohol withdrawal. *N Engl J Med,* 348(18): 1786-1795.

RCT = Randomized Controlled (Clinical) Trial, **NIC** = Nursing Interventions Classification, **NOC** = Nursing Outcomes Classification

Lohr R. (2005). Acute alcohol intoxication and alcohol withdrawal. In Wachter RM, Goldman L, Hollander H (Eds). *Hospital medicine.* Philadelphia: Lippincott Williams & Wilkins, pp. 1243-1250.

Mayo-Smith MF, Beecher LH, Fischer TL, Gorelick DA, Guillaume JL, Hill A, et al. (2004). Management of alcohol withdrawal delirium. An evidenced-based practice guideline. *Arch Intern Med,* 164(13):1405-1412.

McKay A, Koranda A, Axen D. (2004). Using a symptom-triggered approach to manage patients in acute alcohol withdrawal. *Medsurg Nurs,* 13(1):15-20, 31.

Moorhead S, Johnson M, Mass M (Eds). (2004). *Nursing Outcomes Classification (NOC),* 3rd ed. St Louis: Mosby.

Ntais C, Pakos E, Kyzas P, Ioannidis JP. (2005). Benzodiazepines for alcohol withdrawal. *Cochrane Database Syst Rev,* (3):CD005063.

Patch PB, Phelps GL, Cowan G. (1997). Alcohol withdrawal in a medical-surgical setting: The 'too little too late' phenomenon. *Medsurg Nurs,* 6(2):79-85, 88-89, 94.

Polycarpou A, Papanikolaou P, Ioannidis JP, Contopoulos-Ioannidis DG. (2005). Anticonvulsants for alcohol withdrawal. *Cochrane Database Syst Rev,* (3):CD005064.

Saitz R, Mayo-Smith MF, Roberts MS, Redmond HA, Bernard DR, Calkins DR. (1994). Individualized treatment for alcohol withdrawal. A randomized double-blind controlled trial. *JAMA,* 272(7):519-523.

Shaw JM, Kolesar GS, Sellers EM, Kaplan HL, Sandor P. (1981). Development of optimal treatment tactics for alcohol withdrawal. I. Assessment and effectiveness of supportive care. *J Clin Psychopharmacol,* 1(6):382-387.

Stanley KM, Worrall CL, Lunsford SL, Simpson KN, Miller JG, Spencer AP; Department of Therapeutic Services, Medical University of South Carolina. (2005). Experience with an adult alcohol withdrawal syndrome practice guideline in internal medicine patients. *Pharmacotherapy,* 25(8):1073-1083.

Trevisan LA, Boutros N, Petrakis IL, Krystal JH. (1998). Complications of alcohol withdrawal: Pathophysiological insights. *Alcohol Health Res World,* 22(1):61-66.

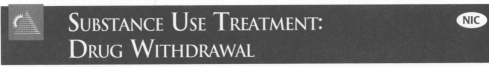

SUBSTANCE USE TREATMENT: DRUG WITHDRAWAL

NIC

Rita Ray-Mihm, MS, APRN-BC

NIC **Definition:** Care of a patient experiencing drug detoxification (Dochterman & Bulechek, 2004).

NURSING ACTIVITIES

Effective

■ **NIC** **SP** *Determine history of substance use.* **LOE = VII**

EO Screen for a history of substance abuse at every health maintenance examination or during an initial pregnancy visit using a validated screening tool (MQIC, 2005).

EO The substances that a patient has been abusing must be assessed for early during treatment related to significant differences in the severity of complications and in the management of withdrawal from alcohol, sedatives, opiates, and stimulants. The initial symptoms of withdrawal, including dysphoria, insomnia, anxiety, nausea, agitation, tachycardia, hypertension, and irritability, are similar for opiates, stimulants, alcohol, and sedatives (Kosten & O'Connor, 2003).

NR = Nursing Research, **MR** = Multidisciplinary Research, **SP** = Standard of Practice, **EO** = Expert Opinion, **LOE** = Level of Evidence

■ **NIC** SP *Discuss with the patient the role that drugs play in his or her life.* **LOE = I**

MR A multisite RCT ($N = 423$ substance users entering outpatient treatment in five community-based treatment settings) randomized substance users to receive either standard intake/evaluation or a session involving motivational interviewing techniques and strategies. Subjects who were assigned to motivational interviewing had significantly better retention through the 28-day follow-up than those who were assigned standard intervention, but no significant effects of motivational interviewing on substance use outcomes were found at 28-day or 84-day follow-up (Carroll et al., 2006).

MR A systematic review of 29 RCTs of motivational interviewing found substantial evidence that motivational interviewing was effective as a substance abuse intervention when used by clinicians who were nonspecialists in substance abuse treatment, particularly when this type of interviewing was related to entry into and engaging in treatment (Dunn et al., 2001).

EO Assess the relationship of substance use to current presenting medical concerns or psychosocial problems, patient readiness to change, and negotiating goals and strategies for reducing consumption and other changes (MQIC, 2005).

■ **NIC** SP *Assist the patient to identify other means of relieving frustrations and increasing self-esteem.* **LOE = IV**

MR A controlled study ($N = 39$) suggested that minor stressors and the perceived severity of these events were significant predictors of cravings. Social support moderated the impact of stress (Ames & Roitzsch, 2000).

MR A descriptive study ($N = 433$ men and 314 women) looking at gender differences with regard to coping and impact on length of stay in treatment provided evidence for identifying and decreasing the use of emotional discharge early in treatment through the possible use of intervention strategies such as anger management, cognitive restructuring, motivational interviewing, and encouraging participation in alternative activities. Few clinically significant differences in coping were noted between men and women entering chemical dependence treatment, but the overall amount of coping strategies used by both men and women in the sample was far less than what was found in the general population (Kohn et al., 2002).

■ **NIC** SP *Monitor for body image distortions and anorexia.* **LOE = VI**

MR A prospective study of women who were diagnosed with anorexia nervosa ($N = 136$) or bulimia nervosa ($N = 110$) assessed these women for drug use disorder. Forty-two (17%) of the women had a lifetime history of drug use disorder, with the most commonly used drugs being amphetamines, cocaine, and marijuana (Herzog et al., 2006).

■ **NIC** SP *Monitor for depression and/or suicidal tendencies.* **LOE = V**

MR A controlled study ($N = 449$ outpatients of Veterans Affairs hospitals who were dependent on either opiates or cocaine) found that patients who attempted suicide ($N = 175$) were younger than patients who had never attempted suicide ($N = 274$). Significantly more patients who attempted suicide were female, had a family history of suicide, had a lifetime history of major depression, received antidepressant medication, and had a history of alcoholism (Roy, 2003).

MR A review of the literature indicated that heroin users had death rates that were 13 times that of their peers and that deaths among heroin users ranged from 3% to 35%. Heroin users were 14 times more likely to die from suicide than their peers (Darke & Ross, 2002).

RCT = Randomized Controlled (Clinical) Trial, **NIC** = Nursing Interventions Classification, **NOC** = Nursing Outcomes Classification

■ **NIC** **SP** *Medicate to relieve symptoms during withdrawal as appropriate.* **LOE = I**

MR A Cochrane systematic review that assessed the effectiveness of interventions involving the use of alpha-2 adrenergic agonists to manage heroin or methadone withdrawal found no significant difference in efficacy between treatment regimens based on alpha-2 adrenergic agonists (clonidine and lofexidine) and those involving reducing the doses of methadone over a period of approximately 10 days (Gowing et al., 2005c).

EO Institute medication-assisted treatment for opioid addiction with methadone, levo-alpha acetyl methadol, and buprenorphine as appropriate (Batki et al., 2005).

MR A Cochrane systematic review that assessed the effectiveness of opioid antagonists in combination with minimal sedation to induce withdrawal found that the use of opioid antagonists in combination with alpha-2 adrenergic agonists was a feasible approach to the management of opioid withdrawal. Whether this approach decreased the duration of withdrawal or assisted with moving the patient to naltrexone treatment was unclear. Close monitoring was indicated for several hours after the administration of opioid antagonists in the event of vomiting, diarrhea, or delirium (Gowing et al., 2005b).

MR An RCT ($N = 180$) in the Netherlands of three intervention groups (tapering of benzodiazepine medications only, tapering of benzodiazepine plus group cognitive behavioral therapy over 3 months, or no support) indicated that a gradual reduction of benzodiazepines with or without cognitive behavioral therapy increased successful withdrawal rates as compared with no support in long-term users (Voshaar et al., 2003).

MR A Cochrane systematic review assessing the effectiveness of interventions involving the use of buprenorphine to manage opioid withdrawal found that buprenorphine was more effective than clonidine for the management of opioid withdrawal and that there were no differences between buprenorphine and methadone with regard to completion of treatment. Withdrawal symptoms resolved more quickly in patients who had taken buprenorphine (Gowing et al., 2006).

■ **NIC** *Encourage involvement in a support group such as Narcotics Anonymous.* **LOE = II**

MR An RCT ($N = 345$ outpatients of Veterans Affairs hospitals) of individuals with substance use disorders entering a new treatment episode compared a standard referral to an intensive referral-to-self-help condition. The authors concluded that brief intensive referral intervention (giving education in the form of discussion, introducing the 12-step philosophy and providing a handout, giving the patient a resource list of meetings and directions, and arranging a meeting between the patient and a 12-step volunteer) was associated with improved 12-step group involvement and substance use outcomes, even among patients with previous 12-step group exposure and formal treatment (Timko et al., 2006).

MR In an RCT of 24-week behavioral treatments with cocaine-dependent outpatients in the National Institutes on Drug Abuse Collaborative Cocaine Treatment Study ($N = 487$ patients recruited from five sites), 12-step attendance did not predict subsequent drug use, but active 12-step participation during a given month predicted less cocaine use during the next month. Also, active participation in a 12-step group was more important than meeting attendance (Weiss et al., 2005).

MR In a prospective, quasi-experimental comparison of 12-step-based and cognitive-behavioral inpatient treatment using a sample from an ongoing research project ($N = 887$), male substance-dependent patients from each type of treatment program were matched with regard to preintake health care costs ($N = 1774$). Results showed that patients who were treated in 12-step programs had significantly greater involvement in self-help groups at follow-up at 1 year as compared with patients who were treated in cognitive-behavioral programs. In addition, the cognitive-behavioral program patients had twice as many outpatient continuing care visits after discharge and received more days of inpatient care. Patients who used 12-step programs had higher rates of abstinence at follow-up (Humphreys & Moos, 2001).

■ **NIC SP** *Facilitate family support.* **LOE = II**

MR Family members and significant others were randomly assigned to community reinforcement training intervention or a popular 12-step Al-Anon self-help group ($N = 32$ concerned family members and significant others of drug users). Family members and significant others assigned to community reinforcement training were more likely to complete treatment and more likely to have their associated drug users enter treatment, whereas both community reinforcement training and self-help groups showed significant reductions in family member and significant other reports of drug use by drug users (Kirby et al., 1999).

EO Involve family members as appropriate (MQIC, 2005).

Possibly Effective

■ **NIC** *Provide symptom management during the detoxification period.* **LOE = VI**

MR The results of a controlled pilot study of 30 individuals living in Hamburg and having auricular acupuncture as treatment for cocaine, heroin, and alcohol addiction showed a reduction of withdrawal symptoms, a slight improvement of physical and mental state related to a decrease in anxiety and depression, and a reduction of alcohol and cocaine consumption. However, as a result of low sample size related to dropouts, the study results were preliminary (Verthein et al., 2002).

MR A review of the literature suggested that clinical experience supported benefits from acupuncture for helping to relieve withdrawal symptoms. The author found that scientific research with good design was lacking and that there was a need for further research (Otto, 2003).

MR An RCT ($N = 60$ cocaine-dependent users admitted to an intensive outpatient treatment program) compared amantadine with placebo. Amantadine may be effective as a treatment for cocaine-dependent patients with severe cocaine withdrawal symptoms, but it was not efficacious for subjects with less severe cocaine withdrawal symptoms (Kampman et al., 2000).

MR A Cochrane systematic review concluded that considerably more research will be needed before conclusions can be made regarding the effectiveness of managing the withdrawal of opioids by administering opioid antagonists under heavy sedation or anesthesia because of the related risk of vomiting during sedation, respiratory depression, and cardiac irregularities. The use of heavy sedation or anesthesia for opioid withdrawal should be considered experimental, with risks and benefits that are uncertain without further research (Gowing et al., 2005a).

MR An RCT assigned participants ($N = 86$ male heroin addicts) to one of three groups: a qigong treatment group ($N = 34$), a medication group receiving lofexidine hydrochloride ($N = 26$), and a control group receiving no treatment ($N = 26$). A reduction of withdrawal symptoms in the qigong group occurred more quickly than in the other groups; this included lower

RCT = Randomized Controlled (Clinical) Trial, **NIC** = Nursing Interventions Classification, **NOC** = Nursing Outcomes Classification

anxiety scores than both groups, which suggests that qigong may be an effective alternative to heroin detoxification (Li et al., 2002).

(EO) Administer ordered medication to relieve the signs and symptoms of substance withdrawal and to prevent or limit the development of life-threatening withdrawal symptoms (Fortinash & Holoday Worret, 2004).

(EO) Therapeutic interventions should be initiated to treat anxiety and to make the patient comfortable (Stuart & Laraia, 2005).

■ (NIC) *Encourage exercise to stimulate the release of endorphins.* LOE = V

(MR) A review of the literature suggested that exercise suppressed pain, induced sedation, reduced stress, and elevated mood. The authors felt that the endorphin hypothesis lacked scientific support and found that exercise increased serum concentrations of endocannabinoids; they are exploring the endocannabinoid hypothesis (Dietrich & McDaniel, 2004).

■ (NIC) (SP) *Assist the patient to recognize that drugs provide a sense of assertiveness, heightened self-esteem, and frustration tolerance.* LOE = VII

(EO) Substance users who are isolated or anxious in social situations often use drugs to gain self-confidence in social situations (Stuart & Laraia, 2005).

(EO) Substance abusers with higher levels of anxiety, inadequate coping skills, and low frustration tolerance need to relate to others and adjust to life situations without reliance on drugs to cope (Fortinash & Holoday Worret, 2004).

■ (NIC) (SP) *Monitor for paranoia and hesitancy to trust others during the detoxification period.* LOE = VII

(EO) Sensory and perceptual alterations may occur with the use of drugs, thus leading patients to incorrectly interpret stimuli (Stuart & Laraia, 2005).

■ (NIC) (SP) *Provide adequate nutrition.* LOE = VII

(EO) To provide adequate nutrition and hydration, patients will need to be supported to meet nutritional and metabolic needs on the basis of their ability to take in nutrition and retain fluids (Fortinash & Holoday Worret, 2004).

■ (NIC) (SP) *Monitor for hypertension and tachycardia.* LOE = VII

(EO) There is a need to assess the physiological symptoms of withdrawal to address potentially life-threatening problems and to assess the effects of the medications that are prescribed to treat withdrawal symptoms (Fortinash & Holoday Worret, 2004).

■ (NIC) (SP) *Encourage self-disclosure.* LOE = VII

(EO) When gathering information about drug use, the nurse uses a systematic approach of integrating questions into the general history, because substance use may often be denied, minimized, or concealed. It is important to reassure the patient about his or her safety to encourage the development of trust, to decrease anxiety, and to encourage verbalization of symptoms (Fortinash & Holoday Worret, 2004).

■ (SP) *Monitor for nausea, vomiting, and diarrhea as appropriate.* LOE = VII

(EO) Opioid withdrawal symptoms can include anorexia, nausea, vomiting, and diarrhea (Kosten & O'Connor, 2003).

NR = Nursing Research, **MR** = Multidisciplinary Research, **SP** = Standard of Practice, **EO** = Expert Opinion, **LOE** = Level of Evidence

■ ⓈⓅ *Monitor hydration and urinary output as appropriate.* **LOE = VII**

ⒺⓄ The patient will need to be supported in meeting his or her nutritional and metabolic needs to provide adequate hydration either orally or intravenously (Fortinash & Holoday Worret, 2004).

■ ⓈⓅ *Monitor for seizures and initiate seizure precautions as appropriate.* **LOE = VII**

ⒺⓄ Substance withdrawal can lead to seizures, and there is a need to assess and intervene to address life-threatening problems (Fortinash & Holoday Worret, 2004).

■ ⓈⓅ *Assess for fall risk and initiate fall precautions as appropriate.* **LOE = VII**

ⒺⓄ There is a need to maintain the safety of the patient with regard to the potential for overdose, withdrawal symptoms, and the effects of medications prescribed to manage symptoms of withdrawal (Fortinash & Holoday Worret, 2004).

■ ⓈⓅ *Provide an environment with decreased stimulation.* **LOE = VII**

ⒺⓄ Perceptual and sensory stimuli can be interpreted incorrectly and can be frightening to patients. Stimuli can be reduced by keeping a soft light in the room, avoiding loud noises, and having trusted family or friends stay with the patient (Stuart & Laraia, 2005).

■ ⓈⓅ *Assist the patient with identifying healthier coping responses.* **LOE = VII**

ⒺⓄ Denial and rationalization are some of the dysfunctional coping mechanisms that can interfere with behavior change and recovery (Stuart & Laraia, 2005).

■ ⓈⓅ *Use withdrawal scales as appropriate to objectively monitor withdrawal symptoms.* **LOE = VII**

ⒺⓄ Withdrawal charts provide a safer and more effective way to manage substance withdrawal (Bronson et al., 2005).

■ ⓈⓅ *Assess skin integrity related to substance use and nutritional status.* **LOE = VII**

ⒺⓄ Physical signs of substance use can be assessed on physical examination. Skin should be assessed for jaundice, needle tracks, cellulitis, conjunctivitis, poor dentition, and rapid weight loss. There is a need to assess for the physiological signs that are associated with withdrawal (Fortinash & Holoday Worret, 2004).

■ ⓈⓅ *Assist the patient with identifying negative consequences to health and other life areas related to substance use.* **LOE = VII**

ⒺⓄ The patient can be motivated to change by recognizing the consequences of substance-abusing behavior. Recognition of the problem, including predisposing factors and precipitating stressors, must occur before the patient can move on to the development of more adaptive behavioral responses (Stuart & Laraia, 2005).

RCT = Randomized Controlled (Clinical) Trial, **NIC** = Nursing Interventions Classification, **NOC** = Nursing Outcomes Classification

- (SP) *Monitor sleep and provide education about sleep hygiene as appropriate.* **LOE = VII**

  (EO) An outcome of treatment is for the patient to verbalize the ability to sleep without sedation. Providing information about supportive measures to induce sleep, including darkening the sleep environment, white noise, back rubs, and soft music, educates patients about methods to use to help them relax and to avoid using drugs to induce sleep (Fortinash & Holoday Worret, 2004).

- (SP) *Provide pharmacological interventions for sleep as ordered by the primary care provider.* **LOE = VII**

  (EO) Insomnia is one of the symptoms that is associated with substance withdrawal. Providing medications can relieve symptoms of withdrawal (Fortinash & Holoday Worret, 2004).

- (SP) *Promote the use of nonpharmacological supportive measures to decrease pain and anxiety, including deep breathing, relaxation, music therapy, and aromatherapy.* **LOE = VII**

  (EO) It is important to initiate therapeutic interventions that help to treat the withdrawal symptoms of anxiety (Fortinash & Holoday Worret, 2004).

- (SP) *Assist the patient with identifying feelings, behaviors, situations, and events that lead to substance use.* **LOE = VII**

  (EO) Patients must first be able to identify and describe the situations that lead to their substance-abusing behaviors before they can plan and practice more adaptive behavioral responses (Stuart & Laraia, 2005).

- (SP) *Assist the patient with identifying triggers that cause him or her to use and to develop strategies to avoid these situations by developing new routines, leisure activities, and the use of support systems.* **LOE = VII**

  (EO) A goal of treatment is for the patient to establish relationships with nondrinking and nondrugging friends and to take steps to avoid situations that triggered or led to substance use in the past. It is important for the patient to engage in a new lifestyle and to use his or her support network (Fortinash & Holoday Worret, 2004).

- (SP) *Provide education to the patient, family, and/or significant other(s) about the health effects of substance use, including the physical, emotional, and cognitive effects of ongoing substance use and the risks of exposure to HIV, hepatitis, and other infections.* **LOE = VII**

  (EO) The nurse is an advocate and a resource for teaching about prevention and the need for a healthy lifestyle for patients, their families, and their significant others (Fortinash & Holoday Worret, 2004).

- (SP) *Provide information about community resources and treatment centers for the patient and his or her family.* **LOE = VII**

  (EO) The nurse can be a resource person to provide patients and families with information to promote their involvement with recovery groups. Patients and families benefit from participation in support groups to help the patient establish a new lifestyle and to allow family members

NR = Nursing Research, **MR** = Multidisciplinary Research, **SP** = Standard of Practice, **EO** = Expert Opinion, **LOE** = Level of Evidence

to seek out groups that help them to change previous patterns of relating to the patient (Fortinash & Holoday Worret, 2004).

■ **SP** *Provide the patient, family, and or significant other(s) with information about the signs and symptoms of substance abuse, relapse, and treatment.* **LOE = VII**

EO The nurse is an advocate and a resource for teaching about prevention and the need for a healthy lifestyle for patients, their families, and their significant others (Fortinash & Holoday Worret, 2004).

■ **SP** *Monitor for contraband brought in by visitors.* **LOE = VII**

EO A top priority in the detoxification stage of the recovery process is the development of a new support system that does not include drug-taking friends. Seeking out substance-using peers interferes with treatment (Fortinash & Holoday Worret, 2004).

■ **SP** *Encourage the use of a support system or of visits or phone contact with a sponsor.* **LOE = VII**

EO Substance abusers have often been socially isolated, they have alienated significant others, or they have lost meaningful contact. Nurses can support the patient's development of a sober support system (Fortinash & Holoday Worret, 2004).

■ **SP** *Verbalize a belief in the patient's ability to make changes.* **LOE = VII**

EO Nurses can support the patient by consistently offering support and expressing a belief that the patient can make changes and adopt a healthier lifestyle (Stuart & Laraia, 2005).

■ **SP** *Assist the patient with identifying the level of motivation needed to make a change.* **LOE = VII**

EO The patient must identify his or her substance-abusing behavior and the consequences that result in order to assume responsibility for those behaviors. The patient's ability to acknowledge a problem helps the nurse to assess where the patient is in terms of his or her readiness to make behavioral changes (Stuart & Laraia, 2005).

■ **SP** *Monitor the patient's mental status.* **LOE = VII**

EO Mental status is part of a comprehensive health assessment. Patients in withdrawal can experience disturbances in cognitive functioning, sensory and perceptual alterations, and suicidal ideation (Stuart & Laraia, 2005).

Not Effective

■ **NIC** *Medicate to relieve symptoms during withdrawal, as appropriate.* **LOE = I**

MR A Cochrane systematic review of the risks, benefits, and costs of a variety of treatments for the management of amphetamine withdrawal concluded that no available treatment had been demonstrated to be effective for the treatment of amphetamine withdrawal. Amineptine was found to have limited benefits, but, as a result of amineptine abuse, it has been withdrawn from the market (Srisurapanont et al., 2001).

MR A small double-blind sample ($N = 10$) of marijuana smokers was given bupropion or placebo to determine whether bupropion influenced symptoms of marijuana withdrawal.

RCT = Randomized Controlled (Clinical) Trial, **NIC** = Nursing Interventions Classification, **NOC** = Nursing Outcomes Classification

During marijuana withdrawal, ratings of irritability, restlessness, depression, and trouble sleeping were increased by bupropion as compared with placebo (Haney et al., 2001).

(MR) A review of recent research on cannabinoids found that no medication had been shown to alter cannabis self-administration by humans (Hart, 2005).

(MR) A Cochrane review found that current evidence did not support the clinical use of dopamine agonists (amantadine, bromocriptine, and pergolide) for the treatment of cocaine dependence (Soares et al., 2003).

Possibly Harmful

No applicable published research was found in this category.

OUTCOME MEASUREMENT

KNOWLEDGE: SUBSTANCE USE CONTROL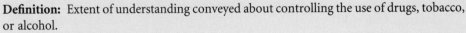

Definition: Extent of understanding conveyed about controlling the use of drugs, tobacco, or alcohol.

Knowledge: Substance Use Control as evidenced by the following selected NOC indicators:

- Description of adverse health effects of substance use
- Description of benefits of eliminating substance use
- Description of dangers of substance use
- Description of social consequences of substance use
- Description of personal responsibility in managing substance use
- Description of support for substance use control
- Description of actions to manage substance use
- Description of potential for relapse in efforts to control substance use
- Description of actions to prevent and manage relapses in substance abuse
- Description of signs of dependence during substance withdrawal

(Rate each indicator of **Knowledge: Substance Use Control:** 1 = none, 2 = limited, 3 = moderate, 4 = substantial, 5 = extensive) (Moorhead et al., 2004).

REFERENCES

Ames SC, Roitzsch JC. (2000). The impact of minor stressful life events and social support on cravings: A study of inpatients receiving treatment for substance dependence. *Addict Behav*, 25(4):539-547.

Antai-Otong D. (2003). *Psychiatric nursing: Biological & behavioral concepts.* Clifton Park, NY: Delmar.

Bailey KP. (2004). Pharmacological treatments for substance use disorders. *J Psychosoc Nurs Ment Health Serv*, 42(8):14-20.

Batki SL, Kauffman JF, Marion I, Parrino MW, Woody GE; Center for Substance Abuse Treatment (CSAT). (2005). Medication-assisted treatment for opioid addiction in opioid treatment programs: Clinical pharmacotherapy. Rockville (MD): Substance Abuse and Mental Health Services Administration (SAMHSA). Available online: http://www.guideline.gov. Retrieved on June 13, 2006.

Bronson M, Swift R, Peers E. (2005). Withdrawal charts: A clinical tool for the management of drug withdrawal symptoms. *Aust Nurs J*, 12(8):19-21.

Carroll KM, Ball SA, Nich C, Martino S, Frankforter TL, Farentinos C, et al. (2006). Motivational interviewing to improve treatment engagement and outcome in individuals seeking treatment for substance abuse: A multisite effectiveness study. *Drug Alcohol Depend*, 81(3):301-312.

Colyar MR, Call-Schmidt T. (2006). Methamphetamine abuse in the primary care patient. *Clinician Reviews*, 16(3):55-60.

Darke S, Ross J. (2002). Suicide among heroin users: Rates, risk factors and methods. *Addiction*, 97(11):1383-1394.

Dietrich A, McDaniel WF. (2004). Endocannabinoids and exercise. *Br J Sports Med*, 38(5):536-541.

Dochterman JM, Bulechek GM (Eds). (2004). *Nursing Interventions Classification (NIC)*, 4th ed. St Louis: Mosby.

Dunn C, Deroo L, Rivara F. (2001). The use of brief interventions adapted from motivational interviewing across behavioral domains: A systematic review. *Addiction*, 96(12):1725-1742.

Fortinash KM, Holoday Worret PA. (2004). *Mental health nursing*, 3rd ed. St Louis: Mosby.

Gowing L, Ali R, White J. (2005a). Opioid antagonists under heavy sedation or anaesthesia for opioid withdrawal. *Cochrane Database Syst Rev*, (2):CD002022.

Gowing L, Ali R, White J. (2005b). Opioid antagonists with minimal sedation for opioid withdrawal. *Cochrane Database Syst Rev*, (1):CD002021.

Gowing L, Ali R, White J. (2006). Buprenorphine for the management of opioid withdrawal. *Cochrane Database Syst Rev*, (2):CD002025.

Gowing L, Farrell M, Ali R, White J. (2005c). Alpha2 adrenergic agonists for the management of opioid withdrawal. *Cochrane Database Syst Rev*, (4):CD002024.

Gorman LM, Raines ML, Sultan DF. (2002). *Psychosocial nursing for general patient care*, 2nd ed. Philadelphia: F.A. Davis.

Haney M, Ward AS, Comer SD, Hart CL, Foltin RW, Fischman MW. (2001). Bupropion SR worsens mood during marijuana withdrawal in humans. *Psychopharmacology*, 155(2):171-179.

Hart C. (2005). Increasing treatment options for cannabis dependence: A review of potential pharmacotherapies. *Drug Alcohol Depend*, 80(2):147-159.

Herzog DB, Franko DL, Dorer DJ, Keel PK, Jackson S, Manzo MP. (2006). Drug abuse in women with eating disorders. *Int J Eat Disord*, 39(5):364-368.

Humphreys K, Moos R. (2001). Can encouraging substance abuse patients to participate in self-help groups reduce demand for health care? A quasi-experimental study. *Alcohol Clin Exp Res*, 25(5): 711-716.

Ignatavicius DD, Workman ML. (2006). *Medical-surgical nursing: Critical thinking for collaborative care*, 5th ed. St Louis: Saunders.

Kampman KM, Volpicelli JR, Alterman AI, Cornish J, O'Brien CP. (2000). Amantadine in the treatment of cocaine-dependent patients with severe withdrawal symptoms. *Am J Psychiatry*, 157(12):2052-2054.

Kirby KC, Marlowe DB, Festinger DS, Garvey KA, La Monaca. (1999). Community reinforcement training for family and significant others of drug abusers: A unilateral intervention to increase treatment entry of drug users. *Drug Alcohol Depend*, 56(1):85-96.

Kohn CS, Mertens JR, Weisner CM. (2002). Coping among individuals seeking private chemical dependence treatment: Gender differences and impact on length of stay in treatment. *Alcohol Clin Exp Res*, 26(8):1228-1233.

Kosten T, O'Connor P. (2003). Management of drug and alcohol withdrawal. *N Engl J Med*, 348(18): 1786-1795.

Li M, Chen K, Mo Z. (2002). Use of qigong therapy in the detoxification of heroin addicts. *Altern Ther*, 8(1):50-54, 56-59.

Michigan Quality Improvement Consortium (MQIC). (2005). Screening and management of substance use disorders. Southfield (MI): Michigan Quality Improvement Consortium. Available online: http://www.guideline.gov. Retrieved on June 28, 2006.

Moorhead S, Johnson M, Maas M (Eds). (2004). *Nursing Outcomes Classification (NOC)*, 3rd ed. St Louis: Mosby.

Newberry L (Ed). (2003). *Sheehy's emergency nursing: Principles and practice*, 5th ed. St Louis: Mosby.

Otto KC. (2003). Acupuncture and substance abuse: A synopsis, with indications for further research. *Am J Addict*, 12(1):43-51.

Roy A. (2003). Characteristics of drug addicts who attempt suicide. *Psychiatry Res*, 121(1):99-103.

Smeltzer SC, Bare BG. (2004). *Brunner & Saddarths' textbook of medical surgical nursing,* 10th ed. New York: Lippincott Williams & Wilkins.

Soares BG, Lima MS, Reisser AA, Farrell M. (2003). Dopamine agonists for cocaine dependence. *Cochrane Database Syst Rev,* (2):CD003352.

Srisurapanont M, Jarusuraisin N, Kittirattanapaiboon P. (2001). Treatment for amphetamine withdrawal. *Cochrane Database Syst Rev,* (4):CD003021.

Stuart GW, Laraia MT. (2005). *Principles and practice of psychiatric nursing,* 8th ed. St. Louis: Mosby.

Timko C, Debenedetti A, Billow R. (2006). Intensive referral to 12-Step self-help groups and 6-month substance use disorder outcomes. *Addiction,* 101(5):678-688.

Verthein U, Haasen C, Krausz M. (2002). Auricular acupuncture as a treatment of cocaine, heroin, and alcohol addiction: A pilot study. *Addict Disord Treat,* 1(1):11-16.

Voshaar RC, Gorgels WJ, Mol AJ, van Balkom AJ, van de Lisdonk EH, Breteler MH, et al. (2003). Tapering off long-term benzodiazepine use with or without group cognitive-behavioural therapy: Three-condition, randomised controlled trial. *Br J Psychiatry,* 182:498-504.

Weiss RD, Griffin ML, Gallop RJ, Najavits LM, Frank A, Crits-Cristoph P, et al. (2005). The effect of 12-step self-help group attendance and participation on drug use outcomes among cocaine-dependent patients. *Drug Alcohol Depend,* 77(2):177-184.

SUBSTANCE USE TREATMENT: OVERDOSE   NIC

Marybeth O'Neil, MS, RN, APRN-BC

NIC **Definition:** Monitoring, treatment, and emotional support of a patient who has ingested prescription or over-the-counter drugs beyond the therapeutic range (Dochterman & Bulecheck, 2004).

NURSING ACTIVITIES

Effective

■ *Assess suicidal intent.* **LOE = V**

 A descriptive study of patients ($N = 2489$) presenting to the hospital after the repetition of self-harm and suicide demonstrated that suicidal intent at the time of overdose was associated with a risk of subsequent suicide (Harriss et al., 2005).

■ **NIC** *Explore the patient's feelings about psychiatric consultation.* **LOE = IV**

 A cohort study of patients ($N = 96$) who presented to the emergency department in a large inner city in the United Kingdom revealed that active follow-up reduced the risk of the repetition of overdose (Kapur et al., 2004).

■ **NIC** **SP** *Provide nonjudgmental support for the conscious patient.* **LOE = VII**

 A nonjudgmental attitude provides unconditional positive regard, which conveys respect for the patient and allows the nurse to develop a rapport with the patient that promotes communication and trust (Townsend, 2006; Taylor et al., 2001).

NR = Nursing Research, **MR** = Multidisciplinary Research, **SP** = Standard of Practice, **EO** = Expert Opinion, **LOE** = Level of Evidence

■ **NIC** *Facilitate follow-up counseling when the diagnosis of overdose is confirmed.* **LOE = II**

MR An RCT of patients ($N = 119$) presenting to the emergency department with deliberate self-poisoning demonstrated that psychotherapy significantly reduced suicidal ideation and repeated suicide attempts (Guthrie et al., 2003).

NR A cohort study of patients ($N = 40$) presenting to a local general acute care hospital after an act of deliberate self-harm demonstrated that solution-focused brief therapy significantly reduced repeated self-harm (Wiseman, 2003).

■ **NIC** *Provide emotional support to the patient and family. Encourage family support of the patient.* **LOE = V**

MR A descriptive study of healthy adults ($N = 201$) demonstrated that daily emotional support was predictive of optimism (Karademas, 2006).

NR A descriptive study of adolescents with cancer ($N = 45$) verified that family is the primary source of emotional support for the patients (Ritchie, 2001).

MR A descriptive study of adults with chronic pain ($N = 275$) showed that patients with supportive families reported significantly less pain intensity, less reliance on medication, and greater activity levels (Jamison & Virts, 1990).

■ **NIC** **SP** *Identify the amount and type of drug or combination of drugs ingested, and the time of ingestion, when possible.* **LOE = VII**

EO One must identify a particular drug or drugs and the time from ingestion to determine the treatment and the use of the appropriate antidote (Criddle, 2003).

■ **NIC** *Administer drug-specific antidotes when the drug that was used is known.* **LOE = V**

MR A descriptive study of patients ($N = 145$) presenting to four poison centers demonstrated that the use of antidote (N-acetylcysteine) and activated charcoal reduced the incidence of liver injury caused by acetaminophen (Spiller et al., 2006).

MR A case series of patients ($N = 27$) admitted to an emergency department of a large hospital in Taiwan with acute acetaminophen poisoning demonstrated that the use of N-acetylcysteine reduced incidence of hepatotoxicity (Tsai et al., 2005).

■ **NIC** **SP** *Monitor respiratory, cardiac, and neurological status.* **LOE = VII**

EO Respiratory and cardiac failure can result in death, and neurological damage may result from seizures (Criddle, 2003).

■ **NIC** **SP** *Monitor fluid and electrolyte levels, liver function tests, blood counts, and arterial blood gas levels.* **LOE = VII**

EO The potential for the systemic effects of toxin warrants the monitoring of all systems (Criddle, 2003).

■ **NIC** **SP** *Monitor for urinary retention and/or renal failure.* **LOE = VII**

EO In cases of overdose, some medications can cause urinary retention, and others may cause renal failure (Criddle, 2003).

RCT = Randomized Controlled (Clinical) Trial, **NIC** = Nursing Interventions Classification, **NOC** = Nursing Outcomes Classification

■ **NIC** **SP** *Monitor for convulsions, seizures, and CNS depression or stimulation.*
LOE = VII

EO Neurological changes can result from overdose, causing seizures, central nervous system depression, or stimulation (Criddle, 2003).

Possibly Effective

■ **NIC** *Administer activated charcoal when the substance used is unknown, as appropriate.* **LOE = II**

MR A descriptive study of patients ($N = 145$) presenting to four poison centers demonstrated that the use of antidote (N-acetylcysteine) and activated charcoal reduced the incidence of liver injury caused by acetaminophen (Spiller et al., 2006).

MR A randomized unblinded study ($N = 13$) of healthy volunteers showed some detoxification benefit 3 hours after overdose (Sato et al., 2003).

MR A randomized controlled four-limb crossover study ($N = 10$) of healthy volunteers did not support the administration of activated charcoal 1 hour after the ingestion of acetaminophen (Green et al., 2001).

MR A randomized controlled crossover study ($N = 12$) of healthy volunteers indicated significant reductions in acetaminophen levels at 1 and 2 hours after ingestion (Christophersen et al., 2002).

MR An RCT of patients ($N = 1479$) who presented to the emergency department with a history of recent oral drug overdose (excluding more than 140 mg/kg of acetaminophen, crack cocaine, mushrooms, volatiles, caustic agents, heavy metals, lithium, or iron preparations) indicated no significant difference between the treatment and control groups with regard to the outcome of treatment, but it did indicate a higher incidence of vomiting with activated charcoal (Merigian & Blaho, 2002).

MR An RCT ($N = 46$) of healthy adults indicated that superactivated charcoal was effective for reducing acetaminophen levels up to 3 hours after ingestion (Sato et al., 2003).

Not Effective

■ **NIC** *Lavage with normal saline using a large-bore gastric tube as appropriate.* **LOE = II**

MR A systematic review demonstrated that gastric lavage did not change the ultimate outcomes of patients (Krenzelok, 2002).

MR A randomized controlled crossover study ($N = 12$) of healthy volunteers indicated no significant difference in acetaminophen levels between gastric lavage and activated charcoal or activated charcoal alone at 1 and 2 hours after ingestion (Christophersen et al., 2002).

Possibly Harmful

■ **NIC** *Administer ipecac as appropriate.* **LOE = I**

MR A systematic review of research including randomized controlled and randomized studies demonstrated that emesis did not change the ultimate outcomes of patients (Krenzelok, 2002).

NR = Nursing Research, **MR** = Multidisciplinary Research, **SP** = Standard of Practice, **EO** = Expert Opinion, **LOE** = Level of Evidence

(MR) A position paper stated that there was no evidence from clinical studies that ipecac improved the outcomes of poisoned patients, and it suggested that the practice should be abandoned (Krenzelok et al., 2004).

OUTCOME MEASUREMENT

COPING (NOC)

Definition: Personal actions to manage stressors that tax an individual's resources.
Coping as evidenced by the following selected NOC indicators:
- Identifies multiple coping strategies
- Uses available social support
- Seeks help from a health care professional as appropriate

(Rate each indicator of **Coping:** 1 = never demonstrated, 2 = rarely demonstrated, 3 = sometimes demonstrated, 4 = often demonstrated, 5 = consistently demonstrated) (Moorhead et al., 2004).

REFERENCES

Christophersen AB, Levin D, Hoegberg LC, Angelo HR, Kampmann JP. (2002). Activated charcoal alone or after gastric lavage: A simulated large paracetamol intoxication. *Br J Clin Pharmacol,* 53(3):312-317.

Criddle LM. (2003). Toxicologic emergencies. In Newberry L (Ed): *Sheehy's emergency nursing: Principles and practice,* 5th ed. St Louis: Mosby.

Dawson A. (2004). Superactivated charcoal. *Am J Emerg Med,* 22(6):496.

Dochterman JM, Bulechek GM (Eds). (2004). *Nursing Interventions Classification (NIC),* 4th ed. St Louis: Mosby.

Green R, Grierson R, Sitar DS, Tenenbein M. (2001). How long after drug ingestion is activated charcoal still effective? *J Toxicol Clin Toxicol,* 39(6):601-605.

Guthrie E, Kapur N, Mackway-Jones K, Chew-Graham C, Moorey J, Mendel E, et al. (2003). Predictors of outcome following brief psychodynamic-interpersonal therapy for deliberate self-poisoning. *Aust N Z J Psychiatry,* 37(5):532-536.

Harriss L, Hawton K, Zahl D. (2005). Value of measuring suicidal intent in the assessment of people attending hospital following self-poisoning or self-injury. *Br J Psychiatry,* 186:60-66.

Jamison RN, Virts K. (1990). The influence of family support on chronic pain. *Behav Res Ther,* 28(4):283-287.

Kapur N, Cooper J, Hiroeh U, May C, Appleby L, House A. (2004). Emergency department management and outcome for self-poisoning: A cohort study. *Gen Hosp Psychiatry,* 26(1):36-41.

Karademas EC. (2006). Self-efficacy, social support and well being: The mediating role of optimism. *Pers Individ Dif,* 40(6):1281-1290.

Krenzelok EP. (2002). New developments in the therapy of intoxications. *Toxicol Lett,* 127(1-3):299-305.

Krenzelok EP, McGuigan M, Lheureux P, Manoguerra AS. (2004). Position paper: Ipecac syrup. *J Toxicol Clin Toxicol,* 42(2):133-143.

Merigian KS, Blaho KE. (2002). Single-dose oral activated charcoal in the treatment of the self-poisoned patient: A prospective, randomized, controlled trial. *Am J Ther,* 9(4):301-308.

Moorhead M, Johnson M, Maas M (Eds). (2004). *Nursing Outcomes Classification (NOC),* 3rd ed. St Louis: Mosby.

Osterhoudt KC, Durbin D, Alpern ER, Henretig FM. (2004). Risk factors for emesis after therapeutic use of activated charcoal in acutely poisoned children. *Pediatrics,* 113(4):806-810.

RCT = Randomized Controlled (Clinical) Trial, **NIC** = Nursing Interventions Classification, **NOC** = Nursing Outcomes Classification

Ritchie MA. (2001). Sources of emotional support for adolescents with cancer. *J Pediatr Oncol Nurs*, 18(3): 105-110.

Sato RL, Wong JJ, Sumida SM, Marn RY, Enoki NR, Yamamoto LG. (2003). Efficacy of superactivated charcoal administered late (3 hours) after acetaminophen overdose. *Am J Emerg Med*, 21(3):189-191.

Spiller HA, Winter ML, Klein-Schwartz W, Bangh SA. (2006). Efficacy of activated charcoal administered more than four hours after acetaminophen overdose. *J Emerg Med*, 30(1):1-5.

Taylor C, Lillis C, MeLone P. (2001). *Fundamentals of nursing: The art and science of nursing care*, 4th ed. Philadelphia: Lippincott Williams & Wilkins.

Townsend M. (2006). *Psychiatric mental health nursing: Concepts of care in evidence-based practice*, 5th ed. Philadelphia: F.A. Davis.

Tsai CL, Chang WT, Weng TI, Fang CC, Walson PD. (2005). A patient-tailored N-acetylcysteine protocol for acute acetaminophen intoxication. *Clin Ther*, 27(3):336-341.

Wiseman S. (2003). Brief intervention: Reducing the repetition of deliberate self-harm. *Nurs Times*, 99(35):34-36.

SUICIDE PREVENTION

Barbara L. Drew, PhD, APRN-BC

NIC **Definition:** Reducing the risk for self-inflicted harm with the intent to end life (Dochterman & Bulechek, 2004).

NURSING ACTIVITIES

Effective

■ **NIC** *Administer medications to decrease anxiety, agitation, or psychosis and to stabilize mood as appropriate.*

MR A systematic review of RCTs indicated that lithium was effective for the prevention of suicide, deliberate self-harm, and death from all causes in patients with mood disorders (Cipriani et al., 2005). **LOE = I**

MR An RCT (*N* = 980) compared the risk for suicidal behavior in patients with schizophrenia or schizoaffective disorder who were treated with clozapine or olanzapine. The clozapine group had significantly fewer incidents of suicidal behavior, subsequent hospitalizations, rescue interventions, or additional treatment with psychotropic medications than patients receiving olanzapine (Meltzer et al., 2003). **LOE = II**

■ **NIC** *Determine if the patient has the available means to follow through with a suicide plan.* **LOE = IV**

MR A case-control study matched 106 gun owners who had experienced an incident in which a child or adolescent used a firearm and shot him- or herself or someone else with 480 gun owners without shooting events. The results determined that 82 of the 106 incidents were suicide attempts (95% fatal) and that 24 were unintentional injuries (52% fatal). Guns from case households were significantly less likely to be stored unloaded, to be stored separately from ammunition, or to have ammunition that was locked, as compared with guns from control households (Grossman et al., 2005).

NR = Nursing Research, **MR** = Multidisciplinary Research, **SP** = Standard of Practice, **EO** = Expert Opinion, **LOE** = Level of Evidence

■ **NIC** *Refer the patient to a mental health care provider (e.g., psychiatrist or psychiatric/mental health advanced practice nurse) for evaluation and treatment of suicidal ideation and behavior as needed.* **LOE = II**

MR An RCT (*N* = 120) compared two groups of adults who were recruited from an emergency department after a suicide attempt. One group was scheduled for 10 outpatient weekly or biweekly cognitive therapy sessions that were specifically designed to prevent suicide, and the second group received standard care. The study demonstrated a significant reduction in the risk of repeat suicide attempts in the experimental group (Brown et al., 2005).

MR An RCT (*N* = 56) in Australia compared two groups of young people who had experienced their first episodes of psychosis and who were assessed to be at high risk for suicide. The first group received standard clinical care, whereas the second group received standard care plus cognitively oriented therapy (LifeSPAN therapy). The study demonstrated that both the treatment and control groups improved over the 6-month study period. The treatment group had a larger drop in suicidal ideation, but the difference was not significant. The treatment group also had a significantly greater decrease in hopelessness and an increase in quality of life, which are characteristics that are indirectly related to suicide (Power et al., 2003).

MR A systematic review indicated that dialectical behavior therapy was effective for reducing suicidal behavior, particularly among people with borderline personality disorder (Koerner & Linehan, 2000).

Possibly Effective

■ **NIC** *Administer medications to decrease anxiety, agitation, or psychosis and to stabilize mood as appropriate.* **LOE = I**

MR Systematic reviews of RCTs have not generally detected reductions in suicidal behavior, although selective serotonin reuptake inhibitors are effective for the treatment of depression and anxiety, both of which are risk factors for suicide (Fergusson et al., 2005; Gunnell et al., 2005; Khan et al., 2003). However, given the methodological constraints of RCTs of an outcome with such low prevalence as suicide, other forms of evidence suggest efficacy, such as correlations of suicide rates with antidepressant prescription rates in the United States (Gibbons et al., 2005).

■ *Educate the public regarding the signs and symptoms of depression in the self and others and also about the steps for responding to suicidal thoughts and behaviors.* **LOE = II**

MR An RCT (post-test only; *N* = 2100) compared two groups of high school students. The first group received a school-based suicide prevention program, whereas the second group received the standard curriculum. Students in the treatment group were 40% less likely to report a suicide attempt 3 months afterward, and they demonstrated modest increases in knowledge about depression and more adaptive attitudes toward depression and suicide. However, there was no statistical difference in help-seeking behavior (Aseltine & DeMartino, 2004).

RCT = Randomized Controlled (Clinical) Trial, **NIC** = Nursing Interventions Classification, **NOC** = Nursing Outcomes Classification

(NR) An RCT ($N = 341$) compared three groups of students who were at risk for dropping out of high school: group 1 received an individual assessment and crisis intervention program (C-CARE), group 2 received a combination of C-CARE and a small group prevention program that consisted of 12 hour-long sessions (CAST), and group 3 was a control group that received a brief assessment interview and typical school interventions. Significant decreases in suicide risk behaviors occurred for all youth, with no differences seen among groups. Participation in both treatment conditions resulted in greater reductions in depression as compared with the control group (Eggert et al., 2002).

■ (NIC) *Provide information about what community resources and outreach programs are available.* **LOE = III**

(MR) A controlled study comparing the numbers of suicides in a nature reserve in England before and after the posting of signs that displayed a phone number for crisis intervention showed that the number of suicides fell significantly from 10 per year to 3.3 per year during the 3-year study period (King & Frost, 2005).

■ *Provide follow-up care after an incident of self-harm.* **LOE = II**

(MR) An RCT ($N = 772$) compared two groups of patients who poisoned themselves. Group 1 was sent a brief greeting from the patient's health care provider on a postcard in a sealed envelope at 1, 2, 3, 4, 6, 8, 10, and 12 months after discharge, whereas the second group received standard care. Group 1 demonstrated a reduction in repetitions of self-poisoning by individuals, but the proportion of individual repeaters was not significantly reduced (Carter et al., 2005).

(MR) An RCT ($N = 843$) compared two groups of patients who had refused ongoing care after hospitalization for depression or suicidality. One group was contacted by letter at least four times per year for 5 years, whereas the second group received no further contact. The study demonstrated a reduction in suicide rate during all 5 years of the study in the treatment group. Further analysis indicated that there was a significantly lower rate of suicide in the treatment group for the first 2 years but that these differences in rates diminished over time, with no differences observed by year 14 (Motto & Bostrom, 2001).

Not Effective

■ (NIC) *Contract (verbally or in writing) with the patient for "no self-harm" for a specified period of time, recontracting at specified time intervals as appropriate.* **LOE = IV**

(NR) A correlational design with a retrospective review of the medical records ($N = 650$) of psychiatric inpatients compared patients with and without no-suicide contracts in terms of whether or not they self-harmed. Patients with contracts were seven times more likely to self-harm than patients without the contracts, which suggested that the staff negotiated contracts with people who were assessed to be at high risk for suicide and that making contracts with them did not prevent self-harm (Drew, 2001).

Possibly Harmful

No applicable published research was found in this category.

NR = Nursing Research, **MR** = Multidisciplinary Research, **SP** = Standard of Practice, **EO** = Expert Opinion, **LOE** = Level of Evidence

OUTCOME MEASUREMENT

SUICIDE SELF-RESTRAINT (NOC)

Definition: Personal actions to refrain from gestures and attempts at killing self.
Suicide Self-Restraint as evidenced by the following selected NOC indicators:
- Refrains from inflicting serious injury
- Maintains connectedness in relationships
- Expresses sense of hope
- Plans for future
- Uses available mental health services

(Rate each indicator of **Suicide Self-Restraint:** 1 = never demonstrated, 2 = rarely demonstrated, 3 = sometimes demonstrated, 4 = often demonstrated, 5 = consistently demonstrated) (Moorhead et al., 2004).

ADDITIONAL ASSESSMENT TOOLS

Self-report instruments to assess risk for suicide include the Beck Hopelessness Scale (Beck et al., 1974); the Scale for Suicide Ideation (Beck et al., 1979); and the Reasons for Living Inventory (Linehan et al., 1983).

REFERENCES

Aseltine RH Jr, DeMartino R. (2004). An outcome evaluation of the SOS Suicide Prevention Program. *Am J Public Health,* 94(3):446-451.

Beck AT, Kovacs M, Weissman A. (1979). Assessment of suicidal intention: The Scale for Suicide Ideation. *J Consult Clin Psychol,* 47(2):343-352.

Beck AT, Weissman A, Lester D, Trexler L. (1974). The measurement of pessimism: The hopelessness scale. *J Consult Clin Psychol,* 42(6):861-865.

Brown GK, Ten Have T, Henriques GR, Xie SX, Hollander JE, Beck AT. (2005). Cognitive therapy for the prevention of suicide attempts: A randomized controlled trial. *JAMA,* 294(5):563-570.

Carter GL, Clover K, Whyte IM, Dawson AH, D'Este C. (2005). Postcards from the EDge project: Randomised controlled trial of an intervention using postcards to reduce repetition of hospital treated deliberate self poisoning. *BMJ,* 331(7520):805-809.

Cipriani A, Pretty H, Hawton K, Geddes JR. (2005). Lithium in the prevention of suicidal behavior and all-cause mortality in patients with mood disorders: A systematic review of randomized trials. *Am J Psychiatry,* 162(10):1805-1819.

Dochterman JM, Bulechek GM (Eds). (2004). *Nursing Interventions Classification (NIC),* 4th ed. St Louis: Mosby.

Drew BL. (2001). Self-harm behavior and no-suicide contracting in psychiatric inpatient settings. *Arch Psychiatr Nurs,* 15(3):99-106.

Eggert LL, Thompson EA, Randell BP, Pike KC. (2002). Preliminary effects of brief school-based prevention approaches for reducing youth suicide—risk behaviors, depression, and drug involvement. *J Child Adolesc Psychiatr Nurs,* 15(2):48-64.

Fergusson D, Doucette S, Glass KC, Shapiro S, Healy D, Hebert P, et al. (2005). Association between suicide attempts and selective serotonin reuptake inhibitors: Systematic review of randomised controlled trials. *BMJ,* 330(7488):396-402.

Gibbons RD, Hur K, Bhaumik DK, Mann JJ. (2005). The relationship between antidepressant medication use and rate of suicide. *Arch Gen Psychiatry,* 62(2):165-172.

Grossman DC, Mueller BA, Riedy C, Dowd MD, Villaveces A, Prodzinski J, et al. (2005). Gun storage practices and risk of youth suicide and unintentional firearm injuries. *JAMA,* 293(6):707-714.

Gunnell D, Saperia J, Ashby D. (2005). Selective serotonin reuptake inhibitors (SSRIs) and suicide in adults: Meta-analysis of drug company data from placebo controlled, randomised controlled trials submitted to the MHRA's safety review. *BMJ*, 330(7488):385-389.

Khan A, Khan S, Kolts R, Brown WA. (2003). Suicide rates in clinical trials of SSRIs, other antidepressants, and placebo: Analysis of FDA reports. *Am J Psychiatry*, 160(4):790-792.

King E, Frost N. (2005). The New Forest Suicide Prevention Initiative (NFSPI). *Crisis*, 26(1):25-33.

Koerner K, Linehan MM. (2000). Research on dialectical behavior therapy for patients with borderline personality disorder. *Psychiatr Clin North Am*, 23(1):151-167.

Linehan MM, Goodstein JL, Nielsen SL, Chiles JA. (1983). Reasons for staying alive when you are thinking of killing yourself: The reasons for living inventory. *J Consult Clin Psychol*, 51(2):276-286.

Meltzer HY, Alphs L, Green AI, Altamura AC, Anand R, Bertoldi A, et al. (2003). Clozapine treatment for suicidality in schizophrenia: International Suicide Prevention Trial (InterSePT). *Arch Gen Psychiatry*, 60(1):82-91.

Moorhead M, Johnson M, Maas M (Eds). (2004). *Nursing Outcomes Classification (NOC)*, 3rd ed. St Louis: Mosby.

Motto JA, Bostrom AG. (2001). A randomized controlled trial of postcrisis suicide prevention. *Psychiatr Serv*, 52(6):828-833.

Power PJ, Bell RJ, Mills R, Herrman-Doig T, Davern M, Henry L, et al. (2003). Suicide prevention in first episode psychosis: The development of a randomised controlled trial of cognitive therapy for acutely suicidal patients with early psychosis. *Aust N Z J Psychiatry*, 37(4):414-420.

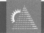 # SURGICAL PREPARATION NIC

Maria Marinelli, BSN, CNOR, RNFA

NIC **Definition:** Providing care to a patient immediately prior to surgery and verifying required procedures/tests and documentation in the clinical record (Dochterman & Bulechek, 2004).

NURSING ACTIVITIES

Effective

■ **NIC** *Ensure that the patient is NPO as appropriate.* **LOE = I**

MR A Cochrane systematic review found that there was no evidence to suggest that a shortened fluid fast of several hours by adult surgical patients results in an increased risk of aspiration, regurgitation, or related morbidity as compared with the standard "nothing by mouth after midnight" fasting policy (Brady et al., 2003).

■ **NIC** *Reinforce preoperative teaching information.* **LOE = I**

MR An RCT ($N = 42$) compared the results of patients who received two episodes of preoperative instruction on stoma education with the result of those who received only postoperative training and found that those who received two episodes demonstrated improved patient outcomes and cost effectiveness (Chaudhri et al., 2005).

NR A Cochrane systematic review found that patients who were involved in a structured preoperative teaching regimen before cataract surgery had decreased anxiety levels. Use of the Spielberger State—Trait Anxiety Inventory enabled the researchers to assess the results of sympathetic nervous system response during the surgical intervention (Morrell, 2001).

NR = Nursing Research, **MR** = Multidisciplinary Research, **SP** = Standard of Practice, **EO** = Expert Opinion, **LOE** = Level of Evidence

■ *Provide preoperative patients with an instructional videotape depicting the breathing and movement skills that they will use during the postoperative period.* **LOE = III**

(NR) A controlled clinical trial (*N* = 70) demonstrated that providing a preoperative intervention videotape depicting breathing and movement skills increased a surgical patient's self-efficacy concepts and provided improvements in postoperative pain and mobility (Heye et al., 2002).

■ *Provide oral preoperative medication to reduce gastric acidity as appropriate.* **LOE = II**

(MR) An RCT (*N* = 60) concluded that oral erythromycin and nizatidine given 1 hour before surgery was effective for reducing gastric pH and volume (Memis et al., 2002).

■ (NIC) (SP) *Administer a surgical shave, scrub, shower, enema, and/or douche as appropriate.* **LOE = VII**

(EO) The surgical site should be free of soil and debris; removing transient microbes, superficial soil, and debris reduces the risk of wound contamination during a surgical procedure (AORN, 2005).

■ *Use clippers to remove hair preoperatively.* **LOE = I**

(EO) The Centers for Disease Control and Prevention Guideline for Prevention of Surgical Site Infection states that using clippers for hair removal immediately before an operation has been shown to be associated with a lower risk of surgical site infection as compared with shaving or clipping performed the night before surgery (Mangram et al., 1999).

(MR) A Cochrane systematic review found that hair removal by clipping was recommended rather than shaving, because microscopic cuts and abrasions often harbor colonizations of microorganisms that may produce surgical site infections (Tanner et al., 2006).

■ *Provide preoperative medication to help relieve the anxiety of surgical patients.* **LOE = I**

(MR) A Cochrane systematic review found that providing premedication for anxiety in adult day care settings helped to alleviate the level of anxiety for surgical patients without delaying discharge from the unit (Smith & Pittaway, 2003).

(MR) An RCT (*N* = 88) demonstrated that administering intravenous midazolam 20 minutes preoperatively provided the surgical patient with an effective anxiolytic result; there was also increased patient satisfaction and a reduction in postoperative nausea and vomiting in the control group (Bauer et al., 2004).

■ (NIC) *Apply sequential compression device sleeves as appropriate.* **LOE = I**

(MR) A meta-analysis concluded that intermittent pneumatic compression devices were more efficacious than graduated compression stockings or mini doses of heparin for the prevention of deep vein thrombosis (Vanek, 1998).

(MR) A literature review concluded that intermittent compression prevented deep vein thrombosis and venous stasis (Morris & Woodcock, 2004).

RCT = Randomized Controlled (Clinical) Trial, **NIC** = Nursing Interventions Classification, **NOC** = Nursing Outcomes Classification

■ *Provide hypnosis to reduce preoperative anxiety.* **LOE = II**

(MR) An RCT ($N = 76$) determined that hypnosis significantly alleviated preoperative anxiety (Saadat et al., 2006).

Possibly Effective

■ *Provide a patient-selected music session in the preoperative holding area.*
LOE = II

(MR) An RCT ($N = 93$) reported that preoperative patients who listened to a 30-minute patient-selected music selection reported lower levels of state anxiety; however, physiological outcomes were not significantly different (Wang et al., 2002).

■ *Provide acupressure to decrease preoperative anxiety.* **LOE = II**

(MR) An RCT ($N = 76$) determined that acupressure was effective for decreasing both preoperative anxiety and bispectral index values; however, these effects were not sustained 30 minutes after the release of the acupressure (Agarwal et al., 2005).

■ *Instruct the patient preoperatively to shower with skin antiseptics to prevent surgical site infection.* **LOE = I**

(MR) A Cochrane systematic review found that there was no benefit for preoperative showering or bathing with chlorhexidine as compared with other wash products for reducing the development of surgical site infections (Webster & Osborne, 2007).

■ (SP) *Whenever possible, leave hair at the surgical site.* **LOE = IV**

(EO) If hair is to be removed, then the following guidelines should be used (AORN, 2005):
• Personnel skilled in hair removal techniques should perform the removal.
• Hair removal should take place as close to the time of surgery as possible.
• Hair removal should take place outside of the room in which the surgery is to be performed.
• Hair removal should be performed in a manner that preserves skin integrity.
(MR) In a case-controlled study ($N = 250$) of neurosurgical patients having craniotomy surgical procedures, 100 patients were shaved and 150 were not shaved. There was no statistical difference in the number of surgical site infections between the two groups (Miller et al., 2001).

Possibly Harmful

■ *Not discontinuing sequential compression devices as recommended; if the patient is mobile, there is an increased risk for patient injury as a result of falls.*
LOE = VII

(EO) Patients wearing sequential compression devices are more than three times as likely to have serious events associated with falls as compared with those without the devices in place (PPSA, 2005).

NR = Nursing Research, **MR** = Multidisciplinary Research, **SP** = Standard of Practice, **EO** = Expert Opinion, **LOE** = Level of Evidence

OUTCOME MEASUREMENT

KNOWLEDGE: TREATMENT PROCEDURE(S) (NOC)

Definition: Extent of understanding conveyed about procedure(s) required as part of a treatment regimen.

Knowledge: Treatment Procedure(s) as evidenced by the following selected NOC indicators:

- Description of treatment procedure(s)
- Explanation of purpose of procedure(s)

(Rate each indicator of **Knowledge: Treatment Procedure(s):** 1 = none, 2 = limited, 3 = moderate, 4 = substantial, 5 = extensive) (Moorhead et al., 2004).

REFERENCES

Agarwal A, Ranjan R, Dhiraaj S, Lakra A, Kumar M, Singh U. (2005). Acupressure for prevention of pre-operative anxiety: A prospective, randomised, placebo controlled study. *Anaesthesia,* 60(10):978-981.

Association of Perioperative Registered Nurses (AORN). (2005). AORN recommended standards of practice for skin preparation of patients. *AORN J* (August) 443-445.

Bauer KP, Dom PM, Ramirez AM, O'Flaherty JE. (2004). Preoperative intravenous midazolam: Benefits beyond anxiolysis. *J Clin Anesth,* 16(3):177-183.

Brady M, Kinn S, Stuart P. (2003). Preoperative fasting for adults to prevent perioperative complications. *Cochrane Database Syst Rev,* (4):CD004423.

Chaudhri S, Brown L, Hassan I, Horgan AF. (2005). Preoperative intensive, community-based vs. traditional stoma education: A randomized, controlled trial. *Dis Colon Rectum,* 48(3):504-509.

Dochterman JM, Bulechek GM (Eds). (2004). *Nursing Interventions Classification (NIC),* 4th ed. St. Louis: Mosby.

Heye ML, Foster L, Bartlett MK, Adkins S. (2002). A preoperative intervention for pain reduction, improved mobility, and self-efficacy. *Appl Nurs Res,* 15(3):174-183.

Mangram AJ, Horan TC, Pearson ML, Silver LC, Jarvis WR. (1999). Guideline for prevention of surgical site infection, 1999. Centers for Disease Control and Prevention (CDC) Hospital Infection Control Practices Advisory Committee. *Am J Infect Control,* 27(2):97-132.

Memis D, Turan A, Karamanlioglu B, Guler T, Yurdakoc A, Pamukcu Z, et al. (2002). Effect of preoperative oral use of erythromycin and nizatidine on gastric pH and volume. *Anaesth Intensive Care,* 30(4):428-432.

Miller JJ, Weber PC, Patel S, Ramey J. (2001). Intracranial surgery: To shave or not to shave? *Otol Neurotol,* 22(6):908-911.

Moorhead M, Johnson M, Maas M (Eds). (2004). *Nursing Outcomes Classification (NOC),* 3rd ed. St Louis: Mosby.

Morrell G. (2001). Effect of structured preoperative teaching on anxiety levels of patients scheduled for cataract surgery. *Insight,* 26(1):4-9.

Morris RJ, Woodcock J. (2004). Evidence-based compression: Prevention of stasis and deep vein thrombosis. *Ann Surg,* 239(2):162-171.

Pennsylvania Patient Safety Advisory (PPSA). (2005). Pennsylvania PSRS Safety Authority 2005 Annual Report. *Patient Safety Advisory,* 2(3):56-57.

Saadat H, Drummond-Lewis J, Maranets I, Kaplan D, Saadat A, Wang SM, et al. (2006). Hypnosis reduces preoperative anxiety in adult patients. *Anesth Analg,* 102(5):1394-1396.

Smith AF, Pittaway AJ. (2003). Premedication for anxiety in adult day surgery. *Cochrane Database Syst Rev,* (1):CD002192.

Tanner J, Woodings D, Moncaster K. (2006). Preoperative hair removal to reduce surgical site infection. *Cochrane Database Syst Rev,* (2):CD004122.

Vanek VW. (1998). Meta-analysis of effectiveness of intermittent pneumatic compression devices with a comparison of thigh-high to knee-high sleeves. *Ann Surg,* 64(11):1050-1058.

RCT = Randomized Controlled (Clinical) Trial, **NIC** = Nursing Interventions Classification, **NOC** = Nursing Outcomes Classification

Wang SM, Kulkarni L, Dolev J, Kain ZN. (2002). Music and preoperative anxiety: A randomized, controlled study. *Anesth Analg,* 94(6):1489-1494.

Webster J, Osborne S. (2007). Preoperative bathing or showering with skin antiseptics to prevent surgical site infection. *Cochrane Database Syst Rev,* (1):CD004985.

 # SWALLOWING THERAPY

Janet C. Mentes, PhD, APRN-BC

> NIC **Definition:** Facilitating swallowing and preventing complications of impaired swallowing (Dochterman & Bulechek, 2004).

NURSING ACTIVITIES

Effective

■ *Ensure that the patient with possible dysphagia receives a formal swallowing evaluation to help reduce the likelihood of aspiration pneumonia.* **LOE = II**

MR An evidenced-based review of the management of dysphagia found that referral for a formal swallowing evaluation was indicated for preventing aspiration pneumonia (Smith Hammond & Goldstein, 2006).

MR A prospective multisite group RCT ($N = 2532$ cases) found that hospitals that used a formal dysphagia screening protocol to treat ischemic stroke patients had a lowered rate of pneumonia (2.4%) as compared with hospitals that did not use a formal protocol (5.4%; Hinchey et al., 2005).

MR In a controlled trial of patients with acute stroke ($N = 124$), early swallow screening and dysphagia management reduced the risk of aspiration pneumonia (Odderson et al., 1995).

■ *Position the patient as recommended from a swallowing evaluation for improved safety during swallowing.* **LOE = III**

EO Compensatory postural strategies, including chin positioning and neck rotation that enables patients with dysphagia to swallow safely, are recommended (Smith Hammond & Goldstein, 2006).

MR In a controlled study ($N = 165$) of the use of postural strategies (chin down, chin up, or head rotated), aspiration was eliminated in 77% of the sample during video fluoroscopy testing (Rasley et al.,1993).

MR A quasi-experimental study ($N = 75$) showed that patients' dysphagia limit (the amount of fluid swallowed safely in one swallow) increased among patients who used chin tucking or head rotation toward their paretic side (Ertekin et al., 2001).

EO Positioning people with dysphagia at an upright 90-degree angle for drinking or eating prevents aspiration (Metheny, 2004).

■ *Use a combination program that includes swallowing exercises/training plus diet modification to promote effective swallowing and to decrease swallowing-related complications.* **LOE = II**

NR A quasi-experimental study ($N = 61$) demonstrated that patients in the experimental group who received an 8-week combination intervention consisting of diet modification,

NR = Nursing Research, **MR** = Multidisciplinary Research, **SP** = Standard of Practice, **EO** = Expert Opinion, **LOE** = Level of Evidence

swallowing exercises, and positioning improved swallowing volumes, mid-arm circumference, and body weight while decreasing episodes of choking as compared with the control group (Lin et al., 2003).

MR An RCT of 306 patients with dysphagia showed that patients who received a high-intensity swallowing intervention as compared with usual care or a low-intensity swallowing intervention were more likely to return to a normal diet and to recover swallowing ability by 6 months (Carnaby et al., 2006).

■ *Add a thickening agent to fluids and use food consistencies as determined by the swallowing evaluation to reduce the risk of aspiration.* **LOE = III**

EO Standardized consistencies of food and fluids to manage dysphagia and reduce the likelihood of aspiration are recommended (ADA, 2002).

MR An evidence-based review recommended the prescription of dietary modifications for stroke patients with dysphagia that could be re-evaluated with testing by offering food and fluids that were consistent with a normal diet during imaging testing (Smith Hammond & Goldstein, 2006).

MR In a prospective observational study ($N = 160$), patients referred for a swallowing evaluation found that aspiration was greater for thin liquids (23.7%) than for ultra thick liquids (5.8%) and that aspiration was more likely with a cup than when fluids were offered by spoon (Kuhlemeier et al., 2001).

Possibly Effective

■ *Encourage patients to perform swallowing exercises as prescribed that can improve swallowing effectiveness.* **LOE = IV**

EO For patients who are generally deconditioned and specifically those who have muscle weakness during swallowing, a variety of exercises with and without electromyographic biofeedback or electric stimulation are promising, but they cannot be recommended (Smith Hammond & Goldstein, 2006).

MR In a single group pre-test/post-test design study ($N = 10$), a progressive lingual resistance exercise program was shown to be effective for improving swallowing pressures and lingual volume (Robbins et al., 2005).

MR In a crossover controlled trial ($N = 27$) of patients with dysphagia of different causes, all patients demonstrated improved upper esophageal opening and laryngeal anterior excursion that resulted in the resumption of oral feeding (Shaker et al., 2002).

MR In a case-control study in which healthy middle-aged and older adults ($N = 64$) completed an effortful swallow, the control exercise improved oral pressures and decreased oral residue, thus indicating a more effective swallow (Hind et al., 2001).

Not Effective

■ *Adding thickening agents to fluids and modifying food consistencies.* **LOE = III**

EO Although modifying the consistency of food and fluids is standard practice for people with swallowing problems, several studies have shown that patients receiving thickened fluids do not meet daily fluid requirements (Finestone et al., 2001; Goulding & Bakheit, 2000).

RCT = Randomized Controlled (Clinical) Trial, **NIC** = Nursing Interventions Classification, **NOC** = Nursing Outcomes Classification

■ *Using a drinking straw for elderly people.* **LOE = VI**

(MR) A comparative descriptive study of healthy older ($N = 18$) and younger ($N = 20$) men found a reduction in airway protection with the use of a straw for drinking among the older men as compared with the younger men (Daniels et al., 2004).

(MR) A comparative controlled study ($N = 11$) demonstrated that increased labial (lip) muscle activity was present with the use of a straw versus the use of a spoon or cup to ingest liquids (Murray et al., 1998).

■ *Using enteral feeding tubes for patients with advanced dementia.* **LOE = V**

(NR) A retrospective medical record review of veterans with dementia who were referred for percutaneous endoscopic gastrostomy (PEG) tubes as compared with those not receiving PEG tubes demonstrated no survival benefit for those who received PEG tubes (Murphy & Lipman, 2003).

(MR) A systematic review of studies examining the effectiveness of tube feedings for patients with advanced dementia found that the use of tube feedings did not prevent aspiration pneumonia, reduce the risk of pressure ulcers, or provide palliation (Finucane et al., 1999).

■ *Providing for the early use of PEG tubes in patients with swallowing difficulties.* **LOE = I**

(MR) In a cohort study ($N = 127$) of patients scheduled for PEG tube insertion, 61 patients received early PEG tube insertion while hospitalized, and 66 patients received PEG tubes 30 days after discharge. Those patients who received PEG tubes after discharge had a 40% lower mortality rate than those who received earlier PEG tube insertion (Abuksis et al., 2004).

(MR) In two arms of a multicenter RCT (83 hospitals in 15 countries) evaluating the use of enteral feeding tubes for patients with dysphagia, the first arm of the trial found that the early use of enteral feeding tubes as compared with avoiding their use improved the survival rate of those using the tubes but also increased poor longer-term outcomes (i.e., functional status, place of residence, method of feeding, quality of life). In the second arm, which examined the use of PEG or nasogastric tubes, PEG tube use was associated with increased mortality and poor longer-term outcomes (Dennis et al., 2005). (Note: In both of these studies, there was a recommendation for the use of a nasogastric tube early during the course of treatment for dysphagia.)

Possibly Harmful

No applicable published research was found in this category.

OUTCOME

SWALLOWING STATUS (NOC)

(Please refer to *Nursing Outcomes Classification* [Moorhead et al., 2004] for the **Swallowing Status** outcome.)

NR = Nursing Research, **MR** = Multidisciplinary Research, **SP** = Standard of Practice, **EO** = Expert Opinion, **LOE** = Level of Evidence

REFERENCES

Abuksis G, Mor M, Plaut S, Fraser G, Niv Y. (2004). Outcome of percutaneous endoscopic gastrostomy (PEG): Comparison of two policies in a 4-year experience. *Clin Nutr*, 23(3):341-346.

American Dietetic Association (ADA). (2002). *National dysphagia diet: Standardization for optimal care.* Chicago: The American Dietetics Association.

Carnaby G, Hankey GJ, Pizzi J. (2006). Behavioural intervention for dysphagia in acute stroke: a randomised controlled trial. *Lancet Neurol*, 5(1):31-37.

Daniels SK, Corey DM, Hadskey LD, Legendre C, Priestly DH, Rosenbek JC, et al. (2004). Mechanism of sequential swallowing during straw drinking in healthy young and older adults. *J Speech Lang Hear Res*, 47(1):33-45.

Dennis MS, Lewis SC, Warlow C; FOOD Trial Collaboration. (2005). Effect of timing and method of enteral tube feeding for dysphagic stroke patients (FOOD): A multicentre randomised controlled trial. *Lancet*, 365(9461):764-772.

Dochterman JM, Bulechek GM (Eds). (2004). *Nursing Interventions Classification (NIC)*, 4th ed. St Louis: Mosby.

Ertekin C, Keskin A, Kiylioglu N, Kirazli Y, On AY, Tarlaci S, et al. (2001). The effect of head and neck positions on oropharyngeal swallowing: A clinical and electrophysiologic study. *Arch Phys Med Rehabil*, 82(9):1255-1260.

Finestone HM, Foley NC, Woodbury MG, Greene-Finestone L. (2001). Quantifying fluid intake in dysphagic stroke patients: A preliminary comparison of oral and nonoral strategies. *Arch Phys Med Rehabil*, 82(12):1744-1746.

Finucane TE, Christmas C, Travis K. (1999). Tube feeding in patients with advanced dementia: A review of the evidence. *JAMA*, 282(14):1365-1370.

Goulding R, Bakheit AM. (2000). Evaluation of the benefits of monitoring fluid thickness in the dietary management of dysphagic stroke patients. *Clin Rehabil*, 14(2):119-124.

Hinchey JA, Shephard T, Furie K, Smith D, Wang D, Tonn S; Stroke Practice Improvement Network Investigators. (2005). Formal dysphagia screening protocols prevent pneumonia. *Stroke*, 36(9):1972-1976.

Hind JA, Nicosia MA, Roecker EB, Carnes ML, Robbins J. (2001). Comparison of effortful and noneffortful swallows in healthy middle-aged and older adults. *Arch Phys Med Rehabil*, 82(12):1661-1665.

Kuhlemeier KV, Palmer JB, Rosenberg D. (2001). Effect of liquid bolus consistency and delivery method on aspiration and pharyngeal retention in dysphagia patients. *Dysphagia*, 16(2):119-122.

Lin LC, Wang SC, Chen SH, Wang TG, Chen MY, Wu SC. (2003). Efficacy of swallowing training for residents following stroke. *J Adv Nurs*, 44(5):469-478.

Metheny N. (2004). Preventing aspiration in older adults with dysphagia. In Boltz M (Ed). *Try this: Best practices in nursing care to older adults.* New York: The Hartford Institute for Geriatric Nursing, Division of Nursing, New York University.

Moorhead M, Johnson M, Maas M (Eds). (2004). *Nursing Outcomes Classification (NOC)*, 3rd ed. St Louis: Mosby.

Murphy LM, Lipman TO. (2003). Percutaneous endoscopic gastrostomy does not prolong survival in patients with dementia. *Arch Intern Med*, 163(11):1351-1353.

Murray KA, Larson CR, Logemann JA. (1998). Electromyographic response of the labial muscles during normal liquid swallows using a spoon, a straw, and a cup. *Dysphagia*, 13(3):160-166.

Odderson IR, Keaton JC, McKenna BS. (1995). Swallow management in patients on an acute stroke pathway: Quality is cost effective. *Arch Phys Med Rehabil*, 76(12):1130-1133.

Rasley A, Logemann JA, Kahrilas PJ, Rademaker AW, Pauloski BR, Dodds WJ. (1993). Prevention of barium aspiration during videofluoroscopic swallowing studies: Value of change in posture. *Am J Roentgenol*, 160(5):1005-1009.

Robbins J, Gangnon RE, Theis SM, Kays SA, Hewitt AL, Hind JA. (2005). The effects of lingual exercise on swallowing in older adults. *J Am Geriatr Soc*, 53(9):1483-1489.

Shaker R, Easterling C, Kern M, Nitschke T, Massey B, Daniels S, et al. (2002). Rehabilitation of swallowing by exercise in tube-fed patients with pharyngeal dysphagia secondary to abnormal UES opening. *Gastroenterology*, 122(5):1314-1321.

Smith Hammond CA, Goldstein LB. (2006). Cough and aspiration of food and liquids due to oral-pharyngeal dysphagia: ACCP evidence-based clinical practice guidelines. *Chest*, 129(1 Suppl):154S-168S.

RCT = Randomized Controlled (Clinical) Trial, **NIC** = Nursing Interventions Classification, **NOC** = Nursing Outcomes Classification

TEACHING: DISEASE PROCESS

Judith Kutzleb, MSN, RN, CCRN, APN-C

NIC **Definition:** Assisting the patient to understand information related to a specific disease process (Dochterman & Bulechek, 2004).
(Note: This guideline focuses on heart failure.)

NURSING ACTIVITIES

Effective

■ *Provide education (nurse directed and/or multidisciplinary) to patients with heart failure, focusing on warning signs of decompensation, diet, medication management, lifestyle changes, and exercise (Kutzleb & Reiner, 2006).* **LOE = I**

EO A nurse-directed patient education treatment strategy significantly improves the patient's role in symptom control and disease self-management (Kutzleb & Reiner, 2006).

NR A prospective quasi-experimental research study ($N = 23$) comparing a nurse-directed care group ($N = 13$) receiving comprehensive disease management education and weekly telephone follow-up with a routine care group ($N = 10$) receiving protocol-driven management demonstrated that nurse-directed patient education was effective for improving patients' roles in symptom control, disease self-management, and quality of life (Kutzleb & Reiner, 2006).

MR A prospective randomized trial ($N = 282$) of intensive patient education, protocol-driven medical therapy, individualized dietary assessment, instruction, and intensive follow-up revealed that rates of reduced hospital admissions and improved quality of life were at least equivalent to those reported with vasodilator therapy, including treatment with angiotensin-converting enzyme inhibitors (Rich et al., 1995).

MR An RCT ($N = 98$) of hospitalized patients with stage IV heart failure found that multidisciplinary care provided essential benefits to patient outcomes (McDonald et al., 2002).

MR An RCT ($N = 98$) found more deaths in a routine care group of hospitalized patients (35.5%) than in a multidisciplinary care group (7.8%) and more rehospitalizations in the routine care group (25.5%) as compared with the multidisciplinary group (3.9%) (McDonald et al., 2002).

Possibly Effective

■ *Instruct patients regarding possible psychological disorders.* **LOE = IV**

EO Depression is found among patients with heart failure (Bennett et al., 1997).

NR A prospective study ($N = 62$) of two groups of adults, one hospitalized and the other outpatient, examined indices of left ventricular function as predictors of hospitalization and showed no specific correlation with rehospitalization. However, heart failure decompensation was presaged by increased anxiety and disorders of mentation (Bennett et al., 1997).

MR A pilot study to diagnose major depressive episodes in heart failure patients ($N = 60$) as a predictor of mortality concluded that there were no differences between the depressed and

NR = Nursing Research, **MR** = Multidisciplinary Research, **SP** = Standard of Practice, **EO** = Expert Opinion, **LOE** = Level of Evidence

nondepressed groups with respect to 3-month readmission and mortality rates among patients who were discharged alive. However, there were trends toward an increased number of inpatient days and higher mortality among the depressed patients (50%) at 3 months than among nondepressed patients (29%) at 1 year. The conclusion was that screening for depression should become a routine part of the medical evaluation of heart failure patients (Freedland et al., 1991).

Not Effective

No applicable published research was found in this category.

Possibly Harmful

No applicable published research was found in this category.

OUTCOME MEASUREMENT

KNOWLEDGE: DISEASE PROCESS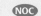

(Please refer to *Nursing Outcomes Classification* [Moorhead et al., 2004] for the **Knowledge: Disease Process** outcome.)

(Note: This outcome requires multiple assessments regarding the ability to validate the patient's understanding of disease-specific education by the patient's demonstration or verbalization of provided nurse-directed education.)

REFERENCES

Bennett SJ, Pressler ML, Hays L, Firestine L, Huster GA. (1997). Psychosocial variables and hospitalizations in persons with chronic heart failure. *Prog Cardiovasc Nurs*, 12(4):4-11.

Dochterman JM, Bulechek GM (Eds). (2004). *Nursing Interventions Classification (NIC)*, 4th ed. St Louis: Mosby.

Freedland KE, Carney RM, Rich MW. (1991). Depression in elderly patients with congestive heart failure. *J Geriatr Psychol Neurol*, 24(1):59-71.

Kutzleb J, Reiner D. (2006). The impact of nurse-directed patient education on quality of life and functional capacity in people with heart failure. *J Am Acad Nurse Pract*, 18(3):116-123.

McDonald K, Ledwidge M, Cahill J, Quigley P, Maurer B, Travers B, et al. (2002). Heart failure management: Multidisciplinary care has intrinsic benefit above the optimization of medical care. *J Card Fail*, 8(3):142-148.

Moorhead M, Johnson M, Maas M (Eds). (2004). *Nursing Outcomes Classification (NOC)*, 3rd ed. St Louis: Mosby.

Rich MW, Beckham V, Wittenberg C, Leven CL, Freedland KE, Carney RM. (1995). A multidisciplinary intervention to prevent readmission of elderly patients with congestive heart failure. *N Engl J Med*, 333(18):1190-1195.

 # TEACHING: FOOT CARE

Deborah L. Gentile, MSN, RN-BC

NIC **Definition:** Preparing a patient at risk and/or significant other to provide preventive foot care (Dochterman & Bulechek, 2004).

RCT = Randomized Controlled (Clinical) Trial, **NIC** = Nursing Interventions Classification, **NOC** = Nursing Outcomes Classification

NURSING ACTIVITIES

Effective

■ **NIC** *Determine current level of knowledge and skills related to foot care.*
LOE = II

NR A randomized prospective study ($N = 40$) designed to improve foot care among home health patients with diabetes used the Foot Care Practices Questionnaire to assess participants' current foot care practices, developed a Foot Care Self-Efficacy Questionnaire, and implemented an educational intervention to improve foot care knowledge and self-efficacy in foot care self-practices. The intervention improved patients' knowledge about foot care and improved self-care practices, such as washing the feet correctly and wearing proper footwear (Corbett, 2003).

MR An RCT involving patients ($N = 1939$) and health care professionals ($N = 150$) assessed knowledge of foot care in both groups. An integrated foot care model was implemented and resulted in increased foot care knowledge for both health care professionals and patients (Donohoe et al., 2000).

MR A systematic review of RCTs ($N = 8$) found that patient education may have a positive but short-lived effect on foot care knowledge and the behavior of patients. Studies reported possible reductions in foot ulceration and amputations, especially among high-risk patients. The poor quality of the studies was cited as a limitation in this review (Valk et al., 2002).

■ **NIC** *Determine current foot care practices.* **LOE = VII**

EO Practice guidelines endorsed by the Diabetes Committee of the American Orthopaedic Foot and Ankle Society are not based on randomized clinical trials, and they include citations from literature that demonstrates a low level of evidence. This article provides guidelines for screening patients who are at risk for developing diabetic foot complications, components of screening and follow-up foot examinations, guidelines for patient education about diabetic foot care, basic treatment guidelines, and guidelines for making referrals to specialists such as orthopedic specialists, endocrinologists, infectious disease experts, and radiologists (Pinzur et al., 2005).

MR An RCT ($N = 276$) demonstrated that the use of Promogran wound dressing (a topical dressing with collagen and oxidized regenerated cellulose materials) resulted in similar wound healing of diabetic foot ulcers as compared with moistened gauze dressings (Veves et al., 2002).

MR A randomized, double-blind, placebo-controlled study ($N = 36$) compared nerve growth factor with conventional topical treatments for noninfected foot ulcers. The treatment group showed a statistically significant acceleration of the healing process (Landi et al., 2003).

MR A randomized study ($N = 8$) compared five patients in a treatment group with three control patients regarding an intervention using lavender and chamomile essential oil to treat grade II and III foot ulcers. Quicker healing was reported for the treatment group (Hartman & Coetzee, 2002).

■ **NIC** *Provide information related to the level of risk for injury.* **LOE = VII**

MR A cross-sectional comparative study ($N = 92$) of plantar sensory levels in diabetic subjects with and without ulceration tested plantar sensory threshold at five sites on the sole of each

---

NR = Nursing Research, **MR** = Multidisciplinary Research, **SP** = Standard of Practice, **EO** = Expert Opinion, **LOE** = Level of Evidence

foot. A 4.5-gram monofilament was applied under the first metatarsal head to determine whether there was any loss of protective sensation. Patients who could not sense the monofilament were considered to be at risk for undetected injury (Saltzman et al., 2004).

(EO) Best practices for the prevention, diagnosis, and treatment of diabetic foot ulcers were drawn from expert opinion, known current clinical practices, and available research (Inlow et al., 2000).

(EO) An overview of the scope of the diabetic foot problem includes the discussion of risk factors for foot ulceration, such as neuropathy, past ulcer history, foot shape, age, and social status. A brief discussion of foot problems and quality of life is presented. The need for screening for diabetes in patients who present with peripheral neuropathy, vascular disease, and foot ulceration is stressed, because these conditions may be the presenting feature of type 2 diabetes. Diabetic foot ulceration is described as largely preventable by providing foot care education and the regular medical review of high-risk patients (Boulton & Vileikyte, 2000).

■ (NIC) *Assist in developing a plan for daily foot assessment and care at home.* LOE = II

(NR) A randomized prospective study ($N = 40$) designed to improve foot care in home health patients with diabetes provided insight into foot care in the home and increased foot care self-efficacy (Corbett, 2003).

(EO) A review of foot care for older adults presented information that was applicable to diabetic and nondiabetic elders. It stressed the importance of foot care for all elderly and the need for foot care as a core competency for nurses who specialize in gerontology (Pattillo, 2004).

■ (NIC) *Determine capacity to carry out foot care (i.e., visual acuity, physical mobility, and judgment).* LOE = II

(MR) An RCT of the self-management of basic foot care among the elderly determined the participants' ability and suitability to manage foot self-care successfully by using a near vision test, a reach test, and a grip strength test. Results showed that patients who were taught to self-manage routine foot care had the same therapeutic results as those who received usual care by a podiatrist. Clinical and cost effectiveness were demonstrated by the self-management program (Waxman et al., 2003).

■ (NIC) *Provide information regarding the relationship between neuropathy, injury, and vascular disease and the risk for ulceration and lower-extremity amputation in persons with diabetes.* LOE = V

(EO) A review presented foot lesions from the epidemiological perspective, including a brief discussion of the epidemiology of foot lesions in diabetes and in diabetic patients with renal disease. Causes of ischemic and neuropathic diabetic foot conditions are compared and contrasted. Assessment and treatment strategies for the diabetic foot are presented for the acute management of the patient with diabetic gangrene and for those in need of revascularization procedures (Schömig et al., 2000).

(NR) A review stressed the role of the nephrology nurse in foot examinations and education aimed at preventing amputations in patients with diabetes and chronic kidney disease. Foot

---

RCT = Randomized Controlled (Clinical) Trial, **NIC** = Nursing Interventions Classification, **NOC** = Nursing Outcomes Classification

examinations were identified as the most fundamental step in reducing the risk of foot ulceration and amputation. Risk factors for ulceration such as vasculopathy, altered biomechanics of the foot (increased plantar pressure, bony abnormalities, and limited joint mobility), and a history of previous ulceration or amputation were discussed. An in-depth review of assessing the diabetic foot provided the basis for practice changes that could lead to the prevention of foot ulceration and amputation (Broersma, 2004).

(MR) A review highlighted the importance of a systematic foot examination and risk stratification for preventing the development of foot ulcers and amputations. Suggestions for essential elements to assess annually for patients at risk were provided. Risk stratification was divided into four groups that were numbered 0 to 3. Recommendations for the frequency of evaluation were as follows: (1) Group 0 was at low risk, had protective sensation in the foot, and should be examined at least annually or at every follow-up visit; (2) Group 1 had lost protective sensation but exhibited no foot deformity and should be evaluated every 4 to 6 months; (3) Group 2 had lost protective sensation and had a foot deformity that required frequent evaluations, perhaps even monthly; and (4) Group 3 had a history of foot ulcer or amputation and should also be evaluated as frequently as every month (Lavery & Gazewood, 2000).

(MR) A review providing a thorough discussion of diabetic neuropathy that included a diagram of causal pathways to foot ulceration emphasized the key role of the patient in the prevention of ulcers (Rathur & Boulton, 2005).

Possibly Effective

No applicable published research was found in this category.

Not Effective

No applicable published research was found in this category.

Possibly Harmful

No applicable published research was found in this category.

OUTCOME MEASUREMENT

KNOWLEDGE: TREATMENT REGIMEN   (NOC)

Definition: Extent of understanding conveyed about a specific treatment regimen.
Knowledge: Treatment Regimen as evidenced by the following selected NOC indicators:
• Description of specific disease process
• Description of rationale for treatment regimen
• Description of self-care responsibilities for ongoing treatment
• Description of self-monitoring techniques
(Rate each indicator of **Knowledge: Treatment Regimen:** 1 = none, 2 = limited, 3 = moderate, 4 = substantial, 5 = extensive) (Moorhead et al., 2004).

REFERENCES

Boulton AJ, Vileikyte L. (2000). The diabetic foot: The scope of the problem. *J Fam Pract*, 49(11 Suppl): S3-S8.

Broersma A. (2004). Preventing amputations in patients with diabetes and chronic kidney disease. *Nephrol Nurs J*, 31(1):53-62.

Corbett CF. (2003). A randomized pilot study of improving foot care in home health patients with diabetes. *Diabetes Educ*, 29(2):273-282.

Dochterman JM, Bulechek GM (Eds). (2004). *Nursing Interventions Classification (NIC)*, 4th ed. St Louis: Mosby.

Donohoe ME, Fletton JA, Hook A, Powell R, Robinson I, Stead JW, et al. (2000). Improving foot care for people with diabetes mellitus—a randomized controlled trial of an integrated care approach. *Diabet Med*, 17(8):581-587.

Hartman D, Coetzee JC. (2002). Two U.S. practitioners' experience of using essential oils for wound care. *J Wound Care*, 11(8):317-320.

Inlow S, Orsted H, Sibbald RG. (2000). Best practices for the prevention, diagnosis, and treatment of diabetic foot ulcers. *Ostomy Wound Manage*, 46(11):55-68.

Landi F, Aloe L, Russo A, Cesari M, Onder G, Bonini S, et al. (2003). Topical treatment of pressure ulcers with nerve growth factor: A randomized clinical trial. *Ann Intern Med*, 139(8):635-641.

Lavery L, Gazewood JD. (2000). Assessing the feet of patients with diabetes. *J Fam Pract*, 49(11 Suppl): S9-S16.

Moorhead M, Johnson M, Maas M (Eds). (2004). *Nursing Outcomes Classification (NOC)*, 3rd ed. St Louis: Mosby.

Pattillo MM. (2004). Therapeutic and healing foot care: A healthy feet clinic for older adults. *J Gerontol Nurs*, 30(12):25-32.

Pinzur MS, Slovenkai MP, Trepman E, Shields NN; Diabetes Committee of American Orthopaedic Foot and Ankle Society. (2005). Guidelines for diabetic foot care: Recommendations endorsed by the Diabetes Committee of the American Orthopaedic Foot and Ankle Society. *Foot Ankle Int*, 26(1): 113-119.

Rathur HM, Boulton AJ. (2005). Recent advances in the diagnosis and management of diabetic neuropathy. *J Bone Joint Surg Br*, 87(12):1605-1610.

Saltzman CL, Rashid R, Hayes A, Fellner C, Fitzpatrick D, Klapach A, et al. (2004). 4.5-gram monofilament sensation beneath both first metatarsal heads indicates protective foot sensation in diabetic patients. *J Bone Joint Surg Am*, 86-A(4):717-723.

Schömig M, Ritz E, Standl E, Allenberg J. (2000). The diabetic foot in the dialyzed patient. *J Am Soc Nephrol*, 11(6):1153-1159.

Valk GD, Kriegsman DM, Assendelft WJ. (2002). Patient education for preventing diabetic foot ulceration: A systematic review. *Endocrinol Metab Clin North Am*, 31(3):633-658.

Veves A, Sheehan P, Pham HT. (2002). A randomized, controlled trial of Promogran (a collagen/oxidized regenerated cellulose dressing) vs. standard treatment of diabetic foot ulcers. *Arch Surg*, 137(7):822-827.

Waxman R, Woodburn H, Powell M, Woodburn J, Blackburn S, Helliwell P. (2003). FOOTSTEP: A randomized controlled trial investigating the clinical and cost effectiveness of a patient self-management program for basic foot care in the elderly. *J Clin Epidemiol*, 56(11):1092-1099.

 # TEACHING: INDIVIDUAL

Judith Kutzleb, MSN, RN, CCRN, APN-C

NIC **Definition:** Planning, implementation, and evaluation of a teaching program designed to address a patient's particular needs (Dochterman & Bulechek, 2004).
(Note: This guideline focuses on heart failure and related medications as well as invasive treatments.)

RCT = Randomized Controlled (Clinical) Trial, **NIC** = Nursing Interventions Classification, **NOC** = Nursing Outcomes Classification

NURSING ACTIVITIES

Effective

■ *Explain the use of angiotensin-converting enzyme (ACE) inhibitors to reduce ischemic events, mortality, and hospital admissions for heart failure (Jessup & Brozena, 2003).* **LOE = I**

(EO) Pharmacotherapy enhances cardiac function and improves quality of life and functional capacity by halting the remodeling processes and inhibiting the neurohormonal responses associated with low ejection fraction in heart failure (Konstam et al., 1996; Eichhorn, 2002).

(MR) In 32 randomized, placebo-controlled trials of patients with mild to severe symptomatic heart failure ($N = 7105$; New York Heart Association classes III and IV), treatment with an ACE inhibitor for a minimum of 8 weeks resulted in a significant 23% reduction in all-cause mortality ($p < .001$) and a 35% reduction in the combined end points of all-cause mortality or hospitalization for worsening heart failure ($p < .001$; Eichhorn, 2002).

(MR) In an RTC, patients with New York Heart Association class III or IV heart failure at randomization who received ACE inhibitor therapy ($N = 651$) had a significantly lower rate of all-cause mortality (24% and 45%, respectively) as compared with those treated with placebo (McMurray et al., 2001).

■ *Explain the use of angiotensin-receptor blockers only in patients who cannot tolerate ACE inhibitors because of cough or angioedema (Hunt et al., 2001).* **LOE = II**

(MR) In a double-blind RCT of patients with essential hypertension and left ventricular hypertrophy ($N = 9193$), treatment with the angiotensin-receptor blocker losartan yielded improvements in cardiovascular morbidity and survival as well as decreases in the incidence of new-onset diabetes as compared with treatment with the beta-blocker atenolol (Dahlof et al., 2002).

■ *Explain the use of beta-blockers to counteract the harmful effects of the sympathetic nervous system that are activated during heart failure (Eichhorn, 2002).* **LOE = I**

(MR) In an RCT ($N = 67$) of patients who were randomly assigned to receive either carvedilol or metoprolol, results demonstrated the beneficial effects of beta-blockers among patients with heart failure from various causes and of all stages (Jessup & Brozena, 2003).

(MR) In an RCT of hospitalized decompensated patients ($N = 1010$), the effects of beta-blockers demonstrated improvements in survival, morbidity, ejection fraction, remodeling, quality of life, the rate of hospitalization, and the incidence of sudden cardiac death (Foody et al., 2002).

■ *Explain the use of diuretics to control symptoms of congestion during the treatment and management of volume overload (Ellison, 1994).* **LOE = I**

(EO) Heart failure is a salt-avid syndrome that results in intravascular overload; diuretics are a mainstay for controlling the symptoms of congestion (Brater, 1998).

NR = Nursing Research, **MR** = Multidisciplinary Research, **SP** = Standard of Practice, **EO** = Expert Opinion, **LOE** = Level of Evidence

Possibly Effective

■ *Explain the use of cardiac glycosides to strengthen cardiac contractility (Jessup & Brozena, 2003).* **LOE = III**

(EO) The use of digoxin in combination with diuretics and ACE inhibitors improved morbidity among people with heart failure (Jessup & Brozena, 2003).

(MR) In an RCT involving hospitalized functional New York Heart Association class I through II patients ($N = 6800$), there was no difference in mortality between patients receiving digoxin and patients receiving placebo. There were decreases in the digoxin group in the rate of worsening heart failure and hospitalization of more than 37 months as compared with placebo, and the combined outcome of death or hospital admission caused by worsening heart failure was reduced.

■ (EO) *Explain the use of an aldosterone antagonist (spironolactone, eplerenone) to counteract the retention of salt, myocardial hypertrophy, and potassium excretion (Jessup & Brozena, 2003).* **LOE = I**

(MR) An RCT ($N = 1663$) of people with recent myocardial infarction complicated by left ventricular dysfunction and clinical heart failure who were already receiving medical treatment determined that adding an aldosterone antagonist reduced mortality as compared with adding a placebo (Pitt et al., 1999, 2003).

■ *Explain the use of cardiac resynchronization therapy (CRT) to provide electromechanical coordination and improved ventricular synchrony in symptomatic patients who have severe systolic dysfunction and clinically significant intraventricular conduction defects, particularly left bundle-branch block (Jessup & Brozena, 2003).* **LOE = III**

(EO) CRT as adjuvant therapy in patients who remain symptomatic despite optimized medical therapy demonstrates improvements in exercise tolerance, quality of life, and rates of hospitalization (Trupp, 2004).

(MR) An RTC ($N = 1520$) showed that CRT demonstrated reverse remodeling that resulted in decreased heart size and ventricular volumes, improved ejection fraction, and decreased mitral regurgitation. A CRT defibrillator device also reduced the risk of sudden death by 56% as compared with drug therapy (Saxon & De Marco, 2001).

Not Effective

No applicable published research was found in this category.

Possibly Harmful

■ *Explain the possible harm in using intravenous inotropic agents that act through the adrenergic pathway in patients with worsening heart failure to achieve arbitrary hemodynamic targets.* **LOE = I**

(EO) There is very little evidence that such treatment improves symptoms or patient outcomes (Thackray et al., 2002).

RCT = Randomized Controlled (Clinical) Trial, **NIC** = Nursing Interventions Classification, **NOC** = Nursing Outcomes Classification

Six RCTs involving hospitalized decompensated heart failure patients ($N = 8006$) found that nondigitalis inotropes increased mortality as compared with placebo (Gheorghiade et al., 1997).

An RCT studying hospitalized decompensated heart failure patients ($N = 1088$) demonstrated that milrinone significantly increased mortality over 6 months as compared with placebo (168/561 [30%] with milrinone versus 127/527 [24%] with placebo; Packer et al., 1991).

OUTCOME MEASUREMENT

MEDICATION AND INVASIVE TREATMENT

Definition: Knowledge of medication therapy and compliance with self-management.
Medication and Invasive Treatment as evidenced by the following indicators:
• Heart rate within expected range
• Oxygen saturation within expected range
• Respiratory rate within expected range
• Systolic blood pressure maintained within expected range
• Diastolic blood pressure maintained within expected range
• Patient demonstrates knowledge of medication dosage and effects according to planned therapy
(Note: This is not a NOC outcome.)

KNOWLEDGE: MEDICATION   NOC

Definition: Extent of understanding conveyed about the safe use of medication.
Knowledge: Medication as evidenced by the following selected NOC indicators:
• Identification of correct name of medications(s)
• Description of actions of medications(s)
• Description of side effects of medication(s)
• Description of precautions for medications(s)
(Rate each indicator of **Knowledge: Medication:** 1 = none, 2 = limited, 3 = moderate, 4 = substantial, 5 = extensive) (Moorhead et al., 2004).

REFERENCES

Brater DC. (1998). Diuretic therapy. *N Engl J Med,* 339(6):387-395.

Dahlof B, Devereux RB, Kjeldsen SE, Julius S, Beevers G, de Faire U, et al. (2002). Cardiovascular morbidity and mortality in the Losartan Intervention for Endpoint reduction in hypertension study (LIFE): A randomised trial against atenolol. *Lancet,* 359(9311):995-1003.

Dochterman JM, Bulechek GM (Eds). (2004). *Nursing Interventions Classification (NIC),* 4th ed. St Louis: Mosby.

Eichhorn EJ. (2002). Treating patients with severe heart failure. In *Postgrad Medicine: A special report,* November 24-31. Minneapolis, McGraw-Hill.

Ellison D. (1994). Diuretic drugs and the treatment of edema: From clinic to bench and back again. *Am J Kidney Dis,* 23(5):623-643.

Foody JM, Farrell MH, Krumholz HM. (2002). Beta-blocker therapy in heart failure: Scientific review. *JAMA,* 287(7):883-889.

Gheorghiade M, Benatar D, Konstam MA, Stoukides CA, Bonow RO. (1997). Pharmacotherapy for systolic dysfunction: A review of randomized clinical trials. *Am J Cardiol,* 80(8B):14H-27H.

Hunt SA, Baker DW, Chin MH, Cinquegrani MP, Feldman AM, Francis GS, et al. (2001). ACC/AHA guidelines for the evaluation and management of chronic heart failure in the adult: Executive summary. A report of the American College of Cardiology/American Heart Association Task Force on Practice Guidelines (Committee to revise the 1995 Guidelines for the Evaluation and Management of Heart Failure). *J Am Coll Cardiol,* 38(7):2101-2113.

Jessup M, Brozena S. (2003). Heart failure. *N Engl J Med,* 348(20):2007-2018.

Konstam V, Salem D, Pouleur H, Kostis J, Gorkin L, Shumaker S, et al. (1996). Baseline quality of life as a predictor of mortality and hospitalizations in 5,025 patients with congestive heart failure. SOLVD Investigations. Studies of Left Ventricular Dysfunction Investigators. *Am J Cardiol,* 78(8):890-895.

McMurray J, Cohen-Solal A, Dietz R, Eichhorn E, Erhardt L, Hobbs R, et al. (2001). Practical recommendations for the use of ACE inhibitors, beta-blockers and spironolactone in heart failure: Putting guidelines into practice. *Eur J Heart Fail,* 3(4):495-502.

Moorhead M, Johnson M, Maas M (Eds). (2004). *Nursing Outcomes Classification (NOC),* 3rd ed. St Louis: Mosby.

Packer M, Carver JR, Rodeheffer RJ, Ivanhoe RJ, DiBianco R, Zeldis SM, et al. (1991). Effect of oral milrinone on mortality in severe chronic heart failure. The PROMISE Study Research Group. *N Engl J Med,* 325(21):1468-1475.

Pitt B, Remme W, Zannad F, Neaton J, Martinez F, Roniker B, et al. (2003). Eplerenone, a selective aldosterone blocker, in patients with left ventricular dysfunction after myocardial infarction. *N Engl J Med,* 348(14):1309-1321.

Pitt B, Zannad F, Remme WJ, Cody R, Castaigne A, Perez A, et al. (1999). The effect of spironolactone on morbidity and mortality in patients with severe heart failure. Randomized Aldactone Evaluation Study Investigators. *N Engl J Med,* 341(10):709-717.

Saxon LA, De Marco T. (2001). Cardiac resynchronization: A cornerstone in the foundation of device therapy for heart failure. *J Am Coll Cardiol,* 38(7):1971-1973.

Thackray S, Easthaugh J, Freemantle N, Cleland JG. (2002). The effectiveness and relative effectiveness of intravenous inotropic drugs acting through the adrenergic pathway in patients with heart failure—a meta-regression analysis. *Eur J Heart Fail,* 4(4):515-529.

Trupp RJ. (2004). Cardiac resynchronization therapy: Optimizing the device, optimizing the patient. *J Cardiovasc Nurs,* 19(4):223-233.

 # TEACHING: PREOPERATIVE

Cynthia K. Lewis, MSN, RN, APRN-BC

NIC **Definition:** Assisting a patient to understand and mentally prepare for surgery and the postoperative recovery period (Dochterman & Bulechek, 2004).

NURSING ACTIVITIES

Effective

■ *Describe general preoperative information and procedures.* **LOE = I**

NR A meta-analysis (*N* = 49 studies) of the relationships between psychoeducational interventions and the length of postsurgical hospitalization supported three types of interventions used in earlier studies that improved patient outcomes: (1) information: the explanation of expected care, equipment, procedures, events, environments, sensations, discomforts, sequence, and patient role expectations; (2) skills training: turning, cough and deep breathing, leg exercises designed to prevent postoperative complications, and self-controlled ways to decrease discomforts by inducing relaxation; and (3) psychosocial support, the assurance of nurse availability, encouragement to request assistance, problem solving, asking questions, and the reinforcement of accurate expectations (Devine & Cook, 1983).

(NR) A two-group randomized, comparative design that included a preoperative questionnaire administered to elective laparoscopic cholecystectomy patients ($N = 93$) demonstrated that a preadmission education intervention helped reduce postoperative pain levels after the procedure and significantly increased patients' knowledge of self-care and complication management (Blay & Donoghue, 2005).

▪ *Describe the postoperative procedures.* **LOE = I**

(NR) An RCT of laparoscopic cholecystectomy patients ($N = 100$) demonstrated that patients who received information related to the surgical procedure and hospital length of stay requested additional information about postoperative expectations and self-care (Blay & Donoghue, 2005).

(EO) Patients' informational needs generally relate to postoperative expectations about pain management, wound care, and food and fluid intake (Henderson & Zernike, 2001; Mordiffi et al., 2003; Young & O'Connell, 2001).

(NR) A Cochrane systematic review demonstrated that educating patients about postoperative routines may reduce the incidence of postoperative complications (Brady et al., 2003).

(NR) A review of the literature supported that consistent descriptions of preoperative education should include informing clients about their condition, surgery, postoperative care, and treatment regime; discussing physical, technical (what patients could expect to happen), administrative, and procedural aspects (hospital activities, health care team); and providing a preoperative checklist to facilitate the transmission of generic content (Fitzpatrick & Hyde, 2005).

(MR) A review of the literature found that preadmission and preoperative interventions, including preoperative information, details of postoperative care, and exercise and activities upon postoperative discharge, improved care and recovery (Johansson et al., 2004).

▪ *Instruct the patient regarding postoperative symptoms.* **LOE = V**

(NR) A review of the literature demonstrated that best practices for pre- and post-procedure teaching should include specific information about the surgery, admission care, discharge, and what to expect regarding pain and discomfort. The most favorable patient outcomes were associated with nursing care that included preoperative teaching and that acknowledged the uniqueness of patients and their situations (AORN, 2005; ASPAN, 2004; Fitzpatrick & Hyde, 2005).

(MR) A descriptive study of patients who were admitted for open cholecystectomy ($N = 55$) answered one questionnaire both at admission and at discharge. The most requested information was related to anxiety-creating factors such as pain and postoperative symptoms after surgery. Thirty percent of the patients wanted both written and verbal information (Lithner & Zilling, 2000).

NR = Nursing Research, **MR** = Multidisciplinary Research, **SP** = Standard of Practice, **EO** = Expert Opinion, **LOE** = Level of Evidence

■ *Instruct the patient regarding self-care after discharge.* **LOE = II**

(NR) An RCT of laparoscopic cholecystectomy patients ($N = 100$) demonstrated that patients who received information related to the surgical procedure and the hospital length of stay requested additional information about postoperative expectations and self-care (Blay & Donoghue, 2005).

■ *Discuss surgery-related information, including details of the procedure and anesthesia.* **LOE = I**

(NR) A meta-analysis ($N = 49$ studies) of the relationships between psychoeducational interventions and the length of postsurgical hospitalization supported three types of interventions used in earlier studies that improved patient outcomes: (1) information: an explanation of expected care, equipment, procedures, events, environments, sensations, discomforts, sequences, and patient role expectations; (2) skills training: turning, coughing and deep breathing, leg exercises designed to prevent postoperative complications, and self-controlled ways to decrease discomforts by inducing relaxation; and (3) psychosocial support: assurance of nurse availability, encouragement to request assistance, problem solving, asking questions, and reinforcement of accurate expectations (Devine & Cook, 1983).

(NR) In a descriptive, cross-sectional study involving three cohorts (patients, nurses, and physicians; $N = 67$), detailed information about anesthesia was identified as the most important preoperative information for patients by all three cohorts. Patients viewed details about the procedure and information about the operating room environment as being of almost equal importance (Mordiffi et al., 2003).

■ (NIC) *Discuss possible pain-control measures.* **LOE = VI**

(EO) Patients' informational needs generally relate to postoperative expectations about pain management, wound care, and food and fluid intake (Henderson & Zernike, 2001; Mordiffi et al., 2003; Young & O'Connell, 2001).

(MR) A descriptive study of patients who were admitted for open cholecystectomy ($N = 55$) answered one questionnaire both at admission and at discharge. The most requested information was related to anxiety-creating factors such as pain and postoperative symptoms after surgery. Thirty percent of the patients wanted both written and verbal information (Lithner & Zilling, 2000).

■ *Provide psychosocial support.* **LOE = III**

(MR) A quasi-experimental study with a pre-test/post-test design with two comparison measurements demonstrated information gaps in the provision of psychosocial information and support by physicians, nurses, and health educators (Tromp et al., 2004).

(NR) A convenience sample of 116 patients demonstrated significant relationships between income level and preference for situational/procedural information and between gender and the preference for psychosocial support information (Bernier et al., 2003).

(NR) A convenience sample of 159 registered nurses identified that patients needed the following information (in order of importance): psychosocial support, skills training, situational/procedural information, patient role information, and sensation/discomfort information (Bernier et al., 2003).

RCT = Randomized Controlled (Clinical) Trial, **NIC** = Nursing Interventions Classification, **NOC** = Nursing Outcomes Classification

Possibly Effective

■ *Discuss the common and rare complications associated with the procedure.* **LOE = III**

NR A nonrandomized study ($N = 182$ in the intervention group, $N = 156$ in the control group) showed that 72% of the intervention group and 69% of the control group wanted information about both common and rare complications (Ivarrsson et al., 2005).

Not Effective

No applicable published research was found in this category.

Possibly Harmful

No applicable published research was found in this category.

OUTCOME MEASUREMENT

KNOWLEDGE: TREATMENT PROCEDURE(S)   NOC

Definition: Extent of understanding conveyed about procedure(s) required as part of a treatment regimen.

Knowledge: Treatment Procedure(s) as evidenced by the following selected NOC indicators:

• Description of treatment procedure(s)
• Description of steps in procedure(s)
• Explanation of purpose of procedure(s)
• Description of restrictions related to procedure(s)
• Description of appropriate action for complications

(Rate each indicator of **Knowledge: Treatment Procedure(s):** 1 = none, 2 = limited, 3 = moderate, 4 = substantial, 5 = extensive) (Moorhead et al., 2004).

REFERENCES

American Society of PeriAnesthesia Nurses (ASPAN). (2004). ASPAN resource 4 criteria for initial, ongoing, and discharge assessment and management. (2004). In AORN, ASPAN (Eds.): *Standards of perianesthesia nursing practice.* Philadelphia: ASPAN, pp 27-31.

Association of Perioperative Nurses (AORN). (2005). AORN guidance statement: Preoperative patient care in the ambulatory surgery setting. In AORN, ASPAN (Eds.): *Standards, recommended practices and guidelines.* Denver: AORN, pp 179-184.

Bernier MJ, Sanares DC, Owen SV, Newhouse PL. (2003). Preoperative teaching received and valued in a day surgery setting. *AORN J,* 77(3):563-572, 575-578, 581-582.

Blay N, Donoghue J. (2005). The effect of pre-admission education on domiciliary recovery following laparoscopic cholecystectomy. *Aust J Adv Nurs,* 22(4):14-19.

Brady M, Kinn S, Stuart P. (2003). Preoperative fasting for adults to prevent perioperative complications. Cochrane Database Syst Rev, (4):CD004423.

Devine E, Cook T. (1983). A meta-analytic analysis of effects of psychoeducational interventions on length of postsurgical hospital stay. *Nurs Res,* 32(5):267-274.

Dochterman JM, Bulechek GM (Eds). (2004). *Nursing Interventions Classification (NIC),* 4th ed. St Louis: Mosby.

Fitzpatrick E, Hyde A. (2005). What characterizes the "usual" preoperative education in clinical contexts? *Nurs Health Sci,* 7(4):251-258.

Henderson A, Zernike W. (2001). A study of the impact of discharge information for surgical patients. *J Adv Nurs,* 35(3):435-441.

Ivarsson B, Sjöberg T, Larsson S. (2005). Waiting for cardiac surgery—Support experienced by next of kin. *Eur J Cardiovasc Nurs,* 4(2):145-152.

Johansson K, Salantera S, Heikkinen K, Kuusisto A, Virtanen H, Leino-Kilpi H. (2004). Surgical patient education: Assessing the interventions and exploring the outcomes from experimental and quasiexperimental studies from 1990 to 2003. *Clin Eff Nurs,* 8(2):81-92.

Lithner M, Zilling T. (2000). Pre- and postoperative information needs. *Patient Educ Couns,* 40(1):29-37.

Moorhead M, Johnson M, Maas M (Eds). (2004). *Nursing Outcomes Classification (NOC),* 3rd ed. St Louis: Mosby.

Mordiffi SZ, Tan SP, Wong MK. (2003). Information provided to surgical patients versus information needed. *AORN J,* 77(3):546-549, 552-558, 561-562.

Tromp F, Dulmen S, Weert J. (2004). Interdisciplinary preoperative patient education in cardiac surgery. *J Adv Nurs,* 47(2):212-222.

Young J, O'Connell B. (2001). Recovery following laparoscopic cholecystectomy in either a 23 hour or an 8 hour facility. *J Qual Clin Pract,* 21(1-2):2-7.

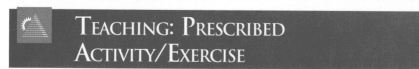

TEACHING: PRESCRIBED ACTIVITY/EXERCISE

NIC

Judith Kutzleb, MSN, RN, CCRN, APN-C

NIC **Definition:** Preparing a patient to achieve and/or maintain a prescribed level of activity (Dochterman & Bulechek, 2004).

(Note: This guideline focuses on prescribed activity/exercise related to heart failure.)

NURSING ACTIVITIES

Effective

■ *Encourage regularly scheduled exercise programs for beneficial effects on symptoms (Coats, 1999).* **LOE = I**

EO Functional capacity in heart failure is a person's ability to carry out the activities of day-to-day life (Wenger, 1989).

NR A prospective, quasi-experimental, multicenter research study ($N = 23$) demonstrated that the 6-minute walk test proved to be an inexpensive and uncomplicated clinical measure of exercise capacity (Kutzleb & Reiner, 2006).

MR An RCT ($N = 134$) of heart failure patients and ($N = 13$) patients with chronic pulmonary disease using the 6-minute walk test were compared with maximal oxygen consumption on the treadmill. The reliability and reproducibility of the walk test was higher than that of the pulmonary function test for predicting functional capacity (Guyatt, 1987; Lipkin et al., 1986).

MR An RCT ($N = 134$) found that the 6-minute walk test was a more sensitive measure of change in the heart failure patient's functional status than conventional exercise tests using cycle ergometry or treadmill techniques (Dracup et al., 1992).

RCT = Randomized Controlled (Clinical) Trial, **NIC** = Nursing Interventions Classification, **NOC** = Nursing Outcomes Classification

Possibly Effective

■ *Consider interventions to improve the quality of life of patients with advanced heart failure that target the reduction of depression and hostility and that increase activity levels.* **LOE = III**

(NR) A quasi-experimental study ($N = 50$) indicated that heart failure patients experienced significant mood disruption that was greater than that reported by other types of cardiac patients and that these patients would benefit from psychosocial interventions (Hawthorne & Hixon, 1994; Richardson, 2003).

(MR) A systematic review of the routine measurement of quality of life and functional capacity both before and after comprehensive medical therapy demonstrated possible benefits of treatment efficacy for the improvement of physical ability and mood disruption (Dracup et al., 1992).

Not Effective

■ *Intermittently counseling patients with regard to exercise, medication management, dietary restriction, and nutritional counseling.* **LOE = III**

(NR) A quasi-experimental study ($N = 50$) of quality of life and functional capacity among patients with heart failure without intensive follow-up demonstrated an increased rate of rehospitalization and an increase in disease uncertainty (Hawthorne & Hixon, 1994).

Possibly Harmful

No applicable published research was found in this category.

OUTCOME MEASUREMENT

FUNCTIONAL CAPACITY AND EXERCISE

Definition: Independent in activities of daily living and mild to moderate exercise.
Functional Capacity and Exercise as evidenced by the following indicators:
• Skin color within expected range in response to activity
• Oxygen saturation within expected range in response to activity
• Respiratory rate within expected range in response to activity
• Activities of daily living performed without evidence of cardiovascular/pulmonary decompensation
• Walking distance gradually increased to improve activity level without evidence of cardiovascular/pulmonary decompensation
(Note: This is not a NOC outcome.)

KNOWLEDGE: PRESCRIBED ACTIVITY   (NOC)

(Please refer to *Nursing Outcomes Classification* [Moorhead et al., 2004] for the **Knowledge: Prescribed Activity** outcome.)

NR = Nursing Research, **MR** = Multidisciplinary Research, **SP** = Standard of Practice, **EO** = Expert Opinion, **LOE** = Level of Evidence

REFERENCES

Coats AJ. (1999). Exercise training for heart failure: Coming of age. *Circulation,* 99(9):1138-1140.

Dochterman JM, Bulechek GM (Eds). (2004). *Nursing Interventions Classification (NIC),* 4th ed. St Louis: Mosby.

Dracup K, Walden JA, Stevenson LW, Brecht ML. (1992). Quality of life in patients with advanced heart failure. *J Heart Lung Transplant,* 11(2 Pt 1):273-279.

Guyatt G. (1987). Use of the six-minute walk test as an outcome measure in clinical trials in chronic heart failure. *Heart Failure,* 3:211-217.

Hawthorne MH, Hixon ME. (1994). Functional status, mood disturbance and quality of life in patients with heart failure. *Prog Cardiovasc Nurs,* 9(1):22-32.

Kutzleb J, Reiner D. (2006). The impact of nurse-directed patient education on quality of life and functional capacity in people with heart failure. *J Am Acad Nurse Pract,* 18(3):116-123.

Lipkin DP, Scriven AJ, Crake T, Poole-Wilson PA. (1986). Six minute walking test for assessing exercise capacity in chronic heart failure. *Br Med J,* 292(6521):653-655.

Moorhead M, Johnson M, Maas M (Eds). (2004). *Nursing Outcomes Classification (NOC),* 3rd ed. St Louis: Mosby.

Richardson LG. (2003). Psychosocial issues in patients with congestive heart failure. *Prog Cardiovasc Nurs,* 18(1):19-27.

Wenger NK. (1989). Quality of life: Can it and should it be assessed in patients with heart failure? *Cardiology,* 76(5):391-398.

TEACHING: PRESCRIBED MEDICATION (NIC)

Barbara J. Olinzock, EdD, MSN, RN; Kathaleen C. Bloom, PhD, CNM

(NIC) **Definition:** Preparing a patient to safely take prescribed medications and monitor for their effects (Dochterman & Bulechek, 2004).

NURSING ACTIVITIES

Effective

- (NIC) *Instruct the patient on the purpose and action of each medication. Instruct the patient on the proper administration/application of each medication.* **LOE = I**

(MR) A Cochrane systematic review found that telling people about their medications was an effective strategy to improve medication compliance both during the short term (<6 months) and the long term (≥6 months). Telling patients about the side effects of medications did not make noncompliance more likely (Haynes et al., 2005).

(NR) A meta-analysis of 25 RCTs investigating interventions for pain in cancer patients found that teaching patients about analgesics and their appropriate use resulted in a decrease in pain levels (Devine, 2003).

- *Assess the likelihood of medication-related problems and noncompliance with the medication regimen.* **LOE = II**

(MR) An RCT (*N* = 194) found that the addition of a five-item questionnaire to the usual teaching regarding medications made it possible to identify 14% more individuals who were at risk for medication-related problems than the usual care practice (Langford et al., 2006).

RCT = Randomized Controlled (Clinical) Trial, **NIC** = Nursing Interventions Classification, **NOC** = Nursing Outcomes Classification

(MR) A validation study ($N = 40$) of a short instrument designed to identify elderly who were at risk for medication-related problems determined that a self-administered questionnaire could be used effectively (Barenholtz Levy, 2003).

(MR) In a descriptive study ($N = 75$) that examined patients' beliefs about anticoagulation therapy and patient satisfaction, researchers were able to correctly predict compliance with warfarin therapy 85% of the time (Orensky & Holdford, 2005).

■ (NIC) *Determine the patient's ability to obtain required medications.* **LOE = V**

(MR) A systematic review of compliance with long-term medication use revealed that a patient's inability to acquire or pay for medications was a significant barrier to adherence (Krueger et al., 2005).

(MR) A systematic review of medication adherence and persistence revealed that adherence was enhanced when the underlying reasons for nonadherence were assessed and addressed (Krueger et al., 2003).

(NR) A case-control study ($N = 97$) that examined medication use among stroke survivors found that patients were often forced to choose between paying bills and buying medication. They often skipped doses to make their medications last longer, bought only a few doses at a time, or went out of the country to obtain their medications more cheaply (Ostwald et al., 2006).

■ *Instruct the patient about self-monitoring and the self-regulation of medications.* **LOE = I**

(MR) A Cochrane systematic review found that comprehensive programs that included self-monitoring and self-regulation were effective for improving medication adherence (Haynes et al., 2005).

(MR) A systematic review of interventions to enhance adherence to medication prescriptions found that the inclusion of self-monitoring and reinforcement within complex interventions was effective for long-term medication adherence (McDonald et al., 2002).

(MR) A systematic review and meta-analysis of 14 trials of self-monitoring and the self-adjustment of oral anticoagulation therapy concluded that self-management resulted in fewer thrombolic events and lower mortality than self-monitoring alone, thus making this strategy preferable for those patients who were capable of self-management (Heneghan et al., 2006).

■ *Provide structured education that is tailored to the individual.* **LOE = I**

(MR) A systematic review of 62 studies of compliance with antihypertensive and lipid-lowering medications revealed that educational interventions that were personalized and that involved frequent contact with the nurse or pharmacist were the most effective (Petrilla et al., 2005).

(NR) A systematic review of 21 RCTs revealed that patients who received structured education involving both verbal and written instructions followed by discussion had greater knowledge and compliance with psychotropic medication therapy (Fernandez et al., 2006).

(NR) In an RCT ($N = 70$) to determine the effect of an intervention to promote the self-care of patients with heart failure, the use of an intervention specifically tailored to perceived benefits and barriers to self-care was found to change the perceived benefits and barriers of these patients (Sethares & Elliott, 2004).

NR = Nursing Research, **MR** = Multidisciplinary Research, **SP** = Standard of Practice, **EO** = Expert Opinion, **LOE** = Level of Evidence

(MR) In a controlled study involving 32 elderly patients with heart failure, patient-centered instructions about familiar and unfamiliar drugs were better recalled and understood than were standard instructions (Morrow et al., 2005).

■ *Provide written educational materials at an appropriate reading level.* **LOE = V**

(MR) A review of studies investigating the use and impact of written drug information revealed that the readability and presentation of the written information influenced knowledge, compliance, and satisfaction (Koo et al., 2003).

(NR) A descriptive correlational study of 62 African American patients taking anticoagulant therapy found that current patient education materials were written at a ninth- to thirteenth-grade level, which was three to four grade levels above the average patient's reading level. In addition, none of the materials was culturally relevant for this population. More than 50% of the study participants were unable to comprehend the written materials provided to them (Wilson et al., 2003).

(MR) A cross-sectional study ($N = 479$) investigating patient factors that influenced the use of written medication information revealed that the patient's health literacy level and health locus of control were predictive both of the patients' reading materials provided to them as well as their seeking of written materials (Koo et al., 2006).

Possibly Effective

■ *Provide for follow-up via telephone.* **LOE = I**

(MR) A Cochrane systematic review found that telephone follow-up was significant during both the short term (<6 months) and the long term (≥6 months) (Haynes et al., 2005).

(MR) An RCT ($N = 294$) of bimonthly telephone counseling by a nurse found that 46% of patients who were nonadherent with their medications at baseline were adherent 6 months into the study as compared with 34% of patients in usual care (Bosworth et al., 2005).

(MR) An RCT ($N = 128$) of a telephone follow-up to improve compliance with antibiotic therapy in patients with tonsillitis or pharyngitis found that an educational intervention that included a telephone call 4 days into the therapy was superior to education alone in terms of the completion of the full course of antibiotic (Urién et al., 2004).

(MR) An RCT ($N = 13,100$) of a telephone follow-up 2 months into therapy for patients taking pravastatin failed to find any benefit in terms of compliance (Guthrie, 2001).

(MR) An RCT ($N = 647$) comparing education alone, education plus a telephone follow-up, and education plus a telephone follow-up and an interactive voice response system failed to find any differences among groups with respect to compliance with antidepressant medications (Stuart et al., 2003).

Not Effective

No applicable published research was found in this category.

Possibly Harmful

No applicable published research was found in this category.

RCT = Randomized Controlled (Clinical) Trial, **NIC** = Nursing Interventions Classification, **NOC** = Nursing Outcomes Classification

OUTCOME MEASUREMENT

KNOWLEDGE: MEDICATION NOC

Definition: Extent of understanding conveyed about the safe use of medication.

Knowledge: Medication as evidenced by the following selected NOC indicators:

- Recognition of need to inform health professional of all medications being taken
- Identification of correct name of medication(s)
- Description of side effects of medication(s)
- Description of potential adverse reactions when taking multiple medications
- Description of self-monitoring techniques

(Rate each indicator of **Knowledge: Medication:** 1 = none, 2 = limited, 3 = moderate, 4 = substantial, 5 = extensive) (Moorhead et al., 2004).

REFERENCES

Barenholtz Levy H. (2003). Self-administered medication-risk questionnaire in an elderly population. *Ann Pharmacother,* 37(7-8):982-987.

Bosworth HB, Olsen MK, Gentry P, Orr M, Dudley T, McCant F, et al. (2005). Nurse administered telephone intervention for blood pressure control: A patient-tailored multifactorial intervention. *Patient Educ Couns,* 57(1):5-14.

Devine EC. (2003). Meta-analysis of the effect of psychoeducational interventions on pain in adults with cancer. *Oncol Nurs Forum,* 30(1):75-89.

Dochterman JM, Bulechek GM (Eds). (2004). *Nursing Interventions Classification (NIC),* 4th ed. St Louis: Mosby.

Fernandez RS, Evans V, Griffiths RD, Mostacchi MS. (2006). Educational interventions for mental health consumers receiving psychotropic medication: A review of the evidence. *Int J Ment Health Nurs,* 15(1):70-80.

Guthrie RM. (2001). The effects of postal and telephone reminders on compliance with pravastatin therapy in a national registry: Results of the first myocardial infarction risk reduction program. *Clin Ther,* 23(6):970-980.

Haynes RB, Yao X, Degani A, Kripalani S, Garg A, McDonald HP. (2005). Interventions to enhance medication adherence. *Cochrane Database Syst Rev,* (4):CD000011.

Heneghan C, Alonso-Coello P, Garcia-Alamino JM, Perera R, Meats E, Glasziou P. (2006). Self-monitoring of oral anticoagulation: A systematic review and meta-analysis. *Lancet,* 367(9508):404-411.

Koo M, Krass I, Aslani P. (2003). Factors influencing consumer use of written drug information. *Ann Pharmacother,* 37(2):259-267.

Koo M, Krass I, Aslani P. (2006). Enhancing patient education about medicines: Factors influencing reading and seeking of written medicine information. *Health Expect,* 9(2):174-187.

Krueger KP, Berger BA, Felkey B. (2005). Medication adherence and persistence: A comprehensive review. *Adv Ther,* 22(4):313-356.

Krueger KP, Felkey BG, Berger BA. (2003). Improving adherence and persistence: A review and assessment of interventions and description of steps toward a national adherence initiative. *J Am Pharm Assoc,* 43(6):668-678.

Langford BJ, Jorgenson D, Kwan D, Papoushek C. (2006). Implementation of a self-administered questionnaire to identify patients at risk for medication-related problems in a family health center. *Pharmacotherapy,* 26(2):260-268.

McDonald HP, Garg AX, Haynes RB. (2002). Interventions to enhance patient adherence to medication prescriptions: Scientific review. *JAMA,* 288(22):2868-2879.

Moorhead M, Johnson M, Maas M (Eds). (2004). *Nursing Outcomes Classification (NOC),* 3rd ed. St Louis: Mosby.

Morrow DG, Weiner M, Young J, Steinley D, Deer M, Murray MD. (2005). Improving medication knowledge among older adults with heart failure: A patient-centered approach to instruction design. *Gerontologist*, 45(4):545-552.

Orensky IA, Holdford DA. (2005). Predictors of noncompliance with warfarin therapy in an outpatient anticoagulation clinic. *Pharmacotherapy*, 25(12):1801-1808.

Ostwald SK, Wasserman J, Davis S. (2006). Medications, comorbidities, and medical complications in stroke survivors: The CAReS study. *Rehabil Nurs*, 31(1):10-14.

Petrilla AA, Benner JS, Battleman DS, Tierce JC, Hazard EH. (2005). Evidence-based interventions to improve patient compliance with antihypertensive and lipid-lowering medications. *Int J Clin Pract*, 59(12):1441-1451.

Sethares KA, Elliott K. (2004). The effect of a tailored message intervention on heart failure readmission rates, quality of life, and benefit and barrier beliefs in persons with heart failure. *Heart Lung*, 33(4):249-260.

Stuart GW, Laraia MT, Ornstein SM, Nietert PJ. (2003). An interactive voice response system to enhance antidepressant medication compliance. *Top Health Inf Manage*, 24(1):15-20.

Urién AM, Guillén VF, Beltran DO, Pinzotas CL, Pérez ER, Arocena MO, et al. (2004). Telephonic back-up improves antibiotic compliance in acute tonsillitis/pharyngitis. *Int J Antimicrob Agents*, 23(2):138-143.

Wilson FL, Racine E, Tekieli V, Williams B. (2003). Literacy, readability and cultural barriers: Critical factors to consider when educating older African Americans about anticoagulation therapy. *J Clin Nurs*, 12(2):275-282.

 ## TEACHING: PROCEDURE/TREATMENT   NIC

Cynthia K. Lewis, MSN, RN, APRN-BC

> **NIC** **Definition:** Preparing a patient to understand and mentally prepare for a prescribed procedure or treatment (Dochterman & Bulechek, 2004).

NURSING ACTIVITIES

Effective

■ *Describe the general procedure, treatment information, and routines.* **LOE = I**

    NR A meta-analysis (*N* = 49 studies) of the relationships between psychoeducational interventions and the length of postsurgical hospitalization supported three types of interventions used in earlier studies that improved patient outcomes: (1) information: an explanation of expected care, equipment, procedures, events, environments, sensations, discomforts, sequences, and patient role expectations; (2) skills training: turning, cough and deep breathing, leg exercises designed to prevent postoperative complications, and self-controlled ways of decreasing discomfort by inducing relaxation; and (3) psychosocial support: assurance of nurse availability, encouragement to request assistance, problem-solving, asking questions, and the reinforcement of accurate expectations (Devine & Cook, 1983).

    NR A two-group, randomized, comparative design that included a preoperative questionnaire that was administered to elective laparoscopic cholecystectomy patients (*N* = 93) demonstrated that a preadmission education intervention helped reduce postoperative pain levels after the procedure and that it significantly increased patients' knowledge of self-care and complication management (Blay & Donoghue, 2005).

RCT = Randomized Controlled (Clinical) Trial, **NIC** = Nursing Interventions Classification, **NOC** = Nursing Outcomes Classification

■ **NIC** *Describe the postprocedure/posttreatment assessments and activities and the rationale for them.* **LOE = I**

NR A review of the literature supported that consistent descriptions of preoperative education should include the following: (1) the process of informing clients about their condition, surgery, postoperative care, and treatment regimen; (2) physical, technical (what patients could expect to happen), administrative, or procedural information (hospital activities, health care team); and (3) a preoperative checklist to facilitate the transmission of generic content (Fitzpatrick & Hyde, 2005).

■ *Instruct the patient about postprocedure and treatment symptoms.* **LOE = V**

NR A review of the literature demonstrated that the best practices for pre- and postprocedure teaching should include specific information regarding what to expect from the surgery, descriptions of admission care and discharge, and what to expect regarding pain and discomfort. The most favorable patient outcomes were associated with nursing care that included preoperative teaching and that acknowledged the uniqueness of patients and their situations (AORN, 2005; ASPAN, 2004; Fitzpatrick & Hyde, 2005).

■ *Instruct the patient regarding self-care after discharge.* **LOE = II**

NR An RCT exploring postoperative expectations and self-care among laparoscopic cholecystectomy patients ($N = 100$) identified the need to receive more information related to the surgical procedure and the length of the hospital stay (Blay & Donoghue, 2005).

■ *Discuss procedure and treatment-related information, including details of the procedure and anesthesia.* **LOE = I**

NR A meta-analysis ($N = 49$ studies) of the relationships between psychoeducational interventions and the length of postsurgical hospitalization supported three types of interventions used in earlier studies that improved patient outcomes: (1) information: an explanation of expected care, equipment, procedures, events, environments, sensations, discomforts, sequences, and patient role expectations; (2) skills training: turning, cough and deep breathing, leg exercises designed to prevent postoperative complications, and self-controlled ways of decreasing discomfort by inducing relaxation; and (3) psychosocial support: assurance of nurse availability, encouragement to request assistance, problem-solving, asking questions, and the reinforcement of accurate expectations (Devine & Cook, 1983).

NR In a descriptive, cross-sectional study involving three cohorts (patients, nurses, and physicians; $N = 67$), details of anesthesia were identified as the most important preoperative information for patients by all three cohorts. Patients viewed details of the procedure and information about the operating room environment as of almost equal importance (Mordiffi et al., 2003).

■ *Discuss possible pain-control measures.* **LOE = VI**

NR A review of the literature revealed patients' informational needs generally related to postoperative expectations about pain management, wound care, and food and fluid intake (Henderson & Zernike, 2001; Mordiffi et al., 2003; Young & O'Connell, 2001).

MR In a descriptive study, patients who were admitted for open cholecystectomy ($N = 55$) answered one questionnaire both at admission and at discharge. The most requested information was related to anxiety-creating factors such as pain and postoperative symptoms after surgery; 30% of patients wanted both written and verbal information (Lithner & Zilling, 2000).

- ■ *Provide psychosocial support.* **LOE = III**

  (MR) A quasi-experimental study ($N = 54$) with a pre-test/post-test design with two comparison measurements demonstrated information gaps in the provision of psychosocial information and support by physicians, nurses, and health educators (Tromp et al., 2004).

  (NR) A convenience sample of patients ($N = 116$) demonstrated significant relationships between income level and the preference for situational/procedural information and between gender and the preference for psychosocial support information (Bernier et al., 2003).

  (NR) A convenience sample of 159 registered nurses identified their perceptions about the informational needs of patients before a procedure. In order of importance, patients' informational needs were determined to be psychosocial support, skills training, situational/procedural information, patient role information, and sensation/discomfort information (Bernier et al., 2003).

Possibly Effective

- ■ *Discuss the common and rare complications associated with the procedure or treatment.* **LOE = III**

  (NR) A nonrandomized study ($N = 182$ members of the intervention group, $N = 156$ members of the control group) showed that 72% of the intervention group and 69% of the control group wanted information about both common and rare complications (Ivarsson et al., 2005).

Not Effective

No applicable published research was found in this category.

Possibly Harmful

No applicable published research was found in this category.

OUTCOME MEASUREMENT

KNOWLEDGE: TREATMENT PROCEDURE(S) (NOC)

Definition: Extent of understanding conveyed about procedure(s) required as part of a treatment regimen.

Knowledge: Treatment Procedure(s) as evidenced by the following selected NOC indicators:

- Description of treatment procedure(s)
- Description of steps in procedure(s)
- Explanation of purpose of procedure(s)
- Description of restrictions related to procedure(s)
- Description of appropriate action for complications

(Rate each indicator of **Knowledge: Treatment Procedure(s):** 1 = none, 2 = limited, 3 = moderate, 4 = substantial, 5 = extensive) (Moorhead et al., 2004).

RCT = Randomized Controlled (Clinical) Trial, **NIC** = Nursing Interventions Classification, **NOC** = Nursing Outcomes Classification

REFERENCES

American Society of Post Anesthesia Nurses (ASPAN). (2004). ASPAN resource 4 criteria for initial, ongoing, and discharge assessment and management. In *Standards of perianesthesia nursing practice*. Philadelphia: ASPAN, pp 27-31.

Association of Perioperative Registered Nurses (AORN). (2005). AORN Guidance Statement: Preoperative patient care in the ambulatory surgery setting. *AORN J*, 81(4):871-878.

Bernier MJ, Sanares DC, Owen SV, Newhouse PL. (2003). Preoperative teaching received and valued in a day surgery setting. *AORN J*, 77(3):563-582.

Blay N, Donoghue J. (2005). The effect of pre-admission education on domiciliary recovery following laparoscopic cholecystectomy. *Aust J Adv Nurs*, 22(4):14-19.

Devine EC, Cook TD. (1983). A meta-analytic analysis of effects of psychoeducational interventions on length of postsurgical hospital stay. *Nurs Res*, 32(5):267-274.

Dochterman JM, Bulechek GM (Eds). (2004). *Nursing Interventions Classification (NIC)*, 4th ed. St Louis: Mosby.

Fitzpatrick E, Hyde A. (2005). What characterizes the 'usual' preoperative education in clinical contexts? *Nurs Health Sci*, 7(4):251-258.

Henderson A, Zernike W. (2001). A study of the impact of discharge information for surgical patients. *J Adv Nurs*, 35(3):435-441.

Ivarsson B, Sjöberg T, Larsson S. (2005). Waiting for cardiac surgery. *Eur J Cardiovasc Nurs*, 4(2):1 45-152.

Lithner M, Zilling T. (2000). Pre- and postoperative information needs. *Patient Educ Couns*, 40(1):29-37.

Moorhead M, Johnson M, Maas M (Eds). (2004). *Nursing Outcomes Classification (NOC)*, 3rd ed. St Louis: Mosby.

Mordiffi SZ, Tan SP, Wong MK. (2003). Information provided to surgical patients versus information needed. *AORN J*, 77(3):546-562.

Showalter A, Burger S, Salyer J. (2000). Patients' and their spouses' needs after total joint arthroplasty: A pilot study. *Orthop Nurs*, 19(1):49-57, 62.

Tromp F, Dulmen S, Weert J. (2004). Interdisciplinary preoperative patient education in cardiac surgery. *J Adv Nurs*, 47(2):212-222.

Young J, O'Connell B. (2001). Recovery following laparoscopic cholecystectomy in either a 23 hour or an 8 hour facility. *J Qual Clin Pract*, 21(1-2):2-7.

 # THERAPEUTIC TOUCH

Eloise Monzillo, PhD, RN, AHN-BC, CPHQ, QTTT

NIC **Definition:** Attuning to the universal healing field, seeking to act as an instrument for healing influence, and using the natural sensitivity of the hands to gently focus and direct the intervention process (Dochterman & Bulechek, 2004).

Therapeutic Touch (TT) is an intentionally directed process of energy exchange during which the nurse uses his or her hands as a focus to facilitate healing (NH-PAI, 2005). This intervention is administered with the intent of enabling an individual to repattern his or her energy field in the direction of health. It consists of centering, assessing, intervention, and evaluation/closure (outlined by NH-PAI, 2005). TT is used as a nursing intervention when nurses discern an energy field disturbance in their patients (Moorhead et al., 2004). TT is employed in conjunction with standardized care (SC).

NURSING ACTIVITIES

Effective

■ *Provide TT for patients who are expressing anxiety.* **LOE = I**

(NR) An RCT ($N = 60$) with a pre-test/post-test, two-group design investigated the effectiveness of TT for reducing State Anxiety in a group of hospitalized adult cardiovascular patients as compared with placebo (that mimicked TT treatment). Analysis revealed that the TT-treated group demonstrated significantly lower post-test anxiety scores than the placebo group (Quinn, 1983).

(NR) An RCT ($N = 105$) with a three-group design investigated the effects of TT for reducing State Anxiety in the institutionalized elderly. TT and back rub was compared with mimicked TT and back rub and SC and back rub. Analysis revealed that those receiving TT and a back rub had significantly lower mean State Anxiety scores than the scores that were obtained from a routine back rub alone (Simington & Laing, 1993).

(NR) An RCT ($N = 31$) with a pre-test/post-test, three-group design investigated the effects of TT and Relaxation Treatment on anxiety and tension in inpatient psychiatric patients. Analysis revealed that both TT and Relaxation Treatment resulted in a significant reduction in anxiety scores after the first treatment (Gagne & Toye, 1994).

(NR) An RCT ($N = 31$) with an explorative, two-group, postintervention design investigated the effects of dialogue and TT on pre- and postoperative anxiety, mood, and postoperative pain in breast cancer surgery patients. Analysis revealed significantly lower state anxiety scores after the preoperative TT treatment as compared with the control group. Postoperatively, there were no statistically significant differences between the TT and control groups (Samarel et al., 1998). **LOE = II**

(NR) An experimental study ($N = 90$) with a pre-test/post-test, three-group design investigated the effectiveness of TT for reducing State Anxiety in a group of hospitalized adult cardiovascular patients as compared with causal-touch and no-touch assigned groups. Analysis revealed that the TT-treated group demonstrated a highly significant difference ($p < .001$). When the TT-treated group was compared with the casual-touch control group, the TT-treated group had significantly lower scores in state anxiety ($p < .01$). When the TT-treated group was compared to the no-touch group, there were significantly lower scores on State Anxiety than the no-touch group ($p < .01$ level of significance) (Heidt, 1981). **LOE = II**

(MR) A study with a nonexperimental, no-comparison-group design ($N = 30$) investigated the effects of TT on heart rate variability through power spectral analysis and anxiety/stress through a visual analog scale measure in healthy people and TT practitioners. Analysis revealed a significant decrease in anxiety/stress scores from before and after for both subject and TT practitioner, with no significant changes in the high/low frequency ratio for either group (Sneed et al., 2001). **LOE = III**

(NR) A qualitative study explored the experience of receiving TT in five postpartum women. Five themes captured the experience of TT: "feeling relaxed, open, cared for, connected, and feeling skeptical." The research concluded that these qualities were all relevant to nursing care (Kiernan, 2002). **LOE = IV**

RCT = Randomized Controlled (Clinical) Trial, **NIC** = Nursing Interventions Classification, **NOC** = Nursing Outcomes Classification

■ *Provide TT for patients who are expressing pain.* **LOE = I**

(NR) An RCT (*N* = 82) with a longitudinal design investigated the effectiveness of TT for decreasing pain in elders with degenerative arthritis. Subjects served as their own control as TT was compared with SC and progressive muscle relaxation. Analysis revealed that both TT and progressive muscle relaxation had similar patterns of differences with respect to visual analog scale scores for pain and distress: between the first and sixth pretreatment ($p \leq .001$ and $p = .004$, respectively); between the first treatment and the sixth post-treatment ($p \leq .001$); and before and after the first treatment ($p \leq .001$; Peck, 1997).

(NR) An RCT (*N* = 60) with a two-group, pre- and post-treatment design investigated the effectiveness of TT for subjects who had been diagnosed with tension headache pain. TT was compared with mimicked TT. Analysis revealed that TT-treated subjects experienced a reduction in headache pain from before to after treatment on all three McGill-Melzack Pain Questionnaire subscales ($p < .0001$). Pain scores 4 hours after the TT intervention were below the pre-test pain scores on all three McGill-Melzack Pain Questionnaire subscales for 28 of the subjects ($p < .0001$; Keller & Bzdek, 1986).

(NR) An RCT (*N* = 108) with a three-group design investigated the effectiveness of TT for postoperative abdominal and pelvic surgery pain. TT was compared with mimicked TT and SC. Analysis revealed that subjects in the TT group waited a significantly longer time before requesting further as-needed analgesic medication as compared with the mimicked TT group ($p \leq .05$; Meehan, 1993).

(MR) In a case study of a subject who experienced phantom-limb pain for 4 years, the application of TT was explored. Pain in this subject typically ranged from 8 to 10 on a self-report VAS, with 10 being the maximum intensity. Pharmaceutical intervention left this patient with unacceptable levels of daytime sedation. The use of self-management techniques reduced the patient pain rate to 7 to 8 on the VAS pain scale. TT-treatment was stated as an adjunct to care. After the TT treatment the patient reported pain rate as 0 on the VAS. This relief lasted until just before the patient's next treatment. Again after a brief treatment the patient's self-report pain rating was 0. At a 6-month follow-up the patient reported 0 to 1 VAS rating (Leskowitz, 2000). **LOE = IV**

■ *Provide TT for patients who are experiencing anxiety and pain.* **LOE = II**

(NR) An RCT (*N* = 99) with a pre-test/post-test, repeated-measure design investigated whether TT compared with sham treatment (mimicked TT) for pain and anxiety reduction in adult burn patients. Analysis revealed that the TT-treated group reported a significantly greater reduction in anxiety than those who received the mimicked TT treatments ($p = 0.031$) and lower pain scores than the mimicked TT group on two of the three subscales in the McGill-Melzack Pain Questionnaire ($p = 0.004$ and $p = 0.005$) (Turner et al., 1998).

(NR) An RCT (*N* = 90) with a pre-test/post-test, three-group design investigated the effectiveness of TT for reducing pain and anxiety in an elderly population of patients. TT was compared with SC and mimicked TT. Analysis revealed that the pain-intensity scores decreased in all groups, with a significant reduction in subjective pain ratings in the TT group as compared with the mimicked TT and SC groups ($p \leq .001$). Anxiety was significantly reduced in the TT-treated group as compared with the mimicked TT and SC control groups ($p < .01$) (Yu Shen & Taylor, 1999).

NR = Nursing Research, **MR** = Multidisciplinary Research, **SP** = Standard of Practice, **EO** = Expert Opinion, **LOE** = Level of Evidence

(NR) A case study explored the experience of receiving TT in an individual who reported to be experiencing pain related to endometriosis "most of the time" and fluctuating feelings of anxiety about her health and pain situation. TT was given as an adjunctive intervention. After the first TT intervention, the subject expressed a feeling of relaxation that lasted the day of the TT treatment and into the next day. The patient said of her experience that "the pain had almost disappeared" and reported a sense of total well-being after the TT intervention (Green, 1998). **LOE = IV**

■ *Provide TT for patients with behavioral symptoms that are associated with dementia.* LOE = II

(NR) An RCT ($N = 57$) with a three-group design investigated the effectiveness of TT for the frequency and intensity of behavioral symptoms of dementia in residents from special care units. Analysis revealed a significant change in overall scores on the behavioral symptoms of dementia in the TT-treated group ($p = .033$). When TT was compared with the control group, there was significant reduction in manual manipulation (restlessness) ($p = .02$) and vocalization ($p = .03$) (Woods et al., 2005).

■ *Provide TT for patients who have experienced an alteration in personal well-being.* LOE = II

(NR) An RCT ($N = 20$) with a two-group design investigated the effectiveness of TT on the perception of well-being in people with terminal cancer who were receiving palliative care. Analysis revealed a significant difference in well-being between TT and control group ($p = .0015$). The TT group demonstrated a mean increase in the sensation of well-being; the control group demonstrated a decrease of well-being. Also, the sensation of well-being improved significantly between times one and four in the TT-treated group ($p = .025$) (Giasson & Bouchard, 1998).

■ *Provide TT for patients with sleeplessness.* LOE = III

(NR) In a case study, a woman with shingles of 8 weeks' duration with unrelenting pain and the inability to sleep for 2 weeks received TT treatment. On the patient's return visit a week after one TT treatment, she reported, "I was so relaxed (after the last treatment) I went to sleep for 2 hours . . . and each night now, I am getting several good hours of sleep, so that when I get up in the morning, I feel as if I have had a night's sleep; this is very different" (Heidt, 1991).

■ *Provide TT for patients with physiological expressions of normal human osteoblasts, fibroblasts, and tenocytes.* LOE = I

(MR) A double-blind, basic science study ($N = 36$ samples from six separate experiments) with a three-group design investigated the effect of TT on normal osteoblasts (bone cells). TT was compared with mimicked TT (placebo) and untreated control. An analysis of proliferation revealed significant differences in the TT-treated osteoblasts as compared with the placebo and control groups, and there were also significant differences in mineralization ($N = 24$ samples from four separate experiments) compared with placebo and control (Gronowicz, 2006).

RCT = Randomized Controlled (Clinical) Trial, **NIC** = Nursing Interventions Classification, **NOC** = Nursing Outcomes Classification

(MR) A double-blind, basic science study ($N = 18$ samples from three separate experiments) with a two-group design demonstrated the effect of TT on normal human fibroblast proliferation. Analysis revealed a significant difference in the TT-treated normal human fibroblasts as compared with those of an untreated control group (Gronowicz, 2006).

(MR) A double-blind, basic science study ($N = 12$ samples from two separate experiments) with a two-group design investigated the effect of TT on normal tenocyte (tendon cells) proliferation. Analysis revealed significance differences in the TT-treated tenocytes as compared with those of an untreated control group (Gronowicz, 2006).

■ *Provide TT for patients with physiological expressions of hemoglobin.* **LOE = II**

(MR) An RCT ($N = 86$) with a three-group design investigated the effects of TT on levels of hemoglobin and hematocrit in women with anemia. TT was compared with mimicked TT and SC. Analysis revealed that mean hemoglobin levels were significantly different between the three groups. The mean hemoglobin level in the TT group was significantly higher than that of the mimicked TT and control groups ($p = .05$ and $p \leq .001$, respectively), with no significant differences between TT and mimicked TT on mean hematocrit levels (Movaffaghi et al., 2006).

■ *Provide TT for patients with physiological expressions of immunity.* **LOE = II**

(MR) An RCT ($N = 20$) with a pre-test/post-test design investigated the effectiveness of TT for reducing the adverse immunological effects of stress in a sample of stressed students. Analysis revealed differences between groups after TT treatments. The TT group revealed significantly less decrement in their immunoglobulin M and A levels ($p = .05$), but not in G levels (Olson et al., 1997).

(NR) An RCT ($N = 11$) with a pre-test/post-test repeated-measure design investigated the effectiveness of TT in reducing State Anxiety and pain and for altering plasma T-lymphocyte concentration in adult burn patients. TT was compared with mimicked TT. Analysis of the immunological component of this study revealed that the greatest difference between the groups was noted for the total CD8+ cell concentration. The total CD8+ cells in the TT-treated group decreased by 13.0% from day 1 to day 6 but increased by 46.5% in the mimicked TT group. Total CD4+ cell concentration increased 15.2% from day 1 to day 6 in the TT group but increased by 48.3% in the mimicked TT group. Total T-lymphocyte count increased 1.1% from day 1 to day 6 for the TT group, and it increased by 38.6% for the MTT group (Turner et al., 1998).

Possibly Effective

■ *Provide TT for patients who are expressing anxiety.* **LOE = III**

(NR) A quasi-experimental repeat session design ($N = 23$) investigated the effectiveness of TT for reducing stress and anxiety in healthy subjects after a natural disaster. Analysis revealed that state anxiety scores reduced significantly from before to after the TT intervention ($p = .05$) (Olson et al., 1992).

■ *Provide TT for patients who are expressing pain.* **LOE = II**

(MR) An RCT ($N = 25$) with a three-group, pre-test/post-test, repeated-measure design investigated the effectiveness of TT on patients with osteoarthritis of the knee. TT was compared

---

NR = Nursing Research, **MR** = Multidisciplinary Research, **SP** = Standard of Practice, **EO** = Expert Opinion, **LOE** = Level of Evidence

with mimicked TT and SC. Analysis revealed significantly decreased pain and improved function in the TT-treated groups as compared with both the mimicked TT ($p = 0.002$) and SC groups ($p = 0.005$) (Gordon et al., 1998).

■ *Provide TT for patients with behavioral symptoms that are associated with dementia.* **LOE = II**

NR A study with a within-subject interrupted time series design ($N = 10$) investigated the effectiveness of TT on the frequency and intensity of agitated behavior in residents in special care units who were diagnosed with moderate to severe Alzheimer's disease. Analysis revealed a decrease in overall agitation behavior ($p = 0.00$). This effect was driven by two behaviors: vocalization and pacing or walking. The overall decrease across time was significant, with the most prominent decrease occurring during treatment. This effect was driven by two behaviors: vocalization ($p = 0.00$) and pacing or walking ($p = 0.00$) (Woods & Dimond, 2002).

■ *Provide TT for patients with alterations in personal well-being.* **LOE = IV**

NR A qualitative study compared the perceptions of 18 women with breast cancer who received TT treatment plus a dialogue nursing intervention as compared with those who experienced quiet time plus dialogue. Content analysis revealed similar perceptions. Women regarded both interventions as positive, and they expressed feelings of calmness, relaxation, security, and comfort (Kelly et al., 2004).

NR A qualitative study ($N = 31$) explored patients' experiences of receiving TT. Content analysis of interview data revealed the emergence of three categories, with one of the three being the experience after a TT treatment. A structural description of this category revealed that the lived experience after a TT treatment is one of physiological, mental/emotional, and spiritual personal change that leads to resonating fulfillment (Samarel, 1992).

■ *Provide TT for patients who are experiencing sleeplessness.* **LOE = III**

NR A study with a time series design ($N = 53$) investigated the effects of TT on physiological responses in critical care patients and the analysis of interview data. Analysis revealed no significant differences in physiological variables. Interview data yielded 25 different words and phrases generated by the subjects' response to their experience of TT. The frequently occurring words were clustered into two categories: one category was that of quiescence—relaxed and sleepy (Cox & Hayes, 1999).

NR In a case study of a 29-year-old female who suffered a traffic accident and then remained hospitalized for 87 days, nurses in the intensive care unit described the woman as "very stressed and agitated, and she was observed as sleeping fitfully for 15 to 20 minutes at a time." Whenever the patient presented as "stressed and restless," TT was administered. After the first TT treatment, the patient reported feeling relaxed and calm. TT was administered to this patient upon request; observations were made that the patient's sleeping patterns improved and that she started sleeping for 4 hours at a time (Cox & Hayes, 1997). **LOE = IV**

RCT = Randomized Controlled (Clinical) Trial, **NIC** = Nursing Interventions Classification, **NOC** = Nursing Outcomes Classification

Not Effective

■ *TT for some patients who are expressing anxiety.* **LOE = II**

(NR) An RCT ($N = 151$) with a pre-test/post-test, three-group design replicated and extended previous research that investigated the effects of TT for reducing state anxiety in a group of hospitalized adult cardiovascular patients. Analysis revealed no significant differences among the groups with regard to post-test scores or the reduction of anxiety, systolic blood pressure, or heart rate. Diastolic blood pressure was significantly decreased in the post-test among the TT group (Quinn, 1989). **LOE = III**

(NR) A quasi-experimental study ($N = 11$) with a repeated measure, pre-test/post-test design investigated the effectiveness and magnitude of the effect of TT on three behavioral measures (one being State and Trait anxiety) and four biological measures as compared with placebo (mimicked TT). Analysis revealed no significant changes in the behavioral measures, except in Time Perception, and no significant change in the biological variables, except in Total Pulse Amplitude. Both time perception and Total Pulse Amplitude significantly decrease during the 10-minute recovery time period after TT treatment, the opposite effects of previous research and clinical reports. The significant decrease in the Total Pulse Amplitude indicated a temporary peripheral vasoconstriction. Vasodilitation, a relaxation response, was expected instead of vasoconstriction. TT may have both adverse and positive outcomes. This effect is an area for additional research (Engle & Graney, 2000).

■ *TT for some patients who are expressing pain.* **LOE = II**

(NR) An RCT ($N = 108$) with a three-group design investigated the effectiveness of TT for postoperative abdominal and pelvic pain in surgical patients. TT was compared with mimicked TT and SC. Analysis revealed no significant difference between groups with regard to the reduction of patients' perception of pain (Meehan, 1993).

OUTCOME MEASUREMENT

ANXIETY LEVEL (NOC)

Definition: Severity of manifested apprehension, tension, or uneasiness arising from an unidentifiable source.
Anxiety Level as evidenced by the following selected NOC indicators:
- Restlessness
- Increased blood pressure
- Increased pulse rate
- Verbalized anxiety
- Verbalized apprehension

(Rate each indicator of **Anxiety Level:** 1 = severe, 2 = substantial, 3 = moderate, 4 = mild, 5 = none) (Moorhead et al., 2004).

PERSONAL WELL-BEING (NOC)

Definition: Extent of positive perception of one's health status and life circumstances.
Personal Well-Being as evidenced by the following selected NOC indicators:

NR = Nursing Research, **MR** = Multidisciplinary Research, **SP** = Standard of Practice, **EO** = Expert Opinion, **LOE** = Level of Evidence

OUTCOME MEASUREMENT—*cont'd*

- Psychological health
- Spiritual life
- Ability to relax
- Ability to cope
- Level of happiness

(Rate each indicator of **Personal Well-Being** 1 = not all satisfied, 2 = somewhat satisfied, 3 = moderately satisfied, 4 = very satisfied, 5 = completely satisfied) (Moorhead et al., 2004).

COMFORT LEVEL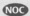

Definition: Extent of positive perception of physical and psychological ease.

Comfort Level as evidenced by the following selected NOC indicators:

- Physical well-being
- Psychological well-being
- Pain control

(Rate each indicator of **Comfort Level:** 1 = not all satisfied, 2 = somewhat satisfied, 3 = moderately satisfied, 4 = very satisfied, 5 = completely satisfied) (Moorhead et al., 2004).

SLEEP   NOC

Definition: Natural periodic suspension of consciousness during which the body is restored.

Sleep as evidenced by the following selected NOC indicators:

- Hours of sleep (at least 5 hr/24 hr)*
- Sleep pattern
- Sleep quality
- Feels rejuvenated after sleep

(Rate each indicator of **Sleep:** 1 = severely compromised, 2 = substantially compromised, 3 = moderately compromised, 4 = mildly compromised, 5 = not compromised) (Moorhead et al., 2004).

*Appropriate for adults.

REFERENCES

Cox C, Hayes J. (1997). Reducing anxiety: The employment of Therapeutic Touch as a nursing intervention. *Complement Ther Nurs Midwifery,* 3(6):163-167.

Cox C, Hayes J. (1999). Physiologic and psychodynamic responses in the administration of therapeutic touch in critical care. *Complement Ther Nurs Midwifery,* 5(4):87-92.

Dochterman JM, Bulechek GM (Eds). (2004). *Nursing Interventions Classification (NIC),* 4th ed. St Louis: Mosby.

EngleVF, Graney MJ. (2000). Biobehavioral effects of therapeutic touch. *J Nurs Scholarsh,* 32(3):287-293.

Fenton M. (2003). Therapeutic touch: A nursing practice. *Altern Ther Health Med,* 9(1):34-36.

Gagne D, Toye R. (1994). The effects of therapeutic touch and relaxation therapy in reducing anxiety. *Arch Psychiatr Nurs,* 8(3):184-189.

RCT = Randomized Controlled (Clinical) Trial, **NIC** = Nursing Interventions Classification, **NOC** = Nursing Outcomes Classification

Giasson M, Bouchard L. (1998). Effect of therapeutic touch on the well being of persons with terminal cancer. *J Holist Nurs,* 16(3):383-398.

Gordon A, Merenstein JH, D'Amico F, Hudgens D. (1998). The effect of therapeutic touch on patients with osteoarthritis of the knee. *J Fam Pract,* 47(4):271-277.

Green C. (1998). Reflection of a therapeutic touch experience: Case study 2. *Complement Ther Nurs Midwifery,* 4(1):17-21.

Gronowicz GA. (2006). Principal investigator, Director of Orthopedic Research, Department of Orthopaedics, University of Connecticut Health Center. Professional communication.

Heidt P. (1981). Effect of therapeutic touch on anxiety levels of hospitalized patients. *Nurs Res,* 30(1):3 2-37.

Heidt P. (1991). Helping patients to rest: Clinical studies in therapeutic touch. *Holist Nurs Pract,* 5(4): 57-66.

Herdtner S. (2000). Using therapeutic touch in nursing practice. *Orthop Nurs,* 19(5):77-82.

Keller E, Bzdek V. (1986). Effects of therapeutic touch on tension headache pain. *Nurs Res,* 35(2):101-106.

Kelly AE, Sullivan P, Fawcett J, Samarel N. (2004). Therapeutic touch, quiet time, and dialogue: Perceptions of women with breast cancer. *Oncol Nurs Forum,* 31(3):625-631.

Kiernan J. (2002). The experience of Therapeutic Touch in the lives of five postpartum women. *Am J Matern Child Nurs,* 27(1):47-53.

Leskowitz ED. (2000). Phantom limb pain treated with therapeutic touch: A case report. *Arch Phys Med Rehabil,* 81(4):522-524.

Meehan TC. (1993). Therapeutic touch and postoperative pain: A Rogerian research study. *Nurs Sci Q,* 6(2):69-78.

Moorhead S, Johnson M, Maas M (Eds). (2004). *Nursing Outcomes Classification (NOC),* 3rd ed. St Louis: Mosby.

Movaffaghi Z, Hasanpoor M, Farsi M, Hooshmand P, Abrishami F. (2006). Effect of therapeutic touch on blood hemoglobin and hematocrit level. *J Holist Nurs,* 24(1):41-48.

Nurse Healers-Professional Associates International (NH-PAI). (2005). Therapeutic touch policy and procedure for health professionals. Available online: www.therapeutic-touch.org. Retrieved on November 6, 2006.

Olson M, Sneed N, Bonadonna R, Ratliff J, Dias J. (1992). Therapeutic touch and post-Hurricane Hugo stress. *J Holist Nurs,* 10(2):120-136.

Olson M, Sneed NV, Virella MG, Bonadonna R, Michel Y. (1997). Stress induced immunosuppression and therapeutic touch. *Altern Ther,* 3(2):68-74.

Peck SD. (1997). The effectiveness of therapeutic touch for decreasing pain in elders with degenerative arthritis. *J Holist Nurs,* 15(2):176-198.

Quinn JF. (1983). Therapeutic touch as energy exchange: Testing the theory. *Adv Nurs Sci,* 6(2):42-49.

Quinn JF. (1989). Therapeutic touch as energy exchange: Replication and extension. *Nurs Sci Q,* 2(2):79-87.

Samarel N. (1992). The experience of receiving therapeutic touch. *J Adv Nur,* 17(6):651-657.

Samarel N, Fawcett J, Davis M, Ryan F. (1998). The effect of dialogue and therapeutic touch on preoperative and postoperative experiences of breast cancer surgery: An exploratory study. *Oncol Nurs Forum,* 25(8):1369-1376.

Simington JA, Laing GP. (1993). The effects of therapeutic touch on anxiety in the institutionalized elderly. *Clin Nurs Res,* 2(4):438-450.

Sneed NV, Olson M, Bubolz B, Finch N. (2001). Influences of a relaxation intervention on perceived stress and power spectral analysis of heart rate variability. *Prog Cardiovasc Nurs,* 16(2):57-64.

Turner JG, Clark AJ, Gauthier DK, Williams M. (1998). The effect of therapeutic touch on pain and anxiety in burn patients. *J Adv Nurs,* 28(1):10-20.

Woods DL, Dimond M. (2002). The effect of therapeutic touch on agitated behavior and cortisol in persons with Alzheimer's disease. *Biol Res Nurs,* 4(2):104-114.

Woods DL, Ruth F, Craven RF, Whitney J. (2005). The effect of therapeutic touch on behavioral symptoms of persons with dementia. *Altern Ther Health Med,* 11(1):66-74.

Yu Shen Lin, Taylor AG. (1999). Effects of therapeutic touch in reducing pain and anxiety in an elderly population. *Integ Med,* 1(4):155-161.

NR = Nursing Research, **MR** = Multidisciplinary Research, **SP** = Standard of Practice, **EO** = Expert Opinion, **LOE** = Level of Evidence

TOBACCO CESSATION ASSISTANCE

Kathleen K. Zarling, MSN, RN, APRN-BC

NIC **Definition:** Helping another to stop using tobacco (Dochterman & Bulechek, 2004).

NURSING ACTIVITIES

Effective

■ **NIC** *Determine the patient's readiness to learn about smoking cessation.*
LOE = I

MR An RCT of 1477 patients showed that the most important finding may have been the experience of hospitalization itself that led to substantial long-term quitting for virtually all categories of hospitalized smokers (Lando et al., 2003).

NR An RCT (*N* = 168) using the Transtheoretical Model found that lower levels of readiness to quit smoking at baseline progressed more readily throughout hospitalization to further stages of change (Chouinard & Robichaud-Ekstrand, 2005).

NR In a cross-sectional survey of staff nurses (*N* = 397) at four hospitals, 63% believed that hospitalization was an ideal time for patients to try to quit smoking and 59% believed that a nurse had an obligation to advise patients to quit smoking (McCarty et al., 2001).

MR In a cohort study of 1021 patients who made quit attempts, findings indicated that stronger efforts should be made to enhance treatment compliance among smokers with indicators of high nicotine dependence and low socioeconomic status (Foulds et al., 2006).

■ **NIC** *Give the smoker clear, consistent advice to quit smoking.* **LOE = I**

NR An RCT (*N* = 250) that involved patients who were daily smokers and were admitted to a Norwegian Vest-Agder Hospital for MI, unstable angina, or for care after coronary artery bypass surgery demonstrated that a smoking-cessation intervention by cardiac nurses with a simple booklet but with no special training achieved a cessation rate of 50% at 12 months (Quist-Paulsen & Gallefoss, 2003).

NR In a Cochrane systematic review, a nursing intervention for smoking cessation in 20 out of 29 studies cited significant increases in "odds of quitting" (Rice & Stead, 2004).

NR A meta-analysis of 34 studies demonstrated that smokers who were offered advice by a nursing professional had an increased likelihood of quitting as compared with smokers without such an intervention (Rice & Stead, 2006).

NR A comprehensive literature review demonstrated nurse-delivered inpatient interventions to be effective from 1996 to 2003, with the purpose being to set a research agenda to strengthen nursing involvement in addressing tobacco use among patient populations (Schultz, 2003).

NR An RCT of a brief nursing intervention after a birth contact (*N* = 238) and eight phone calls over 3 months found a cessation rate of 21% in the treatment group and 18.5% in the control group (Ratner et al., 2000).

RCT = Randomized Controlled (Clinical) Trial, **NIC** = Nursing Interventions Classification, **NOC** = Nursing Outcomes Classification

■ **NIC** *Refer to group programs or individual therapists as appropriate.* **LOE = I**

NR A meta-analysis of 37 RCTs (18 of which were nursing interventions) compared the efficacy of tobacco intervention by provider teams, physicians, dentists, and nurses. Findings revealed that receiving advice from any health care professional increased quit rates, with physicians most effective and nursing interventions comparing favorably with those of multidisciplinary teams and dentists. Additional training in tobacco control for nurses is warranted (Gorin & Heck, 2004).

MR An RCT of 540 smokers hospitalized with myocardial infarction or coronary artery bypass graft demonstrated that interventions comprising several sessions with specialists were shown to be effective, whereas single-session interventions delivered within routine care may have had insufficient power to influence highly dependent smokers (Hajek et al., 2002).

■ **NIC** *Help choose the best method for giving up cigarettes when the patient is ready to quit.* **LOE = I**

EO Tobacco dependence is a chronic condition that often requires repeated interventions, and everyone who uses tobacco should be offered, at the least, a brief intervention. Additional effective treatments include person-to-person contacts, counseling and behavioral therapies, numerous effective pharmacotherapies, and tobacco-dependence treatment programs (Fiore, 2000).

NR In an RCT that was conducted from 1996 to 2001 ($N = 277$) of women diagnosed with cardiovascular disease who were randomly assigned to a usual-care group ($N = 135$) or an intervention group ($N = 142$), it was found that a cognitive-behavioral intervention resulted in a longer average time to the resumption of smoking, with even a brief intervention yielding a high smoking cessation rate over time (Sivarajan Froelicher et al., 2004).

MR In a comprehensive review of the literature regarding pharmacotherapies for tobacco dependence, it was reported that the best hope for improved treatment came from combining existing and new pharmacotherapies together with effective behavioral therapy (Foulds et al., 2004).

MR In a meta-analysis, the effectiveness of multiple traditional and nontraditional treatment modalities for tobacco cessation—along with readiness to change—was explored. Nurses were encouraged to provide the best treatment for addressing the patient's tobacco dependence by first learning the different treatment options and their effectiveness. Findings indicated that knowledge about various treatment options and their efficacy and about the applicability of interventions such as counseling, nicotine replacement therapy, non-nicotine drugs, harm reduction, and acupuncture was a very important prerequisite to choosing the right treatments (Urso, 2003).

■ **NIC** *Manage nicotine-replacement therapy (NRT).* **LOE = I**

MR In two postal surveys of random national samples of general practitioners ($N = 303$) and practicing nurses ($N = 459$), 83% of general practitioners and 74% of nurses recommended NRT to their patients (McEwen & West, 2001).

NR A Cochrane systematic review of 20 nursing interventions for smoking cessation that compared a nursing intervention group with a control group or usual care found that the nursing counseling interventions significantly increased the odds of tobacco cessation. A

NR = Nursing Research, **MR** = Multidisciplinary Research, **SP** = Standard of Practice, **EO** = Expert Opinion, **LOE** = Level of Evidence

challenge exists in making interventions part of standard practice and in including reinforcement and follow-up as part of that standard (Rice & Stead, 2004).

(MR) A Cochrane systematic review found that all forms of NRT made it more likely that a person's attempt to quit smoking would succeed and that these effective NRT strategies increased the odds of quitting by one and a half to two times, regardless of the setting (Silagy et al., 2004).

(MR) In an RCT ($N = 578$), nicotine patch therapy and bupropion were studied in tandem to explore their effectiveness together or as single therapies for tobacco cessation. Bupropion did not reduce relapse to smoking in smokers who stopped smoking with nicotine patch therapy. Also, it did not initiate abstinence among smokers who failed to stop smoking with nicotine patch therapy (Hurt et al., 2003).

■ (NIC) *Arrange to maintain frequent telephone contact with the patient (e.g., to acknowledge that withdrawal is difficult, to reinforce the importance of remaining abstinent, and to offer congratulations on progress).*
LOE = I

(NR) A quasi-experimental study ($N = 102$) resulted in a 46% smoking cessation rate with inpatient intervention and postdischarge telephone follow-up as compared with 31% in the control group at 6 months' follow-up (Deaton & Namasivayam, 2004).

(NR) An RCT ($N = 168$) resulted in a 6-month abstinence rate of 41.5% in the inpatient counseling with telephone follow-up group as compared with 30.2% and 20% in the inpatient counseling and usual care groups, respectively (Chouinard & Robichaud-Ekstrand, 2005).

Possibly Effective

■ (SP) *Implement a registered-nurse-initiated tobacco use intervention protocol upon admission to the hospital to offer both nicotine patch therapy and behavioral intervention. Have the nurse give out written information and advise the patient to cease tobacco use.* **LOE = VII**

(NR) A study across the cardiology wards of five hospitals and involving 85 nurses examined whether or not nurses would use a smoking cessation protocol and what influenced their decisions (e.g., attitudes, social influence, self-efficacy, and user-friendliness). This study found that greater perceived simplicity and advantages of the protocol were associated with increased intentions to continue use, whereas perceived social influences and self-efficacy were not. Nurses who did not intend to continue using the protocol needed to be convinced of the advantages of working with such a protocol and of its user-friendliness (Bolman et al., 2002).

(MR) In a descriptive and evaluative longitudinal study of smoking relapse/reduction intervention for prenatal women that included a detailed review of the literature, four core components were received by all women: (1) home visits by the intervention nurse; (2) follow-up telephone call(s); (3) a resource package; and (4) a letter of congratulations. Participants found the core components of the intervention to be helpful for their smoking cessation goals, particularly the home visit and the resource material. The support groups and the smoking help line were not used (Chalmers et al., 2004).

RCT = Randomized Controlled (Clinical) Trial, **NIC** = Nursing Interventions Classification, **NOC** = Nursing Outcomes Classification

Not Effective

- *Advocating and counseling patients about smoking cessation while continuing to smoke.* **LOE = IV**

  (NR) Serving as nonsmoking role models, nurses can provide an effective intervention while caring for smokers. However, in a recent efficacy study that was focused on smoking cessation interventions that were specific for tobacco-dependent nurses, the authors identified nurses as a special population of tobacco users because of their health knowledge, their position as health educators, and their position as health behavior role models. Further support for tobacco-dependent nurses in their own cessation efforts is needed (Chalmers et al., 2001).

  (NR) Continued smoking among nurses (18% of registered nurses smoke) has been cited as one of the barriers to higher nursing involvement in tobacco cessation efforts. A study of eight focus groups ($N = 60$ registered nurses) in four different states showed that nurses have many of the same misconceptions and difficulties with regard to quitting tobacco as their patients do (Bialous et al., 2004).

  (MR) A survey of nursing students ($N = 126$) and medical students ($N = 397$) who smoked found that providing education for professionals to quit for themselves would enhance their participation in the education and tobacco cessation efforts of their patients (Patkar et al., 2003).

Possibly Harmful

No applicable published research was found in this category.

OUTCOME MEASUREMENT

RISK CONTROL: TOBACCO USE (NOC)

(Please refer to *Nursing Outcomes Classification* [Moorhead et al., 2004] for the **Risk Control: Tobacco Use** outcome.)

FAGERSTROM TEST

The Fagerstrom Test is a validated six-item questionnaire for nicotine dependence to assess the severity of smoking (Fagerstrom & Schneider, 1989).

REFERENCES

Bialous SA, Sarna L, Wewers ME, Froelicher ES, Danao L. (2004). Nurses' perspectives of smoking initiation, addiction, and cessation. *Nurs Res,* 53(6):387-395.

Bolman C, de Vries H, Mesters I. (2002). Factors determining cardiac nurses' intentions to continue using a smoking cessation protocol. *Heart Lung,* 31(1):15-24.

Chalmers K, Bramadat IJ, Cantin B, Murnaghan D, Shuttleworth E, Scott-Findlay S, et al. (2001). A smoking reduction and cessation program with registered nurses: Findings and implications for community health nursing. *J Community Health Nurs,* 18(2):115-134.

Chalmers K, Gupton A, Katz A, Hack T, Hildes-Ripstein E, Brown J, et al. (2004). The description and evaluation of a longitudinal pilot study of a smoking relapse/reduction intervention for perinatal women. *J Adv Nurs*, 45(2):162-171.

Chouinard MC, Robichaud-Ekstrand S. (2005). The effectiveness of a nursing inpatient smoking cessation program in individuals with cardiovascular disease. *Nurs Res*, 54(4):243-254.

Deaton C, Namasivayam S. (2004). Nursing outcomes in coronary heart disease. *J Cardiovasc Nurs*, 19(5):308-315.

Dochterman JM, Bulechek GM (Eds). (2004). *Nursing Interventions Classification (NIC)*, 4th ed. St Louis: Mosby.

Fagerstrom KO, Schneider NG. (1989). Measuring nicotine dependence: A review of the Fagerstrom Tolerance Questionnaire. *J Behav Med*, 12(2):159-182.

Fiore MC. (2000). U.S. public health service clinical practice guideline: Treating tobacco use and dependence. *Respir Care*, 45(10):1200-1262.

Foulds J, Burke M, Steinberg M, Williams JM, Ziedonis DM. (2004). Advances in pharmacotherapy for tobacco dependence. *Expert Opin Emerg Drugs*, 9(1):39-53.

Foulds J, Gandhi KK, Steinberg MB, Richardson DL, Williams JM, Burke MV, et al. (2006). Factors associated with quitting smoking at a tobacco dependence treatment clinic. *Am J Health Behav*, 30(4):400-412.

Gorin SS, Heck JE. (2004). Meta-analysis of the efficacy of tobacco counseling by health care providers. *Cancer Epidemiol Biomarkers Prev*, 13(12):2012-2022.

Hajek P, Taylor TZ, Mills P. (2002). Brief intervention during hospital admission to help patients to give up smoking after myocardial infarction and bypass surgery: Randomized controlled trial. *BMJ*, 324(7329):87-89.

Hurt RD, Krook JE, Croghan IT, Loprinzi CL, Sloan JA, Novotny PJ, et al. (2003). Nicotine patch therapy based on smoking rate followed by bupropion for prevention of relapse to smoking. *J Clin Oncology*, 21(5):914-920.

Lando H, Hennrikus D, McCarty M, Vessey J. (2003). Predictors of quitting in hospitalized smokers. *Nicotine Tob Res*, 5(2):215-222.

McCarty MC, Hennrikus DJ, Lando HA, Vessey JT. (2001). Nurses' attitudes concerning the delivery of brief cessation advice to hospitalized smokers. *Prev Med*, 33(6):674-681.

McEwen A, West R. (2001). Smoking cessation activities by general practitioners and practice nurses. *Tob Control*, 10(1):27-32.

Moorhead M, Johnson M, Maas M (Eds). (2004). *Nursing Outcomes Classification (NOC)*, 3rd ed. St Louis: Mosby.

Patkar AA, Hill K, Batra V, Vergare MJ, Leone FT. (2003). A comparison of smoking habits among medical and nursing students. *Chest*, 124(4):1415-1420.

Quist-Paulsen P, Gallefoss F. (2003). Randomized controlled trial of smoking cessation intervention after admission for coronary heart disease. *BMJ*, 327(7426):1254-1257.

Ratner PA, Johnson JL, Bottorff JL, Dahinten S, Hall W. (2000). Twelve-month follow-up of a smoking relapse prevention intervention for postpartum women. *Addict Behav*, 25(1):81-92.

Rice VH, Stead LF. (2004). Nursing interventions for smoking cessation. *Cochrane Database Syst Rev*, (1): CD001188.

Rice VH, Stead L. (2006). Nursing intervention and smoking cessation: Meta-analysis update. *Heart Lung*, 35(3):147-163.

Schultz AS. (2003). Nursing and tobacco reduction: A review of the literature. *Int J Nurs Stud*, 40(6): 571-586.

Silagy C, Lancaster T, Stead L, Mant D, Fowler G. (2004). Nicotine replacement therapy for smoking cessation. *Cochrane Database Syst Rev*, (3):CD000146.

Sivarajan Froelicher ES, Miller NH, Christopherson DJ, Martin K, Parker KM, Amonetti M, et al. (2004). High rates of sustained smoking cessation in women hospitalized with cardiovascular disease: the Women's Initiative for Nonsmoking (WINS). *Circulation*, 109(5):587-593.

Urso P. (2003). Match the best smoking cessation intervention to your patient. *Nurse Pract*, Suppl:12-16, 18-19, 21.

RCT = Randomized Controlled (Clinical) Trial, **NIC** = Nursing Interventions Classification, **NOC** = Nursing Outcomes Classification

TOTAL PARENTERAL NUTRITION ADMINISTRATION

Lisa Gorski, MS, APRN-BC, CRNI, FAAN

NIC **Definition:** Preparation and delivery of nutrients intravenously and the monitoring of patient responsiveness (Dochterman & Bulechek, 2004).

NURSING ACTIVITIES

Effective

■ *Wash hands using conventional antiseptic soap and water or with waterless alcohol-based gels or foams before and after administering total parenteral nutrition (TPN) to reduce the risk of intravenous (IV)-catheter-related infections.*

EO Good hand hygiene is essential to prevent intravascular catheter infections (O'Grady et al., 2002).
(Refer to the guideline on Infection Control: Hand Hygiene.)

■ *Maintain aseptic technique while performing all TPN-administration-related procedures to reduce the risk of catheter-related bloodstream infection (BSI).* **LOE = I**

(Refer to the guidelines on Infection Control: Hand Hygiene and Infection Protection.)
MR In a review of the literature regarding the critical interventions that are necessary for the reduction of catheter-related BSI, the risk of extraluminal contamination is decreased through skin antisepsis and antimicrobial dressings. The risk of intraluminal contamination is also decreased through hand hygiene, access site disinfection, and antimicrobial flush solutions (Ryder, 2006).
EO Full sterile barrier precautions (e.g., cap, mask, sterile gown, sterile gloves, large sterile drape) should be used during the insertion of central venous catheters (CVCs) to reduce the incidence of BSI (O'Grady et al., 2002).
EO Full-barrier precautions should be used during the insertion of central lines; skin preparation before catheter insertion should be performed using chlorhexidine (ASPEN, 2002).

■ *Use a specialized team to administer and monitor TPN therapy to reduce the risk of complications and the cost of care.* **LOE = II**

EO Specialized "IV teams" have shown unequivocal effectiveness for reducing the incidence of catheter-related infections and their associated complications and costs (O'Grady et al., 2002).
EO Specialized nursing teams should care for venous access devices in patients who are receiving TPN (ASPEN, 2002).
MR In a descriptive study, the formation of a nutritional support team resulted in a significant decrease in the use of inappropriate TPN; indications for the appropriate use of TPN

NR = Nursing Research, **MR** = Multidisciplinary Research, **SP** = Standard of Practice, **EO** = Expert Opinion, **LOE** = Level of Evidence

were based on American Society for Parenteral and Enteral Nutrition guidelines (Saalwachter et al., 2004).

MR A systematic review of studies regarding multidisciplinary TPN teams found that the incidence of total mechanical complications was reduced in patients who were managed by the TPN team. However, the benefit of the TPN team for the reduction of catheter-related sepsis and metabolic and electrolyte complications was inconclusive (Naylor et al., 2004).

■ *Administer TPN through a centrally placed catheter to reduce the risk of phlebitis and the damage to peripheral veins.* LOE = I

EO Parenteral nutrition solutions that contain final concentrations that exceed 10% dextrose and 5% protein, a pH of less than 5 or more than 9, and infusates with an osmolarity of more than 600 mOsm/L should be administered through a central venous access device (INS, 2006).

EO Parenteral nutrition should be delivered through a catheter that is located with its distal tip in the superior vena cava or the right atrium (ASPEN, 2002).

EO The use of antimicrobial-impregnated catheters is recommended for high-risk patients and high-risk care settings (ASPEN, 2002).

EO Peripheral parenteral nutrition solutions in final concentrations of 10% dextrose or lower and 5% protein or lower may be administered peripherally, but they should not be administered for longer than 7 to 10 days unless they are supplemented with oral or enteral nutrition to ensure adequate nutrition (INS, 2006).

■ **SP** *Use a 1.2-micron filter (for three-in-one TPN solutions) or a 0.2-micron filter (for a TPN solution that does not contain lipids) as part of the IV administration set when administering TPN solutions to reduce the risk of infusing particulate matter.* LOE = V

MR In an in vitro study to assess the ability of 1.2-micron filters to filter large fat globules, 1.2-micron filters significantly reduced the total number and concentration of enlarged fat globules and suggested that in-line TPN filtration should be a standard part of nutrition therapy (Driscoll et al., 1996).

EO At least two patient deaths and two cases of respiratory distress occurred after the administration of three-in-one TPN. Autopsies showed microvascular pulmonary emboli that contained calcium phosphate. Because of the risk of particulate matter, a 1.2-micron filter is recommended for all three-in-one TPN solutions (McKinnon, 1996).

EO Use a 0.2-micron filter for TPN solutions that do not contain lipids; use a 1.2-micron filter for three-in-one TPN solutions (INS, 2006; ASPEN, 2002).

EO Appropriate filters should be used during the administration of TPN for patients who are receiving intensive or prolonged TPN, the immunocompromised, neonates, children, and patients receiving home TPN because of the large volumes administered and their increased susceptibility to the detrimental effects of particulate contamination (Bethune et al., 2001).

■ **SP** *Identify the patient and assess for the appropriate formula and rate of infusion before initiating the TPN infusion.* LOE = VII

EO This is the standard practice for safety before beginning a TPN infusion (INS, 2006).

RCT = Randomized Controlled (Clinical) Trial, **NIC** = Nursing Interventions Classification, **NOC** = Nursing Outcomes Classification

■ ⓈⓅ *Administer TPN using an electronic infusion pump.* **LOE = VII**

⒠Ⓞ This is the standard practice for safety to maintain an appropriate rate of administration (INS, 2006).

■ ⓈⓅ *Trace the IV catheter from the point of origin every time an infusion container or device is changed and when a patient is transferred from one setting to another (e.g., the intensive care unit to the medical unit, the medical unit to home care) to reduce the risk of the accidental connection of an infusion to the wrong type of catheter.* **LOE = VII**

⒠Ⓞ Tubing misconnections have resulted in significant adverse events, including patient deaths. Examples include erroneously connecting IV infusions to epidural catheters or feeding tubes or vice versa (Joint Commission, 2006; ISMP, 2004).

■ ⓈⓅ *Infuse TPN solutions that contain lipids (three-in-one solutions) within 24 hours and complete the infusion of lipid emulsions alone within 12 hours of hanging the solution.* **LOE = III**

⒠Ⓞ This is the recommended practice for the administration of TPN (INS, 2006).
⒠Ⓞ Complete the administration of TPN that contains lipids within 24 hours after it is hung, and complete the administration of lipid solutions within 12 hours (O'Grady et al., 2002).

■ *Assess for and consult with the pharmacist regarding the compatibility of medications added to the TPN solution to reduce the risk of precipitate formation; add medications immediately before hanging the solution.* **LOE = VII**

ⓂⓇ An in vitro study tested the compatibility of selected drugs ($N = 106$) with three-in-one TPN solution. Certain drugs may result in precipitate formation or the disruption of the fat emulsion, such as oil separation (Trissel et al., 1999).
⒠Ⓞ The coadministration of an admixture of medications that are known to be incompatible with TPN should be prevented (ASPEN, 2002).
⒠Ⓞ Medications added to TPN solutions should be documented on the label that is affixed to the TPN bag (INS, 2006).
⒠Ⓞ Medications should not be added to the TPN solution after it is actively infusing (INS, 2006).

■ ⓈⓅ *Maintain TPN administration through a dedicated and separate administration set using a dedicated lumen of the patient's CVC.* **LOE = VII**

⒠Ⓞ Using a dedicated administration set and the same lumen for TPN administration reduces the risk for incompatible fluids or drugs forming a precipitate (Weinstein, 2006; INS, 2006).

■ *Change IV administration sets* for TPN solutions that do not contain lipids every 72 hours.* **LOE = II**

⒠Ⓞ It is common practice to administer lipids into the last port of the TPN tubing. Because of this, it is also common practice to change the TPN tubing every 24 hours.

---

*The administration set is defined as including the IV tubing and any add-on devices, such as extension sets, filters, and the needleless connector.

NR = Nursing Research, **MR** = Multidisciplinary Research, **SP** = Standard of Practice, **EO** = Expert Opinion, **LOE** = Level of Evidence

(MR) A systematic review of all randomized or systematically allocated controlled trials that addressed IV administration set frequency and included outcome measures of infusate colonization, infusate-related BSI, catheter colonization, catheter-related BSI, and mortality was performed to determine the optimal time interval for IV tubing replacement. There were insufficient data regarding the incidence of infusate-related BSI and catheter-related BSI among patients who were receiving parenteral nutrition (particularly lipid-containing TPN) to make recommendations for optimal IV tubing replacement (Gillies et al., 2004).

(MR) Patients with cancer who required infusion therapy were randomized to IV tubing changes every 3 days ($N = 280$) or within 4 to 7 days ($N = 232$). Although the subset analysis of high-risk patients was lacking in power, there was a trend toward a higher frequency and degree of contamination of infusate in patients receiving TPN who had tubing changes within 4 to 7 days. The authors suggested that it may not be safe to extend tubing changes beyond 72 hours (Raad et al., 2001).

(EO) Replace administration sets no more than every 72 hours unless administering blood, blood products, or lipid emulsions (O'Grady et al., 2002).

(EO) Change primary and secondary administration continuous administration sets no more than every 72 hours and immediately upon suspected contamination or when the integrity of the product or system has been compromised (INS, 2006).

■ *Change IV administration sets for IV fat emulsions—administered either separately or as part of a three-in-one TPN solution—every 24 hours, because lipid solutions are known to enhance microbial growth.* **LOE = II**

(MR) A systematic review of all randomized or systematically allocated controlled trials ($N = 18$) that addressed IV administration set frequency found no evidence to suggest that administration sets including lipids should be changed more often than every 24 hours (Gillies et al., 2004).

(EO) Replace administration sets used to administer lipid emulsions within 24 hours of initiating the infusion (O'Grady et al., 2002).

■ *Initiate an infusion of dextrose 5% in water solution at the same rate as the TPN if the TPN must be abruptly stopped (e.g., if the CVC is occluded).* **LOE = VIII**

(EO) Initiating an infusion of dextrose 5% in water reduces the risk of rebound hypoglycemia (Weinstein, 2006).

■ *Administer TPN in the home setting when comprehensive discharge planning involves the assessment of the patient's condition and his or her readiness for discharge, patient/caregiver willingness to learn home TPN administration and monitoring, home environment issues and needs, and reimbursement.* **LOE = IV**

(MR) A retrospective study that looked at 5 years of outcomes for patients receiving home TPN from one home TPN provider found that catheter infection and occlusion rates are generally low and that time on home TPN therapy had increased (Ireton-Jones & DeLegge, 2005).

(EO) Factors to address when transitioning a patient to home TPN include the assessment of the patient's clinical stability with regard to the TPN, such as fluid volume status, blood

RCT = Randomized Controlled (Clinical) Trial, **NIC** = Nursing Interventions Classification, **NOC** = Nursing Outcomes Classification

glucose levels, serum electrolytes, nutritional goals, the willingness and ability of the patient/ caregiver to participate in the home care plan, the adequacy of the home environment (cleanliness, refrigeration), and reimbursement (Gorski, 2005).

(EO) A smooth transition to home requires discharge planning and interdisciplinary care that involves the home infusion provider and the home nutrition support team (Ireton-Jones et al., 2003).

(EO) Patient education should address adverse reactions, side effects, risks and benefits, and self-care practices, and it should include the validation of understanding of how to and the ability to safely perform infusion-related procedures (INS, 2006).

■ *Transition the patient to a cyclic TPN infusion when planning for home care to allow for a more normal lifestyle; this also provides physiological benefits.*
LOE = V

(EO) Long-term continuous TPN may result in fatty liver, elevated liver enzymes, and hepatomegaly caused by hyperinsulinism. Cyclic TPN is used more often for long-term TPN (Hammond et al., 2001).

(MR) A sleep study was performed on patients who were dependent on TPN for an average of 23 months ($N = 5$) and found that, although sleep quality was reduced in patients who were receiving TPN as compared with aged-matched controls, sleep quality did not seem to be negatively affected by cyclic TPN infusion (Scolapio et al., 2002).

(EO) Cyclic TPN is usually run over 12 to 16 hours during the nighttime to allow patients daytime freedom from carrying an infusion pump and thus the experience of a more normal lifestyle (Ireton-Jones et al., 2003).

(EO) Cycling the TPN infusion from 24 hours per day to 12 to 16 hours per day is usually done over several days by gradually reducing the infusion by 4 hours at a time until the goal time is achieved. The patient is monitored for fluid volume status and blood glucose alterations as the cycling time is reduced (Weinstein, 2006).

■ *Monitor the patient for signs and symptoms of metabolic-related complications and electrolyte imbalance including daily weights, intake and output, and blood glucose levels every 6 hours until stabilized at a level of less than 200 mg/dL.*
LOE = VI

(MR) A retrospective analysis of medical records for patients receiving TPN ($N = 111$) found that increased blood glucose levels were significantly associated with poorer outcomes, including cardiac, infectious, and renal complications as well as death, thus providing support for the need for tight glycemic control (Cheung et al., 2005).

(EO) Metabolic complications may result from glucose intolerance, overfeeding, electrolyte shifts, and fluid imbalance (Lyman, 2002).

(EO) Monitor the serum glucose, electrolyte, blood urea nitrogen, creatinine, magnesium, and phosphorus levels weekly until stable. Monitor the complete blood cell count, serum protein level, and serum triglyceride level every month for 3 months. Monitor the serum glucose, blood urea nitrogen, creatinine, magnesium, phosphorus, and calcium levels every month for 3 months and then every other month. Monitor the serum albumin, aspartate aminotransferase, alkaline phosphatase, total bilirubin, and international normalized ratio levels every 3 months, and monitor micronutrient levels as clinically necessary (ASPEN, 1998).

NR = Nursing Research, **MR** = Multidisciplinary Research, **SP** = Standard of Practice, **EO** = Expert Opinion, **LOE** = Level of Evidence

(EO) Blood glucose levels should be maintained in the 100 to 200 mg/dL range in hospitalized patients with diabetes mellitus (ASPEN, 2002).

■ *Monitor the patient and the infusion access device for signs and symptoms of catheter-related BSI, which is the most common complication among patients receiving TPN in the hospital or home setting.* **LOE = III**

(MR) Outcome data were collected prospectively to evaluate the incidence of complications during a 90-day period for patients who were discharged home requiring TPN ($N = 97$). One third of patients experienced a complication; more than 50% of complications were infectious, with the most common being a catheter-related BSI (de Burgoa et al., 2006).

(MR) Patients with CVCs in an acute care hospital were prospectively followed for the development of CVC-related infection ($N = 153$). Parenteral nutrition was found to be an independent risk factor for CVC-related infection (Beghetto et al., 2005).

(NR) A retrospective descriptive study of CVC outcomes in a home care agency over a 7-year period ($N = 551$ CVCs representing 20,879 catheter days) found that TPN administration was a statistically significant risk factor for CVC-related sepsis (Gorski, 2004).

(MR) A prospective cohort study of patients receiving home infusion therapy ($N = 827$) was conducted and found five probable risk factors associated with the increased risk of catheter-related infection; one of the five risk factors was TPN administration (Tokars et al., 1999).

Possibly Effective

■ *Use an antiseptic barrier cap over the needleless device to reduce the risk of catheter-related BSI.* **LOE = II**

(MR) An in vitro study consisted of the bacterial contamination of three different types of needleless caps and a comparison of the conventional 3- to 5-second disinfection of the needleless cap with 70% alcohol with the use of an antiseptic barrier cap (containing 2% chlorhexidine in 70% alcohol) left in place for 10 minutes followed by removal and allowing the needleless cap septum to dry. Sixty-seven percent of alcohol-disinfected caps showed the transmission of microorganisms, whereas only 1.6% of barrier caps showed any transmission; this technology should be studied in a clinical trial (Menyhay & Maki, 2006).

(MR) A prospective randomized multicenter study in which surgical intensive care unit patients with nontunneled CVCs for 6 or more days' duration ($N = 230$) were randomized to either a standard Luer-Lock cap or a hub with a 3% iodinated alcohol chamber found a significant decrease in culture-positive catheter hubs and catheter-related BSI in the antiseptic hub chamber group (Leon et al., 2003).

Not Effective

No applicable published research was found in this category.

Possibly Harmful

No applicable published research was found in this category.

RCT = Randomized Controlled (Clinical) Trial, **NIC** = Nursing Interventions Classification, **NOC** = Nursing Outcomes Classification

OUTCOME MEASUREMENT

FREE OF BLOOD STREAM INFECTION (BSI)

Definition: Free of localized or generalized signs of BSI.

Free of BSI as evidenced by the following indicators:

- IV site condition
- Skin around IV insertion
- Swelling around IV site
- Swelling in involved extremity
- Drainage around IV site
- White blood cell count
- Temperature

(Note: This is not a NOC outcome.)

REFERENCES

American Society for Parenteral and Enteral Nutrition (ASPEN). (2002). Guidelines for the use of parenteral and enteral nutrition support in adult and pediatric patients. *JPEN*, 26(Suppl 1):1SA-138SA.

American Society for Parenteral and Enteral Nutrition (ASPEN). (1998). *Clinical pathways and algorithms for delivery of parenteral and enteral nutrition support in adults.* Silver Spring, MD: ASPEN.

Beghetto MG, Victorino J, Teixeira L, de Azevedo MJ. (2005). Parenteral nutrition as a risk factor for central venous catheter related infection. *JPEN*, 29(5):367-373.

Bethune K, Allwood M, Grainger C, Wormleighton C. (2001). Use of filters during the preparation and administration of parenteral nutrition: Position paper and guidelines prepared by a British pharmaceutical nutrition group working party. *Nutrition*, 17(5):403-408.

Cheung NW, Napier B, Zaccaria C, Fletcher JP. (2005). Hyperglycemia is associated with adverse outcomes in patients receiving total parenteral nutrition. *Diabetes Care*, 28(10):2367-2371.

de Burgoa LJ, Seidner D, Hamilton C, Stafford J, Steiger E. (2006). Examination of factors that lead to complications for new home parenteral nutrition patients. *J Infus Nurs*, 29(2):74-80.

Dochterman JM, Bulechek GM (Eds). (2004). *Nursing Interventions Classification (NIC)*, 4th ed. St Louis: Mosby.

Driscoll DF, Bacon MN, Bistrian BR. (1996). Effects of in-line filtration on lipid particle size distribution in total nutrient admixtures. *JPEN*, 20(4):296-301.

Gillies D, O'Riordan L, Wallen M, Rankin K, Morrison A, Nagy S. (2004). Timing of intravenous administration set changes: A systematic review. *Infect Control Hosp Epidemiol*, 25(3):240-250.

Gorski LA. (2004). Central venous access device outcomes in a homecare agency: A 7-year study. *J Infus Nurs*, 27(2):104-111.

Gorski LA. (2005). Hospital to home care: Discharge planning for the patient requiring home infusion therapy. *Topics Advance Pract Nurs eJournal*, 5(3). Available online: http://www.medscape.com/viewarticle/507906. Retrieved on July 7, 2007.

Hammond KA, Szesycki E, Pfister D. (2001). Transitioning to home and other alternate sites. In Gottschlich MM (Ed): *The science and practice of nutritional support: A case based core curriculum.* Dubuque, IA: Kendall/Hunt, pp 701-726.

Infusion Nurses Society (INS). (2006). Infusion nursing standards of practice. *J Infus Nurs*, 29(1 Suppl): S1-S92.

Ireton-Jones C, DeLegge M, Epperson LA, Alexander J. (2003). Management of the home parenteral nutrition patient. *Nutr Clin Pract*, 18(4):310-317.

Ireton-Jones C, DeLegge M. (2005). Home parenteral nutrition registry: A five year retrospective evaluation of outcomes of patients receiving home parenteral nutrition support. *Nutrition*, 21(2):156-160.

The Joint Commission. (2006). Tubing misconnections—a persistent and potentially deadly occurrence. *Sentinel Event Alert*, 36:1-3.

Institute for Safe Medication Practices (ISMP). (2004). Problems persist with life threatening tubing misconnections. *ISMP Medication Safety Alert*. Available online: http://www.ismp.org. Retrieved on July 7, 2007.

Leon C, Alvarez-Lerma F, Ruiz-Santana S, Gonzalez V, de la Torre MV, Sierra R, et al. (2003). Antiseptic chamber-containing hub reduces central venous catheter related infection: A prospective, randomized study. *Crit Care Med*, 31(5):1318-1324.

Lyman B. (2002). Metabolic complications associated with parenteral nutrition. *J Infus Nurs*, 25(1):36-44.

McKinnon BT. (1996). FDA safety alert: Hazards of precipitation associated with parenteral nutrition. *Nutr Clin Pract*, 11(2):59-65.

Menyhay SZ, Maki DG. (2006). Disinfection of needleless catheter connectors and access ports with alcohol may not prevent microbial entry: The promise of a novel antiseptic-barrier cap. *Infect Control Hosp Epidemiol*, 27(1):23-27.

Naylor CJ, Griffiths RD, Fernandez RS. (2004). Does a multidisciplinary total parenteral nutrition team improve patient outcomes? A systematic review. *JPEN*, 28(4):251-258.

O'Grady NP, Alexander M, Dellinger EP, Gerberding JL, Heard SO, Maki DG, et al. (2002). Guidelines for the prevention of intravascular catheter-related infections. Centers for Disease Control and Prevention. *MMWR Recomm Rep*, 51(RR-10):1-32.

Raad I, Hanna HA, Awad A, Alrahwan A, Bivins C, Khan A, et al. (2001). Optimal frequency of changing intravenous administration sets: Is it safe to prolong use beyond 72 hours? *Infect Control Hosp Epidemiol*, 22(3):136-139.

Ryder M. (2006). Evidence-based practice in the management of vascular access devices for home parenteral nutrition therapy. *JPEN*, 30(1 Suppl):S82-S93, S98-S99.

Saalwachter AR, Evans HL, Willcutts KF, O'Donnell KB, Radigan AE, McElearney ST, et al. (2004). A nutrition support team led by general surgeons decreases inappropriate use of total parenteral nutrition on a surgical service. *Am Surg*, 70(12):1107-1111.

Scolapio JS, Savoy AD, Kaplan J, Burger CD, Lin SC. (2002). Sleep patterns of cyclic parenteral nutrition, a pilot study: Are there sleepless nights? *JPEN*, 26(3):214-217.

Tokars JI, Cookson ST, McArthur MA, Boyer CL, McGeer AJ, Jarvis WR. (1999). Prospective evaluation of risk factors for bloodstream infection in patients receiving home infusion therapy. *Ann Intern Med*, 131(5):340-347.

Trissel LA, Gilbert DL, Martinez JF, Baker MB, Walter WV, Mirtallo JM. (1999). Compatibility of medications with 3-in-1 parenteral nutrition solutions. *JPEN*, 23(2):67-74.

Weinstein SM. (2006). *Plumer's principles and practice of intravenous therapy*, 8th ed. Philadelphia: Lippincott Williams & Wilkins.

 # TOUCH   **NIC**

Alicia Huckstadt, PhD, APRN-BC, FNP, GNP

NIC Definition: Providing comfort and communication through purposeful tactile contact (Dochterman & Bulechek, 2004).

NURSING ACTIVITIES

Effective

No applicable published research was found in this category.

Possibly Effective

■ *Provide touch to relieve anxiety.* **LOE = II**

(NR) An experimental study of cataract surgery patients under local anesthesia ($N = 62$) assessed the effectiveness of handholding on subjective and objective measures of anxiety, including a visual analog scale, pulse rate, systolic and diastolic blood pressure, serum epinephrine, norepinephrine, cortisol, neutrophils, lymphocytes, and natural killer cells. Reported decreased anxiety and significantly lower epinephrine levels were found in the experimental group (Moon & Cho, 2001).

■ *Provide touch as massage for comfort and psychological/biological factors.* **LOE = II**

(NR) An experimental study of bone marrow transplant patients ($N = 88$) that examined the effectiveness of massage or therapeutic touch on the engraftment time, complications, and perceived benefits of therapy demonstrated that the massage group had significantly lower scores for central nervous system or neurological complications as compared with the therapeutic touch and control groups. In addition, patient perceptions of the benefits of therapy were significantly higher in the massage group than in the control group. Comfort scores were significantly higher in both the massage and therapeutic touch groups as compared with the control group (Smith et al., 2003).

■ *Provide touch to enhance biobehavioral effects on preterm infants.* **LOE = II**

(NR) An experimental study examined the use of gentle human touch on the physiological and behavioral measures (caloric intake, motor activity and inactivity, sleep, behavioral distress cues, heart rate, oxygen saturation, number of days on supplemental oxygen, number of blood transfusions, number of days on phototherapy, length of hospitalization, discharge weight) of 20 medically fragile preterm infants. Findings revealed that touch was not aversive or stressful to preterm infants. Furthermore, touch had positive beneficial effects, promoting physiological adaptation as evidenced by heart rate and oxygen saturation stability during and after the touch intervention. Touch also promoted behaviors that reflected adaptation, such as decreased motor activity during touch, decreased behavioral distress cues, more quiet sleep, and less drowsiness during and after touch (Modrcin-Talbott et al., 2003).

(MR) An experimental study examining the effects of auditory, tactile, visual, and vestibular (ATVV) interventions on the length of hospitalization, alertness, and feeding progression of 37 preterm infants revealed increased alertness, faster transition to complete nipple feeding, and decreased length of stay in the ATVV group as compared with the control group (White-Traut et al., 2002a).

(MR) A prospective design with the random assignment of 45 drug-exposed and 72 nonexposed newborns to ATVV intervention or control groups demonstrated increased alertness and less quiet sleep in both drug-exposed and nonexposed newborns that received ATVV as compared with the control infants (White-Traut et al., 2002b).

■ (NIC) *Encourage parents to touch newborn or ill child.* **LOE = II**

(MR) A randomized group experimental study ($N = 176$) compared the temperatures of newborns who experienced skin-to-skin contact with their mothers' chests (skin-to-skin group), newborns who were held in their mothers' arms while being either swaddled or clothed (mother's arms group), or newborns who were kept in a cot in the nursery while being either swaddled or clothed (nursery group). The results revealed that postnatal skin-to-skin contact may reverse labor-stress-related effects on the newborn's circulation (Bystrova et al., 2003).

(MR) An experimental study of 146 premature infants that examined parenting outcomes and preterm infant development with skin-to-skin (kangaroo) and traditional care found that, after kangaroo care, mothers showed more positive affect, touch, and adaptation to infant cues, and infants showed more alertness and less gaze aversion. The researchers concluded that skin-to-skin contact had a significant positive impact on the infant's perceptual-cognitive and motor development and on the parenting process (Feldman et al., 2002).

(MR) A Cochrane review of skin-to-skin (kangaroo) mother care and the morbidity and mortality of low-birth-weight infants in three studies ($N = 1362$) concluded that skin-to-skin contact appeared to reduce severe infant morbidity without any serious deleterious effects. However, but there was still insufficient evidence to recommend its routine use with low-birth-weight infants (Conde-Agudelo et al., 2003).

▪ *Provide touch to create positive interpersonal relationships.* LOE = V

(NR) A qualitative study of 12 health care workers that explored the meanings of giving touch as part of the nursing care of older patients revealed that a friendly, calm, and humane relationship was created between the caregiver and patient when touch was given and that the relationship transcended the moment of touch and influenced the caregiver's way of caring (Edvardsson et al., 2003).

(NR) A qualitative study with four patients who had been treated for psychosis investigated the meaning of physical contact and revealed that touching meant "to be in need," "to yearn," and "to belong" and that it communicated feelings of acknowledgement as a human being (Salzmann-Erikson & Eriksson, 2005).

(NR) Through a concept development process, 39 adult health care professionals, inpatients, and healthy people were interviewed to develop a conceptual structure of physical touch in caring. The concept of physical touch emerged as a complex phenomenon that had meanings in different dimensions. The conceptual structure included five goals: (1) promoting physical comfort; (2) promoting emotional comfort; (3) promoting mind-body comfort; (4) performing a social role; and (5) sharing spirituality (Chang, 2001).

▪ *Provide touch to encourage communication.* LOE = VI

(NR) A literature review of the use of touch with older people experiencing dementia supported that touch was a special type of nonverbal communication and that emotions were formed through the physical, psychological, and spiritual effects of touch. In observational studies of nurses' touch, patient perceptions revealed comfort, reassurance, and caring (Gleeson & Timmins, 2004b).

(NR) A literature review of the use of touch to enhance the nursing care of older people concluded that empiric evidence was needed to further describe the categorization and occurrence of touch in nursing situations and that the benefits of touch and ethical issues required further examination, especially in patients with cognitive impairment (Gleeson & Timmins, 2004a).

▪ *Use touch with patients who are experiencing nausea and vomiting.* LOE = VI

(NR) Using a phenomenological method, tactile massage and its effect on severe nausea and vomiting during pregnancy with 10 women revealed that tactile massage promoted relaxation (Agren & Berg, 2006).

RCT = Randomized Controlled (Clinical) Trial, **NIC** = Nursing Interventions Classification, **NOC** = Nursing Outcomes Classification

■ *Encourage touch with older adults.* **LOE = V**

(NR) A literature review of research on touch and older adults reported the paucity of rigorous studies examining the efficacy of touch, but it concluded that touch had the potential to benefit older adults in several ways, including comfort enhancement among dying persons and their caregivers and the modest improvement of confusional symptoms among the cognitively impaired (Bush, 2001).

(NR) A theoretical model on the use of touch with Alzheimer's patients was formulated through theory synthesis of research findings. This Touch-Stress model can guide future nursing research and practice interventions for Alzheimer's patients with behavioral and emotional problems (Kim & Buschmann, 2004).

Not Effective

■ *Using touch to improve developmental outcomes.* **LOE = VII**

(MR) A Cochrane database review revealed that the evidence of the benefits of massage for preterm infants with regard to developmental outcomes was weak and that it did not warrant the wider use of preterm infant massage. Future research should assess the effects of massage interventions on clinical outcomes and process-of-care measures (Vickers et al., 2004).

Possibly Harmful

■ *Using touch and sexualization.* **LOE = VI**

(NR) A qualitative study exploring the experiences of eight male nurses and the ways that gender affected their caring for patients revealed that stereotypes of men as sexual aggressors and male nurses as gay could stigmatize touch and men's roles as nurses, thereby creating complex and contradictory situations of acceptance, rejection, and suspicion of men as nurturers and caregivers (Evans, 2002).

OUTCOME MEASUREMENT

PERSONAL WELL-BEING   (NOC)

Definition: Extent of positive perception of one's health status and life circumstances.
Personal Well-Being as evidenced by the following selected NOC indicators:
• Physical health
• Psychological health
• Ability to cope
• Ability to relax
• Social relationships
• Level of happiness
(Rate each indicator of **Personal Well-Being:** 1 = not at all satisfied, 2 = somewhat satisfied, 3 = moderately satisfied, 4 = very satisfied, 5 = completely satisfied) (Moorhead et al., 2004).

REFERENCES

Agren A, Berg M. (2006). Tactile massage and severe nausea and vomiting during pregnancy—women's experiences. *Scand J Caring Sci,* 20(2):169-176.

Bush E. (2001). The use of human touch to improve the well-being of older adults. A holistic nursing intervention. *J Holist Nurs,* 19(3):256-270.

Bystrova K, Widstrom AM, Matthiesen AS, Ransjo-Arvidson AB, Welles-Nystrom B, Wassberg C, et al. (2003). Skin-to-skin contact may reduce negative consequences of "the stress of being born": A study on temperature in newborn infants, subjected to different ward routines in St. Petersburg. *Acta Paediatr,* 92(3):320-326.

Chang SO. (2001). The conceptual structure of physical touch in caring. *J Adv Nurs,* 33(6):820-827.

Conde-Agudelo A, Diaz-Rossello JL, Belizan JM. (2003). Kangaroo mother care to reduce morbidity and mortality in low birthweight infants. *Cochrane Database Syst Rev,* (2):CD002771.

Dochterman JM, Bulechek GM (Eds). (2004). *Nursing Interventions Classification (NIC),* 4th ed. St Louis: Mosby.

Edvardsson JD, Sandman PO, Rasmussen BH. (2003). Meanings of giving touch in the care of older patients: Becoming a valuable person and professional. *J Clin Nurs,* 12(4):601-609.

Evans JA. (2002). Cautious caregivers: Gender stereotypes and the sexualization of men nurses' touch. *J Adv Nurs,* 40(4):441-448.

Feldman R, Eidelman AI, Sirota L, Weller A. (2002). Comparison of skin-to-skin (kangaroo) and traditional care: Parenting outcomes and preterm infant development. *Pediatrics,* 110(1 Pt 1):16-26.

Gleeson M, Timmins F. (2004a). The use of touch to enhance nursing care of older person in long-term mental health care facilities. *J Psychiatr Ment Health Nurs,* 11(5):541-545.

Gleeson M, Timmins F. (2004b). Touch: A fundamental aspect of communication with older people experiencing dementia. *Nurs Older People,* 16(2):18-21.

Kim EJ, Buschmann MT. (2004). Touch-stress model and Alzheimer's disease: Using touch intervention to alleviate patients' stress. *J Gerontol Nurs,* 30(12):33-39.

Modrcin-Talbott MA, Harrison LL, Groer MW, Younger MS. (2003). The biobehavioral effects of gentle human touch on preterm infants. *Nurs Sci Q,* 16(1):60-67.

Moon JS, Cho KS. (2001). The effects of handholding on anxiety in cataract surgery patients under local anaesthesia. *J Adv Nurs,* 35(3):407-415.

Moorhead M, Johnson M, Maas M (Eds). (2004). *Nursing Outcomes Classification (NOC),* 3rd ed. St Louis: Mosby.

Salzmann-Erikson M, Eriksson H. (2005). Encouraging touch: A path to affinity in psychiatric care. *Issues Ment Health Nurs,* 26(8):843-852.

Smith MC, Reeder F, Daniel L, Baramee J, Hagman J. (2003). Outcomes of touch therapies during bone marrow transplant. *Altern Ther Health Med,* 9(1):40-49.

Vickers A, Ohlsson A, Lacy JB, Horsley A. (2004). Massage for promoting growth and development of preterm and/or low birth-weight infants. *Cochrane Database Syst Rev,* (2):CD000390.

White-Traut RC, Nelson MN, Silvestri JM, Vasan U, Littau S, Meleedy-Rey P, et al. (2002a). Effect of auditory, tactile, visual, and vestibular intervention on length of stay, alertness, and feeding progression in preterm infants. *Dev Med Child Neurol,* 44(2):91-97.

White-Traut R, Studer T, Meleedy-Rey P, Murray P, Labovsky S, Kahn J. (2002b). Pulse rate and behavioral state correlates after auditory, tactile, visual, and vestibular intervention in drug-exposed neonates. *J Perinatol,* 22(4):291-299.

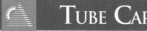

TUBE CARE: CHEST NIC

Kathleen Higgins, RN, CCRN, CS, MSN, CRNP

> **NIC** **Definition:** Management of a patient with an external water-seal drainage device exiting the chest cavity (Dochterman & Bulechek, 2004).

RCT = Randomized Controlled (Clinical) Trial, **NIC** = Nursing Interventions Classification, **NOC** = Nursing Outcomes Classification

NURSING ACTIVITIES

Effective

- **NIC** *Monitor for signs and symptoms of pneumothorax.* **LOE = VII**

  EO It is essential to patient safety to recognize the signs and symptoms of pneumothorax, which include pleuritic chest pain, dyspnea, anxiety, tachypnea, respiratory distress cyanosis, and agitation; a delay in treatment increases mortality (Marini & Wheeler, 2006).

- **NIC** *Ensure that all tubing connections are securely attached and taped.* **LOE = VII**

  EO Monitor for secure connections between the chest tube and the drainage system to avoid air leaks (Lancey, 2003).

- **NIC** *Keep the drainage container below chest level.* **LOE = VII**

  EO Monitor the tubing system for kinks, which obstruct flow, increase negative pressure, and maintain tubing in a dependent position (Lancey, 2003).

  EO A chest tube drainage system is to be maintained below the patient's chest level to ensure proper drainage and to prevent air and fluid from reentering the chest cavity (Rothrock et al., 2003).

- **NIC** *Anchor the tubing securely.* **LOE = VII**

  MR A retrospective case-control study that took place over 12 months ($N = 134$ patients) demonstrated that contributing factors for subcutaneous emphysema included nursing-related care issues such as poor drainage, poor tube placement, tube blockage, and side-port migration, which increase morbidity and mortality (Jones et al., 2001).

  EO A chest tube drainage system uses a Y connector to connect two chest tubes to drain into a drainage container; all connections should be banded or otherwise secured with taping at the end of the connection (Rothrock et al., 2003).

- **NIC** *Monitor x-ray reports for tube position.* **LOE = VI**

  EO Monitor x-ray reports for an increase or decrease in pneumothorax or subcutaneous emphysema (Lancey, 2003).

  MR A prospective case study ($N = 75$ patients) over 1 year demonstrated that obtaining a chest x-ray within 1 to 3 hours after chest tube removal in mechanical ventilation patients was safe and effective to monitor for pneumothorax (Pizano et al., 2002).

  EO The British Thoracic Society guidelines state that a chest x-ray should be performed and reviewed after the initial insertion of a chest tube drainage system (Laws et al., 2003).

- **NIC** *Monitor chest tube tidaling/output and air leaks.* **LOE = VII**

  EO The health care provider should monitor the drainage amount and type and report drainage of more than 200 mL/hour (Verrier & Hampton, 2002).

  EO The American Association of Critical Care Nurses (AACCN) states that the chest tube drainage system should be evaluated for fluctuation in the water-seal chamber, because persistent bubbling can indicate an air leak in the system (Lawrence, 2005a).

NR = Nursing Research, **MR** = Multidisciplinary Research, **SP** = Standard of Practice, **EO** = Expert Opinion, **LOE** = Level of Evidence

■ **NIC** *Observe for signs of infection.* **LOE = VII**

EO Monitor the drainage type and amount; if drainage is thick or empyema is present, antibiotic therapy should be considered (Marini & Wheeler, 2006).

EO Monitor the drainage amount and remove the chest tube when drainage is less than 50 mL per 24 hours (Marini & Wheeler, 2006).

EO Never advance an established chest tube into the pleural space, because this may dislodge the tube placement or introduce bacteria into the chest cavity (Lancey, 2003).

EO The AACCN procedure manual states that the chest tube drainage site and the surrounding skin should be assessed for the presence of subcutaneous air and signs of infection or inflammation with each dressing change or every day (Lawrence, 2005b).

■ *Remove the chest tube system as indicated.* **LOE = III**

MR A prospective case-control study randomized patients with chest tubes ($N = 102$) to two methods of removal (end of expiration or end of inspiration) and demonstrated that both methods were equally effective (Bell et al., 2001).

■ **SP** *Apply suction to the water-seal system.* **LOE = VII**

EO Suction should be applied to a water-seal system if the lung does not quickly re-expand without suction (Baumann et al., 2001).

■ **NIC** *Monitor for bubbling of the suction chamber of the chest tube drainage system and tidaling in the water-seal chamber.* **LOE = VII**

EO The nurse should monitor the water-seal chamber for persistent bubbling, which can indicate an air leak in the system in the lung, the tubing, or the connection (Marini & Wheeler, 2006).

EO Monitor the water-seal chamber for tidal variations, which indicate a change in optimal intrapleural pressure. An abrupt increase in tidaling magnitude indicates a problem within the system that may include air leak, lobar atelectasis, upper airway obstruction, impaired secretion clearance, and hyperpnea. The absence of tidaling indicates tube obstruction (Marini & Wheeler, 2006).

■ **NIC** *Use petroleum jelly gauze for dressing change.* **LOE = VII**

EO The AACN procedure manual states that a petrolatum gauze dressing should be placed around the chest tube site with split sponges around the tube and covered with gauze dressing and tape or that treatment should occur in accordance with institutional standards (Lawrence, 2005a, b).

Possibly Effective

■ **NIC** *Monitor the patency of the chest tube by stripping and milking the tube.* **LOE = I**

MR A Cochrane systematic review found that there was no evidence to support or refute the efficacy of varying levels of suction or suction in combination with milking, stripping, fanfolding, and tapping the chest drains (Wallen et al., 2004).

NR A systematic review of the literature about the nursing management of chest drains demonstrated that chest drainage systems remained patent with or without milking or strip-

---

RCT = Randomized Controlled (Clinical) Trial, **NIC** = Nursing Interventions Classification, **NOC** = Nursing Outcomes Classification

ping; however, the total drainage was increased when the tubes were stripped or milked (Charnock & Evans, 2001).

(NR) A randomized controlled study ($N = 200$ patients) examined two methods of clot clearance from a chest system in postoperative myocardial revascularization patients and found no difference in outcomes when comparing stripping or milking methods (Pierce et al., 1991).

■ (NIC) *Monitor for crepitus around the chest tube site.* **LOE = IV**

(MR) A retrospective case-control study that lasted for 12 months ($N = 134$ patients) reviewed patients with chest tubes who developed subcutaneous emphysema and noted that subcutaneous emphysema was associated with trauma, bronchopleural fistulae, large and bilateral pneumothoraces, mechanical ventilation, poor drainage, poor tube placement, tube blockage, and side-port migration (Jones et al., 2001).

(EO) Monitor for subcutaneous emphysema under the chest wall and at the tube insertion site (Marini & Wheeler, 2006).

■ *Maintain the chest tube system to water seal.* **LOE = IV**

(MR) A retrospective case-control study ($N = 838$ patients) placed postoperative elective pulmonary resection patients with known air leak and pneumothorax chest tube systems to water seal and monitored for signs and symptoms of water-seal failure (symptomatic increasing pneumothorax or subcutaneous emphysema). The results demonstrated that water seal is safe for most patients with an air leak and pneumothorax, unless the leak or pneumothorax is large (Cerfolio et al., 2005).

■ *Monitor and administer pain management therapy upon chest tube removal.* **LOE = II**

(NR) A randomized controlled study ($N = 74$ patients) investigated four methods of pain management associated with chest tube removal: (1) intravenous (IV) morphine and education; (2) IV ketorolac and education; (3) IV morphine plus education and sensory information; and (4) IV ketorolac plus education and sensory. No significant differences were found among the groups (Puntillo & Ley, 2004).

Not Effective

■ *Assisting the patient with bronchial hygiene, including cough, deep breathing, turning every 2 hours, and using incentive spirometry.* **LOE = I**

(MR) A Cochrane systematic review demonstrated that there was not enough evidence to recommend the use of bronchial hygiene (postural drainage, chest percussion, vibration, chest shaking, direct coughing, or forced exhalation technique) for patients with chronic obstructive pulmonary disease and bronchiectasis (Jones & Rowe, 2000).

(MR) A Cochrane systematic review demonstrated that there was not enough evidence to support conventional chest physiotherapy techniques over other airway clearance techniques for improved respiratory function (Main et al., 2005).

(MR) A systematic review of the literature demonstrated that there was no evidence to support the use of incentive spirometry for the postoperative cardiac or abdominal patient to decrease postoperative pulmonary complications (Overend et al., 2001).

NR = Nursing Research, **MR** = Multidisciplinary Research, **SP** = Standard of Practice, **EO** = Expert Opinion, **LOE** = Level of Evidence

■ *Administering morphine during chest tube removal.* **LOE = V**

(NR) A review of the literature was conducted to analyze the effectiveness of nonpharmacological and pharmacological methods of pain management during chest tube removal. It was demonstrated that morphine alone was not effective for pain management and that further research in this area is needed (Bruce et al., 2006).

(NR) A qualitative study looked at methods to reduce pain upon chest removal and showed that analgesics and relaxation exercise techniques were not more effective than analgesics without relaxation exercise techniques for reducing the pain associated with chest tube removal (Houston & Jesurum, 1999).

■ *Using nonpharmacological pain management therapy during chest tube removal.*
LOE = II

(MR) A Cochrane systematic review of two RCTs ($N = 23$)demonstrated that patients who listened to music could reduce pain intensity and decrease opioid requirements; however, the decrease in intensity was not significant (Cepeda et al., 2006).

■ *Monitoring chest x-ray (CXR) reports for tube position.* **LOE = IV**

(MR) A retrospective case-control study ($N = 1021$) compared postoperative coronary artery bypass/valve replacement patients who had routine postoperative chest tube removal CXRs and patients who did not have CXRs. The study demonstrated that routine CXR after chest tube removal was not necessary. CXRs should be based on patients' symptoms (McCormick et al., 2002).

Possibly Harmful

■ *Clamping a chest tube.* **LOE = VII**

(EO) A bubbling chest tube system should not be clamped. A clamped chest tube system should be immediately opened if the patient becomes breathless or develops subcutaneous emphysema, and a chest tube system that is not bubbling should not usually be clamped (Henry et al., 2003).

OUTCOME MEASUREMENT

RESPIRATORY STATUS: VENTILATION

Definition: Movement of air in and out of the lungs.
Respiratory Status: Ventilation as evidenced by the following selected NOC indicators:
• Respiratory rate
• Ease of breathing
• Auscultated breath sounds
(Rate each indicator of **Respiratory Status: Ventilation:** 1 = severely compromised, 2 = substantially compromised, 3 = moderately compromised, 4 = mildly compromised, 5 = not compromised) (Moorhead et al., 2004).

RCT = Randomized Controlled (Clinical) Trial, **NIC** = Nursing Interventions Classification, **NOC** = Nursing Outcomes Classification

REFERENCES

Baumann MH, Strange C, Heffner JE, Light R, Kirby TJ, Klein J, et al. (2001). Management of spontaneous pneumothorax: An American College of Chest Physicians Delphi consensus statement. *Chest*, 119(2):590-602.

Bell RL, Ovadia P, Abdullah F, Spector S, Rabinovici R. (2001). Chest tube removal: End-inspiration or end-expiration? *J Trauma*, 50(4):674-677.

Bruce EA, Howard RF, Franck LS. (2006). Chest drain removal pain and its management: A literature review. *J Clin Nurs*, 15(2):145-154.

Cepeda MS, Carr DB, Lau J, Alvarez H. (2006). Music for pain relief. *Cochrane Database Syst Rev*, (2): CD004843.

Cerfolio RJ, Bryant AS, Singh S, Bass CS, Bartolucci AA. (2005). The management of chest tubes in patients with a pneumothorax and an air leak after pulmonary resection. *Chest*, 128(2):816-820.

Charnock Y, Evans D. (2001). Nursing management of chest drains: A systematic review. *Aust Crit Care*, 14(4):156-160.

Dochterman JM, Bulechek GM (Eds). (2004). *Nursing Interventions Classification (NIC)*, 4th ed. St Louis: Mosby.

Henry M, Arnold T, Harvey J; Pleural Diseases Group, Standards of Care Committee, British Thoracic Society. (2003). BTS guidelines for the management of spontaneous pneumothorax. *Thorax*, 58(Suppl 2):ii39-ii52.

Houston S, Jesurum J. (1999). The quick relaxation technique: Effect on pain associated with chest tube removal. *Appl Nurs Res*, 12(4):196-205.

Jones PM, Hewer RD, Wolfenden HD, Thomas PS. (2001). Subcutaneous emphysema associated chest tube drainage. *Respirology*, 6(2):87-89.

Jones AP, Rowe BH. (2000). Bronchopulmonary hygiene physical therapy for chronic obstructive pulmonary disease and bronchiectasis. *Cochrane Database Syst Rev*, (2):CD00045.

Lancey RA. (2003). Chest tube insertion and care. In Irwin RS, Rippe JM, Curley FJ, Heard SO (Eds). *Procedures and techniques in intensive care medicine*, 3rd ed. Philadelphia: Lippincott Williams & Wilkins, pp 127-135.

Lawrence DM. (2005a). Chest tube placement (perform). In Wiegand DJ, Carlson KK (Eds): *AACN procedure manual for critical care*, 5th ed. St Louis: WB Saunders.

Lawrence DM. (2005b). Chest tube placement (assist). In Wiegand DJ, Carlson KK (Eds): *AACN procedure manual for critical care*, 5th ed. St Louis: WB Saunders.

Laws D, Neville E, Duffy J; Pleural Diseases Group, Standards of Care Committee, British Thoracic Society. (2003). BTS guidelines for the insertion of a chest drain. *Thorax*, 58(Suppl 2):ii53-ii59.

Main E, Prasad A, Schans C. (2005). Conventional chest physiotherapy compared to other airway clearance techniques for cystic fibrosis. *Cochrane Database Syst Rev*, (1):CD002011.

Marini JJ, Wheeler AP. (2006). *Critical care medicine*, 3rd ed. Philadelphia: Lippincott Williams & Wilkins.

McCormick JT, O'Mara MS, Papasavas PK, Caushaj PF. (2002). The use of routine chest x-ray films after chest tube removal in postoperative cardiac patients. *Ann Thorac Surg*, 74(6):2161-2164.

Moorhead M, Johnson M, Maas M (Eds). (2004). *Nursing Outcomes Classification (NOC)*, 3rd ed. St Louis: Mosby.

Overend TJ, Anderson CM, Lucy SD, Bhatia C, Jonsson BI, Timmermans C. (2001). The effect of incentive spirometry on postoperative pulmonary complications: A systematic review. *Chest*, 120(3): 971-978.

Pierce JD, Piazza D, Naftel DC. (1991). Effects of two chest tube clearance protocols on drainage in patients after myocardial revascularization surgery. *Heart Lung*, 20(2):125-130.

Pizano LR, Houghton DE, Cohn SM, Frisch MS, Grogan RH. (2002). When should a chest radiograph be obtained after chest tube removal in mechanically ventilated patients? A prospective study. *J Trauma*, 53(6):1073-1077.

Puntillo K, Ley SJ. (2004). Appropriately timed analgesics control pain due to chest tube removal. *Am J Crit Care*, 13(4):292-301.

Rothrock JC, Smith DA, McEwen DR. (2003). *Alexander's care of the patient in surgery*, 12th ed. St Louis: Mosby.

Verrier ED, Hampton CR. (2002). Cardiothoracic surgery. In Bongard FS, Sue DY (Eds): *Current critical care, diagnosis & treatment,* 2nd ed. New York: McGraw Hill, pp 551-572.

Wallen M, Morrison A, O'Riordan E, Bridge C, Stoddart F. (2004). Mediastinal chest drain clearance for cardiac surgery. *Cochrane Database Syst Rev,* (2):CD003042.

 ## TUBE CARE: GASTROSTOMY

Kathleen A. Fitzgerald, PhD, RN

NIC **Definition:** Management of a patient with a gastrointestinal tube (Dochterman & Bulechek, 2004).

Gastrostomy tubes (G-tubes) are placed through the skin into the stomach. They can be inserted surgically, endoscopically, radiographically, and per oral image-guided gastrostomy (Laasch et al., 2003).

NURSING ACTIVITIES

Effective

■ **SP** *Stabilize the G-tube to prevent the dislodgement and/or migration of the tube until the tract is healed.* **LOE = VII**

EO The G-tube should come straight out of the tract to prevent the development of a pressure ulcer on the skin from the tube being taped to the skin. If there is not a bumper in place, a dressing or tube holder should be used to prevent the movement of the tube back into the stomach or the migration of the tube out of the tract. Sideways movement may create a larger hole, thus resulting in leakage. There are a variety of commercial products available to aid in stabilization. A nipple from an infant bottle or a gauze dressing may also be fashioned to stabilize the tube (Crawley-Coha, 2004).

EO A major institution set up a protocol to follow for routine gastrostomy or jejunostomy tube care that consists of tube stabilization, the treatment of peritubular skin irritation, and the containment of drainage from the tube site. The outcomes of the implementation of a protocol, including guidelines for tube stabilization, were a decrease in tube dislodgement and peritubular skin irritation (Bryant & Fleiser, 2006).

EO Percutaneous G-tubes should not be removed for at least 14 days to allow a fibrous tract to develop. It is important at this time to maintain tube stability and to not create a tract that is larger than the tube, because this may result in leakage (Stroud et al., 2003).

■ **SP** *Check the placement of the G-tube by first pulling gently on the tube until resistance is met and then marking the spot at the exit site with a permanent marker. This marking should be observed before the administration of a tube feeding or medications.* **LOE = VII**

EO G-tube migration is a potential complication of an unsecured tube. The tube should be anchored. Migration of the tube within the stomach can cause lodgment in the esophagus or the pylorus, thereby causing obstruction (Borkowski & Rogers, 2004).

■ **SP** *Cleanse the skin surrounding the G-tube with soap and water.* **LOE = VII**

RCT = Randomized Controlled (Clinical) Trial, **NIC** = Nursing Interventions Classification, **NOC** = Nursing Outcomes Classification

(EO) A mild antibacterial soap or simple soap and water used daily are sufficient to keep the G-tube site clean (McClave & Neff, 2006).

(EO) After the G-tube site matures, soap and water may be used to clean the area. It is important to dry the area around the tube tract thoroughly to keep the skin dry and the tube stabilized. A dressing is not necessary, and it may cause undue pressure on the bumper (Tracey & Patterson, 2006).

■ (SP) *Place a surgical drain sponge or an absorbent dressing around the drain site only if there is leakage of gastrointestinal contents. Change the dressing as needed to maintain dry and intact skin.* **LOE = VII**

(EO) It is normal for a small amount of bleeding or mucus to be present immediately after a percutaneous endoscopic gastrostomy (PEG) tube or G-tube is placed. The site should be kept dry to protect the skin from moisture (Overstreet, 2004).

(EO) Persistent or increasing gastrointestinal drainage at the tube site may indicate a dislodgement of the tube and should be reported to the physician immediately (Tracey & Patterson, 2006).

■ (SP) *If the skin surrounding the G-tube becomes irritated or denuded, determine the cause.* **LOE = VII**

(EO) Cutaneous candidiasis may occur when there is drainage around the tube, leakage of formula, or moisture under the bumper. Candidiasis infection may be mild and consist of erythema and a few pustules, or it can be severe with extensive erythema, maceration, and excoriation of the skin. Mild, localized candidiasis can be treated with topical antifungal powder and greater attention to maintaining a dry surface surrounding the tube. Severe candidal infection may require oral systemic treatment (Crawley-Coha, 2004).

(EO) Cellulitis is characterized by spreading erythema, induration, fever, tenderness or pain, and purulent discharge. The cause may be chemical irritation from the leakage of gastric contents or infection. Systemic antibiotic therapy is most frequently used (Goldberg et al., 2005).

■ (SP) *Watch for the formation of hypergranulation tissue, which occurs when there is an inflammatory reaction to the tube that causes the appearance of mucosa-like tissue outside the tract.* **LOE = VII**

(EO) The actual cause of hypergranulation tissue is unknown, but it is suspected to be caused by excess tube movement, ill-fitting low profile or skin-level devices, or excessive drainage. This tissue is a proliferation of capillaries that can be painful to touch, that may bleed easily, and that can have more drainage (Borkowski, 2005; Goldberg et al., 2005).

(EO) The excessive tissue is frequently chemically cauterized with silver nitrate sticks, which causes the tissue to turn gray and slough off. This can be painful to the patient. Other options include steroid cream applied to the tissue. Stoma adhesive powder and absorptive dressings such as foam may also be applied to the granulation tissue to absorb the drainage (Borkowski, 2005; Goldberg et al., 2005).

(EO) To protect the skin when there is draining hypergranulation tissue, apply a skin barrier such as petroleum jelly or skin sealant. If the skin becomes irritated, apply a skin barrier product such as zinc oxide ointment. A pectin-based wafer can be cut to fit the peristomal skin, and it will then act to protect the skin (Borkowski, 2005).

NR = Nursing Research, **MR** = Multidisciplinary Research, **SP** = Standard of Practice, **EO** = Expert Opinion, **LOE** = Level of Evidence

■ (SP) *Flush the G-tube with a 30-mL or larger syringe to prevent excess pressure and possible rupture of the tube. Flush volumes should be determined on the basis of maintaining the patency of the tube and the hydration requirements of the patient. The G-tube should be flushed before and after the administration of medications and feedings.* LOE = VII

(EO) A literature search of journals and nursing textbooks and a survey of 19 Indiana hospitals revealed water as the flushing fluid that is most consistently recommended. Recommended irrigation flush volumes varied from 20 to 100 mL for patients receiving continuous feedings. The frequency of flushing was from every 4 to 8 hours. In patients receiving intermittent feedings, the amount of fluid for flushing ranged from 15 to 100 mL before and after each feeding. It is recommended by most sources to flush before and after medications to maintain the patency of the tubes. Many of the clogging problems are thought to be related to medication administration. There are no specific guidelines regarding the amount of flush to use (Reising & Neal, 2005).

■ (SP) *If it is necessary to use the tube for decompression of the stomach, use gravity drainage only.* LOE = VII

(EO) G-tubes are used for the gastric decompression of palliative patients, thus improving the quality of their lives. Because the tube is not vented, gravity drainage is recommended for decompression to protect the stomach from mucosal erosion from the suction. The tubes may require flushing, depending on the thickness of the drainage (McClave & Ritchie, 2006).

(EO) A review article described the successful use of percutaneous G-tubes for decompression during palliative care (McClave & Ritchie, 2006).

Possibly Effective

No applicable published research was found in this category.

Not Effective

■ *Using antibiotics to treat yellow-brown crusty drainage.* LOE = VII

(EO) Yellow-brown crusty drainage commonly seen around the G-tube site is not considered an infection and should not be treated with systemic or local antibiotics (Goldberg et al., 2005).

Possibly Harmful

■ *Allowing the external bumper to be very tight on the skin, thereby applying traction to the skin.* LOE = III

(MR) In a controlled study ($N = 8$ dogs) to determine the best length at which a PEG tube bolster or bumper should be secured at the skin, eight mongrel dogs had tubes placed and bolsters secured at 0 cm, 1 cm, and 4 cm. The bolsters that were placed at 0 cm had one wound infection and one internal bolster migration, and five had severe tissue inflammation at the skin site. Two dogs had severe tissue irritation at 1 cm, and there were no problems reported at 4 cm. The study concluded that the apposition of the external bolster against the skin was not necessary for the formation of the PEG tube tract and that

RCT = Randomized Controlled (Clinical) Trial, **NIC** = Nursing Interventions Classification, **NOC** = Nursing Outcomes Classification

the tighter bolster may cause more problems than would a looser bolster (DeLegge et al., 2006).

(MR) A prospective controlled study was conducted that compared abdominal wound healing after PEG placement. Complications were compared between patients ($N = 67$) who had traction placed on the external bolster (tract length, 4.9 ± 1.1 cm) and patients ($N = 47$) who had no traction placed on the external bolster (tract length, 11.6 ± 2.3 cm). There were 11 patients with traction on the external bolster who had problems with peristomal leakage, cellulitis, tube extrusion, and gastric mucosal bleeding. Only one patient with the nontraction bolster had a complication. The authors concluded that traction on the external bolster was not necessary but that it may cause problems (Chung & Schertzer, 1990).

(EO) A letter to the editor by a nurse specialist described mucosal erosion or ulceration when the external bumper is too tight against the skin (Borne, 2005).

■ *Cleansing the G-tube site with hydrogen peroxide.* **LOE = VII**

(EO) Hydrogen peroxide is effective for reducing bacterial colonization and wound infection, but it is corrosive to the skin and therefore not recommended as a cleansing agent. It will dry the skin and the tissue of the gastrostomy tract, thus causing a disruption of healing of the tube tract (McClave & Neff, 2006).

OUTCOME MEASUREMENT

GASTROSTOMY FUNCTION

Definition: Condition of the skin around the insertion site and the patency of the tube.
Gastrostomy Function as evidenced by the following indicators:
• Skin condition around the insertion site
• Signs of infection around the insertion site
• Positioning of the external bolster
(Note: This is not a NOC outcome.)

REFERENCES

Borkowski S. (2005). G tube care: Managing hypergranulation tissue. *Nursing,* 35(8):24.
Borkowski S, Rogers VE. (2004). Similar gastrostomy peristomal skin irritations in three pediatric patients. *J Wound Ostomy Continence Nurs,* 31(4):201-205.
Borne S. (2005). PEG tube problems. *Nursing,* 35(9):12.
Bryant D, Fleiser I. (2006). Simple to complex: strategies for preventing and managing tube-related complications. *J Wound Ostomy Continence Nurs,* 33(3 Suppl):S29-S30.
Chung RS, Schertzer M. (1990). Pathogenesis of complications of percutaneous endoscopic gastrostomy. A lesson in surgical principles. *Am Surg,* 56(3):134-137.
Crawley-Coha T. (2004). A practical guide for the management of pediatric gastrostomy tubes based on 14 years of experience. *J Wound Ostomy Continence Nurs,* 31(4)193-200.
DeLegge M, DeLegge R, Brady C. (2006). External bolster placement after percutaneous endoscopic gastrostomy tube insertion: Is looser better? *J Parenter Enteral Nutr,* 30(1):16-20.
Dochterman JM, Bulechek GM (Eds). (2004). *Nursing Interventions Classification (NIC),* 4th ed. St. Louis: Mosby.
Goldberg E, Kaye R, Yaworski J, Liacouras C. (2005). Gastrostomy tubes: Facts, fallacies, fistulas, and false tracts. *Gastroenterol Nurs,* 28(6):485-493.

Laasch HU, Wilbraham L, Bullen K, Marriott A, Lawrance JA, Johnson RJ, et al. (2003). Gastrostomy insertion: Comparing the options—PEG, RIG or PIG? *Clin Radiol*, 58(5):398-405.

McClave SA, Neff RL. (2006). Care and long-term maintenance of percutaneous endoscopic gastrostomy tubes. *J Parenter Enteral Nutr*, 30(1 Suppl):S27-S38.

McClave SA, Ritchie CS. (2006). The role of endoscopically placed feeding or decompression tubes. *Gastroenterol Clin North Am*, 35(1):83-100.

Overstreet M. (2004). How does a PEG tube stay in? *Nursing*, 34(6):21.

Reising DL, Neal RS. (2005). Enteral tube flushing. *Am J Nurs*, 105(3):58-63.

Stroud M, Duncan H, Nightingale J; British Society of Gastroenterology. (2003). Guidelines for enteral feeding in adult hospital patients. *Gut*, 52(Suppl 7):vii1-vii12.

Tracey DL, Patterson GE. (2006). Care of the gastrostomy tube in the home. *Home Healthc Nurse*, 24(6): 381-386.

 # TUBE CARE: URINARY

Katherine N. Moore, PhD, RN, CCCN; Betty J. Ackley, MSN, EdS, RN

NIC **Definition:** Management of a patient with urinary drainage equipment (Dochterman & Bulechek, 2004).

NURSING ACTIVITIES

Effective

■ **NIC** *Maintain a closed urinary drainage system.* **LOE = I**

EO The principles of catheter care and urinary tract infection put forward by the Centers for Disease Control and Prevention (CDC) guidelines in 1981 remain current today: the CDC guidelines recommend that the urinary drainage system be kept closed (Wong & Hooton, 1981).

NR A systematic review recommends the use of sealed (taped) drainage systems to help prevent bacteriuria (Joanna Briggs Institute, 2000).

MR A randomized controlled pilot study (*N* = 82) of postoperative catheterized surgical patients testing the intervention of the administration of an antibiotic found that the study requirements of maintaining a closed urinary drainage system resulted in a low incidence of infection for the control group receiving a placebo (Esposito et al., 2006).

MR Review articles stressed the importance of maintaining a closed urinary drainage system as an effective way to prevent catheter-related urinary tract infections (Ha & Cho, 2006; Drinka, 2006; Nicolle, 2005).

■ **SP** *Wash hands immediately before and immediately after any manipulation of the catheter site or of the bag, such as emptying the bag.* **LOE = VII**

EO The CDC guidelines recommend that the hands be washed both before and after all catheter care (Wong & Hooten, 1981).

EO Universal precautions from the World Health Organization (2006) recommend washing the hands before and after procedures.

RCT = Randomized Controlled (Clinical) Trial, **NIC** = Nursing Interventions Classification, **NOC** = Nursing Outcomes Classification

■ (SP) *Don clean gloves before emptying a catheter bag, and remove them afterward.* **LOE = VII**

(EO) Universal precautions from the World Health Organization (2006) recommend wearing gloves when in contact with body fluids.

■ (SP) *Secure the catheter to the patient's thigh or lower abdomen.* **LOE = VII**

(NR) A systematic review of the literature revealed an absence of experimental studies that evaluated the effectiveness of securing the catheter (Gray, 2004).

(EO) Securing the catheter to the thigh or abdomen helps decrease the risk of trauma, bleeding, necrosis of the meatus, and bladder spasms from pressure and traction on the catheter (SUNA, 2006).

(NR) A descriptive exploratory study demonstrated that nurses ($N = 82$) in a community medical center indicated that securing indwelling urinary catheters was a necessary part of nursing care. However, when a prevalence study was conducted, only 4.4% of the indwelling catheters were stabilized (Siegel, 2006).

■ *If a diagnostic urine specimen is needed from a catheterized patient, insert a new catheter, and then obtain a urine specimen. If this is not possible, use a sterile syringe to collect the specimen from the sample port.* **LOE = III**

(MR) In a controlled study ($N = 85$ spinal cord injury patients), withdrawing a sample from the catheter in situ in the control group resulted in a contaminated sample from organisms resting within the catheter lumen (sessile organisms) rather than from the planktonic (floating) organisms that can be treated with antibiotics that were found in the experimental group (Shah et al., 2005).

(EO) If it is not possible to change the catheter or if the catheter has been in situ for only a few days, the CDC guidelines recommend that the specimen be obtained using a sterile needle and syringe after cleansing the sampling port on the tubing with an antiseptic (Wong & Hooton, 1981).

■ *Schedule the removal of the catheter from a surgical patient between 10 PM and 12 midnight rather than in the morning.* **LOE = II**

(NR) A systematic review of research by the Joanna Briggs Institute demonstrated that the removal of the catheter at midnight versus in the morning resulted in a reduced mean hospital stay (Joanna Briggs Institute, 2006).

(NR) An RCT of general medical surgical patients ($N = 210$) demonstrated that there was no difference in the length of stay if the catheter was removed in the evening as compared with the usual morning removal time. If only the surgical patients were examined, the catheter removal did result in a shortened hospital stay, but the results were not statistically significant (Webster et al., 2006).

(MR) A Cochrane systematic review demonstrated that the removal of the catheter earlier versus later resulted in a decreased length of the hospital stay; the evidence was suggestive but not conclusive (Griffiths & Fernandez, 2005).

(MR) A prospective, randomized study ($N = 84$) of patients who had transurethral resection of the prostate demonstrated an increased incidence of sleep disturbances in the group who received midnight catheter removal versus morning catheter removal (Ganta et al., 2005).

NR = Nursing Research, **MR** = Multidisciplinary Research, **SP** = Standard of Practice, **EO** = Expert Opinion, **LOE** = Level of Evidence

Possibly Effective

■ *Ensure that patients with a urinary catheter do not have roommates with an infection, including a urinary tract infection associated with a catheter.* **LOE = VII**

(EO) The CDC guidelines recommend that there be a distance kept between patients with catheters to decrease the chances of cross infection; they should not be in the same room or in adjacent beds (Wong & Hooton, 1981).

Not Effective

■ *Providing daily special meatal care using povidone-iodine solution, chlorhexidine gluconate, or silver sulfadiazine cream.* **LOE = II**

(MR) An RCT ($N = 229$) of both male and female patients with indwelling catheters examined the rate of bacteriuria in three groups: (1) meatal care with povidone-iodine twice a day and the use of the povidone-iodine ointment; (2) washing with green soap and water; and (3) no meatal care. The results demonstrated no benefit of meatal cleaning in any of the groups (Burke et al., 1981).

(NR) In a nonrandomized study ($N = 130$), patients in the intensive care unit were divided into groups that received meatal care of chlorhexidine gluconate, povidone-iodine, or control care once or twice daily. The antiseptics proved to be of no benefit for decreasing the rate of bacteriuria (Koskeroglu et al., 2004).

(MR) An RCT of 696 patients evaluating the effectiveness of 1% silver sulfadiazine cream applied twice daily to the urethral meatus found that the meatal care did not prevent the development of catheter-associated bacteriuria (Huth et al., 1992).

■ *Using antibacterial solutions added to drainage bags or antibacterial irrigations.* **LOE = I**

(NR) A systematic review found that the use of antibacterial solutions in drainage bags had no effect in reducing the incidence of catheter-associated infections (Joanna Briggs Institute, 2000).

Possibly Harmful

■ *Disconnecting the closed urinary drainage system.* **LOE = I**

(EO) The CDC guidelines recommend that the urinary drainage system be kept closed (Wong & Hooton, 1981).

(NR) A systematic review recommended the use of sealed (taped) drainage systems to help prevent bacteruria (Joanna Briggs Institute, 2000).

■ *Using a clamp-and-release protocol before removing a catheter.* **LOE = I**

(NR) A systematic review of the literature found that research on clamping indwelling catheters before removal was equivocal because of the quality of the studies. However, on the basis of the review, clamping is not recommended (Fernandez & Griffiths, 2005).

(NR) A systematic review found that there was limited evidence to support clamping before removal; instead, removal of the catheter without clamping is recommended (Joanna Briggs Institute, 2006).

RCT = Randomized Controlled (Clinical) Trial, **NIC** = Nursing Interventions Classification, **NOC** = Nursing Outcomes Classification

OUTCOME MEASUREMENT

URINARY ELIMINATION (NOC)

Definition: Collection and discharge of urine.

Urinary Elimination as evidenced by the following selected NOC indicators:

- Urine odor
- Urine amount
- Urine color
- Urine clarity
- Adequate fluid intake

(Rate each indicator of **Urinary Elimination:** 1 = severely compromised, 2 = substantially compromised, 3 = moderately compromised, 4 = mildly compromised, 5 = not compromised) (Moorhead et al., 2004).

REFERENCES

Burke JP, Garibaldi RA, Britt MR, Jacobson JA, Conti M, Alling DW. (1981). Prevention of catheter-associated urinary tract infections. Efficacy of daily meatal care regimens. *Am J Med*, 70(3):655-658.

Dochterman JM, Bulechek GM (Eds). (2004). *Nursing Interventions Classification (NIC)*, 4th ed. St Louis: Mosby.

Drinka PJ. (2006). Complications of chronic indwelling urinary catheters. *J Am Med Dir Assoc*, 7(6): 388-392.

Esposito S, Noviello S, Leone S, Marvaso A, Drago L, Marchetti F, et al. (2006). A pilot study on prevention of catheter-related urinary tract infections with fluoroquinolones. *J Chemother*, 18(5):494-501.

Fernandez RS, Griffiths RD. (2005). Clamping short-term indwelling catheters: A systematic review of the evidence. *J Wound Ostomy Continence Nurs*, 32(5):329-336.

Ganta SB, Chakravarti A, Somani B, Jones MA, Kadow K. (2005). Removal of catheter at midnight versus early morning: The patients' perspective. *Urol Int*, 75(1):26-29.

Gray M. (2004). What nursing interventions reduce the risk of symptomatic urinary infections in the patient with an indwelling catheter. *J WOCN*, 31(1):3-13.

Griffiths R, Fernandez R. (2005). Policies for the removal of short-term indwelling urethral catheters. *Cochrane Database Syst Rev*, (1):CD004011.

Ha US, Cho YH. (2006). Catheter-associated urinary tract infections: New aspects of novel urinary catheters. *Int J Antimicrob Agents*, 28(6):485-490.

Huth TS, Burke JP, Larsen RA, Classen DC, Stevens LE. (1992). Randomized trial of meatal care with silver sulfadiazine cream for the prevention of catheter-associated bacteriuria. *J Infect Dis*, 165(1):14-18.

Joanna Briggs Institute. (2000). Management of short term indwelling urethral catheters to prevent urinary tract infections. *Best Practice*, 4(1):1-6.

Joanna Briggs Institute. (2006). Removal of short term indwelling urethral catheters. *Best Practice*, 10(3):1-4.

Koskeroglu N, Durmaz G, Bahar M, Kural M, Yelken B. (2004). The role of meatal disinfection in preventing catheter-related bacteriuria in an intensive care unit: A pilot study in Turkey. *J Hosp Infect*, 56(3): 236-238.

Moorhead M, Johnson M, Maas M (Eds). (2004). *Nursing Outcomes Classification (NOC)*, 3rd ed. St Louis: Mosby.

Nicolle LE. (2005). Catheter-related urinary tract infection. *Drugs Aging*, 22(8):627-639.

Shah P, Cannon J, Sullivan C, Nemchausky B, Pachucki C. (2005). Controlling antimicrobial use and decreasing microbiological laboratory tests for urinary tract infections in spinal-cord-injury patients with chronic indwelling catheters. *Am J Health Syst Pharm*, 62(1):74-77.

NR = Nursing Research, **MR** = Multidisciplinary Research, **SP** = Standard of Practice, **EO** = Expert Opinion, **LOE** = Level of Evidence

Siegel TJ. (2006). Do registered nurses perceive the anchoring of indwelling urinary catheters as a necessary aspect of nursing care? A pilot study. *J Wound Ostomy Continence Nurs,* 33(2):140-144.

Society of Urologic Nurses and Associates (SUNA) Clinical Practice Guidelines Task Force. (2006). Care of the patient with an indwelling catheter. *Urol Nurs,* 26(1):80-81.

Webster J, Osborne S, Woollett K, Shearer J, Courtney M, Anderson D. (2006). Does evening removal of urinary catheters shorten hospital stay among general hospital patients? A randomized controlled trial. *J Wound Ostomy Continence Nurs,* 33(2):156-163.

Wong ES, Hooton TM. (1981). Guideline for prevention of catheter-associated urinary tract infections. Department of Health, Centers for Disease Control and Prevention. Available online: http://www.cdc.gov/. Retrieved on July 7, 2007.

World Health Organization. (2006). Universal Precautions, including injection safety. Available online: http://www.who.int/. Retrieved on July 7, 2007.

TUBE FEEDING (ENTERAL)

Kathleen A. Fitzgerald, PhD, RN; Betty J. Ackley, MSN, EdS, RN

NIC **Definition:** Delivering nutrients and water through a gastrointestinal tube (Dochterman & Bulechek, 2004).

NURSING ACTIVITIES

Effective

■ **NIC** *Elevate the head of the bed 30 to 45 degrees during feedings.* **LOE = II**

NR A prospective descriptive study ($N = 360$) of aspiration during tube feedings among critically ill patients identified multiple factors associated with high risk for aspiration. A bed backrest elevation <30 degrees was significantly associated with patients with a high risk of aspiration (Metheny et al., 2006).

NR A review of aspiration in mechanically ventilated patients receiving tube feedings was conducted with the goal of designing an algorithm for care. Six studies supported a decrease in aspiration risk when the head of the bed was elevated at least 30 degrees (Bowman et al., 2005).

NR A controlled study ($N = 30$) of mechanically ventilated patients receiving tube feedings demonstrated an increase of the presence of pepsin (from gastric contents) in pulmonary secretions if the patient was in a flat position versus being positioned with the head elevated (Metheny et al., 2002a).

MR In an RCT of mechanically ventilated patients ($N = 86$) receiving tube feedings, patients were randomly assigned to either a supine or semirecumbent position in bed. The trial was stopped because the results demonstrated a significant association between the supine position and nosocomial pneumonia (Drakulovic et al., 1999).

■ **NIC** **SP** *Confirm tube placement by x-ray examination prior to administering feedings or medications via the tube per agency protocol.* **LOE = VII**

MR A review of complications associated with the bedside placement of feeding tubes noted that most institutions required that feeding tube placement be confirmed by chest x-ray to

RCT = Randomized Controlled (Clinical) Trial, **NIC** = Nursing Interventions Classification, **NOC** = Nursing Outcomes Classification

avoid complications of inadvertent bronchial, pleural, or lung placement and to rule out the placement of the tube in the esophagus (Baskin, 2006).

(EO) Because of the possibility of tube malposition in the tracheobronchial tree, radiographic confirmation of the position of the feeding tube tip is recommended (ASPEN, 2002).

■ *Use a closed versus an open enteral delivery system of tube feeding, if possible. If an open system is used, aseptic technique is necessary for handling the feeding tube, the formula, the feeding tube set, the connection hub, and the ports for medication use. The feeding tube set is changed every 24 hours.*
LOE = III

(NR) A controlled study of rinsing feeding tube sets was conducted to determine whether rinsing would increase the contamination of the set. Trials were conducted with 52 sets in a laboratory and 32 critically ill patients with variable rinse times. There was no significant difference in bacteria counts in the formula at 24 hours no matter how frequently the sets were rinsed (Kohn-Keeth et al., 1996).

(MR) A controlled study demonstrated that the closed delivery system did not result in the contamination of the feedings. The use of the open bags resulted in several tube feeding formulas becoming contaminated (Vanek, 2000).

(MR) A simulated study was performed that mimicked the clinical environment. The study compared the use of a closed delivery system (feeding and tubing were preprepared) and an open system in which the feeding formula was poured into the feeding bag. The open method, when prepared with aseptic technique using clean gloves, was minimally contaminated with bacteria, and the closed system was not contaminated. When the trial was repeated with contaminated hands, the closed system was not contaminated, whereas the open system method was heavily contaminated. Closed delivery systems were the preferred route to minimize the bacterial contamination. Following aseptic technique and wearing clean gloves minimized the contamination of the open delivery systems (Beattie & Anderton, 2001).

(MR) In a prospective study involving the swabbing of the enteral tube hub (i.e., the connection point of the feeding system with the feeding tube) both externally and internally to determine contamination with bacteria, the tubing hub was found to be contaminated both inside and outside with enteric bacteria and nonenteric bacteria (Staphylococci and Pseudomonas). Two specific types of bacteria were found on adjacent nursing units, which indicates the possibility of cross-contamination by health care workers. It was determined as a result of this study that the hub contamination was caused by the improper technique of health care workers and that aseptic procedures should be followed when preparing enteral feedings that include the decontamination of the tubing hub (Matlow et al., 2006).

(NR) A summary article recommended the following practices for enteral feeding: using a closed system versus an open system; washing the hands or using an alcohol rub before handling any part of the system; using nonsterile gloves; using prepackaged formula; discarding or covering and refrigerating opened formula containers; using tap water for irrigation unless contraindicated; replacing delivery sets every 24 hours and assembling the feeding system on a disinfected surface; disinfecting the opening and rim of the can with alcohol; and disinfecting the hub of the tubing before and after disconnecting or giving medications. Formula should be hanging for only 12 hours in an open system (Padula et al., 2004).

NR = Nursing Research, **MR** = Multidisciplinary Research, **SP** = Standard of Practice, **EO** = Expert Opinion, **LOE** = Level of Evidence

Possibly Effective

■ *Use a pump to administer the tube feeding in patients who have postpyloric feedings or who are bedridden.* **LOE = II**

MR A prospective randomized crossover study of bedridden patients ($N = 100$) with percutaneous endoscopic gastrostomy tubes was conducted to determine whether pump or gravity-assisted tube feedings were safer. Participating patients suffered neurological disorders and were dependent on full care from caregivers. All patients had received percutaneous endoscopic gastrostomy feedings for at least 6 months before the study, so their tolerance of feeding was well established. The pump-assisted feedings were during the night over a median time of 7.4 hours. The gravity drip feedings were infused over a median time of 5.1 hours, with a standard deviation of 3.5 hours. Nurses and caregivers evaluated the duration of the nutrition, regurgitation, vomiting, bowel movements, quality of feces, episodes of aspiration, and the rate of pneumonia diagnosed by radiograph. The subjects receiving the pump-assisted feedings had a lower rate of side effects. Only the subjects receiving gravity-assisted feedings had pneumonia (Shang et al., 2004).

EO Gastric feedings do not necessarily require a feeding pump for the delivery of formula. In the presence of adequate gastric emptying, the stomach acts as a reservoir, releasing formula into the duodenum gradually. Small bowel feedings require continuous infusion, because a large bolus of formula may cause gastrointestinal discomfort and complications (Kirby et al., 1998).

■ **SP** *Provide oral care at least two times per day.* **LOE = VI**

MR In a comparison study of nursing home patients ($N = 215$ subjects), the nasogastric tube–fed patients had 81% pathogenic bacteria in mouth, the PEG patients had 51% pathogenic bacteria in the mouth, and the orally fed patients had 17.5% pathogenic bacteria (Leibovitz et al., 2003).

■ *Flush the tube with at least 30 mL of warm water every 4 hours during continuous feedings, before and after administering a medication through the tube, before and after administering a bolus feeding, and after checking gastric residual.* **LOE = VII**

EO A project querying 19 hospitals and the nursing and medical literature to determine the standard practice of enteral tube flushing found very little evidence to determine the frequency, the timing related to medication, and the volume of flush. Two studies found that flushing with water was effective for decreasing the occlusion of the tub. On the basis of current practices described in textbooks and in the 19 hospitals, the following recommendations were made: flush a tube with continuous feeding every 4 hours; before, between, and after medication administration; and before and after checking gastric residuals. Use a 30-mL syringe, flush with at least 30 mL of warm water, and establish a standard protocol for the facility (Reising & Neal, 2005; Kohn-Keeth, 2000).

NR An experimental study using polyurethane ($N = 54$) and silicone ($N = 54$) feeding tubes was conducted to compare the efficacy of water, cranberry juice, and carbonated cola for maintaining tube patency. The results indicated that the polyurethane tubes were superior to the silicone and that water and carbonated cola were superior to cranberry juice for maintaining tube patency (Metheny et al., 1988).

RCT = Randomized Controlled (Clinical) Trial, **NIC** = Nursing Interventions Classification, **NOC** = Nursing Outcomes Classification

(MR) A study comparing the effects of water versus cranberry juice found water to be a more effective flushing agent; cranberry juice was associated with more clogged tubes (Wilson & Haynes-Johnson, 1987).

■ *Recognize that postpyloric feeding tube placement may decrease the risk of tracheobronchial aspiration among patients who have significantly delayed gastric emptying.* **LOE = I**

(NR) A prospective descriptive study using pepsin as a marker for gastric contents determined risk factors for tracheobronchial aspiration. Tube location (gastric versus small bowel) was a significant factor in aspiration, with a significantly higher percentage of pepsin-positive tracheal secretions in the patients with gastric tube placement (Metheny, 2006).

(MR) A randomized trial was conducted to determine whether nasogastric tube feedings versus nasojejunal tube feedings posed a greater risk of gastrointestinal complications and nosocomial pneumonia among intensive care unit patients. The results indicated less gastrointestinal complications in the nasojejunal-tube-fed patients but no difference in the occurrence of nosocomial pneumonia (Montejo et al., 2002).

(MR) A systematic review of nine prospective RCTs of patients with nasogastric versus nasojejunal tube feedings was conducted to determine the incidence of nosocomial pneumonia among other outcomes. The risk of pneumonia was reported in seven studies, and it was concluded that there was no significant difference in the incidence of pneumonia between the two groups (Marik & Zaloga, 2003).

■ *Use a large-diameter tube with multiple ports to measure gastric residual volumes; using a small bore tube is less accurate.* **LOE = IV**

(NR) A controlled trial was conducted to determine the ability to accurately measure tube feeding formula aspirated from small-bore (10 F) feeding tubes. Both small-bore tubes and large-bore (14 or 18 F) nasogastric tubes were placed in 62 critically ill patients. There were 645 aspirations from the small-bore tubes followed by 645 aspirations from the large-bore tubes. The results indicated that the aspirations from the large-bore tubes were about 1.5 times greater than the amount obtained from the small bore tubes (Metheny et al., 2005).

Possibly Effective

■ *Measure gastric residual volume to predict the risk for aspiration.* **LOE = IV**

(NR) In a prospective study of 244 critically ill gastric-fed patients, a comparison was made between gastric residual volumes (GRVs) and aspiration as assessed by the presence of pepsin in tracheal-bronchial secretions (Metheny et al., 2005). More than 3000 tracheal GRVs were measured. It was found that aspiration occurred significantly more often when patients had two or more GRVs of 150 mL or more over a 3-day study period as compared with patients whose GRVs were consistently less than 100 mL. However, despite a higher incidence of aspiration among patients with high GRVs, aspiration occurred at a relatively high rate among patients whose GRVs were consistently low. The investigators concluded that high GRVs increased aspiration risk; however, the absence of high GRVs did not preclude aspiration, possibly because of measurement error (Metheny, 2006).

NR = Nursing Research, **MR** = Multidisciplinary Research, **SP** = Standard of Practice, **EO** = Expert Opinion, **LOE** = Level of Evidence

(MR) A prospective study of critically ill patients was conducted to determine whether GRVs accurately predicted the risk for aspiration and the most appropriate GRV at which tube feedings should be stopped. Forty patients were evaluated by 1118 oral or tracheal-suctioned specimens. The frequency of regurgitation and aspiration did not vary significantly over a range of residual volumes from 0 to 400 mL. The study results did not support the use of residual volumes as a clinical marker for the risk of aspiration, and they cannot support holding tube feeding for a specific residual volume (McClave et al., 2005). In a recent review, a problem with this study was emphasized: only 6.2% of the GRVs were greater than 150 mL, and only 1.5% were greater than 400 mL. Therefore, there was likely inadequate statistical power to determine the relationship between large GRVs and aspiration.

(EO) Until more definitive research is available, it is prudent to consider guidelines issued by expert panels. For example, one set of guidelines indicates that the feeding regimen should be reviewed if a GRV is greater than 200 mL (Stroud et al., 2003). Another set of guidelines indicate that GRVs should be checked frequently when feedings are started and that the feedings should be held if residual volumes exceed 200 mL on two successive assessments (ASPEN, 2002).

Not Effective

- **Measuring the pH of the aspirate when the patient is receiving continuous feedings. LOE = VI**

(EO) When the patient is receiving continuous feedings, the formula generally buffers the secretions to near neutral levels. Measuring the pH can be effective when the feeding has been held for several hours (Metheny, 2006).

(NR) A descriptive study measured the efficacy of using pH testing to confirm the placement of nasogastric tubes. In 29% of the patients with nasogastric tubes, the pH was not accurate for determining placement, because the patient was receiving histamine-2 blockers and proton-pump inhibitors, which produced false readings. In addition, some brands of pH strips were inaccurate or their results were misinterpreted by staff (Taylor & Clemente, 2005).

- **Using the auscultation method to differentiate between the respiratory or gastric placement of a feeding tube. LOE = VI**

(NR) A descriptive study of 85 acutely ill patients and 123 taped auscultations was conducted to determine whether air insufflated through feeding tubes ending in the esophagus, stomach, duodenum, and proximal jejunum would produce a different pitch and volume of sounds. Expert raters listened to the sounds and recorded their impressions. X-rays were taken to verify the feeding tube tip placement. Overall results revealed correct classifications of the tapes 34.4% of the time, thus indicating that air insufflation was an inaccurate procedure to use to verify feeding tube placement (Metheny et al., 1990).

(EO) There have been multiple case reports of small-bore feeding tubes being inserted into the lung after the use of the auscultation method to check placement. This has also happened with a large-bore feeding tube (Metheny, 2006). Several publications recommend that the auscultatory method be abandoned, because it can indicate that blindly placed tubes are correctly positioned, even when they are actually in the lung or esophagus (AACN, 2005; NPSA, 2005).

RCT = Randomized Controlled (Clinical) Trial, **NIC** = Nursing Interventions Classification, **NOC** = Nursing Outcomes Classification

Possibly Harmful

■ *Using blue dye in tube feeding to detect aspiration associated with tube feedings.*
LOE = III

EO A U.S. Food and Drug Administration (FDA) Public Health Advisory reported adverse occurrences in at least 20 patients and 12 deaths from the use of blue dye in the enteral feeding. The FDA warns that the safety of blue dye used for the detection of aspiration has not been established; that patients with risk factors such as increased intestinal permeability, sepsis, burns, trauma, shock, renal failure, and inflammatory bowel disease may absorb the dye and experience adverse events; and that the blue-tinted enteral feedings may give false-positive results on hemoccult stool tests (Acheson, 2003).

NR An experimental study ($N = 30$) using white rabbits and gastric juice was conducted to determine whether the aspiration of blue-dye-stained enteral formula was a useful marker for aspiration in humans. Dye was visible in only 46.3% of suctioned tracheal secretions, thereby indicating that the use of dye in tube feedings was inadequate to detect tracheal aspiration (Metheny et al., 2002b).

MR Multiple cases have been reported in which food dye placed in feeding tubes was systemically absorbed, sometimes causing fatal outcomes (Maloney et al., 2000).

EO Most institutions have banned the use of food dye because it is insensitive for detecting aspiration and may result in harm (Maloney et al., 2002).

OUTCOME MEASUREMENT

NUTRITIONAL STATUS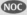

Definition: Extent to which nutrients are available to meet metabolic needs.
Nutritional Status as evidenced by the following selected NOC indicators:
• Nutrient intake
• Weight/height ratio
• Hematocrit
• Hydration
(Rate each indicator of **Nutritional Status:** 1 = severe deviation from normal range, 2 = substantial deviation from normal range, 3 = moderate deviation from normal range, 4 = mild deviation from normal range, 5 = no deviation from normal range) (Moorhead et al., 2004).

REFERENCES

Acheson DW. (2003). Reports of blue discoloration and death in patients receiving enteral feedings tinted with the dye, FD&C Blue No. 1. *FDA Public Health Advisory*, September 29, 2003, pp 1-3.

American Association of Critical-Care Nurses (AACN). (2005). Practice alert: Verification of feeding tube placement. Available online: http://www.aacn.org. Retrieved on July 7, 2007.

American Society for Parenteral and Enteral Nutrition (ASPEN) Board of Directors. (2002). Section VIII: Access for administration of nutritional support. *J Parenter Enteral Nutr*, 26(1 Suppl):33SA-35SA.

Baskin WN. (2006). Acute complications associated with bedside placement of feeding tubes. *Nutr Clin Pract*, 21(1):40-55.

NR = Nursing Research, **MR** = Multidisciplinary Research, **SP** = Standard of Practice, **EO** = Expert Opinion, **LOE** = Level of Evidence

Beattie TK, Anderton A. (2001). Decanting versus sterile pre-filled nutrient containers—the microbiological risks in enteral feeding. *Int J Environ Health Res*, 11(1):81-93.

Bowman A, Greiner JE, Doerschug KC, Little SB, Bombei CL, Comried LM. (2005). Implementation of an evidenced-based feeding protocol and aspiration risk reduction algorithm. *Crit Care Nurs Q*, 28(4):324-333.

Dochterman JM, Bulechek GM (Eds). (2004). *Nursing Interventions Classification (NIC)*, 4th ed. St Louis: Mosby.

Drakulovic MB, Torres A, Bauer TT, Nicolas JM, Nogue S, Ferrer M. (1999). Supine body position as a risk factor for nosocomial pneumonia in mechanically ventilated patients: A randomised trial. *Lancet*, 353(9193):1851-1858.

Kirby DF, Minard G, Kohn-Keeth C. (1998). Enteral access and infusion equipment. In American Society for Parenteral and Enteral Nutrition (ASPEN) (Ed): *The ASPEN nutritional support manual.* Colorado: ASPEN.

Kohn-Keeth C. (2000). How to keep feeding tubes flowing freely. *Nursing*, 30(3):58-59.

Kohn-Keeth C, Shott S, Olree K. (1996). The effects of rinsing enteral delivery sets on formula contamination. *Nutr Clin Pract*, 11(6):269-273.

Leibovitz A, Plotnikov G, Habot B, Rosenberg M, Segal R. (2003). Pathogenic colonization of oral flora in frail elderly patients fed by nasogastric tube or percutaneous enterogastric tube. *J Gerontol A Biol Sci Med Sci*, 58(1):52-55.

Maloney JP, Halbower AC, Fouty BF, Fagan KA, Balasubramaniam V, Pike AW, et al. (2000). Systemic absorption of food dye in patients with sepsis. *N Engl J Med*, 343(14):1047-1048.

Maloney JP, Ryan TA, Brasel KJ, Binion DG, Johnson DR, Halbower AC, et al. (2002). Food dye use in enteral feedings: A review and a call for a moratorium. *Nutr Clin Pract*, 17(3):169-181.

Marik PE, Zaloga GP. (2003). Gastric versus post-pyloric feeding: A systematic review. *Crit Care*, 7(3): R46-R51.

Matlow A, Jacobson M, Wray R, Goldman C, Streitenberger L, Freeman R, et al. (2006). Enteral tube hub as a reservoir for transmissible enteric bacteria. *Am J Infect Control*, 34(3):131-133.

McClave SA, Lukan JK, Stefater JA, Lowen CC, Looney SW, Matheson PJ, et al. (2005). Poor validity of residual volumes as a marker for risk of aspiration in critically ill patients. *Crit Care Med*, 33(2): 324-330.

Metheny NA. (2006). Preventing respiratory complications of tube feedings: Evidence-based practice. *Am J Crit Care*, 15(4):360-369.

Metheny NA, Chang Y, Ye JS, Edwards SJ, Defer J, Dahms TE, et al. (2002a). Pepsin as a marker for pulmonary aspiration. *Am J Crit Care*, 11(2):150-154.

Metheny NA, Clouse RE, Chang Y, Stewart BJ, Oliver DA, Kollef MH. (2006). Tracheobronchial aspiration of gastric contents in critically ill tube-fed patients: Frequency, outcomes, and risk factors. *Crit Care Med*, 34(4):1007-1015.

Metheny NA, Dahms TE, Stewart BJ, Stone KS, Edwards SJ, Defer JE, et al. (2002b). Efficacy of dye-stained enteral formula in detecting pulmonary aspiration. *Chest*, 122(1):276-281.

Metheny N, Eisenberg P, McSweeney M. (1988). Effect of feeding tube properties and three irrigants on clogging rates. *Nurs Res*, 37(3):165-169.

Metheny N, McSweeney M, Wehrle MA, Wiersema L. (1990). Effectiveness of the auscultatory method in predicting feeding tube location. *Nurs Res*, 39(5):262-267.

Metheny NA, Stewart J, Nuetzel G, Oliver D, Clouse RE. (2005). Effect of feeding-tube properties on residual volume measurements in tube-fed patients. *J Parenter Enteral Nutr*, 29(3):192-197.

Montejo JC, Grau T, Acosta J, Ruiz-Santana S, Planas M, Garcia-de-Lorenzo A, et al. (2002). Multicenter, prospective, randomized, single-blind study comparing the efficacy and gastrointestinal complications of early jejunal feeding with early gastric feeding in critically ill patients. *Crit Care Med*, 30(4): 796-800.

Moorhead M, Johnson M, Maas M (Eds). (2004). *Nursing Outcomes Classification (NOC)*, 3rd ed. St Louis: Mosby.

National Patient Safety Agency (NPSA). (2005). Patient safety alert: Reducing the harm caused by misplaced naso and orogastric feeding tubes in babies under the care of neonatal units. Available online: http://www.npsa.nhs.uk. Retrieved on July 7, 2007.

Padula CA, Kenny A, Planchon C, Lamoureux C. (2004). Enteral feedings: What the evidence says. *Am J Nurs*, 104(7):62-69.

Reising DL, Neal RS. (2005). Enteral tube flushing. *Am J Nurs,* 105(3):58-63.

Shang E, Geiger N, Sturm JW, Post S. (2004). Pump-assisted enteral nutrition can prevent aspiration in bedridden percutaneous endoscopic gastrostomy patients. *J Parenter Enteral Nutr,* 28(3):180-183.

Stroud M, Duncan H, Nightingale J; British Society of Gastroenterology. (2003). Guidelines for enteral feeding in adult hospital patients. *Gut,* 52(Suppl 7):vii1-vii12.

Taylor SJ, Clemente R. (2005). Confirmation of nasogastric tube position by pH testing. *J Hum Nutr Diet,* 18(5):371-375.

Vanek VW. (2000). Closed versus enteral delivery systems: A quality improvement study. *Nutr Clin Pract,* 15(5):234-243.

Wilson M, Haynes-Johnson V. (1987). Cranberry juice or water? A comparison of feeding-tube irrigants. *Nutr Supp Serv,* 7(7):23-24.

 # UNILATERAL NEGLECT MANAGEMENT

Lori M. Rhudy, PhD, RN, CNRN, CRRN, APRN-BC

> **NIC** **Definition:** Protecting and safely reintegrating the affected part of the body while helping the patient adapt to disturbed perceptual abilities (Dochterman & Bulechek, 2004).

NURSING ACTIVITIES

Effective

■ **SP** *Assess for sensory, visual, auditory, cognitive, and communication impairments.* **LOE = VII**

> **EO** All patients should be screened for motor, sensory, cognitive, and communication deficits (VHA, 2003).
>
> **EO** All patients should be screened for cognitive deficits as soon as it is practical; this should be a standard practice in the care of stroke patients (ISWP, 2004).

■ **NIC** **SP** *Instruct caregivers on the cause, mechanisms, and treatment of unilateral neglect.* **LOE = VII**

> **EO** Families should be involved in decision making; this should be a standard practice in the care of stroke patients (ISWP, 2004; McGovern & Rudd, 2003).

■ **NIC** *Consult with occupational and physical therapists concerning the timing and strategies to facilitate the reintegration of neglected body parts and function.* **LOE = I**

> **EO** Poststroke care should be delivered in a setting in which rehabilitation care by a multidisciplinary team is coordinated and organized (VHA, 2003).
>
> **EO** Patients with persisting neglect should receive therapy (ISWP, 2004).
>
> **MR** A systematic review concluded that there was strong evidence that rehabilitation interventions that were specifically designed to treat unilateral neglect resulted in significant improvements in neglect scores (Jutai et al., 2003).

NR = Nursing Research, **MR** = Multidisciplinary Research, **SP** = Standard of Practice, **EO** = Expert Opinion, **LOE** = Level of Evidence

■ **NIC** **SP** *Ensure that the affected extremities are properly and safely positioned.* **LOE = V**

EO Stretching and mobilization techniques are recommended to improve range of motion as a means to prevent frozen shoulder and shoulder-hand pain syndrome (VHA, 2003).

MR In a controlled study of 10 consecutive patients (five each with right and left side hemiparesis) in the preclinical (community) setting, no differences in the vital parameters of oxygen saturation, mean arterial blood pressure, breathing pattern, or electrocardiogram were found in stroke patients positioned on the affected side as compared with the unaffected side. As a result, it was concluded that patients should be positioned on the affected side to prevent aspiration and to have the unaffected arm free to enhance communication with emergency care providers (Brainin et al., 2004).

NR In a seminal article, a review of positioning recommendations for a variety of positions for both unaffected and affected sides concluded that attendance to posture was one way to promote physical recovery 24 hours a day while at the same time preventing complications of stroke (particularly poststroke spasticity) that could contribute to contractures and limit mobility and/or other functional activities (Carr & Kenney, 1992).

■ **NIC** **SP** *Rearrange the environment to use the right or left visual field; position personal items, television, or reading materials within view on the unaffected side.* **LOE = VII**

EO Positioning the call light and personal items on the patient's unaffected side is a standard nursing intervention for unilateral neglect in right hemisphere stroke (Hinkle et al., 2004).

EO Placing items to accommodate visual field cuts is a standard nursing intervention for the management of sensory and visual perceptual problems in stroke patients (Howard, 2000).

Possibly Effective

■ **NIC** *Instruct the patient to scan from left to right.* **LOE = V**

MR A Cochrane review evaluating the effects of cognitive rehabilitation in spatial neglect after stroke found that, although patients showed improved performance on neuropsychological tests, the effect on disability was inconclusive (Bowen et al., 2002).

MR In recent systematic reviews, it was concluded that there was strong evidence that treatment using primarily enhanced visual scanning technique improved visual neglect after a stroke with associated improvements in function. However, even with treatment, unilateral neglect was a negative prognostic factor (Jutai et al., 2003; Teasell et al., 2005).

EO Treatments focused on functional adaptation, such as visual scanning, environmental cues, and environmental adaptation, may be useful for stroke patients with sensory perceptual problems (VHA, 2003).

EO Rehabilitation techniques such as cueing, scanning, and environmental adaptations should be used for patients with persistent and disabling impairment from neglect (ISWP, 2004; Bowen et al., 2002).

EO Nursing and therapy sessions for activities such as shoulder pain, postural control, and feeding should be modified to cue attention to the impaired side (ISWP, 2004).

RCT = Randomized Controlled (Clinical) Trial, **NIC** = Nursing Interventions Classification, **NOC** = Nursing Outcomes Classification

■ **NIC** *Focus tactile and verbal stimuli on the affected side as the patient demonstrates an ability to compensate for neglect.* **LOE = V**

MR Systematic reviews of stroke rehabilitation research concluded that there was conflicting evidence regarding the effect of external sensory stimulation interventions on the treatment of neglect. Interventions in the studies reviewed ranged from the use of treatment glasses to various combinations of tactile, auditory, nonverbal, and unilateral versus bilateral stimulation (Jutai et al., 2003; Teasell et al., 2005).

MR A qualitative phenomenological study of the experiences of four women recovering from unilateral neglect concluded that it was important for caregivers to understand the changing experience of neglect and to adjust support as necessary (Tham & Kielhofner, 2003).

MR A quasi-experimental study of 31 brain injury patients in a day rehabilitation program found that the use of systematic cueing for the use of visual imagery improved performance on attention and verbal cancellation tasks. Tactile stimuli such as a shoulder tap on the affected side were provided in addition to the verbal cues, but the influence of tactile stimuli was not evaluated (Niemeier, 1998).

MR Twenty patients in a matched control crossover study demonstrated lasting improvement with a combined treatment of contralesional (affected) side neck vibration and visual exploration training as compared with visual exploration therapy alone. In addition, these patients demonstrated improvements in self-care, reaching and grasping, and spatial orientation as compared with visual exploration training alone (Schindler et al., 2002).

Not Effective

No applicable published research was found in this category.

Possibly Harmful

No applicable published research was found in this category.

OUTCOME MEASUREMENT

ADAPTATION TO PHYSICAL DISABILITY   **NOC**

Definition: Adaptive response to a significant functional challenge due to a physical disability.

Adaptation to Physical Disability as evidenced by the following selected NOC indicators:

• Adapts to functional limitations
• Verbalizes reconciliation to disability
• Modifies lifestyle to accommodate disability
• Identifies risk of complications associated with disability
• Modifies lifestyle to accommodate disability
• Seeks professional help as appropriate

(Rate each indicator of **Adaptation to Physical Disability:** 1 = never demonstrated, 2 = rarely demonstrated, 3 = sometimes demonstrated, 4 = often demonstrated, 5 = consistently demonstrated) (Moorhead et al., 2004).

NR = Nursing Research, **MR** = Multidisciplinary Research, **SP** = Standard of Practice, **EO** = Expert Opinion, **LOE** = Level of Evidence

REFERENCES

Bowen A, Lincoln NB, Dewey M. (2002). Cognitive rehabilitation for spatial neglect following stroke. *Cochrane Database Syst Rev*, (2):CD003586.

Brainin M, Funk G, Dachenhausen A, Huber G, Matz K, Eckhardt R. (2004). Stroke emergency: Evidence favours laying the patient on the paretic side. *Wien Med Wochenschr*, 154(23-24):568-570.

Carr EK, Kenney FD. (1992). Positioning of the stroke patient: A review of the literature. *Int J Nurs Stud*, 29(4):355-369.

Dochterman JM, Bulechek GM (Eds). (2004). *Nursing Interventions Classification (NIC)*, 4th ed. St Louis: Mosby.

Hinkle JL, Guanci MM, Bowman L, Hermann L, McGinty LB, Rose J. (2004). Cerebrovascular events of the nervous system. In Bader MK, Littlejohns LR (Eds): *AANN core curriculum for neuroscience nursing*. St. Louis: WB Saunders.

Howard CJ. (2000). Stroke. In Edwards PA (Ed): *The specialty practice of rehabilitation nursing: A core curriculum*, 4th ed. Glenview, IL: Association of Rehabilitation Nurses.

Intercollegiate Stroke Working Party (ISWP). (2004). *National clinical guidelines for stroke*, 2nd ed. London: Royal College of Physicians of London.

Jutai JW, Bhogal SK, Foley NC, Bayley M, Teasell RW, Speechley MR. (2003). Treatment of visual perceptual disorders post stroke. *Top Stroke Rehabil*, 10(2):77-106.

McGovern R, Rudd A. (2003). Management of stroke. *Postgrad Med J*, 79(928):87-92.

Moorhead M, Johnson M, Maas M (Eds). (2004). *Nursing Outcomes Classification (NOC)*, 3rd ed. St Louis: Mosby.

Niemeier JP. (1998). The Lighthouse Strategy: Use of a visual imagery technique to treat visual inattention in stroke patients. *Brain Inj*, 12(5):399-406.

Schindler I, Kerkhoff G, Karnath HO, Keller I, Goldenberg G. (2002). Neck muscle vibration induces lasting recovery in spatial neglect. *J Neurol Neurosurg Psychiatry*, 73(4):412-419.

Teasell R, Salter K, Bitensky J, Bhogal S, Foley N, Menon A, et al. (2005). *Evidence-based review of stroke rehabilitation. Module 13: Perceptual disorders*. Available online: http://www.ebrsr.com. Retrieved on July 7, 2007.

Tham K, Kielhofner G. (2003). Impact of the social environment on occupational experience and performance among persons with unilateral neglect. *Am J Occup Ther*, 57(4):403-412.

Veterans Health Administration (VHA), Department of Defense. (2003). *VA/DOD clinical practice guideline for the management of stroke rehabilitation in the primary care setting*. Washington (DC): Department of Veteran Affairs.

URINARY CATHETERIZATION   NIC

Betty J. Ackley, MSN, EdS, RN; Katherine N. Moore, PhD, RN, CCCN

NIC **Definition:** Insertion of a catheter into the bladder for the temporary or permanent drainage of urine (Dochterman & Bulechek, 2004).

NURSING ACTIVITIES

Effective

■ **SP** *Use catheters only when necessary, and avoid them if possible.* **LOE = VII**

NR A descriptive study (*N* = 285) of randomly selected patients who were 65 years old or older demonstrated that only half of the patients who received a catheter had appropriate reasons for the insertion of a catheter and that, in 33% of these patients' charts, there was no order for catheterization (Gokula et al., 2004).

EO The Centers for Disease Control and Prevention (CDC) guidelines recommend that catheters be inserted only when necessary and removed as soon as possible when they are no longer needed (Wong & Hooton, 1981).

■ *Wash hands before beginning to catheterize and also after finishing the procedure.* **LOE = I**

(Please refer to the guideline on Infection Control: Hand Hygiene.)

■ **SP** *If the female perineum or the male penis is visibly dirty or has an odor, wash the area first to decrease organisms in the area.* **LOE = VII**

EO In the male patient, retract the foreskin and wash the penis with soap and water before beginning catheterization to decrease the incidence of infection (Doherty, 2006).

■ **SP** *Retract the foreskin before catheterization if the male patient is not circumcised, and replace the foreskin after catheterization to ensure that the foreskin is brought back down over the glans.* **LOE = VII**

EO Retract the foreskin as needed and reduce/reposition the foreskin after catheterization. If the foreskin is not properly replaced, paraphimosis will occur, during which the foreskin constricts the glans and causes painful vascular dilatation and swelling. The swelling and pain may necessitate an emergency surgical procedure to resolve them (Gerber & Brendler, 2002).

■ **NIC** **SP** *Maintain strict aseptic technique.* **LOE = VII**

EO The CDC guidelines recommend that catheters be inserted with aseptic technique using sterile equipment (Wong & Hooton, 1981).

MR An RCT comparing sterile technique (scrubbing hands and arms for 4 minutes and cleansing with cetrimide) and clean technique (usual handwashing, clean gloves, and cleansing with sterile water) for catheter insertion ($N = 156$) found that aseptic technique did not result in decreased bacteriuria within a 3-day period (Carapeti et al., 1996).

■ *Use lidocaine gel as ordered for the insertion of a catheter into a male patient.* **LOE = II**

MR In an RCT of males requiring catheterization ($N = 36$), those receiving 15 mL topical 2% lidocaine gel injected into the urethra and held in place for 15 minutes versus 15 mL surgical lubricant had decreased pain with catheter insertion (Siderias et al., 2004).

MR In an RCT of females requiring catheterization ($N = 100$), half received 5 mL 2% lidocaine injected into the meatus 1 minute before catheterization, and the other half received plain lubricant. The study demonstrated no difference in pain levels, but a limitation of the study was the 1-minute wait time for the lidocaine to become effective (Tanabe et al., 2004).

EO In the male patient, instill 5 to 10 mL of 2% lidocaine jelly into the urethra using a catheter-tipped syringe to decrease pain, dilate the urethra, and lubricate the passage (Senese, 2004).

EO Lidocaine is likely to be more effective for decreasing pain if it is left in the male urethra for 5 to 10 minutes before catheterization (Canes, 2006).

NR = Nursing Research, **MR** = Multidisciplinary Research, **SP** = Standard of Practice, **EO** = Expert Opinion, **LOE** = Level of Evidence

■ (SP) *Insert the catheter in a male patient to the Y junction.* **LOE = V**

(MR) In a descriptive study ($N = 10$), male patients had catheters inserted 8 inches into the penis as recommended in most procedure manuals and textbooks. Fluoroscopy indicated that not all of the catheters were in the bladder but rather were in the prostatic urethra or bladder neck. Inserting the catheter to the Y bifurcation is recommended (Daneshgari et al., 2002).

■ (SP) *Use 10 mL of sterile water to fill the balloon of a 5-cc Foley catheter balloon. Do not use normal saline.* **LOE = VII**

(EO) Using 10 mL fills the 5-mL balloon symmetrically, thus promoting better drainage from the bladder. Saline can crystallize and make the catheter more difficult to remove (SUNA, 2006).

(EO) With gentle pressure, inflate the 5-mL balloon with 10 mL of sterile water; use 35 mL of sterile water to inflate the 30-mL balloon (Bard, 1999).

■ (SP) *Secure the catheter to the patient's thigh or lower abdomen.* **LOE = VII**

(EO) The CDC guidelines recommend that catheters be secured after insertion to decrease movement and pulling on the urethra (Wong & Hooton, 1981).

(NR) A systematic review of the literature demonstrated no experimental studies that evaluated the effectiveness of securing the catheter in one position or another (Gray et al., 2004).

(EO) Securing the catheter to the thigh or lower abdomen helps decrease the risk of trauma, bleeding, necrosis of the meatus, and bladder spasms from pressure and traction on the catheter (SUNA, 2006).

(NR) A descriptive exploratory study demonstrated that nurses ($N = 82$) in a community medical center indicated that securing indwelling urinary catheters was a necessary part of nursing care. However, when a prevalence study was conducted, only 4.4% of the indwelling catheters were stabilized (Siegel, 2006).

Possibly Effective

■ *Use a silver-alloy-coated Foley catheter to prevent infection.* **LOE = III**

(MR) A systematic review found that more RCTs are needed to determine whether silver-coated urinary catheters are effective for decreasing urinary tract infections (Niel-Weise et al., 2002).

(MR) In a prospective crossover study ($N = 3036$) of patients receiving either a silicone-based silver-coated catheter or a silicone-based hydrogel-coated catheter, there was no difference in urinary tract infection (Srinivasan et al., 2006). The authors did note that the study groups were different. There were more men, a shorter duration of catheterization, and fewer urine cultures in the silver-coated catheter group.

(EO) A review of the literature found that silver-alloy hydrogel catheters may reduce catheter-associated urinary tract infections in select patients with short-term indwelling catheters (Davenport & Keeley, 2005).

Not Effective

No applicable published research was found in this category.

RCT = Randomized Controlled (Clinical) Trial, **NIC** = Nursing Interventions Classification, **NOC** = Nursing Outcomes Classification

Possibly Harmful

■ *Disconnecting the closed urinary drainage system.* **LOE = I**

(EO) The CDC guidelines recommend that the urinary drainage system be kept closed (Wong & Hooton, 1981).

(NR) A systematic review recommends the use of sealed (taped) drainage systems to help prevent bacteriuria (Joanna Briggs Institute, 2000).

(MR) Review articles stressed the importance of maintaining a closed urinary drainage system as an effective way to prevent catheter-related urinary tract infections (Ha & Cho, 2006; Drinka, 2006; Nicolle et al., 2005).

(Note: Refer to the guideline on Tube Care: Urinary for more information about the care of the patient after catheterization.)

OUTCOME MEASUREMENT

URINARY ELIMINATION   (NOC)

Definition: Collection and discharge of urine.
Urinary Elimination as evidenced by the following selected NOC indicators:
• Urine odor
• Urine amount
• Urine color
• Urine clarity
• Adequate fluid intake
(Rate each indicator of **Urinary Elimination:** 1 = severely compromised, 2 = substantially compromised, 3 = moderately compromised, 4 = mildly compromised, 5 = not compromised) (Moorhead et al., 2004).

REFERENCES

Bard, Inc. (1999). Bard Foley Catheter inflation/deflation guidelines. Covington, GA.

Canes D. (2006). Male urethral catheterization. *N Engl J Med*, 355(11):1178-1179.

Carapeti EA, Andrews SM, Bentley PG. (1996). Randomised study of sterile versus non-sterile urethral catheterisation. *Ann R Coll Surg Engl*, 78(1):59-60.

Daneshgari F, Krugman M, Bahn A, Lee RS. (2002). Evidence-based multidisciplinary practice: improving the safety and standards of male bladder catheterization, *Medsurg Nurs*, 11(5):236-241, 246.

Davenport K, Keeley FX. (2005). Evidence for the use of silver-alloy-coated urethral catheters. *J Hosp Infect*, 60(4):298-303.

Dochterman JM, Bulechek GM (Eds). (2004). *Nursing Interventions Classification (NIC)*, 4th ed. St Louis: Mosby.

Doherty W. (2006). Male urinary catheterisation. *Nurs Stand*, 20(35):57-63.

Drinka PJ. (2006). Complications of chronic indwelling urinary catheters. *J Am Med Dir Assoc*, 7(6):388-392.

Gerber GS, Brendler CB. (2002). Evaluation of the urologic patient: History, physical examination, and urinalysis. In Walsh PC, Retick AB, Vaughan ED, Wein AJ (Eds): *Campbell's urology*, 8th ed. Philadelphia: Saunders, pp 83-110.

Gokula RR, Hickner JA, Smith MA. (2004). Inappropriate use of urinary catheters in elderly patients at a midwestern community teaching hospital. *Am J Infect Control*, 32(4):196-199.

NR = Nursing Research, **MR** = Multidisciplinary Research, **SP** = Standard of Practice, **EO** = Expert Opinion, **LOE** = Level of Evidence

Gray M; Center for Clinical Investigation. (2004). What nursing interventions reduce the risk of symptomatic urinary tract infection in the patient with an indwelling catheter? *J Wound Ostomy Continence Nurs,* 31(1):3-13.

Ha US, Cho YH. (2006). Catheter-associated urinary tract infections: New aspects of novel urinary catheters. *Int J Antimicrob Agents,* 28(6):485-490.

Joanna Briggs Institute. (2000). Management of short term indwelling urethral catheters to prevent urinary tract infections. *Best Practice,* 4(1):1-6.

Moorhead M, Johnson M, Maas M (Eds). (2004). *Nursing Outcomes Classification (NOC),* 3rd ed. St Louis: Mosby.

Nicolle LE, Bradley S, Colgan R, Rice JC, Schaeffer A, Hooton TM, et al. (2005). Infectious Diseases Society of America guidelines for the diagnosis and treatment of asymptomatic bacteriuria in adults. *Clin Infect Dis,* 40(5):643-654.

Niel-Weise BS, Arend SM, van den Broek PJ. (2002). Is there evidence for recommending silver-coated urinary catheters in guidelines? *J Hosp Infect,* 52(2):81-87.

Senese V. (2004). Secrets revealed for male catheterization. *Urol Nurs,* 24(2):78.

Siderias J, Guadio F, Singer AJ. (2004). Comparison of topical anesthetics and lubricants prior to urethral catheterization in males: A randomized controlled trial. *Acad Emerg Med,* 11(6):703-706.

Siegel TJ. (2006). Do registered nurses perceive the anchoring of indwelling urinary catheters as a necessary aspect of nursing care? A pilot study. *J Wound Ostomy Continence Nurs,* 33(2):140-144.

Society of Urologic Nurses and Associates (SUNA) Clinical Practice Guidelines Task Force. (2006). Care of the patient with an indwelling catheter. *Urol Nurs,* 26(1):80-81.

Srinivasan A, Karchmer T, Richards A, Song X, Perl TM. (2006). A prospective trial of a novel, silicone-based, silver-coated Foley catheter for the prevention of nosocomial urinary tract infections. *Infect Control Hosp Epidemiol,* 27(1):38-43.

Tanabe P, Steinmann R, Anderson J, Johnson D, Metcalf S, Ring-Hurn E. (2004). Factors affecting pain scores during female urethral catheterization. *Acad Emerg Med,* 11(6):699-702.

Wong ES, Hooton TM. (1981). Guideline for prevention of catheter-associated urinary tract infections. Department of Health, Centers for Disease Control and Prevention. Available online: http://www.cdc.gov/. Retrieved on July 7, 2007.

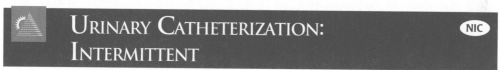

URINARY CATHETERIZATION: INTERMITTENT

NIC

Katherine N. Moore, PhD, RN, CCCN

NIC **Definition:** Regular periodic use of a catheter to empty the bladder (Dochterman & Bulechek, 2004).

NURSING ACTIVITIES

Effective

■ **SP** *Use intermittent catheterization to achieve bladder emptying; this is associated with fewer urological complications than indwelling catheters or condom drainage.* **LOE = IV**

EO Intermittent catheterization causes fewer complications than indwelling catheters or condom drainage (NIDRR, 1992).

MR A comprehensive review of the existing literature supported the benefit of intermittent catheterization over indwelling catheter or condom drainage. It also identified the need for further well-designed studies to address the many questions concerning sterile versus clean technique or hydrophilic versus polyvinylchloride (PVC) catheters (Hedlund et al., 2001).

■ ⬤ SP *Establish the catheterization schedule on the basis of several issues: urodynamics (particularly bladder pressures with filling), the presence of detrusor sphincter dyssynergia or vesicoureteral reflux, functional bladder capacity, and a fluid intake diary recorded for 24 to 48 hours.* **LOE = VII**

⬤ EO It is accepted that maintaining a bladder volume between 400 and 500 mL is optimal. Schedules will vary depending on the issues identified previously as well as fluid intake, physical activity, air temperature, and bladder and renal risk factors (Schaffer, 2002).

■ ⬤ SP *Watch for symptoms of a urinary tract infection (UTI), which may occur at the initiation of intermittent catheterization or at any time during treatment.* **LOE = VII**

⬤ EO Symptoms of a UTI are positive urine culture, the presence of leukocytes in the urine on microscopy (pyuria), and one or more of the following symptoms: suprapubic discomfort or flank pain, increased temperature, hematuria (gross), increased spasticity, autonomic dysreflexia, excessively cloudy or odorous urine, malaise, and lethargy (NIDRR, 1992).

Possibly Effective

■ *Use sterile single-use catheters with sterile technique to prevent UTIs in intermittent catheterization users versus sterile single-use catheters with clean technique during rehabilitation.* **LOE = II**

⬤ NR A randomized study in recent spinal cord injured adults ($N = 36$) compared sterile technique versus clean technique (clean gloves and a clean disposable collection container) with single-use PVC catheters in both groups and found no difference in time to the onset of UTI (Moore et al., 2006). All of the patients were catheterized by a nurse. Thirty-six participants had complete data, with the study end point being a symptomatic UTI as per National Institute on Disability and Rehabilitation Research definition. There were no significant differences in symptomatic UTIs between the clean group and the sterile group (37% versus 43%), with a mean time to onset of 4.6 weeks for the clean group and 4.3 weeks for the sterile group. Further research is recommended to confirm these results.

■ *Use sterile uncoated catheters with sterile technique to prevent UTIs in intermittent catheterization users versus clean uncoated catheters with clean technique during rehabilitation.* **LOE = II**

⬤ NR In a prospective study in three long-term care facilities, men ($N = 80$) were randomized to sterile technique or catheters washed with soap and water and reused for approximately 1 week. UTI was defined as $\leq 10^5$ colony-forming units per mL plus symptoms or >10 white blood cells per high-power field. The intent was to follow participants for 90 days, but a high dropout rate meant that complete data were only available for day 15. Overall for all participants, 20 out of 38 in the clean group and 22 out of 42 in the sterile group had UTIs. There was no difference in days to first treatment of UTI (24.4 days with a standard deviation of 21.2 days in the clean group versus 21.84 days with a standard deviation of 21.9 days in the sterile group; Duffy et al., 1995).

NR = Nursing Research, **MR** = Multidisciplinary Research, **SP** = Standard of Practice, **EO** = Expert Opinion, **LOE** = Level of Evidence

(MR) In an RCT, participants ($N = 46$) with spinal cord injury used sterile or clean catheters washed with bar soap. The primary outcome was UTI defined as $\geq 10^4$ colony-forming units per L plus clinical symptoms. Five UTIs occurred in the clean group (mean days to onset, 7.9 with a standard deviation of 6.1), and three occurred in the sterile group (mean days to onset, 8.8 with a standard deviation of 7.4; King et al., 1992).

Note: Both studies were limited by high attrition rates, low sample size, and heterogeneity, so it is difficult to draw conclusions on the use of clean intermittent catheterization in continuing care facilities. However, the days to onset of symptomatic UTIs did not seem to differ between the sterile and clean groups.

■ *Use sterile uncoated catheters with clean technique to prevent UTIs in intermittent catheterization users versus clean reused catheters.* **LOE = III**

(MR) In a crossover trial ($N = 10$), children with spina bifida were randomized to sterile single-use PVC catheters or reused PVC catheters that were boiled for 3 minutes. Over the 8-month study, two subjects in each group developed a symptomatic UTI ($>10^4$ colony-forming units per L plus symptoms); 76% of the clean and 73% of the sterile catheter participants had positive cultures (Schlager et al., 2001).

(NR) In a randomized crossover trial ($N = 30$), children with spina bifida were enrolled to sterile catheters or clean reused catheters (washed with soap and water and air dried). Children were followed for 1 year with monthly urine cultures but no microscopy. Thirty-eight percent of the participants in both groups had positive cultures, but symptoms of UTI were not reported, and several took prophylactic antibiotics. This trial and the preceding trial were limited by sample size and the concomitant use of antibiotics, so it is difficult to state with confidence that there is no difference in the incidence of symptomatic UTI between the two procedures (Moore et al., 1993).

■ *Use sterile coated catheters (hydrophilic) with clean technique to prevent UTIs in intermittent catheterization users versus clean uncoated catheters with clean technique.* **LOE = II**

(MR) In a prospective study, 32 men with prostate enlargement were randomized to clean catheters (soap and water and reused for 24 hours) or sterile hydrophilic catheters. At the end of the 3-week study, 51% of the sterile group and 63% of the clean group had positive cultures but no symptomatic UTIs (Pachler & Frimodt-Möller, 1999).

(MR) In a prospective study, boys with neurogenic bladders ($N = 33$) were randomized to an 8-week protocol of hydrophilic or clean PVC catheters (cleaning not described). Results reported that no group differences were found in symptomatic UTI or asymptomatic bacteriuria, although a higher percentage of the PVC noncoated group had microscopic hematuria (Sutherland et al., 1996).

(MR) In a study comparing UTIs in participants using hydrophilic coated catheters or clean reused PVC catheters, participants were followed for a total of 12 months, with a urinalysis and culture every 3 months. There were no differences in pyuria, bacteriuria, or clinical UTI between the two groups at any of the follow-up points; the incidence at 12 months was 0.14 for the coated catheter group and 0.13 for the uncoated clean catheter group (Vapnek et al., 2003).

When comparing the three studies in this section, all authors checked hematuria as an evaluation of urethral irritation, expecting that the hydrophilic coating on the coated catheter

RCT = Randomized Controlled (Clinical) Trial, **NIC** = Nursing Interventions Classification, **NOC** = Nursing Outcomes Classification

would protect the urethra as compared with the uncoated PVC catheter. There was a lower incidence of microscopic hematuria in two of the coated catheter groups: 0.31 versus 0.65 (Vapnek et al., 2003); 6 out of 14 (43%) versus 11 out of 14 (78%) (Sutherland et al., 1996), and two subjects in each group with "transient" bleeding (Pachler & Frimodt-Möller, 1999). Subject preference for the two products was somewhat more positive for the hydrophilic catheter. All of these studies were limited by sample size, types of subjects (boys, men with prostate disease, patients with spinal cord injuries), and length of follow-up. Thus, it is difficult to say whether there was a clinically relevant difference between hydrophilic or clean reused catheter users in terms of UTI. Hematuria appears to be lower in the hydrophilic users, but the clinical significance of this finding is limited by the short-term follow-up of the study participants.

■ Use sterile coated catheters (hydrophilic) with clean technique to prevent UTIs in intermittent catheterization users versus sterile uncoated catheters with clean technique. LOE = III

(MR) In a study comparing single-use hydrophilic coated catheters with single-use PVC catheters and clean technique, men with spinal cord injuries (≤6 months since injury) were followed at day 15 and then monthly for 12 months with urine microscopy and culture. At the study conclusion, there were no group differences in pyuria, bacteriuria, or hematuria; patient-reported diaries recorded more incidences of UTI in the clean uncoated group (82%) as compared with the sterile coated group (64%), but these subjective ratings were not confirmed by laboratory analysis. Twenty-two percent of the uncoated group and 33% of the coated group were "very satisfied" with the catheter to which they were randomized (De Ridder et al., 2005).

Note: As with the three studies described previously, it is not possible to state with certainty that hydrophilic catheter users have fewer UTIs. Most participants were pleased with the hydrophilic catheter and found it to be comfortable to use. On the basis of the current research, the hydrophilic or PVC catheters appear to be similar in terms of clinical outcomes.

■ Use sterile coated catheters with sterile technique (catheter and bag system) to prevent UTIs in intermittent catheterization users versus sterile uncoated catheters with sterile technique. LOE = III

(NR) An RCT randomly assigned 30 spinal cord injury patients or stroke patients to an integrated catheter and bag system or to a sterile catheter and tray. After 4 days, one patient in the clean group and one in the sterile catheter group developed UTIs as demonstrated by $>10^5$ colony-forming units per mL (Quigley & Riggin, 1993).

(NR) In an RCT feasibility study with 11 patients participating for a total of only 24 hours, no patients in the closed system and two in the open sterile system developed a positive colony count (Day et al., 2003). This study, as well as the study by Quigley & Riggin (1993) mentioned previously, was limited by a very small sample and a short follow-up duration. No interpretation about the effectiveness with respect to the prevention of UTI could be made about the closed system.

(MR) A randomized crossover trial assessed 18 men with spinal cord injuries for a total of 7 weeks evaluating PVC catheters and prelubricated, no-touch catheters. UTI was defined as clinical symptoms plus pyuria. At 7 weeks, four patients in the coated catheter group (7.4%) and 12 (22.2%) in the uncoated group had UTIs. The number of days to the onset of UTI was not recorded, and it is not clear whether patients were treated and re-entered. It is not

---

NR = Nursing Research, **MR** = Multidisciplinary Research, **SP** = Standard of Practice, **EO** = Expert Opinion, **LOE** = Level of Evidence

possible to draw conclusions about the effectiveness of one method as compared with the other in this group (Giannantoni et al., 2001).

■ *Use sterile coated catheters with sterile technique (integrated catheter and bag system) to prevent UTIs in intermittent catheterization users versus clean uncoated catheters with clean technique.* **LOE = III**

(NR) In an RCT, 29 patients were randomly assigned to the integrated system or to reused red rubber catheters that were washed with soap and water and used for 1 week. Weekly urinalysis was conducted for a total of 4 weeks. In the integrated system, nine patients had a symptomatic UTI ($>10^5$ colony-forming units per L plus pyuria and symptoms) as compared to eight in the clean group. Patients with UTIs were treated and then re-entered into the study (Prieto-Fingerhut et al., 1997).

Note: Although this was an RCT, design issues weaken the study.

Not Effective

■ *Performing routine urinalysis for people using intermittent catheterization.* **LOE = VII**

(EO) It is not unusual for individuals using intermittent catheterization to have a positive culture. However, unless they are symptomatic, they should not be treated. The treatment of people who have asymptomatic bacteriuria places the individual at risk for antibiotic resistance (Schaffer, 2002). It is recommended that people using intermittent catheterization have annual follow-up visits with a health care professional so that risks for renal or bladder health deterioration can be identified.

■ *Using antibiotics prophylactically to prevent UTIs, except in special situations.* **LOE = VII**

(EO) The value of prophylaxis is not established for beginning intermittent catheterization. People should be taught the signs and symptoms of UTIs and to contact their nurse practitioner or family physician if symptoms occur (Nicolle et al., 2005).

Possibly Harmful

No applicable published research was found in this category.

Note: Although all studies in the above review are RCTs and were well-designed for their time, by the current standard for evidence-based practice, the majority are limited because of imprecise outcome measures, small heterogeneous samples, and short-term follow-up. Thus, it is difficult to draw conclusions about the efficacy of the interventions. On the basis of the current evidence, there appears to be no difference with regard to clean or sterile technique during rehabilitation, no difference between clean reused or sterile catheters in the community, no difference between hydrophilic or sterile PVC (or reused) in the community, and no difference between integrated sterile systems and a standard sterile catheter system. Of note is that hematuria may be reduced among people who are using hydrophilic catheters, but longer follow-up is needed to determine the clinical significance of microscopic hematuria. The current findings could change with further, better-designed studies. Finally, it is not known whether there is a subset of individuals who would benefit from sterile single-use catheters as compared with clean catheters, and further research in this area is also

RCT = Randomized Controlled (Clinical) Trial, **NIC** = Nursing Interventions Classification, **NOC** = Nursing Outcomes Classification

required. Intermittent catheterization urgently requires additional systematic study to guide practice.

OUTCOME MEASUREMENT

URINARY ELIMINATION   NOC

Definition: Collection and discharge of urine.

Urinary Elimination as evidenced by the following selected NOC indicators:

- Urine odor
- Urine amount
- Urine color
- Urine clarity

(Rate each indicator of **Urinary Elimination:** 1 = severely compromised, 2 = substantially compromised, 3 = moderately compromised, 4 = mildly compromised, 5 = not compromised) (Moorhead et al., 2004).

Additional non-NOC indicators:

- Results of urine culture
- Presence of white blood cells in urine
- Presence of blood in urine
- Temperature
- Presence of suprapubic pain

REFERENCES

Day RA, Moore KN, Albers MK. (2003). A pilot study comparing two methods of intermittent catheterization: Limitations and challenges. *Urol Nurs,* 23(2):143-147, 158.

De Ridder DJ, Everaert K, Fernandez LG, Valero JV, Duran AB, Abrisqueta ML, et al. (2005). Intermittent catheterisation with hydrophilic-coated catheters (SpeediCath) reduces the risk of clinical urinary tract infection in spinal cord injured patients: A prospective randomised parallel comparative trial. *Eur Urol,* 48(6):991-995.

Dochterman JM, Bulechek GM (Eds). (2004). *Nursing Interventions Classification (NIC),* 4th ed. St Louis: Mosby.

Duffy LM, Cleary J, Ahern S, Kuskowski MA, West M, Wheeler L, et al. (1995). Clean intermittent catheterization: Cost-effective bladder management for male residents of VA nursing homes. *J Am Geriatr Soc,* 43(8):865-870.

Giannantoni A, Di Stasi SM, Scivoletto G, Virgili G, Dolci S, Porena M. (2001). Intermittent catheterization with a prelubricated catheter in spinal cord injured patients: A prospective randomized crossover study. *J Urol,* 166(1):130-133.

Hedlund H, Hjelmas K, Jonsson O, Klarskov P, Talja M. (2001). Hydrophilic versus non-coated catheters for intermittent catheterization. *Scand J Urol Nephrol,* 35(1):49-53.

King RB, Carlson CE, Mervine J, Wu Y, Yarkony GM. (1992). Clean and sterile intermittent catheterization methods in hospitalized patients with spinal cord injury. *Arch Phys Med Rehabil,* 73(9):798-802.

Moore KN, Burt J, Voaklander DC. (2006). Intermittent catheterization in the rehabilitation setting: A comparison of clean and sterile technique. *Clin Rehabil,* 20(6):461-468.

Moore KN, Kelm M, Sinclair O, Cadrain G. (1993). Bacteriuria in intermittent catheterization users: The effect of sterile versus clean reused catheters. *Rehabil Nurs,* 18(5):306-309.

Moorhead M, Johnson M, Maas M (Eds). (2004). *Nursing Outcomes Classification (NOC),* 3rd ed. St Louis: Mosby.

National Institute on Disability and Rehabilitation Research (NIDRR). (1992). The prevention and management of urinary tract infections among people with spinal cord injuries. National Institute on Disability and Rehabilitation Research Consensus Statement. *J Am Paraplegia Soc,* 15(3):194-204.

NR = Nursing Research, **MR** = Multidisciplinary Research, **SP** = Standard of Practice, **EO** = Expert Opinion, **LOE** = Level of Evidence

Nicolle LE, Bradley S, Colgan R, Rice JC, Schaeffer A, Hooton TM, et al. (2005). Infectious Diseases Society of America guidelines for the diagnosis and treatment of asymptomatic bacteriuria in adults. *Clin Infect Dis,* 40(5):643-654.

Pachler J, Frimodt-Möller C. (1999). A comparison of prelubricated hydrophilic and non-hydrophilic polyvinyl chloride catheters for urethral catheterization. *BJU Int,* 83(7):767-769.

Prieto-Fingerhut T, Banovac K, Lynne CM. (1997). A study comparing sterile and nonsterile urethral catheterization in patients with spinal cord injury. *Rehabil Nurs,* 22(6):299-302.

Quigley PA, Riggin OZ. (1993). A comparison of open and closed catheterization techniques in rehabilitation patients. *Rehabil Nurs,* 18(1):26-29, 33.

Schaffer AJ. (2002). Infections of the urinary tract. In Walsh PC, Retik AB, Vaughan ED: *Campbell's urology,* 8th ed, Volume 1. Philadelphia: WB Saunders, pp 515-602.

Schlager TA, Clark M, Anderson S. (2001). Effect of a single-use sterile catheter for each void on the frequency of bacteriuria in children with neurogenic bladder on intermittent catheterization for bladder emptying. *Pediatrics,* 108(4):E71.

Sutherland RS, Kogan BA, Baskin LS, Mevorach RA. (1996). Clean intermittent catheterization in boys using the LoFric catheter. *J Urol,* 156(6):2041-2043.

Vapnek JM, Maynard FM, Kim J. (2003). A prospective randomized trial of the LoFric hydrophilic coated catheter versus conventional plastic catheter for clean intermittent catheterization. *J Urol,* 169(3):994-998.

URINARY HABIT TRAINING

Jean F. Wyman, PhD, APRN-BC, GNP, FAAN

NIC Definition: Establishing a predictable pattern of bladder emptying to prevent incontinence for persons with limited cognitive ability who have urge, stress, or functional incontinence (Dochterman & Bulechek, 2004).

NURSING ACTIVITIES

Effective

■ *Use an individualized habit retraining program either alone or in combination with other methods, such as the education to staff/caregivers, fluid manipulation, toileting prompts, continent reinforcement, and environmental modifications.* **LOE = II**

(MR) A Cochrane systematic review concluded that there was insufficient evidence to reach firm conclusions for practice. The few trials on habit training that met inclusion criteria did not demonstrate statistical differences in the incidence and volume of urinary incontinence among groups. However, within-group analysis did show some improvements (Ostaszkiewicz et al., 2004).

(MR) An International Consultation on Incontinence systematic review was unable to determine the treatment effect of habit training among frail older people (Fonda et al., 2005).

(NR) An RCT (*N* = 118) demonstrated that an individualized scheduled toileting program was more effective for reducing urinary incontinence in memory-impaired elderly care recipients and their caregivers at home as compared with the results seen in a usual care control group (Jirovec & Templin, 2001).

(NR) A study with a quasi-experimental design that tested a 12-week program of individualized habit training using an electronic monitoring device for cognitively or physically impaired nursing home residents ($N = 113$) found a reduction in incontinence frequency but not in incontinence volume in the group using the device (Colling et al., 1992).

(NR) An RCT demonstrated that an individualized habit training program using an electronic monitoring device in community-dwelling frail older adults ($N = 78$) was more effective than usual care for reducing incontinence frequency and volume and for improving skin rashes and breakdown. It did not have an effect on reducing urinary tract infections (Colling et al., 2003).

(NR) An RCT comparing elderly patients in acute care rehabilitation wards ($N = 41$) did not find within or between group differences in self-reported or caregiver-reported incontinence frequency among those who received habit training with the use of an electronic monitoring device as compared with those who received standard habit training (Nikoletti et al., 2004).

■ (SP) *Establish a fixed toileting schedule (e.g., every 2 hours).* **LOE = VI**

(MR) A case series found a reduction of incontinence episodes after 2 weeks using a fixed 2-hour toilet schedule in nursing home patients ($N = 13$) with detrusor overactivity (Ouslander et al., 1988).

Note: Using a voiding diary that includes space to record the times of voluntary voiding and incontinence episodes is very helpful when initiating care for incontinence. Other information that could be collected would be fluid intake, precipitating circumstances of incontinence, amount of leakage, whether an urge was present at the time of voiding, whether a request to toilet was made, and/or pad changes.

Possibly Effective

No applicable published research was found in this category.

Not Effective

No applicable published research was found in this category.

Possibly Harmful

No applicable published research was found in this category.

OUTCOME MEASUREMENT

URINARY CONTINENCE   (NOC)

Definition: Control of the elimination of urine from the bladder.
Urinary Continence as evidenced by the following selected NOC indicators:
• Maintains predictable pattern of voiding
• Gets to toilet between urge and passage of urine
• Recognizes urge to void
• Urine leakage between voidings
• Wets underclothing during day
(Rate each indicator of **Urinary Continence:** 1 = never demonstrated, 2 = rarely demonstrated, 3 = sometimes demonstrated, 4 = often demonstrated, 5 = consistently demonstrated) (Moorhead et al., 2004).

NR = Nursing Research, **MR** = Multidisciplinary Research, **SP** = Standard of Practice, **EO** = Expert Opinion, **LOE** = Level of Evidence

REFERENCES

Colling J, Ouslander J, Hadley BJ, Eisch J, Campbell E. (1992). The effects of patterned urge-response toileting (PURT) on urinary incontinence among nursing home residents. *J Am Geriatr Soc,* 40(2): 135-141.

Colling J, Owen TR, McCreedy M, Newman D. (2003). The effects of a continence program on frail community-dwelling elderly persons. *Urol Nurs,* 23(2):117-122, 127-131.

Dochterman JM, Bulechek GM (Eds). (2004). *Nursing Interventions Classification (NIC),* 4th ed. St Louis: Mosby.

Fonda D, DuBeau CE, Harari D, Ouslander JG, Palmer M, Roe B. (2005). Incontinence in the frail elderly. In Abrams P, Cardozo L, Khoury S, Wein A (Eds): *Incontinence: Management.* Volume 2. Paris: Health Publication Ltd, pp 1163-1240.

Jirovec MM, Templin T. (2001). Predicting success using individualized scheduled toileting for memory-impaired elders at home. *Res Nurs Health,* 24(1):1-8.

Moorhead M, Johnson M, Maas M (Eds). (2004). *Nursing Outcomes Classification (NOC),* 3rd ed. St Louis: Mosby.

Nikoletti S, Young J, King M. (2004). Evaluation of an electronic monitoring device for urinary incontinence in elderly patients in an acute care setting. *J Wound Ostomy Continence Nurs,* 31(3):138-149.

Ostaszkiewicz J, Johnston L, Roe B. (2004). Habit retraining for the management of urinary incontinence in adults. *Cochrane Database Syst Rev,* (2):CD002801.

Ouslander JG, Blaustein J, Connor A, Pitt A. (1988). Habit training and oxybutynin for incontinence in nursing home patients: A placebo-controlled trial. *J Am Geriatr Soc,* 36(1):40-46.

URINARY STRESS INCONTINENCE CARE

Jean F. Wyman, PhD, APRN-BC, GNP, FAAN

NIC   **Definition:** Assistance in promoting continence and maintaining perineal skin integrity (Dochterman & Bulechek, 2004).
(Note: This guideline focuses on stress incontinence.)

NURSING ACTIVITIES

Effective

■ *Institute weight reduction programs for moderately and morbidly overweight adults.* **LOE = I**

MR   A systematic review concluded that there was evidence that weight loss in morbidly obese women decreased incontinence and scant evidence that moderately obese women who lost weight had less incontinence than those who did not. There was no available evidence to assess the effectiveness of weight loss in incontinent men (Wilson et al., 2005).

MR   An RCT of a liquid diet weight reduction program in overweight and obese women (*N* = 47) demonstrated a significant reduction in stress urinary incontinent episodes in the intervention group as compared with the wait-listed control group. The authors concluded that a weight loss of 5% to 10% was efficacious (Subak et al., 2005).

MR   An RCT found that an intensive lifestyle intervention involving weight loss and exercise in overweight women (*N* = 1957) reduced the prevalence of incontinent episodes in those with stress incontinence more than metformin alone and more than placebo with standard

RCT = Randomized Controlled (Clinical) Trial, **NIC** = Nursing Interventions Classification, **NOC** = Nursing Outcomes Classification

lifestyle advice. Weight loss was the most important mediator of the beneficial effect; increased physical activity did not appear to have an effect (Brown et al., 2006).

■ *Encourage pelvic floor muscle exercises in postpartum women.* **LOE = I**

(MR) A systematic review reported that pelvic floor muscle training for women who had symptoms of urinary incontinence at 3 months postpartum was a more effective treatment than standard postnatal care (Wilson et al., 2005).

■ *Encourage pelvic floor muscle exercises in all other women.* **LOE = I**

(MR) A systematic review reported that women who performed pelvic floor muscle exercises were more likely to report cure or improvement and to have approximately two fewer incontinent episodes per 3 days as compared with controls (Wilson et al., 2005).

(MR) A Cochrane systematic review found that women with stress incontinence who performed pelvic floor muscle exercises were more likely to report that they were cured or improved than those who did not (Hay-Smith & Dumoulin, 2006).

■ *Encourage pelvic floor muscle training in men who are undergoing prostatectomy.* **LOE = I**

(MR) A systematic review reported that it was unclear whether knowledge and practice of pelvic floor muscle exercises before radical prostatectomy surgery improved continence recovery. However, there was modest support found for its effectiveness when it was taught after radical prostatectomy as compared with no active intervention for reducing incontinence. There was some evidence that pelvic floor muscle training after transurethral prostatectomy may reduce incontinence during the first 3 postoperative weeks, but this effect was not sustained (Wilson et al., 2005).

(MR) An RCT found that a biofeedback-assisted pelvic floor muscle exercise training program implemented 2 to 4 weeks before radical prostatectomy surgery and resumed after urethral catheter removal ($N = 100$) did not improve the rate of return of urinary control or overall continence as compared with a control group that received written and brief verbal instructions before and after surgery (Bales et al., 2000).

(MR) An RCT demonstrated that preoperative behavioral training (pelvic floor muscle control and pelvic floor muscle exercises) in men after radical prostatectomy surgery ($N = 125$) was more effective for decreasing the time to continence and the proportion of patients with severe leakage at 6 months as compared with usual care (Burgio et al., 2006).

■ *Use biofeedback-assisted pelvic floor muscle exercises in women.* **LOE = I**

(NR) A systematic review concluded that there did not appear to be any post-treatment benefit of biofeedback-assisted pelvic floor muscle exercises (at home or in a clinic) as compared with pelvic floor muscle exercises alone in women (Wilson et al., 2005).

(NR) An RCT comparing an 8-week program of biofeedback-assisted pelvic floor muscle exercises, pelvic floor muscle exercises alone, and no treatment in older women with stress incontinence ($N = 135$) demonstrated that biofeedback-assisted and non-biofeedback-assisted pelvic floor muscle exercises were equally effective for reducing incontinent episodes as compared with the control group (Burns et al., 1993).

(NR) An RCT found that a biofeedback-assisted pelvic floor training program in older homebound adults ($N = 85$) was more effective for reducing stress incontinence episodes than usual care (McDowell et al., 1999).

NR = Nursing Research, **MR** = Multidisciplinary Research, **SP** = Standard of Practice, **EO** = Expert Opinion, **LOE** = Level of Evidence

■ *Use biofeedback-assisted pelvic floor muscle exercises in men after prostatectomy.* **LOE = I**

(MR) A Cochrane systematic review found that pelvic floor muscle training with biofeedback may be better than no treatment or sham treatment for the short term for men after radical prostatectomy. However, there were insufficient data to derive conclusions for those undergoing transurethral prostatectomy (Hunter et al., 2004).

(MR) A systematic review concluded that the addition of biofeedback to pelvic floor muscle exercises did not appear to improve the outcomes of men after radical prostatectomy (Wilson et al., 2005).

■ *Use bladder training in adults.* **LOE = I**

(MR) A systematic review reported that there was scant evidence that bladder training as compared with no treatment may be effective for women with stress and mixed incontinence. However, there were insufficient data to derive conclusions for its use in men with stress incontinence (Wilson et al., 2005).

(MR) An RCT of a 6-week bladder training program in older women ($N = 123$) found that bladder training was more effective than no treatment and that women with stress incontinence had similar reductions in incontinence episodes and quality of life as compared with women with detrusor overactivity, with effects maintained over 6 months (Fantl et al., 1991; Wyman et al., 1997).

■ *Use conservative management programs in adults, including lifestyle interventions, pelvic floor muscle exercises, and/or bladder training.* **LOE = I**

(MR) A systematic review concluded that conservative management packages were more effective for reducing incontinent episodes and daytime micturitions and for improving quality of life as compared with control treatments for women with stress incontinence (Wilson et al., 2005).

Note: Using a voiding diary that includes space to record times of voluntary voiding and incontinence episodes is very helpful when initiating care for stress incontinence. Other information that could be collected would be fluid intake, precipitating circumstances of the incontinence episode, the amount of leakage, and pad use.

Possibly Effective

■ *Encourage smoking cessation.* **LOE = VII**

(MR) A systematic review found that smoking appeared to increase the risk of more severe urinary incontinence in women. However, data were not available to determine whether smoking cessation resolved incontinence in either women or men (Wilson et al., 2005).

■ *Encourage caffeine reduction.* **LOE = III**

(MR) A systematic review reported that there was scant evidence demonstrating that caffeine reduction improved continence (Wilson et al., 2005).

(MR) A randomized crossover study found that caffeine restriction alone did not reduce urinary symptoms (pad weights, incontinent episodes) or improve quality of life in women with stress incontinence ($N = 39$). However, caffeine restriction and decreased fluids did reduce incontinent episodes (Swithinbank et al., 2005).

RCT = Randomized Controlled (Clinical) Trial, **NIC** = Nursing Interventions Classification, **NOC** = Nursing Outcomes Classification

■ *Employ constipation prevention.* **LOE = VII**

(MR) A systematic review reported that chronic straining to empty the bowel may be a risk factor for the development of urinary incontinence. However, there were no clinical trials examining the impact of constipation prevention on urinary incontinence (Wilson et al., 2005).

■ *Use vaginal cones/balls.* **LOE = V**

(MR) A systematic review found inconclusive evidence regarding whether vaginal cones were better than control treatments for postnatal women with stress incontinence. They also noted that vaginal cones were not suitable for some women because of adverse events (Wilson et al., 2005).

■ *Use electrical stimulation in adults.* **LOE = II**

(MR) A systematic review reported that there was insufficient evidence to determine whether electrical stimulation was better than no treatment or placebo treatment for women and men with stress incontinence. There did not seem to be any benefit to adding electrical stimulation to pelvic floor muscle exercise (Wilson et al., 2005).

(MR) A double-blinded RCT found that a 15-week program of home electrical stimulation in women with stress incontinence ($N = 35$) was more effective for reducing incontinence episodes and pad test weights and for improving vaginal muscle strength than a sham device (Sand et al., 1995).

(MR) A double-blinded RCT found that a 4-week program of home electrical stimulation in women and men with stress incontinence ($N = 29$) was more effective than sham stimulation for reducing incontinent episodes, with more patients cured or showing significant improvement (Yamanishi et al., 1997).

(MR) An RCT found that a biofeedback-assisted behavioral training program (pelvic floor muscle control and exercises) with home pelvic floor stimulation was more effective for reducing incontinent episodes than self-administered behavioral treatment using a self-help booklet in women with stress incontinence ($N = 200$; Goode et al., 2003).

■ *Use magnetic stimulation in adults.* **LOE = I**

(MR) A systematic review reported that magnetic stimulation may be effective for the treatment of stress incontinence in women. However, there was insufficient evidence to determine its efficacy in men (Wilson et al., 2005).

■ *Use a penile compression device in men.* **LOE = IV**

(NR) A study involving a crossover design using a Latin square found that the Cunningham clamp was more effective for reducing urine loss and that it was more acceptable to cognitively intact men 6 months after radical prostatectomy ($N = 12$) than the Timms C3 or U-Tex device. However, it lowered cavernosal artery blood flow velocity even at its loosest setting. The authors concluded that individualized instruction was necessary to ensure appropriate application, comfort, and fit (Moore et al., 2004).

Not Effective

No applicable published research was found in this category.

NR = Nursing Research, **MR** = Multidisciplinary Research, **SP** = Standard of Practice, **EO** = Expert Opinion, **LOE** = Level of Evidence

Possibly Harmful

No applicable published research was found in this category.

OUTCOME MEASUREMENT

URINARY CONTINENCE   NOC

Definition: Control of the elimination of urine from the bladder.

Urinary Continence as evidenced by the following selected NOC indicators:
- Urine leakage with increased abdominal pressure (e.g., sneezing, laughing, lifting)
- Maintains predictable pattern of voiding
- Voids >150 cc each time
- Urine leakage between voidings
- Wets underclothing during day

(Rate each indicator of **Urinary Continence:** 1 = never demonstrated, 2 = rarely demonstrated, 3 = sometimes demonstrated, 4 = often demonstrated, 5 = consistently demonstrated) (Moorhead et al., 2004.)

INCONTINENCE IMPACT QUESTIONNAIRE

Condition-specific quality of life instrument (Uebersax et al., 1995).

REFERENCES

Bales GT, Gerber GS, Minor TX, Mhoon DA, McFarland JM, Kim HL, et al. (2000). Effect of preoperative biofeedback/pelvic floor training on continence in men undergoing radical prostatectomy. *Urology,* 56(4):627-630.

Brown JS, Wing R, Barrett-Connor E, Nyberg LM, Kusek JW, Orchard TJ, et al. (2006). Lifestyle intervention is associated with lower prevalence of urinary incontinence. The Diabetes Prevention Program. *Diabetes Care,* 29(2):385-390.

Burgio KL, Goode PS, Urban DA, Umlauf MG, Locher JL, Bueschen A, et al. (2006). Preoperative biofeedback assisted behavioral training to decrease post-prostatectomy incontinence: A randomized, controlled trial. *J Urol,* 175(1):196-201.

Burns PA, Pranikoff K, Nochajski TH, Hadley EC, Levy KJ, Ory MG. (1993). A comparison of effectiveness of biofeedback and pelvic muscle exercise treatment of stress incontinence in older community-dwelling women. *J Gerontol,* 48(4):M167-M174.

Dochterman JM, Bulechek GM (Eds). (2004). *Nursing Interventions Classification (NIC),* 4th ed. St Louis: Mosby.

Fantl JA, Wyman JF, McClish DK, Harkins SW, Elswick RK, Taylor JR, et al. (1991). Efficacy of bladder training in older women with urinary incontinence. *JAMA,* 265(5):609-613.

Goode PS, Burgio KL, Locher JL, Roth DL, Umlauf MG, Richter HE, et al. (2003). Effect of behavioral training with or without pelvic floor electrical stimulation on stress incontinence in women: A randomized controlled trial. *JAMA,* 290(3):345-352.

Hay-Smith EJ, Dumoulin C. (2006). Pelvic floor muscle training versus no treatment, or inactive control treatments, for urinary incontinence in women. *Cochrane Database Syst Rev,* (1):CD005654.

Hunter KF, Moore KN, Cody DJ, Glazener CM. (2004). Conservative management for postprostatectomy urinary incontinence. *Cochrane Database Syst Rev,* (2):CD001843.

McDowell BJ, Engberg S, Sereika S, Donovan N, Jubeck ME, Weber E, et al. (1999). Effectiveness of behavioral therapy to treat incontinence in homebound older adults. *J Am Geriatr Soc,* 47(3):309-318.

Moore KN, Schieman S, Ackerman T, Dzus HY, Metcalfe JB, Voaklander DC. (2004). Assessing comfort, safety, and patient satisfaction with three commonly used penile compression devices. *Urology*, 63(1): 150-154.

Moorhead M, Johnson M, Maas M (Eds). (2004). *Nursing Outcomes Classification (NOC)*, 3rd ed. St Louis: Mosby.

Sand PK, Richardson DA, Staskin DR, Swift SE, Appell RA, Whitmore KE, et al. (1995). Pelvic floor electrical stimulation in the treatment of genuine stress incontinence: A multicenter, placebo-controlled trial. *Am J Obstet Gynecol*, 173(1):72-79.

Subak LL, Whitcomb E, Shen H, Saxton J, Vittinghoff E, Brown JS. (2005). Weight loss: A novel and effective treatment for urinary incontinence. *J Urol*, 174(1):190-195.

Swithinbank L, Hashim H, Abrams P. (2005). The effect of fluid intake on urinary symptoms in women. *J Urol*, 174(1):187-189.

Uebersax JS, Wyman JF, Shumaker SA, McClish DK, Fantl JA. (1995). Short forms to assess life quality and symptom distress for urinary incontinence in women: The Incontinence Impact Questionnaire and the Urogenital Distress Inventory. Continence Program for Women Research Group. *Neurourol Urodyn*, 14(2):131-139.

Wilson PD, Hay-Smith J, Wyman J, Yamanishi T, Berghmans B et al. (2005). Adult conservative management. In Abrams P, Cardozo L, Khoury S, Wein A (Eds): *Incontinence: Management*, Volume 2. Paris: Health Publication Ltd, pp 855-964.

Wyman JF, Fantl JA, McClish DK, Harkins SW, Uebersax JS, Ory MG. (1997). Quality of life following bladder training in older women with urinary incontinence. *Int Urogynecol J Pelvic Floor Dysfunct*, 8(4):223-229.

Yamanishi T, Yasuda K, Sakakibara R, Hattori T, Ito H, Murakami S. (1997). Pelvic floor electrical simulation in the treatment of stress incontinence: An investigational study and a placebo controlled double-blind trial. *J Urol*, 158(6):2127-2131.

URINARY URGE INCONTINENCE CARE

Jean F. Wyman, PhD, APRN-BC, GNP, FAAN

> **NIC** **Definition:** Assistance with promoting continence and maintaining perineal skin integrity (Dochterman & Bulechek, 2004).
> (Note: This guideline focuses on urge incontinence.)

NURSING ACTIVITIES

Effective

■ *Use weight reduction programs for moderately and morbidly overweight adults.*
LOE = I

> (MR) A systematic review concluded that weight loss among morbidly obese women decreased incontinence, and it found scant evidence that moderately obese women who lost weight had less incontinence than those who did not. There was no available evidence to assess the effectiveness of weight loss among incontinent men (Wilson et al., 2005).

> (MR) An RCT of a liquid diet weight reduction program for overweight and obese women (*N* = 47) found a significant reduction in urge urinary incontinence episodes in the intervention group as compared with the wait-listed control group. The authors concluded that a weight loss of 5% to 10% is efficacious (Subak et al., 2005).

NR = Nursing Research, **MR** = Multidisciplinary Research, **SP** = Standard of Practice, **EO** = Expert Opinion, **LOE** = Level of Evidence

(MR) An RCT of an intensive lifestyle intervention involving weight loss and exercise among overweight women ($N = 1957$) did not reduce the prevalence of urge incontinence more than metformin alone and placebo with standard lifestyle advice (Brown et al., 2006).

■ *Use bladder training in adults.* **LOE = I**

(MR) A Cochrane systematic review reported that the evidence favored the effectiveness of bladder training versus no treatment in women but that this conclusion was tentative. There were no studies in men (Wallace et al., 2004).

(MR) A systematic review reported that there was scant evidence that bladder training may be effective for women with urge and mixed incontinence as compared with no treatment. However, there were insufficient data to derive conclusions for its use in men with urge or mixed incontinence (Wilson et al., 2005).

(MR) An RCT of a 6-week bladder training program among women 55 years old and older ($N = 123$) found that bladder training was more effective than no treatment for reducing incontinent episodes and pad weights and for improving the quality of life of those with detrusor overactivity, with effects maintained over 6 months (Fantl et al., 1991; Wyman et al., 1997).

(NR) A quasi-experimental study of a 4-week bladder training program with telephone monitoring in older women ($N = 19$) demonstrated a reduction of incontinent episodes immediately after treatment which was maintained 6 months later (Publicover & Bear, 1997).

(NR) An RCT of an 8-week bladder training program in women ($N = 31$) demonstrated that those undergoing bladder training had a greater reduction in urinary frequency and increased voiding volumes but no differences in urine loss as compared with a control group (Yoon et al., 2003).

■ *Use behavioral treatment programs that involve a combination of lifestyle interventions, pelvic floor muscle exercises, and bladder training in women.* **LOE = I**

(MR) A systematic review concluded that a conservative management package (pelvic floor muscle exercises, bladder training for those with urge symptoms, and lifestyle interventions) was better than no treatment in women for reducing incontinence episodes (Wilson et al., 2005).

(NR) An RCT of a multicomponent intervention was implemented that consisted of lifestyle intervention (caffeine, fluid intake, and bowel management advice), bladder training, and pelvic floor muscle exercises. It was found to be more effective for reducing incontinence episodes and pad test weights and for improving quality of life in women ($N = 218$; 92.5% with urge or mixed incontinence) as compared with a control group. The interventions were implemented in a stepwise fashion on the basis of the women's goals (Dougherty et al., 2002).

(NR) An RCT of an 8-week program of diet and fluid advice, bladder training, pelvic floor awareness, and lifestyle advice delivered by specially trained nurses found that the intervention group had greater improvements in incontinent episodes and urinary urgency and frequency and reported higher patient satisfaction than the control group, which received usual care ($N = 3746$ [2299 women and 1447 men]; Williams et al., 2006).

■ *Encourage pelvic floor muscle exercises in adults.* **LOE = I**

(MR) A systematic review reported some evidence that women with detrusor overactivity with or without concomitant urge incontinence were more likely to report cure or improvement and to have reduced incontinence episodes after a pelvic floor muscle treating program as

RCT = Randomized Controlled (Clinical) Trial, **NIC** = Nursing Interventions Classification, **NOC** = Nursing Outcomes Classification

compared with women in a no-treatment control group. There was no evidence to draw similar conclusions for men (Wilson et al., 2005).

(MR) A Cochrane systematic review found that women with urge and mixed incontinence who performed pelvic floor muscle exercises were more likely to report that they were cured or improved than those who did not do the exercises (Hay-Smith & Dumoulin, 2006).

(MR) An RCT found that a behavioral training program (pelvic floor muscle training with verbal feedback of exercise performance based on vaginal palpitation) had similar efficacy as a self-administered behavioral treatment using a self-help booklet for reducing incontinence episodes in women with urge incontinence ($N = 149$), although the group who received the verbal feedback and assisted behavioral training had higher treatment satisfaction (Burgio et al., 2002).

■ *Encourage biofeedback-assisted pelvic floor muscle exercises.* **LOE = I**

(MR) A systematic review concluded that there did not appear to be any post-treatment benefit of biofeedback-assisted (clinic) pelvic floor muscle exercises as compared with pelvic floor muscle exercises alone. Both treatments reduced incontinent episodes similarly (Wilson et al., 2005).

(NR) An RCT found that a biofeedback-assisted pelvic floor training program in older home-bound adults ($N = 85$) was more effective for reducing urge incontinence episodes, nocturia, and daytime micturitions as compared with usual care (McDowell et al., 1999).

(MR) An RCT found that a biofeedback-assisted behavioral training program (pelvic floor muscle control and exercises) had similar efficacy for reducing incontinence episodes among women with urge incontinence ($N = 222$) as a behavioral training program using verbal feedback based on vaginal palpitation and a self-administered behavioral treatment using self-help (Burgio et al., 2002).

Note: Using a voiding diary that includes space to record times of voluntary voiding and incontinence episodes is very helpful when initiating care for urge incontinence. Other information that could be collected would be fluid intake, precipitating circumstances of the incontinence, the amount of leakage, whether an urge was present at the time of voiding, whether a request to toilet was made, and/or pad changes.

Possibly Effective

■ *Encourage caffeine reduction.* **LOE = III**

(MR) A systematic review found conflicting data regarding the role of caffeine intake and urinary incontinence and reported that there was scant evidence demonstrating that decreasing caffeine improves continence (Wilson et al., 2005).

(MR) A randomized crossover study found that caffeine restriction did not reduce incontinent episodes in women ($N = 30$) with detrusor overactivity (Swithinbank et al., 2005).

(NR) An RCT found that a caffeine reduction education and bladder training program in adults ($N = 74$) led to less urinary urgency and frequency, with a trend toward fewer incontinence episodes than bladder training alone (Byrant et al., 2002).

■ *Encourage fluid modifications.* **LOE = III**

(MR) A systematic review found that fluid intake played a minor (if any) role in the pathogenesis of incontinence. Consuming carbonated drinks appeared to increase the risk of overactive bladder (Wilson et al., 2005).

NR = Nursing Research, **MR** = Multidisciplinary Research, **SP** = Standard of Practice, **EO** = Expert Opinion, **LOE** = Level of Evidence

(NR) An RCT did not find differences in incontinent episodes among women ($N = 32$) who increased their fluid intake by 500 mL, who maintained their baseline fluid intake, or who decreased their fluid intake by 300 mL. However, adherence to fluid intake protocols was poor, which may have influenced results (Dowd et al., 1996).

(MR) A randomized crossover study found that reducing fluid intake decreased voiding frequency, urgency, and improved quality of life among women ($N = 30$) with detrusor overactivity and that increasing fluid intake increased voiding frequency and urgency (Swithinbank et al., 2005).

■ *Encourage constipation prevention.* **LOE = VII**

(MR) A systematic review reported that chronic straining to empty the bowel may be a risk factor for the development of urinary incontinence. However, there were no clinical trials examining the impact of constipation prevention on urinary incontinence (Wilson et al., 2005).

■ *Use lifestyle interventions that combine caffeine reduction education, fluid modifications, bowel management strategies, and toileting advice.* **LOE = II**

(NR) An RCT of a self-monitoring intervention that included caffeine, fluid intake, and bowel management advice among older women with urinary incontinence ($N = 41$ with 92.7% with urge and mixed incontinence) resulted in a greater reduction of incontinence episodes and pad test weights as compared with a control group (Dougherty et al., 2002).

■ *Use electrical stimulation in adults.* **LOE = II**

(MR) A systematic review found that there was insufficient evidence to determine whether electrical stimulation is better than no treatment for women and men with detrusor overactivity. There was some evidence that favored electrical stimulation over placebo stimulation for women with detrusor overactivity (Wilson et al., 2005).

(MR) A double-blinded RCT found that a 4-week treatment of electrical stimulation (15 minutes twice a day) was more effective for reducing incontinence episodes, nocturia, and pad use and for improving quality of life scores than sham stimulation in female ($N = 39$) and male ($N = 29$) patients with urinary incontinence as a result of detrusor overactivity (Yamanishi et al., 2000).

■ *Use magnetic stimulation in adults.* **LOE = V**

(MR) A systematic review reported that there was insufficient evidence to derive a conclusion about the effect of magnetic stimulation as compared with no treatment, placebo, or control treatment in women or men (Wilson et al., 2005).

Not Effective

No applicable published research was found in this category.

Possibly Harmful

No applicable published research was found in this category.

RCT = Randomized Controlled (Clinical) Trial, **NIC** = Nursing Interventions Classification, **NOC** = Nursing Outcomes Classification

OUTCOME MEASUREMENT

URINARY CONTINENCE (NOC)

Definition: Control of the elimination of urine from the bladder.

Urinary Continence as evidenced by the following selected NOC indicators:

- Maintains predictable pattern of voiding
- Responds to urge in timely manner
- Gets to toilet between urge and passage of urine
- Voids >150 cc each time
- Recognizes urge to void
- Urine leakage between voidings
- Wets underclothing or bedding during night

(Rate each indicator of **Urinary Continence:** 1 = never demonstrated, 2 = rarely demonstrated, 3 = sometimes demonstrated, 4 = often demonstrated, 5 = consistently demonstrated) (Moorhead et al., 2004).

CONDITION-SPECIFIC QUALITY OF LIFE MEASUREMENT INSTRUMENTS

Incontinence Impact Questionnaire (Uebersax et al., 1995); Overactive Bladder Questionnaire (OAB-q) (Coyne et al., 2002; 2005).

REFERENCES

Brown JS, Wing R, Barrett-Connor E, Nyberg LM, Kusek JW, Orchard TJ, et al. (2006). Lifestyle intervention is associated with lower prevalence of urinary incontinence: The Diabetes Prevention Program. *Diabetes Care,* 29(2):385-390.

Bryant CM, Dowell CJ, Fairbrother G. (2002). Caffeine reduction education to improve urinary symptoms. *Br J Nurs,* 11(8):560-565.

Burgio KL, Goode PS, Locher JL, Umlauf MG, Roth DL, Richter HE, et al. (2002). Behavioral training with and without biofeedback in the treatment of urge incontinence in older women: A randomized controlled trial. *JAMA,* 288(18):2293-2299.

Coyne KS, Matza LS, Thompson CL. (2005). The responsiveness of the Overactive Bladder Questionnaire (OAB-q). *Qual Life Res,* 14(3):849-855.

Coyne K, Revicki D, Hunt T, Corey R, Stewart W, Bentkover J, et al. (2002). Psychometric validation of an overactive bladder symptom and health-related quality of life questionnaire: The OAB-q. *Qual Life Res,* 11(6):563-574.

Dochterman JM, Bulechek GM (Eds). (2004). *Nursing Interventions Classification (NIC),* 4th ed. St Louis: Mosby.

Dougherty MC, Dwyer JW, Pendergast JF, Boyington AR, Tomlinson BU, Coward RT, et al. (2002). A randomized trial of behavioral management for continence with older rural women. *Res Nurs Health,* 25(1):3-13.

Dowd TT, Campbell JM, Jones JA. (1996). Fluid intake and urinary incontinence in older community-dwelling women. *J Community Health Nurs,* 13(3):179-186.

Fantl JA, Wyman JF, McClish DK, Harkins SW, Elswick RK, Taylor JR, et al. (1991). Efficacy of bladder training in older women with urinary incontinence. *JAMA,* 265(5):609-613.

Hay-Smith EJ, Dumoulin C. (2006). Pelvic floor muscle training versus no treatment, or inactive control treatments, for urinary incontinence in women. *Cochrane Database Syst Rev,* (1):CD005654.

McDowell BJ, Engberg S, Sereika S, Donovan N, Jubeck ME, Weber E, et al. (1999). Effectiveness of behavioral therapy to treat incontinence in homebound older adults. *J Am Geriatr Soc,* 47(3):309-318.

NR = Nursing Research, **MR** = Multidisciplinary Research, **SP** = Standard of Practice, **EO** = Expert Opinion, **LOE** = Level of Evidence

Moorhead M, Johnson M, Maas M (Eds). (2004). *Nursing Outcomes Classification (NOC)*, 3rd ed. St Louis: Mosby.

Publicover C, Bear M. (1997). The effect of bladder training on urinary incontinence in community-dwelling older women. *J Wound Ostomy Continence Nurs*, 24(6):319-324.

Subak LL, Whitcomb E, Shen H, Saxton J, Vittinghoff E, Brown JS. (2005). Weight loss: A novel and effective treatment for urinary incontinence. *J Urol*, 174(1):190-195.

Swithinbank L, Hashim H, Abrams P. (2005). The effect of fluid intake on urinary symptoms in women. *J Urol*, 174(1):187-189.

Uebersax JS, Wyman JF, Shumaker SA, McClish DK, Fantl JA. (1995). Short forms to assess life quality and symptom distress for urinary incontinence in women: The Incontinence Impact Questionnaire and the Urogenital Distress Inventory. Continence Program for Women Research Group. *Neurourol Urodyn*, 14(2):131-139.

Wallace SA, Roe B, Williams K, Palmer M. (2004). Bladder training for urinary incontinence in adults. *Cochrane Database Syst Rev*, (1):CD001308.

Williams KS, Assassa RP, Cooper NJ, Turner DA, Shaw C, Abrams KR, Mayne C, Jagger C, Matthews R, Clarke M, McGrother CW; The Leicestershire MRC Incontinence Study Team. (2006). Clinical and cost-effectiveness of a new nurse-led continence service: A randomised controlled trial. *Evid Based Nurs*, 9(3):85.

Wilson PD, Hay-Smith J, Wyman J, Yamanishi T, Berghmans B, et al. (2005). Adult conservative management. In Abrams P, Cardozo L, Khoury S, Wein A (Eds): *Incontinence: Management*, Volume 2. Paris: Health Publication Ltd, pp 855-964.

Wyman JF, Fantl JA, McClish DK, Harkins SW, Uebersax JS, Ory MG. (1997). Quality of life following bladder training in older women with urinary incontinence. *Int Urogynecol J Pelvic Floor Dysfunct*, 8(4):223-229.

Yamanishi T, Yasuda K, Sakakibara R, Hattori T, Suda S. (2000). Randomized, double-blind study of electrical stimulation for urinary incontinence due to detrusor overactivity. *Urology*, 55(3):353-357.

Yoon HS, Song HH, Ro YJ. (2003). A comparison of effectiveness of bladder training and pelvic muscle exercise on female urinary incontinence. *Int J Nurs Stud*, 40(1):45-50.

VALIDATION THERAPY

Dorothy A. Forbes, PhD, RN

Definition: A way of communicating with people suffering from dementia in which the recognition and validation of emotions using an empathic approach is central (Finnema et al., 2000). Empathizing with the feelings and meanings behind their confused speech and behavior is more important than the person's orientation to the present (Douglas et al., 2004). Validation therapy (VT) aims to restore self-worth and reduce stress by validating emotional ties to the past (APA, 1997). VT was developed by Naomi Feil (1993).

NURSING ACTIVITIES

Effective

No applicable published research was found in this category.

Possibly Effective

No applicable published research was found in this category.

RCT = Randomized Controlled (Clinical) Trial, **NIC** = Nursing Interventions Classification, **NOC** = Nursing Outcomes Classification

Not Effective

■ *Using VT to improve disturbing behaviors.* **LOE = I**

(NR) A Cochrane review concluded that there was insufficient evidence to support the efficacy of VT. One study ($N = 26$) found an improvement in disturbing behaviors in residents with physical and mental problems at 6 weeks when the experimental group was compared with the usual care group. VT included a discussion of a topic of mutual interest, singing and movement activity, a closing ritual, refreshments, and group work as outlined by Feil (1982) (Neal & Briggs, 2003; Peoples, 1982).

(MR) A recent RCT ($N = 151$ patients in 16 nursing homes) investigated the effects of emotion-oriented care on elderly people with cognitive impairment and behavioral problems. This approach was mainly based on VT. No statistically significant or clinically relevant effects on the behavioral outcome measures were observed in favor of the intervention as compared with usual care (Schrijnemaekers et al., 2002).

■ *Using VT to improve mood.* **LOE = III**

(MR) A Cochrane review found that one study ($N = 54$) that included residents with moderate to severe dementia who displayed problem behaviors demonstrated that these patients displayed a significant improvement in depression only at 12 months after VT when the experimental group was compared with the social contacts group. VT offered for 30 minutes four times a week for 52 weeks included greetings, singing a song or poetry, interaction about a topic of interest, refreshments, and individual goodbyes (Neal & Briggs, 2003; Toseland et al., 1997).

(NR) A clinical controlled trial ($N = 34$) compared three groups of residents with dementia who received VT, reality orientation, or no formal therapy. The study found no significant differences in depression, functional status, and cognition among the groups. The groups were offered for 30 minutes five times a week over 4 months and were lead by a registered nurse with a background in psychotherapy (Scanland & Emershaw, 1993).

■ *Using VT to improve cognition.* **LOE = I**

(MR) A Cochrane review examined changes in cognition but found no statistically significant differences between the treatment group and those who received social contact, reality orientation, or usual therapy (Neal & Briggs, 2003).

■ *Using VT to improve activities of daily living.* **LOE = I**

(MR) A Cochrane review examined changes in activities of daily living and found no statistically significant differences between VT and social contact or VT and usual therapy (Neal & Briggs, 2003).

Possibly Harmful

No applicable published research was found in this category.

NR = Nursing Research, **MR** = Multidisciplinary Research, **SP** = Standard of Practice, **EO** = Expert Opinion, **LOE** = Level of Evidence

OUTCOME MEASUREMENT

ANXIETY LEVEL NOC

Definition: Severity of manifested apprehension, tension, or uneasiness arising from an unidentifiable source.

Anxiety Level as evidenced by the following selected NOC indicators:

- Restlessness
- Pacing
- Distress
- Irritability
- Outbursts of anger

(Rate each indicator of **Anxiety Level:** 1 = severe, 2 = substantial, 3 = moderate, 4 = mild, 5 = none) (Moorhead et al., 2004).

REFERENCES

American Psychiatric Association (APA). (1997). Practice guideline for the treatment of patients with Alzheimer's disease and other dementias of late life. *Am J Psychiatry,* 154(5 Suppl):1-39.

Douglas S, James I, Ballard C. (2004). Non-pharmacological interventions in dementia. *Adv Psychiatr Treat,* 10(3):171-177.

Feil N. (1982). *Validation the Feil method: How to help the disorientated old-old.* Cleveland, OH: Feil Productions.

Feil N. (1993). *The validation breakthrough: Simple techniques for communicating with people with "Alzheimer's-type dementia."* Baltimore: Health Promotion Press.

Finnema E, Droes RM, Ribbe M, van Tilburg W. (2000). The effects of emotion-oriented approaches in the care for persons suffering from dementia: A review of the literature. *Int J Geriatr Psychiatry,* 15(2):141-161.

Moorhead M, Johnson M, Maas M (Eds). (2004). *Nursing Outcomes Classification (NOC),* 3rd ed. St Louis: Mosby.

Neal M, Briggs M. (2003). Validation therapy for dementia. *Cochrane Database Syst Rev,* (3): CD001394.

Peoples M. (1982). *Validation therapy versus reality orientation as treatment for disorientated institutionalized elderly.* Masters dissertation, College of Nursing, University of Akron.

Scanland SG, Emershaw LE. (1993). Reality orientation and validation therapy. Dementia, depression, and functional status. *J Gerontol Nurs,* 19(6):7-11.

Schrijnemaekers V, van Rossum E, Candel M, Frederiks C, Derix M, Sielhorst H, et al. (2002). Effects of emotion-oriented care on elderly people with cognitive impairment and behavioral problems. *Int J Geriatr Psychiatry,* 17(10):926-937.

Toseland RW, Diehl M, Freeman K, Manzanares T, Naleppa M, McCallion P. (1997). The impact of validation group therapy on nursing home residents with dementia. *J Appl Gerontol,* 16(1):31-50.

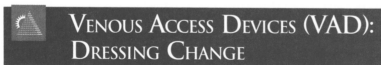

VENOUS ACCESS DEVICES (VAD): DRESSING CHANGE

Kathleen Higgins, RN, CCRN, CS, MSN, CRNP

Definition: Dressing changes for the patient with prolonged venous access.

RCT = Randomized Controlled (Clinical) Trial, **NIC** = Nursing Interventions Classification, **NOC** = Nursing Outcomes Classification

NURSING ACTIVITIES

Effective

■ *Use chlorhexidine for the skin cleansing of venous access devices for antisepsis while performing a dressing change.* **LOE = I**

(MR) A meta-analysis comparing chlorhexidine gluconate and povidone-iodine for the skin preparation of 4143 central venous catheters demonstrated that the use of chlorhexidine gluconate rather than povidone-iodine for vascular catheter site care was statistically significant in the reduction in catheter colonization and bloodstream infections (Chaiyakunapruk et al., 2002).

(MR) A prospective randomized study ($N = 688$) revealed that chlorhexidine was superior to povidone-iodine for the prevention of infections associated with central venous catheters (Maki et al., 1991).

■ (SP) *Change dressings using aseptic technique and Universal Precautions.* **LOE = VII**

(Refer to the guideline on Infection Control.)

■ *Use either gauze squares or a transparent dressing in accordance with patient preference for the occlusive dressing of a venous access device.* **LOE = I**

(MR) A Cochrane systematic review found that there was no evidence of any difference in the incidence of infectious complications among any of the dressing types compared in the review (Gillies et al., 2003).

(MR) A review article reported that the use of polyurethane dressings could increase the risk of colonization as compared with regular gauze dressing (Polderman & Girbes, 2002) and that increased colonization may indirectly lead to an increased risk of infection (Hota, 2004).

■ (SP) *Change venous access device dressings every 7 days if using a transparent dressing or when the dressing is no longer intact and every 48 hours if using a gauze dressing.* **LOE = VII**

(EO) Gauze dressings that prevent visualization of the insertion site should be changed routinely every 48 hours on peripheral and central catheter sites and immediately if the integrity of the dressing is compromised (INS, 2006).

■ (SP) *When changing the dressing, ensure that the catheter is secured and stabilized to prevent accidental dislodgement.* **LOE = V**

(EO) Catheters should be stabilized using a method that does not interfere with the assessment and monitoring of the access site or impede vascular circulation or the delivery of the prescribed therapy (INS, 2006).

■ *Identify the signs and symptoms associated with catheter-related infection, including redness, swelling, tenderness, fever, and malaise.* **LOE = V**

(MR) A review article reported that the use of polyurethane dressings could increase the risk of colonization as compared with regular gauze dressing (Polderman & Girbes, 2002).

NR = Nursing Research, **MR** = Multidisciplinary Research, **SP** = Standard of Practice, **EO** = Expert Opinion, **LOE** = Level of Evidence

Possibly Effective

No applicable published research was found in this category.

Not Effective

No applicable published research was found in this category.

Possibly Harmful

■ *Using antimicrobial ointment at the insertion site when changing dressings.*
LOE = IV

 The Centers for Disease Control and Prevention guidelines for the prevention of intra-vascular-catheter-related infections recommend that antimicrobial ointment should not be used; studies addressing the application of the antimicrobial ointments have been contradictory, and there is concern that fungal infections may be associated with the use of these ointments (O'Grady et al., 2002).

OUTCOME MEASUREMENT

KNOWLEDGE: INFECTION CONTROL (NOC)

Definition: Extent of understanding conveyed about the prevention and control of infection.

Knowledge: Infection Control as evidenced by the following selected NOC indicators:
• Description of practices that reduce transmission
• Description of signs and symptoms
• Description of monitoring procedures
(Rate each indicator of **Knowledge: Infection Control:** 1 = none, 2 = limited, 3 = moderate, 4 = substantial, 5 = extensive) (Moorhead et al., 2004).

REFERENCES

Chaiyakunapruk N, Veenstra DL, Lipsky B, Saint S. (2002). Chlorhexidine compared with povidone-iodine solution for vascular catheter-site care: A meta-analysis. *Ann Intern Med,* 136(11):792-801.

Gillies D, O'Riordan E, Carr D, O'Brien I, Frost J, Gunning R. (2003). Central venous catheter dressings: A systematic review. *J Adv Nurs,* 44(6):623-632.

Hoffmann KK, Weber DJ, Samsa GP, Rutala WA. (1992). Transparent polyurethane film as an intravenous catheter dressing: A meta-analysis of the infection risks. *JAMA,* 267(15):2072-2076.

Hota B. (2004). Contamination, disinfection, and cross-colonization: Are hospital surfaces reservoirs for nosocomial infection? *Clin Infect Dis,* 39(8):1182-1189.

Infusion Nurses Society (INS). (2006). Infusion nursing standards of practice. *J Infus Nurs,* 29(1 Suppl): S1-S92.

Maki DG, Ringer M, Alvarado CJ. (1991). Prospective randomised trial of povidone-iodine, alcohol, and chlorhexidine for prevention of infection associated with central venous and arterial catheters. *Lancet,* 338(8763):339-343.

Moorhead M, Johnson M, Maas M (Eds). (2004). *Nursing Outcomes Classification (NOC),* 3rd ed. St Louis: Mosby.

RCT = Randomized Controlled (Clinical) Trial, **NIC** = Nursing Interventions Classification, **NOC** = Nursing Outcomes Classification

O'Grady NP, Alexander M, Dellinger EP, Gerberding JL, Heard SO, Maki DG, et al. (2002). Guidelines for the prevention of intravascular catheter-related infections. Centers for Disease Control and Prevention. *MMWR Recomm Rep*, 51(RR-10):1-29.

Polderman KH, Girbes AR. (2002). Central venous catheter use. Part 2: Infectious complications. *Intensive Care Med*, 28(1):18-28.

VENOUS ACCESS DEVICES (VAD): FLUSHING

Kathleen Higgins, RN, CCRN, CS, MSN, CRNP

Definition: Flushing the venous access device (VAD) of the patient with prolonged venous access.

NURSING ACTIVITIES

Effective

■ *Accessing and maintaining the VAD should be done by a nurse with validated competency in these areas.* **LOE = VII**

EO The accessing and maintaining of an implantable port or pump should be performed by a nurse with validated competency as established by organizational policies and procedures as well as practice guidelines and in accordance with the state's Nurse Practice Act rules and regulations promulgated by the state Board of Nursing (INS, 2006).

■ *Establish a mechanism to flush the VAD (i.e., by using a positive displacement technique or technology), and flush the central VAD at regular intervals.* **LOE = VII**

EO VADs should be flushed at established intervals to promote and maintain patency and to prevent the mixing of incompatible medications and solutions (INS, 2006).

EO Positive fluid displacement should be used in accordance with administration system requirements (INS, 2006).

EO Flush with preservative-free 0.9% sodium chloride or another solution as indicated by infusate compatibility before and after the administration of medications and solutions (INS, 2006).

EO Flushing with a heparin flush solution to maintain the patency of an intermittently used central VAD should be performed at established intervals (INS, 2006).

EO To prevent catheter damage, use a large-bore syringe. Small-barrel syringes appear to create a greater pressure of pounds per square inch (INS, 2006).

■ SP *Use sterile technique along with specially designed noncoring needles when accessing an implanted port or pump.* **LOE = VII**

EO Specially-designed noncoring safety needles should be used to access an implanted port or pump, and the manufacturer's instructions for use should be followed. This type of needle is designed with a deflected bevel that will slice through the dense port septum rather than core it out. Using a regular needle will cause coring of this septum that will subsequently lead to port failure (Hadaway, 2006).

NR = Nursing Research, **MR** = Multidisciplinary Research, **SP** = Standard of Practice, **EO** = Expert Opinion, **LOE** = Level of Evidence

■ *Use fibrinolytic agents to restore patency to an occluded VAD when thrombotic occlusion is suspected.* **LOE = I**

(MR) A phase III multicenter trial ($N = 955$) evaluating the safety and efficacy of alteplase for restoring function to occluded central venous catheters demonstrated the restoration of flow in 90% of the central venous catheters (Deitcher et al., 2002).

(EO) A system that makes use of negative pressure is recommended, because this enables the instillation of a fibrinolytic agent without increasing pressure within the catheter (Dougherty, 2000).

■ *Disinfect injection caps with a chlorhexidine/alcohol solution or povidone-iodine both before and after flushing to reduce the risk of catheter-related infection.* **LOE = II**

(MR) An RCT comparing the microbial contamination rate of standard injection caps and a needleless positive-pressure valve ($N = 77$ patients) demonstrated that the disinfection of needless connectors with either chlorhexidine/alcohol or povidone-iodine significantly reduced external microbial contamination, with the lowest contamination rate seen when the ports were disinfected both before and after manipulation (Casey et al., 2003).

Possibly Effective

No applicable published research was found in this category.

Not Effective

No applicable published research was found in this category.

Possibly Harmful

■ *Attempting to force an intravenous flush if resistance occurs.* **LOE = VII**

(EO) When too much pressure is applied, the catheter may expand and allow fluid around a clot, thus enabling dislodgement into the venous system (Dougherty, 2000). In addition, increased pressure can result in rupture of the catheter and the catheter being forced into the venous system (Hadaway, 1998).

OUTCOME MEASUREMENT

KNOWLEDGE: INFECTION CONTROL   (NOC)

Definition: Extent of understanding conveyed about the prevention and control of infection.

Knowledge: Infection Control as evidenced by the following selected NOC indicators:
• Description of practices that reduce transmission
• Description of signs and symptoms
• Description of monitoring procedures

(Rate each indicator of **Knowledge: Infection Control:** 1 = none, 2 = limited, 3 = moderate, 4 = substantial, 5 = extensive) (Moorhead et al., 2004).

RCT = Randomized Controlled (Clinical) Trial, **NIC** = Nursing Interventions Classification, **NOC** = Nursing Outcomes Classification

REFERENCES

Casey AL, Worthington T, Lambert PA, Quinn D, Faroqui MH, Elliott TS. (2003). A randomized, prospective clinical trial to assess the potential infection risk associated with the PosiFlow needleless connector. *J Hosp Infect,* 54(4):288-293.

Deitcher SR, Fesen MR, Kiproff PM, Hill PA, Li X, McCluskey ER, et al. (2002). Safety and efficacy of alteplase for restoring function in occluded central venous catheters: Results of the cardiovascular thrombolytic to open occluded lines trial. *J Clin Oncol,* 20(1):317-324.

Dochterman JM, Bulechek GM (Eds). (2004). *Nursing Interventions Classification (NIC),* 4th ed. St Louis: Mosby.

Dougherty L. (2000). Central venous access devices. *Nurs Stand,* 14(43):45-50.

Hadaway L. (1998). Catheter connection. *J Vasc Access Devices,* 3(3):40.

Hadaway L. (2006). Accessing port-a-caths without using a noncoring needle. *The Patient Safety Discussion Forum.* March 7, 2006. Personal communication.

Infusion Nurses Society (INS). (2006). Infusion nursing standards of practice. *J Infus Nurs,* 29(1 Suppl): S1-92.

Moorhead M, Johnson M, Maas M (Eds). (2004). *Nursing Outcomes Classification (NOC),* 3rd ed. St Louis: Mosby.

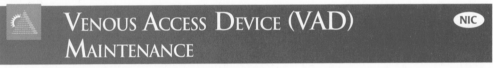

VENOUS ACCESS DEVICE (VAD) MAINTENANCE NIC

Kathleen Higgins, RN, CCRN, CS, MSN, CRNP

NIC **Definition:** Management of the patient with prolonged venous access via tunneled and nontunneled (percutaneous) catheters and implanted ports (Dochterman & Bulechek, 2004).

NURSING ACTIVITIES

Effective

■ *Use chlorhexidine for the skin preparation of venous access devices (VADs) for antisepsis.* **LOE = I**

MR A randomized control study (*N* = 125 patients) of patients undergoing foot and ankle surgery compared iodine and isopropyl alcohol preparation with chloroxylenol preparation and with chlorhexidine gluconate and isopropyl alcohol preparation and found that the culture specimens from the chlorhexidine gluconate and isopropyl alcohol preparation group were significantly lower than those found for the other two groups (Ostrander et al., 2005).

MR A meta-analysis comparing chlorhexidine gluconate and povidone-iodine for the skin preparation of 4143 central venous catheters demonstrated that the use of chlorhexidine gluconate rather than povidone-iodine for vascular catheter site care was statistically significant for a reduction in catheter colonization and bloodstream infections (Chaiyakunapruk et al., 2002).

■ **SP** *Accessing and maintaining the VAD should be performed by a nurse with validated competency in these areas.* **LOE = VII**

EO Accessing and maintaining an implantable port or pump should be performed by a nurse with validated competency as established by organizational policies and procedures and

NR = Nursing Research, **MR** = Multidisciplinary Research, **SP** = Standard of Practice, **EO** = Expert Opinion, **LOE** = Level of Evidence

practice guidelines and in accordance with the state's Nurse Practice Act rules and regulations promulgated by the state Board of Nursing (INS, 2006).

■ **NIC** **SP** *Verify infusate orders as applicable.* **LOE = VII**

EO The nurse should verify that the physician's or authorized prescriber's order is clear, concise, legible, and complete before the initiation of therapy (INS, 2006).

■ **SP** *Appropriately identify the patient before therapy.* **LOE = VII**

EO The nurse should identify the patient before the initiation of therapy or a procedure using at least two methods of identification (INS, 2006).

■ **SP** *Educate the patient and family.* **LOE = VII**

EO The nurse should educate the patient, caregiver, or legally authorized representative regarding the prescribed infusion therapy and plan of care, including (but not limited to) potential complications associated with the treatment or therapy, the risks, and the benefits (INS, 2006).

■ **NIC** **SP** *Change tubing, dressings, and caps according to agency policy.* **LOE = VII**

EO Aseptic technique and Standard Precautions should be used to change tubing dressings and caps. Caps should be changed at least every 7 days (INS, 2006), and tubing should be changed at least every 96 hours (O'Grady et al., 2002).

■ **NIC** *Maintain universal precautions.* **LOE = VII**

Note: Refer to the guideline on Infection Control.

■ **SP** *Confirm the placement of a central VAD with an x-ray report after the initial insertion and before beginning therapy.* **LOE = VII**

EO Pneumothorax is one of the most serious and potentially life-threatening complications of central venous catheter insertion. All patients, regardless of whether they have symptoms, should have a chest x-ray after the insertion of a central venous catheter (Drewett, 2000).

■ **NIC** **SP** *Maintain aseptic technique whenever the VAD is manipulated.* **LOE = I**

MR An RCT compared the microbial contamination rate of standard injection caps and a needleless positive-pressure valve ($N = 77$ patients) and demonstrated that the disinfection of needless connectors with either chlorhexidine/alcohol or povidone-iodine significantly reduced external microbial contamination, with the lowest contamination rate seen when the ports were disinfected both before and after manipulation (Casey et al., 2003).

MR A prospective cohort study in 357 central venous catheters indicated that certain manipulations, blood sampling, and the disconnection of the catheter increased the risk of catheter-associated bloodstream infection among neonatal intensive care patients (Mahieu et al., 2001).

EO Sterile technique should be used when accessing an implanted port or pump (INS, 2006).

EO Gloves should be worn during all infusion procedures that will potentially expose the nurse to blood and body fluids (INS, 2006).

RCT = Randomized Controlled (Clinical) Trial, **NIC** = Nursing Interventions Classification, **NOC** = Nursing Outcomes Classification

(EO) Acceptable hand hygiene techniques should be employed before and after all clinical procedures (INS, 2006).

(EO) The use of aseptic and sterile techniques, the observation of Standard Precautions, and the maintenance of product sterility should be required for all infusion procedures (INS, 2006).

(EO) Maximal sterile barrier precautions (i.e., sterile gown, powder-free sterile gloves, caps, mask, protective eyewear, and large sterile drapes and towels) should be used for midline and peripherally inserted central catheters and all types of central VADs (INS, 2006).

(EO) The nurse should prepare the intended insertion site with antiseptic solution(s) using aseptic or sterile technique as appropriate (INS, 2006).

■ *Minimize interruptions of the intravenous system to reduce the risk of infection.* **LOE = IV**

(MR) A prospective cohort study in 357 central venous catheters indicated that certain manipulations, blood sampling, and the disconnection of the catheter increased the risk of catheter-associated bloodstream infection among neonatal intensive care patients (Mahieu et al., 2001).

■ (NIC) (SP) *Monitor for signs and symptoms associated with local and systemic infection (e.g., redness, swelling, tenderness, fever, malaise).* **LOE = IV**

(EO) The nurse should use appropriate infection control measures, including aseptic technique, while accessing the VAD, administering medications or fluids, and flushing infusion access devices to reduce the risk of infusion and catheter-related infection (INS, 2006).

(EO) Catheters should be stabilized using a method that does not interfere with the assessment and monitoring of the access site or impede the vascular circulation or the delivery of the prescribed therapy (INS, 2006).

■ (NIC) (SP) *Monitor for signs of catheter occlusion.* **LOE = VII**

(EO) Proper primary assessment steps for central venous catheter occlusions include screening for extrinsic compression from clamps, sutures, and kinked catheter tubing; checking catheter function in terms of infusion and blood aspiration; assessing whether the occlusion is relieved by postural changes such as raising the ipsilateral arm and shrugging the shoulders forward; determining the history of what was recently infused through the catheter, including any recent blood sampling; and assessing the patient for physical signs of edema, redness, pain, or dilated vessels (Krzywda et al., 2006).

Possibly Effective

No applicable published research was found in this category.

Not Effective

No applicable published research was found in this category.

Possibly Harmful

No applicable published research was found in this category.

NR = Nursing Research, **MR** = Multidisciplinary Research, **SP** = Standard of Practice, **EO** = Expert Opinion, **LOE** = Level of Evidence

OUTCOME MEASUREMENT

KNOWLEDGE: INFECTION CONTROL

Definition: Extent of understanding conveyed about the prevention and control of infection.

Knowledge: Infection Control as evidenced by the following selected NOC indicators:
- Description of practices that reduce transmission
- Description of signs and symptoms
- Description of monitoring procedures

(Rate each indicator of **Knowledge: Infection Control:** 1 = none, 2 = limited, 3 = moderate, 4 = substantial, 5 = extensive) (Moorhead et al., 2004).

REFERENCES

Casey AL, Worthington T, Lambert PA, Quinn D, Faroqui MH, Elliott TS. (2003). A randomized, prospective clinical trial to assess the potential infection risk associated with the PosiFlow needleless connector. *J Hosp Infect,* 54(4):288-293.

Chaiyakunapruk N, Veenstra DL, Lipsky B, Saint S. (2002). Chlorhexidine compared with povidone-iodine solution for vascular catheter-site care: A meta-analysis. *Ann Intern Med,* 136(11):792-801.

Dochterman JM, Bulechek GM (Eds). (2004). *Nursing Interventions Classification (NIC),* 4th ed. St Louis: Mosby.

Drewett SR. (2000). Complications of central venous catheters: Nursing care. *Br J Nurs,* 9(8):466-468, 470-478.

Infusion Nurses Society (INS). (2006). Infusion nursing standards of practice. *J Infus Nurs,* 29(1 Suppl): S1-S92.

Krzywda EA, Andris DA, Edmiston CE, Wallace JR. (2006). Parenteral access devices. In Gottschlich MM (Ed). *ASPEN Core Curriculum. American Society for Parental and Enteral Nutrition.* Silver Spring, MD: Aspen.

Mahieu LM, De Dooy JJ, Lenaerts AE, Ieven MM, De Muynck AO. (2001). Catheter manipulations and the risk of catheter-associated bloodstream infection in neonatal intensive care unit patients. *J Hosp Infect,* 48(1):20-26.

Moorhead M, Johnson M, Maas M (Eds). (2004). *Nursing Outcomes Classification (NOC),* 3rd ed. St Louis: Mosby.

O'Grady NP, Alexander M, Dellinger EP, Gerberding JL, Heard SO, Maki DG, et al. (2002). Guidelines for the prevention of intravascular catheter-related infections. Centers for Disease Control and Prevention. *MMWR Recomm Rep,* 51(RR-10):1-29.

Ostrander RV, Botte MJ, Brage ME. (2005). Efficacy of surgical preparation solutions in foot and ankle surgery. *J Bone Joint Surg Am,* 87(5):980-985.

 # VISITATION FACILITATION

Mary Muth, MS, RN, APNP, CEN; Mary Kay Jiricka, MSN, RN, APN-BC, CCRN

NIC **Definition:** Promoting beneficial visits by family and friends (Dochterman & Bulechek, 2004).

NURSING ACTIVITIES

Effective

■ *Maintain visitation hours that are liberalized, open, and flexible.* **LOE = II**

(MR) In a randomized study, two visiting policies were randomly alternated in an intensive care unit. Results of the study demonstrated that liberalizing visitation did not increase septic complications and that it may reduce cardiovascular complications, possibly as a result of decreased anxiety (Fumagalli et al., 2006).

(NR) A research use project that expanded on the work of Molter's research showed that family visitation guidelines, policies, and procedures were developed to facilitate a family member's visitation experience. During the evaluation phase, it was determined that the change in practice had a positive effect on nursing staff and family members (Lopez-Fagin, 1995).

(NR) An exploratory study investigated the importance of the visiting needs of family members who had a relative hospitalized in an intensive care unit. Family members identified that visiting hours should be open and flexible (Stillwell, 1984).

■ *Adjust visitation according to the patient's condition.* **LOE = VI**

(NR) A two-phase descriptive study examined the perceptions of visitation needs during the medical intensive care unit experience from the perspectives of cardiac patients and their family members. Results implied that nurses should adjust visitation according to individual patients' conditions (Boykoff, 1986).

■ *Provide information about the hospitalized family member and the bedside environment.* **LOE = VI**

(NR) A retrospective, descriptive, qualitative study reported that family members needed to receive information about their critically ill family member before the first visit and on an ongoing basis. Family members needed to be oriented to the intensive care unit environment and routine (Jamerson et al., 1996).

(NR) A literature review described the special needs of the elderly when visiting a critically ill family member. Nurses needed to provide information about the critical event as soon as possible. Elderly family members often had chronic health problems that they were dealing with, and special attention needed to be focused on their health needs (e.g., taking of medications, adherence to eating on a regular basis, obtaining adequate rest periods). Information was best processed if it was presented in small, frequent increments while speaking at a slow pace. Elderly family members may want to stay for extended periods at the bedside to be near the family member (Leske & Heidrich, 1996).

■ *Provide family members with interventions and actions that will be helpful to the ill family member.* **LOE = V**

(NR) A literature review described the needs and experiences of family members when care is being provided to hospitalized family members. Family members reported that they wanted to speak daily to a physician about the condition and prognosis of the patient. Family members also reported that they expected nurses to explain to them about the care that the patient was receiving, about the hospital environment, and about what they could do for the patient (Verhaeghe et al., 2005).

NR = Nursing Research, **MR** = Multidisciplinary Research, **SP** = Standard of Practice, **EO** = Expert Opinion, **LOE** = Level of Evidence

(NR) A repeat-measures research design examined the relationships between the variables of closeness, helpfulness, and optimism with emotional outcomes. Research participants reported the following interventions as being helpful: (1) visiting the patient; (2) being at the bedside; (3) passive and active touching; (4) assisting with activities of daily living; and (5) doing things for the patient (e.g., getting water, assisting with meals; Eldredge, 2004).

(NR) A prospective multicenter survey that was designed to elicit opinions and experiences about family members participating in direct patient care found that 88% of intensive care unit caregivers were willing to invite family members to participate in patient care but that only 33% of family members wanted to participate in care. One possible explanation for this disparity is that family members felt that they did not receive adequate information about what participation entailed (Azoulay et al., 2003).

(NR) A literature review presented nursing actions that facilitated family visitation in the intensive care unit. Nurse behaviors that were identified by family members as being helpful included the following: (1) providing information about what to expect at the bedside; (2) providing information about the patient's condition, the intensive care unit environment, and the current plan of care; (3) coaching and role modeling methods of communication with the patient; and (4) providing anticipatory guidance to family members, especially regarding the patient's appearance, level of consciousness, and the equipment being used at the bedside (Clarke, 1995).

(MR) A prospective single-cohort descriptive study measured and contrasted family member expectations in an intensive care unit as compared with a general ward. Family members of intensive care unit patients reported the following needs: (1) directions from the staff regarding what to do at the bedside; (2) more support from their own family members; (3) a place to be alone; (4) advance notice of any transfer plans; and (5) flexibility in visitation times (Foss & Tenholder, 1993).

■ (NIC) *Inform visitors, including children, what they may expect to see and hear before their first hospital visitation, as appropriate.* **LOE = IV**

(NR) A controlled study of intensive care unit patients' family members (N = 66) showed a significant reduction of anxiety when the family was provided with information sessions regarding what to expect (Chiu et al., 2004).

(MR) An exploratory study examining family members' experiences in the intensive care unit (N = 13) as compared with registered nurses' perceptions of family member experiences demonstrated that family members responded very positively to communication preparation regarding what they would see, hear, and feel as well as to information regarding the patient's condition before visits (Hughes et al., 2005).

(NR) A descriptive study (N = 30) that examined the unmet needs of relatives in an intensive care unit waiting room found that family members felt unprepared for the intensive care environment before the first visit (Browning & Warren, 2006).

(EO) "Anticipatory guidance" helps guide relatives through visitation, because it provides a mechanism to share with the visitor what to expect, including what the patient's condition is, what will be seen and heard, and what type of equipment will be in the room (Clarke, 1995).

■ *Facilitate open communication between health care providers and family members regarding the patient's condition and the plan of care.* **LOE = V**

(MR) A descriptive study in Belgium (N = 200) found that the most important need for families of patients in an intensive care unit was information (Delva et al., 2002).

RCT = Randomized Controlled (Clinical) Trial, **NIC** = Nursing Interventions Classification, **NOC** = Nursing Outcomes Classification

(NR) An exploratory study ($N = 92$) to identify and assess the family needs of patients in an intensive care unit demonstrated that the top six most important needs were related to communication, having questions answered, and being updated about the patient's condition (Forrester et al., 1990).

(NR) A descriptive study of patients ($N = 20$) and family members that explored perceptions of visitation needs identified that both the patients and their family members ranked explaining the patient's condition to visitors as being of the highest importance (Boykoff, 1986).

(MR) A descriptive study ($N = 55$) demonstrated that 86.5% of family members of trauma patients felt that scheduled family rounds with the primary registered nurse, a surgeon, or another health care team member helped to increase communication (Mangram et al., 2005).

(NR) A controlled study ($N = 40$) of patients who were admitted to two different postanesthesia care units (one that allowed visitors and one did not allow visitors) demonstrated that there was a decrease in anxiety among the patients who had a relative visit during their stay in the unit (Poole, 1993).

Possibly Effective

No applicable published research was found in this category.

Not Effective

No applicable published research was found in this category.

Possibly Harmful

No applicable published research was found in this category.

OUTCOME MEASUREMENT

FAMILY SUPPORT DURING TREATMENT   (NOC)

Definition: Family presence and emotional support for an individual undergoing treatment.

Family Support During Treatment as evidenced by the following selected NOC indicators:

• Members express desire to support ill member
• Members express feelings and emotions of concern for ill member
• Members ask how they may assist
• Collaborates with health care providers in determining care

(Rate each indicator of **Family Support During Treatment:** 1 = never demonstrated, 2 = rarely demonstrated, 3 = sometimes demonstrated, 4 = often demonstrated, 5 = consistently demonstrated) (Moorhead et al., 2004).

REFERENCES

Azoulay E, Pochard F, Chevret S, Arich C, Brivet F, Brun F, et al. (2003). Family participation in care to the critically ill: Opinions of families and staff. *Intensive Care Med,* 29(9):1498-1504.

Boykoff SL. (1986). Visitation needs reported by patients with cardiac disease and their families. *Heart Lung*, 15(6):573-578.

Browning G, Warren NA. (2006). Unmet needs of family members in the medical intensive care waiting room. *Crit Care Nurs Q*, 29(1):86-95.

Chiu Y, Chien W, Lam L. (2004). Effectiveness of a needs-based education programme for families with critically ill relative in an intensive care unit. *J Clin Nurs*, 13(5):655-656.

Clarke SP. (1995). Increasing the quality of family visits to the ICU. *Dimens Crit Care Nurs*, 14(4):200-212.

Delva D, Vanoost S, Bijttebier P, Lauwers P, Wilmer A. (2002). Needs and feelings of anxiety of relatives of patients hospitalized in intensive care units: Implications for social work. *Soc Work Health Care*, 35(4):21-40.

Dochterman JM, Bulechek GM (Eds). (2004). *Nursing Interventions Classifications (NIC)*, 4th ed. St Louis: Mosby.

Eldredge D. (2004). Helping at the bedside: Spouses' preferences for helping critically ill patients. *Res Nurs Health*, 27(5):307-321.

Forrester DA, Murphy PA, Price DM, Monaghan JF. (1990). Critical care family needs: Nurse-family member confederate pairs. *Heart Lung*, 19(6):655-661.

Foss KR, Tenholder MF. (1993). Expectations and needs of persons with family members in an intensive care unit as opposed to a general ward. *South Med J*, 86(4):380-384.

Fumagalli S, Boncinelli L, Lo Nostro A, Valoti P, Baldereschi G, Di Bari M, et al. (2006). Reduced cardiocirculatory complications with unrestrictive visiting policy in an intensive care unit: Results from a pilot, randomized trial. *Circulation*, 113(7):946-952.

Hughes F, Bryan K, Robbins I. (2005). Relatives' experiences of critical care. *Nurs Crit Care*, 10(1):23-30.

Jamerson P, Scheibmeir M, Bott MJ, Crighton F, Hinton RH, Cobb AK. (1996). The experiences of families with a relative in the intensive care unit. *Heart Lung*, 25(6):467-474.

Leske JS, Heidrich SM. (1996). Interventions for aged family members. *Crit Care Nurs Clin North Am*, 8(1):91-102.

Lopez-Fagin L. (1995). Critical Care Family Needs Inventory: A cognitive research utilization approach. *Crit Care Nurse*, 15(4):21, 23-26.

Mangram AJ, McCauley T, Villarreal D, Berne J, Howard D, Dolly A, et al. (2005). Families' perception of the value of timed daily "family rounds" in a trauma ICU. *Am Surg*, 71(10):886-891.

Moorhead M, Johnson M, Maas M (Eds). (2004). *Nursing Outcomes Classification (NOC)*, 3rd ed. St Louis: Mosby.

Poole EL. (1993). The effects of postanesthesia care unit visits on anxiety in surgical patients. *J Post Anesth Nurs*, 8(6):386-394.

Stillwell SB. (1984). Importance of visiting needs as perceived by family members of patients in the intensive care unit. *Heart Lung*, 13(3):238-242.

Verhaeghe S, Defloor T, Van Zuuren F, Duijnstee M, Grypdonck M. (2005). The needs and experiences of family members of adult patients in an intensive care unit: A review of the literature. *J Clin Nurs*, 14(4):501-509.

 # VITAL SIGNS MONITORING

Mary E. Hagle, PhD, RN, AOCN

NIC **Definition:** Collection and analysis of cardiovascular, respiratory, and body temperature data to determine and prevent complications (Dochterman & Bulechek, 2004).

NURSING ACTIVITIES

Cardiovascular Data

Effective

■ *Count the heart rate, using the radial pulse, for either 30 seconds and multiply by 2 or for 60 seconds; when the heart rate is rapid as it is during atrial fibrillation or in infants or when the radial pulse is difficult to count, use an apical pulse rate with a stethoscope.* **LOE = II**

(NR) An RCT was conducted with a sample of 206 healthy young adults. Findings revealed that there was significantly more accuracy when the radial pulse was counted for 30 or 60 seconds rather than 15 seconds, and that the count should start from "1" rather than "0" (Hwu et al., 2000).

(MR) A systematic review conducted by a collaborating center of the Joanna Briggs Institute and using a standard search strategy with the evaluation of each study concluded that shorter times for counting pulse rates were less accurate. Few studies are available that relate to pulse rate measurement (Lockwood et al., 2004).

■ *Use a standard method and technique for blood pressure measurement, and indicate which method is used.* **LOE = V**

(MR) A systematic review conducted by a collaborating center of the Joanna Briggs Institute and using a standard search strategy with the evaluation of each study concluded that many factors affected blood pressure measurement, including the position of the person and the extremity, the cuff, the technique, auscultation, and the specific Korotkoff sounds used. Additionally, health care workers did not adhere to procedural guidelines, thus contributing to inaccuracy (Lockwood et al., 2004).

(NR) A narrative review of nurse-authored research included 54 studies from 1990 through 1999. The authors concluded that the method used for blood pressure measurement was not always documented, thus leading to inaccurate comparisons over time for the same patient (Thomas et al., 2002).

■ *Use the upper arm and support the arm at about heart level while the person is resting or, preferably, sitting.* **LOE = V**

(MR) A systematic review conducted by a collaborating center of the Joanna Briggs Institute and using a standard search strategy with the evaluation of each study found from two early studies that arm position changes influenced both systolic and diastolic measurement by as much as 11 to 20 mm Hg. A body of literature addressed the influence of anxiety and activity on blood pressure measurement (Lockwood et al., 2004).

(NR) In a narrative review of nurse-authored research that included 54 studies from 1990 through 1999, several studies found that activity increased blood pressure readings for both values by as much as 19 mm Hg (Thomas et al., 2002).

■ *Use a 12-cm wide cuff for most adults, but base the final cuff choice on arm circumference.* **LOE = V**

(MR) A systematic review conducted by a collaborating center of the Joanna Briggs Institute and using a standard search strategy with the evaluation of each study cited several studies of the influence of cuff size on blood pressure measures. A cuff that was too large decreased the final value, whereas a cuff that was too small increased the final value (Lockwood et al., 2004).

■ *Use trended blood pressure measurements for clinical decisions.* **LOE = V**

(MR) A systematic review conducted by a collaborating center of the Joanna Briggs Institute and using a standard search strategy with the evaluation of each study emphasized the importance of using serial blood pressure measures, which may overcome the anxiety associated with the test or situation (Lockwood et al., 2004).

Possibly Effective

■ *Have the patient sit with his or her feet flat on the floor during blood pressure measurement.* **LOE = V**

(NR) A controlled study of 100 ambulatory hypertensive males revealed that legs that were crossed at the knee during blood pressure measurement significantly increased blood pressure readings ($p < .0001$) for both systolic and diastolic values (Foster-Fitzpatrick et al., 1999).

(NR) An RCT of 103 ambulatory seniors and strict blood pressure measurement techniques found that legs that were crossed at the knee significantly ($p < .001$) increased both systolic and diastolic blood pressure readings (Keele-Smith & Price-Daniel, 2001).

(NR) A controlled study of 238 ambulatory patients revealed that crossing the legs at the knee significantly ($p < .001$) increased blood pressure measurements by 8.5 mm Hg for systolic blood pressure reading and by 5.7 mm Hg for the diastolic reading (Pinar et al., 2004).

Not Effective

■ *Monitoring orthostatic or postural changes to blood pressure in adults as an indicator of intravascular blood volume.* **LOE = V**

(MR) A systematic review conducted by a collaborating center of the Joanna Briggs Institute and using a standard search strategy with the evaluation of each study concluded that orthostatic blood pressure changes were unreliable for detecting reduced intravascular blood volume. Orthostatic blood pressure changes were significant if systolic blood pressure decreased by more than 10 mm Hg or if diastolic blood pressure decreased by more than 10 mm Hg (Lockwood et al., 2004).

Possibly Harmful

No applicable published research was found in this category.

Respiratory Data

Effective

■ *Count respirations for 1 full minute and when the patient is at rest; avoid counting during periods of agitation and distress.* **LOE = IV**

(MR) A systematic review conducted by a collaborating center of the Joanna Briggs Institute and using a standard search strategy with the evaluation of each study concluded that

RCT = Randomized Controlled (Clinical) Trial, **NIC** = Nursing Interventions Classification, **NOC** = Nursing Outcomes Classification

counting respirations for less than 30 seconds resulted in high variability (Lockwood et al., 2004).

(MR) A controlled study of 12,096 emergency department patients identified that a rate of 20 breaths per minute (±4 breaths) was usual, which is a rate that is higher than the frequently reported "normal" respiratory rate (Mower et al., 1996).

■ *Use the respiratory rate and its trends in conjunction with other physiological measures, such as oxygen saturation, to assess physiological deterioration.*
LOE = V

(NR) A narrative review of a variety of research papers identified the relationship of respiratory dysfunction with adverse events. It also found that the early identification and reversal of the dysfunction improved mortality. Increased respiratory rate (>30 breaths per minute) was the most common and significant alteration found in five studies of 1859 patients; 37% of 2202 patients were hypoxemic (with a saturation of peripheral oxygen of less than 90%) before an adverse event (Considine, 2005).

(MR) A systematic review conducted by a collaborating center of the Joanna Briggs Institute and using a standard search strategy with the evaluation of each study concluded that respiratory rate alone and without sequential measures was not effective in an acute situation (Lockwood et al., 2004).

(NR) A narrative review summarized expert opinions about the importance of trending the respiratory rate over several hours from the patient's baseline to detect respiratory depression; the rate may not be below a "normal" threshold (Hagle et al., 2004).

■ *Monitor oxygen saturation using pulse oximetry when accurate assessment is critical or for the detection of physiological deterioration.* **LOE = I**

(MR) A systematic review conducted by a collaborating center of the Joanna Briggs Institute and using a standard search strategy with the evaluation of each study concluded that pulse oximetry monitoring was recommended for patients during invasive procedures and for patients who were acutely ill in the emergency department. Pulse oximetry results reduced the frequency of sampling for arterial blood gas and changed treatment decisions (Lockwood et al., 2004).

(MR) A Cochrane systematic review of four RCTs that included 21,773 patients during the perioperative period revealed that pulse oximetry detected hypoxemia and related adverse events from anesthesia but that there was no significant difference with regard to complications, length of stay, or deaths when pulse oximetry was not used (Pedersen et al., 2003).

■ *Identify alterations from normal oxygen saturation measured via pulse oximetry.*
LOE = VII

(EO) Oxygen saturation as measured from a pulse oximeter is reported as the saturation of peripheral oxygen; normal values are 95% to 100%, and values of less than 85% to 90% require further evaluation and/or intervention (Smeltzer & Bare, 2004).

(NR) In a narrative review, some researchers defined respiratory depression as oxygen saturation of less than 85% or of less than 90% for more than 1 minute (Hagle et al., 2004).

NR = Nursing Research, **MR** = Multidisciplinary Research, **SP** = Standard of Practice, **EO** = Expert Opinion, **LOE** = Level of Evidence

Possibly Effective

■ *Use pulse oximetry rather than respiratory rate to assess oxygen saturation and desaturation.* **LOE = VI**

(MR) A descriptive study of 1466 postoperative patients using patient-controlled analgesia reported that respiratory depression was identified in six patients with a respiratory rate of less than 10 breaths per minutes, whereas 19 patients had respiratory depression that was identified with oxygen saturation of less than 90% for more than 1 minute (Tsui et al., 1997).

(MR) A controlled study of 12,096 consecutive adult emergency department patients in the United States revealed low correlations between auscultated respiratory rates measured for 1 minute and pulse oximetry; only 33% of patients with oxygen saturations of less than 90% had an increased respiratory rate (Mower et al., 1996).

■ *Obtain clinical knowledge and skills education about the use, application, and interpretation of pulse oximetry equipment and its results.* **LOE = VI**

(NR) A study with a pre-test/post-test design measured changes in pulse oximetry knowledge using 17 questions for nurses, physicians, and respiratory therapists in the United States after an educational intervention. The pre-test was completed by 442 staff members, with 66% of answers being correct; 252 staff members completed the post-test, with 82% of answers being correct ($p < .01$; Attin et al., 2002).

(MR) A descriptive survey of 63 nurses and physicians in New Zealand using an investigator-developed tool revealed a fair to good understanding of pulse oximetry, although only 16% of respondents received formal training; 65% requested more training (Davies et al., 2003).

(NR) A descriptive survey of 551 critical care nurses at a professional conference in the United States that addressed their knowledge of pulse oximetry using six investigator-developed questions revealed moderate levels of knowledge (Giuliano & Liu, 2006).

(NR) A descriptive survey of 50 trained and untrained nurses and medical staff in the United Kingdom addressed their knowledge of pulse oximetry using an investigator-developed tool and revealed a knowledge deficit; training was undertaken (Howell, 2002).

Not Effective

No applicable published research was found in this category.

Possibly Harmful

No applicable published research was found in this category.

Temperature Data

Effective

■ *Position oral thermometers in the left or right posterior sublingual pocket for 7 minutes, and use the same site and device for serial patient temperatures.* **LOE = V**

(NR) A controlled study using a repeated measures design with 257 adult surgical patients supported the use of either oral or tympanic temperatures. Although there were no statistically significant differences between the measurements, 34% of the differences were clinically significant, and researchers supported the consistent use of the same device and site for each patient when performing serial measurements (Gilbert et al., 2002).

(MR) A systematic review conducted by a collaborating center of the Joanna Briggs Institute and using a standard search strategy with the evaluation of each study concluded that this position and dwell time were more accurate for oral measurement (Lockwood et al., 2004).

■ *Take accurate oral temperatures even with oxygen therapy in place and with varying breathing patterns; wait at least 15 minutes to take an oral temperature if the patient has consumed hot or cold oral fluids.* **LOE = V**

(MR) A systematic review conducted by a collaborating center of the Joanna Briggs Institute and using a standard search strategy with the evaluation of each study concluded from a series of studies that oxygen therapy did not affect the accuracy of oral temperatures when proper positioning of the thermometer was used (Lockwood et al., 2004).

■ *Use the ear tug method and avoid cerumen-impacted ears when taking tympanic temperatures.* **LOE = V**

(MR) A systematic review conducted by a collaborating center of the Joanna Briggs Institute and using a standard search strategy with the evaluation of each study concluded from a series of studies that the proper positioning of the ear improved tympanic measurement and that impacted cerumen decreased temperature accuracy (Lockwood et al., 2004).

Possibly Effective

■ *Replace glass mercury thermometers with Galinstan-in-glass thermometers.* **LOE = VI**

(NR) A descriptive study with a convenience sample of 120 adult patients compared oral, axillary, groin, and rectal temperatures using glass mercury and glass mercury-free thermometers. No significant differences were found between the thermometers (Smith, 2003).

■ *Identify normal temperature parameters for the site of measurement.* **LOE = V**

(NR) A narrative review of a variety of published studies from 1935 to 1999 identified a wider range of normal temperatures than is usually reported. This report used an evidence classification schema to rate studies for inclusion; 27 studies were analyzed to provide sample sizes ranging from 347 to 2749 for a mean oral temperature of 36.4°C, a mean rectal temperature of 36.5°C, and a mean tympanic temperature of 36.5°C, with total ranges from 33.2°C to 38.2°C (Sund-Levander et al., 2002).

Not Effective

No applicable published research was found in this category.

Possibly Harmful

■ *Using glass mercury thermometers may increase the risk of rectal perforation during rectal use or the risk of tissue injury and mercury exposure as a result of a broken thermometer during oral or rectal use.* **LOE = V**

(MR) A systematic review conducted by a collaborating center of the Joanna Briggs Institute and using a standard search strategy with the evaluation of each study concluded that

NR = Nursing Research, **MR** = Multidisciplinary Research, **SP** = Standard of Practice, **EO** = Expert Opinion, **LOE** = Level of Evidence

glass mercury thermometers had been associated with adverse events (Lockwood et al., 2004).

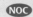 The Agency for Toxic Substances and Disease Registry in the Centers for Disease Control and Prevention recommends the proper disposal of glass mercury thermometers and the use of alternative thermometers to reduce harmful exposure to mercury during adverse events (1999).

OUTCOME MEASUREMENT

VITAL SIGNS   NOC

(Please refer to *Nursing Outcomes Classification* [Moorhead et al., 2004] for the **Vital Signs** outcome.)

REFERENCES

Agency for Toxic Substances and Disease Registry (ATSDR). (1999). *Toxicological profile for mercury.* Atlanta, GA: US Department of Health and Human Services, Public Health Service.

Attin M, Cardin S, Dee V, Doering L, Dunn D, Ellstrom K, et al. (2002). An educational project to improve knowledge related to pulse oximetry. *Am J Crit Care,* 11(6):529-534.

Considine J. (2005). The role of nurses in preventing adverse events related to respiratory dysfunction: Literature review. *J Adv Nurs,* 49(6):624-633.

Davies G, Gibson AM, Swanney M, Murray D, Beckert L. (2003). Understanding of pulse oximetry among hospital staff. *N Z Med J,* 116(1168):U297.

Dochterman JM, Bulechek GM (Eds). (2004). *Nursing Interventions Classifications (NIC),* 4th ed. St Louis: Mosby.

Foster-Fitzpatrick L, Ortiz A, Sibilano H, Marcantonio R, Braun LT. (1999). The effects of crossed leg on blood pressure measurement. *Nurs Res,* 48(2):105-108.

Gilbert M, Barton AJ, Counsell CM. (2002). Comparison of oral and tympanic temperatures in adult surgical patients. *Appl Nurs Res,* 15(1):42-47.

Giuliano KK, Liu LM. (2006). Knowledge of pulse oximetry among critical care nurses. *Dimens Crit Care Nurs,* 25(1):44-49.

Hagle ME, Lehr VT, Brubakken K, Shippee A. (2004). Respiratory depression in adult patients with intravenous patient-controlled analgesia. *Orthop Nurs,* 23(1):18-27.

Howell M. (2002). Pulse oximetry: An audit of nursing and medical staff understanding. *Br J Nurs,* 11(3): 191-197.

Hwu YJ, Coates VE, Lin FY. (2000). A study of the effectiveness of different measuring times and counting methods of human radial pulse rates. *J Clin Nurs,* 9(1):146-152.

Keele-Smith R, Price-Daniel C. (2001). Effects of crossing legs on blood pressure measurement. *Clin Nurs Res,* 10(2):202-213.

Lockwood C, Conroy-Hiller T, Page T. (2004). Vital signs. *JBI Reports,* 2(6):207-230.

Moorhead M, Johnson M, Maas M (Eds). (2004). *Nursing Outcomes Classification (NOC),* 3rd ed. St Louis: Mosby.

Mower WR, Sachs C, Nicklin EL, Safa P, Baraff LJ. (1996). A comparison of pulse oximetry and respiratory rate in patient screening. *Respir Med,* 90(10):593-599.

Pedersen T, Dyrlund Pedersen B, Moller AM. (2003). Pulse oximetry for perioperative monitoring. *Cochrane Database Syst Rev,* (3):CD002013.

Pinar R, Sabuncu N, Oksay A. (2004). Effects of crossed leg on blood pressure. *Blood Press,* 13(4):252-254.

Smeltzer SC, Bare BG. (2004). *Brunner & Suddarth's textbook of medical-surgical nursing,* 10th ed. Philadelphia: Lippincott Williams and Wilkins.

Smith LS. (2003). Reexamining age, race, site, and thermometer type as variables affecting temperature measurement in adults—a comparison study. *BMC Nurs,* 2(1):1-14.

RCT = Randomized Controlled (Clinical) Trial, **NIC** = Nursing Interventions Classification, **NOC** = Nursing Outcomes Classification

Sund-Levander M, Forsberg C, Wahren LK. (2002). Normal oral, rectal, tympanic and axillary body temperature in adult men and women: A systematic literature review. *Scand J Caring Sci*, 16(2):122-128.

Thomas SA, Liehr P, DeKeyser F, Frazier L, Friedmann E. (2002). A review of nursing research on blood pressure. *J Nurs Scholarsh*, 34(4):313-321.

Tsui SL, Irwin MG, Wong CM, Fung SK, Hui TW, Ng KF, et al. (1997). An audit of the safety of an acute pain service. *Anaesthesia*, 52(11):1042-1047.

WEIGHT GAIN ASSISTANCE

Carolyn Thompson Martin, PhD, RN, CFNP; Sandra F. Simmons, PhD

(NIC) **Definition:** Facilitating gain of body weight (Dochterman & Bulechek, 2004).

NURSING ACTIVITIES

Effective

- ◼ *Offer additional foods and fluids between meals.* **LOE = I**

  (MR) A controlled study (*N* = 134 nursing home residents) showed that 44% of residents with low oral food and fluid consumption during meals significantly increased their daily caloric intake when offered additional foods and fluids three times per day between meals (Simmons & Schnelle, 2004).

  (MR) An RCT (*N* = 68 nursing home residents) with patients who were at risk for poor nutritional status showed that the daily provision of additional calories via supplement or snack delivery three times per day for 6 weeks resulted in significant gains in daily caloric intake and weight for both the supplement and snack intervention groups as compared with a control group (Turic et al., 1998).

  (MR) An RCT (*N* = 63 incontinent nursing home residents) showed that 78% of residents increased their daily fluid intake and improved their hydration status in response to an intervention that included multiple prompts per day to consume fluids between meals, the availability of fluid choices, and consistent toileting assistance (Simmons et al., 2001a).

  (MR) A descriptive study (*N* = 25) demonstrated that, to optimize the nutritional status of nursing home residents with dementia (age >77 years), efforts must be directed toward the morning, when those with behavior difficulties and/or increased cognitive impairment are most responsive to food being provided (Young et al., 2001).

  (MR) A systematic literature review reported that regular presentations of fluids to older adults helped maintain adequate hydration and that the daily oral intake of fluids should be not less than 1600 mL per 24 hours. A simple oral fluid intake sheet and/or a bedside urine specific gravity test are the best methods for monitoring daily fluid intake (Hodgkinson et al., 2003).

- ◼ *Provide oral liquid nutritional supplements between meals to promote adequate nutrient intake.* **LOE = I**

  (Note: It is very important that the patients receive the ordered supplements and that they receive assistance with ingesting them as needed for this activity to be effective.)

NR = Nursing Research, **MR** = Multidisciplinary Research, **SP** = Standard of Practice, **EO** = Expert Opinion, **LOE** = Level of Evidence

(MR) A Cochrane review found that supplementation with protein and energy supplements in the elderly resulted in a small but consistent weight gain among older people (Milne et al., 2005).

(MR) A systematic review of 24 studies ($N = 2135$) demonstrated that patients receiving supplements gained more weight (or lost less weight) than those who received dietary advice (Baldwin & Parsons, 2004).

(MR) A descriptive study ($N = 132$) showed that less than 10% of nursing home residents received supplements that were consistent with their orders in daily care practice. In addition, supplements were often provided with regularly scheduled meals instead of between meals, and staff provided little to no assistance with encouraging consumption (Simmons & Patel, 2006).

(MR) A descriptive study ($N = 40$) showed that compliance with oral liquid nutritional supplements among hospitalized and community-dwelling geriatric patients was low as a result of personal preferences and the palatability of supplements (Lad et al., 2005).

(MR) An RCT ($N = 34$ nursing home residents, age >83 years) recommended that the provision of a nutrient supplement as a midmorning snack was an effective way to enhance energy intake among institutionalized seniors with dementia (Young et al., 2004).

(MR) A descriptive study ($N = 15$ elderly patients, age >70 years) suggested that older adults with low energy intakes after liquid dietary supplementation may increase their consumption if supplements with lower fat content are substituted. The supplements were given between meals and ≥1 hour before the next meal (Wilson et al., 2002).

(MR) A descriptive study ($N = 143$ nursing home residents, age >59 years) reported that it was possible to increase weight and maintain the protein status of debilitated elderly patients in nursing homes by using a simple, inexpensive, in-house formula (a high-protein, milk-based, formula with vitamin and mineral supplementation) for total nutritional support (Levinson et al., 2005).

Additional research: Lauque et al., 2004.

■ *Use social stimulation, enhanced environment, verbal cueing, and physical guidance to enhance self-feeding ability, oral food and fluid consumption, and quality of life.* **LOE = II**

(MR) A controlled study ($N = 74$ nursing home residents) showed that the use of a graduated-prompting protocol that included social stimulation, verbal cueing, and physical guidance enhanced self-feeding ability and oral food and fluid consumption during meals for 50% of patients with oral intake problems (Simmons et al., 2001b).

(MR) A controlled study ($N = 134$ nursing home residents) showed that the use of a graduated-prompting protocol that included social stimulation, verbal cueing, and physical guidance enhanced self-feeding ability and oral food and fluid consumption during meals for 46% of the patients with oral intake problems. These findings replicated a previous study (Simmons & Schnelle, 2004).

(MR) A descriptive study ($N = 400$ nursing home residents, age >62 years) reported that nursing homes with a lower prevalence of weight loss (as reported in the minimum data set weight-loss quality indicator) had staff who provided verbal prompting and social interaction to more residents during meals (Simmons et al., 2003a).

(MR) A descriptive study ($N = 50$, age >59 years) suggested that a way to increase caloric intake in homebound older adults was to arrange for family members and caregivers to eat with them. The simple presence of a family member and a caregiver at meals did not increase caloric intake (Locher et al., 2005).

(NR) An RCT ($N = 24$ female nursing home residents, age >67 years) demonstrated that verbal prompts and the positive reinforcement of elderly nursing home patients with dementia improved eating behaviors. These elders retained treatment at both post-tests. The dementia diagnosis should not preclude the possibility that eating skills may be reacquired (Coyne & Hoskins, 1997).

(NR) A controlled study ($N = 20$) showed that the use of physical touch and verbal cueing provided by nurse aides resulted in a significant increase in oral intake among hospitalized elderly patients with severe cognitive impairment (Lange-Alberts & Shott, 1994).

Additional research: Musson et al., 1990; Ragneskog et al., 1996; McDaniel et al., 2001.

▪ *Assess and treat symptoms of depression using a standardized interview protocol.* LOE = II

(MR) A cross-sectional study ($N = 396$ nursing home residents) showed that the prevalence of depressive symptoms among patients was significantly higher according to a standardized interview (Geriatric Depression Scale) than the prevalence reported on the basis of medical record information. The treatment and management of depression required improvement for all patients (Simmons et al., 2004).

(MR) A qualitative study (grounded theory) showed that psychological well-being greatly affected appetite among older adults ($N = 15$). Stress from social conditions such as bereavement, depression, isolation, and a lack of control over one's life had been found to reduce nutrient intake among the elderly (Wikby & Fagerskiold, 2004).

(MR) An RCT ($N = 56$ primary care patients, age >65 years) demonstrated that older adults could accurately self-report overall changes in their depressive symptoms. A patient's report of at least "much improved" could be used as an estimate of at least a 50% response to depression treatment (Datto et al., 2006).

(MR) A descriptive study ($N = 30$ nursing home residents, age >64 years) showed that measuring and monitoring patients' everyday emotions may be an important innovative strategy for improving the food intake of elderly patients in institutions (Paquet et al., 2003).

(MR) A controlled study ($N = 68$, age >67 years) reported that the 10-item Center for Epidemological Studies Depression Scale had excellent properties for use as a screening instrument for the identification of major depression among older adults (Irwin et al., 1999).

Additional research: Morley & Kraenzle, 1994; Thomas et al., 2000; Blaum et al., 1995; Burrows et al., 1995.

▪ (SP) *Assess patient preferences related to nutritional care using a standardized interview such as the FoodEx-LTC (Long-Term Care).* LOE = V

(MR) A descriptive study ($N = 105$) showed that family members of nursing home residents preferred that noninvasive nutrition interventions, such as improvements in food quality and staff assistance, be attempted before the use of oral liquid supplements or appetite-stimulant medications (Simmons et al., 2003b).

(MR) A descriptive study ($N = 75$) showed that the medical record documentation (minimum data set) of residents' oral food and fluid intake and food complaints was inaccurate as compared with independent assessments by research staff using standardized direct observation (oral intake) and interview (food complaints) protocols. A total of 47% of the participants expressed stable complaints about some aspect of the nursing home's food service (e.g., variety, appearance, temperature; Simmons et al., 2002).

(NR) The FoodEx-LTC is a 44-item questionnaire for cognitively intact to mildly impaired nursing home residents to assess their satisfaction with the food and food service (Crogan et al., 2004).

(EO) A standardized brief 7-item interview developed to assess nursing home residents' dining location preferences and satisfaction with the food service can be conducted with nursing home residents who have mild to moderate cognitive impairment. Criteria for how to select residents who are appropriate for interview is also provided (BCGR, 2007).

Possibly Effective

■ *Re-evaluate the need for restricted and/or modified-texture diets for malnourished patients.* **LOE = IV**

(MR) A descriptive chart review study (*N* = 217 nursing home residents) showed that a restricted diet (i.e., altered texture and/or reduced sodium, sugar, or calorie) may contribute to malnutrition among nursing home residents (Buckler et al., 1994).

(MR) A review article suggested that the liberalization of dietary restrictions may help to increase caloric intake and prevent malnutrition among elderly patients (Aldrich & Massey, 1999).

(MR) A descriptive chart review and an observation-based study (*N* = 212 nursing home residents) showed that many residents may be inappropriately placed or maintained on altered-texture diets and that patients should be re-evaluated for feeding and swallowing skills and the appropriateness of the diet order (Groher & McKaig, 1995).

(MR) A cohort study (*N* = 2805, age >59 years) reported that monitoring cholesterol was unnecessary after the age of 70 years, because there is no evidence to support that coronary heart disease and stroke can be prevented with treatment after this age (Simons et al., 2001).

(MR) Nutritional therapy must balance medical needs and elders' desires and maintain their quality of life. Unacceptable or unpalatable diets can lead to poor food and fluid intake, which results in weight loss, malnutrition, and a spiral of negative health effects (Niedert et al., 2005).

■ *Use a red tray for patients who need help and support from staff to eat.* **LOE = VI**

(NR) An evaluation study demonstrated that using the red tray to flag patients in a hospital who needed additional time and support to eat resulted in patients being better identified and supported with their meals (Bradley & Rees, 2003).

■ *Ensure that nursing home patients who are at risk for malnutrition and/or in need of staff assistance are taken to the dining room or other common area for most meals.* **LOE = IV**

(MR) A descriptive study (*N* = 407 residents) of dementia patients in assisted-living and nursing home facilities showed that more than half had low food and fluid intake and that having meals in a public dining area and the provision of staff monitoring were associated with higher food and fluid intake (Reed et al., 2005).

(MR) A cross-sectional study (*N* = 761 nursing home residents) showed that nutritional care quality was significantly better according to two of four care process measures when patients ate meals in the dining room as compared with eating in their rooms. First, patients who were rated by staff as requiring assistance to eat were more likely to receive assistance in the dining room as compared with eating in their rooms. Second, staff medical record documentation of oral food and fluid consumption was more accurate when residents ate in the dining room (Simmons & Levy-Storms, 2005).

(MR) A controlled study (N = 48 nursing home residents) reported that food intake was improved when residents ate together in a supervised dining room (Wright et al., 2006).

▣ *Ensure that nursing home patients who are at risk for malnutrition have optimal oral status.* **LOE = IV**

(MR) A descriptive study (N = 120 nursing home residents, age >72 years) showed that poor oral status increased difficulty with eating hard foods, increased mashed food consumption, decreased eating pleasure, and placed institutionalized subjects at a higher risk of malnutrition (Lamy et al., 1999).

(MR) A descriptive study (N = 97 hospitalized patients, age >69 years) reported that oral candidiasis resulting from treatment with antibiotics, poor oral hygiene, denture wearing, and vitamin C deficiency was related to malnutrition. Oral candidiasis causes mucosal lesions that have a negative impact on energy intake, which may subsequently worsen nutritional status (Paillaud et al., 2004).

(MR) A cohort study (N = 147 long-term care residents, age >80 years) demonstrated that there were considerable unmet dental needs with significant oral disease and poor levels of oral and denture hygiene among the elderly who were living in institutions (Samaranayake et al., 1995).

(MR) A descriptive study (N = 260 long-term care residents, age >59 years) reported that oral cleanliness and dental care should be improved with regard to dentures and teeth among the institutionalized elderly (Peltola et al., 2004).

Not Effective

No applicable published research was found in this category.

Possibly Harmful

▣ *Using feeding tubes in the patient with dementia.* **LOE = I**

(MR) A comprehensive literature review showed no evidence that tube feeding improved clinical outcomes (e.g., survival, aspiration pneumonia, pressure sores) for patients with advanced dementia. In fact, the review showed much evidence of substantial risks being associated with tube feedings (Finucane et al., 1999).

(MR) A descriptive study with surrogate decision makers (N = 58) for elderly patients showed that, after 5 weeks of use, 84% stated that they would repeat the decision to place a feeding tube for their relative. However, almost one third felt that the patient would not want the tube. A greater emphasis may need to be placed on the wishes of the patient before placing feeding tubes (McNabney et al., 1994).

(MR) A descriptive study with nursing home residents (N = 379) who were deemed capable of making decisions showed that 33% would prefer a feeding tube if they were no longer able to eat as a result of brain damage. However, 25% changed their minds about wanting a tube when they were told that physical restraints are sometimes used during the feeding process. Providers need to ensure that decisions to place a feeding tube are based on comprehensive information about the care practices and the potential risks and benefits (O'Brien et al., 1997).

 Two editorial articles suggested that there may be a financial incentive for nursing homes to place feeding tubes in patients with advanced dementia as a result of a higher per diem from Medicaid and a reduction in the staff time necessary for feeding assistance care provision. The clinical appropriateness of feeding tube placement as a nutritional intervention should be carefully considered in light of these financial and staff resource incentives (Mitchell, 2003; Simmons et al., 2003b).

OUTCOME MEASUREMENT

NUTRITIONAL STATUS   NOC

Definition: Extent to which nutrients are available to meet metabolic needs.
Nutritional Status as evidenced by the following selected NOC indicators:
- Food intake
- Fluid intake
- Energy
- Weight/height ratio
- Hydration

(Rate each indicator of **Nutritional Status:** 1 = severe deviation from normal range, 2 = substantial deviation from normal range, 3 = moderate deviation from normal range, 4 = mild deviation from normal range, 5 = no deviation from normal range) (Moorhead et al., 2004).

REFERENCES

Aldrich JK, Massey LK. (1999). A liberalized geriatric diet fits most dietary prescriptions for long-term care patients. *J Am Diet Assoc*, 99(4):478-480.

Baldwin C, Parsons TJ. (2004). Dietary advice and nutritional supplements in the management of illness-related malnutrition: Systematic review. *Clin Nutr*, 23(6):1267-1279.

Blaum CS, Fries BE, Fiatarone MA. (1995). Factors associated with low body mass index and weight loss in nursing home residents. *J Gerontol A Biol Sci Med Sci*, 50(3):M162-M168.

Borun Center for Gerontological Research (BCGR). (2007). Weight loss prevention. Step 1 assessment: Nutrition and food complaints. Available online: http://borun.medsch.ucla.edu. Retrieved on July 7, 2007.

Bradley L, Rees C. (2003). Reducing nutritional risk in hospital: the red tray. *Nurs Stand*, 17(26):33-37.

Buckler DA, Kelber ST, Goodwin JS. (1994). The use of dietary restrictions in malnourished nursing home patients. *J Am Geriatr Soc*, 42(10):1100-1102.

Burrows AB, Satlin A, Salzman C, Nobel K, Lipsitz LA. (1995). Depression in a long-term care facility: Clinical features and discordance between nursing assessment and patient interviews. *J Am Geriatr Soc*, 43(10):1118-1122.

Coyne ML, Hoskins L. (1997). Improving eating behaviors in dementia using behavioral strategies. *Clin Nurs Res*, 6(3):275-290.

Crogan NL, Evans B, Velasquez D. (2004). Measuring nursing home resident satisfaction with food and food service: Initial testing of the FoodEx-LTC. *J Gerontol A Biol Sci Med Sci*, 59(4):370-377.

Datto CJ, Thompson R, Knott K, Katz IR. (2006). Older adult report of change in depressive symptoms as a treatment decision tool. *J Am Geriatr Soc*, 54(4):627-631.

Dochterman JM, Bulechek GM (Eds). (2004). *Nursing Interventions Classification (NIC)*, 4th ed. St Louis: Mosby.

Finucane TE, Christmas C, Travis K. (1999). Tube feeding in patients with advanced dementia: A review of the evidence. *JAMA*, 282(14):1365-1370.

Groher ME, McKaig TN. (1995). Dysphagia and dietary levels in skilled nursing facilities. *J Am Geriatr Soc*, 43(5):528-532.

Hodgkinson B, Evans D, Wood J. (2003). Maintaining oral hydration in older adults: A systematic review. *Int J Nurs Pract*, 9(3):S19-S28.

Irwin M, Artin KH, Oxman MN. (1999). Screening of depression in the older adult: Criterion validity of the 10-item Center for Epidemiological Studies Depression Scale (CES-D). *Arch Intern Med*, 159(15): 1701-1704.

Lad H, Gott M, Gariballa S. (2005). Elderly patients compliance and elderly patients and health professional's views and attitudes towards prescribed sip-feed supplements. *J Nutr Health Aging*, 9(5):310-314.

Lamy M, Mojon P, Kalykakis G, Legrand R, Butz-Jorgensen E. (1999). Oral status and nutrition in the institutionalized elderly. *J Dent*, 27(6):443-448.

Lange-Alberts ME, Shott S. (1994). Nutritional intake. Use of touch and verbal cueing. *J Gerontol Nurs*, 20(2):36-40.

Lauque S, Arnaud-Battandier F, Gillette S, Plaze JM, Andrieu S, Cantet C, et al. (2004). Improvement in weight and fat-free mass with oral nutritional supplementation in patients with Alzheimer's disease at risk of malnutrition: A prospective randomized study. *J Am Geriatr Soc*, 52(10):1702-1707.

Levinson Y, Dwolatzky T, Epstein A, Adler B, Epstein L. (2005). Is it possible to increase weight and maintain the protein status of debilitated elderly residents of nursing homes? *J Gerontol A Biol Sci Med Sci*, 60(7):878-881.

Locher JL, Robinson CO, Roth DL, Ritchie CS, Burgio KL. (2005). The effect of the presence of others on the caloric intake in homebound older adults. *J Gerontol A Biol Sci Med Sci*, 60(11):1475-1478.

McDaniel JH, Hunt A, Hackes B, Pope JF. (2001). Impact of dining room environment on nutritional intake of Alzheimer's residents: A case study. *Am J Alzheimers Dis Other Demen*, 16(5):297-302.

McNabney MK, Beers MH, Siebens H. (1994). Surrogate decision-makers' satisfaction with the placement of feeding tubes in elderly patients. *J Am Geriatr Soc*, 42(2):161-168.

Milne AC, Potter J, Avenell A. (2005). Protein and energy supplementation in elderly people at risk from malnutrition. *Cochrane Database Syst Rev*, (2):CD003288.

Mitchell S. (2003). Financial incentives for placing feeding tubes in nursing home residents with advanced dementia. *J Am Geriatr Soc*, 51(1):129-131.

Moorhead M, Johnson M, Maas M (Eds). (2004). *Nursing Outcomes Classification (NOC)*, 3rd ed. St Louis: Mosby.

Morley JE, Kraenzle D. (1994). Causes of weight loss in a community nursing home. *J Am Geriatr Soc*, 42(6):583-585.

Musson ND, Kincaid J, Ryan P, Glussman B, Varone L, Gamarra N, et al. (1990). Nature, nurture, nutrition: Interdisciplinary programs to address the prevention of malnutrition and dehydration. *Dysphagia*, 5(2):96-101.

Niedert KC; American Dietetic Association (ADA). (2005). Position of the American Dietetic Association: Liberalization of the diet prescription improved quality of life for older adults in long-term care. *J Am Diet Assoc*, 105(12):1955-1965.

O'Brien LA, Siegert EA, Grisso JA, Maislin GM, LaPann K, Evans LK, et al. (1997). Tube feeding preferences among nursing home residents. *J Gen Intern Med*, 12(6):364-371.

Paillaud E, Merlier I, Dupeyron C, Scherman E, Poupon J, Bories PN. (2004). Oral candidiasis and nutritional deficiencies in elderly hospitalized patients. *Br J Nutr*, 92(5):861-867.

Paquet C, St.-Arnaud-McKenzie D, Kergoat M, Ferland G, Dube L. (2003). Direct and indirect effects of everyday emotions on food intake of elderly patients in institutions. *J Gerontol A Biol Sci Med Sci*, 58(2):153-158.

Peltola P, Vehkalahti MM, Wuolijoki-Saaristo K. (2004). Oral health and treatment needs of long-term hospitalized elderly. *Gerodontology*, 21(2):93-99.

Ragneskog H, Kihlgren M, Karlsson I, Norberg A. (1996). Dinner music for demented patients: Analysis of video-recorded observations. *Clin Nurs Res*, 5(3):262-277; discussion 278-282.

NR = Nursing Research, **MR** = Multidisciplinary Research, **SP** = Standard of Practice, **EO** = Expert Opinion, **LOE** = Level of Evidence

Reed PS, Zimmerman S, Sloane PD, Williams CS, Boustani M. (2005). Characteristics associated with low food and fluid intake in long-term care residents with dementia. *Gerontologist,* 45 Spec No 1(1):74-80.

Samaranayake LP, Wilkieson CA, Lamey PJ, MacFarlane TW. (1995). Oral disease in the elderly in long-term hospitals care. *Oral Dis,* 1(3):147-151.

Simmons SF, Alessi C, Schnelle JF. (2001a). An intervention to increase fluid intake in nursing home residents: Prompting and preference compliance. *J Am Geriatr Soc,* 49(7):926-933.

Simmons SF, Cadogan MP, Cabrera GR, Al-Samarrai NR, Jorge JS, Levy-Storms L, et al. (2004). The minimum data set depression quality indicator: Does it reflect differences in care processes? *Gerontologist,* 44(4):554-564.

Simmons SF, Garcia ET, Cadogan MP, Al-Samarrai NR, Levy-Storms LF, Osterweil D, et al. (2003a). The minimum data set weight-loss quality indicator: Does it reflect differences in care processes related to weight loss? *J Am Geriatr Soc,* 51(10):1410-1418.

Simmons SF, Lam H, Rao G, Schnelle JF. (2003b). Family members' preferences for nutrition interventions to improve nursing home residents' oral food and fluid intake. *J Am Geriatr Soc,* 51(1):69-74.

Simmons SF, Levy-Storms L. (2005). The effect of dining location on nutritional care quality in nursing homes. *J Nutr Health Aging,* 9(6):434-439.

Simmons SF, Lim B, Schnelle JF. (2002). Accuracy of minimum data set in identifying residents at risk for undernutrition: Oral intake and food complaints. *J Am Med Dir Assoc,* 3(3):140-145.

Simmons SF, Osterweil D, Schnelle JF. (2001b). Improving food intake in nursing home residents with feeding assistance: A staffing analysis. *J Gerontol A Biol Sci Med Sci,* 56(12):M790-M794.

Simmons SF, Patel AV. (2006). Nursing home staff delivery of oral liquid nutritional supplements to residents at risk for unintentional weight loss. *J Am Geriatr Soc,* 54(9):1372-1376.

Simmons SF, Schnelle JF. (2004). Individualized feeding assistance care for nursing home residents: Staffing requirements to implement two interventions. *J Gerontol A Biol Sci Med Sci,* 59(9):M966-M973.

Simons LA, Simons J, Friedlander Y, McCallum J. (2001). Cholesterol and other lipids predict coronary heart disease and ischaemic stroke in the elderly, but only in those below 70 years. *Atherosclerosis,* 159(1):201-208.

Thomas DR, Ashmen W, Morley JE, Evans WJ. (2000). Nutritional management in long term care: Development of a clinical guideline. Council for Nutritional Strategies in Long-Term Care. *J Gerontol A Biol Sci Med Sci,* 55(12):M725-M734.

Turic A, Gordon KL, Craig LD, Ataya DG, Voss AC. (1998). Nutrition supplementation enables elderly residents of long-term care facilities to meet or exceed RDAs without displacing energy or nutrient intakes from meals. *J Am Diet Assoc,* 98(12):1457-1459.

Wikby K, Fagerskiold A. (2004). The willingness to eat. An investigation of the appetite among elderly people. *Scand J Caring Sci,* 18(2):120-127.

Wilson MM, Purushothaman R, Morley JE. (2002). Effects of liquid dietary supplements on energy intake in the elderly. *Am J Clin Nutr,* 75(5):944-947.

Wright L, Hickson M, Frost G. (2006). Eating together is important: Using a dining room in an acute elderly medical ward increases energy intake. *J Hum Nutr Diet,* 19(1):23-26.

Young KW, Binns MA, Greenwood CE. (2001). Meal delivery practices do not meet needs of Alzheimer patients with increased cognitive and behavioral difficulties in long-term care facilities. *J Gerontol A Biol Sci Med Sci,* 56(10):M656-M661.

Young KW, Greenwood CE, van Reekum R, Binns MA. (2004). Providing nutrient supplements to institutionalized seniors with probable Alzheimer's disease is least beneficial in those with low body weight status. *J Am Geriatr Soc,* 52(8):1305-1312.

 # WEIGHT REDUCTION ASSISTANCE

Marina Martinez-Kratz, MS, RN; Betty J. Ackley, MSN, EdS, RN

NIC **Definition:** Facilitating the loss of weight and/or body fat (Dochterman & Bulechek, 2004).

RCT = Randomized Controlled (Clinical) Trial, **NIC** = Nursing Interventions Classification, **NOC** = Nursing Outcomes Classification

NURSING ACTIVITIES

Effective

- *Use a low-calorie diet to enhance weight loss.* **LOE = I**

  (MR) A systematic review demonstrated that safe choices for weight loss included low-calorie diets such as the Dietary Approach to Stop Hypertension diet or a Weight Watchers type of diet (Strychar, 2006).

  (MR) A descriptive study of the National Weight Control Registry members ($N = 4800$) who had maintained a weight loss of at least 33 kg for more than 5 years indicated that eating a low-calorie, low-fat diet was one of many factors associated with maintenance of the weight loss (Wing & Phelan, 2005).

- *Perform moderate-intensity physical activity for 30 to 60 minutes most days of the week.* **LOE = III**

  (MR) A Cochrane review found evidence that exercise resulted in weight loss, especially when exercise was combined with a change in diet (Shaw et al., 2006).

  (MR) A controlled clinical trial ($N = 56$) suggested that 30 minutes of walking on most days of the week may be as beneficial as 60 minutes (in combination with diet) for promoting weight loss (Bond Brill et al., 2002).

  (MR) A descriptive study of the National Weight Control Registry members ($N = 4800$) who had maintained a weight loss of at least 33 kg for more than 5 years indicated that exercising 1 hour per day was one of many factors associated with maintenance of the weight loss (Wing & Phelan, 2005).

  (EO) Exercise lasting 60 to 90 minutes per day is needed for many to lose weight, but significant health benefits can be obtained by exercising for 30 minutes per day (Jakicic & Otto, 2006).

  (MR) A controlled study ($N = 3$) demonstrated that the use of a pedometer along with brief e-counseling resulted in two times the usual amount of activity and weight loss among over-weight adults (VanWormer, 2004).

  (MR) A controlled study ($N = 80$) demonstrated that middle-aged women who walked more had lower body mass indices (BMIs) and that women who walked 10,000 or more steps per day were in the normal range for BMI (Thompson et al., 2004).

- *Use a primarily plant-based or vegetarian diet to lose weight.* **LOE = I**

  (NR) A systematic review of 40 studies demonstrated that the weight and BMI of vegetarians was on average 3% to 20% lower than that of nonvegetarians (Berkow & Barnard, 2006).

  (MR) An RCT called the Prefer Study ($N = 197$) demonstrated that people who voluntarily chose a lacto-ovo-vegetarian diet as part of weight loss treatment were able to continue with the diet for 18 months (Burke et al., 2006).

- *Teach appropriate food portion sizes.* **LOE = II**

  (MR) An RCT ($N = 76$) found that group training was effective for teaching individuals to accurately estimate and measure food portion sizes (Ayala, 2006).

  (MR) A controlled study ($N = 177$) of young adults who self-selected portion sizes for breakfast and dinner demonstrated significantly increased portion sizes than those recommended, which predisposed these individuals to weight gain (Schwartz & Byrd-Bredbenner, 2006).

NR = Nursing Research, **MR** = Multidisciplinary Research, **SP** = Standard of Practice, **EO** = Expert Opinion, **LOE** = Level of Evidence

■ *Incorporate behavior modification techniques.* LOE = I

(MR) A Cochrane review found that cognitive-behavioral therapy in combination with a diet and exercise intervention resulted in more weight loss than diet and exercise alone. Behavioral therapy used independently as a standalone therapy also resulted in significant weight loss (Shaw et al., 2005).

(MR) A Cochrane review found that weight loss methods including dietary, exercise, or behavioral interventions resulted in significant weight loss among people with prediabetes and in a decrease in the development of diabetes (Norris et al., 2005).

(MR) An RCT ($N = 92$) demonstrated that adding e-counseling to a basic Internet weight loss intervention program significantly improved weight loss (Tate et al., 2003).

■ *Use combination approaches to weight loss.* LOE = I

(MR) A systematic review of RCTs demonstrated that adding behavior therapy or exercise to diet improved weight loss (Avenell et al., 2004).

Possibly Effective

■ *Recommend the eating of a healthy breakfast every morning.* LOE = III

(MR) An observational study ($N = 867$) demonstrated that people who skipped breakfast were more likely to overeat in the evening and that eating late at night resulted in an increased calorie intake (deCastro, 2004).

(MR) A controlled study ($N = 499$) demonstrated that people who skipped breakfast were 450 times more likely to be obese (Ma et al., 2003).

(MR) A descriptive study of people who binge ate ($N = 173$) found that less than half of the people ate breakfast (43%) and that those who did weighed less than those who did not (Masheb & Grilo, 2006).

(MR) A descriptive study of the National Weight Control Registry members ($N = 4800$) who had maintained a weight loss of at least 33 kg for more than 5 years indicated that eating breakfast regularly was one of many factors associated with maintenance of the weight loss (Wing & Phelan, 2005).

■ *Use self-help weight loss programs.* LOE = II

(MR) An RCT ($N = 423$) that compared two groups—those using a commercial weight loss program and those using a self-help weight loss program—demonstrated that the self-help group was able to lose weight and maintain the weight loss for approximately 1 year (Heshka et al., 2003).

Not Effective

■ *Using a low-carbohydrate diet to lose weight.* LOE = II

(MR) A systematic review of 107 studies demonstrated that there was insufficient evidence to make recommendations for or against the use of a low-carbohydrate diet for weight loss (Bravata et al., 2003).

(MR) A systematic review demonstrated that safe choices for weight loss did not include a low-carbohydrate diet (Strychar, 2006).

RCT = Randomized Controlled (Clinical) Trial, **NIC** = Nursing Interventions Classification, **NOC** = Nursing Outcomes Classification

Possibly Harmful

■ *Using a severely restricted low-carbohydrate diet with high fat and protein intake.* **LOE = VII**

(EO) Diets that are severely restricted in carbohydrates and high in fat may cause the formation of atherosclerosis in blood vessels, and they may also predispose individuals to hypertension and cancer (Strychar, 2006).

■ *Using very-low-calorie diets (modified fasts).* **LOE = VII**

(EO) These diets are indicated only for the obese. They have been associated with complications including cholelithiasis, loss of muscle, ketosis, increased serum uric acid, and sudden death (Strychar, 2006).

OUTCOME MEASUREMENT

WEIGHT CONTROL (NOC)

(Please refer to *Nursing Outcomes Classification* [Moorhead et al., 2004] for the **Weight Control** outcome.)

REFERENCES

Avenell A, Brown TJ, McGee MA, Campbell MK, Grant AM, Broom J, et al. (2004). What interventions should we add to weight reducing diets in adults with obesity? A systematic review of randomized controlled trials of adding drug therapy, exercise, behaviour therapy or combinations of these interventions. *J Hum Nutr Diet,* 17(4):293-316.

Ayala GX. (2006). An experimental evaluation of a group- versus computer-based intervention to improve food portion size estimation skills. *Health Educ Res,* 21(1):133-145.

Berkow SE, Barnard N. (2006). Vegetarian diets and weight status. *Nutr Rev,* 64(4):175-188.

Bond Brill J, Perry AC, Parker L, Robinson A, Burnett K. (2002). Dose-response effect of walking exercise on weight loss. How much is enough? *Int J Obes Relat Metab Disord,* 26(11):1484-1493.

Bravata DM, Sanders L, Huang J, Krumholz HM, Olkin I, Gardner CD, et al. (2003). Efficacy and safety of low-carbohydrate diets: A systematic review. *JAMA,* 289(14):1837-1850.

Burke LE, Choo J, Music E, Warziski M, Styn MA, Kim Y, et al. (2006). PREFER study: A randomized clinical trial testing treatment preference and two dietary options in behavioral weight management–rationale, design and baseline characteristics. *Contemp Clin Trials,* 27(1):34-48.

deCastro JM. (2004). The time of day of food intake influences overall intake in humans. *J Nutr,* 134(1):104-111.

Dochterman JM, Bulechek GM (Eds). (2004). *Nursing Interventions Classification (NIC),* 4th ed. St Louis: Mosby.

Heshka S, Anderson JW, Atkinson RL, Greenway FL, Hill JO, Phinney SD, et al. (2003). Weight loss with self-help compared with a structured commercial program: A randomized trial. *JAMA,* 289(14): 1792-1798.

Jakicic JM, Otto AD. (2006). Treatment and prevention of obesity: What is the role of exercise? *Nutr Rev,* 64(2 Pt 2):S57-S61.

Ma Y, Bertone ER, Stanek EJ III, Reed GW, Hebert JR, Cohen NL, et al. (2003). Association between eating patterns and obesity in a free-living US adult population. *Am J Epidemiol,* 158(1):85-92.

Masheb RM, Grilo CM. (2006). Eating patterns and breakfast consumption in obese patients with binge eating disorder. *Behav Res Ther,* 44(11):1545-1553.

Moorhead M, Johnson M, Maas M (Eds). (2004). *Nursing Outcomes Classification (NOC)*, 3rd ed. St Louis: Mosby.

Norris SL, Zhang X, Avenell, Gregg E, Schmid CH, Lau J. (2005). Long-term non-pharmacological weight loss interventions for adults with prediabetes. *Cochrane Database Syst Rev*, (2):CD005270.

Schwartz J, Byrd-Bredbenner C. (2006). Portion distortion: Typical portion sizes selected by young adults. *J Am Diet Assoc*, 106(9):1412-1418.

Shaw K, Gennat H, O'Rourke P, Del Mar C. (2006). Exercise for overweight or obesity. *Cochrane Database Syst Rev*, (4):CD003817.

Shaw K, O'Rourke P, Del Mar C, Kenardy J. (2005). Psychological interventions for overweight or obesity. *Cochrane Database Syst Rev*, (2):CD003818.

Strychar I. (2006). Diet in the management of weight loss. *CMAJ*, 174(1):56-63.

Tate DF, Jackvony EH, Wing RR. (2003). Effects of Internet behavioral counseling on weight loss in adults at risk for type 2 diabetes: A randomized trial. *JAMA*, 289(14):1833-1836.

Thompson DL, Rakow J, Perdue SM. (2004). Relationship between accumulated walking and body composition in middle-aged women. *Med Sci Sports Exerc*, 36(5):911-914.

VanWormer JJ. (2004). Pedometers and brief e-counseling: Increasing physical activity for overweight adults. *J Appl Behav Anal*, 37(3):421-425.

Wing RR, Phelan S. (2005). Long-term weight loss maintenance. *Am J Clin Nutr*, 82(1 Suppl):222S-225S.

WOUND CARE   NIC

Mary E. Hagle, PhD, RN, AOCN; Kathleen M. Kochanski, BSN, RN-BC;
Deborah L. Gentile, MSN, RN-BC; Jan Avakian-Kopatich, BSN, RN, CWON

NIC **Definition:** Prevention of wound complications and the promotion of wound healing (Dochterman & Bulechek, 2004).

NURSING ACTIVITIES

Effective

■ *Use standard assessment criteria and a measurement protocol to evaluate wound status and treatment effectiveness (healing), including the following: location; type of tissue at wound base or visible (e.g., granulated, necrotic, eschar); size, shape, and depth of wound; presence of undermining or tunneling; exudate (i.e., amount, type, character, odor); presence or absence of infection; wound edges (e.g., open or closed, macerated, indurated, rashy); stage of pressure ulcer, if appropriate; and condition of periwound skin. Document this information.* **LOE = V**

EO A narrative review of the literature critically evaluated wound measurement techniques and components of a measurement protocol, including the use of a digital planimeter (Flanagan, 2003).

NR A retrospective descriptive study evaluated the quality and accuracy of the documentation of pressure ulcers and interventions for 413 patients as compared with previous patient physical examinations. Pressure ulcer prevalence was underrepresented by 19% when

RCT = Randomized Controlled (Clinical) Trial, **NIC** = Nursing Interventions Classification, **NOC** = Nursing Outcomes Classification

documentation was used versus physical examination, and the quality of pressure ulcer description was poor (Gunningberg & Ehrenberg, 2004).

(EO) Effectively communicate and evaluate wound assessment and intervention by using risk assessment tools, wound assessment tools, and photography (Hess, 2005).

(NR) A systematic review supported the Agency for Health Care Policy and Research Clinical Practice Guideline of 1999 for pressure ulcer wound assessment criteria (WOCN, 2003).

■ *Reassess wounds for noticeable deterioration at each dressing change, when a patient returns from the operating room, when a wound develops an odor or purulent exudates, or when there are other significant changes. Reassess and measure a wound every 7 days or upon discharge, admission, or transfer between facilities. Document this information.* **LOE = V**

(EO) Recommendations for skin and wound assessment and reassessment parameters and frequency are based on normal tissue and wound healing anatomy and physiology in addition to expected patient outcomes on the basis of the care setting (Doughty, 2004).

(NR) A systematic review critically evaluated five types of wound measurement techniques for aspects of measurement, including wound area and depth, monitoring healing, and predicting healing. On the basis of the analysis of published studies, the recommendation was made for evaluating venous leg ulcer therapy based on a percentage of wound healing over a specified time period (Flanagan, 2003).

(NR) On the basis of a systematic review of the literature, clinical practice guidelines were developed for the prevention and management of pressure ulcers. One of the recommendations included the frequency for conducting wound assessment and reassessment (WOCN, 2003).

■ *Assess for initial healing after 1 week of treatment and then weekly; reduction in the measured wound area by at least 15% per week represents normal healing.* **LOE = V**

(EO) If healing does not progress as expected, a change in therapy is recommended (Attinger et al., 2006).

(MR) A prospective descriptive study of long-term care, long-term acute care, and home care identified healing times for 433 patients with 767 wounds when standardized protocols were used and found that stage II pressure ulcers or partial-thickness venous ulcers healed in an average of 29 to 31 days. About one third of full-thickness chronic wounds healed in an average of 62 days (Bolton et al., 2004).

(EO) A healing rate reduction of less than 20% to 40% over the initial 2 to 4 weeks indicates that healing is not progressing (Flanagan, 2003).

(MR) A narrative review evaluating 28 articles about methods of measuring wound healing and comparing three formulas for assessing the rate of healing recommended a standard formula to evaluate wound healing, and it also recommended assessing wound healing at 2 and 4 weeks and setting benchmarks at 4-week intervals (Jessup, 2006).

(EO) Partial-thickness pressure ulcers (stage II) should show evidence of healing within 1 to 2 weeks. Reduction in wound size after 2 weeks of therapy for stage III and IV pressure ulcers may predict healing (WOCN, 2003).

■ **Assess for and correct, when possible, comorbid conditions, immobility, nutritional status, and medications that may affect healing in addition to the underlying causes of tissue damage. LOE = V**

(MR) A systematic review of a variety of studies provided an algorithm for the treatment of chronic wounds that focused on three components: "treating the cause, providing local wound care, and addressing patient-centered concerns." Thirteen evidence-based recommendations were made that addressed each of the components (Sibbald et al., 2000).

(NR) A systematic review supported the Agency for Health Care Policy and Research Clinical Practice Guideline of 1999 recommendation to assess for factors that may hamper healing, such as malignancy, diabetes, cerebral vascular accident, heart failure, renal failure, pneumonia, immobility, and malnutrition, and for the medications that may impair healing, including steroids, immunosuppressive agents, and antineoplastic agents (WOCN, 2003).

■ **Assess for acute and chronic pain associated with wounds and wound care. LOE = VI**

(NR) A systematic review of the literature ($N = 13$ publications) indicated the McGill Pain Questionnaire, a visual analog scale, and the Faces Rating Scale were useful for assessing pressure ulcer pain (de Laat et al., 2005).

(MR) In a comprehensive review of the anatomy and physiology of pain and how it relates to wound pain, the physiological evidence guided the type of assessment parameters that were recommended and the need for the multidimensional assessment of wound pain (Popescu & Salcido, 2004).

(NR) A prospective descriptive study ($N = 5957$) identified the pain behaviors associated with six procedures that were commonly performed in acute care settings, including turning, central venous catheter insertion, wound drain removal, wound care, tracheal suctioning, and femoral catheter removal. This evaluation of an instrument that was designed to describe facial responses to pain, verbal and body movement behaviors, pain intensity, and procedural distress explained only 33% of the variance in behavioral activity during painful procedures. Behaviors that inferred procedural pain included grimace, rigidity, wincing, closed eyes, and verbal complaints. The recognition of pain behaviors was proposed as a way to identify the need for analgesic interventions when patients were unable to verbally describe their pain (Puntillo et al., 2004).

(NR) A comparative descriptive study ($N = 28$) compared the pain experienced at rest and during a dressing change by patients with stage II, III, and IV pressure ulcers. A number of design flaws, such as a small sample size, a lack of control for analgesics, pressure reduction devices, and types of dressings used resulted in a failure to support any of the study hypotheses concerning pain intensity related to pressure ulcer stage, rest versus dressing change, or rest versus dressing change at each stage of ulcer. The study concluded that the majority of patients with pressure ulcers experienced pain at rest and during dressing changes (Szor & Bourguignon, 1999).

■ **Manage pain during wound care. LOE = V**

(NR) A systematic review of the literature ($N = 13$ publications) reported effective wound pain relief using the local application of morphine gel or benzydamine gel (de Laat et al., 2005).

RCT = Randomized Controlled (Clinical) Trial, **NIC** = Nursing Interventions Classification, **NOC** = Nursing Outcomes Classification

(EO) Treatment options for wound pain resulting from pressure ulcers include systemic analgesia, lidocaine patches, and a variety of nonpharmacological interventions (Popescu & Salcido, 2004).

(MR) A descriptive study ($N = 50$) concluded that mild to moderate pain experienced during wound care was relieved by medications and positioning. Quality-of-life variables such as physical activity and social functioning were also affected by wound pain (Shukla et al., 2005).

■ *Prepare the wound bed for optimal healing by removing foreign bodies and necrotic or abnormal tissue and reducing the amount of exudates and the bacterial load. This is done through debridement methods, including autolytic, enzymatic, biodebridement, mechanical, surgical, conservative sharp, and laser; no one method is optimal.* **LOE = VII**

(EO) An overview article stated that wound bed preparation was a multistep process used to accelerate the patient's tissue healing and to facilitate the effectiveness of other treatments (Hess & Kirsner, 2003).

(MR) A systematic review of a variety of studies provided an algorithm with a feedback loop for debridement and the treatment of chronic wounds. It identified the best treatment for specific wounds and addressed other components of treatment, such as the cause of the wound and wound bed viability (Sibbald et al., 2000).

(NR) On the basis of a systematic review of the literature, clinical practice guidelines were developed for the management of pressure ulcers. Using an evidence rating based on the type of study design, specific debridement methods were reviewed and recommended in addition to identifying debridement methods that needed further research (WOCN, 2003).

■ *Use dressings that retain moisture, remove exudates, promote gas exchange, provide insulation, and protect the wound from bacteria and contaminants.* **LOE = VII**

(MR) A comprehensive and critical review of current wound care techniques identified key functions for wound dressings and which type of dressing was recommended on the basis of wound characteristics (Attinger et al., 2006).

■ *Use compression for the treatment of venous stasis leg ulcers.* **LOE = V**

(MR) A systematic review of research supported a 1997 systematic review recommendation of compression treatment for the underlying cause of venous leg ulcers (Sibbald et al., 2000).

Possibly Effective

■ *Assess for odor after the wound is cleaned; excessive, foul, pungent, fecal, strong, or musty odor may indicate bacterial colonization or infection.* **LOE = VII**

(EO) Odor helps identify the presence of bacteria or infection in the wound and possibly the type of bacteria (Hess & Kirsner, 2003).

■ *Use topical negative pressure wound treatment (NPWT) for stage III and IV pressure ulcers, diabetic wounds, surgical wounds, and other wounds.* **LOE = VII**

(MR) A systematic review concluded that NPWT may be more effective than wet saline gauze dressings to assist with the healing of specific wounds, but the evidence is cautionary.

NR = Nursing Research, **MR** = Multidisciplinary Research, **SP** = Standard of Practice, **EO** = Expert Opinion, **LOE** = Level of Evidence

This conclusion is based on two RCTs having sample sizes of 10 and 24 patients with chronic or diabetic wounds and comparing NPWT to wet saline gauze dressings (Evans & Land, 2001).

(EO) A narrative review of the literature on NPWT recommended NPWT for many types of wounds, including acute, chronic, traumatic, and dehisced wounds; pressure and diabetic ulcers; and flaps, grafts, and partial-thickness burns. Contraindications to NPWT, an algorithm for the use of NPWT, and care procedures were also presented (Gupta et al., 2004).

(NR) A systematic review recommended NPWT as an adjunctive therapy for consideration (WOCN, 2003).

(EO) NPWT is effective both clinically and economically (Kaufman & Pahl, 2003).

(MR) In a retrospective, descriptive study, NPWT was effective for healing a variety of wounds in 51 pediatric patients (Caniano et al., 2005).

▪ Use silver-based dressings for chronic leg wounds. LOE = VI

(NR) A prospective descriptive study of 30 patients with various types of chronic wounds evaluated a silver-based Hydrofiber dressing for 4 weeks for wound healing. Wound size decreased 27% in half of the subjects. No statistical evaluation was done, and no control group was used (Coutts & Sibbald, 2005).

(MR) A health-economic analysis was done using six studies that addressed four types of wound care protocols, including a silver-based foam dressing, for chronic leg wounds. Two protocols were clinically and equally effective; however, the economic analysis identified that one of the clinically effective protocols was financially superior and thus recommended for use (Scanlon et al., 2005).

▪ Use noncontact normothermic wound therapy (radiant heat). LOE = II

(MR) A prospective RCT was conducted in one acute care hospital and seven long-term–care settings with 40 patients having stage III and IV pressure ulcers. The healing rate was significantly greater in the treatment group ($p < .02$), and a trend was seen in the incidence of closure during the trial period (Kloth et al., 2002).

▪ Use topical hyperbaric oxygen therapy (THOT) as primary treatment or as an adjunctive therapy for numerous chronic wounds. LOE = I

(MR) A systematic review concluded that the use of THOT for patients with chronic foot ulcers may significantly reduce the risk of amputation and may improve the probability of healing within a 1-year length of time. The summary, which was based on five trials and included 147 patients, should be interpreted cautiously as a result of numerous limitations (Kranke et al., 2004).

(MR) A systematic review of more than 2000 patients concluded that THOT may be effective for the treatment of compromised skin grafts, osteoradionecrosis, soft-tissue radionecrosis, gas gangrene, progressive necrotizing fasciitis, and chronic nonhealing diabetic wounds. The review also identified potentially serious side effects of THOT, including barotraumatic otitis, seizures, pneumothorax, and pulmonary edema (Wang et al., 2003).

RCT = Randomized Controlled (Clinical) Trial, **NIC** = Nursing Interventions Classification, **NOC** = Nursing Outcomes Classification

Not Effective

■ *Using silver-based wound dressings and topical agents for diabetic foot ulcers.* **LOE = I**

(MR) A systematic review revealed no RCTs or controlled clinical trials with which to evaluate the use of silver-based dressings or topical agents for diabetic foot infections or ulcers (Bergin & Wraight, 2006).

■ *Using therapeutic touch for healing acute wounds.* **LOE = I**

(MR) A systematic review of four RCTs used therapeutic touch as the treatment for experimentally induced wounds made with a skin biopsy instrument. There was insufficient evidence to support the use of therapeutic touch to promote acute wound healing (O'Mathuna & Ashford, 2003).

Possibly Harmful

■ *Attaching NPWT sponges and equipment to wall suction.* **LOE = VII**

(MR) A summary review of articles and studies from 1996 to 2006 identified the indications and complications of topical NPWT. Several adverse events resulted from attaching the equipment to wall suction, from failing to activate the suction on the equipment, and from residual sponges in the wound (Argenta et al., 2006).

■ *Using topical agents that are toxic to cells (antiseptic) to heal wounds when the agent is applied as part of wound care (e.g., a gel) and not as an irrigating solution (refer to the guideline on Wound Irrigation). Such agents include povidone-iodine, chlorhexidine, and hydrogen peroxide.* **LOE = VII**

(EO) For wound bed preparation and the use of topical agents, topical antiseptic agents are not selective with regard to their antimicrobial action, and they damage all cells on contact (Warriner & Burrell, 2005).

OUTCOME MEASUREMENT

WOUND HEALING: PRIMARY INTENTION   (NOC)

Definition: Extent of the regeneration of cells and tissues following intentional closure.
Wound Healing: Primary Intention as evidenced by the following selected NOC indicators:
• Skin approximation
• Wound edge approximation
(Rate each indicator of **Wound Healing: Primary Intention:** 1 = none, 2 = limited, 3 = moderate, 4 = substantial, 5 = extensive) (Moorhead et al., 2004).

REFERENCES

Argenta LC, Morykwas MJ, Marks MW, DeFranzo AJ, Molnar JA, David LR. (2006). Vacuum-assisted closure: State of clinic art. *Plast Reconstr Surg*, 117(7 Suppl):127S-142S.

NR = Nursing Research, **MR** = Multidisciplinary Research, **SP** = Standard of Practice, **EO** = Expert Opinion, **LOE** = Level of Evidence

Attinger CE, Janis JE, Steinberg J, Schwartz J, Al-Attar A, Couch K. (2006). Clinical approach to wounds: Debridement and wound bed preparation including the use of dressings and wound-healing adjuvants. *Plast Reconstr Surg,* 117(7 Suppl):72S-109S.

Bergin SM, Wraight P. (2006). Silver based wound dressings and topical agents for treating diabetic foot ulcers. *Cochrane Database Syst Rev,* (1):CD005082.

Bolton L, McNees P, van Rijswijk L, de Leon J, Lyder C, Kobza L, et al. (2004). Wound-healing outcomes using standardized assessment and care in clinical practice. *J Wound Ostomy Continence Nurs,* 31(2): 65-71.

Caniano D, Ruth B, Teich S. (2005). Wound management with vacuum-assisted closure: Experience in 51 pediatric patients. *J Pediatr Surg,* 40(1):128-132.

Coutts P, Sibbald RG. (2005). The effect of a silver-containing Hydrofiber® dressing on superficial wound bed and bacterial balance of chronic wounds. *Int Wound J,* 2(4):348-356.

de Laat EH, Scholte op Reimer WJ, van Achterberg T. (2005). Pressure ulcers: Diagnostics and interventions aimed at wound-related complaints: A review of the literature. *J Clin Nurs,* 14(4):464-472.

Dochterman JM, Bulechek GM (Eds). (2004). *Nursing Interventions Classification (NIC),* 4th ed. St Louis: Mosby.

Doughty D. (2004). Wound assessment: Tips and techniques. *Adv Skin Wound Care,* 17(7):369-372.

Evans D, Land L. (2001). Topical negative pressure for treating chronic wounds. *Cochrane Database Syst Rev,* (1):CD001898.

Flanagan M. (2003). Improving accuracy of wound measurement in clinical practice. *Ostomy Wound Manage,* 49(10):28-40.

Gunningberg L, Ehrenberg A. (2004). Accuracy and quality in the nursing documentation of pressure ulcers: A comparison of record content and patient examination. *J Wound Ostomy Continence Nurs,* 31(6):328-335.

Gupta S, Baharestani M, Baranoski S, de Leon J, Engel SJ, Mendez-Eastman S, et al. (2004). Guidelines for managing pressure ulcers with negative pressure wound therapy. *Adv Skin Wound Care,* 17(Suppl 2):1-16.

Hess CT. (2005). The art of skin and wound care documentation. *Adv Skin Wound Care,* 18(1):43-53.

Hess CT, Kirsner RS. (2003). Orchestrating the wound healing: Assessing and preparing the wound bed. *Adv Skin Wound Care,* 16(5):246-259.

Jessup R. (2006). What is the best method for assessing the rate of wound healing? A comparison of 3 mathematical formulas. *Adv Skin Wound Care,* 19(3):138-147.

Kaufman MW, Pahl DW. (2003). Vacuum-assisted closure therapy: Wound care and nursing implications. *Dermatol Nurs,* 15(4):317-20, 323-325.

Kloth LC, Berman JE, Nett M, Papanek PE, Dumit-Minkel S. (2002). A randomized controlled clinical trial to evaluate the effects of noncontact normothermic wound therapy on chronic full-thickness pressure ulcers. Adv Skin Wound Care, 15(6):270-276.

Kranke P, Bennett M, Roeckl-Wiedmann I, Debus S. (2004). Hyperbaric oxygen therapy for chronic wounds. *Cochrane Database Syst Rev,* (2):CD004123.

Moorhead M, Johnson M, Maas M (Eds). (2004). *Nursing Outcomes Classification (NOC),* 3rd ed. St Louis: Mosby.

O'Mathuna DP, Ashford RL. (2003). Therapeutic touch for healing acute wounds. *Cochrane Database Syst Rev,* (4):CD002766.

Popescu A, Salcido R. (2004). Wound pain: a challenge for the patient and the wound care specialist. *Adv Skin Wound Care,* 17(1):14-20.

Puntillo KA, Morris AB, Thompson CL, Stanik-Hutt J, White CA, Wild LR. (2004). Pain behaviors observed during six common procedures: results from Thunder Project II. *Crit Care Med,* 32(2): 421-427.

Scanlon E, Karlsmark T, Leaper D, Carter K, Poulsen P, Hart-Hansen K, et al. (2005). Cost-effective faster wound healing with a sustained silver-releasing foam dressing in delayed healing leg ulcers—a health-economic analysis. *Int Wound J,* 2(2):150-160.

Shukla D, Tripathi AK, Agrawal S, Ansari MA, Rastogi A, Shukla VK. (2005). Pain in acute and chronic wounds: A descriptive study. *Ostomy Wound Manage,* 51(11):47-51.

Sibbald RG, Williamson D, Orsted H, Campbell K, Keast D, Krasner D, et al. (2000). Preparing the wound bed—debridement, bacterial balance, and moisture balance. *Ostomy Wound Manage,* 46(11): 14-35.

RCT = Randomized Controlled (Clinical) Trial, **NIC** = Nursing Interventions Classification, **NOC** = Nursing Outcomes Classification

Szor JK, Bourguignon C. (1999). Description of pressure ulcer pain at rest and at dressing change. *J Wound Ostomy Continence Nurs*, 26(3):115-120.

Wang C, Schwaitzberg S, Berliner E, Zarin DA, Lau J. (2003). Hyperbaric oxygen for treating wounds: A systematic review of the literature. *Arch Surg*, 138(3):272-279.

Warriner R, Burrell R. (2005). Infection and the chronic wound: A focus on silver. *Adv Skin Wound Care*, 18(Suppl 1):2-12.

Wound, Ostomy and Continence Nurses Society (WOCN). (2003). *Guideline for prevention and management of pressure ulcers.* Glenview, IL: WOCN.

 # WOUND IRRIGATION

Mary E. Hagle, PhD, RN, AOCN; Jan Avakian-Kopatich, BSN, RN, CWON

NIC **Definition:** Flushing of an open wound to cleanse and remove debris and excessive drainage (Dochterman & Bulechek, 2004).

NURSING ACTIVITIES

Effective

No applicable published research was found in this category.

Possibly Effective

■ *For adults, use tap water in the shower 24 to 48 hours after surgery to cleanse the wound with or without an additional cleansing agent or keep the wound dry until it is healed.* **LOE = V**

(Note: Before using tap water, it is particularly important to evaluate the water quality, the nature of the wound, and the patient's age and general condition, including immunosuppression and other comorbidities.)

(NR) A systematic review declared that there was insufficient evidence to support or discount tap water for wound cleansing. However, the review evaluated three quasi-experimental studies of adult patients after surgery or with sutured soft-tissue lacerations. Sample sizes were 200, 121, and 817 patients, and outcomes measured infection and wound healing. No statistically significant differences were found between the use of tap water and not cleansing with regard to the incidence of infection or delayed wound healing. Patients who could shower reported feelings of well-being. Consider water quality and other factors before using tap water as an irrigation solution (Fernandez et al., 2002).

(NR) One quasi-experimental study of 705 patients evaluated by a systematic review found some support for lower infection rates when wounds were cleansed with tap water versus normal saline ($p = .04$), although the cleansing agents were different temperatures (Fernandez et al., 2002).

(NR) In a review of the literature, four RCTs with a total of 483 surgical patients found no significant differences in infection or healing when data were pooled (JBI, 2003).

■ *Use 1% povidone-iodine to cleanse contaminated wounds.* **LOE = II**

(EO) A solution of 1% povidone-iodine is recommended to cleanse contaminated wounds (JBI, 2003).

NR = Nursing Research, **MR** = Multidisciplinary Research, **SP** = Standard of Practice, **EO** = Expert Opinion, **LOE** = Level of Evidence

(NR) A systematic review recommended 1% povidone-iodine rather than normal saline to cleanse contaminated wounds in adults on the basis of a well-designed RCT with 56 patients having both contaminated and clean wounds that demonstrated a significant difference in reduction of infection ($p<.01$) and improved wound healing ($p<.005$). A quasi-experimental study with 531 patients having various wounds reported no difference in infection rates between povidone-iodine, normal saline, or Shur-Clens (pluronic F-68). Two small controlled studies also supported the use of 1% povidone-iodine for the treatment of contaminated wounds (Fernandez et al., 2004).

(MR) A systematic review of research on the use of povidone-iodine supported its continued use for wound cleansing. The review evaluated each study on a rating system and used only the results from the higher-rated studies, which provided strong support for povidone-iodine (Banwell, 2006).

■ *Use irrigation at pressures between 8 and 15 pounds per square inch (psi) to cleanse wounds; 13 psi is recommended. Pressure irrigation removes microbes and loose debris without damaging tissue.* **LOE = II**

(NR) A systematic review recommended 13 psi for irrigation pressure for adults and children with traumatic wounds on the basis of one RCT with a sample size of 335 and significant reductions in inflammation and infection. Another RCT with 208 patients found similar infection rates (1% and 4%, not significant) with two irrigation devices that delivered the solution in less than 4 minutes and with 1.5 and 2 psi. The amount and rate of irrigation still need study (Fernandez et al., 2004).

(EO) An international expert panel summarized best practices for wound care and recommended irrigation pressures of 8 to 15 psi (Schultz et al., 2003).

(EO) A 30-mL syringe and a 19-gauge needle are recommended to achieve sufficient pressure (8 psi) for effective irrigation; 60 mL/cm of wound length is one suggestion for the amount of irrigating fluid, although this requires further study (Howell & Chisholm, 1997).

■ *Use Vulnopur (a saline spray that contains aloe vera, silver chloride, and decyl glucoside) for pressure ulcer wound cleansing.* **LOE = II**

(NR) A systematic review cautiously recommended Vulnopur on the basis of an RCT with 133 patients and improved wound healing using a valid and reliable tool (Moore & Cowman, 2005).

■ *Use warmed irrigating solutions when possible for cleaning wounds; adhere to standard infection control and warming guidelines.* **LOE = II**

(MR) An RCT with 38 patients serving as their own controls studied warmed sterile saline versus room temperature saline and found that patients preferred warmed saline (difference, 34%; 95% confidence interval, 6 to 63; Ernst et al., 2003).

Not Effective

■ *Using boiled, cooled water or distilled water.* **LOE = I**

(NR) A systematic review concluded that there was insufficient evidence available to draw conclusions regarding the type of water to use in wound cleansing and for which type of wounds. Sample sizes from studies were 35 and 86 divided into three arms (Fernandez et al., 2002).

RCT = Randomized Controlled (Clinical) Trial, **NIC** = Nursing Interventions Classification, **NOC** = Nursing Outcomes Classification

■ *Using cleansing, whirlpool, or water or saline versus no cleansing or no whirlpool.* **LOE = I**

(EO) The use of cleansing, whirlpool, or water or saline versus no cleansing or no whirlpool could not be supported as a result of a lack of sound research (Moore & Cowman, 2005).

Possibly Harmful

■ *Using hydrogen peroxide to irrigate wounds.* **LOE = V**

(MR) A systematic review of hydrogen peroxide use and inadvertent administration concluded that its use for wound irrigation was potentially dangerous (Watt et al., 2004).

■ *Using high pressure (≥20 psi) for wound irrigation with or without pulsatile lavage.* **LOE = IV**

(MR) A case-control study in a 1000-bed hospital concluded that an infectious outbreak in 11 patients within 2 months was associated with pulsatile lavage therapy. Infection control precautions are needed with lavage therapy (Maragakis et al., 2004).

(EO) The use of high-pressure pulsatile lavage is cautioned for all types of wounds; the Agency for Health Care Policy and Research Guideline pressures of 4 to 15 psi for wound irrigation are recommended. Early studies support pulsatile lavage for wound cleansing, but more RCTs are needed (Luedtke-Hoffmann & Schafer, 2000).

OUTCOME MEASUREMENT

WOUND HEALING: SECONDARY INTENTION   (NOC)

Definition: Extent of regeneration of cells and tissues in an open wound.
Wound Healing: Secondary Intention as evidenced by the following selected NOC indicators:
• Granulation
• Scar formation
• Decreased wound size
(Rate each indicator of **Wound Healing: Secondary Intention:** 1 = none, 2 = limited, 3 = moderate, 4 = substantial, 5 = extensive) (Moorhead et al., 2004).

REFERENCES

Banwell H. (2006). What is the evidence for tissue regeneration impairment when using a formulation of PVP-I antiseptic on open wounds? *Dermatology,* 212(Suppl 1):66-76.
Dochterman JM, Bulechek GM (Eds). (2004). *Nursing Interventions Classification (NIC),* 4th ed. St Louis: Mosby.
Ernst AA, Gershoff L, Miller P, Tilden E, Weiss S. (2003). Warmed versus room temperature saline for laceration irrigation: A randomized clinical trial. *South Med J,* 96(5):436-439.
Fernandez R, Griffiths R, Ussia C. (2002). Water for wound cleansing. *Cochrane Database Syst Rev,* (4): CD003861.
Fernandez R, Griffiths R, Ussia C. (2004). Effectiveness of solutions, techniques and pressure in wound cleansing. *JBI Reports,* 2(7):231-270.
Howell JM, Chisholm CD. (1997). Wound care. *Emerg Med Clin North Am,* 15(2):417-425.

Joanna Briggs Institute (JBI). (2003). Solutions, techniques and pressure for wound cleansing. *Best Pract,* 7(1):3.

Luedtke-Hoffmann KA, Schafer DS. (2000). Pulsed lavage in wound cleansing. *Phys Ther,* 80(3):292-300.

Maragakis LL, Cosgrove S, Song X, Kim D, Rosenbaum P, Ciesla N, et al. (2004). An outbreak of multi-drug-resistant *Acinetobacter baumannii* associated with pulsatile lavage wound treatment. *JAMA,* 292(24):3006-3011.

Moore ZE, Cowman S. (2005). Wound cleansing for pressure ulcers. *Cochrane Database Syst Rev,* (4): CD004983.

Moorhead M, Johnson M, Maas M (Eds). (2004). *Nursing Outcomes Classification (NOC),* 3rd ed. St Louis: Mosby.

Schultz GS, Sibbald RG, Falanga V, Ayello E, Dowsett C, Harding K, et al. (2003). Wound bed preparation: A systematic approach to wound management. *Wound Repair Regen,* 11(Suppl 1):S1-S28.

Watt BE, Proudfoot A, Vale J. (2004). Hydrogen peroxide poisoning. *Toxicol Rev,* 23(1):51-57.

INDEX